AF522515

Clinical Implantology

Clinical Implantology

AJAY VIKRAM SINGH
BDS, PG Cert Dental Implant, DICOI
Founder and Director
International Implant Training Centre
Agra, India

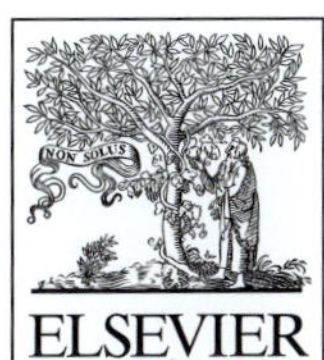

ELSEVIER
A division of
RELX India Private Limited
(Formerly Reed Elsevier India Private Limited)

Clinical Implantology
Singh

ELSEVIER
A division of
RELX India Private Limited (Formerly Reed Elsevier India Private Limited)

Mosby, Saunders, Churchill Livingstone, Butterworth-Heinemann and Hanley & Belfus are the Health Science imprints of Elsevier.

ISBN: 978-81-312-3324-5
First Printed in India 2013, Reprinted 2014, 2020

Published by Elsevier, a division of RELX India Private Limited
Registered Office: 818, Indraprakash Building, 8th Floor, 21, Barakhamba Road, New Delhi-110001
Corporate Office: 14th Floor, Buiding No. 10B, DLF Cyber City, Phase II, Gurgaon, Haryana - 122 002.

Sr. Commissioning Editor: Nimisha Goswami
Sr. Managing Editor (Development): Anand K Jha
Copy Editor: TNQ
Publishing Operations Manager: K Sunil Kumar
Project Manager: Karthikeyan Murthy
Production Manager: NC Pant
Cover Designer: Raman Kumar

Typeset by TNQ, Chennai

Printed and bound in India at EIH Ltd.-Unit Printing Press, IMT Manesar (Haryana).

Dedicated to my parents, lovely wife Sunita and my wonderful son Palin whose continued love and support made possible to write this book

Contributors

AJAY VIKRAM SINGH, BDS, PG Cert Dental Implant, DICOI

Founder and Director
International Implant Training Centre
Agra, India

ANGELO TROEDHAN, MD, DMD, PhD

Visiting Professor, Health Science University
Faculty of Dentistry, Vientiane
Center for Facial Esthetics, Vienna
Health Science University, Faculty of Dentistry, Vientiane
Brauhausgasse 12-14
1050 Vienna, Austria

JUN SHIMADA, DDS, PhD

Professor, Division of Oral and Maxillofacial Surgery
Department of Diagnostic and Therapeutic Sciences
Meikai University School of Dentistry, Japan

STEFAN KA IHDE, DDS

International Implant Foundation
Munich Head, Dental Implant Faculty
Leopoldstr. 116
DE-80802 Munich, Germany

AMIR GAZMAWE, DMD, BSc

Prosthodontist
Private practice, Osishkin Street
Ramat Hasharon, Israel

TETSU TAKAHASHI, DDS, PhD

Professor and Head
Division of Oral and Maxillofacial Surgery
Department of Oral Medicine and Surgery
Tohoku University Graduate School of Dentistry
4-1, Seiryo-machi, Aoba-ku, Sendai
Miyagi, Japan

LEN TOLSTUNOV, DDS, DABOMS, DABOI/ID, DICOI, FAAOMS, FCALOMS

Assistant Clinical Professor
Department of Oral and Maxillofacial Surgery
UOP (Pacific)
School of Dentistry, San Francisco, CA (USA)
Founder and Director "The Implant Team"
advanced implant
seminars in San Francisco

FRÉDÉRIC JOACHIM, DDS, MSc

Private practice, Lille, France

ISSAM JOACHIM-SAMAHA, DDS, MSc

Private practice, Villeneuve d'Ascq, France

JACQUES CHARON, DDS, MSc

Private practice, Lille, France

PETER RANDELZHOFER, DDS

Private practice, Weinstr, Munchen
Germany

SHLOMO BIRSHAN, DMD, DICOI

Private practice, Tel Aviv, Israel

SUNITA SINGH, BDS, MIAO

Private practice, Agra
Director, International Implant Training Centre
Dr Ajay Dental Clinic and Research Centre
Agra, India

TERRY D WHITTEN, DDS

Private practice, Sabetha
Northeast Kansas (USA)

RAMI JANDALI, DMD, MS

Chief Operations Officer
Global Implant Solutions, Bedford
Massachusetts (USA)

ATA GARAJEI, DMD

Assistant Professor of Oral and Maxillofacial Surgery
Department of Head and Neck Surgical Oncology
and Reconstructive Surgery
The Cancer Institute, School of Medicine
Tehran University of Medical Sciences
Tehran, Iran
The Cancer Institute, Imam Hospital Complex, Keshavarz
Blvd., Tehran, Iran

SAÂD ZEMMOURI, DDS

Private practice, Casablanca, Morocco

SUNG-MIN CHUNG, DDS, MSD, PhD

Well Dental Clinic, Seoul, Korea

SANG-WAN SHIN, DDS, MPH, PhD

Advanced Prosthodontics
Institute for Clinical Dental Research
Graduate School of Clinical Dentistry
Korea University
Seoul, Korea

ANTONINA IHDE, DDS

Private practice, Lindenstr. 68
CH-8738 Uetliburg, Switzerland

HIMANSHU JOSHI, BDS

Private practice, Jaipur, India

AMIN YAMANI, DDS

Private practice, Tehran, Iran
Former Assistant Professor
Zahedan University, Zahedan
Iran

Preface

Since Prof PI Branemark described the concept of osseointegration, the dental implantology has evolved tremendously over the past 35 years. Thanks to all the past and current researchers and clinicians in the field of implantology whose continued efforts have brought this science to a great level of success. Today, the implant is sought to be the most successful and reliable option for the missing tooth replacement and also to retain the loose dentures.

In the last 35 years, the various modifications in the implant designs and surface have been made to improvise the pace and quality of osseointegration. After practising the conventional implant treatment protocol for several years, the implant researchers and clinicians have successfully developed several modifications such as immediate implant, immediate restoration, etc. to provide a desired level of implant treatment to the patients. Further, development of bone augmentation procedures made the high level of possibilities with a greater success to provide implant therapy in the patients with ridge deficiencies and bone defects.

Several textbooks have been published so far presenting detailed description of the literatures and studies on the implants. These books have definitely been providing detailed knowledge of the literature in the field of implantology and have been playing a very important role in the success of any implant dentist including the author of this book, but many dentists especially clinicians feel difficult to go through all that time-consuming literatures. Moreover, most of the textbooks on implantology do not adequately describe diagrammatically all the clinical implant procedures but give most of the description in the text supported with only a few diagrams not showing all steps of the procedure. Thus, the clinicians find it difficult to understand the way with which they can correctly perform any particular procedure. Keeping this in mind, few clinical books have been recently published which have beautifully presented the step-by-step procedures but most of these books present only few implant techniques such as bone augmentation, all-on-four procedures, etc.

The purpose of this book is to diagrammatically present all the basic to advance level implant procedures along with basic science and diagnosis and treatment planning. The author and the contributors have tried to describe all the implant procedures which are currently being practised worldwide along with the recent advances. The initial chapters of this book describe basic science, implant dentistry tools, diagnosis and treatment planning, and step-by-step basic implant surgical and prosthetic procedures. The rest of the chapters describe all the advanced bone and soft tissue augmentation procedures such as sinus grafting, nasal floor grafting, ridge splitting, block grafting and soft tissue grafting along with graft less immediate loading all-on-four/all-on-six techniques. This book can be seen as a complete implant dentistry book covering all the basic as well as advanced level of clinical implantology. All the procedures have been described with important and very concise text with step-by-step diagrammatic presentation making it easy to understand for the clinicians and undergraduate and postgraduate dental students. Several clinical cases are presented with high resolution pictures in various chapters of this book. The author has first tried to describe the techniques using high resolution and beautifully drawn diagrams followed by presentation of same technique with step-by-step clinical pictures. More than 3,000 high resolution coloured clinical pictures and diagrams are published in this book which are definitely going to help the novice as well as experienced implant dentists to comprehend easily basic to advanced level implantology.

Ajay Vikram Singh

Acknowledgements

At the outset I would like to express sincere gratitude to my parents for their unconditional love and support throughout my life.

Further, I would like to thank my lifelong companion and lovely wife Sunita and my son Palin for their unconditional love, support and immense contribution to this book by sacrificing their precious time during preparation of this manuscript for which I worked all day and night on my implant patients and then on computer for approximately 3 years.

In addition, I would like to express my sincere gratitude to all my teachers and mentors for providing me up-to-date knowledge. Without their continuous and unselfish guidance, inspiration and education, this book would not have been possible.

I would also like to thank all my friends around the globe for their precious contribution in the book. The implant cases as well as the literature they contributed have tremendously helped in making this a complete implant book.

Further, I would also like to thank various companies in the field of implantology including Nobel Biocare, Alpha Bio, Osseolink, Salvin Dental Specialties, bredent, BOI, Dentium, Straumann, Setlec, Amron and Adin for contributing the illustrations of their implants, inventories and armamentaria which tremendously helped me in presenting the component science and methodology of the basic as well as advanced implantology.

I would like to thank the entire editorial and marketing team of Elsevier India especially Mr Anand K Jha, Ms Ritu Sharma, Ms Nimisha Goswami and Mr Karthikeyan Murthy for their extraordinary approach and hard work to publish this book.

Last but not the least, I would like to thank the entire team of my centre, Dr Ajay Dental Clinic and Research Centre, Agra for assisting me in performing and documenting several implant cases presented in this book. I would also like to thank all my implant patients for their cooperation during the documentation of the procedures.

At the end, I would like to thank all my students at International Implant Training Centre (IITC), Agra. It is always a pleasure and an honour to share my knowledge and implant expertise in dental implantology. I have always enjoyed spreading my implant expertise to the dentists who come to receive training at my centre.

Contents

Introduction and fundamental science

1

Ajay Vikram Singh

CHAPTER CONTENTS HD

Introduction

Teeth are designed for the lifetime but often patients lose teeth partially or completely because of causes such as dental caries, periodontal problems, accidental trauma, etc. Replacing missing teeth is important to the patient's general health as well as to the health of his/her other teeth. Not only does the patient lose chewing ability when a tooth is lost, but if it is not replaced, it can cause other teeth to be lost, tipped or crowded and create subsequent problems. Moreover, there are the obvious problems of poor appearance and loss of self-esteem caused by one or more missing teeth.

With advancement in dental science and public awareness of better dental treatment options, the dental implant should always be considered as an option to replace a failing or missing tooth. The replacement of lost teeth with dental implants has been in use for more than 50 years and is recognized as an effective treatment choice. Many studies and clinical trials worldwide have shown that the dental implant is considered more predictable than conventional bridgework, resin-bonded bridges and endodontic therapy. Often, the patient faces a difficult decision in choosing to insert dental implants to replace one or more missing teeth. However, clinical studies have shown a very high success rate for dental implants of around 90–95%, on average. These figures do vary according to the part of the mouth that is being treated. Because of reasons like lower bone density, facial cantilevering, and sinus pneumatization, the upper jaw has been and continues to be, more difficult to treat than the lower jaw and this is reflected in the success rates.

Definition of dental implant

"Dental implant is an alloplastic and biocompatible material placed into (endosseous) or onto (subperiosteal) the jawbone to support a fixed prosthesis, or to stabilize removable prosthesis."

Implant success rate

Backed by worldwide studies, research, clinical trials and documentation, over more than 50 years, the dental implant has been established as a full-fledged tooth replacement option. The success rate of the implant varies from case to case, depending on several factors like bone volume, bone density, soft tissues, force factors, treatment planning and the skill of the implant surgeon and restoring dentist. Generally, implant therapy is a little more successful in the mandible than in the maxilla. The lower success of the implant in the maxilla compared to the mandible, is because the maxilla shows poor bone density to stabilize the implant, lower bone volume because of vertical as well as lateral bone resorption and sinus pneumatization and facial cantilevering. Approximate success rate of the implant in the four regions of jaws – anterior maxilla: 90–95%; anterior mandible: 95–98%; posterior mandible: 85–95%; posterior maxilla: 85–90%.

Benefits of dental implants

Dental implants offer several benefits over conventional tooth replacement options like the dental bridge and removable partial to complete dentures.

1. It prevents bone loss because the implant anchors (osseointegrates) the jawbone and thus prevents further bone loss (Fig 1.1).
2. It restores the function and aesthetics of the overall maxillofacial prosthesis.
3. It offers best and most preferred option for stabilizing loose dentures (Fig 1.2).
4. It is thought to be the only option to deliver the fixed prosthesis where the conventional bridge is not possible (Fig 1.3).
5. It is the strongest and long-lasting treatment for the replacement of missing teeth.
6. The deep flanges and palatal extension of complete dentures, which cause substantial discomfort to patients, can be avoided once the denture is retained over the implants.

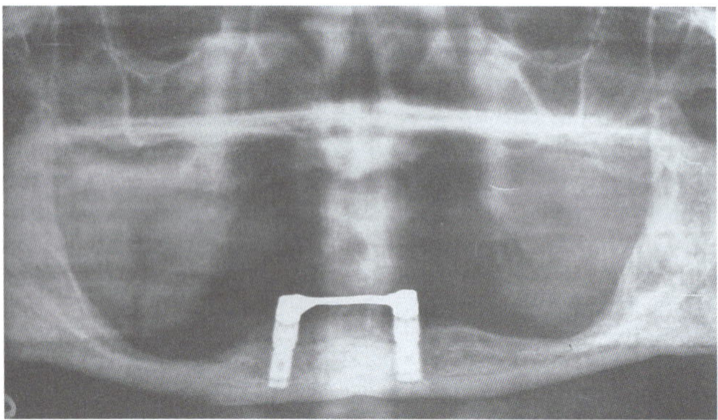

Fig 1.1 Two implants inserted 20 years back in the anterior mandible have maintained the bone volume and prevented the further bone loss in the region while in the other part of the jaw, the patient has lost most of the bony ridge.

History of dental implants

The history of dental implants is believed to have begun as far back as in the seventh century. In the 1930s, dental implants (in their original form, made of seashells) were found in Mayan burial archeological sites, placed in a young woman's jawbone.

Modern implants had their origin in the discovery by a Swedish professor of Orthopaedics named Branemark, who found that titanium (a very strong and noncorrosive metal) attached itself to a bone when it was implanted into it. During one of his experiments, he embedded titanium devices into rabbit's leg bones to study bone healing. After a few months, he tried to remove these expensive devices and when he could not, he noticed that the bone had attached itself to the metal. He eventually decided that the mouth was far more practical than the leg for his experiments, as it was easier to watch the progress and there were more toothless people than people with serious joint problems. He called the attachment of the titanium to the bone 'osseointegration' and in 1965 he used the first titanium dental implant in a human volunteer.

Over the next few years, he published a lot of research on the use of titanium dental implants, and in 1978 he commercialized the development and marketing of his titanium dental implants. Over 7 million implants under his brand name have been placed. Needless to say, there are other dental implant companies that have used his patent.

Looking at the technology involved and the high success rates of dental implants, it is hard to believe that the history of dental implants goes back only 40 years.

It did not take long to realize the enormous potential of this technique. Dr Branemark began focussing on how he could use osseointegration, to help humans. During his studies, he found that titanium screws could serve as bone anchors for teeth.

Titanium, researchers came to realize, was the only consistently successful material for dental implants. Before Dr Branemark's work, other doctors had been toying with the idea of dental implants for years. A most of other metals, including silver and gold, had failed. Even human teeth (from donors) were tried.

Dr Branemark continued his studies for nearly three decades. His fellow scientists were sceptical, so he

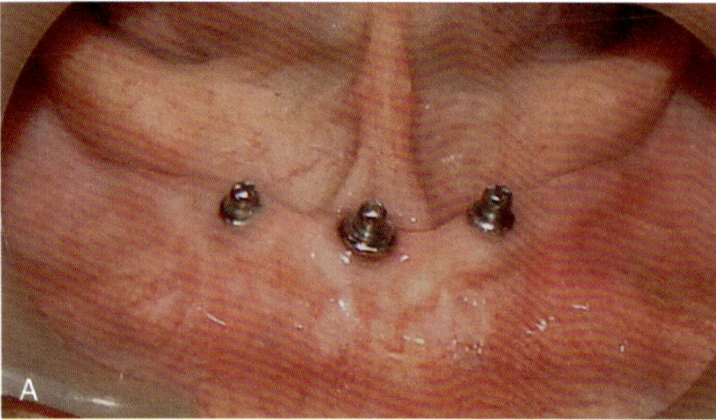

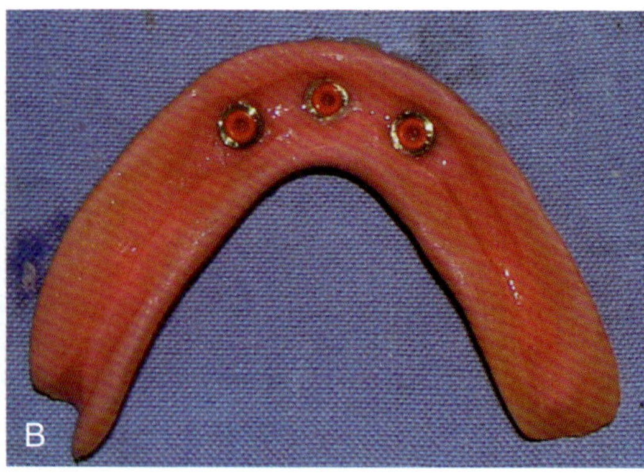

Fig 1.2 (A and B) Dental implants are the most successful and preferred option to retain the loose dentures.

conducted numerous tests, including some on humans, before he published his findings in 1981.

After scientific scrutiny of Dr Branemark's paper, medical confidence in the procedure grew. Guidelines for implantology were set during the Toronto Conference in Clinical Dentistry in 1982. The standardization of the process during the conference proved to be the jump-start that the dental implant needed. The public began to accept that dental implants were safe.

Commercial oral implantology grew during the 1980s. Osseointegration was being used to permanently fix an individual tooth into the patient's mouth. Implants proved to be successful in over 90% of cases. The modern dental implant had arrived!

Over the next two decades, technology continued to improve the process. For instance, slight modifications to the titanium used decreased healing time. As time goes by and as the practice of dentistry advances, patients will continue to see dental implants becoming quicker, easier, and less painful.

Fundamental science

Definition of osseointegration

PI Branemark and associates in 1986 defined the osseointegration of the implant as "direct structural and functional connection between ordered, living bone and the surface of a load-carrying implant."

SG Steinemann and associates in 1986 simplified the definition of osseointegration as "direct contact between bone and an implant surface."

Phases of implant osseointegration

Immediately after the implant is inserted into the jawbone, the peri-implant bone passes step by step, through different phases of histological change, to reach the final stage of osseointegration of the implant with the surrounding bone (Fig 1.4). In the author's experience, the clinician should be aware of these histological changes, as all these can be deciding factors in the modification of the conventional two-stage implant treatment protocol to one-stage, immediate or early loading of the implant.

Clinical evidence of successful osseointegration

- Implant is not mobile when tested clinically
- Implant is asymptomatic – absence of persistent signs and symptoms, such as pain, infections, etc.
- Stable crestal bone levels – annual rate of bone loss should be less than 0.2 mm after the first year in function
- Increasing mineralization of the newly-formed bone at the implant surface
- Healthy soft tissues
- Absence of peri-implant radiolucency.

Enhancement of rate and degree of osseointegration

Several research studies have been performed to find an optimal surface treatment to increase mechanical stability and to improve the contact between bone and implant. Many studies provide conclusive scientific evidence that

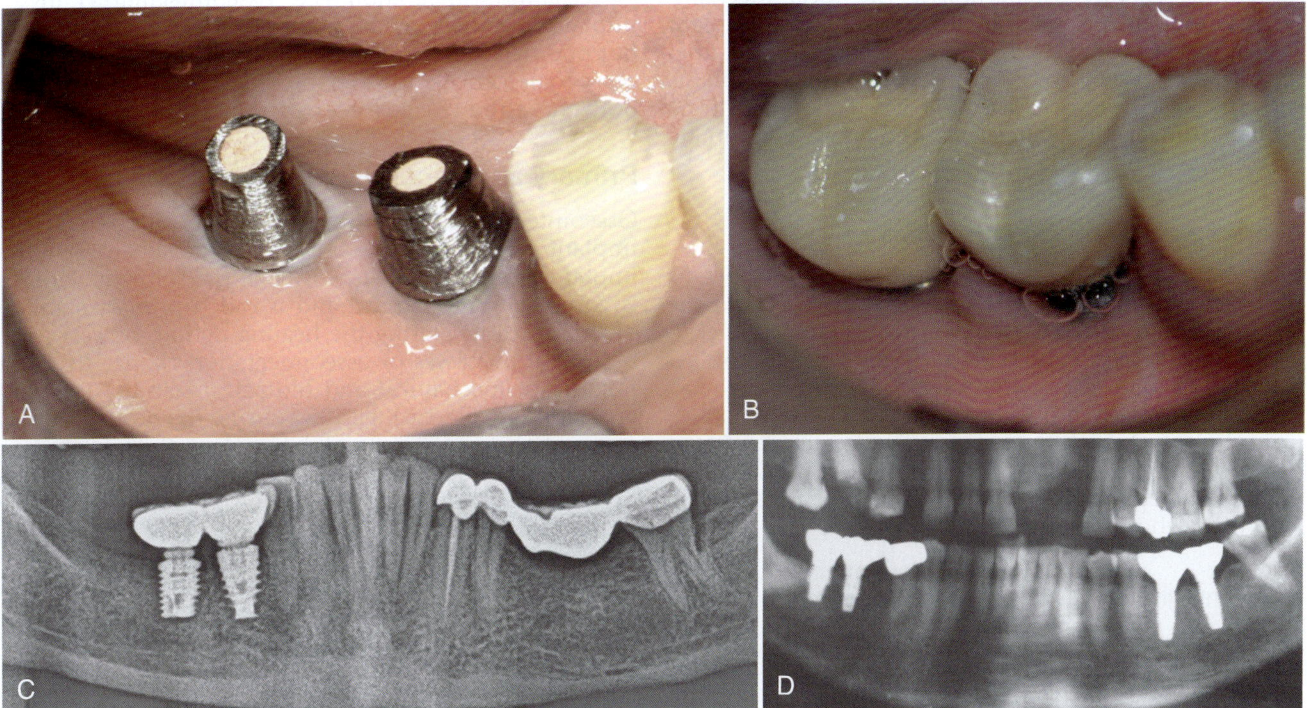

Fig 1.3 (A–C) In cases where no teeth or no firm teeth are available to be used as the abutments to support the conventional fixed bridge, the implant is the only option to deliver a fixed prosthesis. (D) Even in the cases where the dental bridge is possible, the implant prosthesis should be preferred as it does not need to cut down adjacent healthy teeth and also prevents further ridge loss.

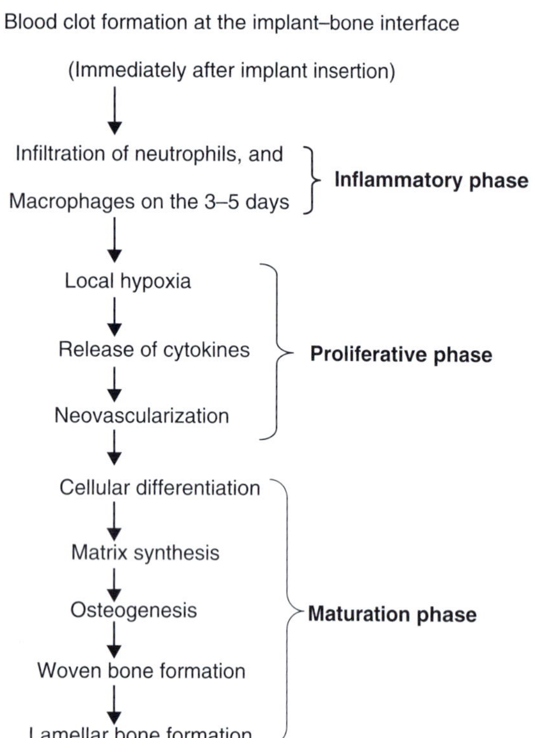

Fig 1.4 Flowchart showing the sequential phases of osseointegration.

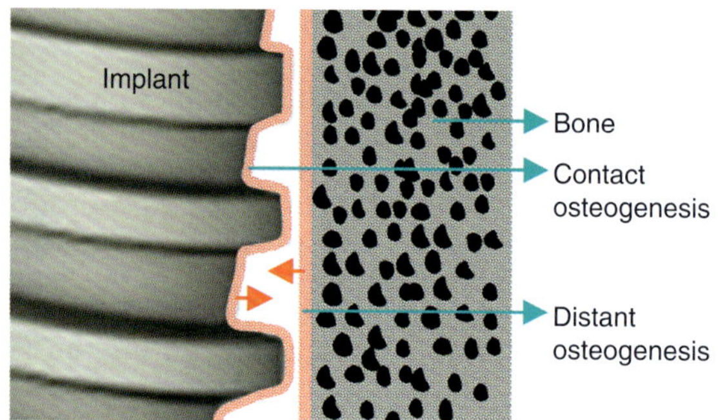

Fig 1.5 Diagrammatic presentation of contact and distant osteogenesis at the implant surface–host bone interface.

a roughened titanium implant surface improves bone anchoring compared to conventionally machined titanium surfaces. The rough surface facilitates migration of osteogenic cells to the implant surface for *de novo* bone formation (contact osteogenesis). The local mechanical environment provided by the rough-surface implant also influences cellular differentiation and tissue synthesis (distance osteogenesis). The rough-surface implants show increased removal forces, greater and earlier bone implant contact (BIC) percentage, and improved ultimate osseointegration.

Contact and distant osteogenesis

After implant insertion, new bone formation begins simultaneously at the prepared osteotomy wall and the implant surface. The new bone synthesis (osteogenesis) which begins at the implant surface is called 'contact osteogenesis' and other synthesis which simultaneously begins at the osteotomy wall is called 'distant osteogenesis'. Completion of both osteogenesis processes results in complete new bone synthesis at the implant – host–bone interface which is finally called 'implant osseointegration' with the jawbone (Fig 1.5).

Osseointegration versus osseocoalescence

The term 'osseointegration' is commonly used in conjunction with dental implants. Osseointegration means that there is no relative movement between the implant and the surrounding bone. Although some investigators believe that there is a chemical integration between bone and the surface of titanium implants, osseointegration largely refers to the physical integration or mechanical fixation of an implant in the bone. With purely physical interaction, the interface would be able to withstand shear forces; however, the interface would not be able to withstand even moderate tensile forces. The term 'osseocoalescence' refers specifically to the chemical integration of implants in bone tissue. The term applies to surface-reactive materials, such as calcium phosphates and bioactive glasses, which undergo reactions that lead to chemical bonding between bone and biomaterial. With these materials, the tissues effectively coalesce with the implant. An example of qualitative evidence of chemical bonding is that fracture lines propagate through either the implant or the tissue but not along the interface. Osseocoalesced implants exhibit resistance to both shear and tensile loads. Unfortunately, the term has not found widespread use and osseointegration still is often used when describing interactions between bioactive materials and bone.

Mechanical integration (i.e. osseointegration) of an implant in bone provides good resistance to shear forces but poor resistance to tension. Chemical integration (i.e. osseocoalescence) however provides good resistance to both shear and tensile forces.

Primary and secondary implant stability

Osseointegration requires bone apposition on the implant surface without any micromovement. During implant insertion, the stability that the implant achieves is completely mechanical and is called primary stability of the implant. During the healing period, however, the biological processes of osseointegration change this to a mixture of mechanical and biological stability (secondary stability) (Fig 1.6). Further, during the biological processes of osseointegration of the implant, the surrounding bone physiologically changes during the multiple phases of bone resorption and new bone apposition over the implant surface. Any micromovement of the implant during this phase may lead to the failure of implant osseointegration with the bone. The primary or mechanical stability changes to secondary or biological stability, once the osseointegration of the implant is completed. According to different studies, this process may take 4–6 months.

Soft tissue integration

Soft tissue integration around implant superstructures like transmucosal healing abutment, final abutment,

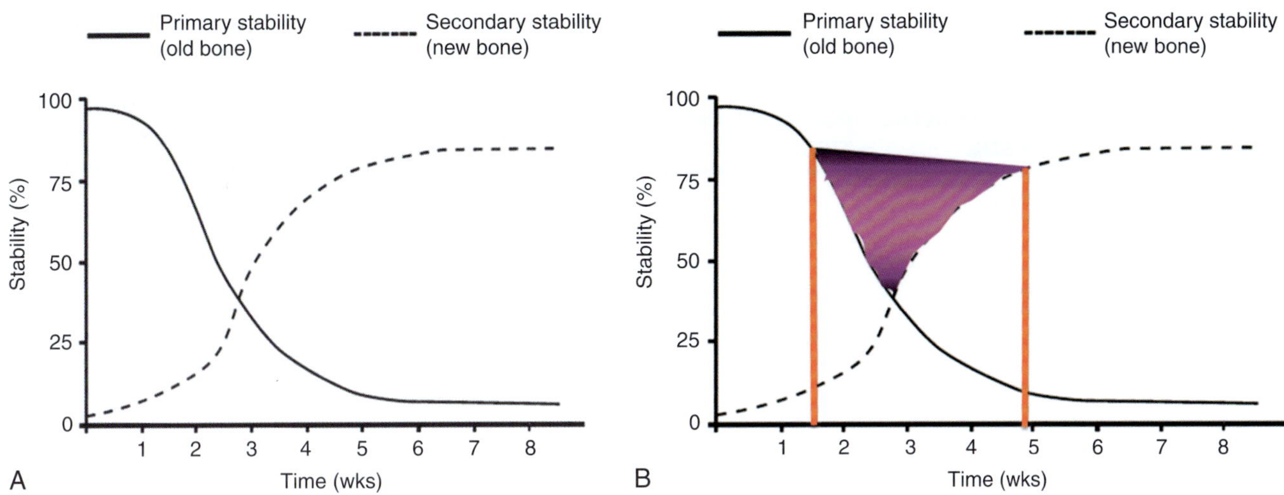

Fig 1.6 (A and B) Primary and secondary stability curves of an implant during the transition period when the implant remains at higher risk of micromovement and fails to osseointegrate (*Courtesy: Raghavendra et al. Int J Oral Maxillofac Implants. 2000;20:425-431*).

etc. can be defined as "biologic processes that occur during the formation and maturation of the structural relationship between the soft tissues and the transmucosal implant superstructures."

"The establishment of an adequate zone of attached and keratinized soft tissue with intimate adaptation to transmucosal implant superstructures is critical for long-term success of the restored implants." The epithelial and connective tissue elements are organized to form a protective soft tissue seal around the implant superstructures, which serves to resist bacterial and mechanical challenges encountered in the oral cavity. "The functional soft tissue – implant interface is equally as important as osseointegration for the long-term success of implant-supported prosthesis." Thus, a careful manipulation and preservation of existing soft tissue is paramount for long-term implant success. If the area is devoid of attached and keratinized soft tissue, soft tissue grafting procedures should be performed to regenerate a healthy, thick, attached, and keratinized zone of marginal soft tissue (minimum of 3 mm), around the implant superstructures (Fig 1.7).

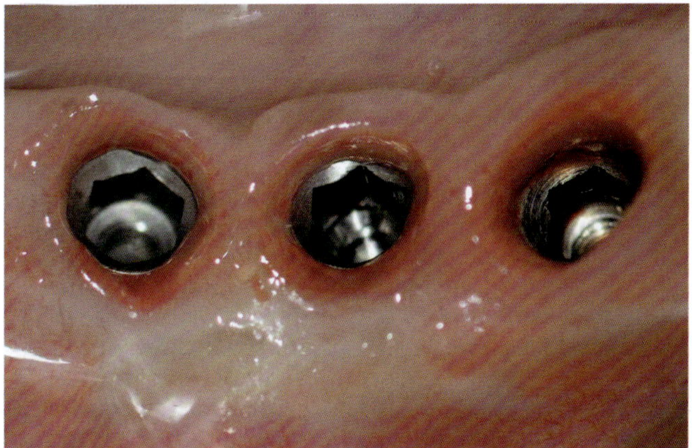

Fig 1.7 The establishment of an adequate zone of attached and keratinized soft tissue with intimate adaptation to transmucosal implant superstructures is critical for long-term success of restored implants.

Comparative anatomy of the natural tooth and the osseointegrated implant

Although the dental implant clinically looks like the natural tooth after restoration, the bone and soft tissue integration to the implant surface and to its superstructures shows several biological differences compared to the natural tooth (Fig 1.8). The doctor and the patient should be aware of these differences to achieve a predictable implant therapy and long-term maintenance practices (Table 1.1). The natural tooth possesses periodontal ligament space which not only provides additional nutrient supply to the periodontal hard and soft tissues for their maintenance and long-term survival, but also acts as the shock absorber against undue forces over the tooth. The implant which gets directly osseointegrated with the bone and shows no structure like the periodontal ligament, only possesses limited sources of nutrient supply to the peri-implant tissue and also transverses all the occlusal forces directly to the bone. This often can be the cause of bone resorption

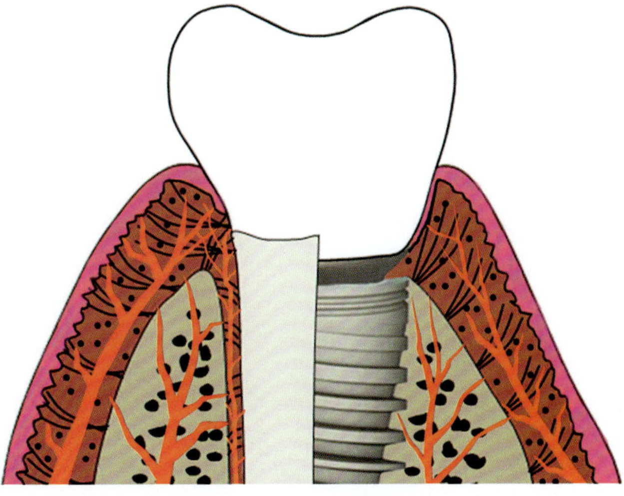

Fig 1.8 Diagrammatic presentation of comparative anatomy of periodontal and peri-implant bone and soft tissue.

Table 1.1 Comparative anatomic features of periodontal and peri-implant bone and soft tissue

FEATURES	PERIODONTAL TISSUE	PERI-IMPLANT TISSUE
Periodontal ligaments	Present	Not present
Sulcular epithelium	Present	Present
Junctional epithelium	Present	Present
Basal lamina	Present	Present
Hemidesmosomes	Present	Present
Glycoprotein adhesion	Present	Present
Connective tissue attachment	Present	Not present
Soft tissue circulation	Three sources	Two sources
Surrounding connective tissue zone	Vascular and cellular	Hypovascular and hypocellular
Sulcular probing	Indicated	Not indicated

around the implant. Another difference which the doctor should know is that the peri-implant soft tissue does not show any connective tissue attachments to the implant collar and its superstructures like the natural tooth, and thus any physical or chemical injury to the soft tissue sulcus may directly affect the peri-implant crestal bone and may cause crestal bone resorption. For this reason, deliberate sulcular probing around the implant is not recommended. One point the author would like to emphasize here is that as described earlier, the peri-implant tissues (bone as well as soft tissue) receive blood supply from only two sources – from the periosteum and from the basal bone. They do not have the third source of blood supply like the natural tooth, which receives blood supply from the periodontal ligament also; thus, the peri-implant tissue with limited thickness may find it difficult to survive and may get resorbed.

Summary

The dental implant definitely offers several advantages over the conventional dental bridge and partial or complete dentures for patients with partial to complete edentulism; but before he/she starts offering the implant to his/her patients, the clinician should know basic implant science and how the implant is different from the natural tooth. The phases of implant osseointegration and the factors affecting the osseointegration are very important. Protocols like immediate implantation in an extraction socket with open healing, immediate to early loading, etc. are solely dependent on the primary stability and the force factors on the implant during the phase of osseointegration. Thus the surgeon should know the primary and secondary stability of the implant to successfully introduce modifications in conventional techniques. The type of soft tissue and bone volume and quality are key features for long-term implant success. Patients deficient in bone volume and healthy keratinized marginal soft tissue should be encouraged to undertake bone and soft tissue augmentation procedures before or at the time of implant placement. As described in this chapter, the osseointegrated implant does not have any periodontal ligament-like structure or connective tissue attachment to the implant collar and its superstructure. Thus the dentist should be aware of how force factors and mechanical to chemical injuries affect the long-term survival of the implant.

Further Reading

Four Linkow textbooks online.

Natali Arturo N, editor. Dental biomechanics. London/New York: Taylor & Francis; 2003, ISBN 9-780-415-30666-9, pp. 69–87. p. 273.

Zard, et al. Osseointegration. Quintessence; 2009.

Palmer R. Ti-unite dental implant surface may be superior to machined surface in replacement of failed implants. J Evid Based Dent Pract March 2007;7(1):8–9.

Binon PP. Treatment planning complications and surgical miscues. J Oral Maxillofac Surg July 2007;65(7 Suppl. 1): 73–92.

Sclar AG. Soft tissue and esthetic considerations in implant therapy. Quintessence; 2003.

Becker W, Goldstein M, Becker BE, et al. Minimally invasive flapless implant placement: follow-up results from a multicenter study. J Periodontol 2009;80(2):347–52.

Gerds TA, Vogeler M. Endpoints and survival analysis for successful osseointegration of dental implants. Stat Methods Med Res December 2005;14(6):579–90.

Albrektsson T, Zarb GA. Current interpretations of the osseointegrated response: clinical significance. Int J Prosthodont 1993;6(2):95–105.

Kapur SP, Russell TE. Sharpey fiber bone development in surgically implanted dog mandible. Acta Anat 1978;102:260.

Dental implant designs and surfaces

Ajay Vikram Singh

2

CHAPTER CONTENTS HD

Introduction

Based on research and clinical trials, several dental implant designs have been developed and widely used to provide optimal implant therapy to patients. Researchers in the field of implantology have developed a variety of implant designs and surfaces to achieve optimal osseointegration with the bone, ease of placement, immediate placement into extraction sockets, adequate primary stability of the implant, immediate to early loading protocols, and to provide a wide range of prosthetic options. There are several features in implant design and modified implant surfaces that are very important for a clinician to know, in order to choose the correct implant, to learn its placement and restoration protocols, and to provide maintenance for long-term aesthetics and function. Although several implant designs have been developed, implant design continues to be one of the key fields for research oriented towards improving the acceptability and success of the implant.

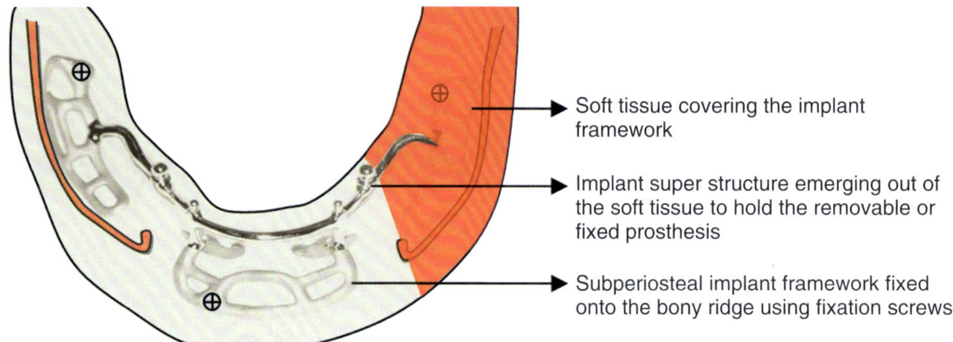

Fig 2.1 Diagrammatic presentation of subperiosteal implant.

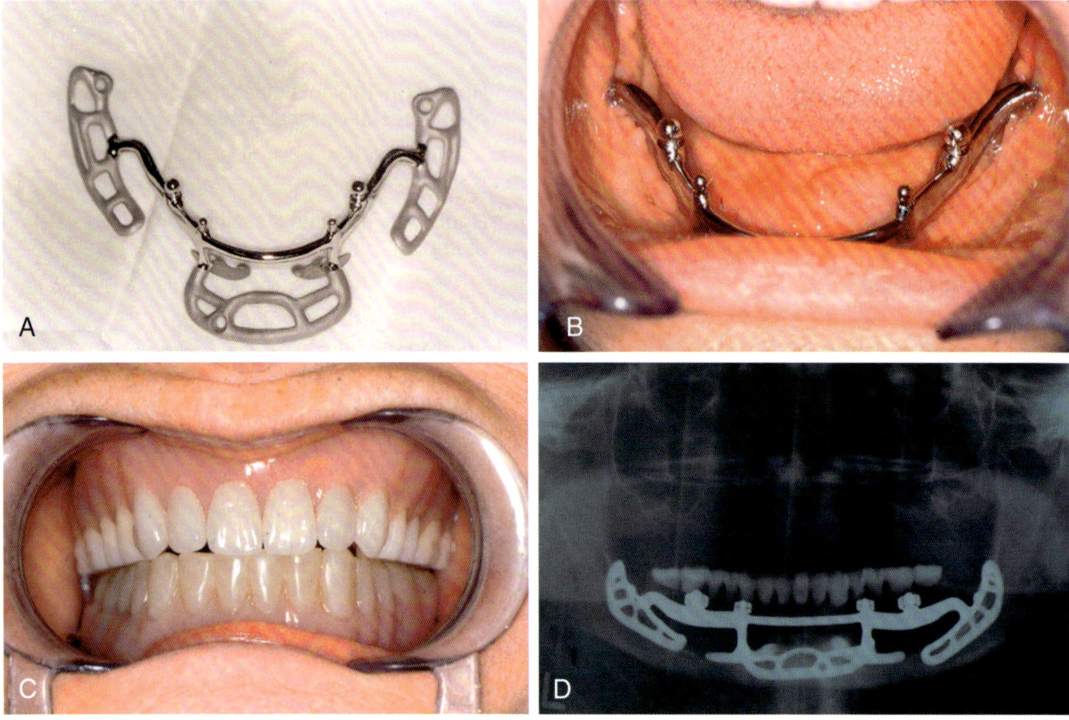

Fig 2.2 (A) Subperiosteal implant (B) placed in the patient's mouth (C) supporting mandibular denture (D) post loading X-ray *(Courtesy: Terry D Whitten, DDS)*.

Subperiosteal implants

The "implants which are placed under the periosteum and fixed over the jaw bone are called subperiosteal implants." These implants are placed under the periosteum on the bony ridge that holds the removable or fixed type of prostheses (Fig 2.1). These implants are preferred in cases of severely resorbed mandibles where endosseous implants are difficult to place, because of the compromised dimensions of the bone and the close proximity of the mandibular canal to the crest of the ridge. The success of the subperiosteal implant in treating partial to completely edentulous patients has been validated by several publications. The first subperiosteal implant was placed in 1949 by Gustav Dahl and has been constantly improved in design since then.

Fabrication. After treatment planning, the buccal and lingual full-thickness flaps are elevated to extend beyond the sulcular depth and an accurate impression of the bony ridge is made, using a hydrophilic impression material (e.g. polyether). The flap is sutured back, the impression is poured with dental stone, and a titanium framework is fabricated over the replica, which has vertical extensions (abutments) emerging out of the soft tissue to hold the prosthesis. After the soft tissue has healed, the full thickness flap is elevated again to the same extent, the titanium framework is placed over the bony ridge and immobilized using fixation screws, and the flap is sutured back with the vertical extensions emerging out of the soft tissue. After a healing period of approximately one-and-half months, the periosteum gets attached to the underlying bone firmly anchoring the framework. An impression of the vertical extensions (abutments) is made and a fixed or removal type of prosthesis is fabricated, and fixed or stabilized over the implant (Fig 2.2).

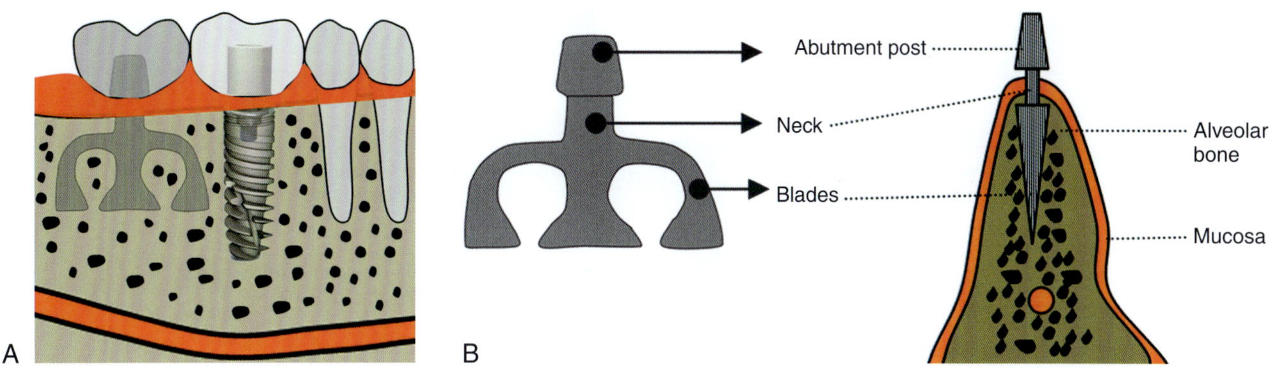

Fig 2.3 (A) Blade and root form implants in the facial view of the alveolar ridge. (B) Blade implant in the cross-section view of the ridge.

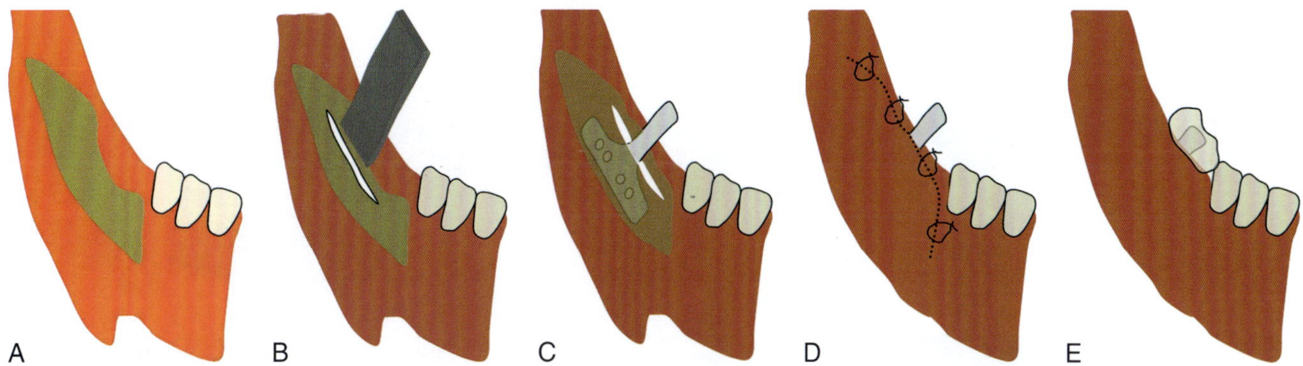

Fig 2.4 (A) To place a blade implant, flap is elevated to expose the ridge crest and (B) a deep mid-crestal horizontal osteotomy is prepared using piezo saw/rotary bur/disc etc. (C) The blade implant with correct dimensions is inserted and tapped to fit into the prepared osteotomy. (D) The flap is sutured back and (E) implant is loaded, once it gets osseointegrated with the bone.

Endosseous implants

The "implants which are placed within the jaw bone are called endosseous implants," e.g. blade implants, root form endosseous implants.

Blade implants

Blade implants, which are very useful for narrow ridge cases, are available prefabricated in the shape of blades with an integrated abutment, which emerges out of the soft tissue to support the prosthesis (Fig 2.3). The endosteal blade implant, was introduced independently in 1967 by Leonard Linkow.

Placement. To place the blade implant, a full thickness flap is elevated to expose the bony ridge and a thin sharp diamond bur/disc/piezo saw is used to prepare a horizontal osteotomy conforming to the size of selected implant. The implant is tapped into the prepared horizontal slot and the flap is sutured back, leaving the abutment emerging out of the soft tissue to hold the future removable or fixed type prosthesis. The blade implants are restored 2 to 3 months after placement (Fig 2.4).

Endosseous root form implants

The two-stage, threaded, titanium root form implant was first invented by Dr Branemark in 1978. These are now the most widely used implants. The root form implant usually has two parts – one part, which is inserted in the bone in the form root, is called the fixture and the other part, which is called the abutment, is immediately or later fixed to the fixture and emerges out of the soft tissue to hold the prosthesis (Fig 2.3).

Transosteal implants

These implants are usually inserted in severely resorbed mandibles where placing the endosseous implant may lead to mandible fracture. They are mostly used to stabilize loose dentures. The posts are inserted through the mandibular basal bone and stabilized with a submandibular metal plate (Fig 2.5). This metal plate also prevents the mandible from getting fractured. These implants are rarely used, as their insertion requires major surgical intervention under general anaesthesia.

Basal osseointegrated implants (BOI)

These implants are integrated to the high-density basal bone or their basal discs are engaged bicortically, to avoid any movement during function. To insert these implants, a lateral bone cutter is used to prepare a lateral slot through the facial cortical plate and an implant of exact size and shape is tapped from the lateral access into the prepared slot. The flap is sutured around the

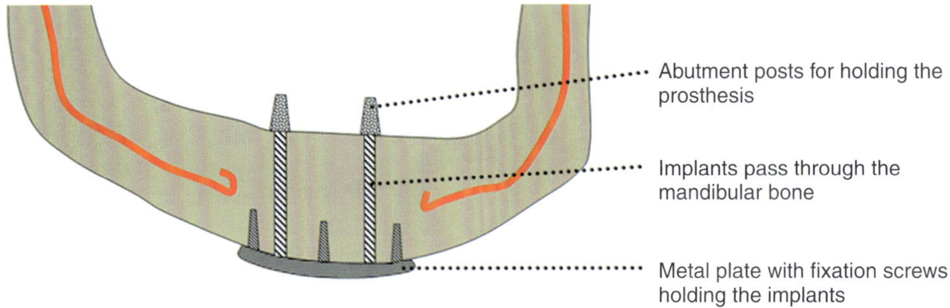

Fig 2.5 Diagrammatic presentation of transosteal implant.

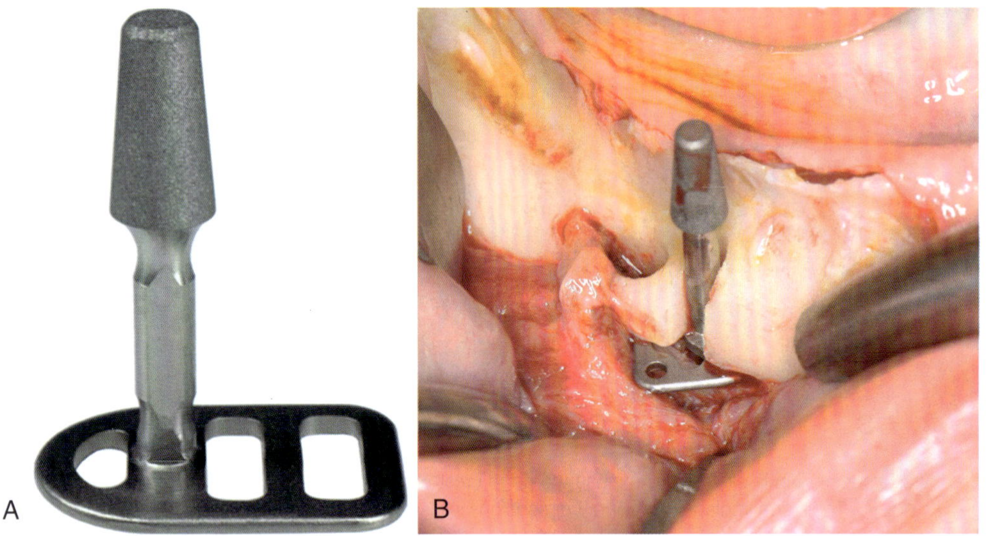

Fig 2.6 (A) Basal osseointegration implant (B) being placed in the posterior mandible *(Courtesy: Prof Dr Stefan KA Ihde, Munich, Germany).*

implant abutment, which emerges out of the soft tissue. These implants usually achieve high initial stability and thus can be restored immediately or soon after implantation. These implants, because they have the advantages of minimum inventories and immediate loading, have gained high popularity and are being widely used by many implant surgeons. These implants are very useful for cases with compromised bone volume, limited bone height above the mandibular canal, sinus pneumatization, etc. The only disadvantage with these implants is that their placement needs the lateral approach (Fig 2.6).

Classification of endosseous root form implants

As described earlier in this chapter, endosseous root form implants are the most widely used implants. Several research projects and clinical trials have been done and continue to be done, to develop an optimal implant design. There are many parameters which differentiate one root form implant from another, and dentists practising or willing to practise clinical implantology should know these features and their benefits to successfully choose the correct implant design. Root form implants can be classified as follows:

Root form implants classified on the basis of surface design

Non-threaded implants

These implants do not have any threads along their body, and thus are tapped into the prepared osteotomy slot. The non-threaded implant offers the advantages of more surface area and more bone implant–surface contact percentage (e.g. the Endopore implant) (Fig 2.7A). The limitations of these implants are that they require technique-sensitive placement and only a conventional two-stage protocol can be practised with these implants.

Threaded implants

These implants are the most widely used and contain threads along the implant body. These implants are screwed into the prepared osteotomy site. (e.g. Biohorizons implants, Nobel Biocare implants, etc.) (Fig 2.7B). Threaded implants offer several advantages over the non-threaded implants including ease of placement, more initial stability even in low-density bone, and the facility to practise non-submerged and immediate to early loading protocols.

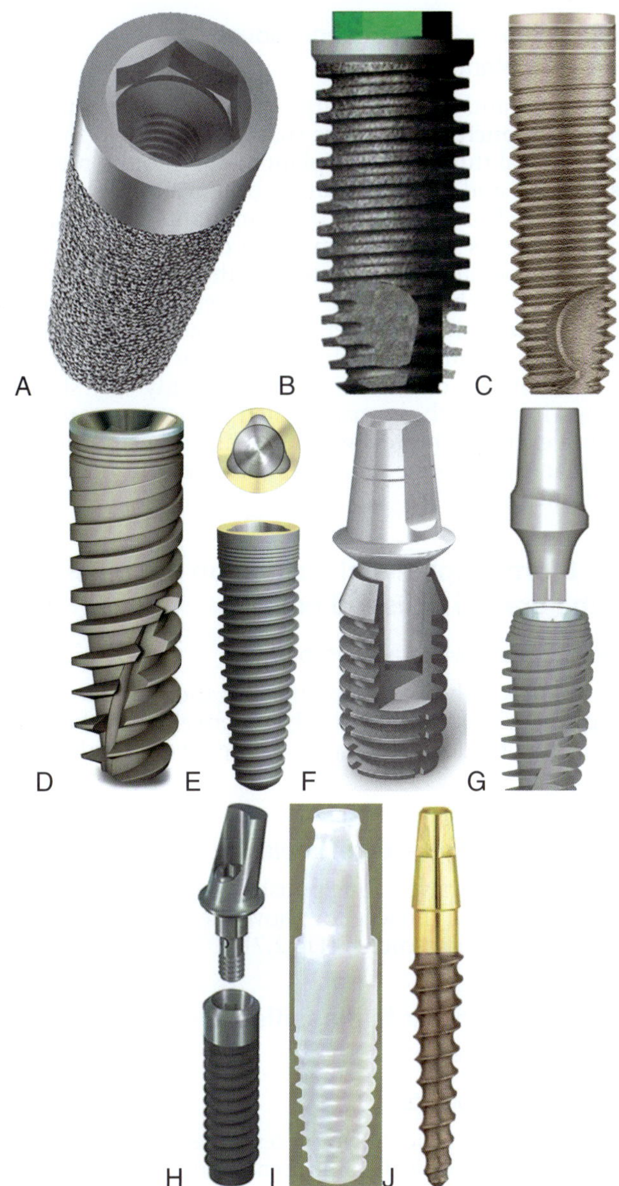

Fig 2.7 Various endosseous root form implants commonly used in practise. (A) Non-threaded implant of Endopore system with hexagonal internal connection. (B) Threaded implant in Maestro, Biohorizons with square threads and hexagonal external connection. (C) Parallel body design of ATID implant with self-tapping thread design from Alpha Bio. (D) Tapered body SPI implant from Alpha Bio with variable thread design. (E) Tapered implant from Nobel Biocare with triangular internal connection. (F) Bicon's locking (cold welded) tapered internal connection implant. (G) WP implant from Adin with Morse taper internal connection. (H) Soft tissue level single-stage implant from Straumann. (I) White sky zirconium implant from Bredent, Germany. (J) ARRP one-piece implant from Alpha Bio, Israel.

Root form implants classified on the basis of body design

Depending on the body taper, root form implants can be parallel or tapered body implants.

Parallel body implants

The bodies of these implants remain almost parallel, without any taper. These implants offer the advantage of more surface area compared to tapered implants of the same diameter. The only disadvantage with these implants is their technique-sensitive placement – if osteotomy for this implant slightly gets widen with the final drill, the primary stability of this implant gets reduced or lost. Further, even in the medium density bone, more no. of drills need to be used for osteotomy preparation when compared to the tapered body implant (Fig 2.7C).

Tapered body implants

The body of this implant tapers as it progresses from the implant platform to the apex. These implants require minimal drilling and achieve high primary stability even in low-density bone. The only disadvantage of these implants is their smaller surface area compared to parallel body implants of similar diameter (Fig 2.7D).

Root form implants classified on the basis of implant connection

Implants can be classified as implants with the external connection and implants with internal connection.

External connection (external hex)

In these implants, the implant connection emerges above the implant platform and acts as the male part, because all the implant components like abutment, healing screw etc. get engaged over and around this connection and are fixed using a connection screw, which is engaged in the prepared threads through the implant connection into the implant body. Conventionally most root form implants carry external connections, and it is claimed that these implants can better withstand the forces and do not get fractured (Fig 2.7B).

Internal connection (internal hex)

These implants show the connection which remains inside the implant body and acts as the female part, because the part of all the implant components goes into the implant connection and get engaged, further the components are fixed using the connection screw (Fig 2.7A).

Root form implants classified on the basis of connection design

The design of the implant connection can vary from system to system.

Triangular design

It has three faces, thus the abutment can be fixed at any of the three oriental positions (Fig 2.7E).

Hexagonal design

It has six faces, thus the abutment can be fixed at any of the six oriental positions (Fig 2.7A).

Octagonal design

It has eight faces, thus the abutment can be fixed at any of the eight oriental positions.

Smooth surface/ non-hex (cold-weld) design

This does not have any faces but is a smooth-surface, tube-in-tube connection. It does not need any connection screw but the abutment gets firmly engaged and cold-welded into the implant connection (Fig 2.7F). It is claimed that this connection forms a tight seal at the implant abutment–connection interface and prevents microbial growth in the connection.

Morse taper connection

This is a combination of both hexed and non-hexed (cold-welded, tube-in-tube) connections. It has the hex in the deepest half of the internal connection as the anti rotational feature, where as the smooth non-hexed surface in the crestal half of the connection makes a tight seal to prevent bacterial growth (Fig 2.7G).

Root form implants classified on the basis of implant material

Titanium alloy implants

Most of the root form implants being currently used are made of pure titanium or titanium alloys (Fig 2.7A–H).

Zirconium implants

Zirconium also osseointegrates with bone like titanium. It offers additional advantages, such as high aesthetics, and can be used in patients with titanium allergy. The only disadvantage with the zirconium implant is that it is made in a single body, because zirconium components which can be screwed to the zirconium body have not yet been developed (Fig 2.7I).

Root form implants classified on the basis of thread design

Implants with various thread designs are available in the market and each design offers some advantages.

Square/U-shaped (non-cutting) thread implants

These threads increase the surface area as well the primary stability of the implant. The only disadvantage of these implants is that a special thread former (bone tap) is used to make threads in the finally prepared osteotomy to incorporate the implant threads into it, especially when the implant is being inserted in high-density bone (Fig 2.7B).

Sharp/V-shaped (cutting) thread (self-tapping) implants

These sharp threads are self-tapping and do not require any additional tool to prepare threads in the bone, because being sharp, they get easily engaged in the bone (Fig 2.7C).

Variable thread (corticocancellous) design implants

These implants contain sharp, self tapping, deep threads with high pitch value (more space between two threads) at the apical third of the implant to tap into the prepared osteotomy and to achieve high primary stability in the cancellous bone. Further, these implants have shallow square threads in the central third of the implant body, which are easily incorporated in the already prepared threads in the bone by the apical deep implant threads. These square threads laterally condense the trabecular bone and enhance the primary stability of the implant. The crestal part of these implants has only very shallow micro-rings, which get easily seated in the osteotomy and do not exert much pressure on the high-density and low-vascular crestal bone. This prevents pressure necrosis of the bone (Fig 2.7D).

Root form implants classified on the basis of the crestal polished collar

Subgingival (two-stage) implants

These are widely used implants and their all part of the fixture is placed within the bony envelop of the ridge with their platform is placed at the level of ridge crest (Fig 2.7A–G).

Transgingival (one-stage) implants

These implants have a long polished collar and their platform is placed at the level or above the level of soft tissue (transgingival placement) (Fig 2.7H).

Root form implants classified on the basis of implant pieces

Two-piece implants

Most implants come in two pieces – the fixture is one part and the other part is the abutment, which is screwed over the fixture to support the prosthesis (Fig 2.7A–H).

One-piece implant

This implant comes with the abutment as an integral part of the fixture (all in one piece). All called single body implants. These implants are used for immediate functional or non-functional restoration after implant placement. The fabrication of the connection in the implants (with narrow diameters below 3.3 mm) is difficult and can weaken the implant body. Initially a few companies started manufacturing these implants in the narrow diameters from 2.5–3 mm for use in tight spaces (e.g. the mandibular incisors and maxillary laterals), and to retain dentures in geriatric patients with narrow edentulous ridges. These implants were also termed 'mini implants' because of their small size. Later, these single-piece implants were manufactured in the regular to wider diameters, for use in cases where adequate bone volume and density was available to place and immediately restore these implants (Fig 2.7I and J).

Implant surfaces

Dental implants with different surface treatments are available in the market, and their manufacturers claim that they are superior to the conventional machined surface titanium implants for predictable quality of osseointegration. As a general rule, roughened surfaces increase the bone–implant contact (BIC) percentage during the initial bone healing process.

Several research studies have been performed to find an optimal surface treatment to increase mechanical stability and improve the contact between bone and implant. Many research projects have provided conclusive scientific evidence that a roughened titanium implant surface improves bone anchoring compared to conventionally machined titanium surfaces. The rough surface facilitates migration of osteogenic cells to the implant surface for *de novo* bone formation (contact osteogenesis). The local mechanical environment provided by the rough surface implant also influences cellular differentiation and tissue synthesis (distance osteogenesis). The local mechanical environment provided by the rough surface implant shows increased removal forces, greater BIC percentage, earlier bone–implant contact , and improved ultimate osseointegration.

The 'osseointegration' phenomenon was first described by Branemark and associates and was defined as the direct contact between living bone and a functionally-loaded implant surface without interposed soft tissue at the light microscope level.

Titanium is the metal widely used for dental implant manufacturing, either in the commercially pure titanium form (cpTi) or as an alloy, because it shows a variety of favourable features like high strength, low weight, high corrosion resistance, low modulus of elasticity, and easy shaping and finishing capability. The titanium alloy (titanium-6 aluminium-4 vanadium [Ti_6Al_4V]) most frequently used for implant manufacturing is composed of 90% titanium, 6% aluminium (decreases the specific weight and improves the elastic modulus) and 4% vanadium (decreases thermal conductivity and increases hardness).

An implant made of pure titanium or titanium alloy, when exposed to the air, immediately forms an 'oxide layer' (titanium dioxide [TiO_2]) over its surface. This layer comes in contact with the bony tissue and plays an important role in corrosion resistance, biocompatibility and osseointegration.

The chemical composition of the implant surface can differ markedly from its bulk composition due to manufacturing processes, such as machining, thermal treatment, blasting, etching, coatings, and even sterilization procedures. Surface contamination introduced by these procedures (e.g. traces of metals, ions, lubricants, and detergents), may alter surface biocompatibility for better or worse, even when it is present in small quantities. Based on these considerations, careful control of the composition of the implant surface becomes a relevant procedure to produce high quality implants.

The following are a few of the most commonly used implant surfaces:

Machined/smooth/turned implant surface

It was the most commonly used surface in the past; however, it is not now very commonly used, because of improved stabilization and larger surface area obtained in roughened surface implants.

Modified implant surface

Conventional machine implant surfaces can be modified with either 'additive methods' (e.g. hydroxyapatite coating, plasma spraying, etc.) or 'subtractive methods' (e.g. acid-etching, sandblasting, etc.), to improve the implant surface and its characteristics, to achieve optimal implant osseointegration with the jawbone.

Sandblasted surface

Titanium metal implants are sandblasted, using agents such as aluminium oxide/alumina (Al_2O_3), titanium dioxide (TiO_2), and calcium phosphate to increase surface roughness. The sandblasting not only improves BIC percentage, but also improves contact osteogenesis by allowing the addition, proliferation, and differentiation of the osteoblasts over the implant surface. The few disadvantages of the sandblasting procedure are the presence of sandblasting material residues on the implant surface, non-uniform surface treatment, and loss of metallic substance from the implant body. A specific method to produce calcium phosphate-blasted implants is also used. The titanium base is submitted to blasting with calcium phosphate, a resorbable blast material (RBM), followed by a passivity procedure to remove the residual calcium phosphate ($CaPO_4$) and it is finally, cleaned. The blast medium is resorbed during these processes, and a surface of pure TiO_2 is produced that is free of contaminants (e.g. PTS™/ OsseoFix™ surface of Adin implants).

Titanium plasma sprayed (TPS) surface

These implants are prepared by spraying molten metal on the titanium base, which results in a surface with irregularly sized and shaped valleys, pores, and crevices, increasing the microscopic surface area by approximately 10 times. One disadvantage of using these implants is the possibility of detachment of titanium after implant insertion (e.g. TPS surface of Friadent implants).

Acid-etched surface

Acid-etching of titanium implants is performed using baths of hydrochloric acid (HCL), nitric acid (HNO_3), and sulphuric acid (H_2SO_4) in specific combinations. A dual acid-etched technique is also being used by a few manufacturers to produce a microtextured implant surface which improves the BIC percentage as well as the reverse torque value of the implant. (e.g. Osseotite surface of 3i implants.)

Sandblasted and acid-etched surface

A few implant manufacturers have started creating this surface by first sandblasting to produce macrotexture, followed by acid-etching to produced a final microtextured surface. This surface shows promising results, as these implants have shown high BIC percentage as well as reverse torque value. Other advantages of this surface are higher rate and degree of osseointegration, better osteoconductive properties, and higher capability to induce cell proliferation. Many studies and clinical trials have claimed that these implants, if inserted in bone with adequate volume and density, can be restored after 6 weeks. In a few clinical situations, after consideration of other parameters, these implants can immediately be loaded (e.g. SLA surface of Straumann implants, FRIADENT® plus surface of ANKYLOS® implants, SLA surface of Alpha Bio implants, etc.)

Anodized surface

This surface is prepared by applying voltage on titanium implants immersed in an electrolyte, which results in a surface with variable diameter micropores. The advantages of this surface are improved cell proliferation and attachment, lack of cytotoxicity, and more removal torque value in the implant (e.g. TiUnite surface of Nobel Biocare implants).

Hydroxyapatite (HA) coated surface

Hydroxyapatite coated implants have shown roughness and functional surface area similar to TPS implants. This surface shows accelerated interfacial bone formation and maturation; hence, the direct bonding between the HA coating and the bone is found to be far superior to the bond between titanium and bone or TPS and bone. An initial implant-to-bone interface contact is essential for a predictable interface to form. The space or gap between the implant and bone may affect the BIC percentage after healing. Gap healing can be enhanced by the HA coating. The HA coating also reduces the corrosion rate of the metal (e.g. the HA coated surface of Biohorizons D4 implants). Some advantages of HA coated implants are increased roughness and surface area, enhanced initial implant stability, increased gap healing between bone and HA coating, less corrosion of metal, faster healing at the bone interface, and stronger bone–implant interface. The disadvantages of HA coating are flaking, cracking or scaling of the coating at implant insertion (especially in high-density bone), increased plaque retention when left exposed to the oral environment or resulted after the crestal bone resorption and marginal soft tissue recession. Coating also increases the cost of the implant. Many studies and clinical trials have shown higher success rates for HA coated implants used in low-density (D4) bone.

Summary

An understanding of the various kinds of implant designs and surfaces described in this chapter can be very helpful to the clinician to evaluate the various implants available in the market. Though subperiosteal implants are not now being widely used, they can be very useful for the vertically resorbed mandible, where inadequate bone is left above the mandibular canal to insert root form implant. Blade implants are also not much in use but can be used in cases with the narrow mandibular ridge, where these implants can easily be placed by making a narrow horizontal slot through the ridge crest. The disadvantage of blade implants is that these implants need greater mesiodistal ridge dimensions to be placed, compared with the root form implants. As described earlier in the chapter transosteal implants have very limited use and need major surgical intervention to be correctly placed. Implants with internal connections offer more ease in practise than those with external connection. For this reason, more manufacturers are switching to the internal connection. The Morse taper connection appears good as it has the anti-rotational feature and also achieves a tight antibacterial seal in the connection. Implants with the square thread design achieve more BIC percentage and more promising results; but a special thread former is needed to seal these implants, especially in high-density bone. The implants with variable thread design and tapered body offer the advantages of ease of placement and high primary stability. The single-stage transgingival implants are good for one-stage implant placement but these implants should be used only in areas where adequate primary stability of the implant can be achieved. Several studies have suggested that the sandblasted plus acid-etched surface implant and the anodized surface implant achieve faster osseointegration and thus can be restored immediately or early in some cases. While the implant with HA surface achieves better and early osseointegration, it should be used only in low-density bone, and thus can be a better option for the low-density posterior maxilla. The single-piece mini implants can be the preferred option to support the fixed prosthesis in tight spaces or narrow ridge and also to retain the overdentures in narrow ridge cases.

Further Reading

Weiss CM, Judy K, Chiarenza A. Precompacted, coined titanium endosteal blade implants. J Oral Implantol 1973;3:4.

Deporter DA, Watson PA, Booker D. Simplifying the treatment of edentulism: a new type of implant. J Am Dent Assoc 1996;127:1343.

Adell R, Lekholm U, Rockler B. A 15-year study of osseointegrated implants in the treatment of the edentulous jaw. Int J Oral Surg 1981;10:387.

Cox JF, Zarb GA. The longitudinal clinical efficacy of osseointegrated dental implants: a 3-year report. Int J Oral Maxillofac Implants 1987;2:91.

Steflik DE, et al. Osteogenesis at the dental implant interface: high-voltage electron microscopic and conventional transmission electron microscopic observations. J Biomed Mater Res 1993;27:791.

Roberts HD, Roberts RA. The ramus endosseous implant. J Calif Dent Assoc 1970;38:57.

Small IA. The mandibular staple bone plate: its use and advantages in reconstructive surgery. Dent Clin North Am 1986;30:175.

Weiss CM, Judy K. Modern surgical and design considerations and clinical indications for subperiosteal implants. Implantologist 1978;1:3.

James RA. Tissue behavior in the environment produced by permucosal devices. The dental implant. Littleton, Mass: PSG Publishing; 1985.

Russell TE, Kapur SP. Bone surfaces adjacent to a subperiosteal implant: a SEM study. J Oral Implantol 1977;8:3.

Weiss CM, Judy K. Intramucosal inserts: conserve edentulous ridges and increase retention and stability of removable maxillary prostheses. Oral Health 1973;63:11.

Castilho Guilherme AA, Martins Maximiliano D, Macedo Waldemar AA. Surface characterization of titanium based dental implants. Braz J Phys September, 2006, vol. 36, no. 3B.

Park JY, Gemmell CH, Davies JE. Platelet interactions with titanium: modulation of platelet activity by surface topography. Biomaterials 2001;22:2671–82.

Ogawa T, Nishimura I. Different bone integration profiles of turned and acid-etched implants associated with modulated expression of extracellular matrix genes. Int J Oral Maxillofac Implant 2003;18:200–10.

Galli C, Guizzardi S, Passeri G, et al. Comparison of human mandibular osteoblasts grown on two commercially available titanium implant surfaces. J Periodontol 2005;76:364–72.

Buser D, Nydegger T, Hirt HP, et al. Removal torque values of titanium implants in the maxillae of miniature pigs. Int J Oral Maxillofac Implant 1998;13:611–9.

Cochran DL, Schenk RK, Lussi A, et al. Bone response to unloaded and loaded titanium implants with a sandblasted and acid-etched surface: a histometric study in the canine mandible. J Biomed Mater Res 1998;40:1–1.

Hayakawa T, Kiba H, Yasuda S, et al. A histologic and histomorphometric evaluation of two type of retrieved human titanium implants. Int J Periodontics Restorative Dent 2002;22:164–71.

Cochran DL, Buser D, ten Bruggenkate CM, et al. The use of reduced healing times on ITI implants with a sandblasted and acid-etched (SLA) surface: early results from clinical trials on ITI SLA implants. Clin Oral Implants Res 2002;13:144–53.

Piattelli M, Scarano A, Paoloantonio M, et al. Bone response to machined and resorbable blast material titanium implants: an experimental study in rabbits. J Oral Implant 2002;28:2–8.

Schwrtz-Arad D, Mardinger O, Levin L, et al. Marginal bone loss pattern around hydroxyapatite – coated versus commercially pure titanium implants after up to 12 years of follow – up. Int J Oral Maxillofac Implants 2005;20:238–44.

Implant inventories and armamentarium 3

Ajay Vikram Singh

CHAPTER CONTENTS HD

Introduction

Various kinds of implant inventories and armamentaria are required to practise basic to advanced implant procedures. The novice implant doctor should know that many implant inventories are used to successfully perform the surgical and prosthetic phases of implantation and these inventories may vary in number, size, and shape, depending on the implant design and manufacturer. Although most implant systems present approximately similar surgical and prosthetic components, most of them remain system specific. This means that the surgical or prosthetic components belonging to one particular implant system, usually, cannot be accurately used in any other system; and often components from one group of implants cannot be used in a different group of implants from the same manufacturer. In various implant systems the prosthetic inventories are implant diameter specific, so that the implant inventories of the implant with 4 mm diameter cannot be used for another implant of smaller or larger diameter. To overcome these problems some implant systems come with a common platform, so that common prosthetic inventories can be fitted to implants of any diameter (mix and match prosthetic inventories) in the range. Dental practitioners should know that beside the implant inventories, they need system-specific surgical kits to place particular implants. In addition, implant motor, which is not system-specific, is required for osteotomy preparation and other associated implant and bone grafting procedures. The author has tried to describe in this chapter, the different kinds of inventories and the armamentarium required for basic implant practise in a step by step simplified manner, but there may be a few variations in specific systems. Thus the author advises implant surgeons to attend the mentoring programmes and read the catalogues of particular systems, to brush up complete knowledge of a particular system and its inventories.

Implant components

As described earlier, a range of implant components are required to practise implantology and these components are described here in the order in which they are used.

1. Implant fixture
2. Implant mount
3. Cover screw
4. Gingival former/healing screw/healing abutment/permucosal extension
5. Impression post/impression transfer abutment
6. Implant analogue
7. Abutment
8. Fixation screw

1. Implant fixture. The term fixture is used synonymously for the implant itself which is inserted and gets osseointegrated with the bone (Fig 3.1). It works as the tooth root, and various kinds of components are used to cover it, make its impression, and retain or fix the prosthesis on top of it. The implant fixture comes in a sterile vial which remains covered further in a non-sterile packaging that shows all the details of the implant such as its manufacturer, diameter, length, batch no., expiry details, etc. (Fig 3.2). The inner sterile vial usually contains the implant fixture, its mount, and a cover screw (Fig 3.3).

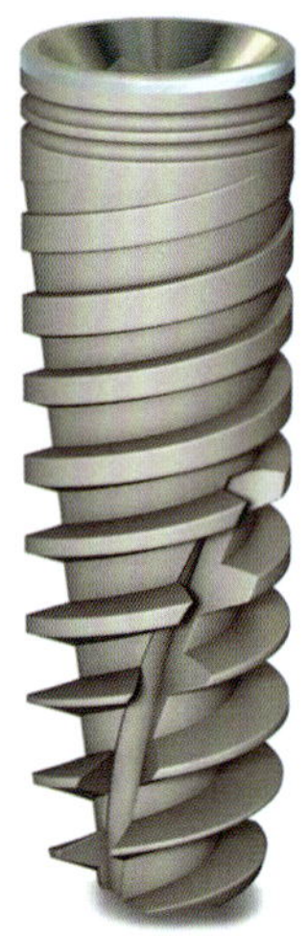

Fig 3.1 Implant fixture.

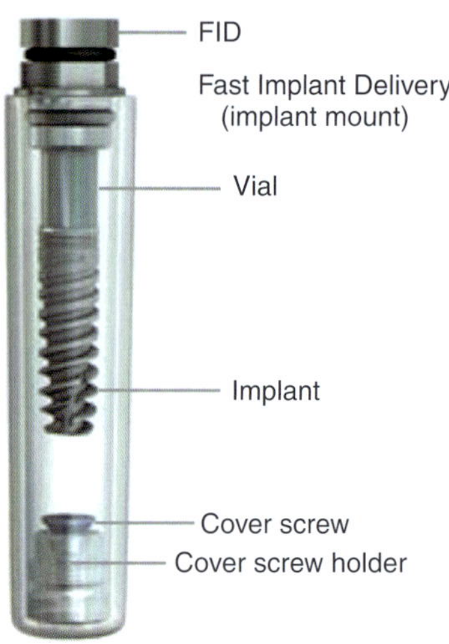

Fig 3.3 Figure showing the implant and its components which the implant packet usually contains.

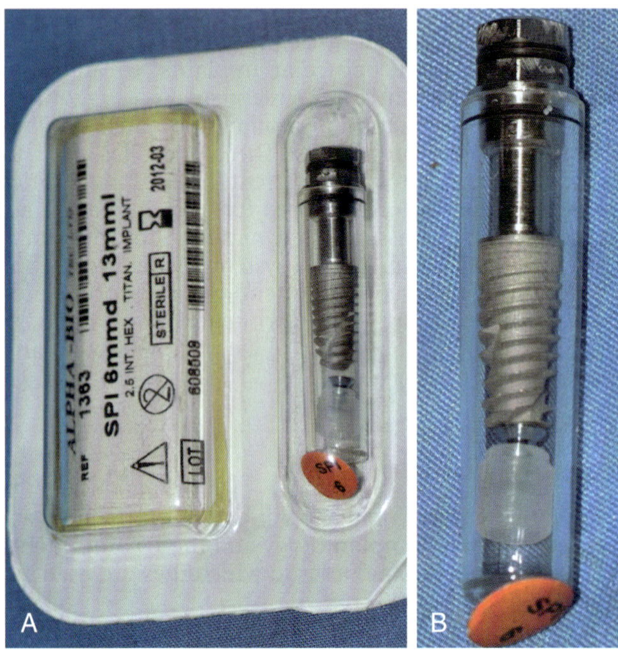

Fig 3.2 (A) The implant fixture comes in a sterile vial which is covered further in a non-sterile packaging which shows all the details of the implant like its make, diameter, length, batch no, expiry, company name, etc. (B) The inner sterile vial contains implant fixture, its mount, and cover screw.

2. Implant mount. The implant mount is a component which usually comes connected with the implant in its vial and it is used to carry the implant from its vial/packaging to the prepared osteotomy site either by hand or with a ratchet/hand piece adaptor. The implant fixture surface being highly sterile should not be touched by the gloved hand or any instrument, to avoid surface contamination. Thus an implant mount is used to carry the implant from its vial to the prepared osteotomy. This mount can be fitted to the ratchet and used to screw the implant in. Once the implant gets adequately engaged in the osteotomy, the mount can be removed and the implant can be further screwed in using a long implant driver (Fig 3.4A–H). In few implant systems, the implant fixture does not carry any mount in its vial, but the implant driver (connected to the hand ratchet or hand piece), which remains available in the implant surgical kit indirectly fitted to implant connection, is used to carry the implant from its vial to the osteotomy site (Fig 3.5).
3. Cover screw. This is the component that is used to cover the implant connection during the submerged healing of the implant (Fig 3.6). It preserves the patency of the connection by preventing any soft tissue ingrowth in the connection (Fig 3.7). This component usually comes with the implant fixture in its sterile vial.
4. Gingival former/healing screw/healing abutment. This is used to form a healthy, aesthetic emergence profile of the soft tissue around the implant prosthesis. When the implant is re-exposed after it is osseointegrated with the bone, the cover screw is removed and replaced with a long gingival former and the site is left to heal for 2 to 3 weeks. After the soft tissue has healed, the removal of the gingival former shows the healed entry to the implant connection through the soft tissue. Gingival formers are available in different heights and shapes and a specific gingival former is selected according to the thickness and emergence profile (straight or divergent) of the soft tissue needed for the future prosthesis (Figs 3.8 and 3.9). In the one-stage (non-submerged) implant healing protocol; the gingival former is inserted over the implant immediately after implant insertion (Fig 3.10).
5. Impression post/impression transfer abutment. The impression post is the component that is used to transfer the implant Hex position and orientation from the mouth to the working cast. Once the soft tissue around the gingival former has healed, the gingival former is removed and impression post is inserted over the implant. An impression is made in silicon impression material (polyether or additional silicon). The post is then removed from the implant, assembled with the implant analogue, and transferred to the impression with the same orientation (Fig 3.11).

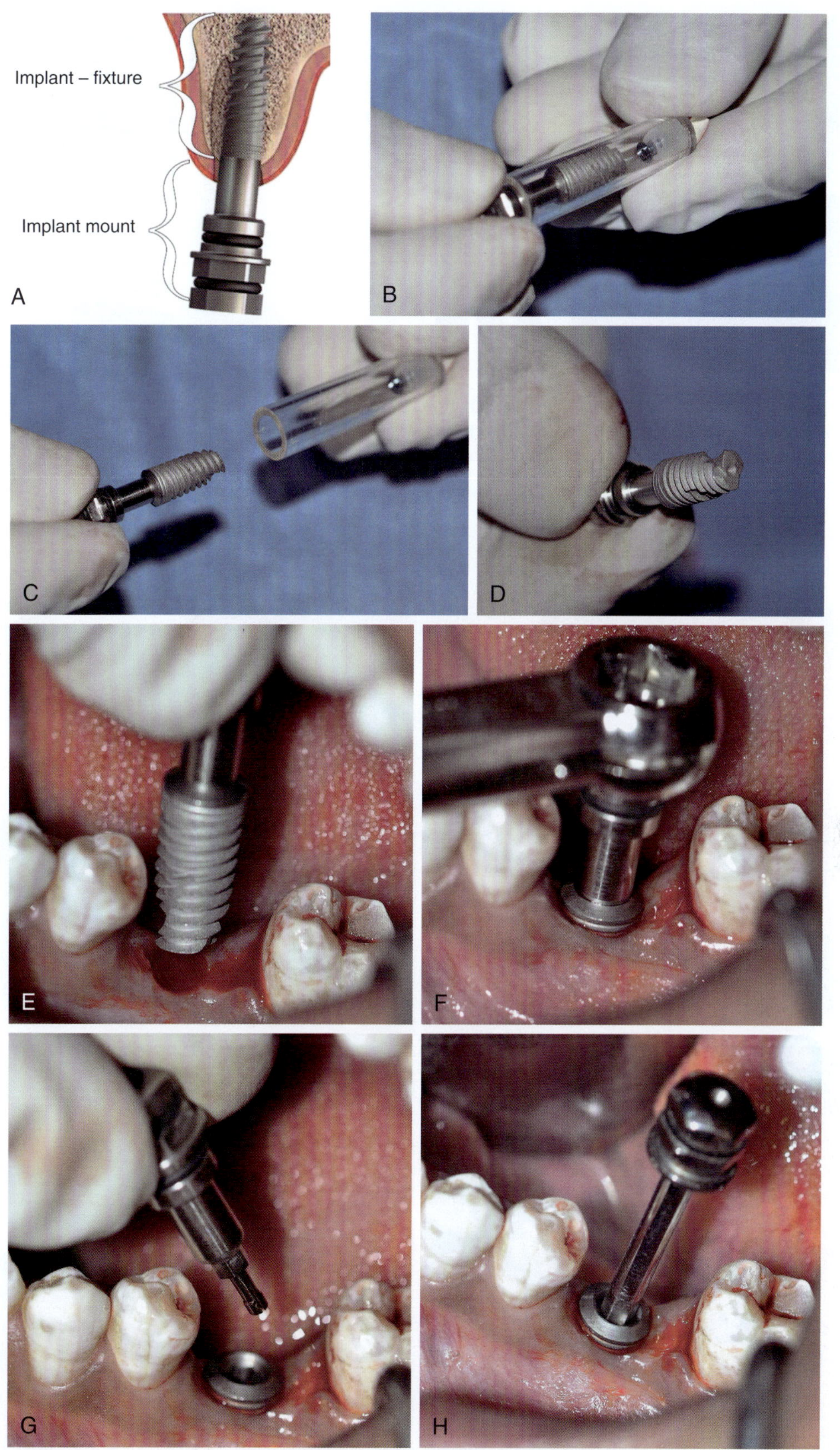

Fig 3.4 (A–H) Implant fixture surface being highly sterile should not be touched with gloved hand or any instrument, to avoid surface contamination. Thus an implant mount is used to carry the implant from its vial to the prepared osteotomy. This mount can be fitted to the ratchet and used to place the implant into the prepared osteotomy. Once the implant gets adequately engaged in the osteotomy, the mount can be removed and the implant can be further screwed in, using a long implant driver.

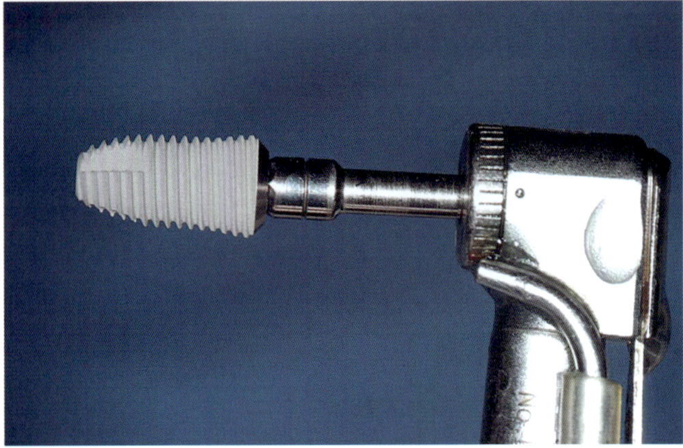

Fig 3.5 A few manufacturers do not provide the implant mount with the implant, but an implant driver from the surgical kit, connected to hand piece, is used to carry the implant from its sterile vial to the prepared osteotomy *(Courtesy: Dentium implants, Seoul, Korea)*.

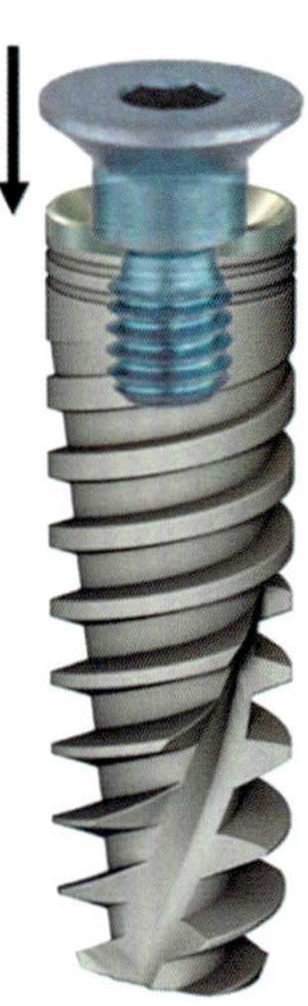

Fig 3.6 The cover screw usually comes with the implant fixture in its sterile vial, and is used to cover the implant connection during its submerged healing period.

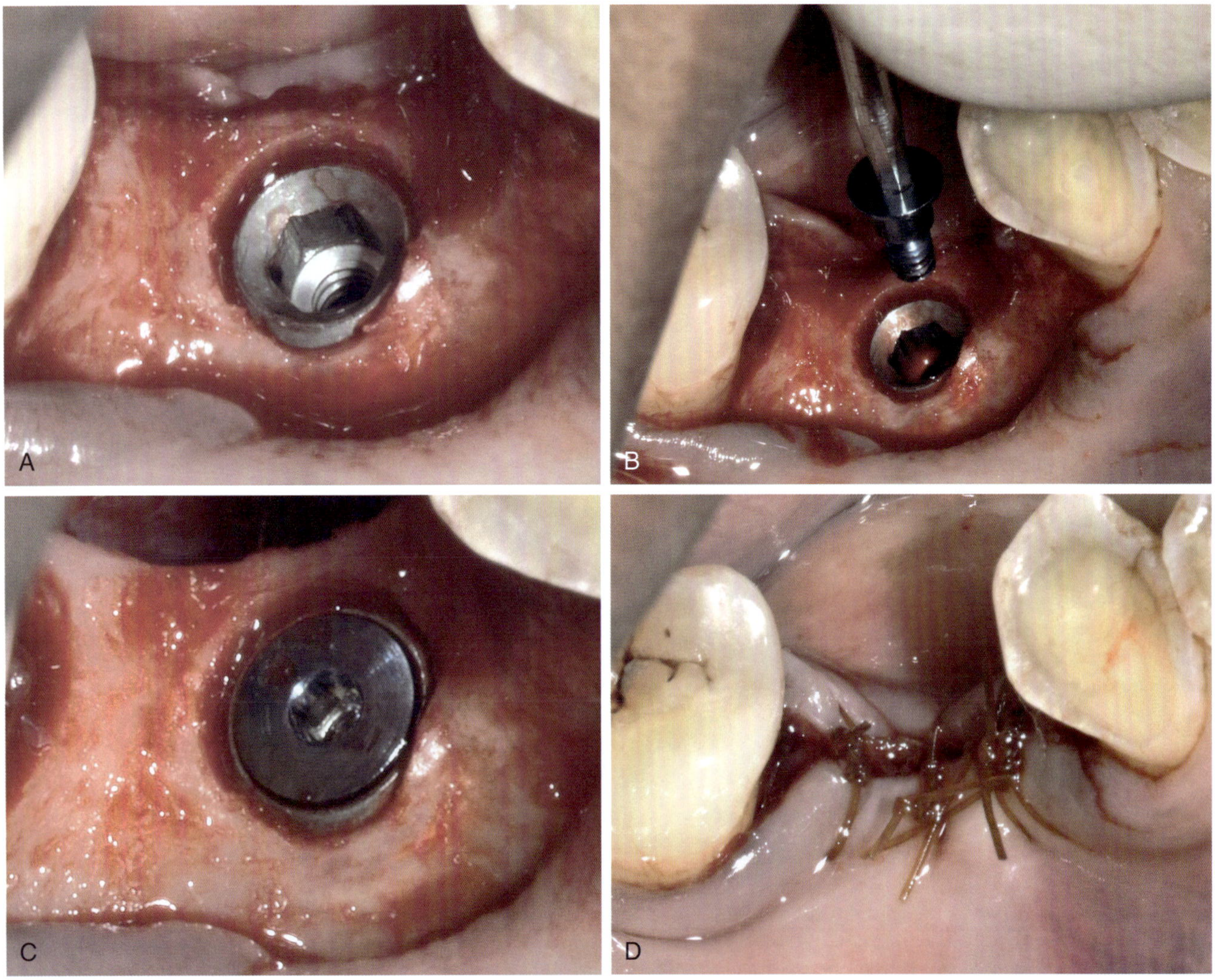

A

B

C

D

Fig 3.7 (A–D) Once the implant is completely seated in the prepared osteotomy, its connection is covered with the cover screw to prevent any soft tissue ingression in the connection. The cover screw is used in the submerged healing protocol, and therefore the flap is sutured back to cover it.

Types of impression posts

1. **Closed tray impression post** poses shallow retention grooves along its body and a short connection screw. It is used in the closed tray impression transfer technique. The complete post remains under the impression and no part of it emerges out of the tray. After making the impression, this post is removed from the implant, assembled to the analogue, and inserted to the impression with the same orientation (Fig 3.12).

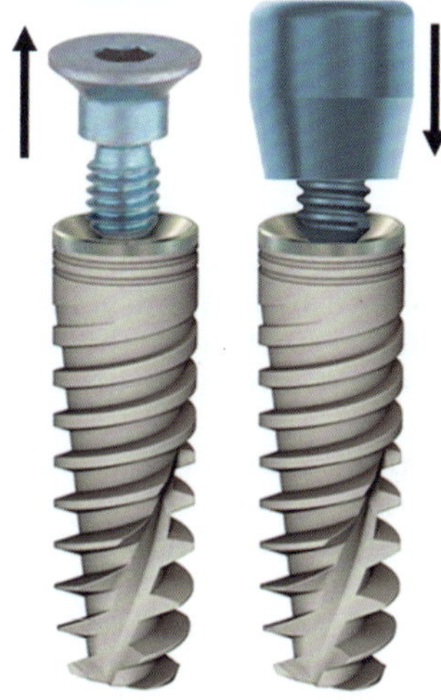

Fig 3.8 The cover screw is replaced with long healing abutment/gingival former to form a healthy entry to the implant through the soft tissue *(Courtesy: Alpha-Bio Implant Systems, Israel)*.

2. **Open tray impression post** poses deep retention grooves along its body and a long connection screw. This post is used in the open tray impression transfer technique. A part of its long screw emerges out of the impression tray, and should be unscrewed before removing the impression from the mouth. This post comes out embedded in the impression. The analogue is assembled with this post on the inner side of the impression, and impression is poured in dia stone (Figs 3.12 and 3.13).

6. Implant analogue is a component which has a different body but its platform and connection are exactly similar to the implant. The analogue is used to replicate the implant platform and connection in the laboratory mode. The impression post is removed from the mouth after the impression is made, and it is assembled with the implant analogue that has its platform and connection design exactly similar to the implant in the mouth. This impression post with analogue is transferred to the impression at the same position and orientation and the impression is poured with dental stone plaster (Figs 3.14 and 3.15).
7. Abutments are, expressed simply, the components that are finally screwed to implants to hold the final prosthesis. Once the dentist has transferred the implant connection position and orientation, using the impression post and analogue, from the patient's mouth to the working cast, an appropriate final abutment is screwed onto the analogue and milled to the required shape and angulation. The prosthesis is fabricated over this abutment in the prosthetic laboratory and sent back to the clinician. The clinician transfers this abutment to the implant in the patient's mouth

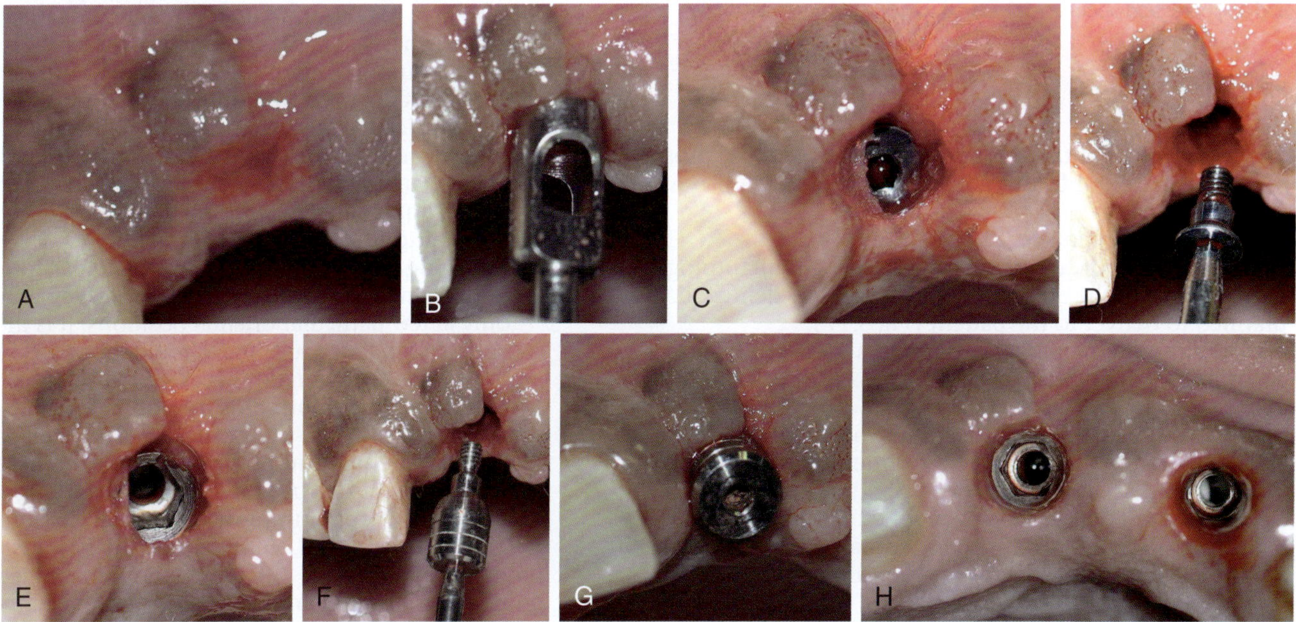

Fig 3.9 (A–H) In the two-stage (submerged healing) implant healing protocol, the implant is uncovered with incision or using a soft tissue punch, after it get osseointegrated with the bone and the cover screw is replaced with a gingival former. The gingival former is left in place for a minimum for 2 to 3 weeks to achieve a healed soft tissue around the implant platform.

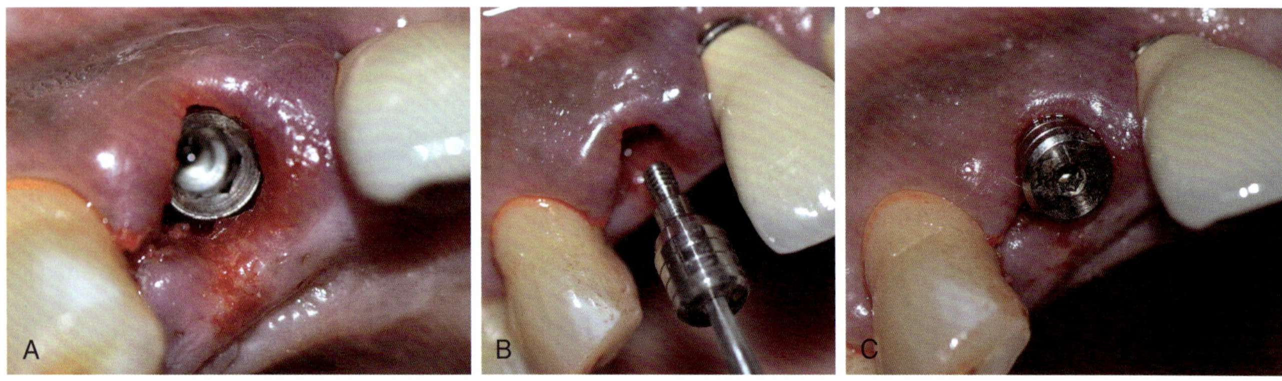

Fig 3.10 (A–C) In the one-stage (non-submerged) implant healing protocol; the gingival former is inserted over the implant immediately after implant insertion.

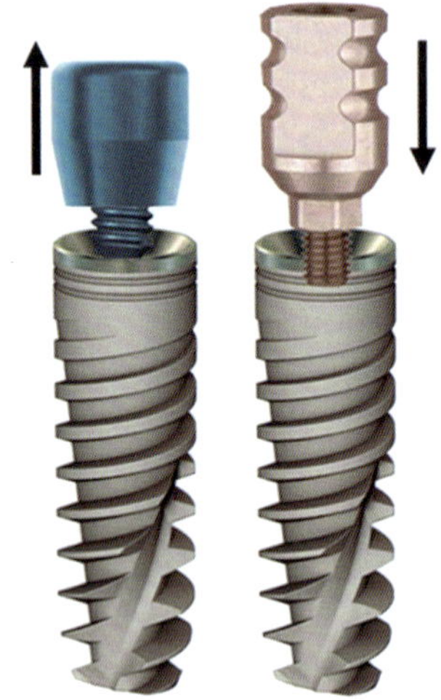

Fig 3.11 Once soft tissue gets healed, the gingival former is removed and an impression abutment is inserted to make the impression.

with same orientation as on the model, and the prosthesis is fixed onto this abutment (Fig 3.16A–F).

Types of Abutments

Various types of abutments are used in implantology depending on the kind of prosthesis, the dentist has planned to deliver to the patient (Fig 3.17).

In a simplified manner, abutments can be classified according to their use.

1. Abutments for ball retained overdentures: used to retain ball retained overdentures (Figs 3.18 and 3.19).
2. Abutments for cement-retained fixed prosthesis:
   a. Straight abutments. Available in different diameters, lengths and soft tissue collar height (Fig 3.19A–D).
   b. Angled abutments. Available with 5°, 15°, 25°, and 30° angulations. Used for prosthetic angulation correction of an implant that is placed at an angle to the prosthetic axis (Fig 3.19 E–G).
   c. **Anatomical/aesthetic abutments.** These abutments have an anatomical finish line to obtain a better aesthetics at the cervical region of the implant prosthesis in the aesthetic region (Fig 3.19F).
   d. **Zirconium abutments.** Used under metal-free zirconium prostheses. They avoid the display of the metal abutment collar through thin marginal soft tissue (Fig 3.19K).
   e. **Temporary abutments.** Used chairside to make a provisional prosthesis over the implant (Fig 3.19J).
3. Plastic/castable abutments for screw-retained fixed prosthesis: These abutments are used to fabricate screw-retained prostheses as they can be cast to make a metal framework that can directly be fixed to the implant. Plastic abutments can be available with or without titanium base. These can be available as straight plastic abutments or angled plastic abutments (Fig 3.19H and I) (Also see Chapter 11).
4. Abutments for abutment level screw-retained fixed prosthesis or bar retained overdentures: These titanium abutments, also called 'abutment for screw' are first screwed onto the implants and used to fabricate screw-retained detachable hybrid prostheses and to fabricate the bar framework for the bar-retained dentures (Fig 3.19L) (Also see Chapter 11 and Chapter 22).
5. Engaging and non-engaging abutments:
   a. **Engaging abutments** have the triangular/hex/octave connection and so can be fixed to implants only at few particular oriental positions. It is the antirotational feature and should be used in most prosthetic situations (Fig 3.19A).
   b. **Non-engaging abutments** do not have any triangular/hex/octave connection and so can be fixed to the implant at any orientation. These abutments can be used in cases of a joint prosthesis fixed over multiple implants (Fig 3.19O).
6. UCLA abutment: The UCLA abutment is a castable abutment. It is offered with a machined gold alloy base or in a fully castable version. It may be used for single- or multiunit screw or cement-retained restorations. It may correct angles up to 30° when cast as a customized abutment (Fig 3.19P).

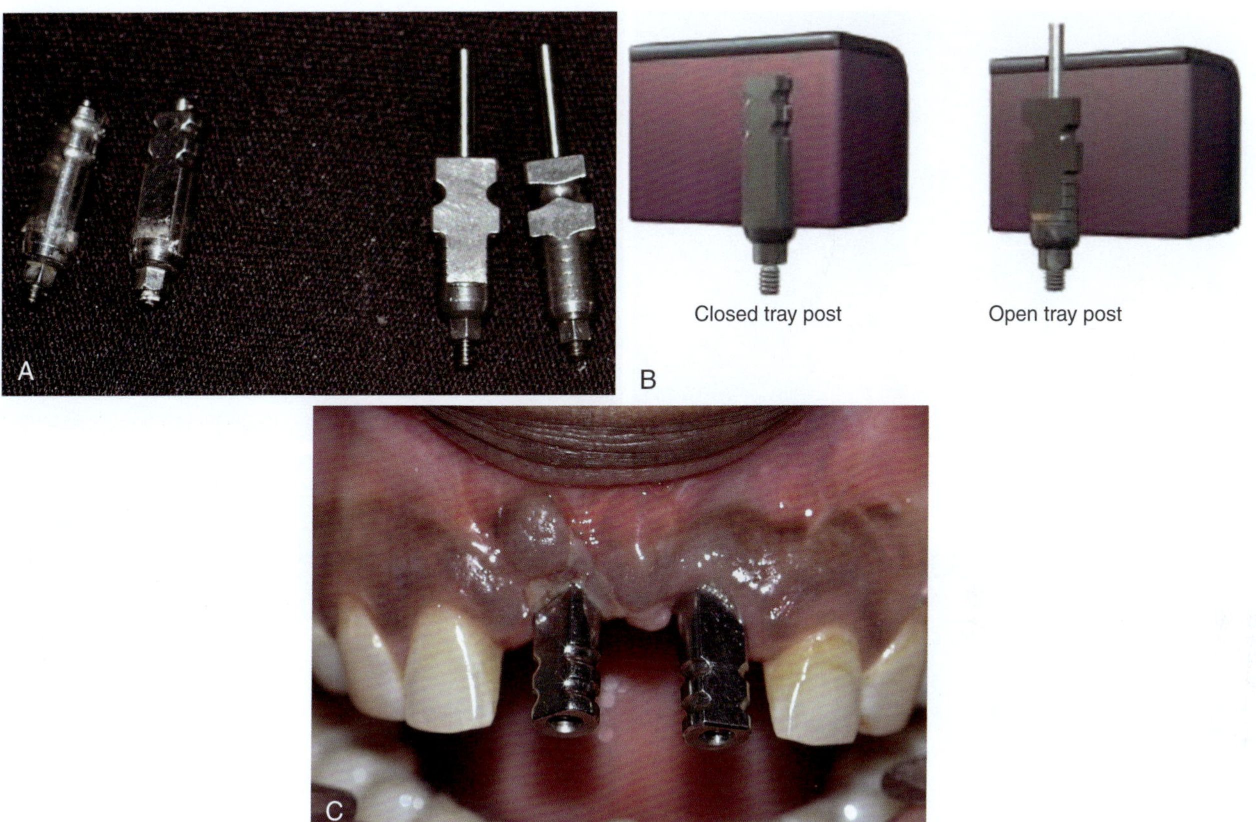

Fig 3.12 (A and B) Closed tray impression posts (left) with shallow retention grooves and short connection screw and open tray impression posts (right) with deep retention grooves and long fixation screws. (C) Closed tray posts connected to implants in the mouth before making impression.

Connection screw. This screw is used to connect any abutment or screw-retained prosthesis to the implant fixture. It comes with all kinds of abutments in the same packaging (Fig 3.19Q).

7. Multiunit abutment: This special abutment is used to correct extreme angulation. It is first connected to the implant with the help of a connection screw and then other prosthetic components of choice can be screwed on top of it. It is available in 17° and 30° angulations. This abutment is widely being used in 'All on 4' and 'All on 6' techniques (Fig 3.20A–C).

Platform switching or the common platform concept

As described earlier, in many systems implant components are implant-diameter specific and the abutment, impression abutment, gingival former, etc. of an implant with a specific diameter cannot be fitted to another implant of a different diameter, even within the same system. These divergent component platforms for implants of different diameters force the clinician to keep stock of several inventories for use in particular diameter implants. The clinician must also keep patient records of all implants inserted, so that he/she can be ready with all the inventories for implants of varying diameters that he/she has used, at every step of the surgical and prosthetic phases. The components for a particular implant that he/she has in stock are not going to fit an implant of a different diameter. To overcome this problem, a few manufacturers started making implants with a similar platform so that any of the components could be fitted to any implant in a particular system, irrespective of diameter. When the smaller diameter abutment is used over the regular to wider diameter implant, it forms an implant–abutment junction narrower than the diameter of the implant, apical to and diameter of abutment occlusal to this junction. When such implants were used, clinicians found that this narrow implant–abutment junction provided stress-free space for the formation of thick bone and soft tissue in the crestal region. Several studies have been done on this platform switching concept and it has been concluded that platform switching may reduce the crestal bone resorption around the loaded implant by as much as 70% (Fig 3.21A and B).

Armamentarium for the practise of implantology

Besides the general dental setup, the dental surgeon needs to have several specific tools to practise basic to advanced dental implant procedures. There are a few basic tools which

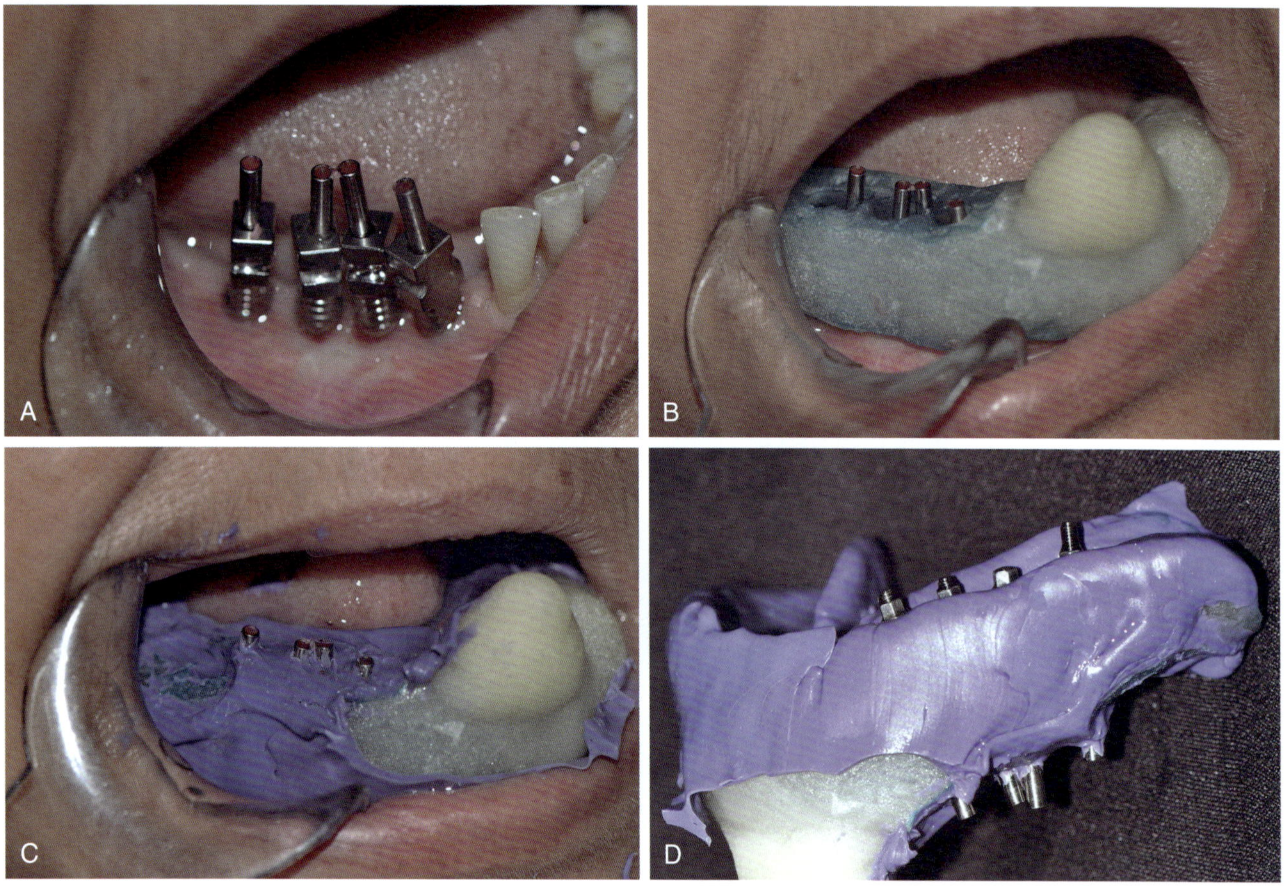

Fig 3.13 (A) Open tray posts inserted to the implants, (B and C) the long connection screws of the posts are emerging out of the impression tray. (D) The connection screws should be unscrewed before removing impression from the implant so that the post comes out embedded in the impression.

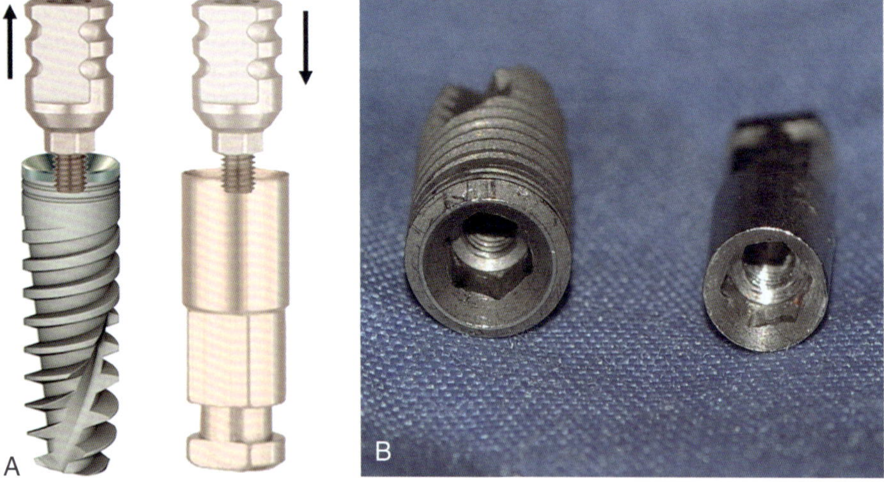

Fig 3.14 (A and B) Impression post is removed from the mouth and assembled with the implant analogue which has different body; but the connection is exactly similar to the implant.

are mandatory for the implant dentist to practise implant procedures and others can be added later depending on the kind of advanced implant procedures the implant surgeon wishes to perform. These tools are described according to their use in particular implant techniques.

A. Inventories used to practise basic implant procedures
   1. Dental implant surgical kit
   2. Implant motor (physiodispensor)
   3. Rotary reduction hand pieces
   4. Basic oral surgery instruments

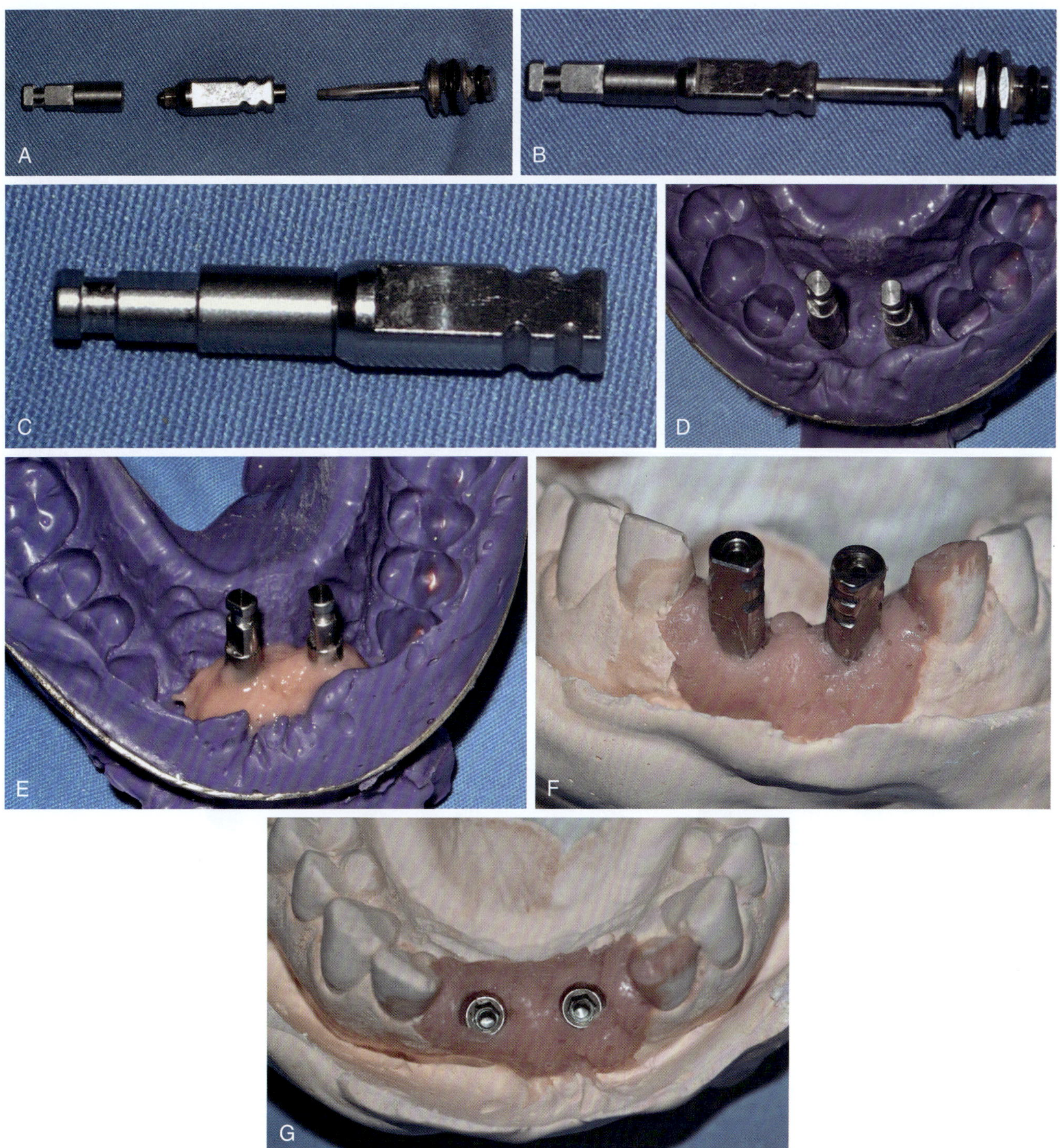

Fig 3.15 (A–G) The post is assembled with the implant analogue and seated into the impression with the same orientation as in the mouth. The impression is first poured with soft tissue replicating material (Gi-Mask) followed by dental stone. The impression post removed from the cast and final abutment of choice is inserted.

5. Surgical draping
6. Cleaning and sterilization equipment

B. Additional inventories for the practise of advanced implant procedures

Inventories required to perform the specific implant procedures like immediate implantation in the fresh extraction socket, guided bone regeneration, the sub-antral and lateral approach of sinus grafting, ridge splitting techniques, block grafting techniques, nerve transposition techniques, distraction osteogenesis, soft tissue grafting, etc. are mentioned in related chapters.

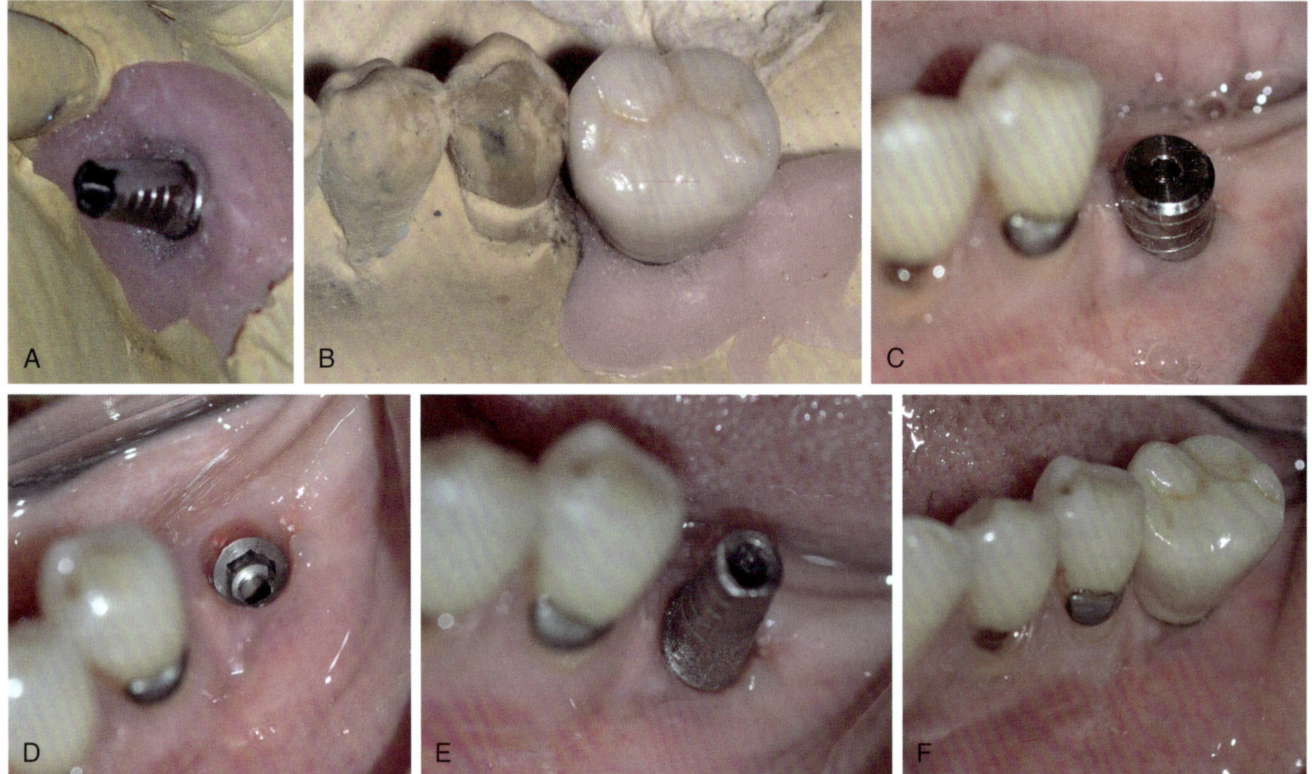

Fig 3.16 (A and B) An appropriate final abutment in inserted to the analogue at the working cast and the prosthesis is fabricated onto it. (C–E) The gingival former is removed from the implant and the final abutment is transferred from the cast to the implant, with the same orientation. (F) The prosthesis is fixed onto it.

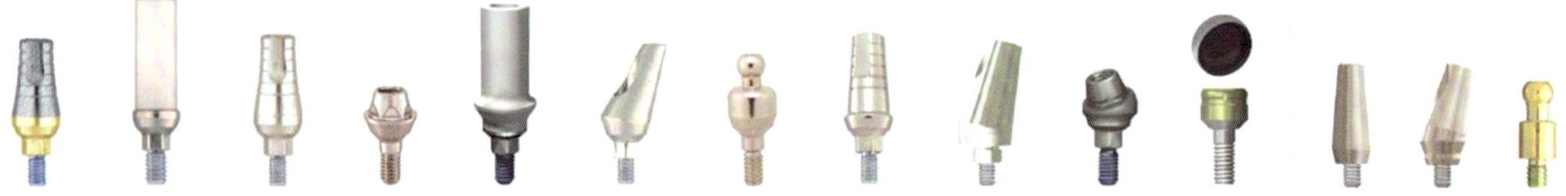

Fig 3.17 Various types of abutments used in implantology for different kinds of implant prostheses *(Courtesy: Alpha-Bio implant system, Israel).*

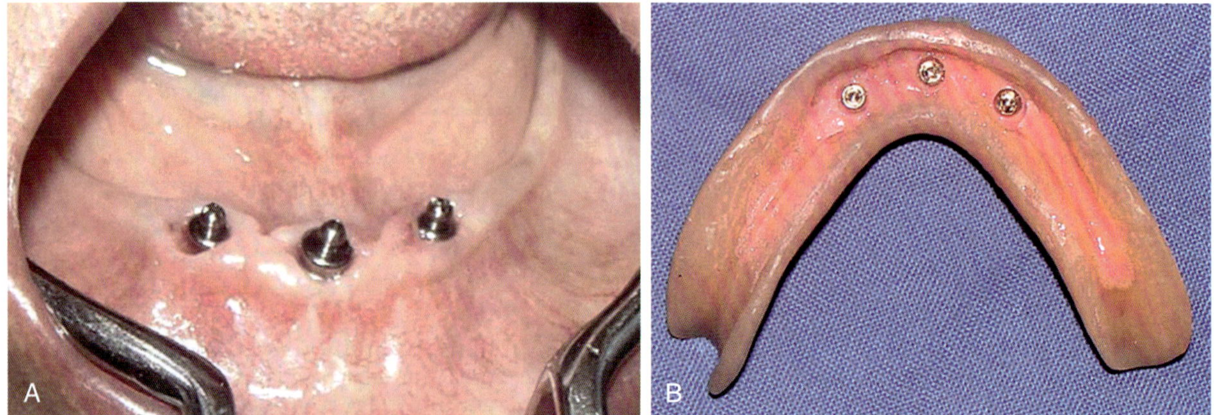

Fig 3.18 (A) Ball abutments are screwed over the implants in the patient's mouth. (B) Metal housings (caps) in the denture. When the overdenture is seated in the mouth, these metal housings get locked over the ball abutments and thus provide adequate retention of the denture.

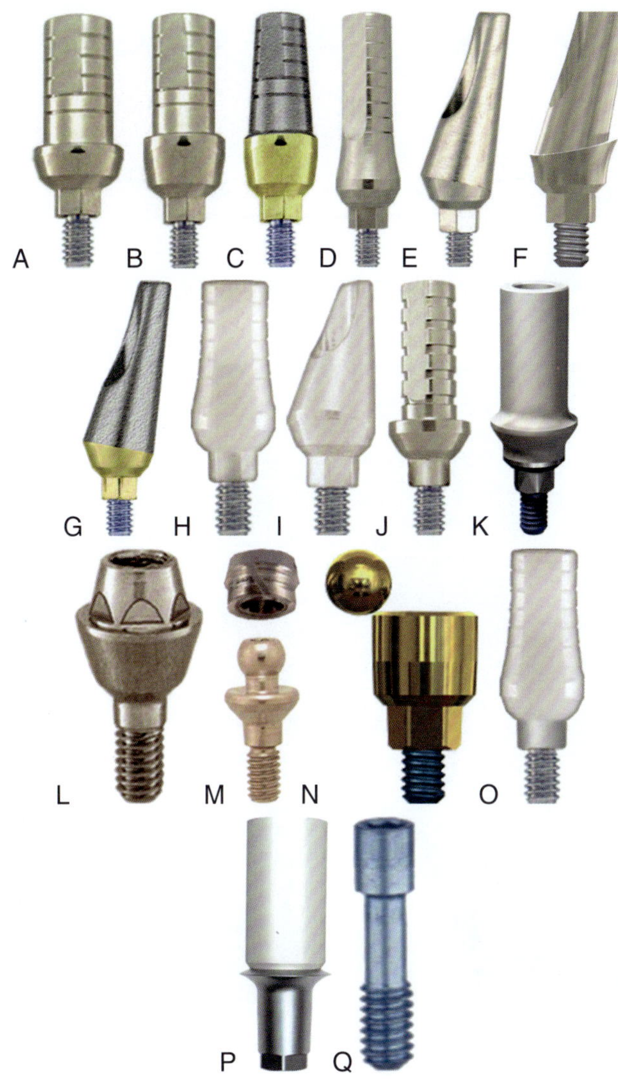

Fig 3.19 Different kinds of abutments and connection screw. (A) Straight abutment with short gingival collar. (B) Straight abutment with long gingival collar for deep seated implants. (C) Straight abutment with long gold-hued gingival collar to avoid see-through of the black metal collar through thin marginal soft tissues. (D) Long straight abutment for long crown height. (E) Angled abutment to correct angulation problem of the implant prosthesis. (F) Anatomical (aesthetic collar) abutment for maxillary anterior implant. (G) Angled abutment with gold-hued aesthetic collar. (H and I) Plastic (castable) abutments (straight and angled) for screw-retained prosthesis. (J) Temporary abutment to immediately temporize the implant. (K) Zirconium abutment for the metal free zirconium prosthesis. (L) TCT abutment for abutment level, screw-retained, fixed prosthesis or bar-retained dentures. (M) Ball abutment for ball retained overdenture (metal cap – above). (N) Angled ball abutment for overdenture to correct angulation problem. (O) Non-engaging abutment. (P) UCLA abutment. (Q) Connection screw *(Courtesy: Alpha-Bio implant system, Israel)*.

Inventories used to practise basic implant procedures

1. Dental implant surgical kit

The dental implant surgical kit contains several surgical tools for implant placement. All dental implant kits are system specific (e.g. for the placement of Biohorizons implants, one cannot use the surgical kit of the Nobel Biocare implant system and vice versa), but in addition, a particular system may also have different kits for different series of implants (e.g. different surgical kits are required to place the Maestro [external hex], tapered, internal, or one-piece implants in the Biohorizons implant system) (Fig 3.22A and B).

Tools in the implant surgical kit. The implant surgical kits of most systems are well designed to make it easy for the dental surgeon to understand and use them during implant placement surgery. The implant kits may contain variable numbers and types of components depending on the particular system, but usually almost all the systems contain the following common inventories:

1. Drills. All implant surgical kits contain a set of surgical drills which are sequentially used for preparation of osteotomies for different diameter implants of a particular system (Fig 3.23). These drills can be of the following types:
   a. Large round carbide bur: specially used to remove bony irregularities and fibrous tissues, and to flatten the sharp and irregular ridge crest before osteotomy preparation for the implant (Fig 3.24A).
   b. Small round carbide bur: Used to mark the implant site and to make an entry through the hard cortical bone at the ridge crest (Fig 3.24B).
   c. Pilot drill: This is the first drill which is used to make an entry to the complete depth. For example, if the length of the planned implant is 13 mm, this drill should be used until 13 mm depth from the ridge crest is achieved. Most systems have a 2 mm diameter pilot drill (Fig 3.24C).
   d. Width-increasing/widening drills: This is a set of the drills sequentially increasing in diameter, used after the pilot drill to widen the osteotomy to the same depth. All the drills (pilot and widening drills) have definitive markings along the length of the drills, representing the lengths of different implants available in a particular system. These markings guide the surgeon during drilling, to drill up to a particular depth marking (Fig 3.24D–H).
2. Parallel guide/depth guide/force direction indicators: The surgical kit may contain multiple numbers of parallel guides (Figs 3.25 and 3.26A). These guides are used for:
   a. accurate measurement of depth in radiographs taken after pilot drilling (called the depth guide).
   b. to visualize the 3-dimensional parallelism during drilling for multiple implants (called the parallel guide).
   c. to visualize the direction of the occlusal force on the future implant (called the force direction indicator).

Parallel and spacing guide: This special guide can be used for precise spacing and parallel placement of multiple implants (Fig 3.26B and C). After the pilot drilling for one implant site, this tool is inserted. The pilot drilling of the next implant is done through the hole in this guide, as shown in the figure.

3. Drill stoppers: These stoppers can be fitted to drills with different diameters to prevent over-drilling,

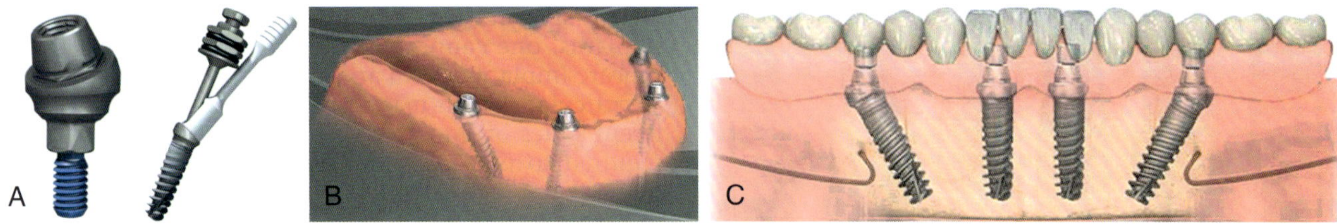

Fig 3.20 (A) Multiunit abutment connected to the implant fixture. (B) TCT abutment is fixed over the multiunit abutment. (C) To deliver a screw-retained prosthesis (all on 4) to the patient *(Courtesy: Alpha-Bio implant system, Israel)*.

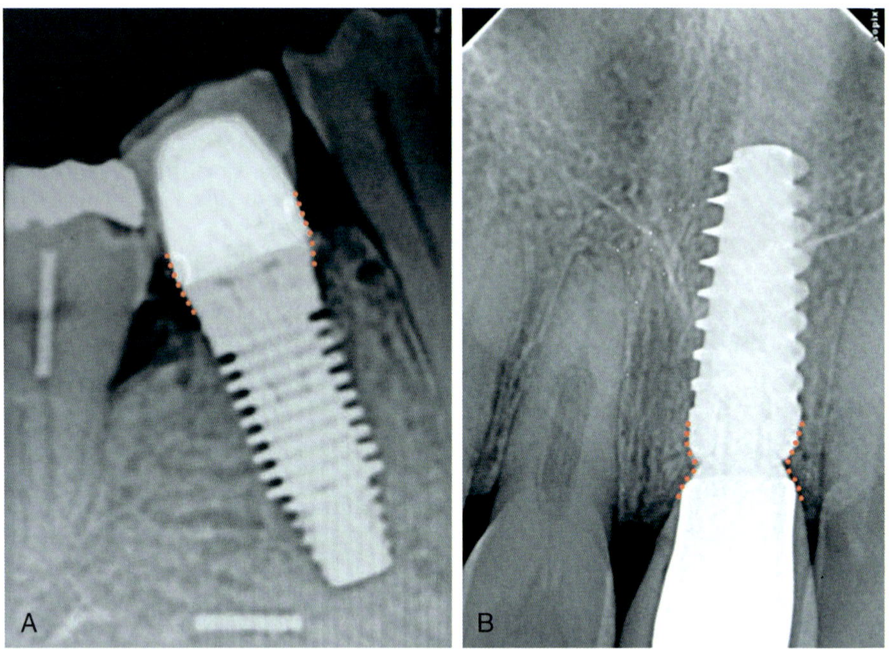

Fig 3.21 (A) Implant without the platform switching feature at implant abutment junction. (B) Implant with the platform switching feature at implant abutment junction.

specially in the area of vital structures like the mandibular canal and the sinus floor (Fig 3.27A and B).

4. Bone tap/thread former: These are the special drills used at very slow speed (20–40 rpm) before implant insertion, to make threads in the bone along the prepared osteotomy walls. These bone taps are implant-design specific and are used when an implant with non-cutting/non self-tapping threads (e.g. Maestro implant from Biohorizons), is inserted in a high-density bone to reduce the chances of pressure necrosis of the bone (Fig 3.28).
5. Crestal bone drill/countersink drill: These are the special drills used at high speed (1500–2000 rpm), before implant insertion limited to the crestal part of the bone to submerge/countersink the wider platform of the implant into the high-density cortical part of the ridge crest (e.g. Maestro implant from Biohorizons) (Fig 3.29).
6. Drill extender: Can be fitted to any drill to extend its length for easy drilling access in narrow spaces between adjacent teeth (Fig 3.30).
7. Implant depth probe: It has definitive markings along its length for depth evaluation of a prepared osteotomy. Its gently rounded apex simplifies depth measurements and provides easy, tactile examination of bone preparation and sinus membrane. Any perforation that may have occurred during osteotomy preparation can also be checked by gently moving its tip along the prepared osteotomy walls (Fig 3.31A and B).
8. Implant insertion tool/implant driver: This tool is used to drive the implant during its insertion in the prepared osteotomy. This can be rotary hand piece driven or hand ratchet driven (Fig 3.32A and B).
9. Ratchet: Ratchets are used to insert implants with the help of the implant driver connected to it. Ratchets can be of two types:
   a. Ratchet wrench: simple ratchet without any torque measurement (Fig 3.33A).
   b. Torque ratchet: allows the clinician to accurately apply the recommended pre-load torque for surgery and prosthetics. The torque level can be adjusted from 0 to 45 Ncm to check the primary stability of the inserted implant and to tighten the connection screw before final prosthetic loading of the implant (Fig 3.33B).
10. Screwdriver/Hex driver: This tool is used to drive the connection screw/cover screw/gingival former, etc. It can be hand driven or rotary hand piece driven (Fig 3.34A and B).

2. Implant motor (physiodispensor)

This is the surgical motor specially used for the implant insertion (Fig 3.35). The physiodispensor is mandatory for dentists to insert dental implants. It should have the following special features:

a. **Torque control.** The implant motor should have torque control from 0 to 50 Ncm, so that the hand piece does not stop rotating during drilling in hard bone and during implant insertion with hand piece at slow speed.
b. **Speed control.** It must be 20 rpm (speed required for implant insertion) to 2500 rpm (speed required for drilling in hard bone) when using a 20:1 speed reduction hand piece.
c. **Saline irrigation control.** It should have a controlled saline flow during osteotomy preparation to reduce the overheating of bone during drilling.
d. **Hand piece selection.** It should offer the option of a range of hand pieces to be connected to it – at least a 1:1 hand piece for osteoplasty, bone harvesting, sinus window preparation, etc. and a 20:1 reduction hand piece for implant osteotomy preparation.
e. **Programmes.** It should have different programmes that can be set for a particular implant procedure to make the surgery easy and comfortable.
f. **Forward and reverse function.** This feature helps in taking the drill/implant out, if it stops in the bone. It is also very useful for removing the cover screw and gingival former from the implant.
g. **Foot control.** The motor should have a foot control with speed, forward, and reverse functions.
h. **Autoclavable implant motor cord.** This is required to maintain the surgical asepsis.

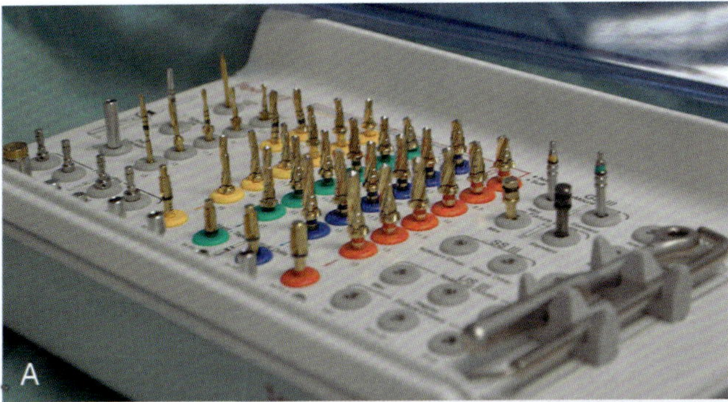

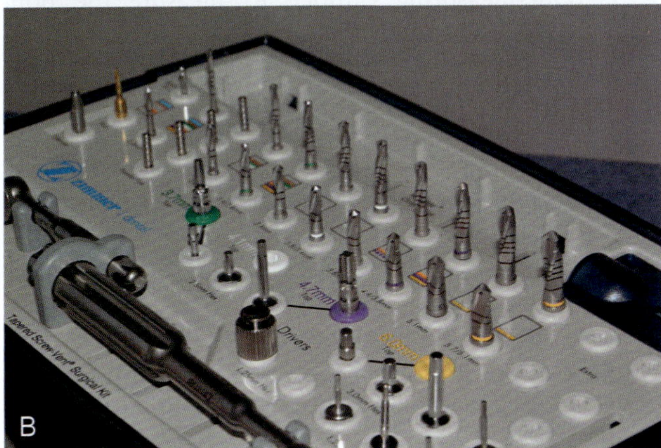

Fig 3.22 (A) Surgical kit of the Osstem implant system. (B) Surgical kit of the Zimmer Dental implant system.

3. Rotary hand pieces

The following hand pieces can be used in implantology

a. **1:1 Straight or contra angle hand piece** can be used for osteoplasty, autogenous bone harvesting, sinus window preparation, etc. (Fig 3.36B and C).
b. **20:1 Speed reduction hand piece** is a standard one, which is used to prepare osteotomy, bone tapping, and implant insertion (Fig 3.36A). Other reduction hand pieces which can also be optionally used for implant osteotomy preparation are 16:1 and 30:1 reduction hand pieces.
c. **Newer generation fibre optic hand pieces** are also available for better visibility during implant insertion procedures (Fig 3.36D).

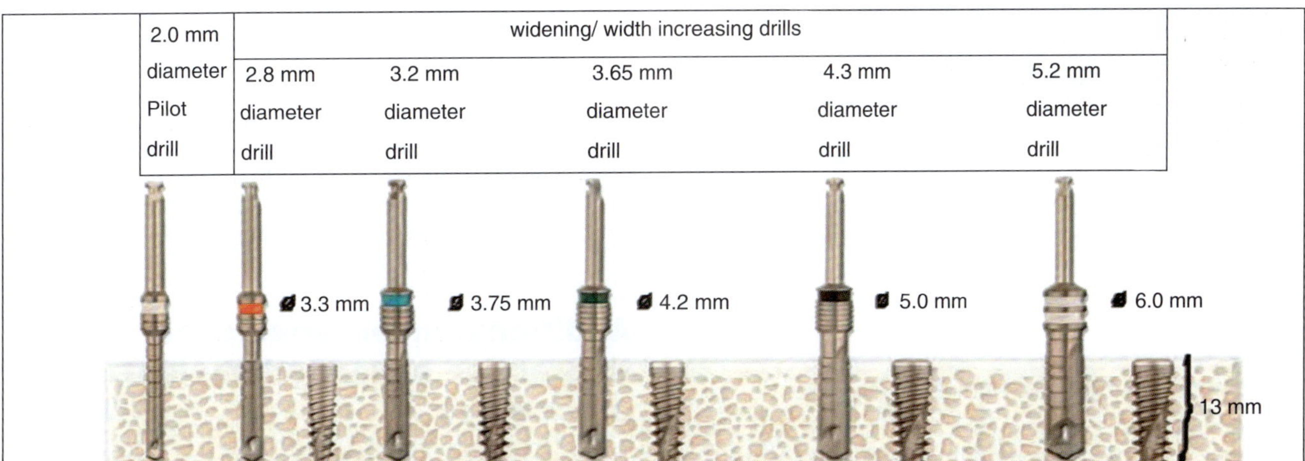

Fig 3.23 Drill sequence for different diameter implants *(Courtesy: Alpha-Bio implant system, Israel).*

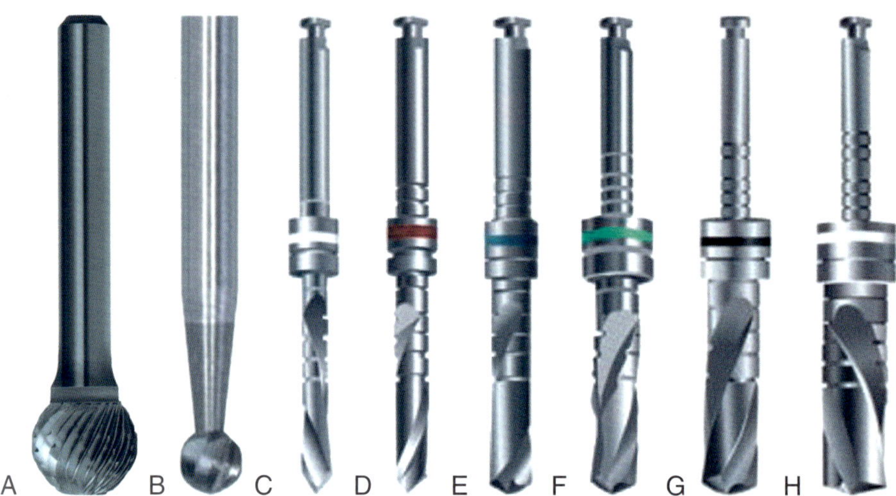

Fig 3.24 (A) Large round carbide bur. (B) Small round carbide bur. (C) Pilot/depth drill. (D–H) Width-increasing/osteotomy-widening drills.

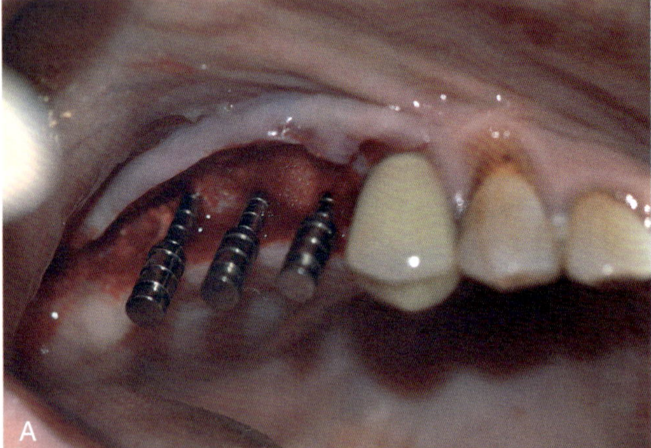

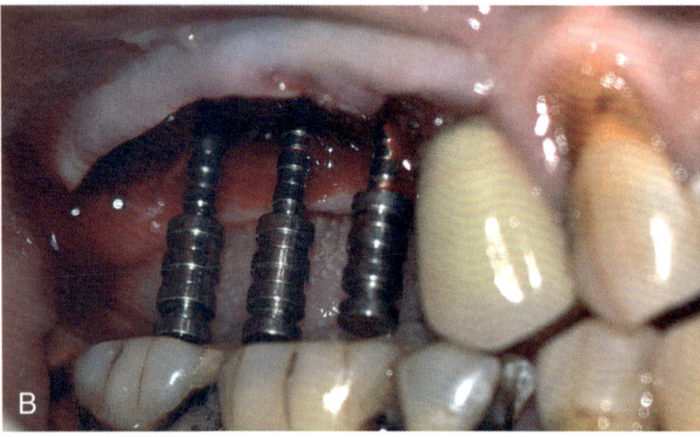

Fig 3.25 (A) Parallel guide pins are used to check for adequate parallelism between future implants as well as to check (B) the direction of occlusal force from the opposing teeth.

4. Basic oral surgery instruments

The dentist needs to have at least the basic oral surgery instruments to perform implant procedures. All of these instruments must be autoclavable. The following instruments are the basic requirement for the implant clinician (Fig 3.37).

a. Lips and cheek retractors for better visibility during surgery.
b. A good set of diagnostic instruments.
c. Bone-measuring calliper, to measure the bone width after raising flap.
d. Bone rongeur, to remove any sharp or irregular bone from the ridge crest. It can also be used to harvest soft cancellous bone from the maxillary tuberosity.
e. Different kinds of periosteal elevators.
f. B.P. handles.
g. A set of good quality needle holders, scissors, artery forceps, etc.

5. Cleaning and sterilization equipment

Implant surgery procedures must be done with high sterility and asepsis to reduce post implantation infections.

a. **Ultra sonic cleaner** All implant drills, drivers, keys, instruments, and other inventories must be cleaned in a good quality ultrasonic cleaner to remove all the blood clots/debris etc. before placing the instruments in the autoclave (Fig 3.38A). The author recommends the ultrasonic cleaning of all instruments every time, before and after implant surgery.
b. **Fumigator** The implant surgery operation theatre/chamber must be fumigated with formalin fumigator to kill all the microorganisms (Fig 3.38B).
c. **Autoclave/steriliser** the author recommends a good quality sterilizer with automatic dry cycles to sterilize all the implant kit and instruments before using them in implant surgery (Fig 3.38C).

Additional Inventories used to practise advanced implant procedures

There are many additional inventories that the implant surgeon should have to practise advanced implant procedures. All the procedure- and technique-specific inventories are described in subsequent related chapters of this book.

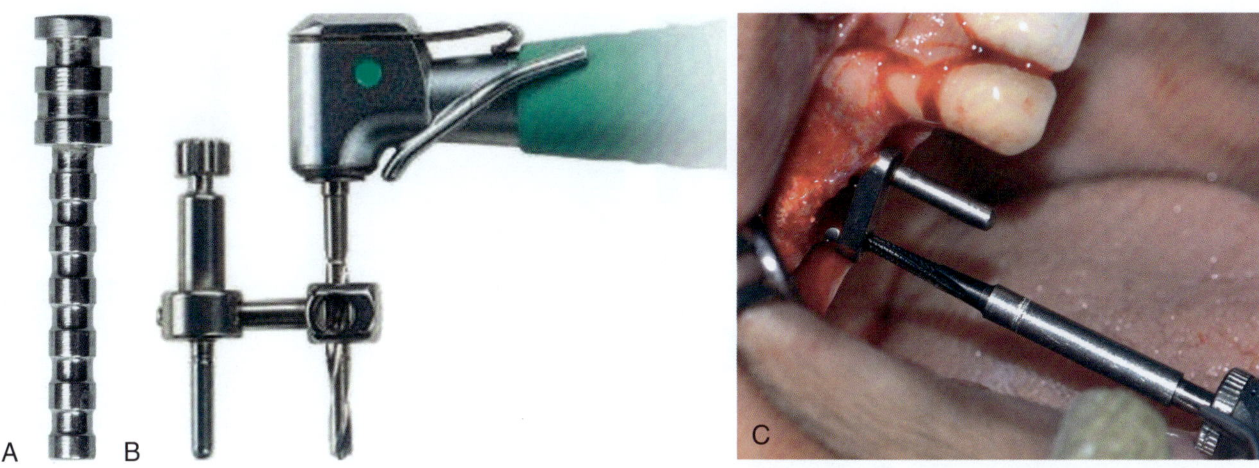

Fig 3.26 (A) Depth guide/parallel pin. (B and C) Spacing guide from the Alpha-Bio implant system, Israel.

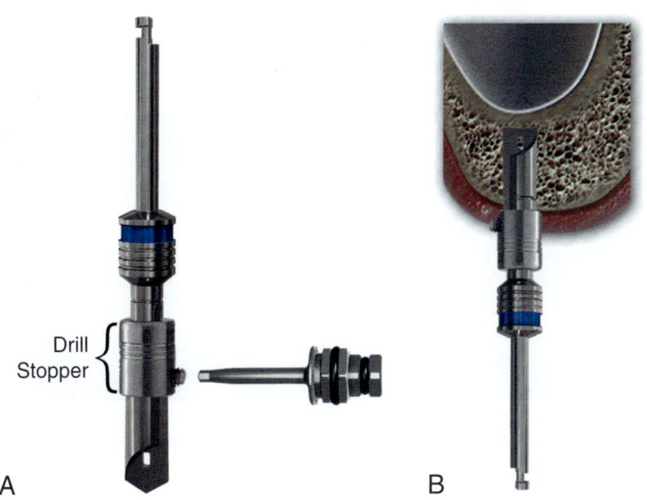

Fig 3.27 (A) Drill stopper fitted to the drill (B) which prevents overdrilling *(Courtesy: Alpha-Bio implant system, Israel)*.

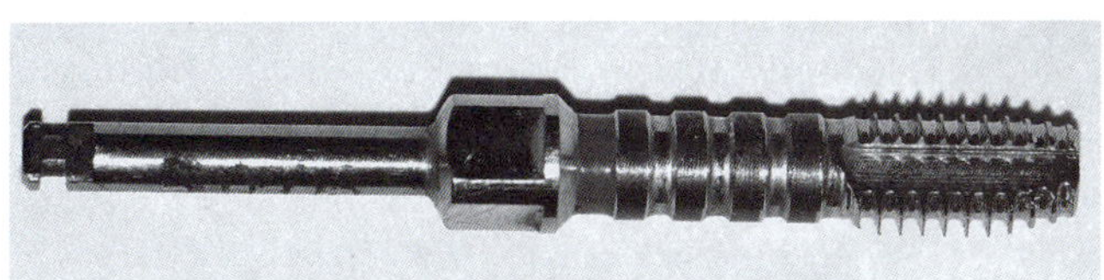

Fig 3.28 Bone tape/thread former for 4 mm diameter (Biohorizons Maestro implant).

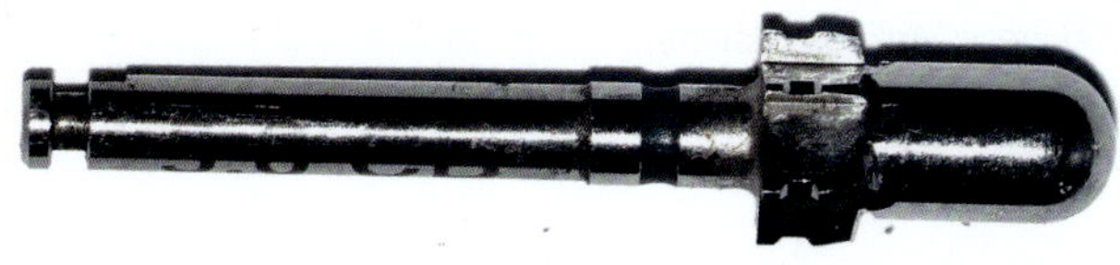

Fig 3.29 Crestal bone drill (CBD) for Biohorizons Maestro implant.

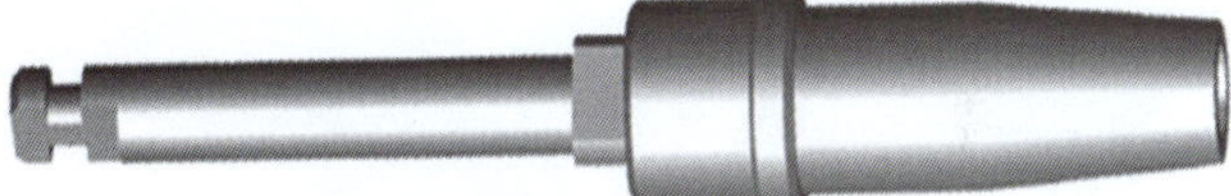

Fig 3.30 Implant drill extender.

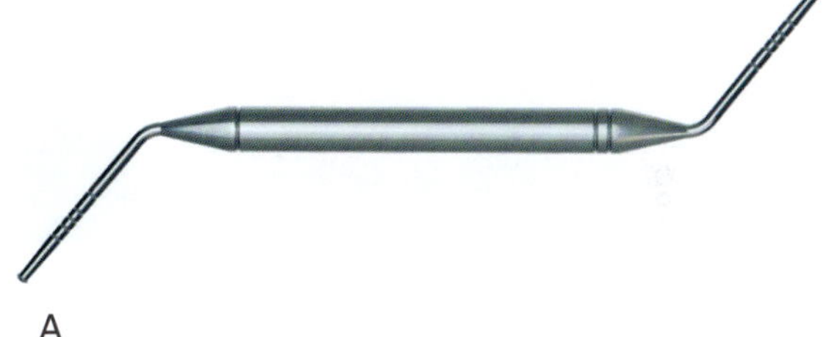

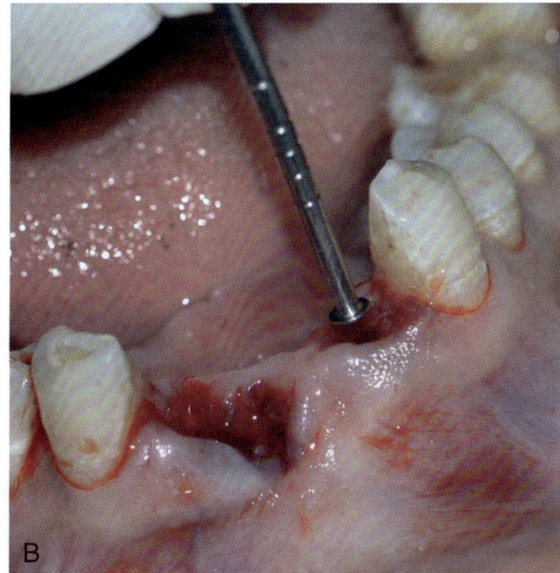

Fig 3.31 (A) IDG Implant depth probe *(Courtesy: Alpha-Bio implant systems, Israel)* is a very useful tool to check any inadvertent perforation (B) that has occurred during osteotomy preparation.

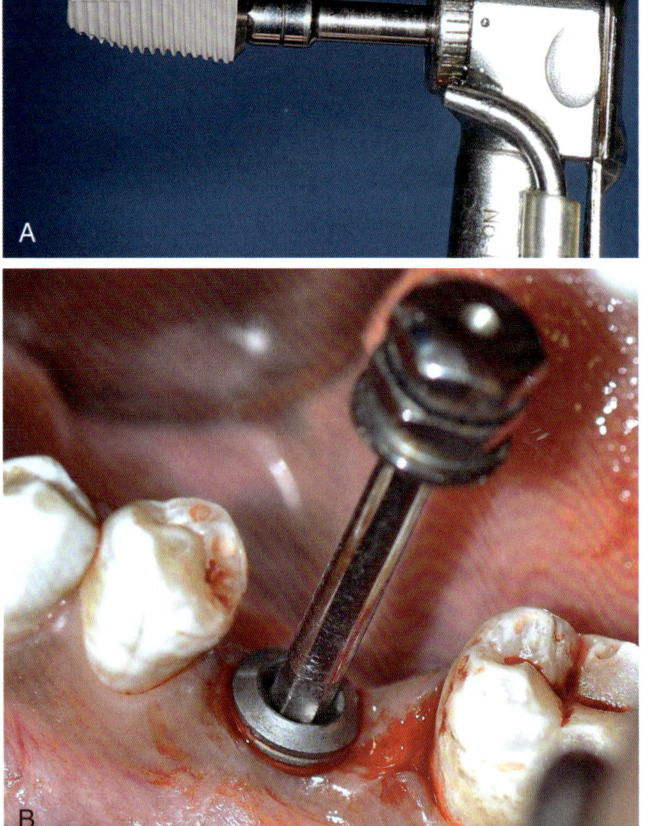

Fig 3.32 (A) Rotary hand piece driven implant driver *(Courtesy: Dentium Co Ltd, Seoul, Korea)*. (B) Hand ratchet-driven implant driver of Alpha-Bio implant system.

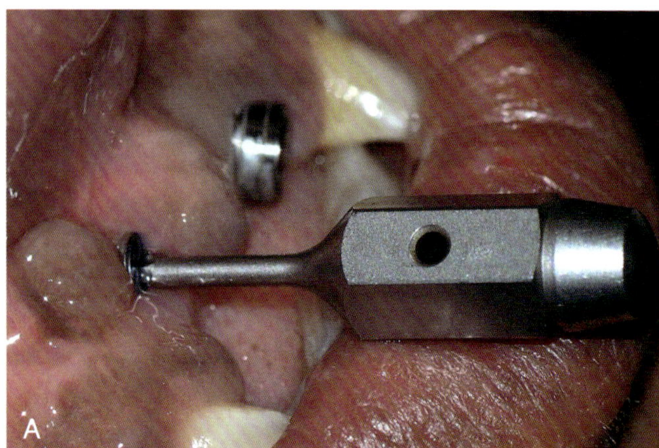

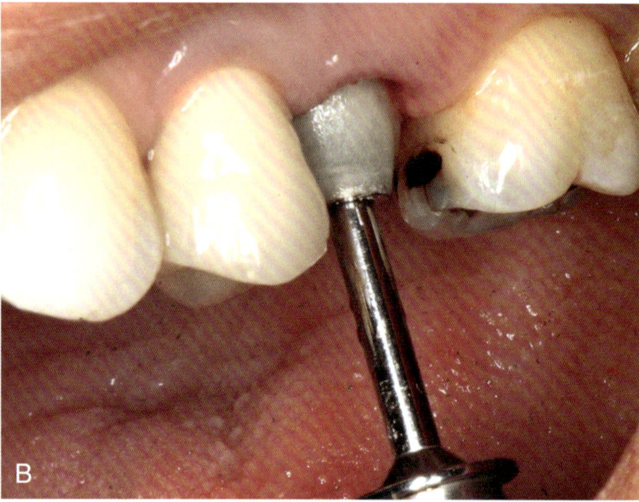

Fig 3.34 (A) A screwdriver being used to drive in the implant cover screw and (B) connection screw of the abutment.

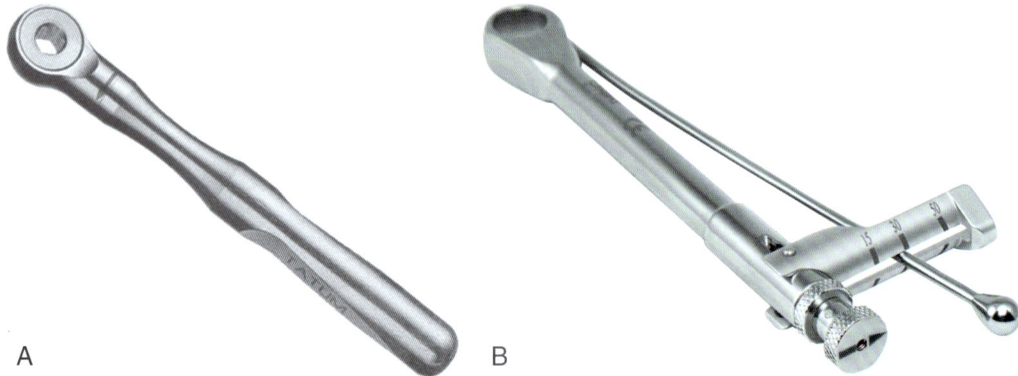

Fig 3.33 (A) Ratchet wrench *(Courtesy: Tatum Surgicals)*. (B) Torque ratchet *(Courtesy: Ankylos system)*.

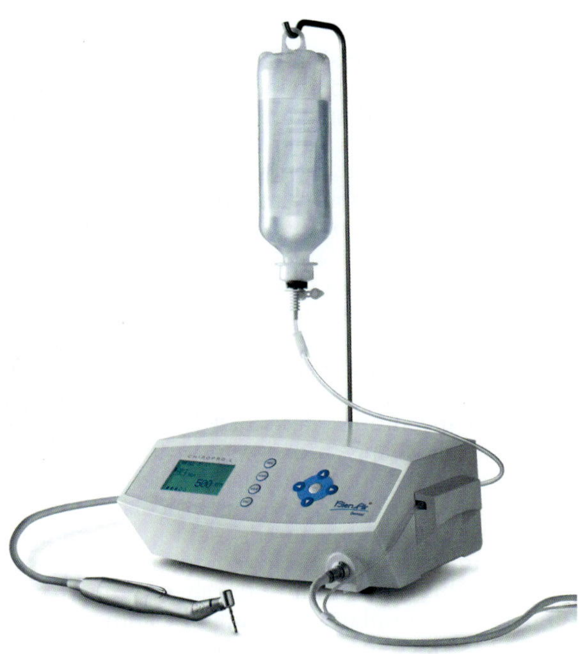

Fig 3.35 Implant motors *(Courtesy: Bein Air)*.

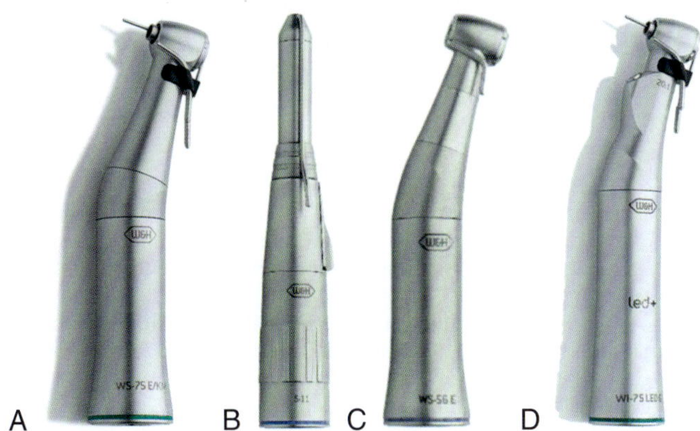

Fig 3.36 (A) 20:1 speed reduction hand piece for implant osteotomy preparation. (B and C) 1:1 straight and contra angle hand pieces for bone modification and harvesting procedures. (D) Newer generation fibre optic 20:1 contra angle hand piece can also be used for better control and visibility during implant osteotomy preparation *(Courtesy: W&H Dental, India)*.

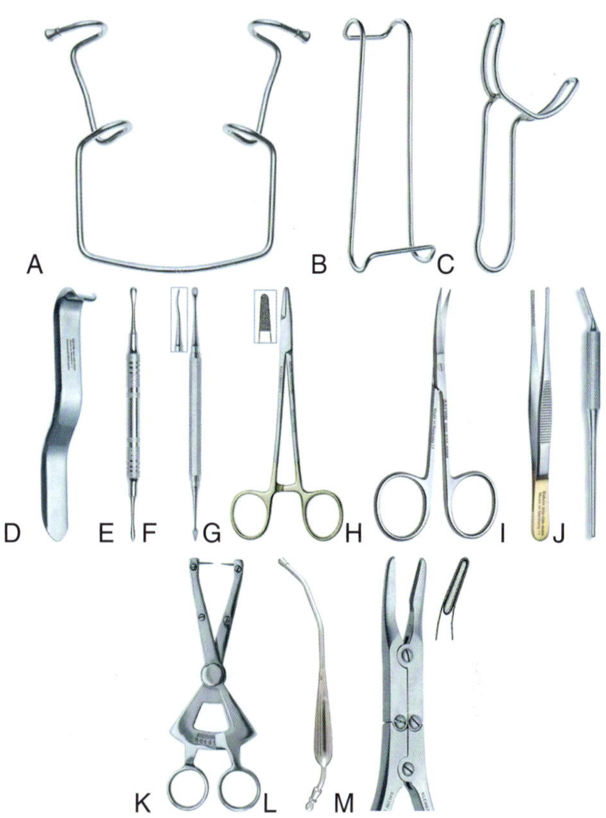

Fig 3.37 (A) Orringer retractor. (B) Columbia lip retractor. (C) Vestibular retractor. (D) Cawood Minnesota retractor. (E) Micro elevator. (F) Buser periosteal elevator. (G) Needle holder. (H) Scissor. (I) Tissue holding forceps. (J) Scalpel handle. (K) Ridge mapping calliper. (L) Autoclavable stainless steel suction tip. (M) Bone rongeur *(Courtesy: Salvin Dental Specialties Inc., 3450 Latrobe Drive, Charlotte, NC 28211, U.S.A. and Amron Instruments, Sark Health Care, India)*.

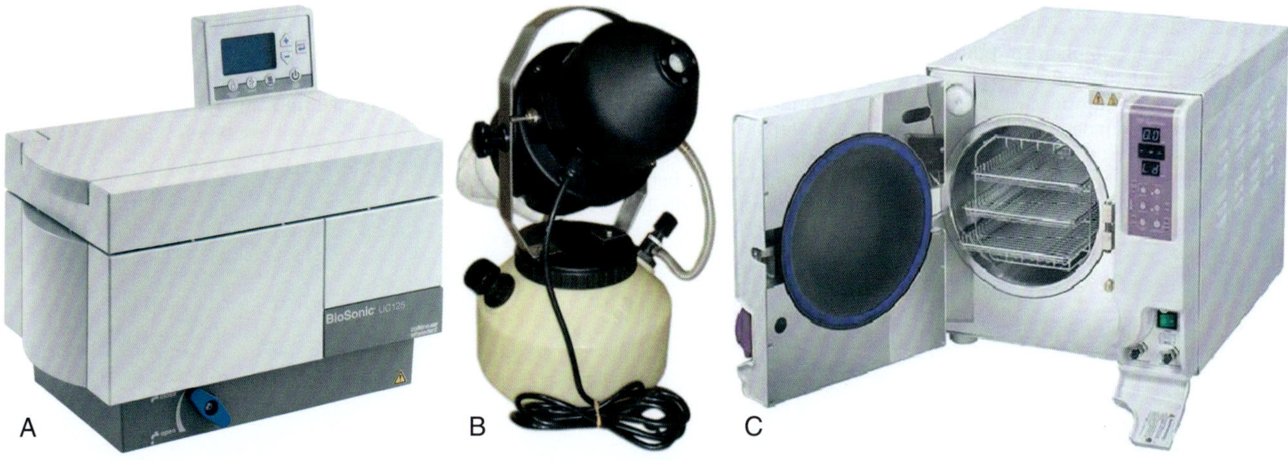

Fig 3.38 (A) Ultrasonic cleaner from Coltene Whaledent. (B) Fumigator. (C) Front loading autoclave with automatic dry cycle.

Summary

The dental implant now has been established as one of the most preferred options for missing tooth replacement and many dentists are already practising this procedure or are willing to incorporate implants in their practise. Further, there are now several implant systems in the market with different implant designs and their specific components. This range and variety may often make it difficult for the novice dentist to understand and use implants and their components. To overcome this problem, a generic terminology has been developed to facilitate easy communication between implant team members and the prosthetic laboratory. Regardless of the implant system used, the generic terms describe the function of the component. During the surgical phase of implant treatment, the fixture or implant is inserted in the bone and covered with the cover screw. Once the implant has osseointegrated with the bone, the implant is uncovered and the cover screw is removed and replaced with a gingival former. The restorative dentist removes the gingival former and places the abutment or makes the implant body impression, using the impression abutment. The implant fixture impression may use the direct or indirect technique. Further, in the indirect technique, the dentist may use the closed tray impression using closed tray posts or the open tray impression using open tray posts. After making the indirect impression, the laboratory uses the implant analogue and assembles it with the post before pouring the impression. After the final working cast has been removed from the impression, the impression post is replaced with an appropriate final abutment and the prosthesis is fabricated onto it. In cases where the dentist has instructed the lab to fabricate the screw retained prosthesis, the laboratory uses the plastic/castable/burn out abutment and fabricates the screw-retained prosthesis. The mechanical torque ratchet is used to evaluate initial implant stability and also to finally tighten the connection screw at 35 Ncm, before fixing the final prosthesis. The implant inventories described in this chapter may vary in number, shape, and size in various implant systems. Therefore, the author strongly suggests that dentists thoroughly read the catalogue of a particular implant system or attend the manufacturer's mentoring programs to completely understand the selected system before using it on patients. This can minimize the chances of errors during and after the implant insertion. The author has compiled and described inventories mostly on the basis of his clinical experience with the various implant systems, but there can be few special inventories in any specific system that readers can only learn of from the particular system's catalogue.

Further Reading

Maestro and Prodigy surgical and prosthetic manuals. Birmingham, AL: Biohorizons Implant Systems; 2005.

Glossary of prosthodontic terms. J Prosthet Dent 1999;81:39–110.

Nobel perfect implant placement/ restorative manual. Gteburg, Sweden: Nobelbiocare AB; 2005.

Canullo L, et al. Platform switching and marginal bone-level alterations: the results of a randomized-controlled trial. Clin Oral Implants Res 2010;21:115–21.

Straumann dental implants product catalog, Andover, MA, 2005.

Baumgarten H, et al. A new implant design for crestal bone preservation: initial observations and case report. Pract Proceed Aesthet Dent 2005;17:735–40.

Misch CE, Misch CM. Generic terminology for endosseous implant prosthodontics. J Prosthet Dent 1992;68:809–12.

Lazzara RJ, et al. Platform switching: a new concept in implant dentistry for controlling postoperative crestal bone levels. Int J Perio Rest Dent 2006;26:9–17.

Screw- vent and advent surgical and prosthetic manuals. Carlsbad, CA: Zimmer Dental; 2005.

Cranin AN. Glossary of implant terms. J oral Implant 1990;16:57–63.

Surgical manual screw internal hex implant system, Alpha-Bio Tec, Israel.

Implants, prosthetics and surgical instrumentations, manual of Alpha-Bio Implants 2011, Israel

Atieh MA, et al. Platform switching for marginal bone preservation around dental implants: a systematic review and meta-analysis. J Perio 2010;81:1350–66.

Sutter F, Weber IIP, Sorenson J, et al. The new restorative concept of the ITI dental implant system: design and engineering. Int J Periodontics Restorative Dent 1993;13:409–31.

Rodríguez-Ciurana X, et al. The effect of interimplant distance on the height of the interimplant bone crest when using platform-switched implants. Int J Perio Rest Dent 2009;29:141–51.

Tarnow DP, et al. The effect of inter-implant distance on the height of the inter-implant bone crest. J Perio 2000;71:546–9.

Vela-Nebot X, et al. Benefits of an implant platform modification technique to reduce crestal bone resorption. Implant Dent 2006;15:313–20.

English CE. Externally hexed implants, abutments, and transfer devices: a comprehensive overview. Implant Den 1992;1:273–83.

Boggan RS, Strong JT, Misch CE, et al. Influence of hex geometry and prosthetic table width on static and fatigue strength of dental implants. J Prosthet Dent 1999;82:436–40.

Soblonsky S, editor: Illustrated dictionary of dentistry. Philadelphia: WB Saunders; 182.

Niznick GA. The implant abutment connection: the key to prosthetic success. Compend Contin Educ Dent 1991;12:932–7.

Jalbout Z, Tbourina G. International congress of oral implantologists: glossary of implant term. Upper Montclair, NJ: ICOI/NYU; 2003.

Adin dental implants - catalog. Israel: Adin Dental Implants System; 2011.

Prosthetic options on implants 4

Ajay Vikram Singh

CHAPTER CONTENTS HD

Introduction

With advances in implant design and implant component technology, many prosthetic options are available in implantology, which the dentist can offer to his/her patients, according to their aesthetic and functional needs and expectations. There can be several factors, like the age of the patient, bone density and bone availability at the implant site, the nature of soft tissue, force factors, the aesthetic and functional demands of the patient, the socioeconomic status of the patient, and the time span available to complete the treatment, that affect the choice of prosthesis. The choice of the implant prosthesis should be made along with diagnosis and treatment planning and there should be a thorough discussion with the patient, well before implant insertion surgery. Here are a few implant prosthetic options that can be offered to patients in different clinical situations.

Implant prosthetic options for partially edentulous patients

The partially edentulous patient can be successfully treated with cement- or screw-retained fixed implant prosthesis. The cement-retained prosthesis is preferred in such cases but the screw-retained prosthesis can be used if there are multiple implants and the exposed screw hole is detrimental in the aesthetic view. The screw-retained prosthesis can also be preferred in cases with limited crown height space, to avoid repeated dislodgement of the implant prosthesis.

1. **Single tooth replacement**
   a. **Cement-retained ceramic prosthesis.** A metal or ceramic abutment is finally screwed over the implant and a metal or ceramic crown is fixed onto it using appropriate luting cement (Fig 4.1A and B). The cement-retained ceramic prosthesis is preferred in most single-tooth implant situations, anterior as well as posterior.
   b. **Screw-retained ceramic prosthesis.** A metal or ceramic crown is fabricated in the laboratory using a castable burnout abutment. The screw-retained crown is directly screwed to the implant using a connection screw and the screw hole is sealed, first using the gutta-percha, followed by a tooth-coloured composite material over it (Fig 4.2A–C).
2. **Multiple tooth replacement.** Depending on the bone density and bone volume available to insert the implant, either an individual implant is inserted for each unit of a prosthesis or a joint prosthesis is given in bridge form over a small number of implants. If adequate amount of bone is available to insert long and wide implants, if bone density at the site is sufficient (e.g. anterior and posterior mandible) or if force factors are minimum (e.g. anterior maxilla and anterior mandible) fewer implants can be inserted to support a multiunit bridge (Fig 4.3). In situations where bone dimensions and bone density are compromised (e.g. posterior maxilla), an implant is inserted to support each individual unit of the prosthesis.
   a. **Individual implant for each tooth (cement- or screw-retained).** If bone dimensions and bone density are compromised and force factors are on the higher side (e.g. posterior maxilla) a minimum of one implant should be inserted to support each prosthesis (Fig 4.4A and B).
   b. **Implant bridge (cement- or screw-retained).** If bone density is higher and force factors are low, the multiunit prosthesis can be supported by fewer implants (Fig 4.5A and B).

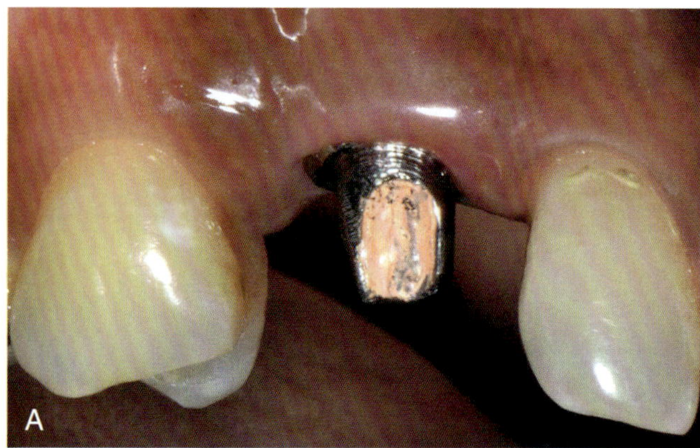

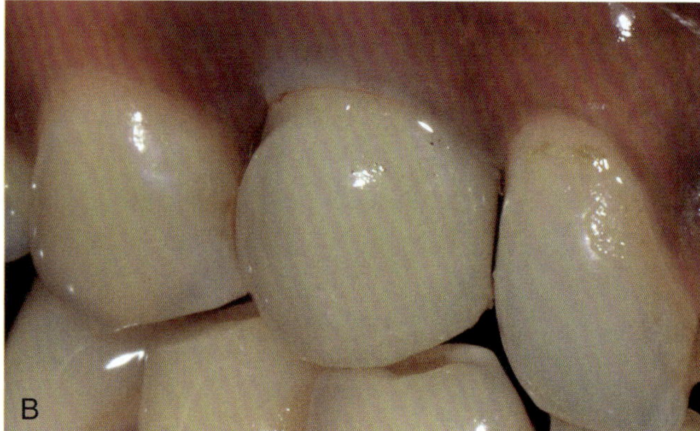

Fig 4.1 (A) Final abutment inserted on implant and (B) ceramic crown fixed over it, using luting cement.

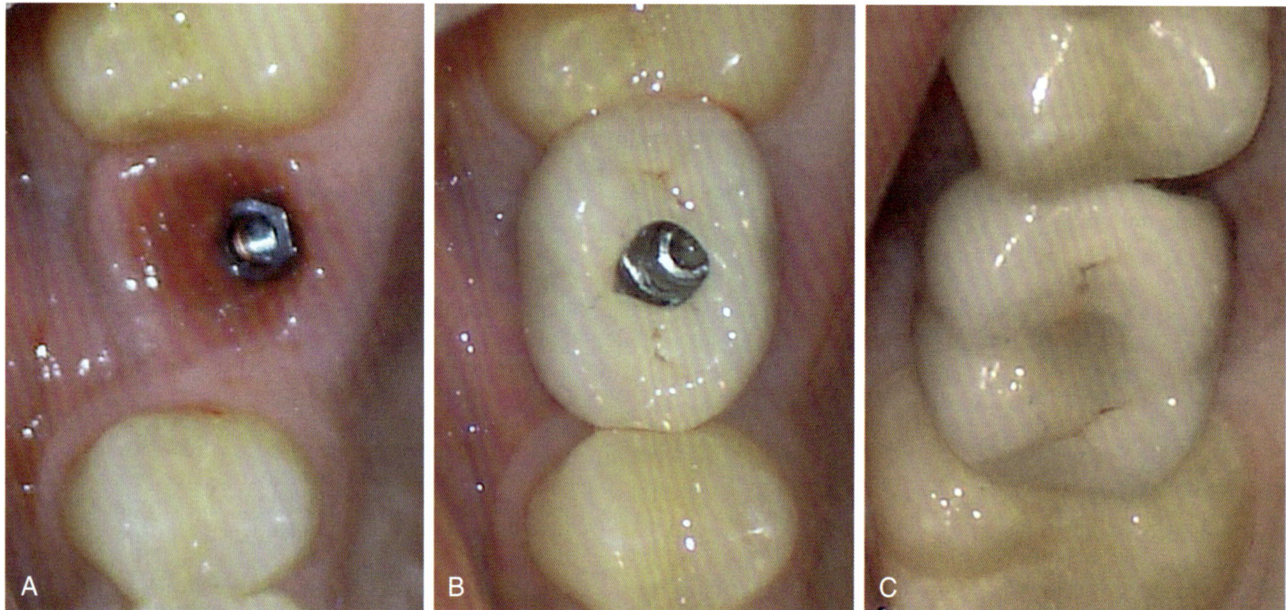

Fig 4.2 (A) Implant before prosthetic loading (mirror image); (B) screw-retained ceramic crown fixed over the implant; (C) screw hole closed using tooth-coloured composite.

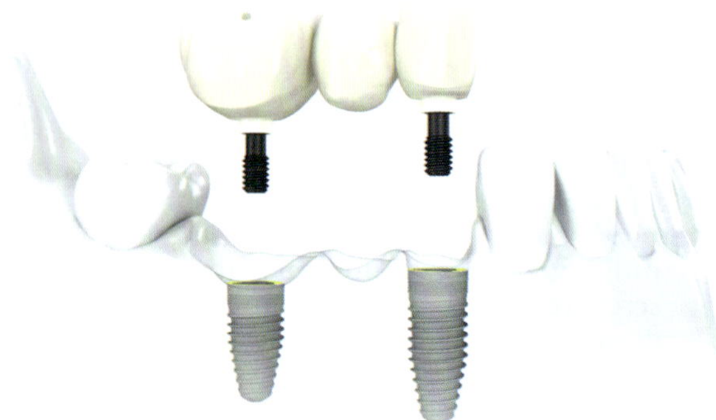

Fig 4.3 If available bone volume and density allow placing longer and adequate diameter implants with adequate amount of primary stability and bone implant contact percentage, a multiple unit bridge can be delivered over a few implants (*Courtesy: Nobel Biocare*).

Implant prosthetic options for completely edentulous patients

For completely edentulous patients, the dental implant is the only option to support a full-arch, fixed prosthesis or to retain loose dentures. Beside the conventional, full-arch, implant-supported prosthesis, advancement in implant component engineering has brought multiple graft-less options ('all on 4'/'all on 6' techniques) for edentulous patients, to deliver fast and fixed prostheses or implants retained overdentures.

1. **Implant-supported removable prosthesis (implant overdenture).** Depending on the dentist's preference and various clinical parameters, usually two types of 'implant overdentures' are delivered to patients.
   a. **Ball-retained overdentures.** Two to four implants are inserted in the anterior mandible while 4–6

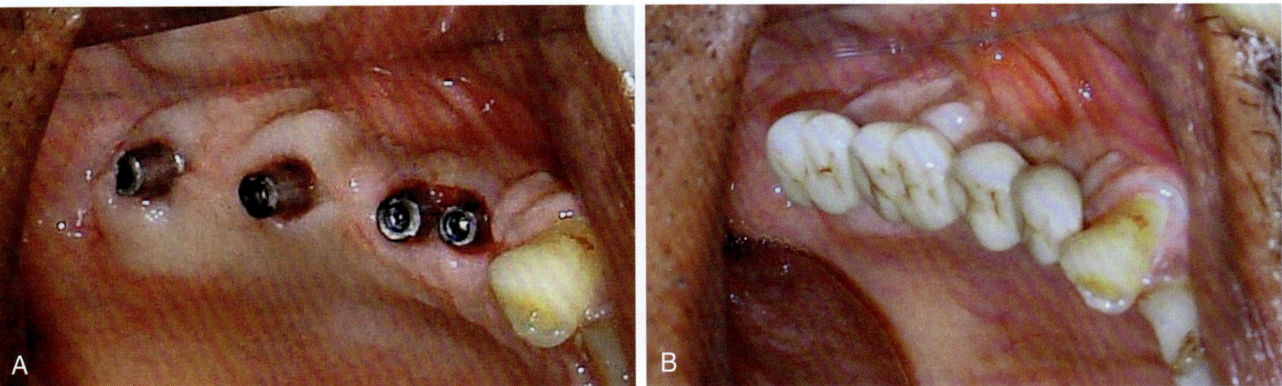

Fig 4.4 (A and B) Four implants are inserted in the posterior maxilla to support a four-unit ceramic prosthesis.

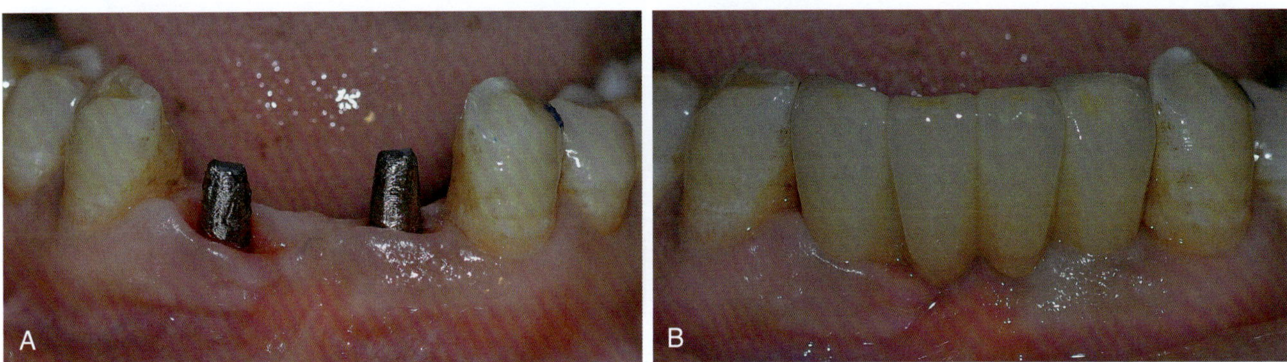

Fig 4.5 (A) Only two implants are inserted to support a four-unit ceramic bridge, (B) in lower anterior region.

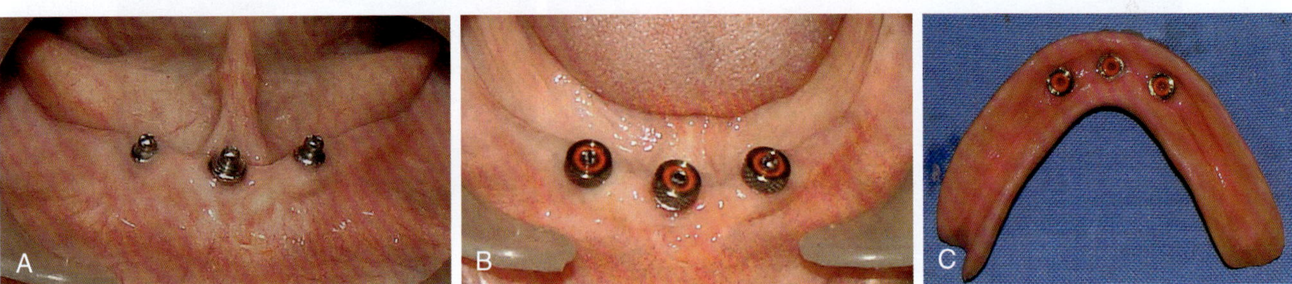

Fig 4.6 (A) Three implants with ball abutments in the anterior mandible, (B) 'O' rings over the ball abutments, (C) 'O' rings transferred to the denture.

implants are inserted in the anterior maxilla; ball abutments or 'locator abutments' are inserted over the implants. The 'O' rings or metal housings are fitted into the tissue surface of the denture and they get locked over the ball abutments or locator abutments, when the dentures are seated in the mouth. These implants provide adequate retention to the dentures (Fig 4.6A–C).

b. **Bar-retained overdentures.** A metal bar is fabricated in the laboratory and fixed over the implants. Special header clips are fixed into the tissue surface of the denture, which gets locked over the bar, when the denture is seated in the mouth. The bar provides adequate retention and stability to the denture (Fig 4.7A–C).

2. **Implant-supported fixed prosthesis.** There are multiple options for the implant-supported fixed prosthesis. Usually a number of implants are inserted in the jawbone and the multiple unit ceramic or hybrid prosthesis is fixed over these implants. The following are different options for the full-arch implant-supported fixed prosthesis:
   a. **Screw or cement-retained ceramic prosthesis.** After thorough diagnosis and treatment planning, several implants (with the best possible dimensions for each implant) are inserted and placed at the best

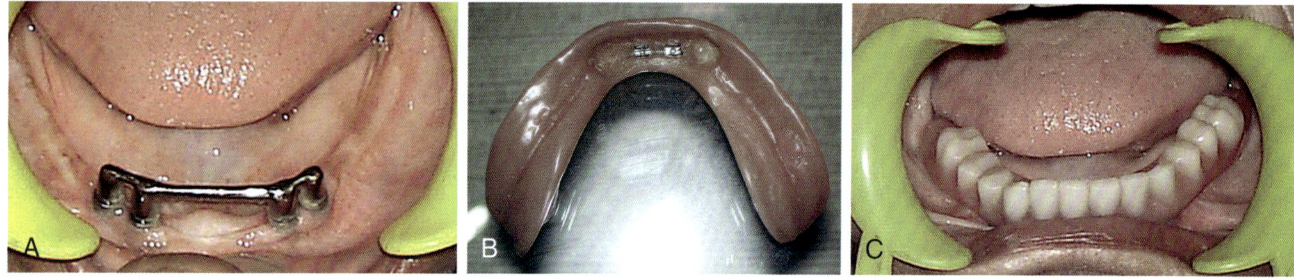

Fig 4.7 (A) A metal bar is fixed over the implants, (B) denture with the header clips fitted into the tissue surface. (C) Overdenture seated over the implants.

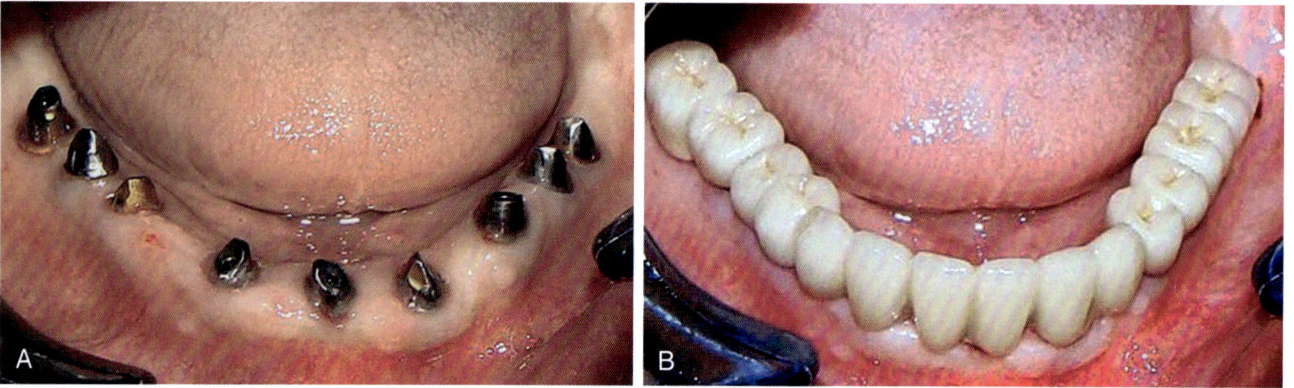

Fig 4.8 (A and B) Full-arch cement-retained ceramic prosthesis is fixed on several implants.

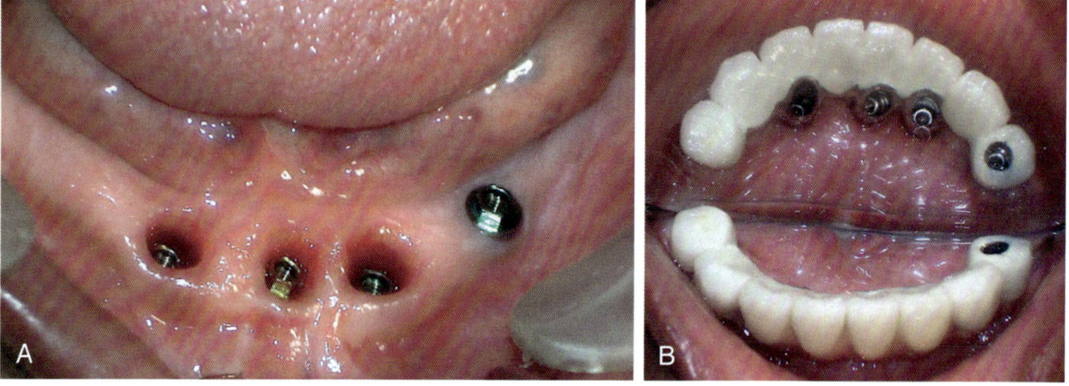

Fig 4.9 (A and B) Screw-retained ceramic prosthesis fixed on four implants.

possible positions in the jawbone, after consideration of prosthetic biomechanics and force factors. The full-arch screw or cement-retained prosthesis is fixed over these implants (Figs 4.8 and 4.9).

b. **Screw or cement-hybrid prosthesis.** Several implants are inserted at the best possible positions in the jawbone. The impression of these implants is made with the indirect technique and a metal framework is fabricated in the dental laboratory, and passively seated over these implants. The tooth setting is done over this framework using prefabricated resin teeth and the prosthesis is acrylized using heat-cured resin. The resulting prosthesis is fixed on the implants using fixation screws (Figs 4.10 and 4.11).

Metal-free zirconium prosthesis

The metal-free zirconium prosthesis can be preferred over the porcelain fused to metal prosthesis, to achieve desired aesthetic results (Figs 4.12 and 4.13).

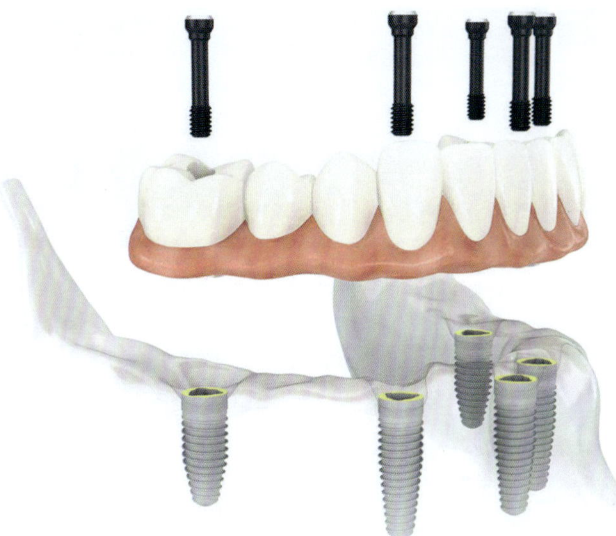

Fig 4.10 Screw-retained hybrid prosthesis can be fixed on multiple implants inserted in the jawbone. The connection screws pass through the prosthesis and fix the prosthesis to the implants. The screw holes of the prosthesis are sealed using either gutta-percha or aesthetic composite (*Courtesy: Nobel Biocare*).

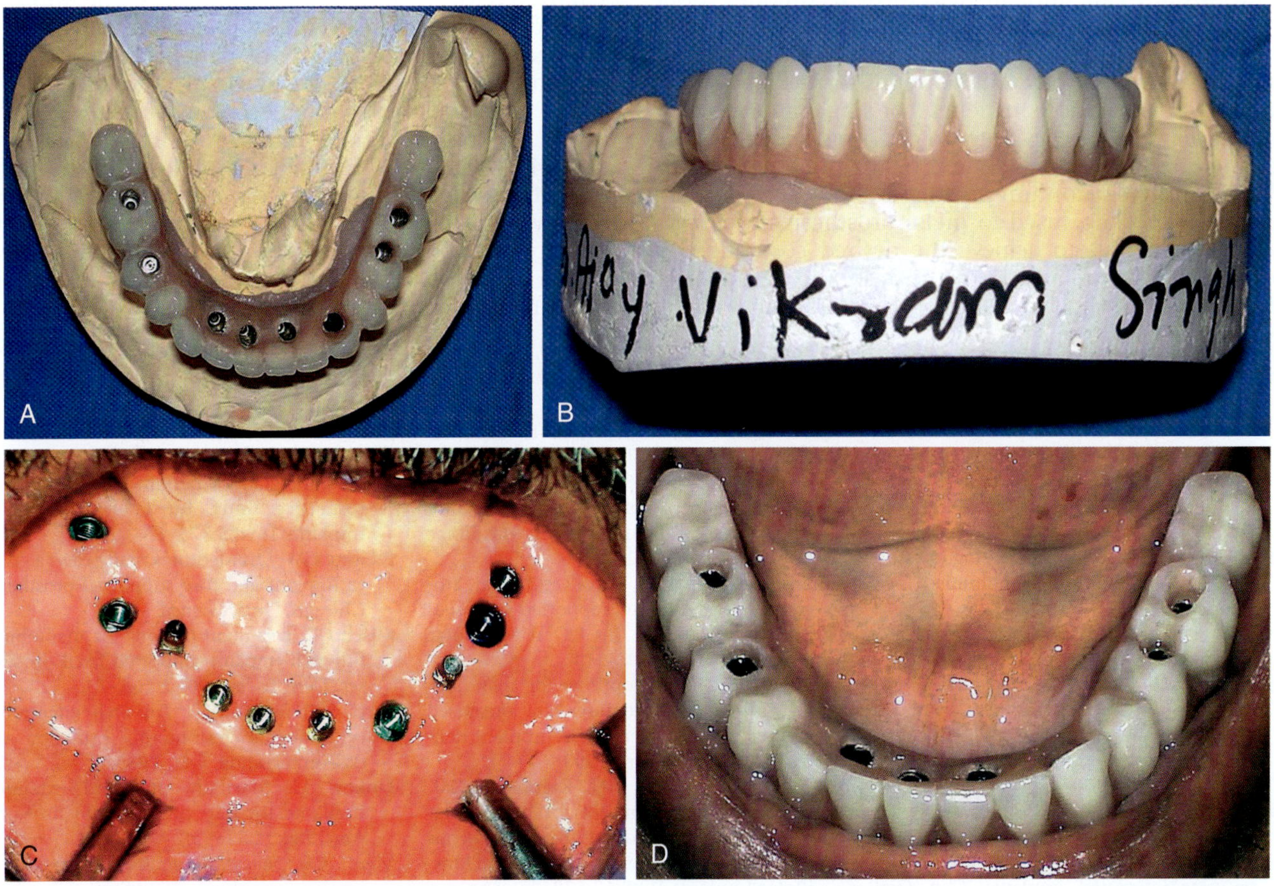

Fig 4.11 (A) Occlusal view of screw-retained hybrid prosthesis on model, (B) frontal view of prosthesis on model, (C) implants in mouth before fixing the screw-retained hybrid prosthesis, (D) prosthesis fixed over the implants. The screw holes can be closed either with gutta-percha or composite.

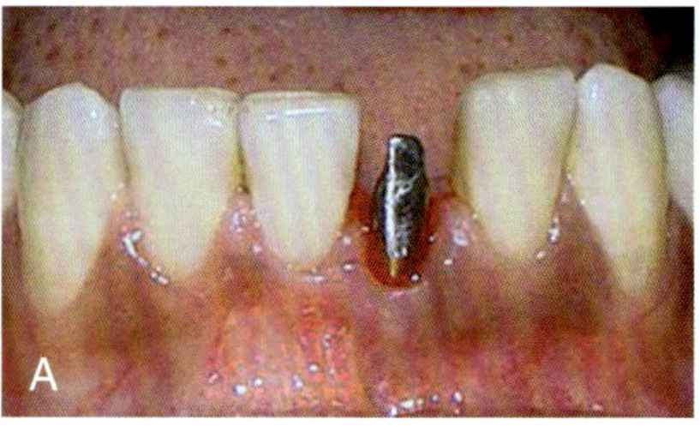

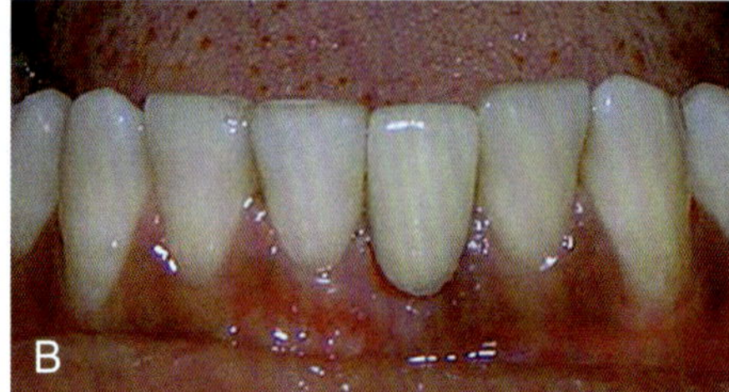

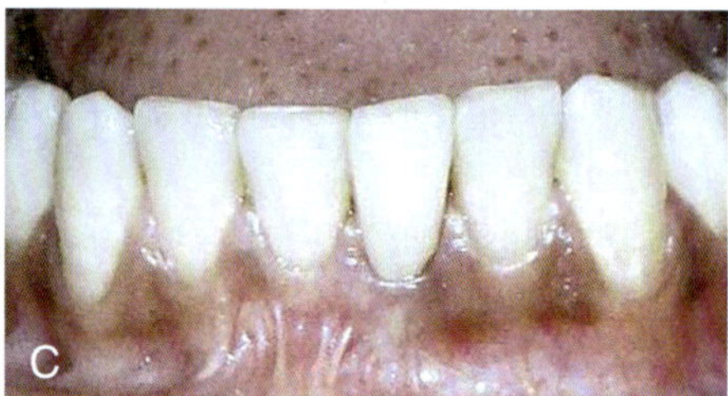

Fig 4.12 (A) Single body implant (B) unaesthetic porcelain fused to metal crown replaced with (C) aesthetic zirconium (Procera) crown.

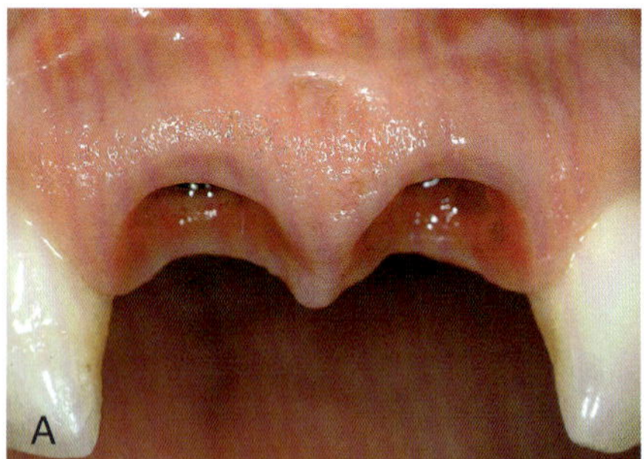

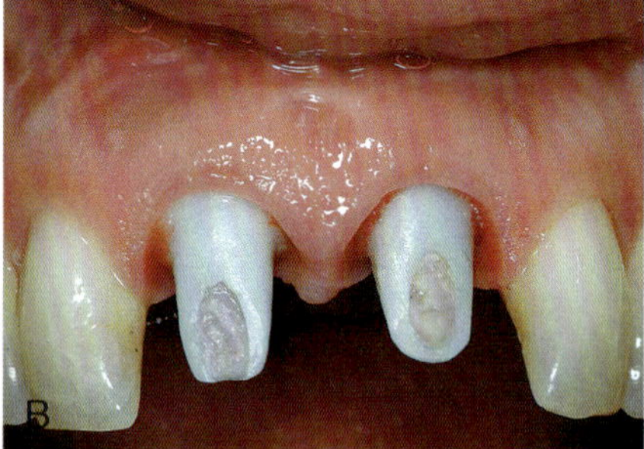

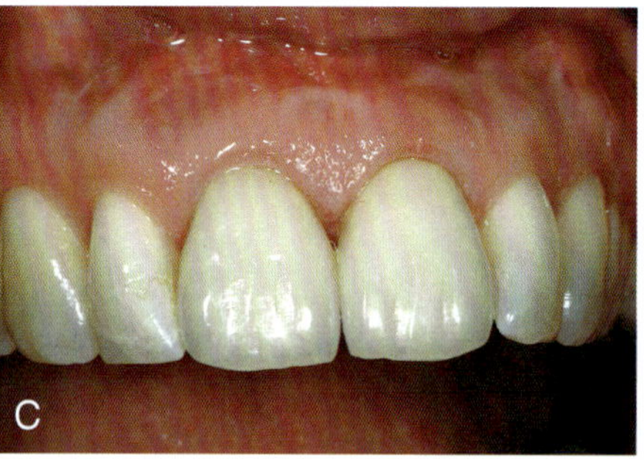

Fig 4.13 (A and B) Zirconium abutments inserted over implants and (C) zirconium prosthesis fixed over the abutments to achieve good aesthetics.

Summary

With advances in implant placement techniques, bone grafting procedures and the availability of several prosthetic components in many of implant systems, there are several implant prosthetic options for the partially to completely edentulous patients. For single and multiple unit implant prostheses, anterior or posterior, the cement-retained fixed prosthesis should be the preferred option. The metal-free zirconium prosthesis should be preferred over the porcelain fused to metal prosthesis at least for aesthetic reasons, to achieve the desired cosmetic outcome. The screw-retained prosthesis should be preferred in cases where the crown height space is less than 8 mm as well as for the full-arch option, because this prosthesis can be retrieved for cleaning or repair purposes. The implants retained overdentures should be preferred over the full-arch, fixed prosthesis for geriatric patients and medically compromised patients, as the placing of several implants for the fixed prosthesis may need long implant surgical sittings and often, bone grafting procedures. The newer 'all on 4' and 'all on 6' implant techniques/tilted implant concepts have gained better acceptance with patients in recent years. They not only save time, and avoid invasive and expensive bone grafting procedures, but also in most cases, a provisional fixed prosthesis can be fixed immediately after implant placement.

Further Reading

Naert I, Quirynen M, van Steenverghe D, et al. A six year prosthodontic study of 509 consecutively inserted implants for the treatment of partial edentulism. J Prosthet Dent 1992;67:236–45.

Misch CE. Maxillary anterior single tooth implant esthetic health compromise. Int J Symp 1995;3:4–9.

Jemt T. Failures and complications in 391 consecutively inserted fixed prosthesis supported by Branemark implants in edentulous jaws: a study of treatment from the time of prosthesis placement to the first annual checkup. Int J Oral Maxillofac Implants 1991;6:270–6.

Smedberg JI, Lothigius E, Bodin I, et al. A clinical and radiological two-year follow up study of maxillary overdentures on osseointegrated implants. Clin Oral Implants 1995;10:303–11.

Van stenverghe D, Lekholm U, Bolender C, et al. The applicability of osseointregated oral implants in the rehabilitation of partial edentulism: a prospective multicenter study on 558 fixtures. Int J Maxillofac Implants 1990;5:272–81.

Anderson B, Odman P, Lidvall AM, et al. Single tooth restorations supported by osseointegrated implants. Int J Oral Maxillofac Implants 1995;10:702–11.

Misch CE. Treatment options for mandibular implant overdenture: an organised approach. In: Contemporary implant dentistry. St Luice: Mosby; 1993.

Batenburg RH, Meijer HH, Raghoebar GM, et al. Treatment concept for mandibular overdentures supported by endosseous implants: a literature review. Int J Oral Maxillofac Implants 1998;13:539–45.

Mericske- Stern R. Clinical evaluation of overdenture restorations supported by osseointegrated titanium implants: a retrospective study. Int J Oral Maxillofac Implants 1990;5:375–83.

Preiskel HW. Overdentures made easy: a guide to implant and root supported prosthesis. Chicago: Quintessence; 1996.

Misch CE. Treatment options for mandibular full-arch implant-supported fixed prostheses. Dent Today 2001;20:68–73.

Parel SM, Sullivan D. Full-arch edentulous ceramometal restoration. Esthetics and osseointegration. OSI; 1989.

Linkow LI. Maxillary pterygoid extension implants: the state of art. Dent Clin North Am 1980;24:535–51.

Misch CE. Maxillary denture opposing an implant prosthesis. In: Misch CE, editor. Contemporary implant dentistry. St Luis: Mosby; 1999.

Bone density for dental implants

5

Ajay Vikram Singh

CHAPTER CONTENTS HD

Introduction

Bone density or quality is the "internal architecture or structure of the bone present at the edentulous site." It is assessed for implant placement through qualitative analysis of the bone present at the edentulous site. It has a major role in the overall success of any implant treatment. Bone density at the edentulous site is one of the main determining factors in treatment planning, implant design, surgical approach for implant placement, and loading protocol during prosthetic reconstruction. Several studies have presented the variable success rates of implants placed in bone with different densities, following standard surgical and prosthetic protocols. Jaffin and Berman reported the excessive loss (44%) of Branemark implant fixtures in the poor density bone of the maxilla, mostly at the stage of implant uncovery. Usually, the jawbone shows different bone densities in different jaw locations – it is highest in the mandibular anterior region and poorest in the posterior maxilla. The other two regions show moderate bone densities. Several studies have shown variable success rates of implants placed in different locations in the jaw. Adell et al reported 10% greater success of implants in the anterior mandible, compared to implants in the anterior maxilla. Schnitmann et al. reported better success rate of implants in the anterior mandible compared with those in the posterior mandible. The survival rate of implants varies with the location but it is directly related to the bone density at the particular location of the jaw. The bone density usually found at different locations of both jaws has been described in this chapter but these densities vary and largely depend on various factors like age of the patient, his/her gender, the presence of local and systemic diseases, hormonal imbalance, whether the patient is on systemic medicines, etc. (e.g. post-menopausal female patients often suffer with osteoporosis and may present with poor density even in the mandible, where the density is usually found at a higher level). Thus the author recommends the evaluation of other relevant parameters besides jaw location at the time of treatment planning, to finally decide the bone density present at the edentulous site and finalize the protocol for implant therapy that achieves a successful outcome. The dental CT scan is a reliable tool for evaluating bone density before performing implant surgery. This chapter provides a scientific rationale for the modification of treatment plans, appropriate implant selection, modifications in surgical protocols, implant-healing and loading protocols, etc. according to the bone density type at the edentulous site. Following these modifications, the clinician can achieve approximately similar success in implants inserted in sites with different bone densities.

Factors related to bone density

The following procedures, which can be affected by bone density, should be modified according to bone density at the edentulous site. Bone density has a major influence on:

1. Treatment planning
2. Drilling speed during osteotomy preparation
3. Saline irrigation flow during osteotomy preparation
4. Implant design with predictable success rate
5. Implant surface for predictable osseointegration
6. Surgical approach for implant insertion
7. Healing protocol (submerged or open)
8. Healing (osseointegration) period for the implant
9. The number of implants required to support multiple unit prostheses
10. Primary stability of the implant
11. Loading protocol – immediate/early/delayed/progressive bone loading.

Lekhom and Zarb classification for jawbone qualities

Lekhom and Zarb described four kinds of bone qualities found in the anteriors of the jawbone (Fig 5.1A–D):

Quality 1 - Homogenous compact bone
Quality 2 - Thick layer of compact bone surrounding a core of dense trabecular bone
Quality 3 - A thin layer of cortical bone surrounding a dense trabecular bone of favourable strength
Quality 4 - A thin layer of cortical bone surrounding a core of low-density trabecular bone.

Misch bone density classification

Carl E Misch defined four bone density types found in all regions of the jaw. The trabecular and cortical parts of these bone types differ at the macroscopic level (Table 5.1). He classified the jawbone regions into four types (Figs 5.2 and 5.3).

1. The anterior maxilla region (second premolar to second premolar), usually has D3 bone, but in few cases it may have D2 bone quality.
2. The posterior maxilla region (molar region) usually has D4 bone but in cases of sinus grafting it may have D3 bone 6 months after grafting.
3. The anterior mandible region (first premolar to first premolar) usually has D2 bone, but the resorbed anterior mandible may have D1 bone quality in approximately 25% of cases, more commonly in males.
4. The posterior mandible region (second premolar and molars) usually has D3 bone, but in some cases it can have D2 bone quality.

Determination of bone density

1. **Computed tomography (CT) scan.** Radiographs give a very limited idea of bone density, but with the help of the dental CT scan (DentaScan), the surgeon can ascertain bone density at the edentulous site before placing the implant. The dental CT scan is frequently used by the implant surgeon in treatment planning, as it gives all the details like three-dimensional bone volume, bone density, any defect present at the site, accurate implant simulation for the best possible prosthesis, etc. well before the actual implant surgery.

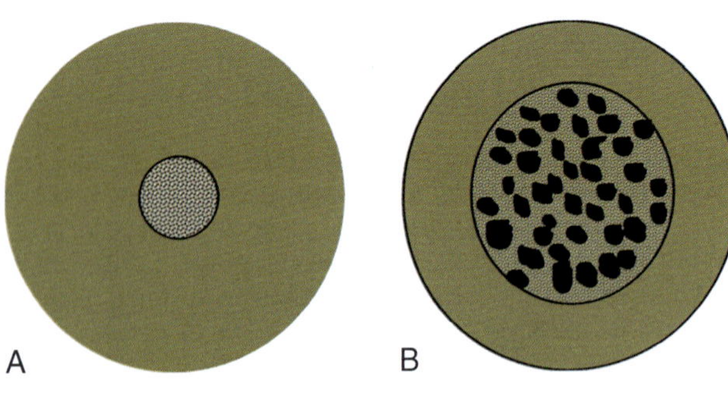

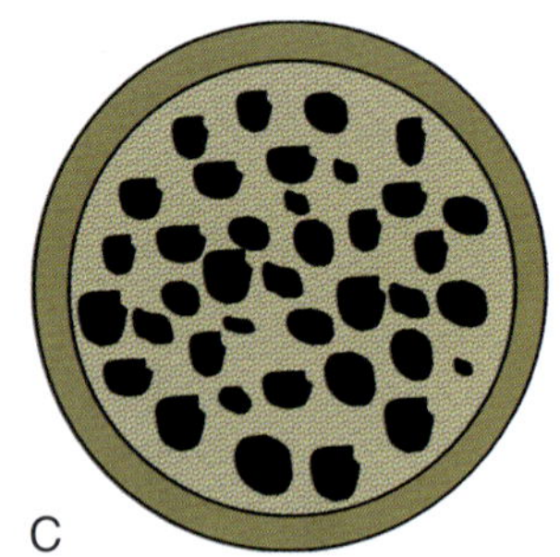

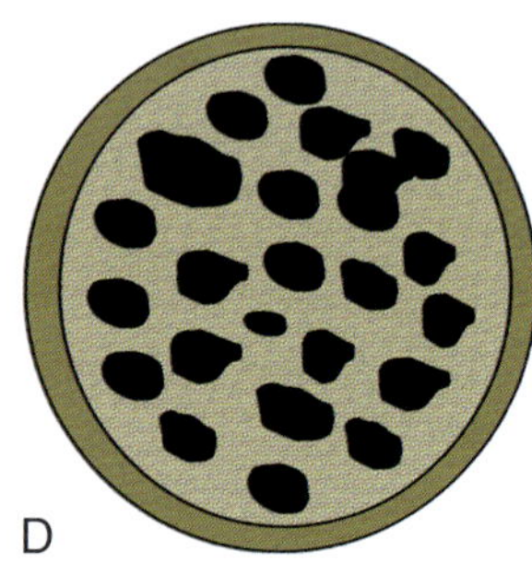

Fig 5.1 Lekhom and Zarb classification of jawbone qualities – (A) quality 1 bone, (B) quality 2 bone, (C) quality 3 bone and (D) quality 4 bone.

Table 5.1 Misch bone density classification

BONE DENSITY	DESCRIPTION	TACTILE ANALOGUE	TYPICAL ANATOMIC LOCATION	HOUNSFIELD UNITS
D1	Dense cortical	Oak/maple	Anterior mandible	>1250
D2	Porous cortical & coarse trabecular	White pine/spruce	Anterior and posterior mandible, anterior maxilla	850–1250
D3	Porous cortical (thin) & fine trabecular	Balsa wood	Posterior mandible, anterior and posterior maxilla	350–850
D4	Fine trabecular	Styrofoam	Posterior maxilla	150–350

Bone density is measured in the CT scan in Hounsfield unit (HU), i.e., denser bones have more Hounsfield units (Table 5.1).

2. **Tactile determination during bone drilling.** As bone density is directly related to bone strength, bone density at the site for implant insertion can be determined by the tactile sensation felt by an experienced implant surgeon during pilot drilling in the bone at the time of osteotomy preparation. Higher speed and more pressure are needed to do pilot drilling in bone with high density. Osteotomy-widening drilling does not give as good an idea of bone density as pilot drilling at the time of osteotomy preparation, because less rigorous drilling is required to widen the osteotomy already prepared by the initial pilot drill.

D1/Type 1 bone (dense cortical bone)

This homogenous compact bone contains almost no trabecular bone. Being dense cortical, it is the hardest bone in the jaw showing the least amount of vascularity. Because of limited blood supply, this bone shows very poor bone regeneration capacity. Osteotomy should be prepared at higher speed and using a new drill, under maximum flow of chilled saline irrigation to reduce heat generation and bone necrosis. This bone type is most commonly found in the mandibular anterior region (Fig 5.4A and B).

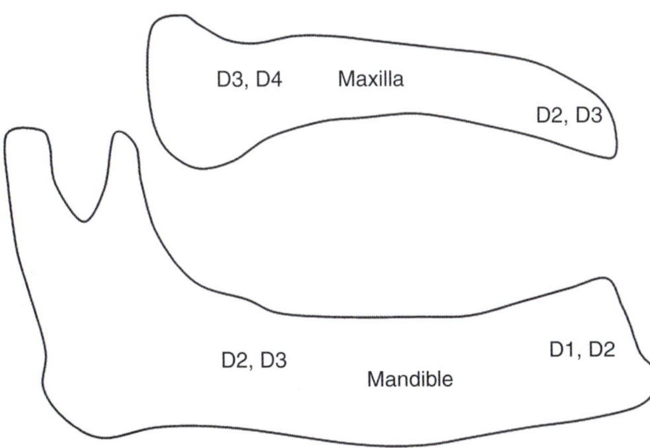

Fig 5.2 Diagrammatic presentation of the jaw sites for possible different bone density types.

Advantages

1. Strongest bone in the mouth
2. Implant achieves highest primary stability
3. Implant achieves higher bone–implant surface contact (BIC) percentage
4. Fewer implants can be inserted to support a multiple unit prosthesis
5. Requires only 3 – 4 months for primary healing of implants (osseointegration)
6. One-stage non-submerged surgical protocol can be practised in most cases
7. Immediate loading protocol can be practised in selective cases
8. Progressive bone loading is not required.

Disadvantages

1. Least amount of vascularity
2. Slow lamellar bone formation
3. Chances of bone overheating during osteotomy preparation are very high and may lead to osteonecrosis
4. Highest rate of failure in implant surgery
5. Longest time taken for implant placement
6. Requires drilling at high speed (2500 rpm) using new drills
7. Requires tapping (thread forming) for implants with non-cutting threads
8. May require crestal bone modification/drilling for the implant with broader platform than the implant body, to reduce incidence of mechanical overload during its insertion at crest.

D2/Type 2 bone

(Porous thick cortical and coarse trabecular) – This bone shows a thick layer of compact bone surrounding a core of dense trabecular bone (Fig 5.5A and B). This bone shows excellent vascularity and osseous healing capacity.

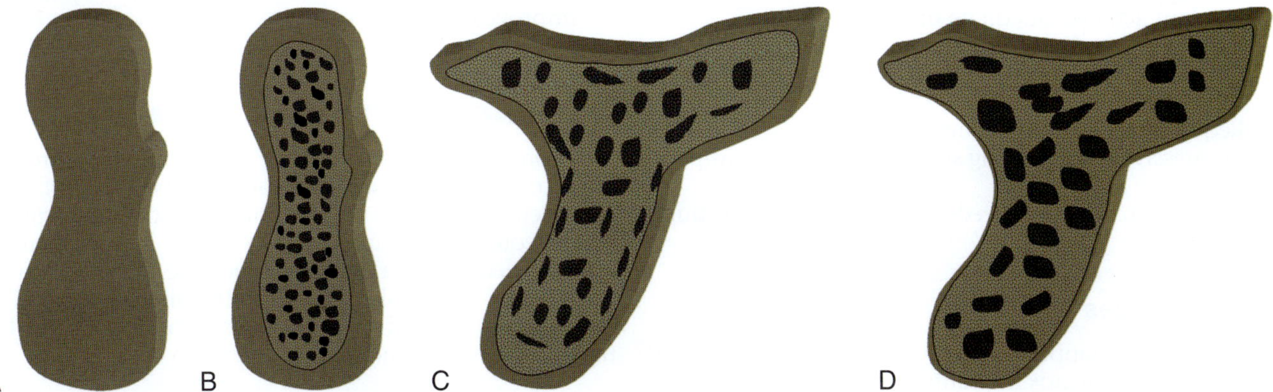

Fig 5.3 Diagrammatic presentation of the four bone density types described by Carl E Misch. (A) D1 bone is dense cortical bone and is the highest in the density, (B) D2 bone is coarse trabecular bone surrounded by thick porous cortical bone, (C) D3 bone is fine trabecular bone surrounded by thin porous cortical bone, and (D) D4 bone is fine trabecular bone with almost no cortical bone.

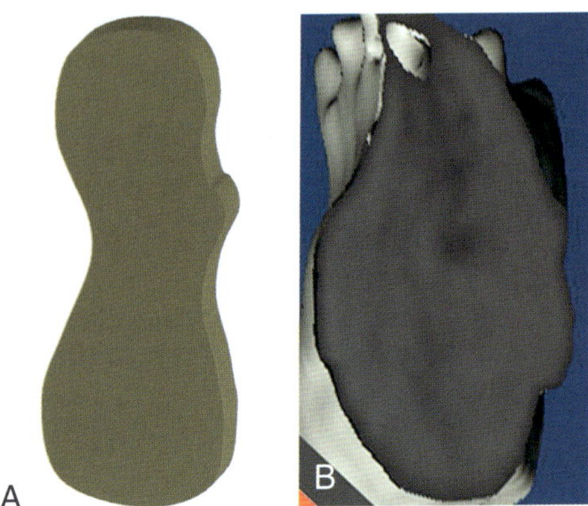

Fig 5.4 Dense cortical or homogenous compact D1 bone, (A) diagrammatic presentation and as seen in (B) 3D cross-section of a dental CT.

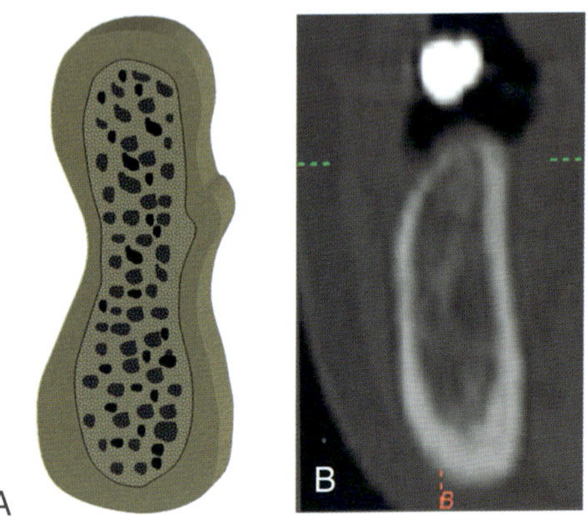

Fig 5.5 Porous cortical and course trabecular D2 bone, (A) diagrammatic presentation and as seen in (B) cross-section of CT scan of a patient's bone.

This bone is most commonly found in the mandibular anterior and posterior regions but may also be present in the maxillary anterior region.

Advantages

1. Strong bone with good regeneration capacity
2. Implant achieves adequate primary stability
3. Excellent vascularity and osseous healing
4. One-stage non-submerged surgical protocol can be followed
5. Requires 4–6 months of healing period
6. Progressive bone loading strengthens the peri-implant bone
7. Fewer implants are needed to support a multiunit prosthesis.

Disadvantages

1. May require tapping for implants with non-cutting/non-cutting threads implants
2. May require crestal bone modification/drilling for the implant with broader platform than the implant body to reduce incidence of mechanical overload during its insertion at the crest.

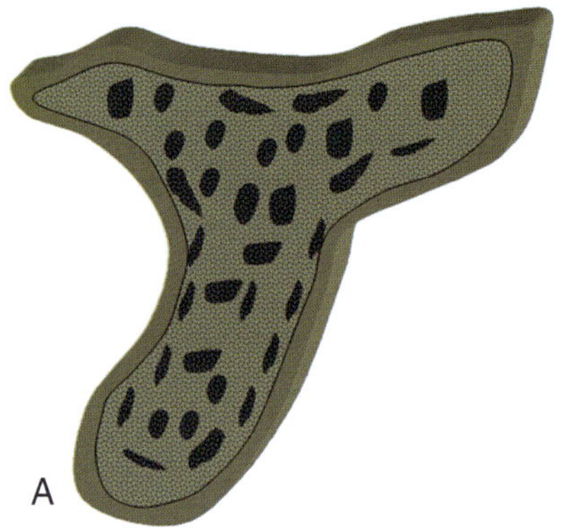

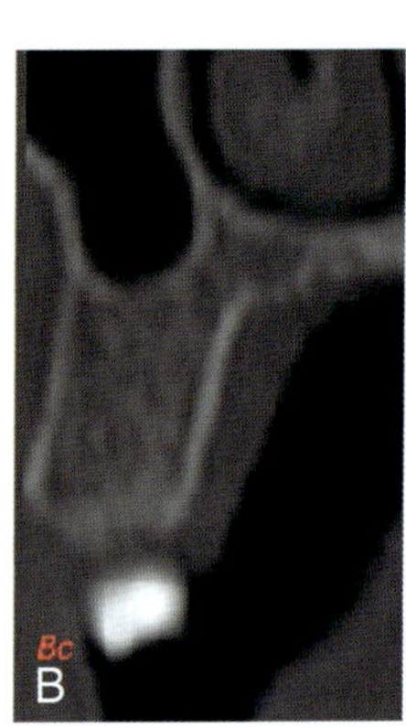

Fig 5.6 Porous cortical (thin) and fine trabecular D3 bone, (A) diagrammatic presentation and as seen in (B) CT scan cross section of a patient's bone.

D3/Type 3 bone (porous cortical [thin] and fine trabecular)

This bone quality shows a thin layer of cortical bone surrounding a dense trabecular bone of favourable strength (Figs 5.6A and B). This bone shows excellent vascularity and osseous healing capacity. This bone is most commonly found in the maxillary anterior region but can be present in the mandibular and maxillary posterior regions.

Advantages

1. Faster osteotomy preparation at slower speed
2. Bone tapping is optional
3. Crestal bone drilling is optional
4. Excellent vascularity
5. Chances of bone overheating are small.

Disadvantages

1. Healing period of 6–8 months
2. Implant may achieve inadequate primary stability
3. More implants are required to be inserted to support multiunit prosthesis
4. Immediate/early bone loading protocol should be avoided
5. Longer progressive loading period is required to improve bone quality.

D4/Type 4 bone (fine trabecular)

This bone shows a very thin layer of cortical bone surrounding a core of low-density, fine trabecular bone of unfavourable strength (Fig 5.7A–C). This bone has excellent vascularity and osseous healing capacity but because it is much compromised in density, it is a challenge to achieve adequate primary stability and favourable osseointegration in the implant. This bone usually shows the highest rate of prosthetic failure. It is most commonly found in the posterior maxilla.

Advantages

1. Only initial or no drilling is done but only osteotomes can be used for osteotomy preparation

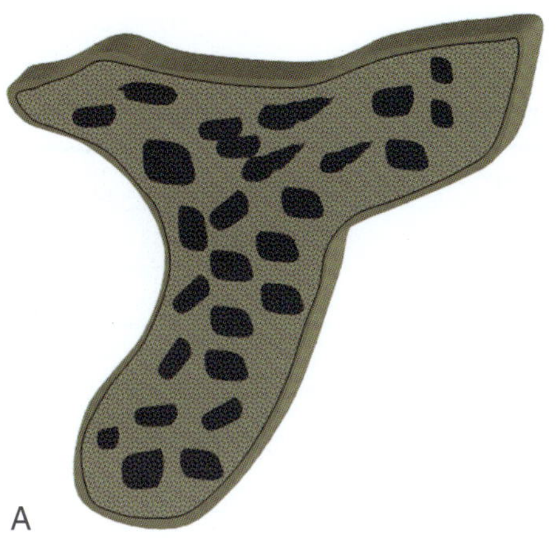

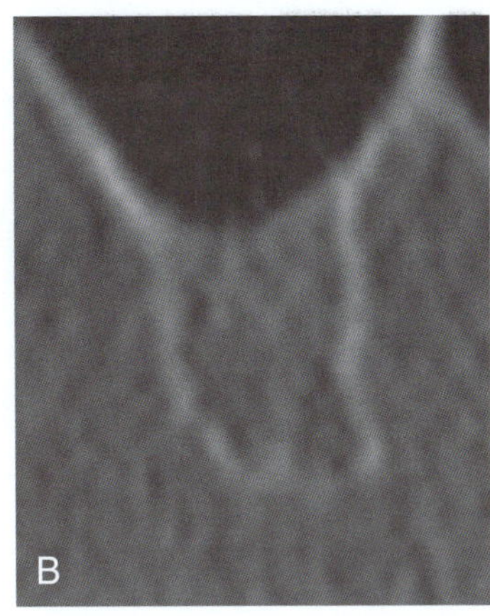

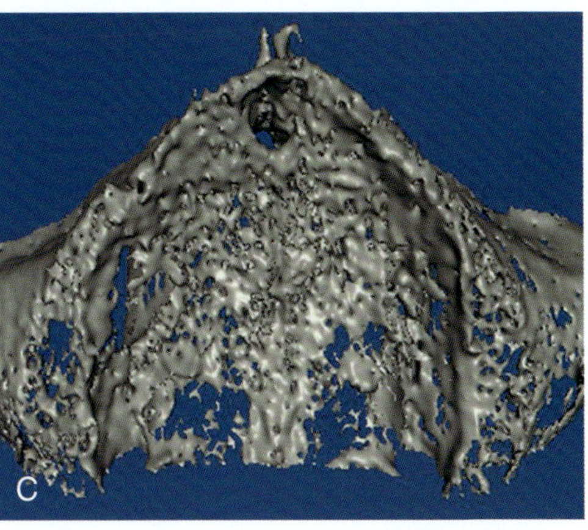

Fig 5.7 Fine trabecular D4 bone, (A) diagrammatic presentation and as seen in (B) CT scan cross-section and (C) 3D view of a patient's bone.

2. No tapping is done
3. No crestal bone preparation is done
4. Least chances of surgical implant failure.

Disadvantages

1. Often difficult to achieve adequate primary stability for the implant
2. Long healing period (8 – 10 months) for implants
3. More implants need to be inserted to support a multiunit prosthesis
4. Long period of progressive loading is required
5. Highest rate of prosthetic implant failure.

Comparative features and clinical differences in four types of bone are given in Table 5.2.

Features increasing the success rate of implants in D4 bone

Carl E Misch suggested few key guidelines to enhance the success of implants in poor density (D4) bone.

1. Wider diameter implants should be used to enhance bone–implant contact surface
2. Implants with more threads should be used
3. Implants with deeper threads should be used
4. Surface textures that increase initial BIC percentage should be used (e.g. HA surface implants [D4 implants] from Biohorizons).
5. Osteotomy site should be prepared using an osteotome for lateral bone condensation. It improves bone density in the peri-implant trabecular bone and the BIC percentage. Thus, the inserted implant achieves adequate primary stability for predictable osseointegration.
6. Bicortical engagement of the implant – the implant collar can be engaged in the relatively high density crestal bone and its apex in the hard sinus floor, by fracturing or grinding up the sinus floor after final osteotomy preparation. For engaging the implant in the sinus floor, a longer 2–3 mm implant, with adequate primary stability, can be inserted (Figs 5.8 and 5.9).
7. The implant should be submerged 0.5–1.0 mm. subcrestal, to prevent micromovement during the healing period (Fig 5.10A and B).
8. Loading of implants in poor density bone like the posterior maxilla shows less (BIC) percentage, even after successful osseointegration. Often, poor osseointegration of the loaded implant with the trabecular bone leads to prosthetic failure. However, if the implant in poor density bone is loaded progressively, it shows progressive strengthening of the peri-implant trabecular bone and a higher BIC percentage, and it successfully withstands occlusal forces without failure after loading (Fig 5.11).

Table 5.2 Comparative features and clinical differences in different types of bone densities

KEY POINTS	D1 BONE	D2 BONE	D3 BONE	D4 BONE
1. Bone density	Very high	High	Low	Very low
2. Bone strength	Very high	High	Low	Very low
3. Vascularity and osseous healing	Poorest	Medium	Good	Highest
4. Heat generation/bone over heating during drilling	Very high	High	Low	Very low
5. Recommended drilling speed	2000–2500 rpm	1500–2000 rpm	1200–1500 rpm	800–1200 rpm
6. Recommended saline/coolant flow during drilling	Maximum	Medium	Medium	Minimum
7. Chances of pressure necrosis of bone	Maximum	Medium	Low	Minimum
8. Bone tapping	Required	Required	Optional	Not required
9. Recommended implant thread design	Implant with shallow threads	Any thread design	Any thread design	Deeper threads with high pitch value
10. Healing period for implant	2–3 months	3–4 months	4–6 months	6–8 months
11. Implant platform positioning	At crestal level	At crestal level	At crestal level	Submerged 0.5–1 mm apical to ridge crest
12. Lateral bone condensation using osteotomes	Not done	Not required	Optional	Mandatory
13. Non-submerged implant placement	Can be done	Can be done	Should be avoided	Contraindicated
14. Primary stability of implant	Highest	Medium	Low	Lowest
15. Immediate/early loading of implant	Can be done	Can be done	Should be avoided	Contraindicated
16. Progressive bone loading	Not required	Optional	Optional	Indicated
17. No. of implants required for multiple unit prosthesis	Minimum no. of implants	Medium no. of implants	More no. of implants	Maximum no. of implants
18. Cantilevered prosthesis	Can be given	Can be given	Should be avoided	Contraindicated
19. Implant failure	Highest surgical failure	Low	Low	Highest prosthetic failure

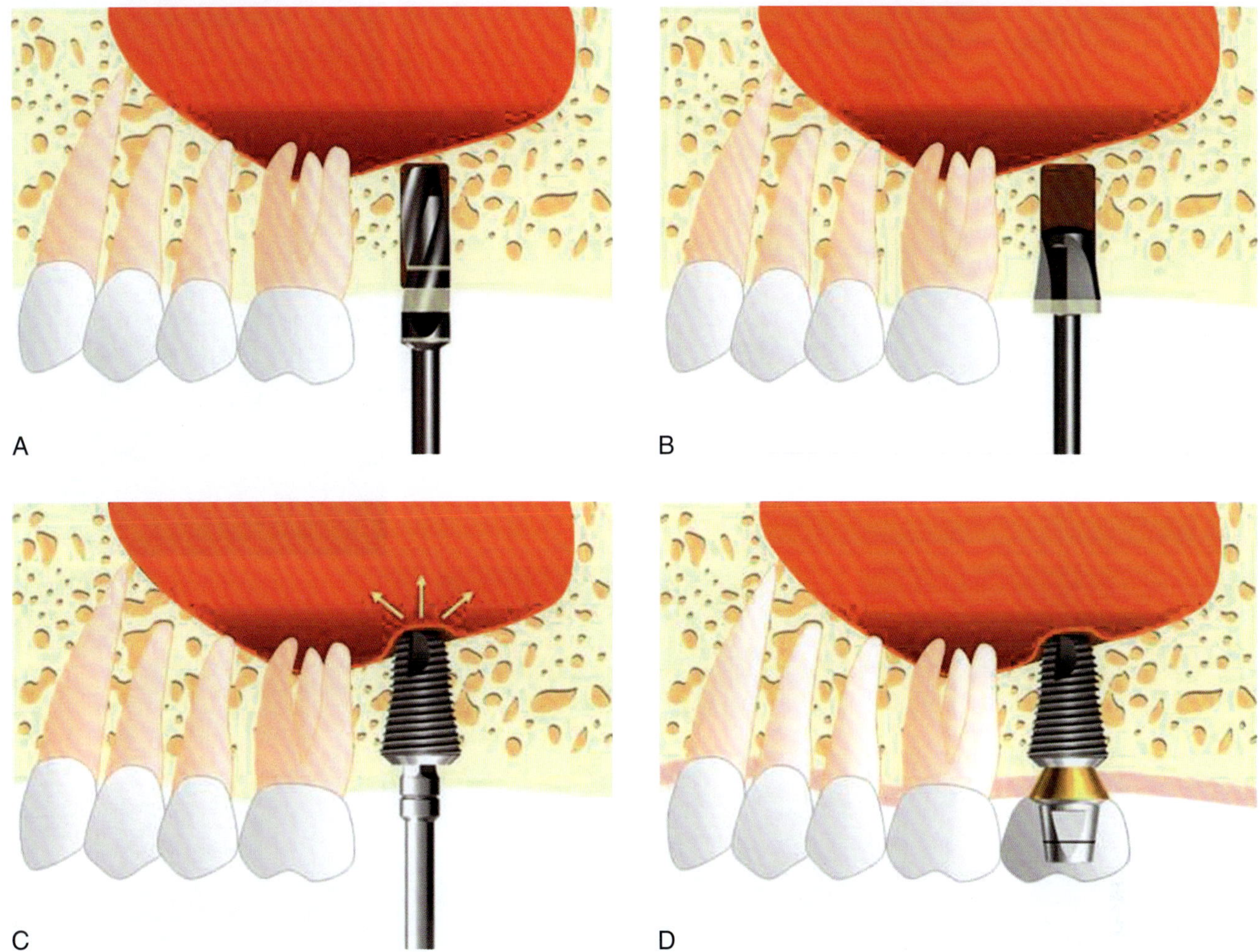

Fig 5.8 Stabilizing implant apex in the high-density sinus floor. (A and B) The implant osteotomy is prepared approximately 1 mm short of the sinus floor, followed by elevating the thin subantral bone using Summer's osteotome or grinding it using a coarse diamond bur (DASK from Dentium, Korea). (C and D) The implant apex is engaged in the hard sinus floor. It results in adequate primary stability of the implant in low-density bone and also allows the placing of a longer 2- to 3-mm implant (*Courtesy: Dentium Implant Co., Seoul, Korea*).

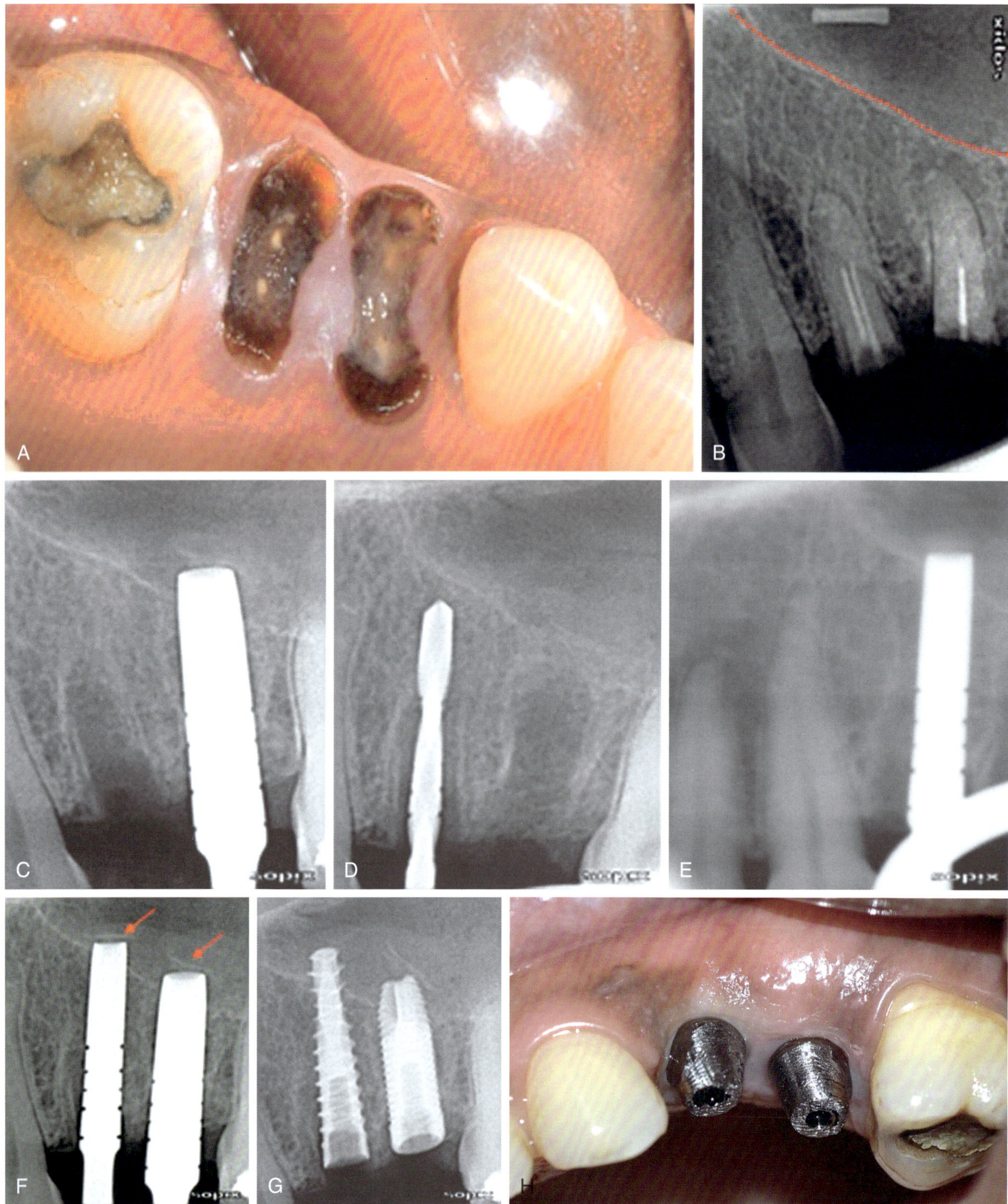

Fig 5.9 (A) Root stumps of left bicuspids planned to be extracted, with immediate implant placement. (B) Dental radiograph showing limited bone height apical to the root stumps (especially in second bicuspid) to adequately engage the immediately inserted implant apex. (C) The root stumps are atraumatically extracted using periotomes, a 4.2-mm-diameter osteotome is inserted into the posterior extraction socket and gently tapped to fracture the hard sinus floor. (D) The implant osteotomy is prepared through the anterior socket only 2 mm short of the sinus floor. (E) Further, a final drill diameter osteotome is used in similar fashion to fracture the sinus floor. (F) Both the osteotomes can be seen in the radiograph reaching beyond the sinus floor with fractured sinus floor bony pieces (red arrows), tenting up the elevated sinus membrane. (G) Both implants are inserted to engage their apex in the hard sinus floor as well as the ridge crest (bicortical engagement) to achieve high initial implant stability (30–35 Ncm) which is quite important for optimal implant success in the low-density posterior maxilla. (H) Successfully osseointegrated implants uncovered after 4 months for prosthetic loading.

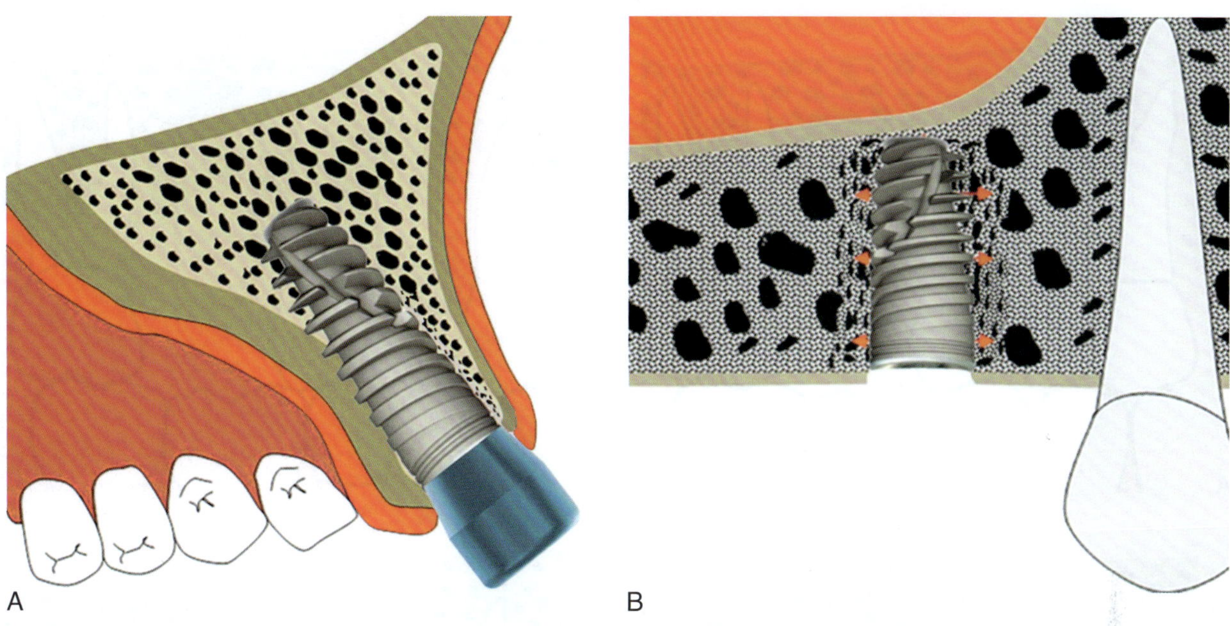

Fig 5.10 (A) The implant can be placed with its platform at the level of the crest with submerged healing, or can be left for non-submerged healing with the immediate insertion of trans gingival abutment in D1 or D2 bone. (B) The implant inserted with its platform submerged 1–2 mm apical to the ridge crest and left to heal with the submerged technique in D4 bone. Submerging the implant apical to the ridge crest prevents any premature loading of the implant during its healing period. The surrounding bone should also be condensed to improve bone density around the implant to achieve adequate primary stability and predictable osseointegration.

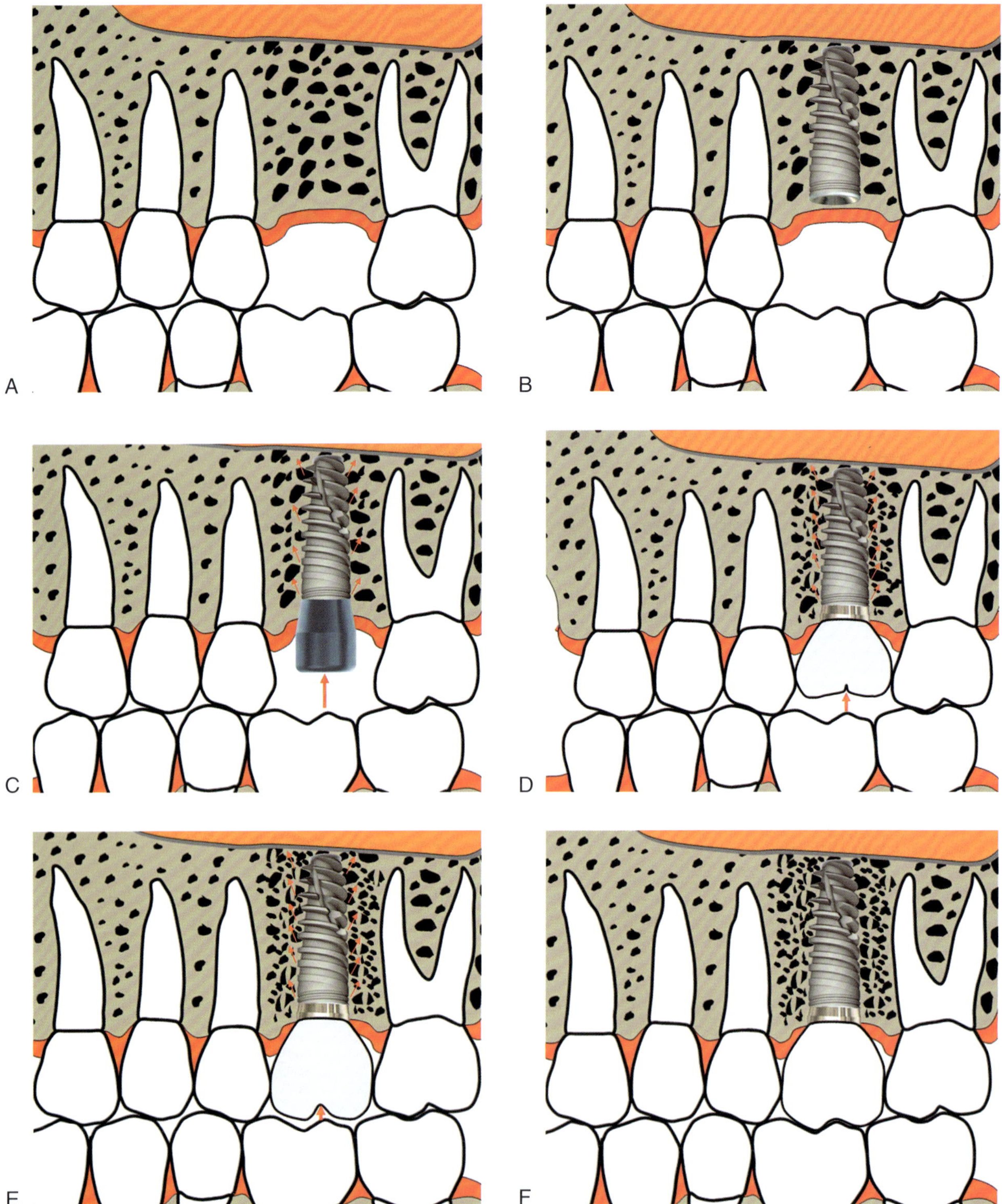

Fig 5.11 (A and B) When placing implant in poor-density bone like the posterior maxilla, the ideal is to submerge the implant 1 mm apical to the ridge crest to avoid premature loading and micromovement during the healing phase. The osseointegrated implant in such bone shows poor amount of trabecular bone attachment to the implant surface (low BIC percentage) which may not provide adequate strength to withstand occlusal forces and often results in implant failure. Thus to strengthen the trabecular bone around the osseointegrated implant, the latter should be progressively loaded. (C) The osseointegrated implant is uncovered and a low profile gingival former is inserted. (D) This gingival former is replaced with a provisional prosthesis which is kept 3–4 mm out of occlusion and the patient is instructed not to chew anything very hard. (E) Further, the material is added to the occlusal surface of the provisional prosthesis at two to three week intervals. The provisional prosthesis should preferably be fabricated with resilient self-cure acrylic. It acts as a shock absorber and, unlike the ceramic prosthesis, it does not immediately transfer occlusal forces to the implant. (F) After the patient has been chewing with the provisional prosthesis for a month, the latter can be replaced with the long-term ceramic prosthesis. Progressive loading results in strengthening of the trabecular bone and increased bone density around the implant.

Summary

Bone density at the edentulous site is the key determinant for endosteal implant success. Bone strength is directly related to bone density. The implant dentist should carefully evaluate bone density at the site, to avoid failures. Treatment planning should be modified, based on bone density at the implant site. The high-density bone should be drilled at higher speed, using new drills, under copious amounts of chilled saline to reduce bone overheating. The placement of the widest and longest possible implants, lateral bone condensation using osteotomes, submerging of the implant 1 mm subcrestal, and progressive bone loading are the key features that should be implemented in cases of poor-density bone. The bone densities at different jaw locations defined by Carl E Misch, can be very helpful to the dentist to predict possible bone density at the edentulous site. The dental CT scan is a very helpful tool for accurately evaluating bone density at the edentulous site.

Further Reading

Adel R, Lekholm U, Rockler B, et al. A 15-year study of osseointegrated implants in the treatment of the edentulous jaw. Int J Oral Sung 1981;6:387–416.

Jaffin RA, Berman CL. The excessive loss of Branemark fixtures in the type IV bone: a 5-year analysis. J Periodontol 1991;62(1):2–4.

Schnitman PA, Rubenstein JE, Whorle PS, et al. Implants for partial edentulism. J Dent Educ 1988;52:725–36.

Minsk L, Polson A, Weisgold A, et al. Outcome failures of endosseous implants from a clinical training center. Compendium 1996;17(9):848–59.

Misch CE, Kircos LT. Diagnostic imaging and techniques. In: Misch CE, editor. Contemporary implant dentistry. 2nd ed. St Luis: Mosby; 1999. pp. 73–87.

Orenstein IH, Synan WJ, Truhlar RS, et al. Bone quality in patients receiving endosseous dental implants, DICRG interim report no. 1. Implant Dent 1994;3(2):90–4.

Higuchi KW, Folmer T, Kultje C. Implant survival rates in partially edentulouos patients: a 3-year prospective multicenter study. J Oral Maxillofac Surg 1995;53:264–8.

Carter DR, Hayes WC. Bone compressive strength: the influence of density and strain rate. Science 1976;194:1174.

Misch CE. Density of bone: effect on treatment plans, surgical approach, healing, and progressive loading. Int J Oral Implantol 1990;6:23–31.

Misch CE, Qu Z, Bidez MW. Mechanical properties of trabecular bone in the human mandible: implications for dental implant treatment planning and surgical placement. J Oral Maxillofac Surg 1999;57:700–6.

Friberg B, Jemt T, Lekholm U. Early failures in 4641 consecutively placed Branemark dental implants: a study from stage I surgery to the connection of completed prosthesis. Int J Oral Maxillofac Implants 1988;3:129–34.

Misch CE, Hoar J, Beck G, et al. A bone quality based implant system: preliminary report of stage I and stage II. Implant Dent 1998;7:35–42.

Lavelle CLB. Biomechanical considerations of prosthodontic therapy: the urgency of research into alveolar bone responses. Int J Oral Maxillofac Implants 1993;8(2):179–84.

Misch CE. Progressive bone loading. Dent Today 1995;12(1):80–3.

Misch CE, Poitras Y, Dietsh-Misch F. Endosteal implants in the edentulous posterior maxilla: rationale and clinical results. Oral Health 2000;90(8):7–16.

Esposito M, Hirsch JM, Lekholm U, et al. Biological factors contributing to failures of osseointegrated oral implants. (II) Etiopathogenesis. Eur J Oral Sci 1998;106:721–64.

Morris HF, Ochi S, Crum P, et al. AICRG, part I: a 6-year multicentred, multidisciplinary clinical study of a new and innovative implant design. J Oral Implantol 2004;30:125–33.

Herrmann I, Lekholm U, Holm S, et al. Evaluation of patient and implant characteristics as potential prognostic factors for oral implant failures. Int J Oral Maxillofac Implants 2005;20:220–30.

Role of available bone in dental implants

6

Ajay Vikram Singh

CHAPTER CONTENTS HD

Introduction

Available bone is a quantitative assessment of the bone suitable for implant placement, which is available at an edentulous site. Bone availability describes "the external architecture and volume of bone in the edentulous area considered for ideal implant placement." It is measured three-dimensionally in buccolingual width, vertical height, mesiodistal dimension of edentulous space, bone angulation, and crown height space for the future prosthesis. If the bone available is inadequate for prosthetically ideal implant insertion, the implant surgeon can perform bone grafting procedures to regenerate lost bone dimensions.

As described in previous chapters, implants are available in different diameters and lengths. The design of a root form implant may vary from one manufacturer to another. The crest module or implant platform of some implants may be wider than the body diameter. For example, the 3.3 mm diameter Adin implant has a 3.75 mm platform. The dentist should be aware that in most clinical situations, the ridge is found to be faciolingually thinnest at the crestal region, which may often make it difficult to place even the narrowest diameter implant without ridge modification. The bone at any edentulous site is considered to be adequate when the implant with adequate dimensions can be placed in such a way that it leaves minimum of 1.5–2 mm of three-dimensional bone all around the implant body and platform (facially, lingually, and apically from vital structures like the sinus floor, mandibular canal, etc.) (Fig 6.1A–D).

Misch and Judy classification of bone availability

In 1985, Misch and Judy presented a classification of available bone for dental implant insertion, which is similar in both arches (Fig 6.2A–D). Bone modification procedures, grafting methods, and prosthodontic-related treatments were suggested for each category.

Division A (abundant bone)

Division A bone is three-dimensionally abundant for the ideal implant insertion (Fig 6.3A and B). According to Misch, bone in this category should be:

a. 5 mm or more in width
b. 12 mm or more in height
c. 7 mm or more in length
d. Less than 30° in angulation
e. 15 mm or less in crown height.

Prosthetic options for Division A bone

The Division A bone:

a. is the best bone for any prosthetic option (Fig 6.4A–I).
b. may need osteoplasty for implant overdentures, to achieve more vertical height space and accommodate the implant suprastructures (ball/bar) under the denture.

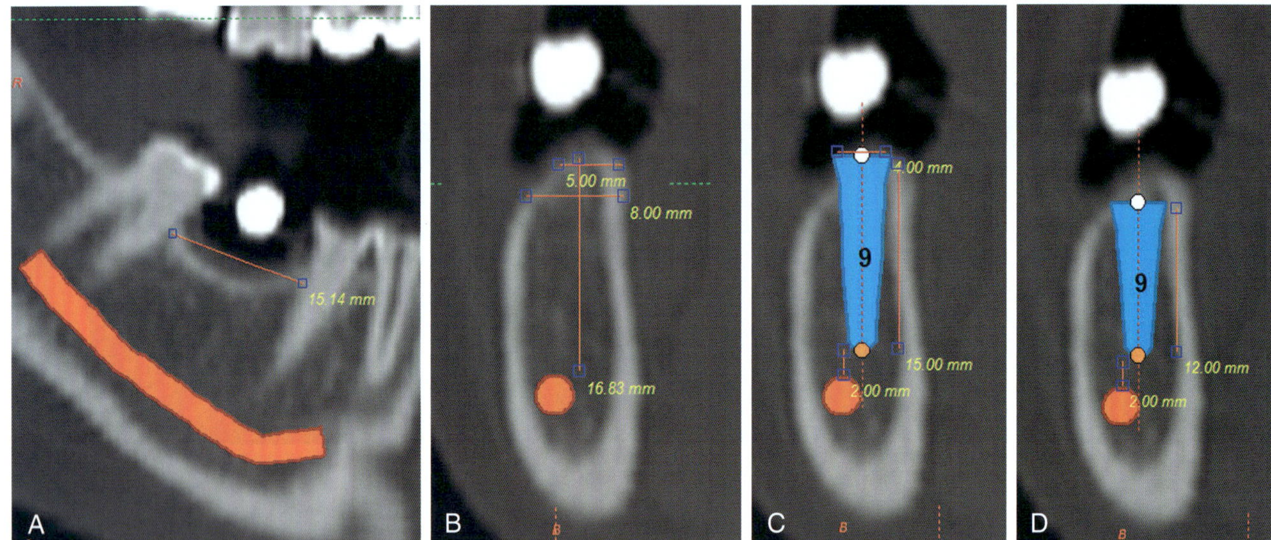

Fig 6.1 (A) Panoramic view of the edentulous mandibular molar site showing adequate bone length availability (15 mm) to place widest implant of any system (B) but the cross-sectional view of the same edentulous region shows inadequate bone availability at the ridge crest (5 mm), which cannot allow placement of even the narrowest implant of any system. The height of the bone above the mandibular canal is adequate (16.83 mm) to place an adequately long implant (14–15 mm long). (C) The implant with 4 mm x 15 mm dimensions can be placed with its platform at the crest level with simultaneous lateral bone augmentation to cover the facially exposed implant threads near the crest. (D) The shorter length (4 mm x 12 mm) implant is placed after 3 mm of osteoplasty, so that the implant platform can be placed at the level of wider subcrestal ridge.

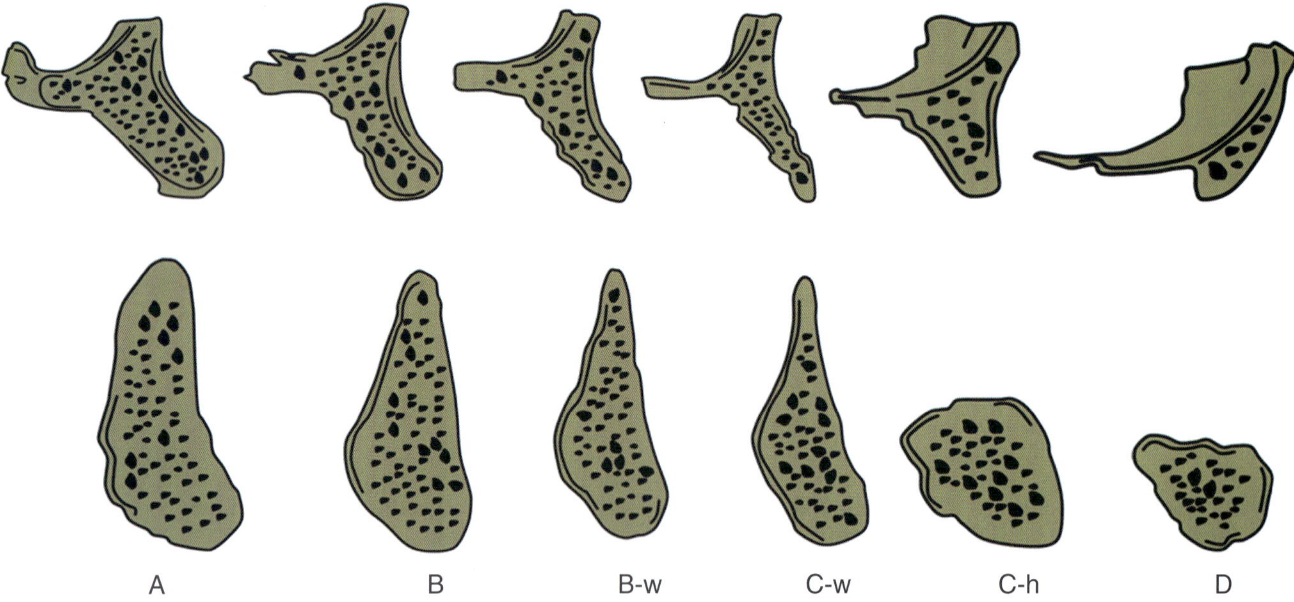

Fig 6.2 Misch and Judy classification of bone availability (Divisions A, B, C and D): Division A (abundant bone), Division B (barely sufficient bone), Division C (compromised bone), Division D (deficient bone), w (width), h (height).

Division B (barely adequate) bone

Bone in this category should be:

a. 2.5–5 mm in width (B+: 4–5 mm; B–: 2.5–4 mm)
b. 12 mm or more in height
c. 6 mm or more in length
d. Less than 20° in angulation
e. 15 mm or less in crown height.

Prosthetic options for Division B bone

The bony ridge with Division B bone may be modified to division A bone by osteoplasty to achieve the wide

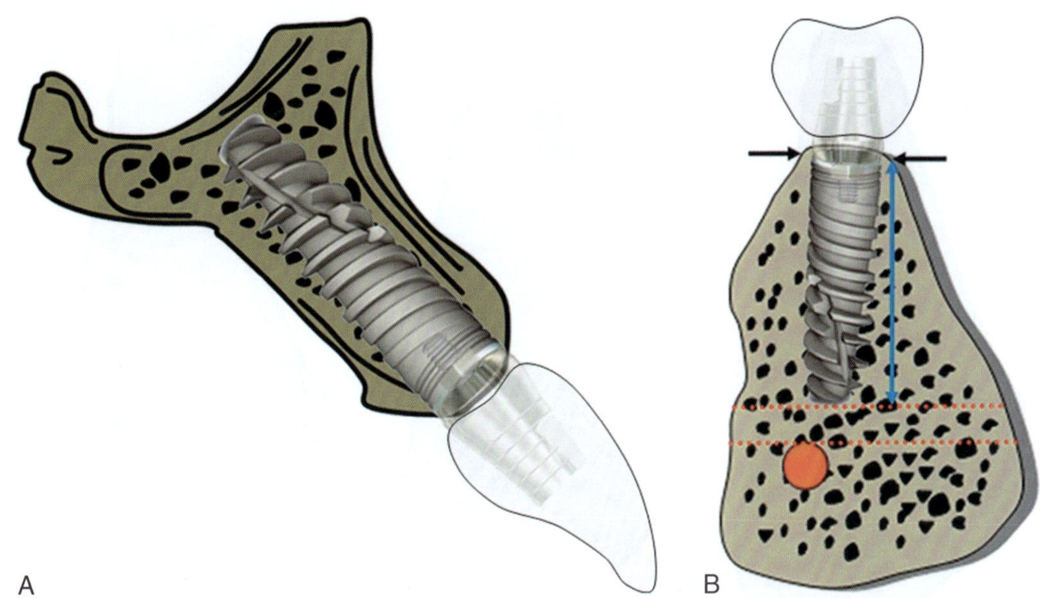

Fig 6.3 (A and B) Abundant bone in the maxilla and mandible suitable for inserting an implant with ideal dimensions.

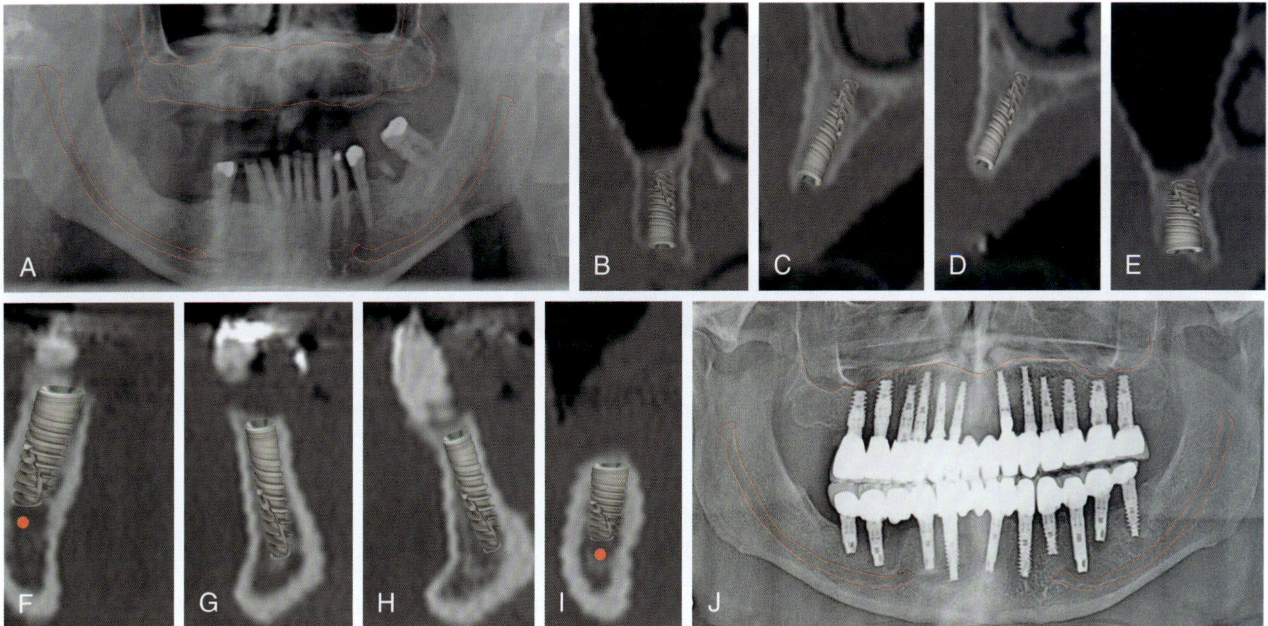

Fig 6.4 (A) Panoramic radiograph and (B–I) CT scan showing cross-sectional views of the maxilla and the mandible, showing the Division A bone (adequate bone) for implant placement without any ridge modification or grafting. (J) The implant-supported, full mouth fixed prosthesis can be seen in the radiograph.

ridge crest required to insert a regular diameter implant (Fig 6.5A–C). Lateral bone augmentation can also be performed before or with implant placement, especially in aesthetic areas where osteoplasty can elongate the clinical crown height (Fig 6.6A–C). This bone may be adequate for any prosthetic option in implant therapy.

Division C (compromised bone)

Bone in Division C category should be:

a. 0–2.5 mm in width (C-w bone)
b. Less than 12 mm in height (C-h bone)
c. More than 30° in angulation (C-a bone)
d. More than 15 mm in crown height.

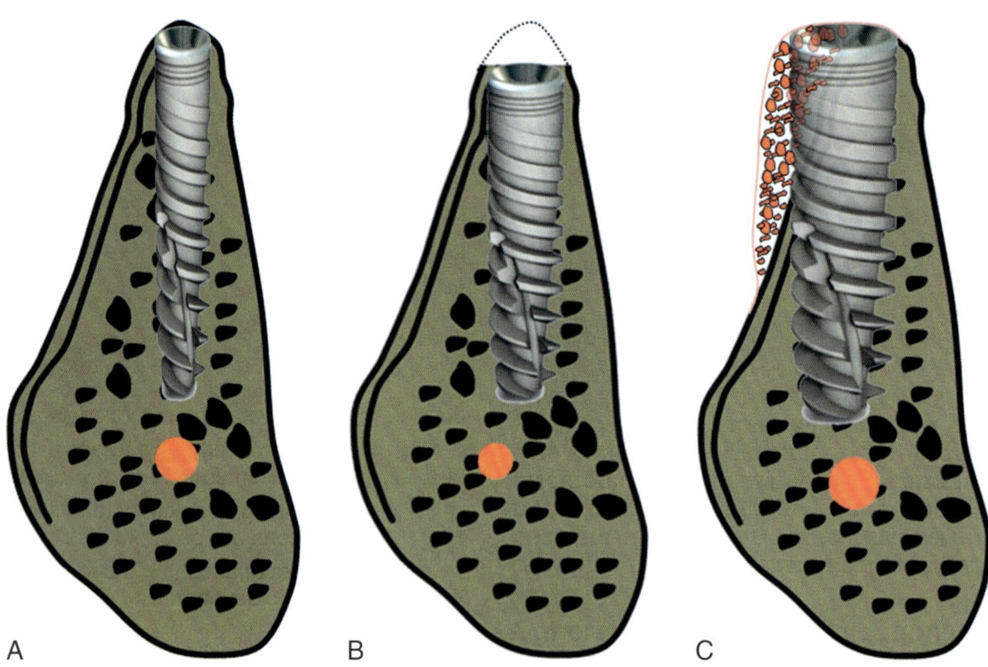

Fig 6.5 (A) Either a narrow diameter implant is inserted or (B) a Division B ridge is converted to Division A bone by vertical ridge osteoplasty or (C) lateral bone augmentation to achieve a wide ridge crest for placement of regular-diameter implant.

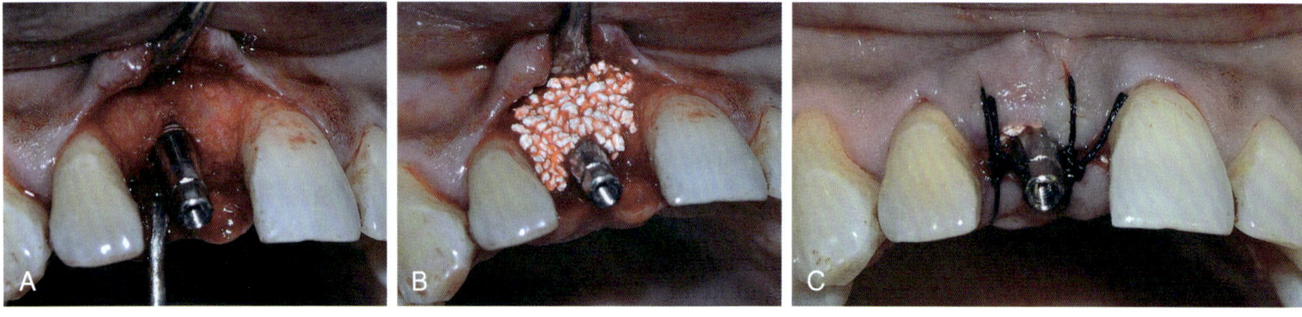

Fig 6.6 (A) Implant placed in the Division B bone, showing implant threads exposed in the crestal region at the facial aspect of ridge. (B and C) Simultaneous lateral bone augmentation is performed to cover the exposed implant threads and also to improve the aesthetic ridge profile.

Treatment options

Osteoplasty can be done in C-w bone to achieve a wider platform to insert the implant, but the preferred option for the C-w bone is lateral bone augmentation before or at the time of implant insertion (Figs 6.7 and 6.8). Either short length root form implants or subperiosteal implants are used in C-h bone. Vertical bone augmentation (Fig 6.9A–C) or inferior alveolar nerve lateralization for posterior mandible and sinus elevation and grafting for posterior maxilla, may be the other options to achieve adequate ridge height for the insertion of long implants (Fig 6.10A–I).

Prosthetic options for Division C bone

a. Implant overdenture.
b. Lateral bone augmentation for C-w bone and vertical bone augmentation for C-h bone are required to deliver fixed, implant- supported prostheses.

Division D bone (deficient bone)

This is the bone with severe atrophy, and it represents as basal bone loss, flat maxilla, and pencil-thin mandible, with more than 20 mm crown height.

Treatment options for the deficient ridge

Bone augmentation like vertical bone block grafting or nerve transpositioning, can be performed to insert adequately long implants in the mandible (Fig 6.11A and B). Vertical bone block grafting and/or sinus/nasal floor elevation and

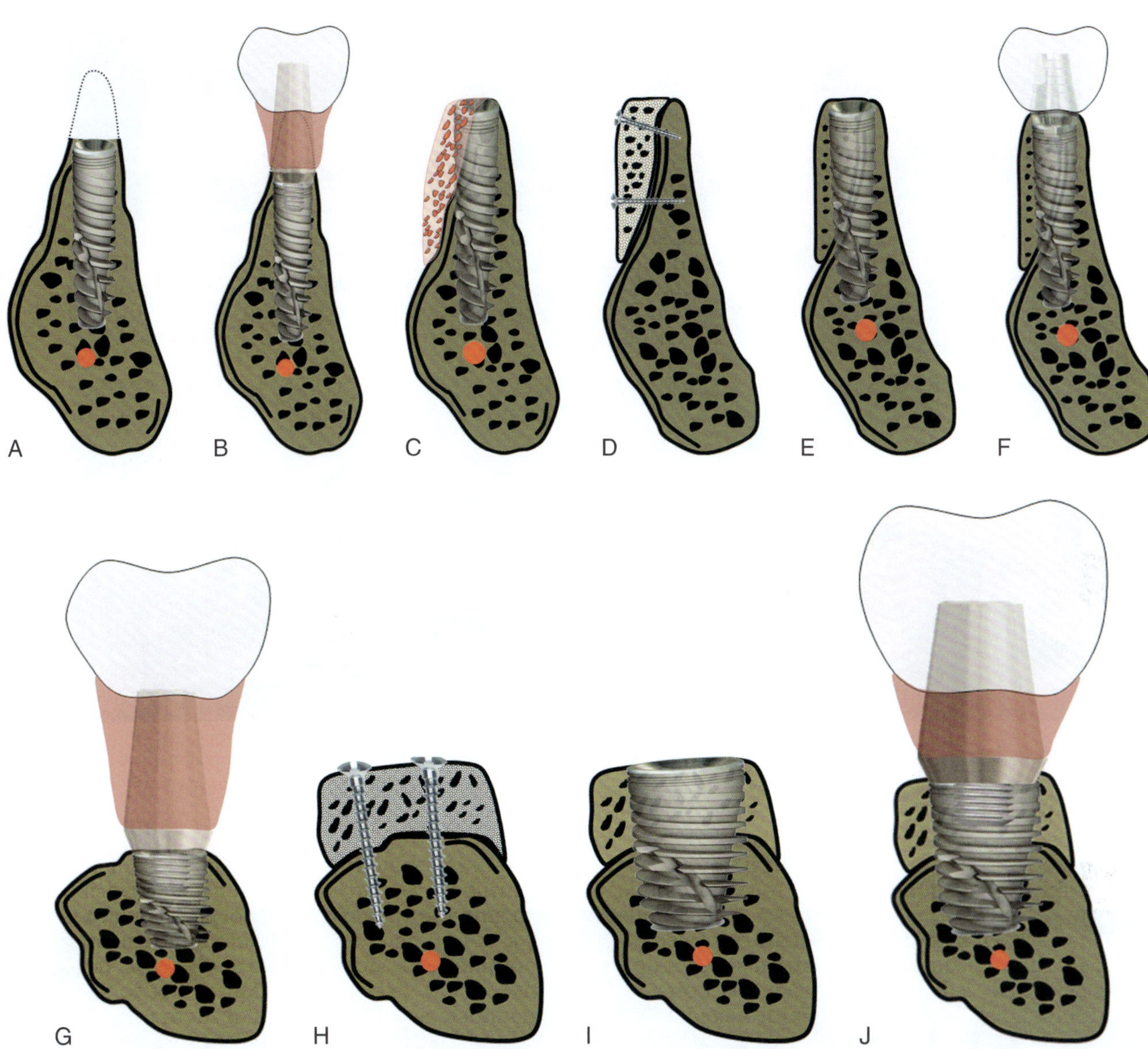

Fig 6.7 (A) Bony ridge in Division C-w bone category needs a large amount of vertical bone reduction to achieve an adequate ridge width for the placement of a narrow-to-regular diameter implant. (B) Osteoplasty not only increases the crown height but also results in increased thick, soft tissue height which may, over time, develop a deep soft tissue pocket that may harbour pathogens and lead to recurrent peri-implantitis. (C) The better option for the Division C-w bone is lateral bone augmentation either at the time of implant insertion or (D) before implant insertion (block grafting) to achieve the wide ridge crest for regular-diameter implant placement (E) for a prosthesis with an (F) ideal crown height. (G) For the Division C-h bone, either the short length implant is inserted or (H) vertical bone augmentation is performed to achieve adequate ridge height for the insertion of an (I) adequately long implant, which further reduces the crown: (J) implant height ratio.

grafting is performed to insert implants in the maxilla, especially if a fixed, implant-supported prosthesis is planned.

Prosthetic options for Division D bone

Implant overdentures should be the treatment of choice for the deficient ridge (Fig 6.12A–D), because implant-supported, fixed prosthesis may need multiple invasive bone grafting procedures like sinus grafting, block grafting, nerve transpositioning, etc. (Fig 6.13A and B). Subperiosteal implants are preferred over endosseous root form implants to avoid problems, such as mandibular fracture in Division D ridge (Fig 6.14A–D).

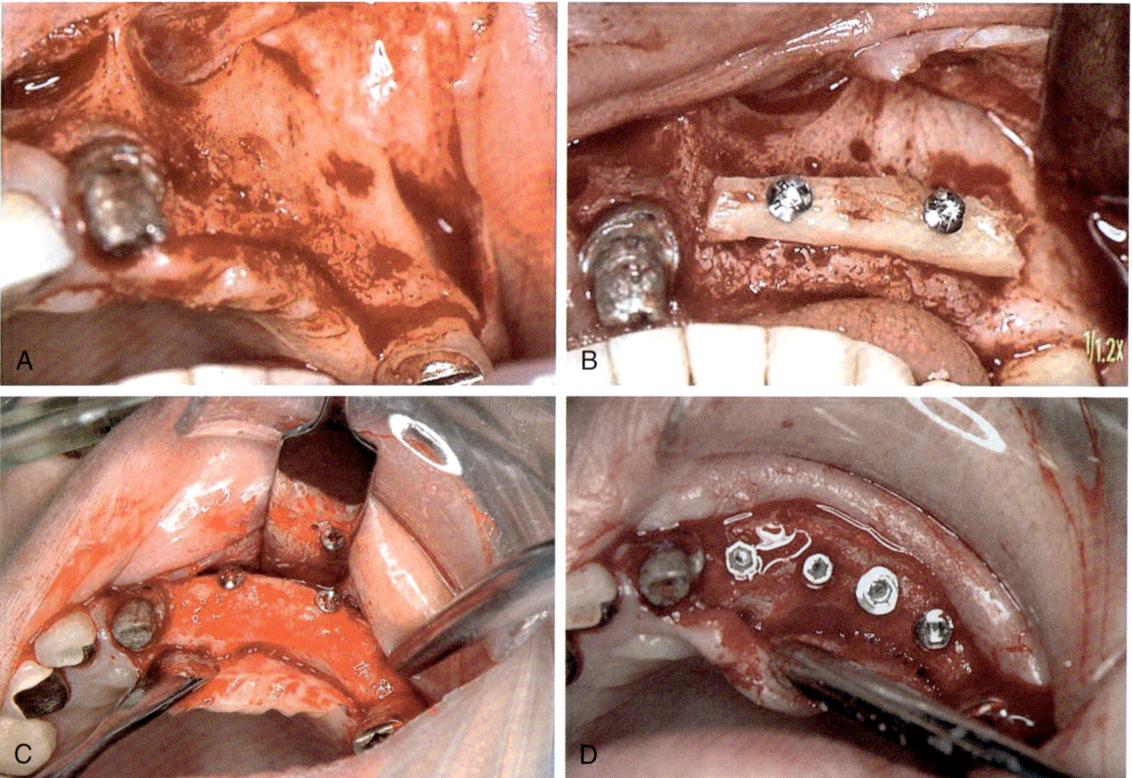

Fig 6.8 (A) Ridge with the C-w type of bone (compromised in width). (B) The lateral bone augmentation is performed using autogenous bone block. (C) Regeneration of new bone dimensions after the site is uncovered after 4 months. (D) Implants are inserted in the bone. (*Courtesy: Jun Shimada, Japan*).

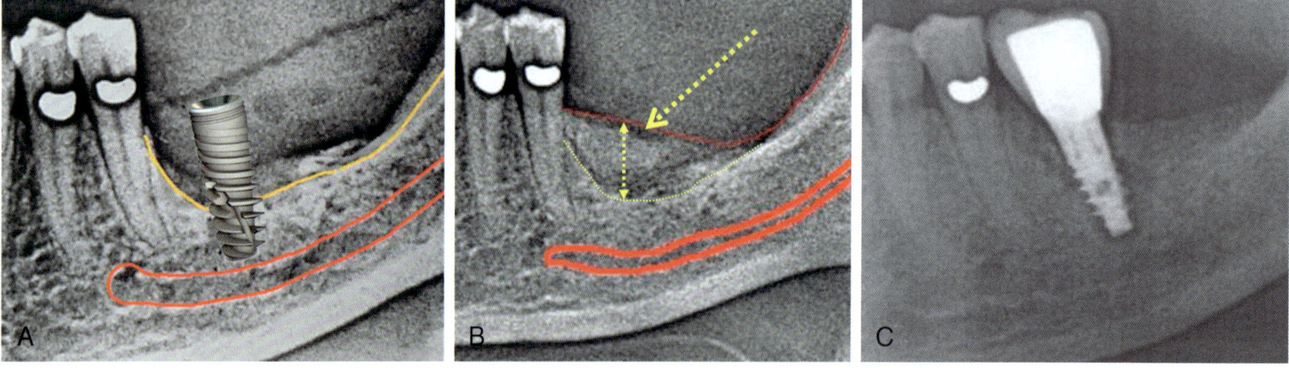

Fig 6.9 (A) Division C-h bone above the mandibular canal, insufficient for placement of adequately long implant, (B) vertical bone augmentation is performed and (C) an adequately long implant is placed in the regenerated bone.

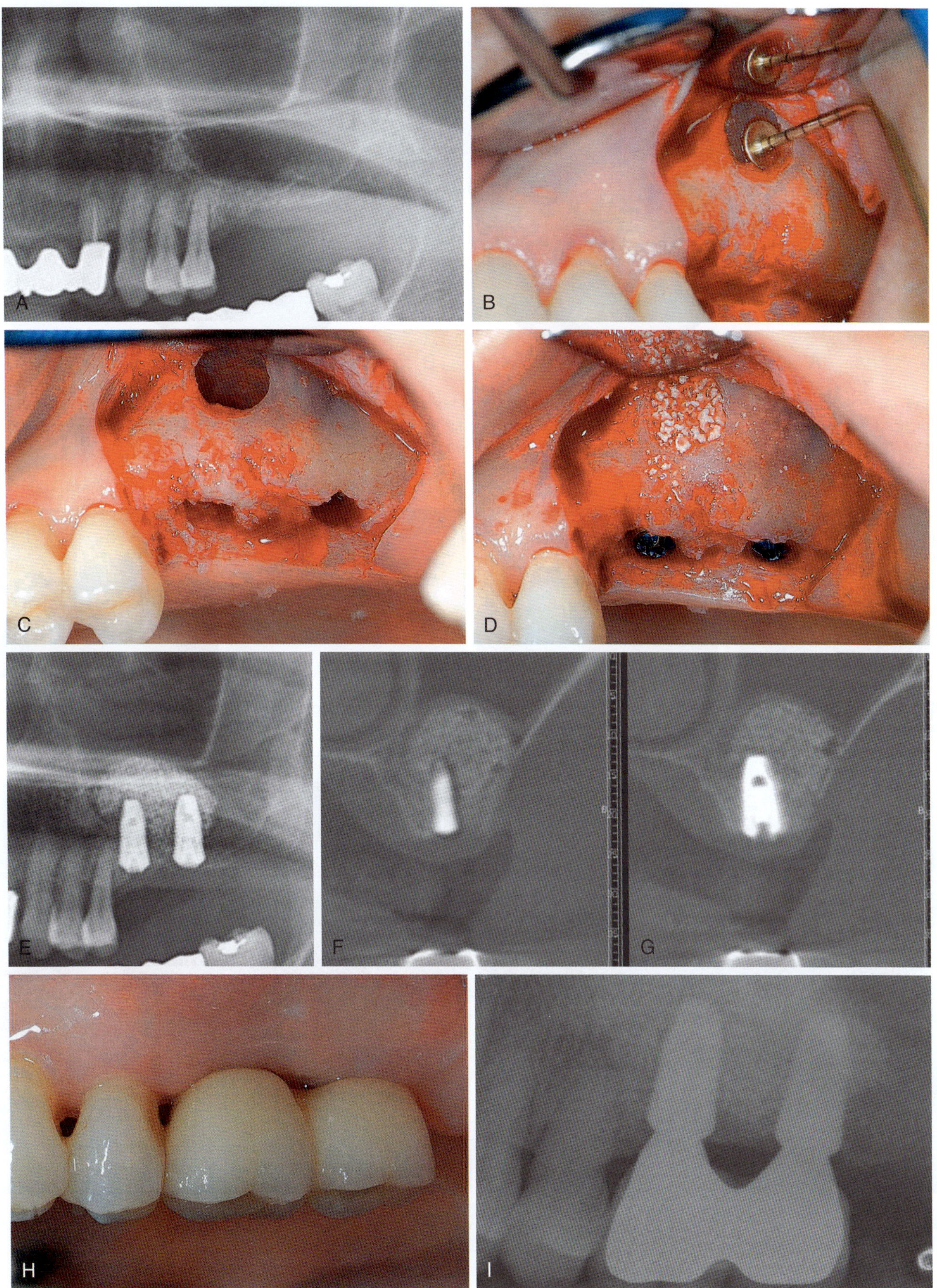

Fig 6.10 (A) Posterior edentulous maxilla with C-h bone (compromised in height). (B and C) The sinus elevation procedure is performed. (D–G) The sinus is grafted with simultaneous implant insertion. (H and I) The implants are uncovered and restored after 6 months (*Courtesy: Dentium Co., Korea*).

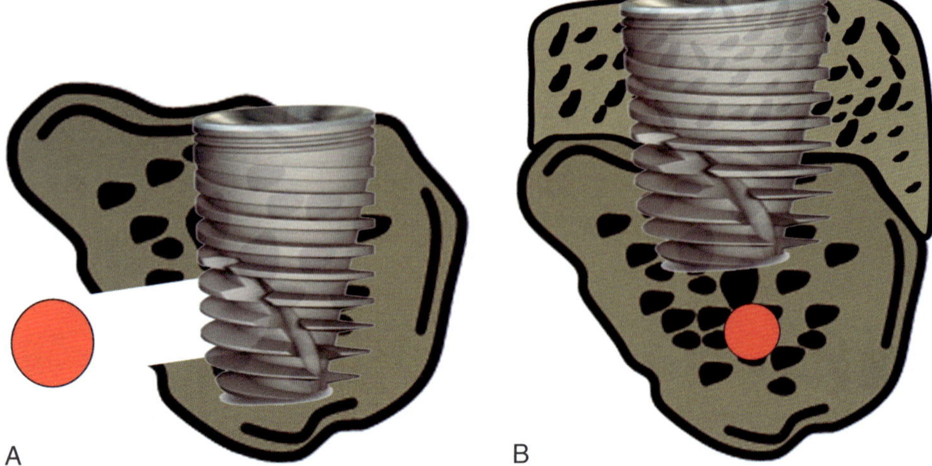

Fig 6.11 (A) With advancements in implant therapy, deficient (Division D) bone has been successfully used for implant placement with multiple approaches like nerve lateralization, sinus grafting, nasal floor grafting, etc. for implant placement; (B) but vertical bone augmentation not only facilitates the placement of adequately long implants but also reduces the long crown height.

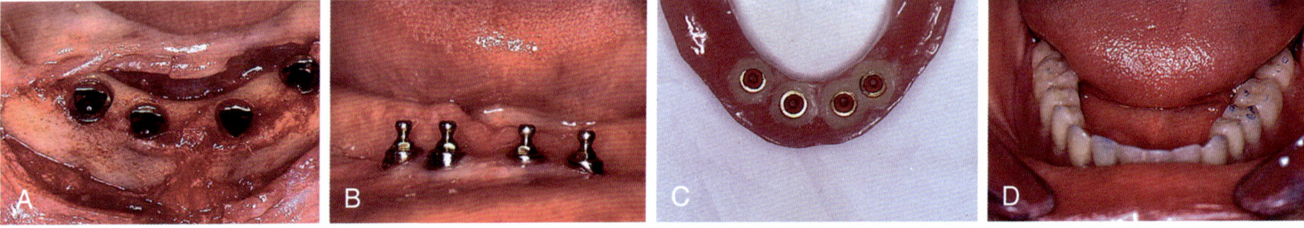

Fig 6.12 Deficient (Division D) mandibular bone with the only basal bone left. (A–D) Four short length implants are placed and an implant overdenture is delivered with ball abutment 'O' ring attachments (*Courtesy: Saad Zemmouri*).

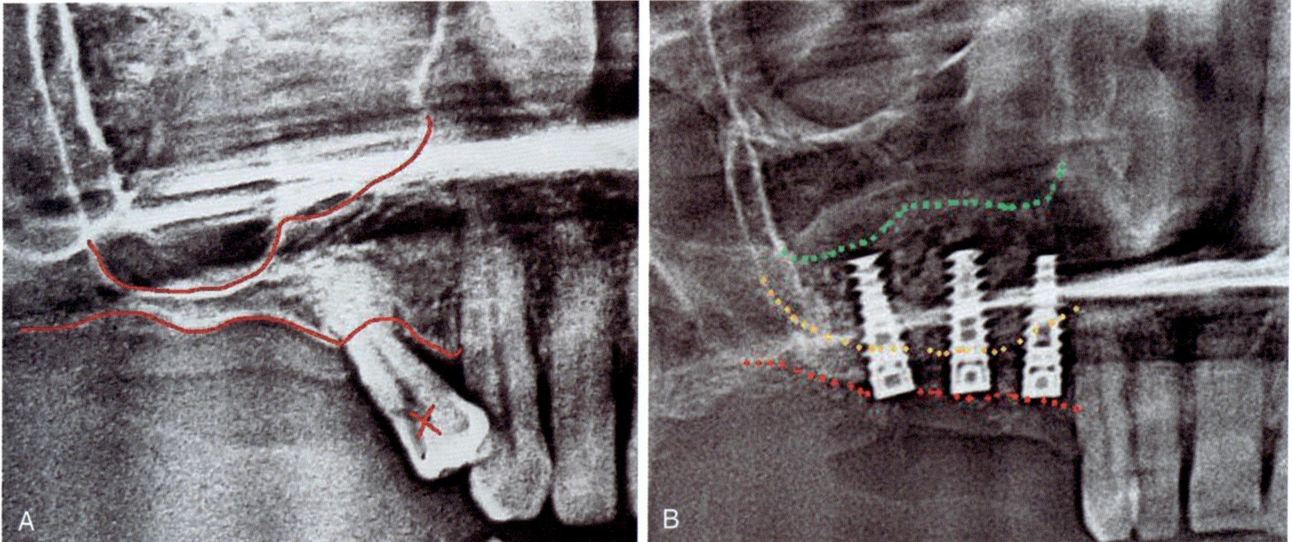

Fig 6.13 (A) Deficient (Division-D) bone in the posterior maxilla caused by vertical ridge resorption and maxillary sinus pneumatization, (B) The sinus elevation and grafting is performed for the insertion of adequately long implants.

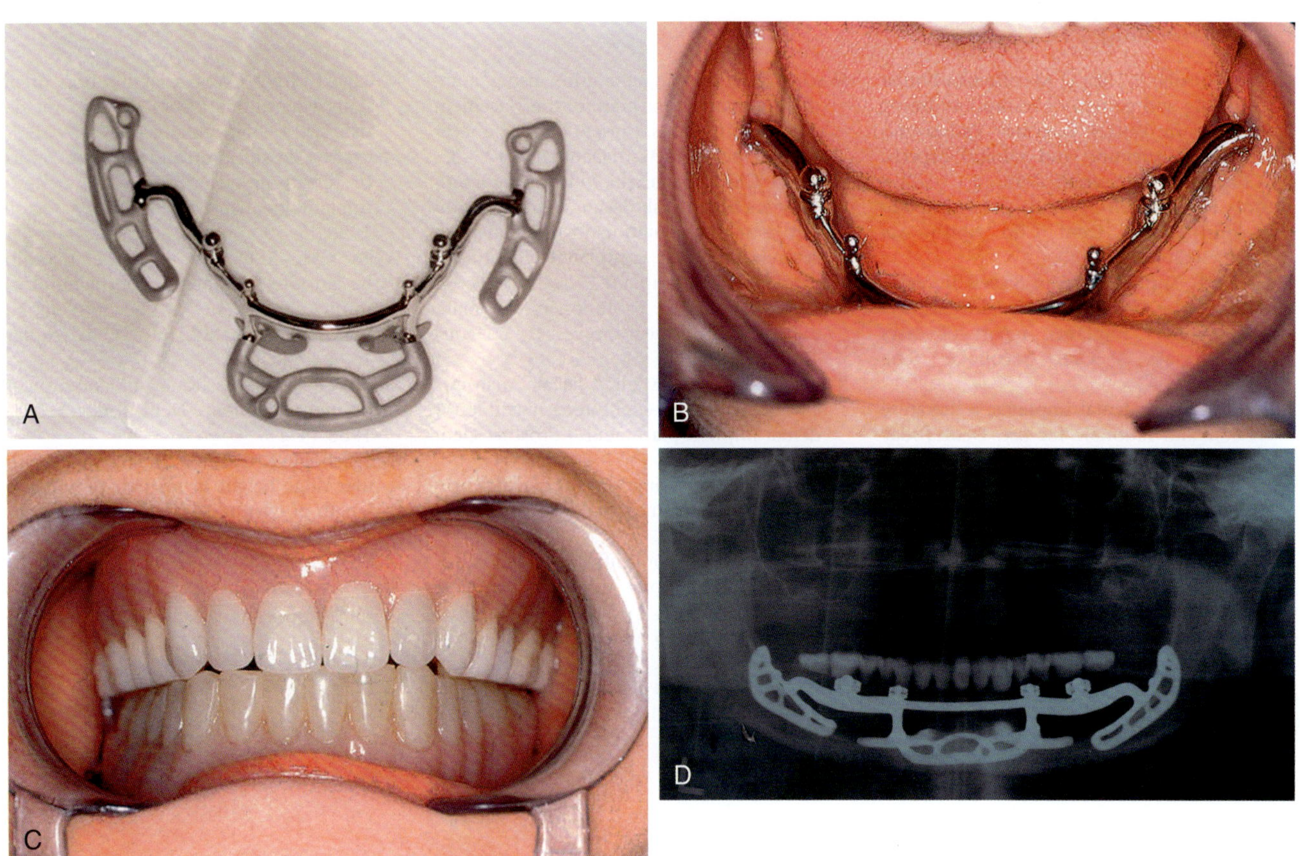

Fig 6.14 The subperiosteal implant can be preferred over the endosseous root form implant to avoid problems such as mandibular fracture in the Division D ridge. (A) Subperiosteal implant (B) placed on the deficient mandibular ridge (C) to support denture. (D) Post-loading radiograph (*Courtesy: Terry D Whitten, DDS*).

Summary

In implant dentistry, the prosthesis is planned before implant insertion and the dimensions, positions, and angulations of implants are decided according to the requirements of the future prosthesis. Considering the various parameters like stress factors, cantilevers etc., and the bone available for the implant insertion plays a key role in the overall implant treatment success. Three-dimensional bone volumes, external architecture, and angulation in relation to the ideal implant axis, are the major factors which should be considered during treatment planning.

The edentulous jawbone available for implant placement has been divided in four types by Carl E Misch, to make it easy to assess patient requirements, plan implant placement, and choose the best prosthesis for long-term success. The Division A type ridge offers adequate bone for the ideal implant insertion to support a prosthesis, with appearance and function approximately similar to the natural tooth. The fixed implant prosthesis is usually preferred for the Division A ridge.

The Division B ridge may provide adequate bone width for narrow diameter implants, but additional implants should be inserted for the multiple unit or full-arch fixed prosthesis. The Division B ridge can be changed to the Division A ridge type with either vertical osteoplasty or lateral bone augmentation to make it adequate in width for regular diameter implant placement. The lateral bone augmentation should be preferred over osteoplasty in the anterior maxilla to deliver aesthetic results. Osteoplasty can be preferred in the anterior mandible as adequate bone height is available to insert long implants and there is not much aesthetic concern. The Division B posterior mandible also usually shows adequate bone height and high density to stabilize short length implants, and thus, osteoplasty can be done in the posterior mandible with Division B ridge. Because of poor bone density and higher stress factors, bone augmentation is preferred over osteoplasty in the posterior maxilla.

Regardless of the location, the Division C-w ridge (ridge compromised in width) should be managed with lateral bone augmentation. While short length implants can be inserted into the Division C-h ridge (ridge compromised in height), vertical bone augmentation is performed to place implants with adequate length.

Deficient bone (Division D) in the mandible can be used to insert multiple short length implants to retain the overdenture, but vertical bone augmentation is required in the deficient maxilla.

Further Reading

Gruber H, Solar P, Ulm C. Maxillomandibular anatomy and pattern of resorption during atrophy. In: Watzek G, editor. Endosseous implants: scientific and clinical aspects. Chicago: Quintessence; 1996.

Tatum HO. Maxillary and sinus implant reconstructions. Dent Clin North Am 1980;30:207–29.

Mason ME, Triplett RG, Van Sickels JE, et al. Mandibular fractures through endosseous cylinder implants: report of cases and review. J Oral Maxillofac Surg 1990;48:311–7.

Misch CE. Short dental implants: a literature review and rationale for use. Dent Today 2005;24:64–8.

Jemt T, Lekholm U. Implant treatment in edentulous maxillae: a 5-year follow-up report on patients with different degrees of jaw resorption. Int J Oral Maxillofac Implants 1995;10:303–11.

Curtis TA, Ware WH, Beirne OR, et al. Autogenous bone grafts for atrophic edentulous mandibles: a final report. J Prosthet Dent 1987;57:73–8.

Misch CE, Wang HL. The procedures, limitations and indications for small diameter implants and a case report. Oral Health August 2004;94:16–26.

Misch CM. Ridge augmentation using mandibular ramus bone graft for the placement of dental implants: presentation of a technique. Pract Perio Aesth Dent 1996:127–35.

Scortecci GM. Immediate function of cortically anchored disk design implants without bone augmentation in moderately to severely resorbed completely edentulous maxillae. J Oral Implant 1999;25:70–9.

Judy KW, Misch CE. Evolution of the mandibular subperiosteal implant. N Y Dent J 1983;53:9–11.

Razavi R, Zena RV, Khan Z, et al. Anatomic site evaluation of edentulous maxillae for dental implant placement. J Prosthet Dent 1995;4:90–4.

Lam RV. Contour changes of the alveolar process following extraction. J Prosthet Dent 1960;10:25–32.

Tallgren A. The continuing reduction of the residual alveolar ridges in complete denture wearers. A mixed longitudinal study covering 25 years. J Prosthet Dent 1972;27:120–32.

Misch CE. Divisions of available bone in implant dentistry. Int J Oral Implants 1990;7:9–17.

Misch CE, Judy KWM. Classification of partially edentulous arches for implant dentistry. Int J Oral Implants 1987;4:7–12.

Misch CE. Classification and treatment options of the completely edentulous arches in implant dentistry. Dent Today October 1990:26–30.

Weiss CM, Judy KWM. Severe mandibular atrophy: biological considerations of routine treatments with complete subperiosteal implants. Int J Oral Implants 1974;4:431–69.

Misch CE. Available bone influences prosthodontic treatment. Dent Today February 1988:44–75.

Karagaclioglu L, Ozkan P. Changes in mandibular ridge height in relation to aging and length of edentulism period. Int J Prosthodont 1994;7:368–71.

Misch CE. Bone classification, training keys to implant success. Dent Today May 1989:39–44.

Patient evaluation and treatment planning

7

Ajay Vikram Singh

CHAPTER CONTENTS HD

Introduction

Patient evaluation and treatment planning are crucial steps in implant treatment and affect the overall success of implant therapy. On the patient's first visit, the implant dentist should carefully evaluate general condition, medical problems, financial situation, intraoral problems, chief complaints and the patient's expectations from the future prosthesis, before committing to implant therapy. Further, the dentist should evaluate ridge type, bone quality and bone availability with the help of dental radiographs and dental CT scans, as well as the soft tissue situation at the implant site and force factors on the future implant prosthesis. After clinical and radiographic evaluation, the dentist should prepare diagnostic models to evaluate the arch form, ridge topography, and fabricate the radiographic template. After clinical evaluation of the patient, and radiographic and model analysis, the dentist must decide what type of implant-supported prosthesis can be provided to the patient. The patient should be recalled and all the possible implant treatment options should be discussed, such as the required number and positions of implants for a particular prosthesis, the surgical and prosthetic steps of the treatment and provisional prosthesis placement, and the total time and expenditure required to complete the therapy. The step by step evaluation and treatment planning of the implant, with the key points related to various clinical and radiographic situations described in this chapter, can be very helpful to the dentist.

Patient evaluation and treatment planning

Treatment planning for implant therapy is known to be the backbone of successful outcome. The author recommends step by step treatment planning even in cases that seem easy and simple, to avoid any post-implantation complications. Special attention is needed during implant insertion, to the mental foramina and mandibular canal in the posterior mandible, and the maxillary sinus in the posterior maxilla. The implant dentist should systematically plan the implant treatment for a patient as follows.

General and medical evaluation

It is paramount to evaluate whether the patient is medically fit for the implant surgical procedure. The following points should be discussed with the patient and evaluated with investigations as needed, to finally decide the fitness of the patient for the implant surgery.

Age

Usually a patient above the age of 18 years is considered to be fit for implant therapy. If the implant is inserted into the adolescent's jawbone, which is still in the growing stage, it may lead to hindered growth on the side and jaw disfigurement. The age of jaw growth completion and hence the minimum age for implant placement, differs in males and females. The minimum age for implant placement in girls is considered to be 16–17 years, whereas in boys it is 17–18 years. Besides minimum age, the patient's age has to be considered key in deciding the type of prosthetic option to be used, e.g. for a young edentulous patient a fixed implant-supported prosthesis is the preferred option but for an older patient the choice should be an implant overdenture, which needs minimal surgical intervention and is easy to maintain and repair.

Medical problems

Diabetes mellitus, hypertension, thyroid disorders, bone diseases, cardiovascular diseases, liver disorders, pregnancy, etc. should be discussed in detail and evaluated with investigations as needed. Usually the patient fit for a surgical extraction is considered to be fit for basic implant surgery. The following medical problems of the patient should be evaluated before commencing implant surgery.

Diabetes mellitus

Diabetes mellitus is one of the diseases which should merely be evaluated and investigated. Diabetes is not an absolute contraindication for implant insertion, and as scientific studies and clinical trials suggest, implant therapy can very successfully be given to the controlled diabetic patient. The patient should be monitored for controlled blood sugar levels for a minimum of 3 weeks before implant insertion and should continue with the same for 4–6 weeks after implant insertion, till the surrounding soft tissues get healed and the implant has achieved initial osseointegration with the bone. Once the implant gets osseointegrated, increased blood sugar levels affect the peri-implant tissues similar to the periodontal tissues in uncontrolled diabetic patients. Thus, a continuous monitoring of such patients is required to maintain the peri-implant tissues in normal health. Oral hygiene maintenance and the earliest treatment of any peri-implant soft tissue infection is paramount for the long-term survival of implants in diabetic patients.

Literature review

Literature 1 – In the past, implant placement was contraindicated in diabetic patients because of increased risk of implant failure and infection. Publications in recent years have shown success rates for dental implants in diabetic patients, resembling those of the general population. Other studies of diabetic patients as well as animal models, have shown an increased risk for implant failure. These results raise the question of whether diabetic patients are suitable for dental implant rehabilitation.[1]

Although a direct relationship with periodontal disease has already been shown, little is known about the results of dental implants in diabetics. The present paper reviews the bibliography linking the effect of diabetes on the osseointegration of implants and the healing of soft tissue. In experimental models of diabetes, a reduced level of bone implant contact (BIC) has been shown, and this can be reversed by means of treatment with insulin. Compared with the general population, a higher failure rate is seen in diabetic patients. Most of these occur during the first year of functional loading, seemingly pointing to the microvascular complications of this condition as a possible causal factor. These complications also compromise the healing of soft tissues. It is necessary to take certain special considerations into account for the placement of implants in diabetic patients. A good control of plasma glycaemia, together with other measures, has been shown to improve the percentages of implant survival in these patients.[2]

It has become increasingly common for controlled diabetic patients to be considered as candidates for dental implants.[3] This study reports the results of placing implants in 34 patients with diabetes who were treated with 227 Branemark implants. At the time of second-stage surgery, 214 of the implants had osseointegrated, a survival rate of 94.3%. Only one failure was identified among the 177 implants followed through to final restoration, a clinical survival rate of 99.9%. Screening for diabetes and efforts to ensure that implant candidates are in metabolic control are recommended to increase the chances of successful osseointegration. Antibiotic protection and avoidance of smoking should also be considered (Implant Dent 1999;8:355–359).

Although the results of this study indicate that excellent results can be obtained when Branemark implants are placed in diabetic patients, certain precautionary measures can increase the likelihood of a successful outcome.

1. Adequate screening is essential. A comprehensive health history should be obtained from every candidate for implant therapy, with attention given to fundamental systemic problems. If the patient has a history of diabetes, additional information should be gathered about his/her current treatment.
2. If the diabetic patient's metabolic control seems to be clinically inadequate, it is best to delay implant therapy until better control is achieved.
3. The doctor should stress to the patient the importance of taking all diabetic medications on the days of surgery and maintaining an acceptable level of metabolic control throughout the healing period.
4. A 10-day regimen of broad-spectrum antibiotics should be started on the day of surgery to reduce the risk of infection.

Conclusion: Dental implants offer significant benefits that require that they be considered for the treatment of a wide spectrum of patients, including the growing number of individuals with diabetes mellitus. Although uncontrolled diabetes has been shown to interfere with various aspects of the healing process, the results of this retrospective study indicate that a high success rate is achievable when dental implants are placed in diabetic patients whose disease is under control.

Literature 2 – Implants in patients with diabetes mellitus.[4]

Diabetes is currently classified as a relative contraindication for implant treatment. Compared with the general population, a higher failure rate has been seen in diabetic patients with adequate metabolic control. In published literature, the survival rate for implants in diabetic patients ranges between 88.8% and 97.3%, 1 year after placement, and 85.6–94.6% in functional terms, 1 year after the prosthesis was inserted. In a retrospective study with 215 implants placed in 40 diabetic patients, 31 failed implants were recorded, 24 of which (11.2%) occurred in the first year of functional loading. This analysis showed an implant survival rate of 85.6% after 6.5 years of functional use. The results obtained show a higher index of failures during the first year after placement of the prosthesis. Another study carried out with 227 implants placed in 34 patients shows a success rate of 94.3% at the time of the second surgery, prior to the insertion of the prosthesis. In a meta-analysis with two implant systems placed in edentulous jaws, failure rates of 3.2% were obtained in the initial stages, whereas in the later stages (from 45 months to 9 years), this figure increased to 5.4%. A prospective study with 89 well-controlled type 2 diabetics in whom a total of 178 implants had been placed, revealed early failure rates of 2.2% (four failures) increasing to 7.3%

[1]Michaeli E, Weinberg I, Nahlieli O. Dental implants in the diabetic patient: systemic and rehabilitative considerations. Quintessence Int 2009 Sep;40[8]:639–45. Review. PubMed PMID: 19639088.

[2]Mellado-Valero A, Ferrer García JC, Herrera-Ballester A, Labaig-Rueda C. Effects of diabetes on the osseointegration of dental implants. Med Oral Patol Oral Cir Bucal 2007 Jan 1;12[1]:E38–43. Review. PubMed PMID: 17195826.

[3]Thomas J. Balshi, DDS, FACP,* Glenn J. Wolfinger, DMD, FACP*. Dental implants in the diabetic patient: a retrospective study.

[4]Mellado-Valero A, Ferrer García JC, Herrera-Ballester A, Labaig-Rueda C. Effects of diabetes on the osseointegration of dental implants. Med Oral Patol Oral Cir Bucal 2007;12:E38–43.© Medicina Oral S. L. C.I.F. B 96689336 - ISSN 1698-6946.

(nine further failures) 1 year after placement, indicating a survival rate of 92.7% within the first year of functional loading. The 5-year survival rate was 90%. The fact that most failures occur after the second-phase surgery and during the first year of functional loading might indicate micro-vascular involvement as one of the factors implicated in implant failures in diabetic patients (Fig 7.1). Most of the articles concluded that, despite the higher risk of failure in diabetic patients, maintaining adequate blood-glucose levels along with other measures, improves the implant survival rates in these patients.

Special considerations for implant therapy in diabetic patients

Healing and risk of postoperative infection: The repercussions of diabetes on the healing of soft tissue depend on the degree of glycaemic control in the perioperative period and the existence of chronic vascular complications. Patients with poor metabolic control have their immune defences impaired: granulocytes have altered functionality with modifications in their movement towards the infection site and deterioration in their microbicide activity, with greater predisposition to infection of the wound. In addition, the high concentration of blood-glucose in body fluids encourages the growth of mycotic pathogens such as candida. The microangiopathy arising as a complication of diabetes may compromise the vascularization of the flap, thus delaying healing, and also acting as a gateway for the infection of soft tissue.

Perioperative measures: In view of the studies revised, high levels of glucose in plasma have a negative influence on healing and bone remodelling processes. In order to ensure osseointegration of the implants (understood as the direct bond of the bone with the surface of the implant subjected to functional loading) and to avoid delays in the healing of gum tissue, it is necessary to maintain good glycaemic control before and after surgery. To measure the status of blood-glucose levels in the previous 6–8 weeks, the HbA1c values have to be known (Table 7.1). A figure of less than 7% for HbA1c is considered a good level of glycaemic control (the normal value for healthy individuals is 3.5–5.5% depending on the laboratory) (Table 7.2).

Table 7.1 Showing the relation of glycosylated Hb% with diabetes

GLYCOSYLATED Hb%	DIABETIC SITUATION	IMPLANT SURGERY
<6%	Non-diabetic	Can be done
6–7%	Excellent control	Can be done
7–8%	Good control	Can be done with regular postoperative blood sugar monitoring
8–10%	Average control	Should be avoided
>10%	Poor control	Contraindicated

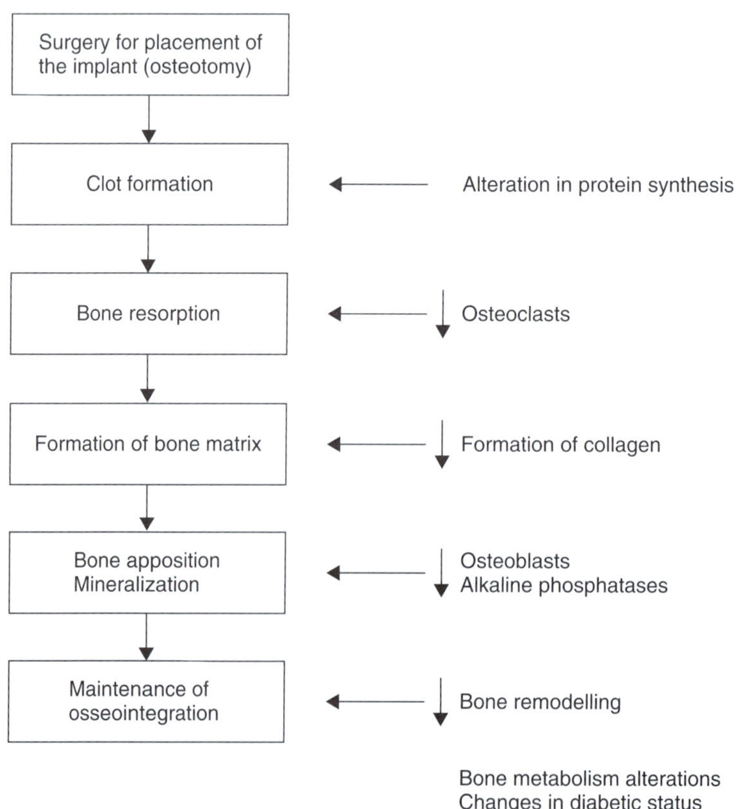

Fig 7.1 Flowchart showing possible alterations in bone healing in diabetic patients.

Although there is some controversy over the use of antibiotics in healthy patients, these are recommended for diabetic patients about to be subjected to implant surgery. The antibiotic of choice is amoxicillin (2 g per os 1 h previously), as the pathogens most frequently causing postoperative complications following the placement of implants, are streptococci, Gram-positive anaerobes and Gram-negative anaerobes. Clindamycin may also be used (600 mg per os 1 h previously), azithromycin or clarithromycin (500 mg per os 1 h previously), and first-generation cephalosporins (cephalexin or cefadroxil: 2 g per os 1 h previously) only if the patient has not had any anaphylactic allergic reaction to penicillin. In addition to antibiotic prophylaxis, the use of 0.12% chlorhexidine mouthwash has shown a clear benefit by reducing the failure rates from 13.5% to 4.4% in type 2 diabetics, during a follow-up period of 36 months. This same study observed a reduction of 10.5% in the failure rate when antibiotics were administered preoperatively.

Conclusion

There is evidence that hyperglycaemia has a negative influence on bone formation and remodelling and reduces osseointegration of implants. Soft tissue is also affected by the microvascular complications deriving from hyperglycaemia – vascularization of the tissue is compromised, healing is delayed and wounds are more predisposed to infection. This entails an increase in the percentage of failures in implant treatment of diabetic patients. The bibliography reviewed recommends good glycaemic control in the perioperative period, in order to improve the survival rates for implants in diabetics. HbA1c figures of less than 7% indicate appropriate glycaemia levels in the preceding 6–8 weeks. Preoperative antibiotic therapy and the use of 0.12% chlorhexidine mouthwash are recommended, as both measures have been shown to reduce the percentage of failures. Although there is a higher risk of failure in diabetic patients, experimental studies have shown that the optimization of glycaemic control improves the degree of osseointegration in implants. Nonetheless, it is necessary to extend the number of prospective studies in humans, in order to clarify the true impact of diabetes on the prognosis for osseointegration.

Hypertension

Hypertensive patients often have the tendency to bleed more than the normal because of high vascular pressure; hence, they should be only operated under controlled blood pressure conditions. A continuous monitoring of the blood pressure is also mandatory during surgical procedures in implantology.

Table 7.2 Recommendations to reduce the risk of implant failure in diabetic patients

1. Good glycaemic control: HbA1c < 7% Baseline and preprandial glycaemia (mg/dl): 80–110 Maximum postprandial level of glycaemia (mg/dl): <180
2. Preoperative antibiotic therapy
3. 0.12% Chlorhexidine mouthwash

Thyroid disorders

Implant therapy can successfully be given to patients with hypothyroidism but hyperthyroidism is a medical problem which requires attention, as excessive production of the thyroxin hormone results in symptoms like increased pulse rate, nervousness, intolerance to heat, excessive sweating, atrial fibrillation, and congestive heart failure. Patients with hyperthyroidism are also sensitive to catecholamines such as epinephrine in local anaesthesia. When such patients are exposed to catecholamines, coupled with the stress often related to implant surgery, an exacerbation of the symptoms of hyperthyroidism may occur during surgery, resulting in thyrotoxicosis or "thyroid storm", which is often life-threatening to the patient. The physician's opinion and the normal range of thyroxin investigation, i.e. the patient who reports normal thyroid function and has had no symptoms of the disease during the preceding 6–8 months, is at low risk and can successfully get the implant surgery done. Patients with hyperthyroidism should receive the implant surgery in a very calm and comfortable operatory environment and if local anaesthesia is used, it should be devoid of adrenalin. Anti-anxiety/sedative drugs should also be avoided in such patients.

Bone disorders

Patients with bone disorders like osteoporosis, which is usually age-related, present with decrease in bone mass, increased micro-architectural deterioration, and susceptibility to bone fractures. This mostly occurs in the patients after the age of 60 but is very common even at an earlier age in postmenopausal women or women who have the history of ovariectomy, because the lack of oestrogen increases the chances of osteoporosis. A recommended dose of calcium, which can be range from 800 to 1500 mg/day and regular exercise is helpful to maintain the bone mass and increase bone strength. Such patients should thoroughly be investigated and treated before implant therapy.

Patients on bisphosphonates

Bisphosphonates are a group of drugs used to treat pathologies, including Paget's disease, osteoporosis, multiple myeloma and metastases associated with breast or prostate cancer. Bisphosphonates act on osteoclasts, inhibiting their chemotaxis and lifespan and hence, they inhibit bone resorption and induce osteonecrosis. There are important differences between bisphosphonates administered intravenously or taken orally. Oral administration of bisphosphonates to postmenopausal women to treat osteoporosis is fairly common. Hence, this group of patients should be investigated for bisphosphonate therapy. The American Association of Oral and Maxillofacial Surgeons does not contraindicate dental implant placement in patients who have been taking bisphosphonates orally for under 3 years prior to surgery, but the drug should be stopped for a minimum of 3 months before carrying out implant surgery and should be restarted only after at least 3 months following implant surgery (Table 7.3). Marx et al A blood test, and the serum C-terminal telopeptide (CTX) test on an empty stomach, are recommended to evaluate the risk of osteonecrosis in patients on bisphosphonate therapy for more than 3 years. If

Table 7.3 Types of oral and intravenous bisphosphonates and their uses

BISPHOS-PHONATES	ACTIVE INGREDIENTS	TRADE NAMES	USED TO TREAT	POSTIMPLANTATION INSERTION OSTEONECROSIS	IMPLANT SURGERY
Oral	Alendronate, Risedronate, Etidronate, Tiludronate, Ibandronate, Clodronate, etc.	Fosamax®, Fosavance®, Actonel®, Osteum®, Difosfen®, Acrel®, Skelid®, Bondronat®, Bonefos®, etc.	Osteoporosis, Paget's disease, Osteogenesis imperfecta etc.	Less common	Can be successfully done
Intravenous	Zoledronate, Clodronate, Ibandronate, Pamidronate, etc.	Zometa®, Aclasta®, Bondronat®, Bonefos®, Aredia®, Linoten®, Pamifos®, Xinsidona®, etc.	To reduce bone pain, malignant hypercalcaemia, skeletal complications suffered by patients with Paget's disease or myeloma, bone metastasis of various cancers, etc.	More common	Should be avoided

values obtained are greater than 150 pg/ml, the implant surgery can be performed with minimum risk and without suspension of medication. When values are lower than 150 pg/ml, medication should be stopped for a period between 4 and 6 months or an alternative treatment option involving other types of prosthesis should be sought. More scientific evidence is required in order to validate CTX testing as the technique for the evaluation of osteonecrosis in these patients. Different studies and clinical trials of implant therapy in patients on bisphosphonate therapy, have found that patients who had taken oral bisphosphonates could successfully be treated with implants. Oral bisphosphonates are stopped 3 months before implant insertion and restarted only after the implant has osseointegrated (3–4 months). As the patients on intravenous bisphosphonates are at high risk of osteonecrosis after implant surgery, other non-surgical prosthetic options should be preferred for such patients.

Oral malignancy and osteoradionecrosis

Any benign or malignant oral lesion should be diagnosed and treated before implant insertion. Patients who are given postsurgical radiotherapy for oral malignant lesions often show degeneration of the osteovascular tissues (osteoradionecrosis); hence the regeneration capacity of the bone is hindered for a minimum of 6 months after radiotherapy is completed. Thus, the implant surgeon should wait for a minimum of 6 months after radiotherapy is completed, to place the implant. Six months after completion of radiotherapy treatment, new vascular tissue starts regenerating inside the bone, which is paramount for predictable quality implant osseointegration with the surrounding bone.

Liver cirrhosis

The major cause for liver cirrhosis is alcohol consumption. The liver synthesizes clotting factors and detoxifies drugs, hence patients with liver disease show reduced synthesis of the clotting factor (thrombocytopaenia) and prolonged bleeding time during implant surgery. The patients with normal liver function test (SMA, CBC, PTT, and PT) values are at low risk and can be treated as normal patients with basic implant procedures. The physician's opinion is highly recommended for these patients before performing the implant surgical procedures.

Angina pectoris

It is a form of coronary heart disease, which causes chest pain or cramp of the cardiac muscles because of temporary myocardial ischaemia (low oxygen supply to the cardiac muscles). Atherosclerosis of the coronary vessels is the most common cause of angina pectoris. When treating such patients, the physician's opinion should be taken before performing implant surgery and nitroglycerin (0.4 mg) tablets should be kept ready in the dental emergency kit. The dental procedure should be done in a stress-free environment and divided into multiple short duration procedures. If the patient complains of chest pain, the procedure should be stopped immediately and the nitroglycerin tablets should be administered sublingually. Local anaesthetics devoid of vasoconstrictors (adrenalin) like xylocard should be used in such patients. Anti-anxiety drugs and prophylactic administration of nitroglycerin tablets are also helpful to reduce the onset of angina in such patients during implant surgery.

Myocardial infarction

Myocardial infarction (MI) is a prolonged ischaemia (lack of oxygen supply) that causes injury to the heart. Such patients complain of severe chest pain in the left precordial area during the MI episode, which radiates to the left arm or mandible. The pain is similar to angina pectoris, but more severe and presents symptoms like cyanosis, cold sweat, weakness, nausea or vomiting, and irregular and increased pulse rate, etc. Being a life-threatening medical problem, the implant surgeon besides taking all the precautions as for angina, should take the opinion of a cardiologist before treating such patients. These patients should preferably be treated in hospital where all the emergency management facilities are available.

Table 7.4 Dose regimen of prophylactic antibiotics administered before dental surgery to patients with history of subacute bacterial endocarditis

PROPHYLACTIC ANTIBIOTICS FOR BACTERIAL ENDOCARDITIS PATIENTS		
Standard antibiotic	Amoxicillin	2 g 1 h before surgical procedure
Patients allergic to penicillin	Clindamycin	600 mg 1 h before surgical procedure

Subacute bacterial endocarditis (SABE)

It is an infection of the heart valves or the endothelial surfaces of the heart. The microorganisms mainly associated with endocarditis following dental treatment, are streptococci and staphylococci, and less frequently, anaerobes. The risk of bacterial endocarditis increases with the amount of intraoral soft tissue trauma. Improvement of oral hygiene with scaling and root planing, and the administration of prophylactic antibiotics before performing any implant surgical procedure, reduce the onset of subacute bacterial endocarditis after dental surgery, to a large extent (Table 7.4).

Pregnancy

Being an elective procedure, implant surgery should be avoided during pregnancy as the radiographs and medications for the implant procedures may adversely affect the growth of the fetus. Moreover, periodontal diseases are often exacerbated during pregnancy.

Smoking

The lower success rate of endosteal implants in smokers is well documented in literature.[1] Tobacco smoking decreases polymorphonuclear leukocyte activity, resulting in a lower rate of chemotactic migration and reduced phagocytic activity, which contribute to decreased resistance to inflammation and infection and impaired wound-healing potential. Smoking also causes decreased calcium absorption, which weakens bone strength. Slower soft tissue healing, bone graft contamination, etc. are common problems in smokers. The patient should be encouraged to avoid smoking at least for a period of 2–3 weeks postimplant surgery till the soft tissue gets healed.

Oral examination

Detailed oral examination of the patient is paramount for diagnosis and treatment planning for successful implant therapy. The following clinical findings should be examined in detail.

Arch form

The arch form influences the number and positions of the implants required in fixed implant prosthesis for the edentulous maxilla and mandible. Three types of dental arch forms are found in patients.

[1]Bain CA, Moy PK. The association between the failure of dental implants and cigarette smoking. Int J Oral Maxillofac Imp 1993;8:609–615.

Square arch: shows minimum facial cantilevered forces; thus minimum number of implants are required to support a full-arch fixed or completely implant-supported removable prosthesis. Only two implants are required at the canine positions to restore the anterior maxillary or mandibular region. Placement of any implant anterior to the canine region is usually not required to restore the full-arch. The full-arch, fixed, implant-supported restoration (12–14 units) can be made possible by placing only six implants (two at canine, two at second premolar, and two at first molar positions) (Fig 7.2A).

Ovoid: shows more facial cantilevered forces on the prosthesis compared to the square arch form, thus one more implant should be added anterior to canines positions (at one of the central incisor positions) to reduce the cantilevered forces on the rest of the implants (Fig 7.2B).

Tapering: has the maximum facial cantilevered forces, thus two more implants should be added anterior to canine positions (one at each central incisor position) to reduce the cantilevered forces on the rest of the implants (Fig 7.2C).

Ridge morphology of edentulous region

Ridge morphology of the edentulous region gives an approximate idea about underlying bone dimensions, positions, and angulations required for implant placement, and also reveals the presence of any severe undercut in ridge morphology, etc.

Soft tissue biotype

A thick biotype that contains a thick connective tissue layer under the keratinized attached epithelium is considered to be favourable for implants. The thick biotype makes a tight seal around the implant prosthesis and is more resistant to the recession and peri-implant infections (Fig 7.3A and B). The thick biotype is also helpful in the aesthetic regions to achieve an aesthetic emergence profile and soft tissue drape around the implant prosthesis. It is easy for the implant surgeon to craft the thick soft tissue biotype as required, to achieve optimal aesthetic outcome in the implant prosthesis in the cervical region. If a thin biotype is found at the edentulous region, the implant surgeon should plan for a connective tissue grafting procedure during the implant insertion, or later at the time of implant uncovery, to convert the thin biotype to the thick biotype.

Width of keratinized soft tissue

A thick band of keratinized soft tissue is paramount around the future implant prosthesis to make it resistant to peri-implant infections. The clinician should evaluate and plan to achieve at least 3 mm of attached keratinized thick marginal soft tissue collar around the implant prosthesis. If a non-keratinized thin and mobile soft tissue is found at the implant site, he/she should plan for soft tissue grafting procedure at the time of implant uncovery, to generate new thick and keratinized soft tissue around the implant prosthesis (Fig 7.4A and B).

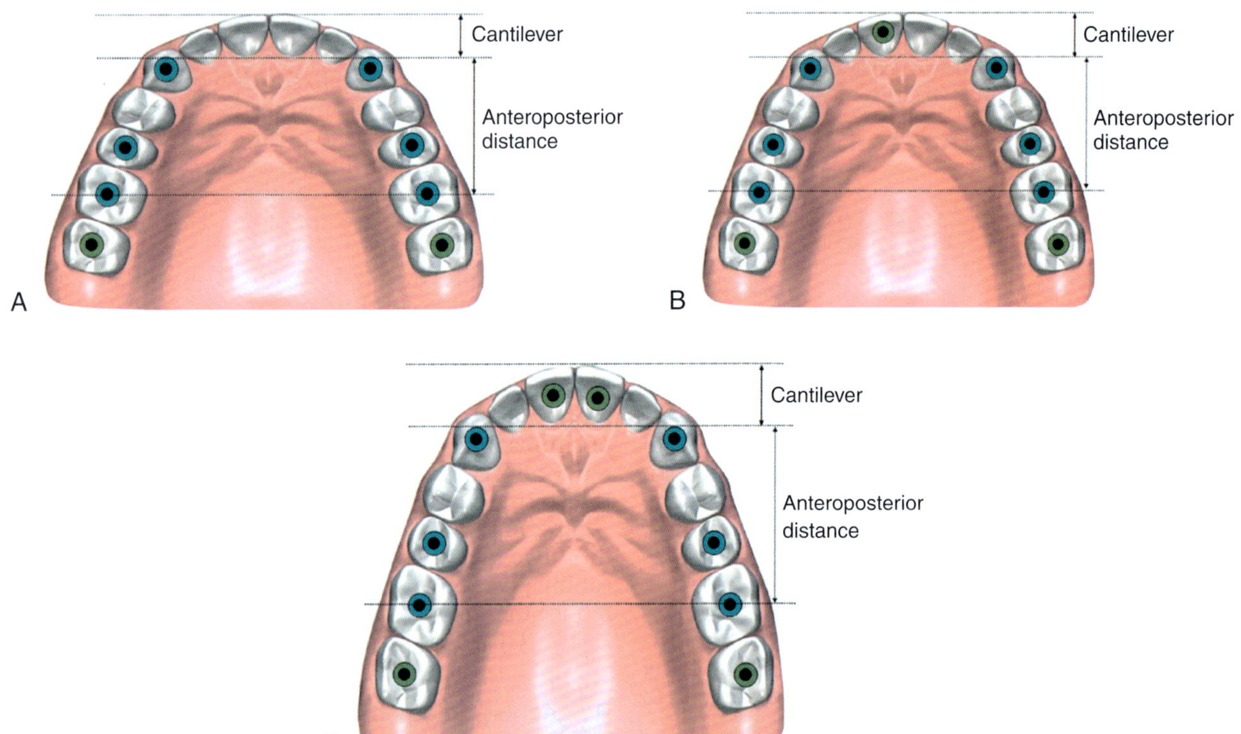

Fig 7.2 The arch form should be evaluated during treatment planning for multiple or full-arch implants. (A) The square arch form shows the least facial cantilever, hence requires least number of implants to restore the maxilla or mandible and no implant is usually required anterior to the canine positions. (B) The oval arch form has more facial cantilevering; hence at least one implant should be added anterior to the canine position to restore such arch. (C) The tapering arch form has the maximum facial cantilevering hence requires two additional implants anterior to the canine positions. If 14-unit fixed prosthesis is planned, two more implants should be added at the second molar positions.

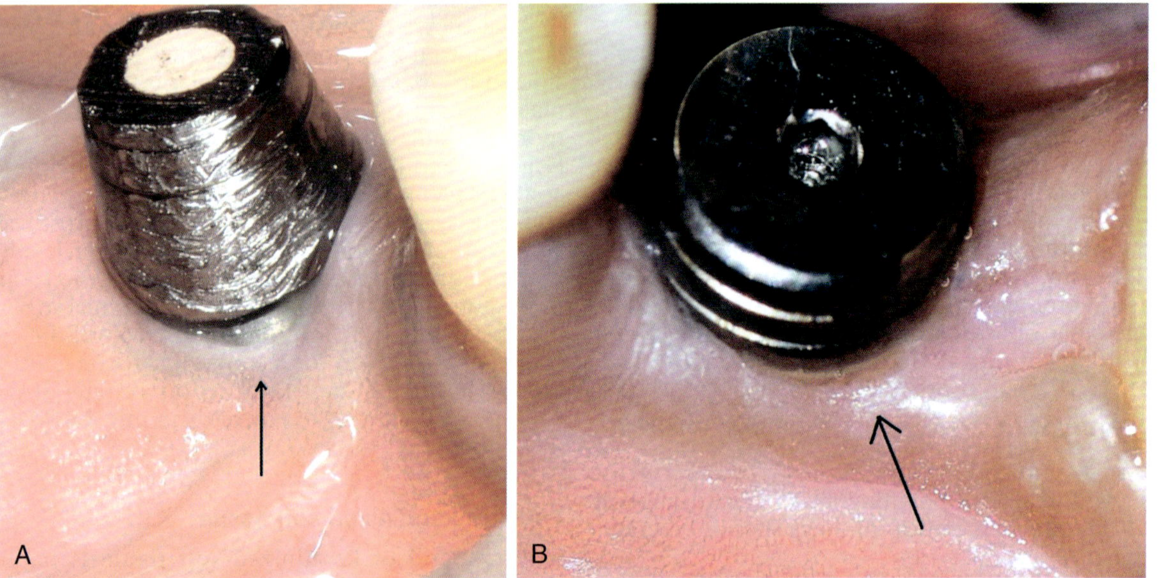

Fig 7.3 (A) Thin biotype, more prone to recession and muscle pull, (B) thick biotype, more resistant to recession.

Papilla at the implant site (intact or flattened)

The careful evaluation of the presence or absence of papilla should be made during treatment planning for the implant in the aesthetic region. If the papillae are intact, the papilla preservation incision is preferred for the implant placement (Fig 7.5A–D).

Periodontal health of adjacent teeth

The teeth adjacent to the edentulous region should be checked for any deep soft tissue pocket, or any periodontal defect with active purulent discharge. Often infection in the adjacent teeth can infect the inserted implant; therefore, all the periodontal problems of the adjacent

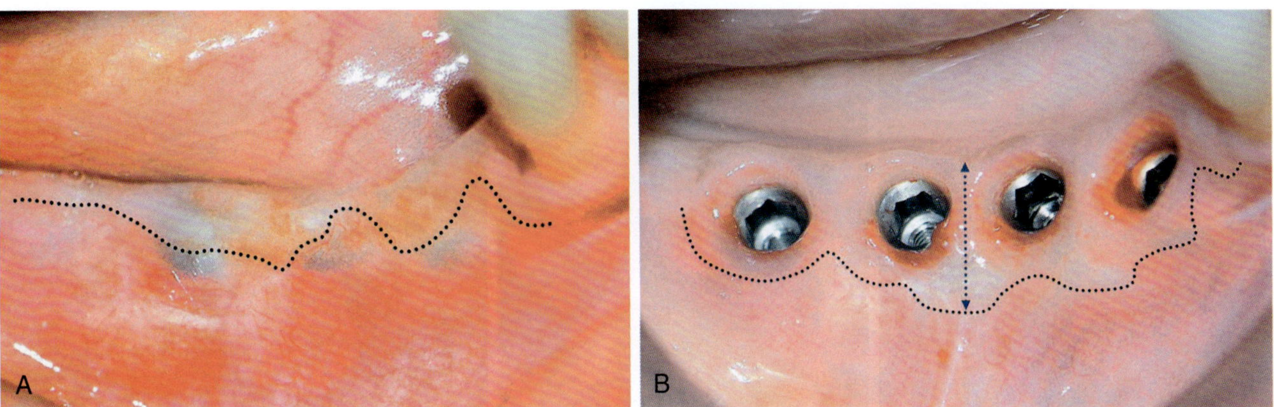

Fig 7.4 (A and B) A thick band of keratinized soft tissue regenerated with soft tissue grafting during implant uncovery to minimize the chances of soft tissue recession and peri-implantitis.

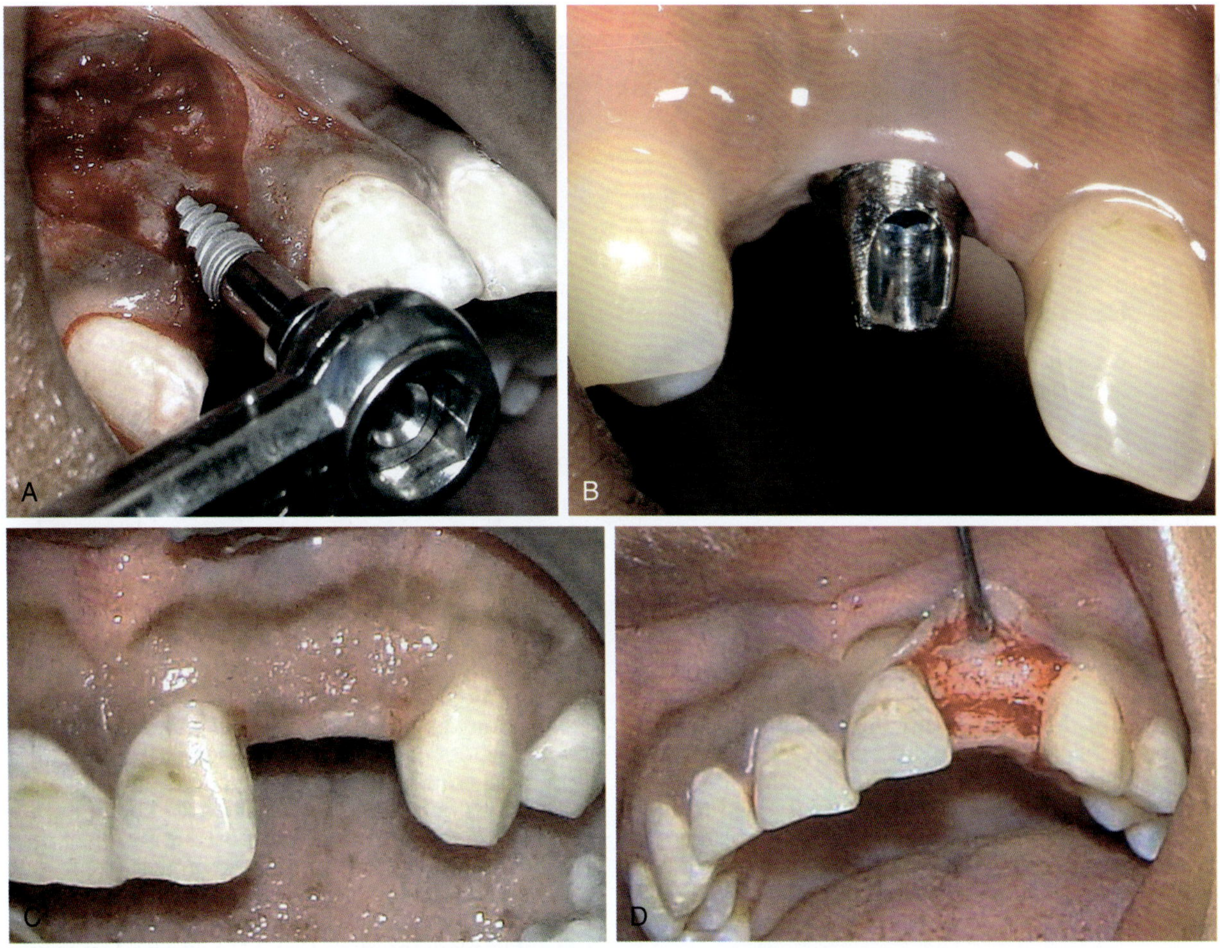

Fig 7.5 Care should be taken to preserve intact papilla in the regions of high aesthetics. (A and B) Papilla preservation incision should be planned in such cases to maintain the papillae for future implant prosthesis. (C and D) Flattened papilla.

teeth should thoroughly be diagnosed and treated before implant insertion (Fig 7.6A–C).

Opposing and adjacent teeth at occlusal position

The teeth adjacent to and opposing the edentulous site should be examined for any supra eruption inclinations, mesial drifting, etc. for prosthetically guided implant insertion (Fig 7.7A–C). Prosthetic planning before implant insertion avoids future problems like unaesthetic prosthesis, recurrent dislodgement of prosthesis, implant component fractures, fractured prosthesis, loosening of the connection screw, implant body fracture, crestal bone resorption, implant failure, etc. after implant is loaded/in function.

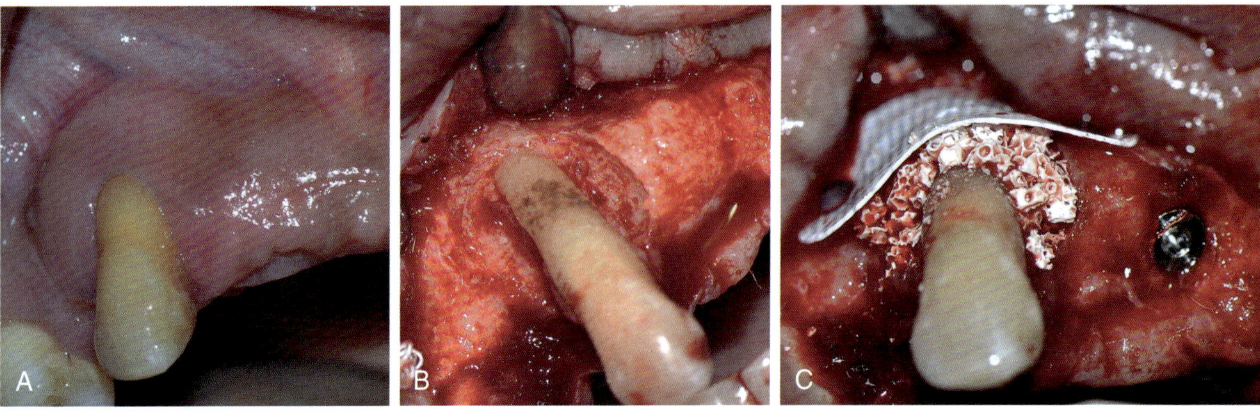

Fig 7.6 (A) Tooth adjacent to the future implant site showing deep periodontal pocket with purulent discharge through a sinus. The infected pocket is treated first with scaling, curettage and antibiotics until it healed and showed no active infection. (B and C) The healed periodontal osseous defect is exposed, cleaned, irrigated with antibiotics and grafted simultaneous to implant placement at the adjacent site.

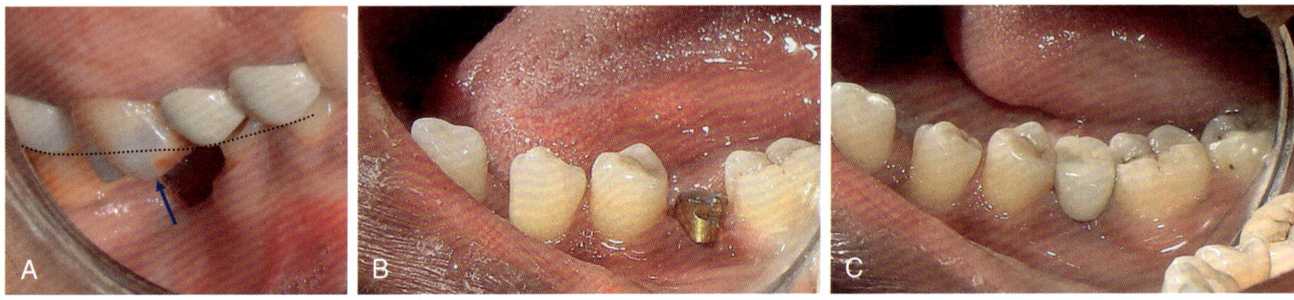

Fig 7.7 (A) Supra-erupted opposing tooth not only result in reduced inter-arch space but also cause undue forces over the implant prosthesis during lateral excursive movements. (B and C) The drifting of adjacent teeth results in reduced mesiodistal dimensions for the implant prosthesis.

These problems usually arise because of offset occlusal forces and extreme angulation of the implant prosthesis with the implant axis.

Oral hygiene of the patient

Oral hygiene maintenance is mandatory to avoid any infection to the inserted implants and also for their long-term survival. Advanced periodontitis should be treated before implant therapy. Scaling and root planing should always be done before implant insertion. Preoperative oral rinses with a 0.12% chlorhexidine digluconate solution has been shown to significantly lower the incidence of postimplantation infectious complications. A preoperative 30-s rinse is recommended, followed by twice daily rinses for 2 weeks following surgery.

Tobacco chewing

Tobacco chewing is often associated with poor oral hygiene and periodontal problems in the remaining teeth. Oral prophylaxis should be done before performing implant therapy and the patient should be encouraged to avoid tobacco chewing and adopt oral hygiene maintenance before placement of implants. Tobacco chewing also causes peri-implantitis in the restored implants; hence the patient should be instructed to avoid tobacco chewing for long-term survival of the implants (Fig 7.8A and B).

Bruxism

The problem of bruxism should be treated before placing implants, to avoid post loading problems, such as the early wearing of the prosthesis, ceramic fractures, component fractures, crestal bone resorption, etc. (Fig 7.9A–D).

History of diseased or lost teeth

The history of tooth loss can be very informative to evaluate the bony tissue present at the planned implant site. The traumatic loss of a tooth often leads to the fracture of the thin facial cortical plate. Either reduced buccolingual bone dimensions or a large osseous defect can be found in such cases, when the bony ridge is exposed for implant insertion (Fig 7.10A–D). The patient, while giving the history of tooth loss because of periodontal infections, usually also presents the osseous defects which need to be grafted before or at the time of implant insertion (Fig 7.11A and B). Teeth with periapical radiolucency or history of apicoectomy often show a medium to large osseous defect at the periapical region during the implant placement (Fig 7.12A and B). For such cases the dentist should plan for bone augmentation procedures during or before the implant placement.

Mouth opening

This is one of the most neglected points when the implant surgeon plans for the implant therapy in the posterior region of the mouth. Often, patients with submucous

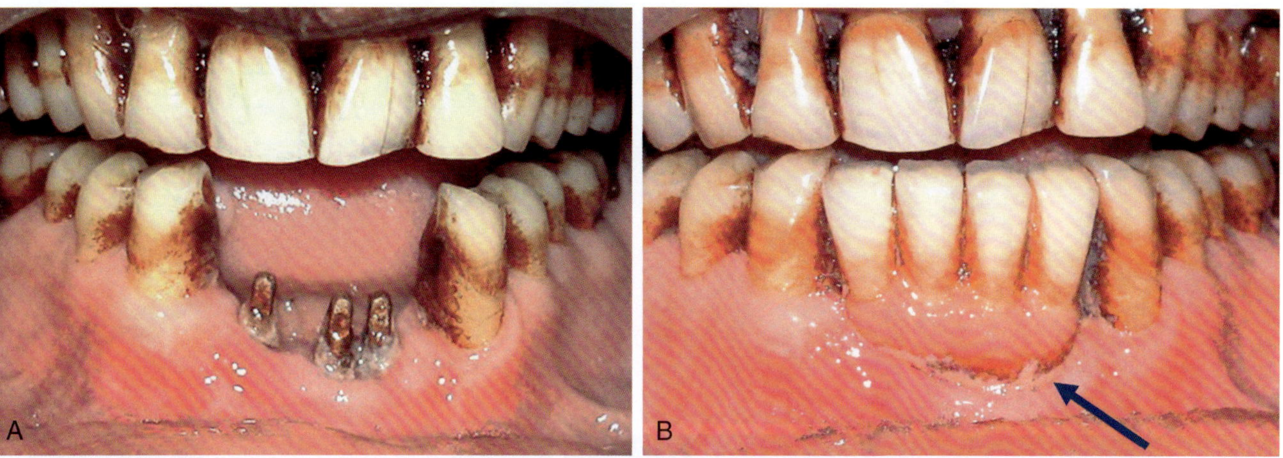

Fig 7.8 (A) Implants if inserted in the patient with the tobacco chewing habit result in (B) recurrent soft tissue infections under the implant prosthesis.

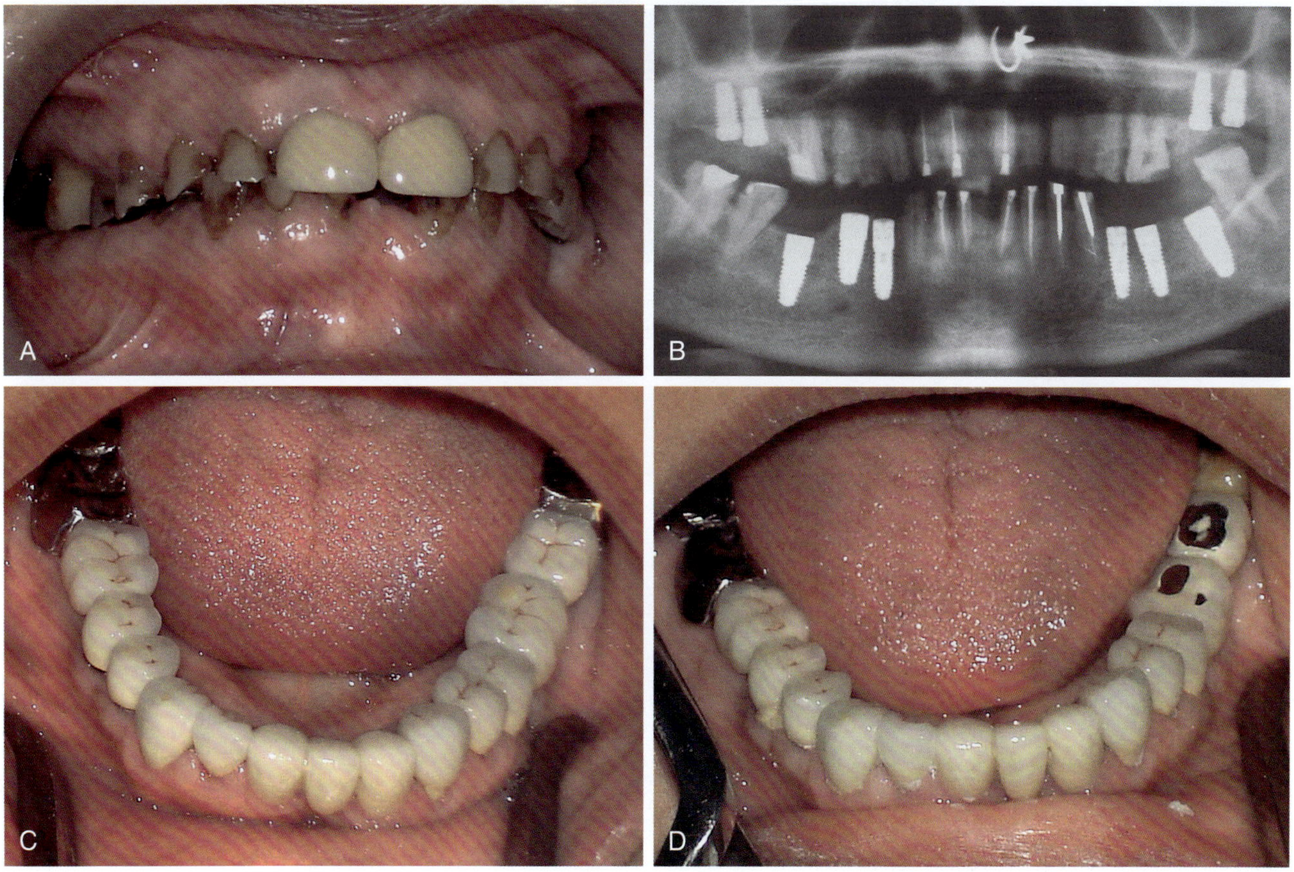

Fig 7.9 (A to D) Full mouth rehabilitation using multiple implants done for a patient who has worn out all the teeth; if proper measures are not taken to treat the bruxism, it may result in wearing out or fracture of the implant prosthesis or its components.

fibrosis or TMJ problems, show limited mouth opening, which can cause problems with osteotomy preparation or other adjuvant procedures like sinus grafting.

Diagnostic (panoramic/periapical) radiographs

Panoramic and periapical radiographs are very useful diagnostic tools to evaluate the edentulous bony ridge and its surrounding structures. These radiographs give ideas about any root remnant, mesiodistal dimensions of the edentulous space, bone height available to insert implant, any root curvature of adjacent teeth, any bone defect, any periodontal or periapical lesion with the adjacent teeth and the position and route of vital structures in the area, like mental foramina, mandibular canal, maxillary sinus floor, nasal floor, etc. However, when the dentist is planning implant therapy, he/she should always keep in mind that the panoramic radiograph may show 10–30%

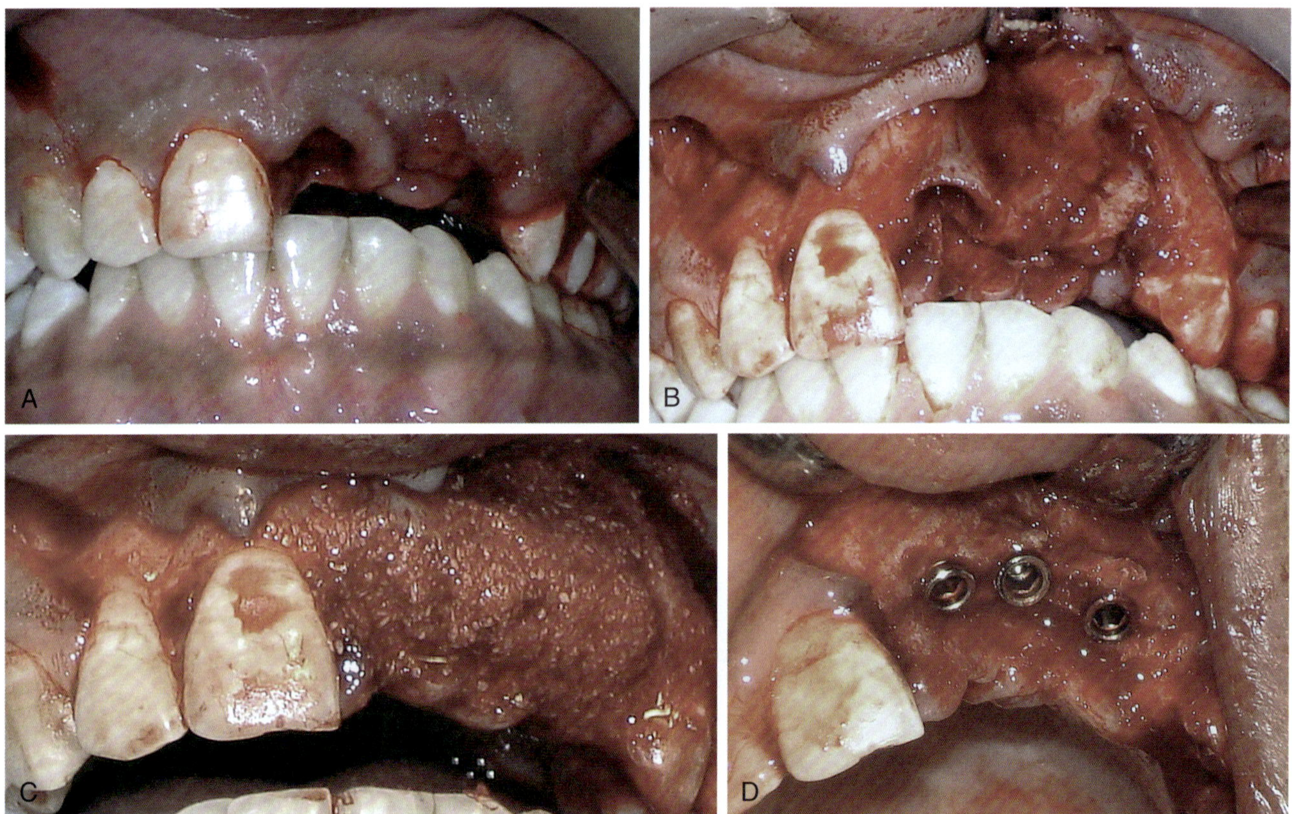

Fig 7.10 (A and B) The traumatic loss of teeth often results in loss of thin facial cortical plate. (C and D) The area should be grafted using bone regeneration material and implant inserted in the new bone dimensions after 4 months.

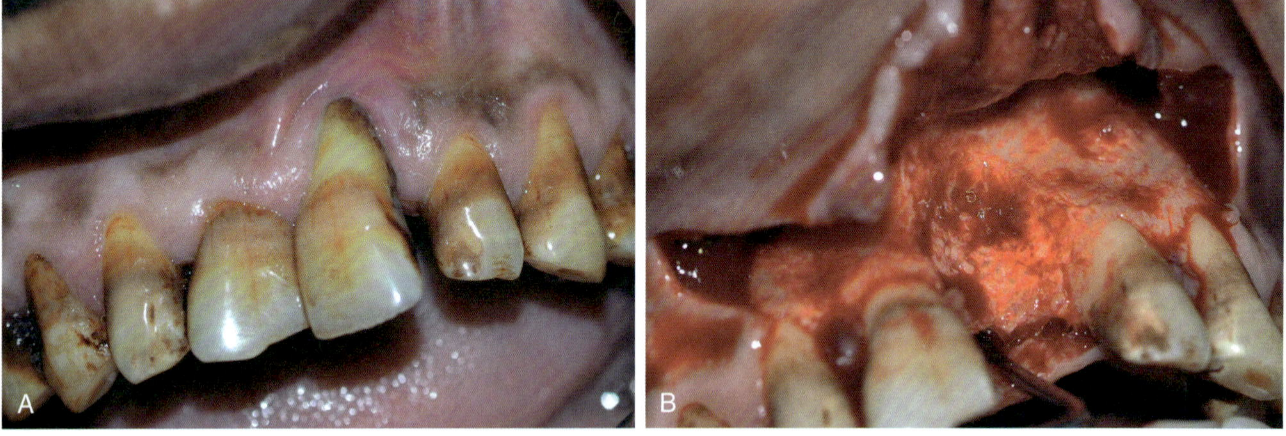

Fig 7.11 (A and B) A large osseous defect can be seen after the extraction of a periodontally compromised tooth.

magnification of hard tissue structures. Whereas, depending on the cone angulation of the radiographic machine, the periapical radiographs show variable amounts of magnification. When planning with these radiographs, a radiographic template with the small metal balls placed above the ridge crest, should be used to calibrate image magnification. If the panoramic radiograph of the patient shows bone dimensions that are more than required, the implant surgeon, to be on the safer side, may plan for the ideal implant size by reducing the radiographic dimensions by 25%. For example, if the panoramic radiograph shows 20 mm bone height above the mandibular canal, it should be reduced by 25% (maximum possible magnification percentage); thus the actual bone height may be 15 mm. Further, leaving 3 mm bone above the canal as a safety guard to avoid nerve injury, the dentist should place only 12 mm long implants. For tight edentulous spaces and limited bone height the bone dimensions can be exactly calibrated using the small metal balls in the radiographic template (e.g. if the metal ball with actual diameter 3 mm is used and shows 4 mm diameter in the radiograph, that means the radiograph is showing 25%

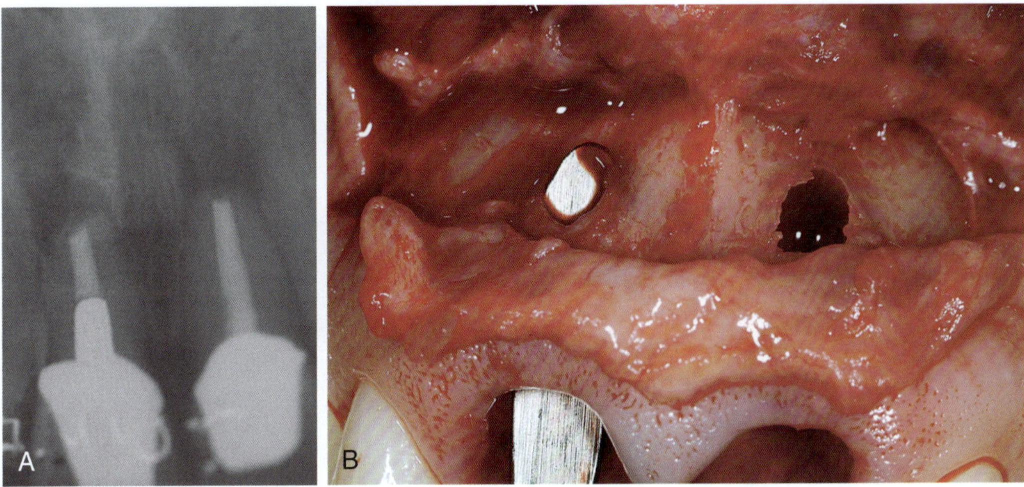

Fig 7.12 (A and B) Teeth with periapical radiolucency or history of apicoectomy often show a medium to large osseous defect during implant placement. For such cases, the dentist should plan bone augmentation during or before implant placement.

magnification). Other disadvantages of these radiographs are that they do not give any idea about bone width and bone density.

Impressions and diagnostic cast preparation

Impression of both the arches should be made using alginate impression material and bite registration should be recorded using an appropriate bite material. Upper and lower diagnostic casts must be articulated in occlusion (for partially edentulous patients) or in centric relation (for completely edentulous patients). These diagnostic casts are used:

a. To evaluate the patient's opposing tooth/teeth, their overeruption, buccal or lingual inclinations, the drifting of adjacent teeth, ridge form, etc.
b. To fabricate a radiographic template (using radiograph or CT scan), which is used for accurate planning of the implant
c. To fabricate the surgical stent for accurate implant placement
d. For the fabrication of an interim prosthesis after implant insertion.

Clinical pictures of the edentulous area

These are used to record:

a. The pre-clinical situation of the case
b. Ridge morphology
c. The width of keratinized soft tissue collar at the implant site
d. The periodontal health of the adjacent teeth
e. Patient's occlusion
f. Patient's smile line
g. Pretreatment maxillofacial prosthesis
h. Any soft tissue lesion.

All these features, which are recorded along with clinical pictures, can be very helpful for treatment planning, as the implant dentist can correlate the hard tissue (bone) situations, which are recorded with the radiographs and CT scan, with the type and amount of soft tissue recorded with the clinical pictures.

Bone mapping

Bone mapping is done to evaluate the buccolingual bone dimensions at the edentulous site, which cannot be recorded with the radiograph. There are different ways of doing bone mapping but the easiest way is using a bone calliper. A surface anaesthetic or a small amount of local infiltration is given at the implant site and the bone calliper tips are pierced through the buccal and lingual soft tissue to reach the underlying bone. The bone calliper shows the reading on its scale. This procedure can be repeated at 2 to 3 points along the ridge height to evaluate the bone width at different points along the bony ridge (Fig 7.13A and B). One can record the bone width dimensions and plan the approximate diameter of the implant which can be used at the particular site. Bone mapping may not give accurate bone dimensions, hence the flaps should be elevated to expose the bony ridge for direct visualization and accurate implant placement. CT planning is considered to be more accurate and the dentist can bypass bone mapping procedure if he/she is doing CT planning for the implant treatment.

Radiographic template fabrication

An ideal provisional prosthesis is fabricated for the edentulous site by setting the teeth in position and in correct occlusion with the opposing dentition or prosthesis. Either radiopaque teeth are used in the template or a radiopaque material like gutta-percha or self-cure resin mixed with radiopaque barium sulphate is filled in the template at the prosthetically accurate, desired implant sites. This template is accurately seated in the patient's mouth and the patient is sent for the dental radiographs and/or dental CT scan. The radiopaque teeth or the radiopaque material filled at the implant site is clearly visible in the dental radiograph or dental CT scan. With reference to these radiopaque sites, which represent the ideal implant positions and three-dimensional orientations for the accurate future prosthesis, the implants with ideal

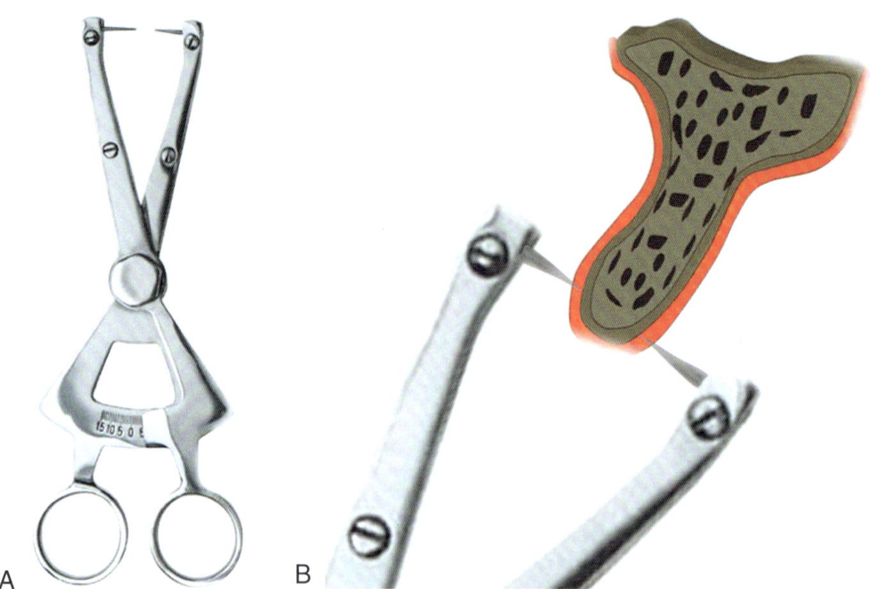

Fig 7.13 (A) Bone mapping calliper (Salvin Dental Specialities, USA). (B) Surface anaesthetic is applied at the site and the buccolingual bone dimensions at different points along the ridge height is measured using the bone calliper. Its sharp and pointed pins punch through the soft tissue to reach the underlying bone and its scale shows the ridge width present at the particular edentulous ridge site.

dimensions, positions, and angulations are planned, executed, and placed accurately for the future prosthesis ('prosthetically guided implant insertion').

Template for radiograph

As described earlier in this chapter, radiographs show some degree of magnification; thus the template with calibrated metal balls should be used in radiographic planning of the implant case, to exactly calculate the percentage of magnification in the radiographic image (Fig 7.14A–E).

Template for dental CT

Using the metal ball in the CT scan template results in the scattering of CT images. Moreover, the dental CT scan does not show any magnification, so ball calibration is also not required; hence any non-metallic, radiopaque material like gutta-percha or self-cure acrylic mixed with barium sulphate can be used in the template to evaluate and plan the desired edentulous ridge sites for three-dimensionally accurate implant placements (Figs 7.15 and 7.16).

Radiographic implant template from the implant system

A few implant systems provide a radiographic template in the form of a transparent sheet showing the actual size images (100%) of all their implants as well as magnified implant images (125%). In planning with the patient's radiograph, the magnified implant image of the template is used to make ideal implant selections for a particular site. However, if the implant surgeon is planning with the dental CT scan which shows no magnification, he/she should use the actual size implant image of the radiographic template for the planning (Fig 7.17A–C).

CT planning

With advancements in diagnostic tools, many implant dentists now prefer to evaluate bone quality and measure three-dimensional ridge dimensions accurately with the help of the dental CT scan (Dentascan). Some implant simulation softwares (Nobel Guide, Implant 3D, etc.) are also available in the market, which can create beautiful axial, panoramic, cross-sections and three-dimensional views of the jawbone using the raw dental CT files (Fig 7.18A–E). They have features for accurate simulation of the implant, graft, and prosthesis. The dental CT scan gives an idea about:

a. Accurate three-dimensional measurement of available bone (buccolingual, mesiodistal, and bone height)
b. Bone density at the implant site
c. Bony ridge morphology
d. Bone angulation
e. Any osseous defect, if present
f. Three-dimensional view of the complete jawbone
g. Three-dimensional paths and architecture of vital structures like the mandibular canal, nasal cavity and its floor, sinus cavity and its floor, etc.
h. Implant simulation for accurate implant selection and its three-dimensional placement orientation for the best possible future prosthesis
i. Volume of the graft required, if any grafting procedure like sinus grafting, block grafting, etc. needs to be performed.

Surgical guide fabrication

As previously mentioned, implant insertion should be guided by the planned future prosthesis. Thus the use of the surgical guide is paramount for the ideal implant insertion. Depending on the technique, there are different ways to fabricate the surgical guide.

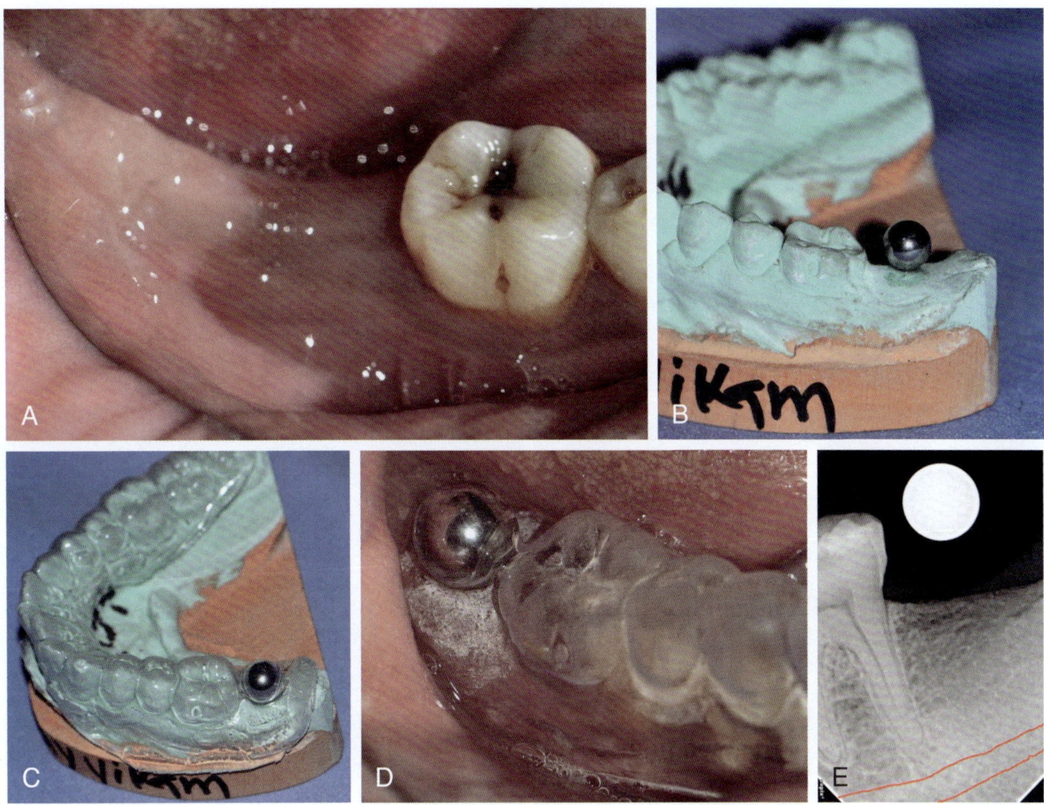

Fig 7.14 (A) Clinical view of missing mandibular second molar. An impression is made and a diagnostic cast is prepared. (B) A metal ball is fixed at the planned implant site on the diagnostic cast, using a glue and (C) a vacuum form tray is adapted over the same. (D) The vacuum form tray carrying the metal ball is seated in the patient's mouth and (E) a radiograph is taken which shows the metal ball as the round white image. Now the diameter of real ball and its white image in radiograph is measured and calibrated to calculate the exact magnification that the radiograph shows. For example, if the diameter of the real ball is 3 mm and its radiographic image shows 4 mm, there is 25% magnification in the radiograph. Thus if the radiograph is showing 16 mm available bone height from crest to mandibular canal for the implant placement, the actual bone height could be only 12 mm (25% less than the radiographic bone height); therefore, the maximum length of the implant that can be inserted is 10 mm (leaving 2 mm as the safety margin from the mandibular canal).

Manual surgical guide

A removable provisional prosthesis is fabricated for the edentulous ridge area and holes are prepared through the teeth of the prosthesis at the desired implant sites. These holes are filled using radiopaque material like heated gutta-percha or self-cure acrylic mixed with radiopaque barium sulphate. The patient is sent for radiography and/or dental CT scan with this template worn in the mouth. The radiographs and different views of the dental CT scan show the radiopaque barium sulphate representing the ideal teeth positions, which are used as the reference for three-dimensionally ideal implant planning. After using this prosthesis as the radiographic template, the barium sulphate is removed from the implant sites and holes are drilled through the same radiographic template. Now before elevating the mucoperiosteal flap, the same radiographic template is seated in the patient's mouth and a small-diameter drill is used to drill the sites through its holes to the partial depth. Bleeding points are noticed at the implant sites after the surgical guide is removed from the mouth. Now the flap is elevated and the osteotomy is prepared for the implants at the same sites with the same directions. The implants are placed at the ideal positions (Fig 7.19A–L). The manual guide is less accurate and can be used only to place the implants at the specific positions and angulations with the open surgical technique. The flapless implant placement technique using this guide, should be avoided especially in cases with limited bone dimensions, as there can be the chances of bone dehiscence or perforation during drilling through the guide.

Computer-assisted surgical guide

With advancement in modern implant dentistry, computer-guided implant placement is one of the preferred methods to obtain the ideal implant insertion with minimum trauma to hard and soft tissue. A radiographic template is fabricated and the dental CT scan of the patient wearing the radiographic template as well as another scan of the template alone (outside the mouth) are done ('dual scan technique'). The implant planning is done using implant simulation software; with reference to both the scans a surgical guide is fabricated using prototyping or CAD/CAM technology. This computer-assisted surgical guide can be soft tissue supported (seated over the soft tissue ridge, with implants inserted with flapless technique) or hard tissue/bone supported (the mucoperiosteal flap is elevated and the guide is seated onto the underlying

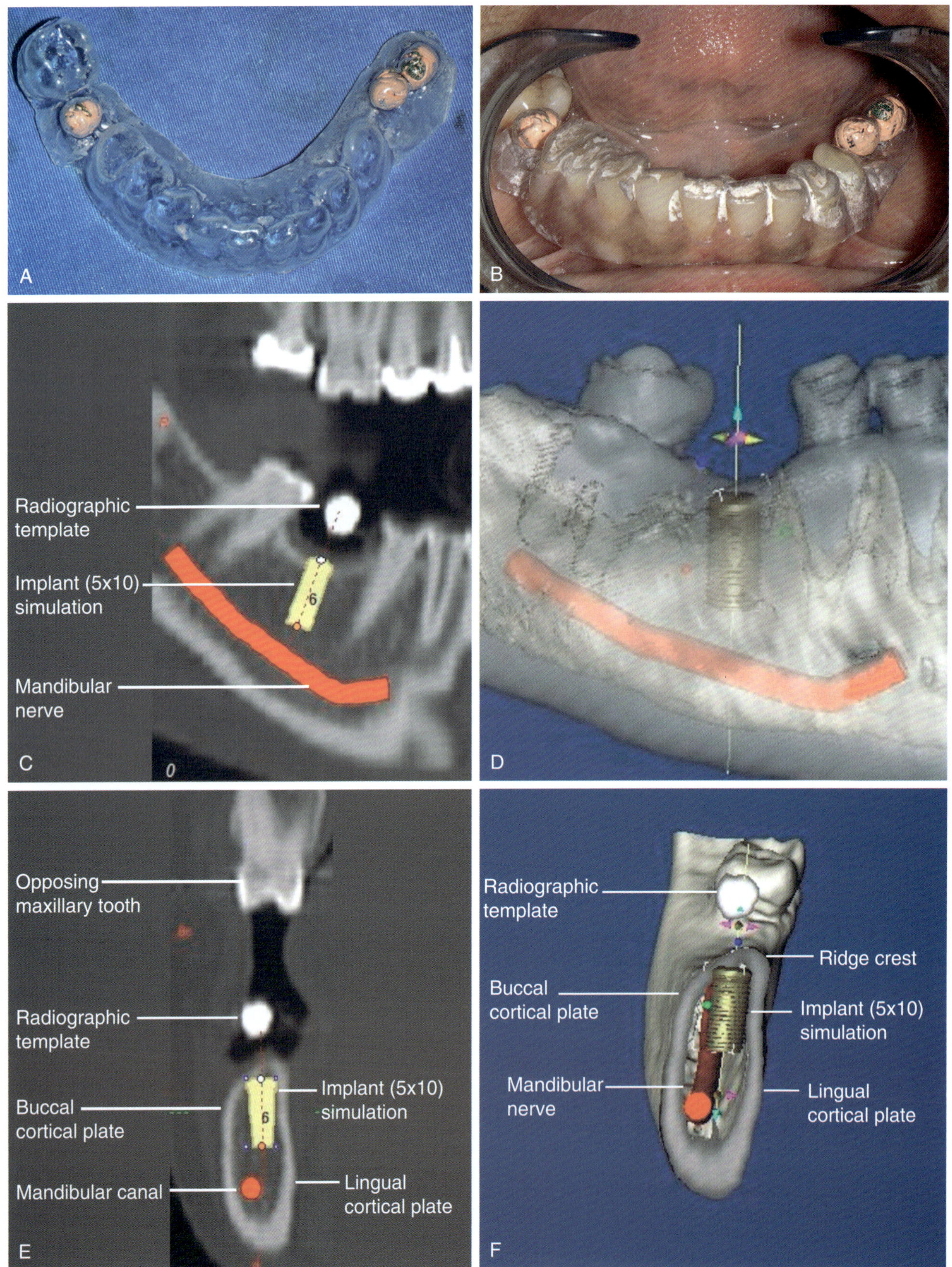

Fig 7.15 (A) The vacuum form tray is fabricated over the gutta-percha placed on the top of the ridge of the diagnostic cast. (B) The patient is sent for the dental CT scan with the vacuum form tray seated in the mouth. (C–F) The gutta-percha balls can be seen in the CT images as a white opaque image, and they are used as the reference point to plan the dimensions and angulation of the implant for the prosthesis.

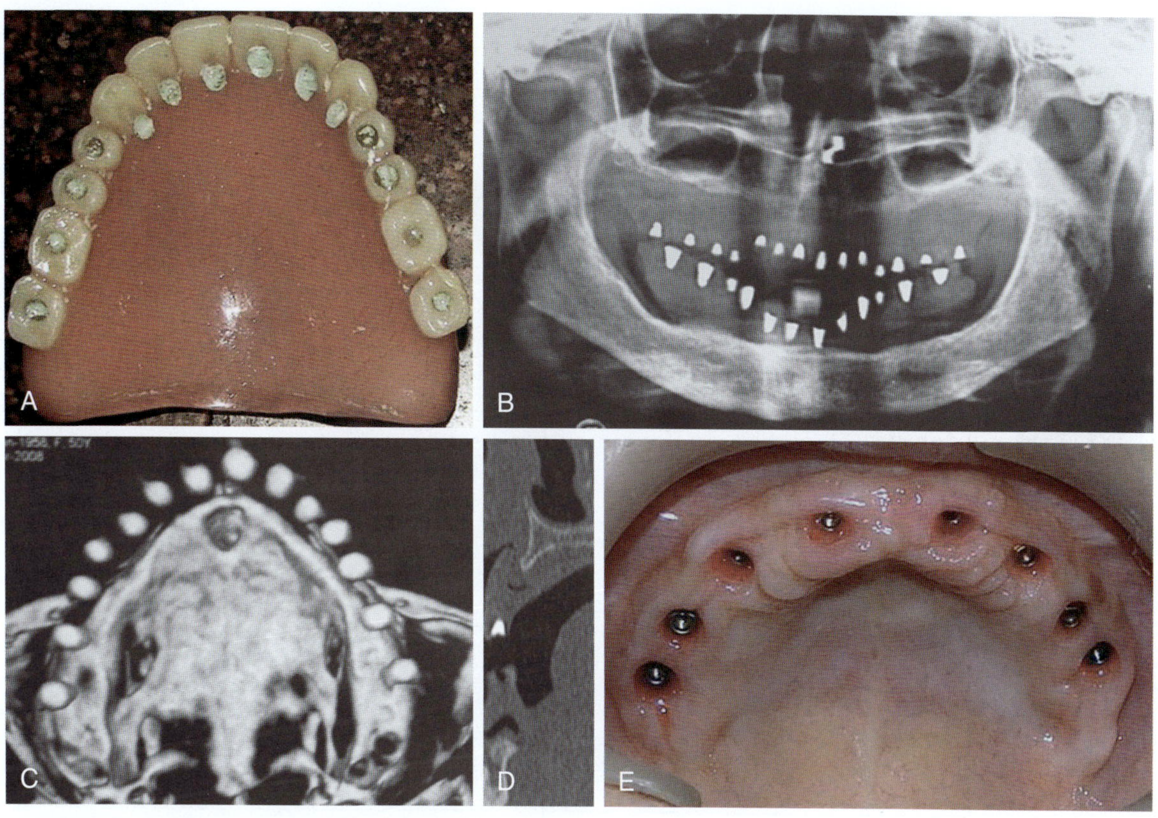

Fig 7.16 (A) Patient's denture teeth are drilled at the ideal implant sites and holes filled with the heated gutta-percha. The patient is sent for radiograph and dental CT scan with the denture in the mouth. (B) The panoramic radiograph, and (C and D) 3D and cross-sectional views of the dental CT scan show the radiopaque GP points. (E) The implants are inserted at the desired site which shows the adequate bone dimensions and are also ideal for the implant prosthesis.

bony ridge for the ideal implant insertion). After seating the guide accurately in the mouth, it is immobilized using fixation screws; and implant osteotomies are prepared through the guide using drill sleeves (Fig 7.20A–H).

Key points of treatment planning for successful implant therapy

Implant diameter selection

An implant with a particular diameter has been conventionally selected according to the bone dimensions available at the edentulous site; but keeping biomechanical parameters in mind, the ideal implant diameter should be chosen to bear occlusal and transverse forces, achieve an aesthetic emergence profile, avoid screw loosening and implant component or body fracture, and facilitate oral hygiene. Thus, when planning placement with radiography, an ideal range of implant diameters for a particular tooth replacement should be kept in mind and correlated with the bone dimensions available. If inadequate bone dimensions are available, either the site should be grafted to regenerate new bone dimensions for the placement of an ideal diameter implant or more number of narrow diameter implants should be inserted and splinted together to distribute the forces when replacing multiple number of teeth or a multi-rooted single molar. If an implant has a diameter that is less than ideal, it should also have additional length to achieve similar amount of bone implant contact. An implant with ideal diameter should be inserted even in cases where a large amount of bone volume is available to insert a bigger diameter implant, because the wider diameter implants have shown many disadvantages with fewer prosthetic advantages.

Advantages of wide diameter implants:

a. Increases bone implant surface contact area.
b. Minimizes the cantilevered offset forces.
c. Decreases screw loosening.
d. Minimizes implant component fracture.
e. Compensates for poor bone density.
f. Improved emergence profile.
g. Facilitates the oral hygiene maintenance.

Disadvantages of wide diameter implant:

a. Decreased amount of surrounding bone thickness may not survive and leads to resorption.
b. More drilling for implant placement causes bone trauma.
c. More chances of bone dehiscence during drilling.
d. Possibility of encroachment to the periodontal ligament of the adjacent teeth.
e. The wider implant does not transfer the sufficient stress to the surrounding bone, which results in disuse atrophy of the bone (similar to the condition when

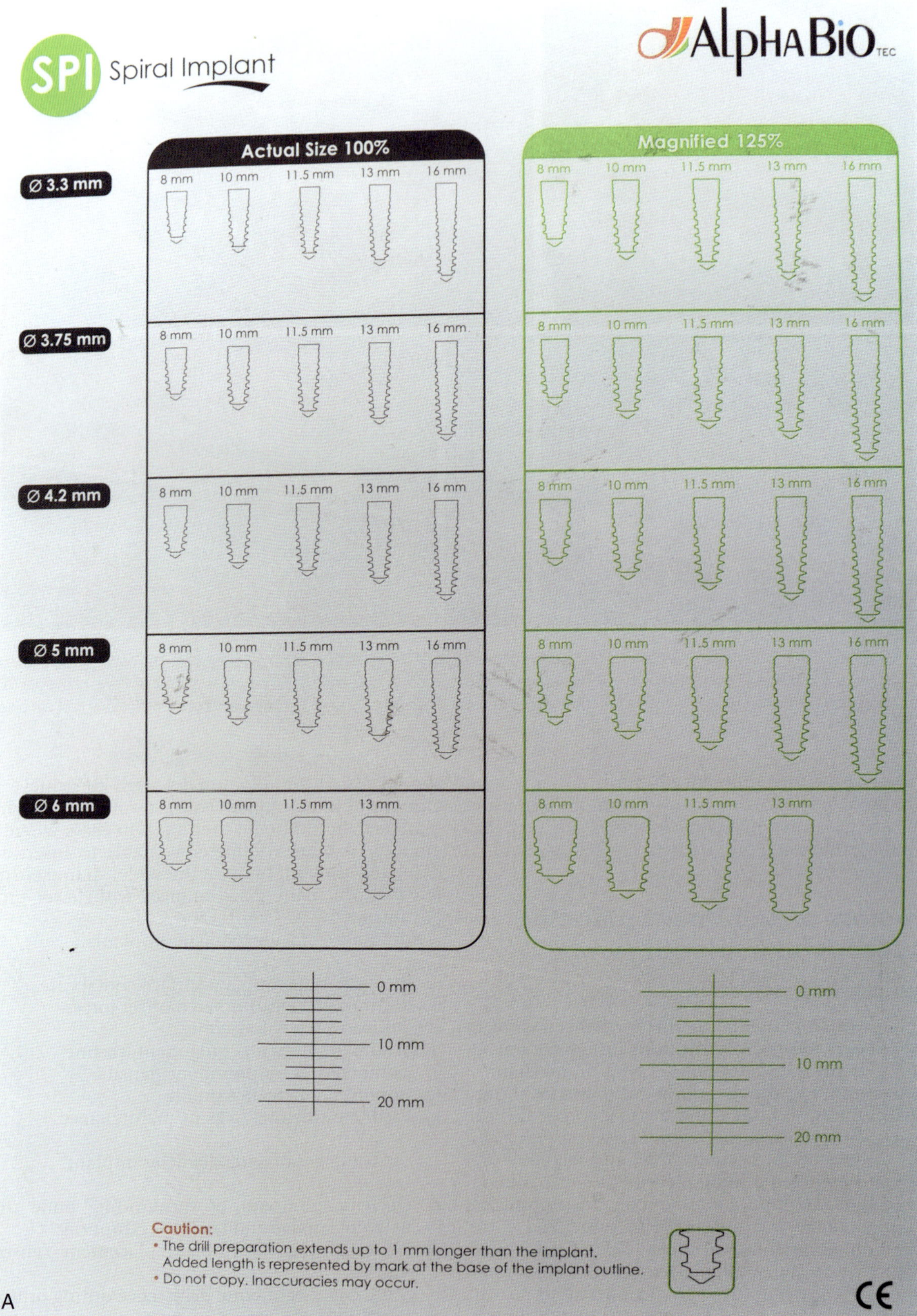

Fig 7.17 (A) The radiographic template sheath of the SPI implant showing actual sizes (100%) of the implants (black images) as well as magnified images (125%) of the same implants (green images).

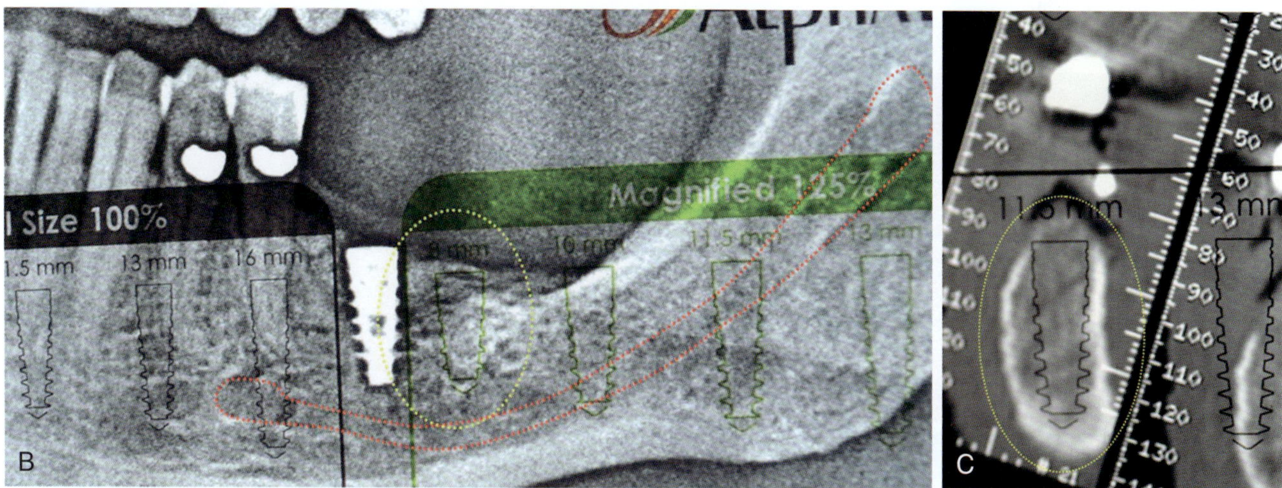

Fig 7.17, con'd (B) When planning with the panoramic radiograph the green coloured magnified image is used for the planning (C) but if planning with the CT scan the black coloured actual size implant image is used for the same.

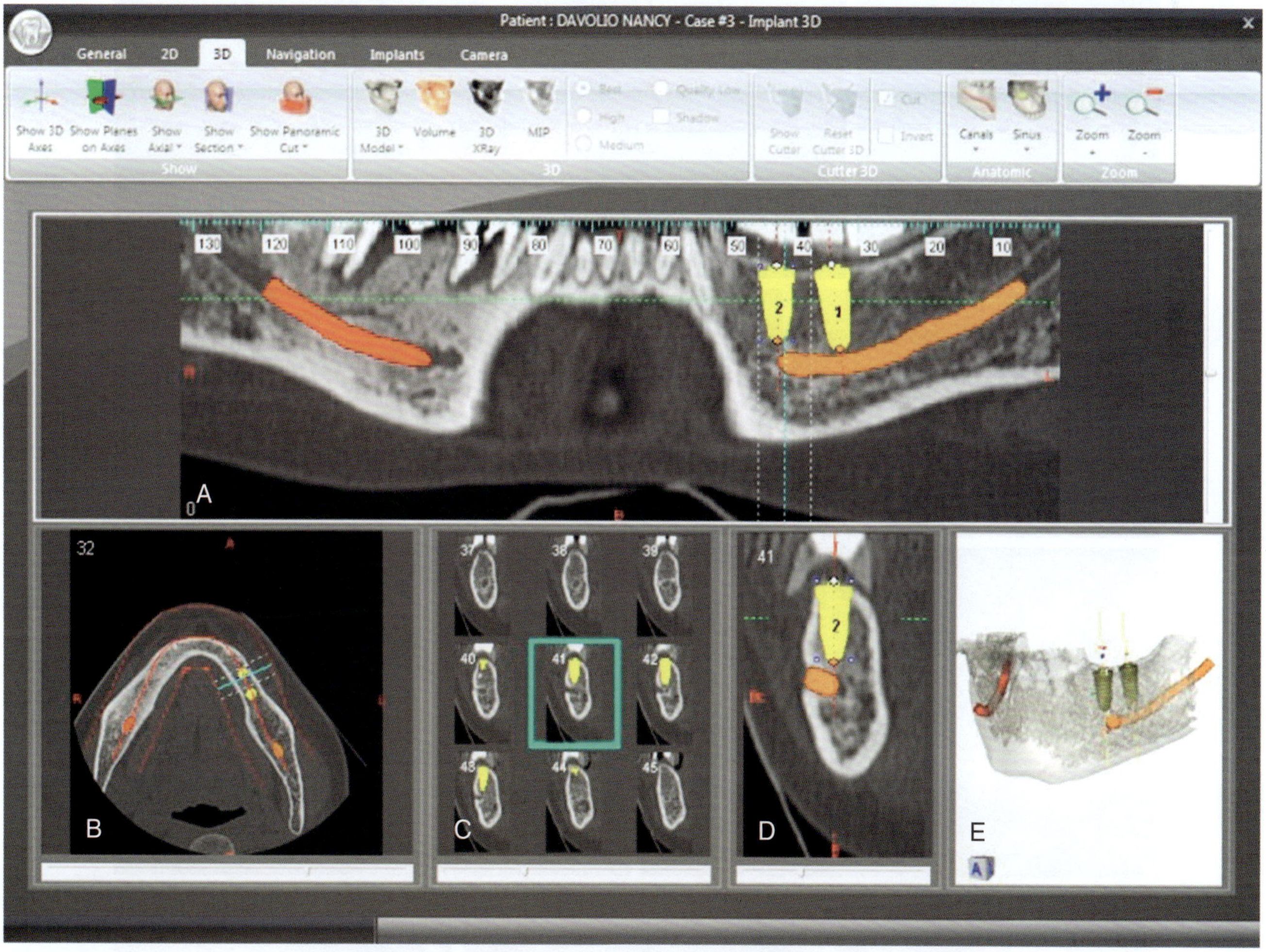

Fig 7.18 (A) CT images created with 3D implant planning software showing panoramic view, (B) axial view, (C and D) cross-sectional views and (E) 3D view with implant simulation, traced nerves, osseous defects and radiographic template.

no strain is transferred to the bone after tooth loss). The bone gets resorbed because of disuse atrophy, if no implant is inserted.

Advantages of narrow diameter implant:

a. Minimal drilling for implant placement causes lesser bone trauma.
b. Better and longer survival of surrounding thicker bone.
c. Less bone modification and grafting are required.

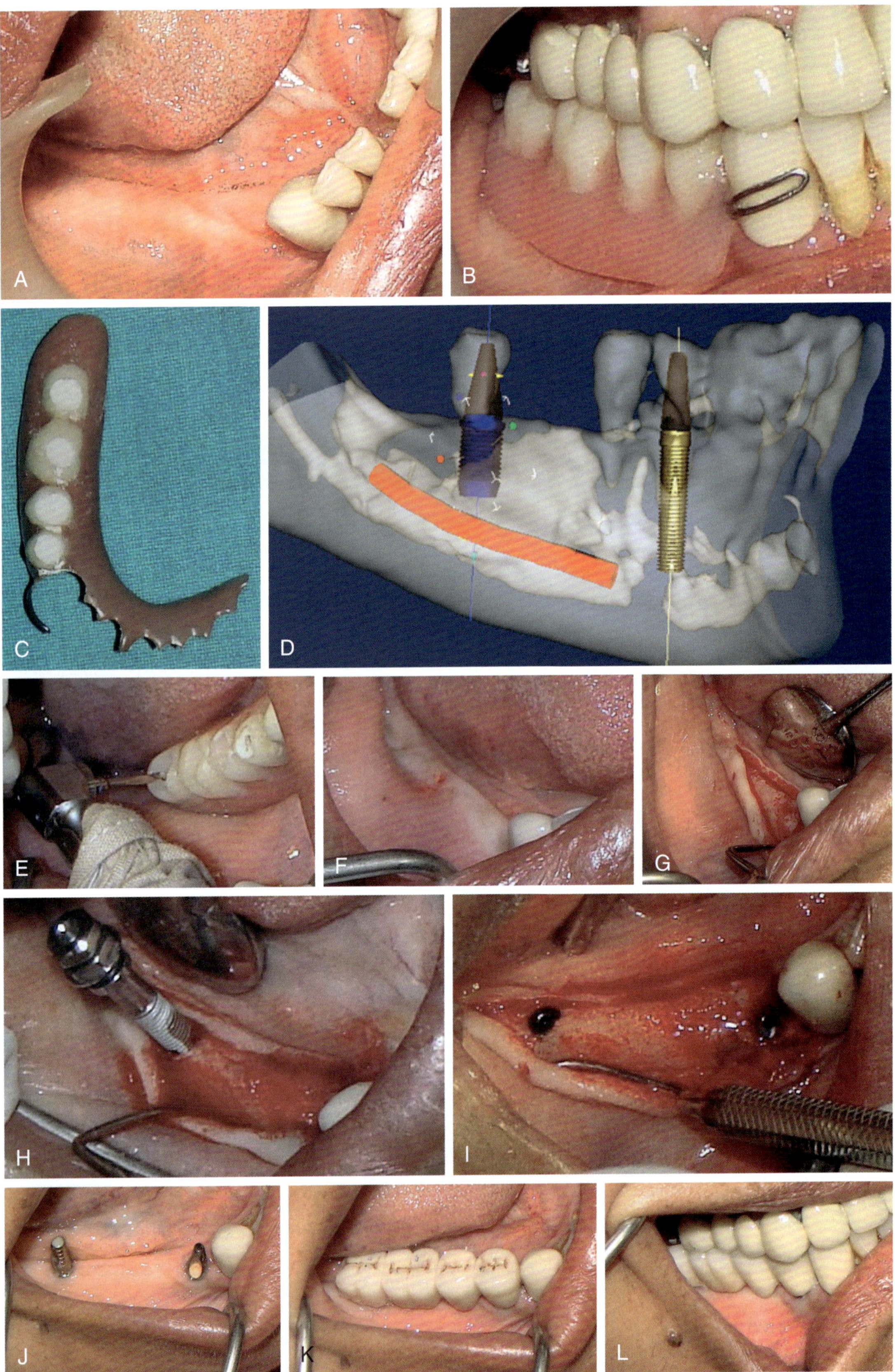
A
B
C
D
E
F
G
H
I
J
K
L

Fig 7.19 (A and B) A removable provisional prosthesis is fabricated for the edentulous area. (C) The teeth are drilled at the ideal implant sites and holes are filled using self-cure acrylic mixed with radiopaque barium sulphate. Patient is sent for the dental CT with the template worn in the mouth. (D) The 3D view of the dental CT is showing the radiopaque barium sulphate representing the ideal teeth positions which are used for implant planning with the planning software by placing the simulated implants in dental CT. The barium sulphate is removed from the implant sites and the holes are drilled through the same radiographic template. (E) Now the radiographic template is seated in the patient's mouth and used as the surgical guide for pilot drilling to partial depth. (F) The bleeding points can be noticed at the implant sites after the surgical guide is removed from the mouth. (G) Now the flap is elevated and the osteotomy is prepared for implants at the same sites with the same directions. (H–J) The implants are placed at the ideal positions to support (K and L) a fixed ceramic prosthesis which is ideal in the form and occlusion.

d. Less chances of bone dehiscence during drilling.
e. In selective cases, can be inserted with flapless or minimal incision technique.

Disadvantages of narrow diameter implant:

a. Screw loosening.
b. Implant body fracture.
c. Component fracture.
d. Inadequate emergence profile.
e. More offset forces when placed for bigger size single tooth prosthesis.
f. Decreased bone implant surface contact area.
g. Problematic for maintenance of oral hygiene.

Usually the diameter of an implant is chosen so that the placement of an implant with selected diameter should leave a minimum 1.5 mm of bone on the facial and lingual sides as well as between the implant and the adjacent tooth, whereas it should be 3.0 mm between two implants (Fig 7.21A and B). But the dentist should keep in mind a minimum and maximum diameter for the implant to replace a particular tooth, to avoid the post-restoration complications described earlier (Fig 7.22A and B).

Implant length selection

An adequately long implant utilizing the maximum amount of available bone, should be inserted to support prosthesis. Using a longer implant increases initial stability and bone implant interface. This may be more advantageous when placing an implant in a fresh extraction socket, followed by an immediate loading protocol. The implant length may also be correlated with the bone density in the area, as weaker bone requires longer implants to achieve adequate primary stability. The longest possible implant should be used in cases where the bone is inadequate in width to insert an adequately wide implant. The compensating length of the implant results in approximately the same amount of bone implant surface contact, despite the inadequate width of bone and implant.

Implant design selection

The internal connection implant is preferred over the external connection implant, except when the large cantilevered bar or fixed prosthesis is placed. The narrow diameter internal connection implant is more prone to fracture under cantilevered forces (e.g. distal-tilted implants in all-on-4 technique). Implants with deeper threads are preferred in low-density bone to achieve adequate primary stability. The implants with shallow threads should be preferred in high-density bone to avoid the deeper threads causing pressure necrosis of the bone. The implant with deeper threads should be chosen for immediate implantation in the extraction socket, because its apex can be adequately secured in the limited bone apical to the socket (Fig 7.23A–D).

Available bone width and height

The available bone width and height should accurately be measured using radiographs and dental CT scan, to select and place the implant with appropriate dimensions. As previously described, implant diameter is selected at least 3 mm smaller than the available bone width, to leave minimum 1.5 mm bone, lingual as well as facial to the implant. Available bone height is calculated after deducting the safety distance (2 mm) for the vital structures. If measured with radiograph, the amount of magnification should be deducted from the total bone height to get the actual bone height. Further, the safety distance should also be deducted from the actual bone height (Fig 7.24).

Bone angulation

Bone angulation should be correlated with the direction of the future implant prosthesis. The implant should be inserted which is more accurate for the prosthesis in spite of placing implant according to the bony ridge angulation (Fig 7.25).

Distance between two adjacent implants

Implants should be inserted so that a minimum 3 mm of bone is left between two adjacent implants. Because the bone between two implants receives blood supply only from the basal bone, it is prone to get vertically resorbed if there is less than 3 mm of bone between adjacent implants (Fig 7.26A).

Distance between implant and adjacent tooth

The minimum bone between the implant surface and the root of the adjacent tooth must be 1.5 mm for long-term survival. The bone between the tooth root and implant surface receives blood supply from the basal bone as well as from the periodontal ligaments of the adjacent root (Fig 7.26B).

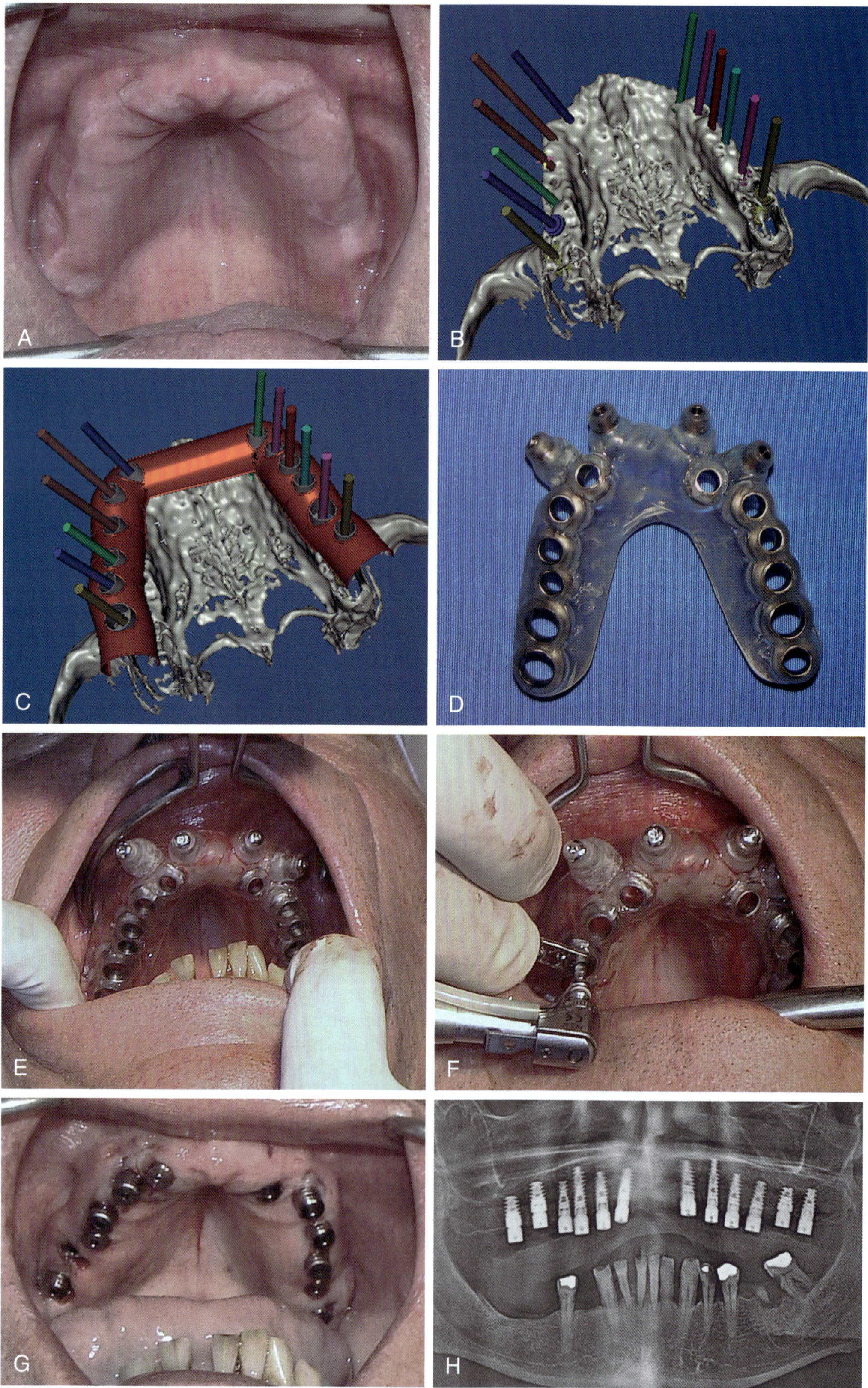

Fig 7.20 (A) Edentulous maxillary ridge. (B) Implant planning using implant simulation software. (C) A surgical guide simulation is done using software. (D) The finally planned CT images are exported to the CAD/CAM system, which fabricates an accurate soft tissue supported surgical guide. (E) Surgical guide is seated over the edentulous ridge and immobilized using fixation screws. (F) The special drill guide sleeves are used to prepare the implant osteotomies through the surgical guide. (G) Clinical and (H) radiographic views immediately after implant insertion.

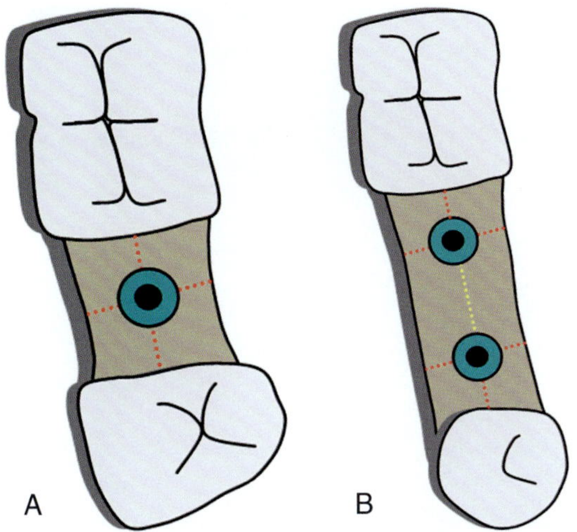

Fig 7.21 (A and B) Placement of an implant with selected diameter should leave minimum 1.5 mm of bone (marked with red lines) on the facial and lingual site as well as between the implant and adjacent tooth, whereas it should be 3 mm (marked with yellow line) between two implants.

Root inclinations of adjacent teeth

The root inclinations of any adjacent tooth must be closely evaluated with the help of radiograph and dental CT scan when placing an implant closer to the tooth root or in tight spaces. The most important areas of concern are the maxillary and mandibular canine regions. The maxillary canine often shows the distal inclination of its root while the mandibular canine shows the mesial inclination of its root. Hence, when placing implant for the maxillary first premolar, the implant apex is often angled distally to remain parallel to the maxillary canine root. A tapered implant is more appropriate for such a situation. While placing an implant for the mandibular lateral incisor, the implant apex is often angled medially to remain parallel to the mandibular canine roots (Fig 7.27A–G). The pilot drilling should be done to a partial depth and a periapical radiograph should be taken from two directions (canine as well as premolar) with the drill in place, to evaluate the direction of drilling in respect of canine root angulation. Further correction in the direction can be done, if required, using a side cutting Lindemann drill.

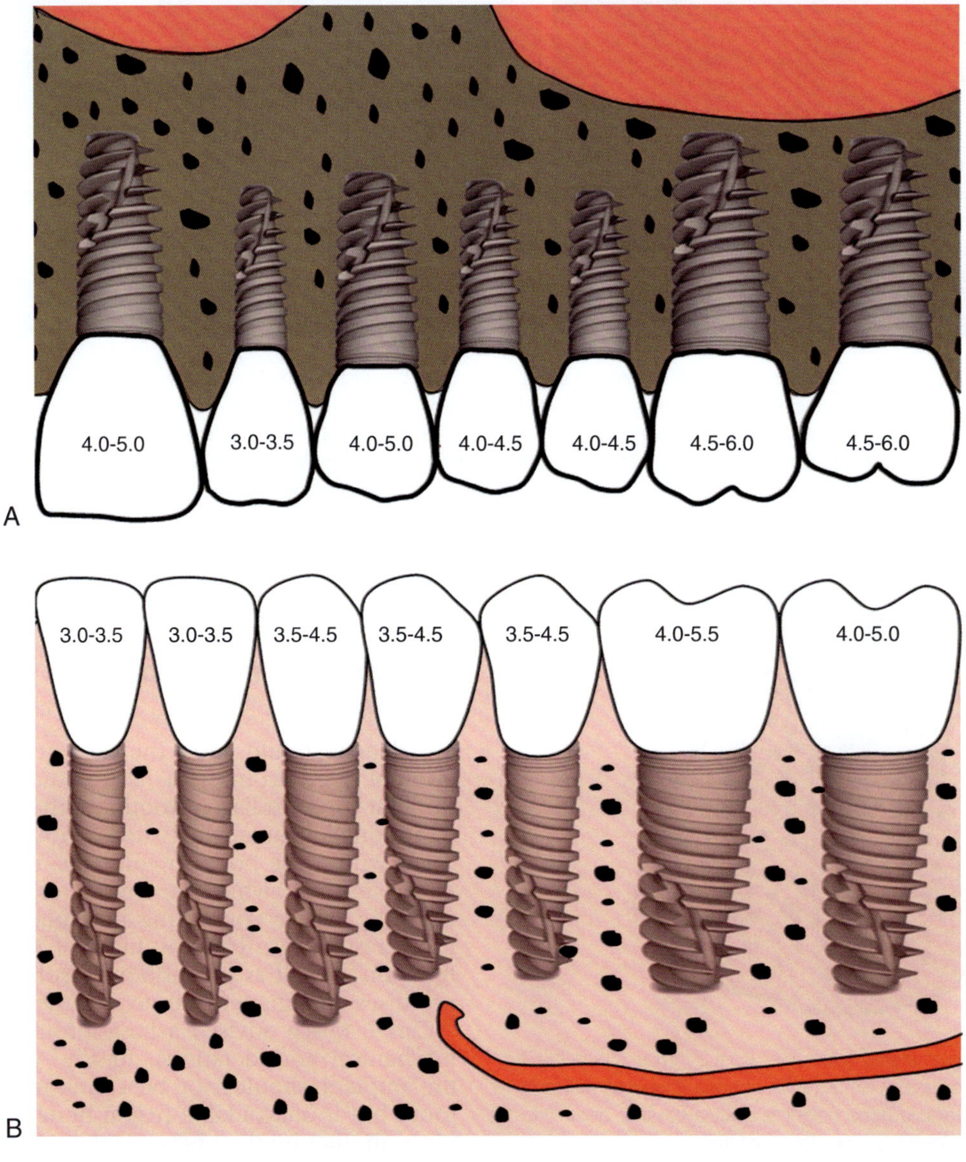

Fig 7.22 (A) The figures show the ideal range of implant diameters which should be selected for replacing any maxillary or (B) mandibular tooth.

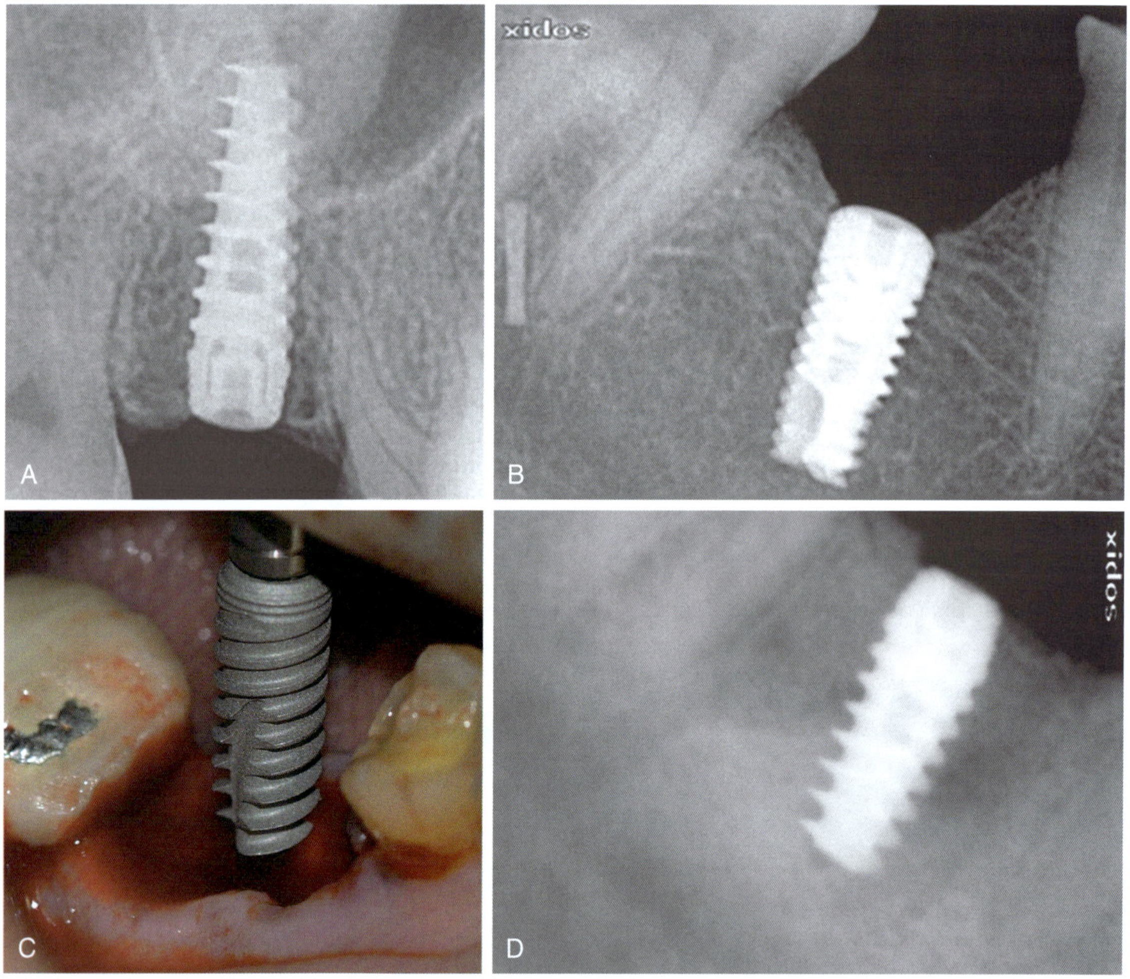

Fig 7.23 (A) The implant with deeper and high pitch (more distance between two threads) threads should be preferred in low density maxillary bone to engage more amount of bone to achieve adequate primary stability for the implant. (B) The implant with shallow and low pitch (less distance between two threads) threads should be preferred in high density mandibular bone to avoid the chances of bone necrosis with deeper threads. (C and D) The implant with shallow and low pitch threads comparatively achieves less primary stability; thus the implant with deeper and high pitch threads can be preferred in immediate implant in extraction socket cases or cases with large osseous defect, to achieve adequate primary stability with low BIC percentage.

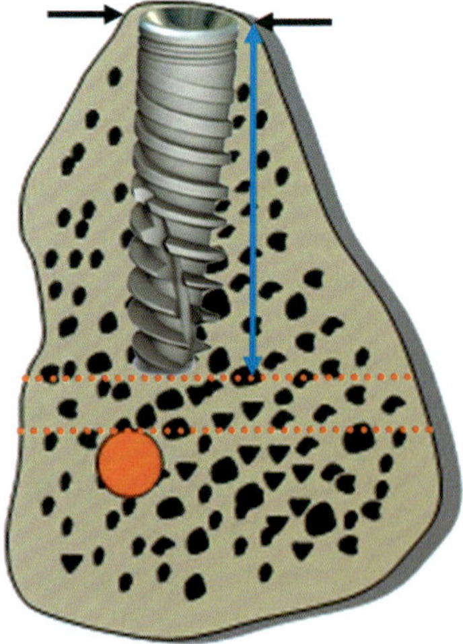

Fig 7.24 Implant diameter is selected at least 3 mm less than the available bone width, to leave minimum 1.5 mm bone, lingual as well as facial, to the implant. Available bone height is calculated after deducting the safety distance (2–3 mm) for the vital structures.

Often the adjacent tooth with extreme angulation that does not allow implant placement, needs to be extracted and replaced with the implant (Fig 7.28A–B).

Connecting implant prosthesis with adjacent tooth/teeth

The dentist should know the basic anatomy of the periodontal and peri-implant hard tissue when connecting implant to any adjacent tooth. As the natural tooth has periodontal ligaments, it shows more degree of movement within the bone in comparison to the osseointegrated implant which is directly osseointegrated with the bone. Hence, connecting an implant with the natural tooth results in micromovement of the implant during function as well as crestal bone resorption, which compromises the long-term survival of the implant.

Carl E Misch advised a basic protocol based on biomechanical considerations. Ideally, whenever possible, the implant should not be connected to the adjacent tooth but if unavoidable (e.g. if bone is not available to place another implant between the tooth and distal-most

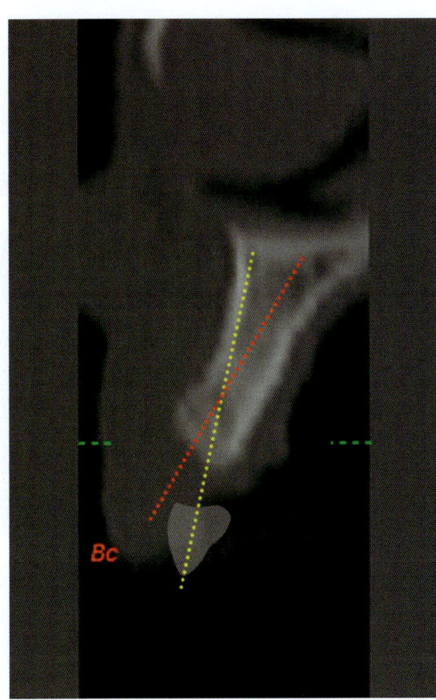

Fig 7.25 Often the bone angulation differs from the ideal tooth position in the prosthesis. Efforts should be made to maximally place the implant along the axis of the prosthesis which often needs ridge modification or guided bone regeneration procedures.

implant site or in the case of a geriatric patient where the least invasive treatment is preferred over the long survival of the implant), one can connect the implant with the adjacent firm immobile tooth. The implant should only be connected with immobile teeth and whenever possible, more firm teeth should be included to minimize the micromovement of the implant during function. If the tooth adjacent to the implant is mobile, the fixed prosthesis should include the firm teeth anterior to the mobile tooth. The implant if placed between two adjacent teeth which need to be crowned, should never be connected with these teeth, as the implant acts as the pier abutment and leads to crestal bone resorption hence, the implant and teeth should be preferred to restore individually.

In the situation where a tooth is present between two implants, either it should be restored separately or it can be used as a pier abutment, as a living pontic between two or more number of implants (Fig 7.29A–F).

Minimum bone buccal or lingual to the inserted implant

As described earlier, a minimum 1.5 mm of bone should left buccal as well as lingual to the inserted implant. Leaving less than 1.5 mm of bone, compromises its blood supply and makes it prone to get resorbed when the implant is restored to function. Either a smaller diameter implant should be placed or the bone which is inadequate in width should be grafted before or during the implant insertion (Fig 7.30A and B).

Implant distance from the mandibular canal

In implant therapy, the mandibular canal is considered to be the most limiting and sensitive structure because injury of the inferior alveolar nerve, which runs through the canal, during osteotomy preparation may cause long-term paraesthesia or dysaesthesia to the patient. The implant surgeon should accurately trace the path of the mandibular canal in radiographs and dental CT scans and should plan to place the implant at least 2 mm short of the mandibular canal. One should keep in mind the magnification shown in the panoramic and dental radiographs, when selecting an implant of the correct length. One should also keep in mind the fact that the drills of few implant systems are 1 mm longer than their marked length. The author recommends use of the CT scan in planning accurate placement of the implant in the mandibular posterior region, especially if bone height above the mandibular canal is limited. The author also recommends pilot drilling to a partial depth and radiographic evaluation, with the drill inserted in the osteotomy, of the bone height available for the further depth-drilling above the mandibular canal (Fig 7.31A and B).

Mental foramina position

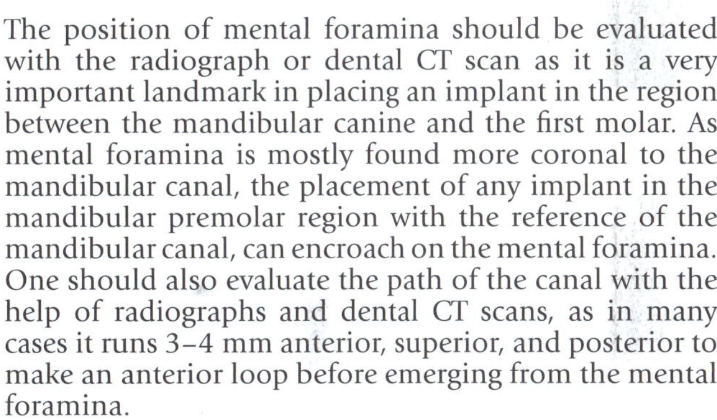

The position of mental foramina should be evaluated with the radiograph or dental CT scan as it is a very important landmark in placing an implant in the region between the mandibular canine and the first molar. As mental foramina is mostly found more coronal to the mandibular canal, the placement of any implant in the mandibular premolar region with the reference of the mandibular canal, can encroach on the mental foramina. One should also evaluate the path of the canal with the help of radiographs and dental CT scans, as in many cases it runs 3–4 mm anterior, superior, and posterior to make an anterior loop before emerging from the mental foramina.

Implant distance from mental foramina (anterior loop)

When placing implant in the mandibular premolar region, the implant apex should end at least 2 mm superior to the mental foramina. If the implant is placed lateral (anterior or posterior) to the mental foramina, the osteotomy is prepared such that the final implant body position remains a minimum of 2 mm away from the mental foramina. While placing implants in the mandibular anterior region (anterior to the mental foramina), the implant body should remain 2 mm anterior to the mental foramina or to the anterior loop, if present. A common mistake which may happen during osteotomy preparation, occurs when the implant surgeon starts the pilot drills 2 mm anterior to the mental foramina; when he/she further widens the osteotomy site and places the implant, it may encroach laterally on to the mental nerve. Hence, the protocol is that if no anterior loop is present, the pilot drilling should begin at the point that is 2 mm plus half of the dimension of the implant diameter; for example, if an implant of 4 mm diameter is planned, drilling should start 4 mm (2.0 mm safety distance + 2 mm cross-section diameter of the implant) anterior to the mental foramina. If the anterior loop is present, an additional 3 mm is added to the safety margin. Hence, to insert a 4 mm diameter

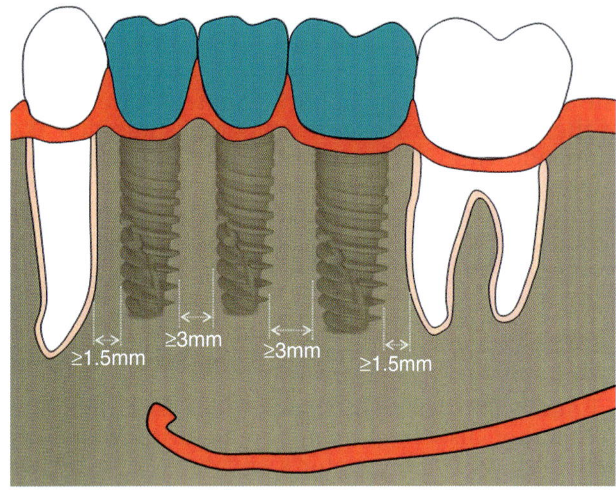

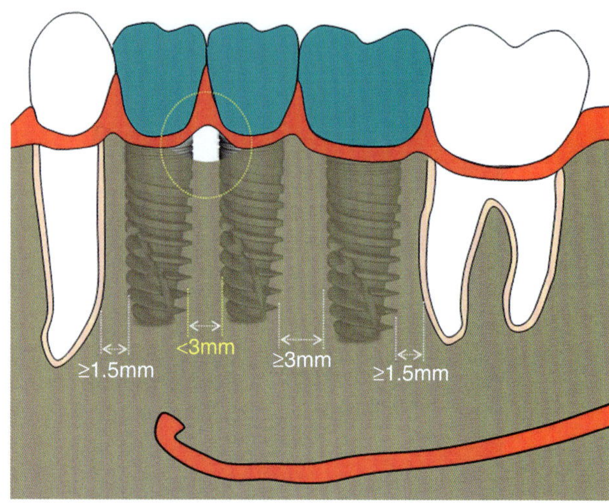

Fig 7.26 (A) Ideally 3 mm or more bone is required between two adjacent implants whereas 1.5 mm or more is required between implant and (B) adjacent tooth root for long-term survival leaving smaller margins may lead to vertical bone resorption.

implant, one should start pilot drilling at 7 mm (2 mm safety distance + 2 mm cross-section diameter of the implant + 3 mm for anterior loop) anterior to the mental foramina (Fig 7.32A–D). The anterior loop can normally be visualized in the radiograph (panoramic) but often it is not so clearly recorded in the radiograph. For such cases, the implant surgeon after elevating the flap, may insert a blunt probe into the mental foramina to evaluate the path of the canal.

Incisive foramen

The incisive foramen, which is found between and palatal to the two maxillary central incisors, contains terminal branches of the nasopalatine nerve, the greater palatine artery and a short mucosal canal (Stensen's organ). A vertical projection is found above the incisive canal along the nasal floor and is called the premaxillary wing. The reflection of the palatal flap rarely results in any bleeding or noticeable postsurgical paraesthesia. Based on findings from different clinical trials, the incisive foramen has also been used as a site for the implant placement in conjunction with placing more number of implants in the posterior region to restore a severely resorbed premaxilla.[1] After reflecting the palatal flap, all the soft tissue is carefully curetted from the metal foramina and implant osteotomy is prepared to insert a wide diameter (5–6 mm) and short length (6–9 mm) implant.

Thin mandibular lingual cortical plate with severe undercut (haemorrhage from the lingual and facial arteries)

Though very rare, a life-threatening haemorrhage can happen with the perforation of lingual cortical plate during drilling for mandibular implants, which may traumatize the two major arteries, the lingual artery (supplying blood to the tongue) and its terminal branches called sublingual arteries (supplying the lingual gingiva and lingual aspects of the anterior cortical plate of the mandible), as well as the facial artery (which runs under the bottom of the mandible in the second molar region). Significant internal bleeding from these arteries in the floor of mouth may result in a life-threatening haemorrhage which causes swelling of the floor of mouth and tongue, and respiratory obstruction. When such haemorrhage is noticed, the dental surgeon should pull out the tongue and place pressure along the inner and inferior aspects of the body of the mandible. He/she should also compress the site with one finger intraorally over the site and other extraorally, compressing the two fingers together. A haemostatic agent should be placed in the osteotomy and the patient should immediately be transported to the hospital, where the team of surgeons can ligate the injured vessels, give an endotracheal intubation or perform an emergency tracheotomy.

Implant distance from sinus floor

The sinus floor can be clearly visualized in dental radiographs and dental CT scans. The implant surgeon usually should place the implant, a minimum of 2 mm short of the sinus floor (Fig 7.33A). If inadequate bone height is present under the sinus floor, he/she should perform sinus elevation and grafting procedure to insert an adequately long implant (see Chapter 18).

Implant distance from nasal floor

The nasal floor can also be clearly visualized in dental radiographs and dental CT scans. The implant surgeon usually should place the implant minimum 2 mm short of the nasal floor (Fig 7.33B). If inadequate bone height is present under the nasal floor, vertical bone augmentation or nasal floor elevation and grafting procedure

[1]Scher ELC. Use of the incisive canal as a recipient site for root form implants: preliminary clinical reports, Implant Dent 1994;3:38–41.

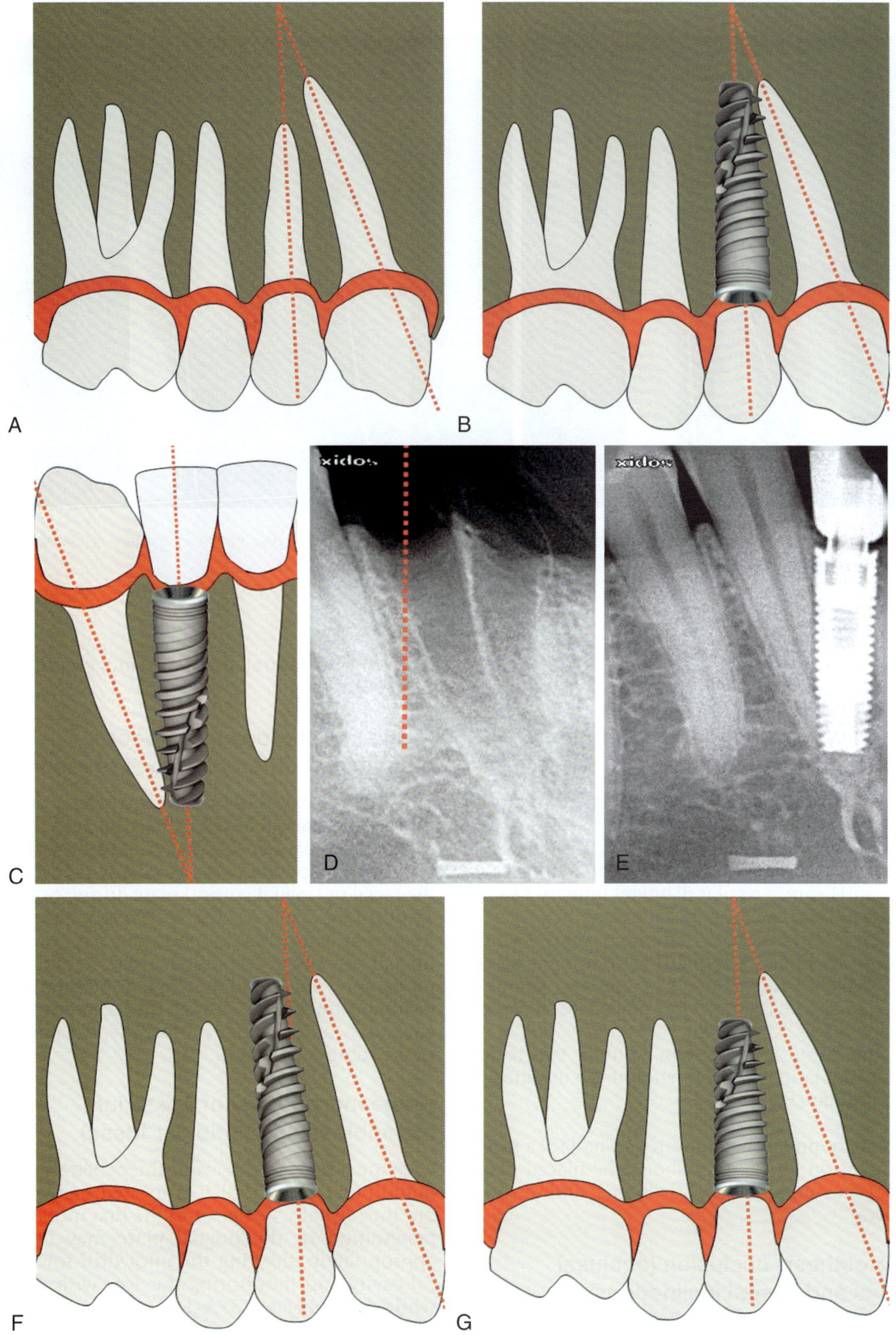

Fig 7.27 When planning for implant placement adjacent to the natural tooth, the implant dentist should always look at the inclination of the root of the adjacent tooth. The maxillary canine often shows distally inclined roots, whereas the mandibular canine often shows mesial root inclinations; hence, placing implants for the maxillary first premolar parallel to the second premolar, may perforate the maxillary canine root apex or encroach the periodontal ligaments of the canine root. (A–C) The same may happen if someone is placing implant at the mandibular lateral incisor position. (D and E) Radiographs showing the mesial inclination of the mandibular canine root, which has resulted in the perforation of the root during drilling and implant placement. (F) For such cases, either the implant should be inclined little away from the root inclination or (G) a short length implant should be inserted to avoid the perforation through the inclined root apex of the adjacent tooth.

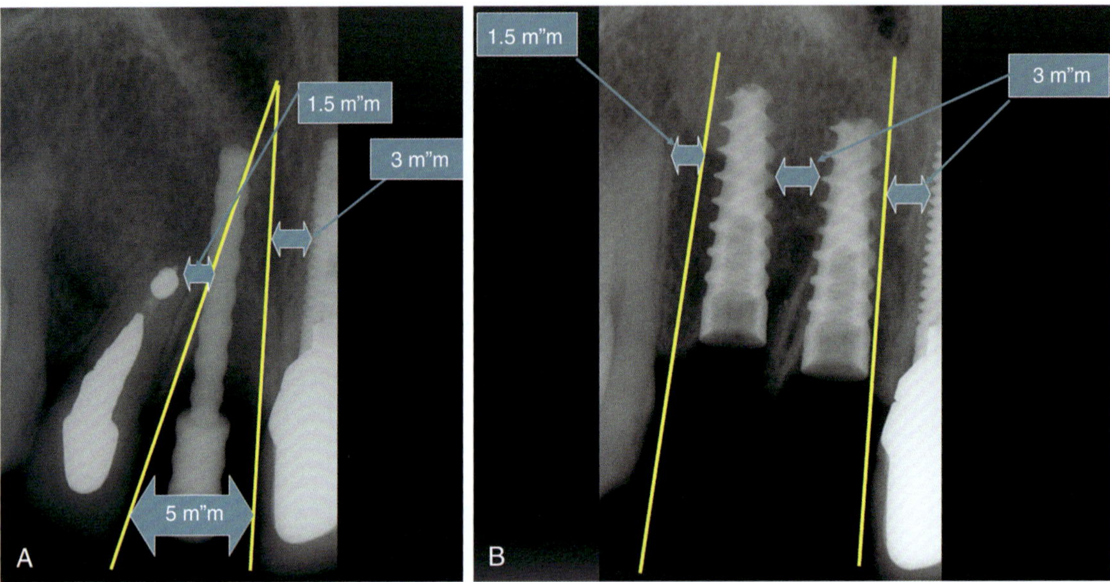

Fig 7.28 (A) Mesial inclination of lateral incisor root causes hindrance to correct osteotomy preparation for implant at central incisor position. (B) Decision is taken to extract the lateral incisor and replace it with an implant.

should be performed, to insert an adequately long implant (see Chapter 19).

Mesiodistal dimension of the edentulous molar site

Carl E Misch advised a protocol for the replacement of a molar which is as follows:

a. If the mesiodistal dimension of a missing molar space is less than 11 mm, a regular diameter implant (4 mm) can be inserted at the mesiodistal midpoint.
b. If the same dimension is between 11 and 13 mm, either a wide diameter implant (5–6 mm) is placed at mesiodistal midpoint or a narrow diameter implant (3.5 mm) should be placed to replace a molar.
c. If this dimension is more than 13 mm, two regular diameter implants (4 mm) should be inserted to replace a molar (Fig 7.34A–D).

Whenever two implants are inserted to replace a molar, if bone dimension allows, they should be placed diagonally so that one implant is slightly lingual and the other slightly buccal.

Implant prosthesis occlusion (occlusal dimensions and cuspal inclinations)

The implant prosthesis for premolars and molars should be fabricated with narrow buccolingual occlusal table to centralize most of the occlusal forces axial to the implant body and to minimize the offset occlusal forces on the prosthesis that may cause crestal bone resorption (Fig 7.35A). The implant prosthesis also should have low cuspal height (minimum cuspal angle) to avoid the tensile forces on the ridge crest during lateral excursive movements of the jaw (Fig 7.35B).

Ridge morphology of anterior mandible at different stages of resorption

The anterior mandible is the area where the bony ridge maximally changes its axial direction at different stages of resorption. The dental surgeon should carefully evaluate bony ridge topography to avoid any dehiscence through the facial or lingual cortical plate during osteotomy preparation (Fig 7.36A–I). The author recommends CT planning or at least intraoral palpation with finger along the lingual part of the edentulous ridge, to evaluate the ridge topography and avoid any lingual perforation, as it may result in (though very rarely), the laceration of the sublingual artery and produce profuse life-threatening bleeding in the sublingual region.

Ridge morphology of posterior mandible (submandibular fossa)

Care must be taken to avoid the penetration of the submandibular fossa, which is located below the mylohyoid line, usually posterior to the first molar. Inadvertent penetration of the lingual plate may be avoided by appropriately directing the pilot drill towards the buccal cavity and monitoring the area with digital contact while drilling (Fig 7.37A–D).

Ridge morphology of premaxilla

The topography of the premaxilla largely depends on the inclination of the maxillary anteriors and the amount of vertical and horizontal bone resorption in the premaxilla. The resorption of the thin facial cortical plate after the loss of the maxillary anteriors results in deficient buccolingual

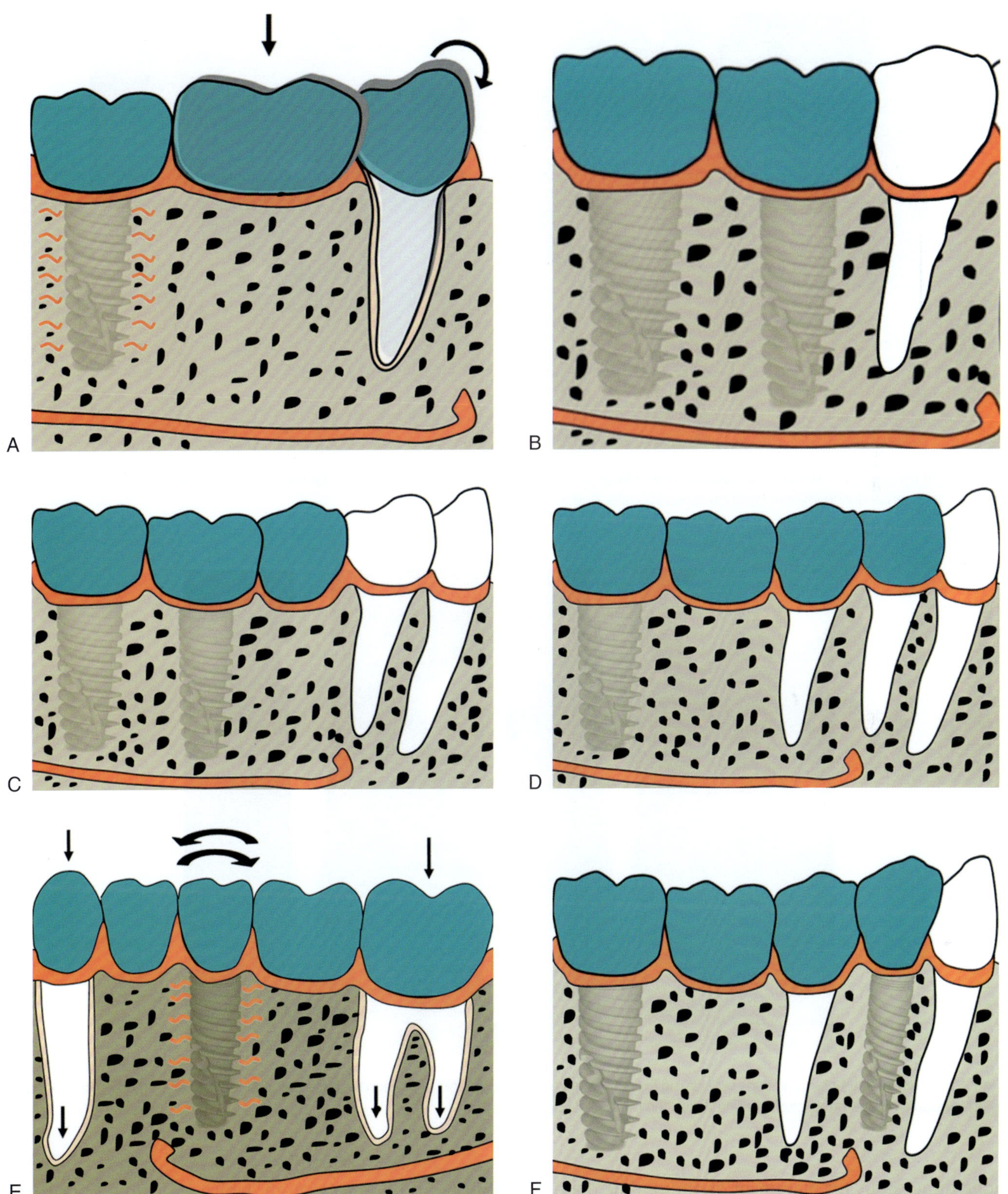

Fig 7.29 Implant if connected with the adjacent tooth may result in crestal bone resorption around the implant and its subsequent loss in future. The tooth has periodontal ligaments and hence shows movement during occlusal and lateral excursive forces, whereas the implant does not have any ligament and is osseointegrated with the bone, and shows very limited or no movement under the compressive forces. (A) Hence, connecting the implant with the adjacent tooth may compromise the implant's life. (B) To avoid such a complication, another implant should be inserted and the prosthesis should be supported only by the implants. (C) Whenever required, anterior cantilevering of the prosthesis is preferred if unavoidable, (D) the implant should be connected with two non-mobile firm teeth to reduce the movement of the implant prosthesis. (E) Using the implant as the pier abutment may also lead to the micromovement of the implant under the prosthesis and subsequently lead to its loss but the (F) natural tooth can be used as a living pontic between two or more implants.

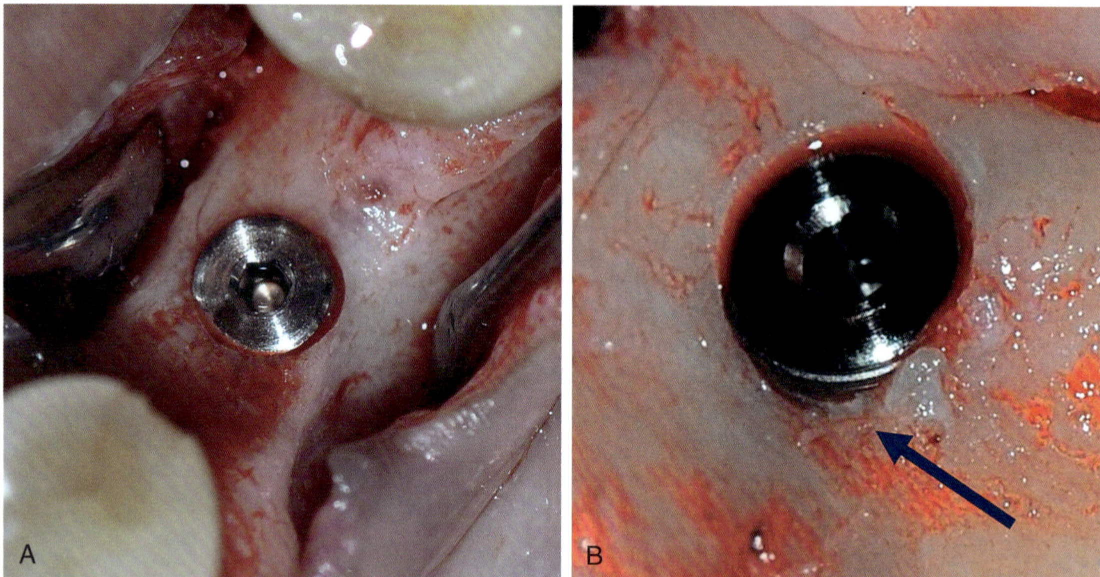

Fig 7.30 (A) Minimum 1.5 mm bone should be present facial or lingual to the finally placed implant. (B) The bone, which is less than 1.5 mm, either leads to dehiscence during implant insertion or resorbs later due to lack of nutrition.

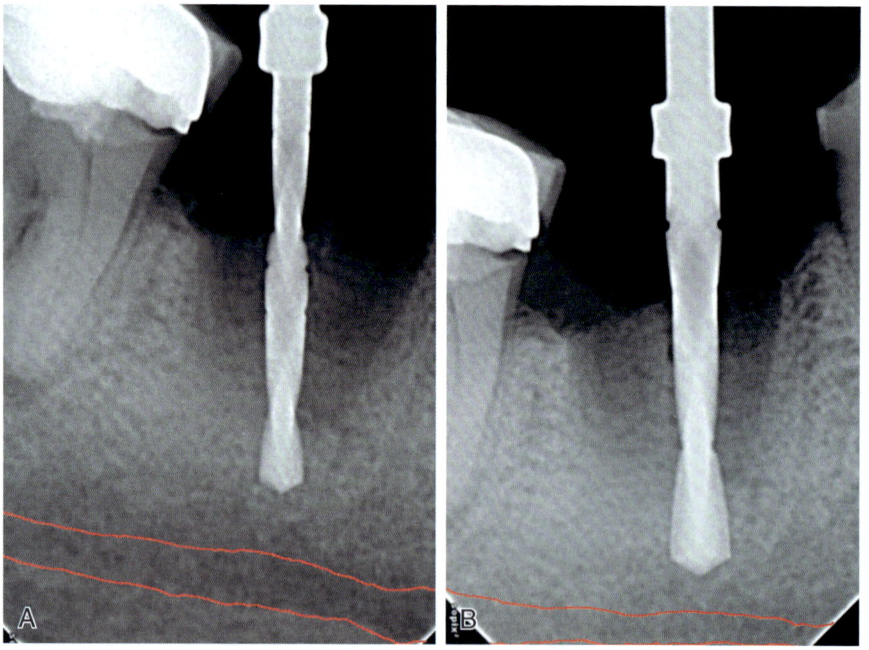

Fig 7.31 (A and B) Author recommends pilot drilling to partial depth and radiographic evaluation (with the drill inserted in the osteotomy), for the bone height available for the further depth drilling above the mandibular canal.

bone dimensions for placement of appropriate diameter implants. The presence of a thick amount of palatal soft tissue often makes it challenging for the implant surgeon to evaluate the topography and dimensions of the buccolingual bony ridge with only clinical evaluation of the edentulous ridge. The dental CT scan is a valuable tool to accurately measure bone dimensions and the topography of the underlying bony ridge. The patient with long time edentulism may be found with a large amount of thin facial bone resorption, which leads to a noticeable amount of facial concavities along the bony ridge. During osteotomy preparation, care must be taken to avoid bone dehiscence through the facial cortical plate in areas of facial concavity. Lateral bone augmentation or ridge splitting procedures often need to be performed for the placement of an implant with an appropriate diameter and at ideal angulation to achieve an aesthetic outcome in premaxillary region (Fig 7.38A–D).

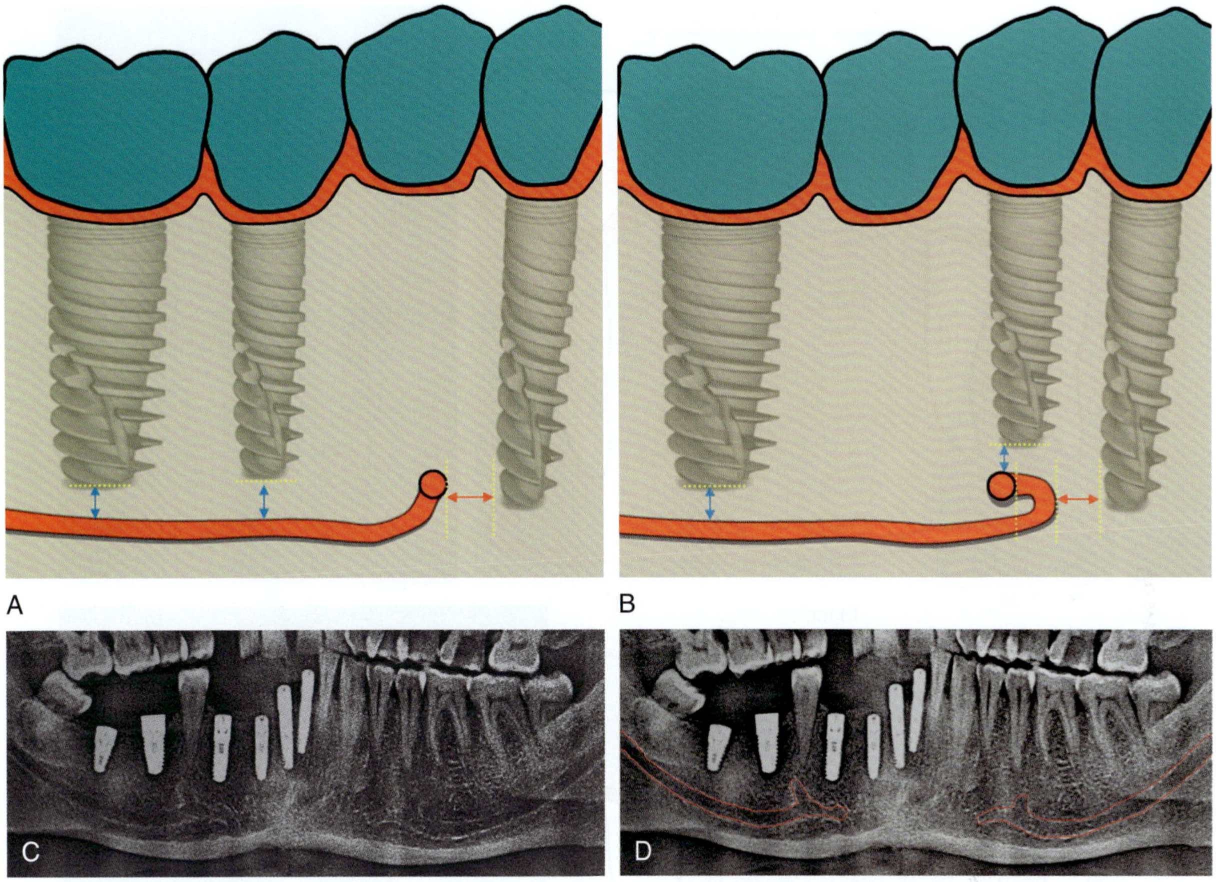

Fig 7.32 (A) Implant apex should end 2 mm short of the mandibular canal. If placed near to the mental foramina it should end 2 mm away (anterior, posterior or superior) to the mental foramina. (B) The anterior loop should closely be evaluated with radiograph, dental CT scan and/or clinical evaluation and if present, the implant apex should be placed minimum 2 mm superior and/or anterior to the loop. (C and D) The panoramic radiograph showing anterior loop of the canal.

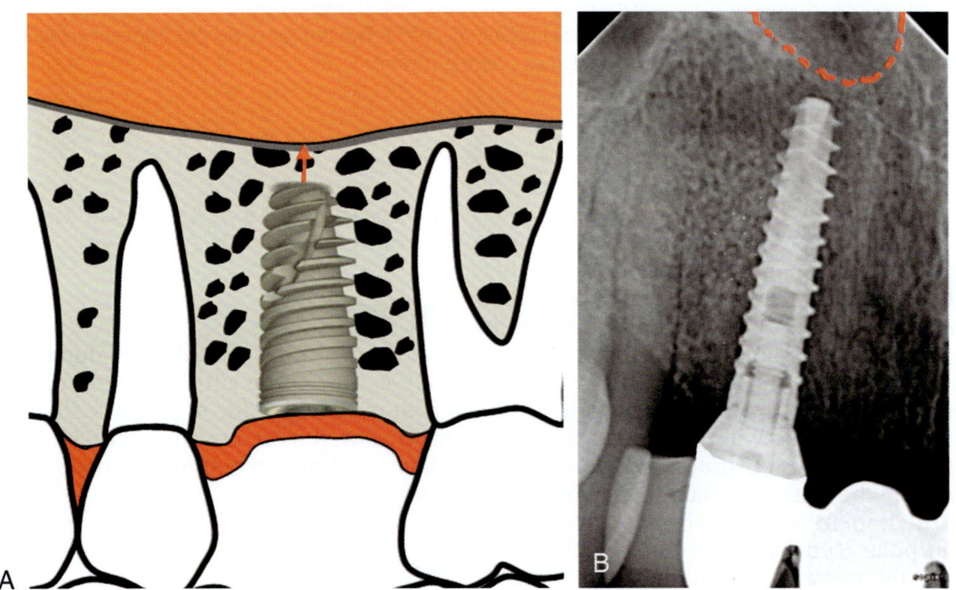

Fig 7.33 (A) On the safer side, the implant should be inserted 2 mm short of vital structures like sinus floor or (B) nasal floor.

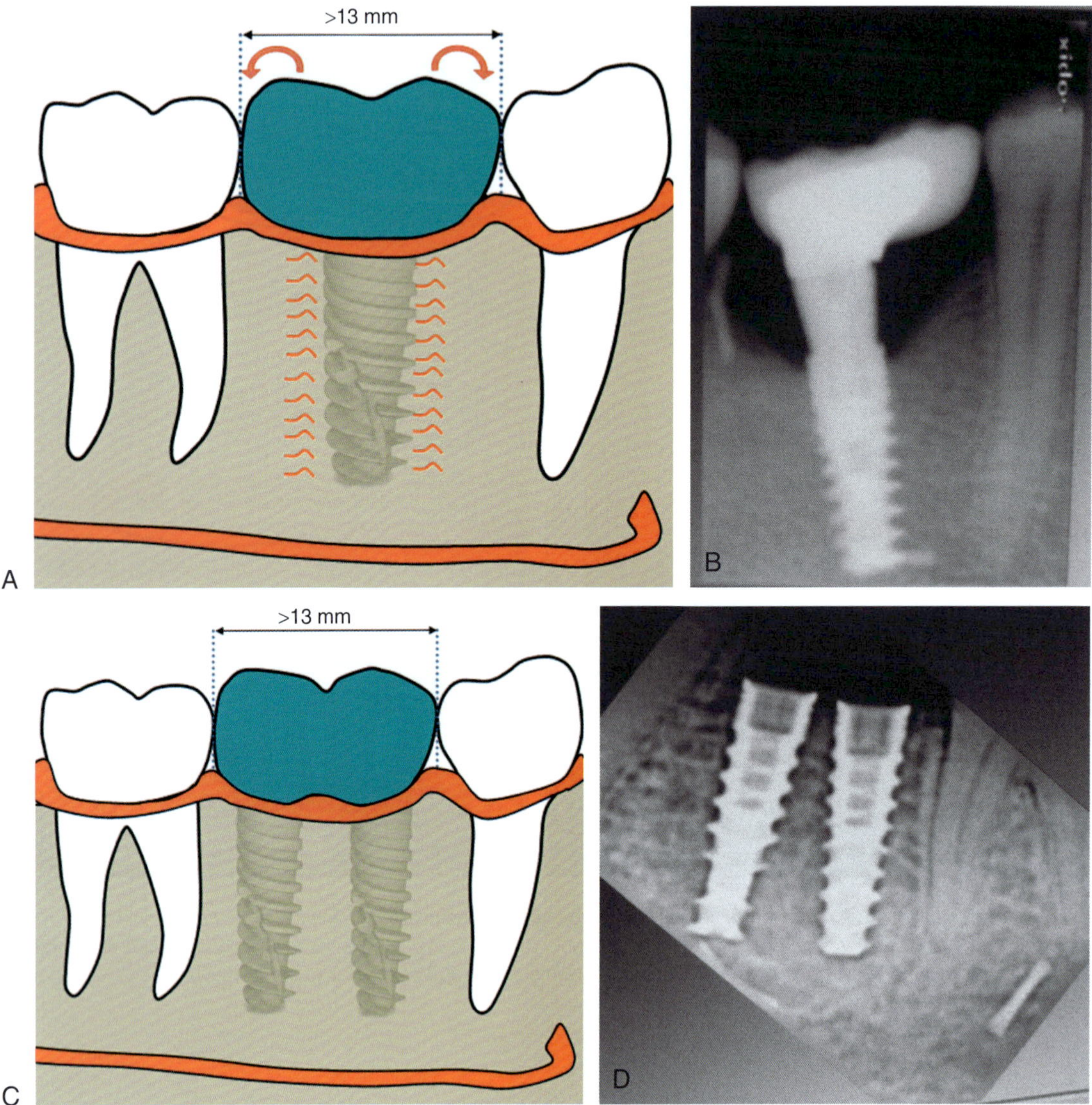

Fig 7.34 (A and B) If mesiodistal dimensions of missing maxillary or mandibular molar is more than 13 mm, it may result in crestal bone loss because of offset forces on the prosthesis supported over a regular size implant. (C and D) Two regular or narrow diameter implants should be inserted to support such prosthesis to overcome the cantilevering offset forces over the implant.

Ridge morphology of posterior maxilla

The bony ridge in the edentulous posterior maxilla resorbs medially and vertically but in most of the cases the implant surgeon gets adequate bone dimensions to insert an appropriate diameter implant. The posterior maxilla does not usually show any facial or palatal concavity but the ridge widens facio-palatally as moves apically. If the available bone dimensions allow it, the dentist can insert an implant with minimum exposure of the bony ridge. As mentioned earlier, the posterior maxilla resorbs medially and hence, the implant surgeon should evaluate the relation of mandibular teeth or prosthesis with the present bony ridge of the posterior maxilla. Often, a lateral hard and soft tissue augmentation is required to insert the implant at the prosthetically correct facio-palatal position and to achieve an aesthetic soft tissue emergence (Figs 7.39 and 7.40).

Lip lines

The lip positions should be evaluated, with lip at rest as well as during the smiling, when the implant therapy is given in the aesthetic region as well as for the full mouth fixed as well as removable implant prosthesis. The maxillary lip lines, when the patient smiles, are of three categories.

Low lip line

It shows no interdental papillae during smiling (Fig 7.41A). These patients are easy to treat as far as dealing

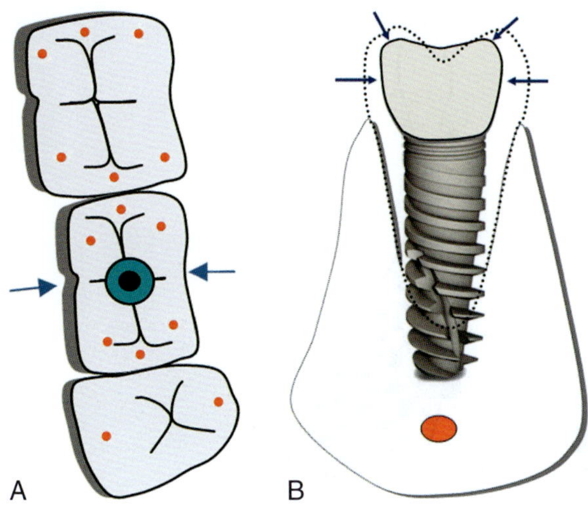

Fig 7.35 (A) The occlusal table of the implant prosthesis should be narrowed buccolingually to avoid distant offset forces over the implant but centralized later along the axis of the implant. (B) The implant prosthesis also should have low cuspal height (minimum cuspal angle) to avoid tensile forces on the bone crest during lateral excursive movements of the jaw.

with their aesthetic demands is concerned. As they do not expose the complete crown height and soft tissue, any prosthesis which looks ideal in the incisor half may satisfy their aesthetic demands. Other procedures, like hard and soft tissue grafting procedures to generate the ideal soft tissue drape around the implant prosthesis, are not usually required in such patients.

Medium lip line (average/ideal)

This type of smile exposes the clinical crown as well as the interdental papillae (Fig 7.41B). As they expose the complete crown as well as the part of the cervical soft tissue, providing aesthetic implant therapy in such patients is a great challenge. All efforts should be made to preserve any existing interdental papillae; if lost, it should be regenerated with the soft tissue manipulation and grafting techniques. Hard and soft tissue regeneration becomes often mandatory in such patients, to achieve an ideal aesthetic soft tissue drape around the implant prosthesis. For the multiple unit prosthesis in the aesthetic region or for the full-arch implant prosthesis, the dentist may also choose a ceramic prosthesis with gingival coloured ceramic to mimic soft tissue. When replacing the full-arch, the vertical ridge reduction during the implant placement, and restoration with hybrid prosthesis is also the treatment of choice to achieve aesthetic results in such patients, as it avoids the display of the transition line between the prosthesis and soft tissue.

High lip line (gummy)

This type of smile exposes the entire clinical crown, the interdental papillae, and the full gingival margin above the teeth (Fig 7.41C). These patients are difficult to treat when they are partially edentulous in the aesthetic region, and all the care should be taken to preserve the entire existing ideal soft tissue profile of the patient. For those patients, who have either lost the same or show any defect, hard and the soft tissue grafting procedures become mandatory to achieve adequate aesthetics. If patients of this category are in the need of full maxillary arch replacement, a considerable amount of vertical ridge reduction during the implant insertion surgery and restoration with either the ceramic prosthesis with a gingival coloured cervical ceramic or a hybrid acrylic prosthesis, is the treatment of choice. Ridge reduction is done to such extent, that the cervical margin of the prosthesis can be placed apical to the smile line to avoid the display of prosthetic base when the patient smiles.

For all three categories, if the patient is completely edentulous, the removable prosthesis over the implant is the treatment of choice to achieve high aesthetic results. The use of pre-fabricated teeth and denture flanges for lip support give a satisfactory maxillofacial aesthetic outcome.

Crown height space

The crown height space is measured from the occlusal plane to the bone level. The crown height space should be closely evaluated to select an implant with appropriate dimensions and implant components, the type of prosthesis, etc. A minimum 8 mm of crown height space is required for a single unit cement-retained ceramic prosthesis. If the crown height space is less than 8 mm, the screw-retained prosthesis should be preferred over the cement-retained one, to avoid the recurrent dislodgement of the prosthesis in the future (Fig 7.42A–F).

Excessive crown height space

Excessive crown height space may result in various long-term problems like stress on the implant, heavy weight in the prosthesis, more chances of screw loosening, implant component or body fracture, etc.

Management

i. Longer implants should be used to minimize the crown-implant height ratio.
ii. More number of implants should be placed.
iii. Regular or wide diameter implants should be used.
iv. Implants with more surface area should be used (parallel-walled implants should be preferred over the tapered implants).
v. Light-weight removable or hybrid prosthesis should be preferred over the fixed ceramic prosthesis for multiple implants or full-arch cases.
vi. Cantilevers should be avoided or shortened to minimize stress on the implant body.
vii. Multiple implants should be splinted together.
viii. Vertical bone augmentation should be done to increase bone height.

Reduced crown height space

Reduced crown height space causes problems like compromised retention of the cement-retained fixed prosthesis, inadequate space for occlusal ceramic layer build-up, prosthesis fracture, dislodgement, unaesthetic prosthesis with structural integrity problems in restoration, etc.

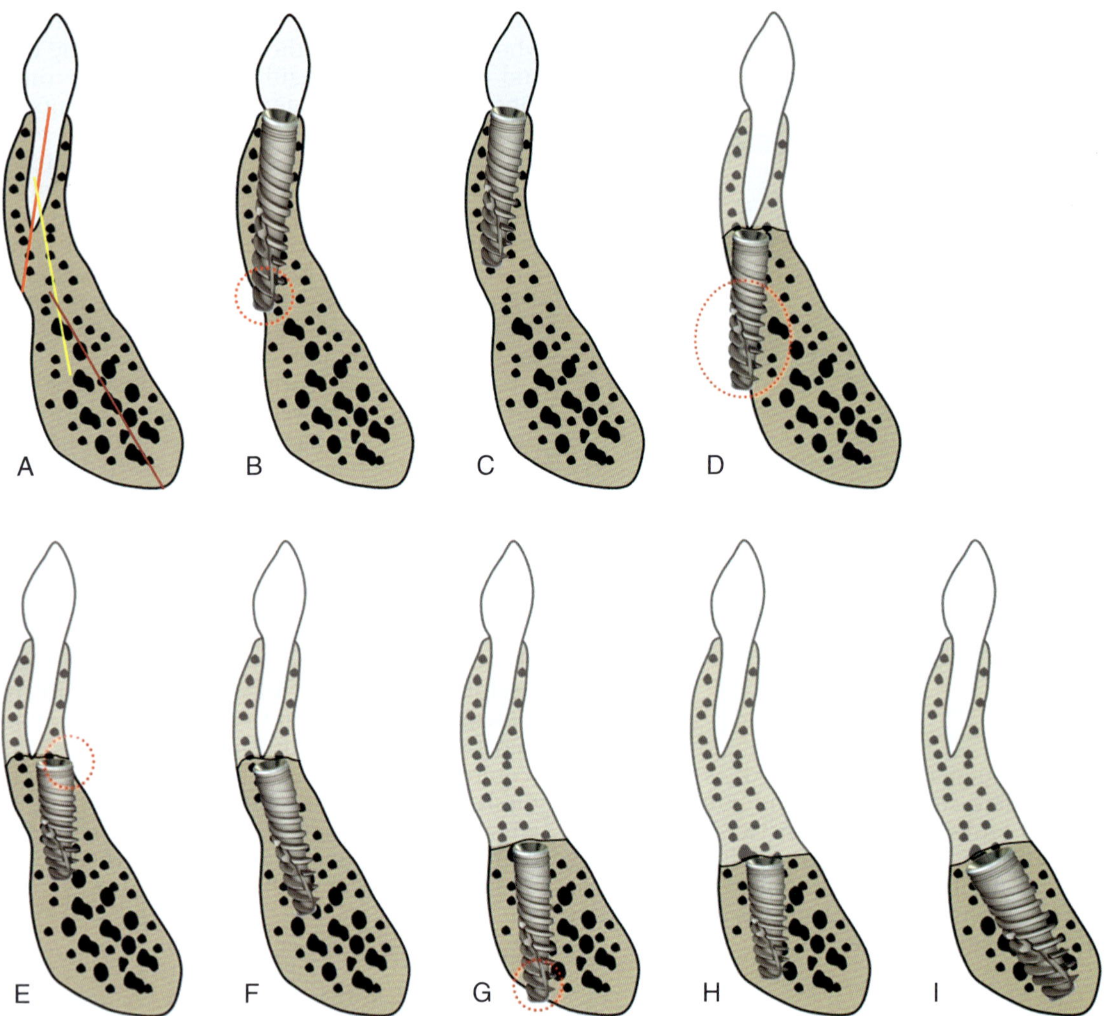

Fig 7.36 The anterior part of the mandible changes its buccolingual bone angulation at the different stages of its resorption. (A) The coronal part of the mandible often shows facial inclination and it changes to lingual inclination as it vertically resorbs towards the basal bone. (B) If a long implant is inserted with the correct prosthetic direction in a non-resorbed anterior mandible, it may result in lingual cortical plate perforation at the lingual undercut area placing a shorter implant (C) however, can avoid this complication. (D) In cases where the coronal one-third of the anterior mandible has vertically resorbed and if the implant is placed with the correct prosthetic inclination, it may result in a large perforation through the lingual cortical plate. (E) Often placing prosthetically correct implant and avoiding this perforation result in dehiscence at the facial cortical plate. (F) The implant should be inserted with little lingual inclination and an angulated abutment used to place the prosthesis with correct axis. (G) Placing the long implant with correct prosthetic axis in a severely resorbed anterior mandible may result in lingual perforation through the basal bone either (H) a short length implant with the correct prosthetic direction or (I) a long implant with little lingual inclination should be placed to avoid such perforation.

Management

- i. Osteoplasty during implant insertion to increase the crown height space.
- ii. Least possible taper in the abutment.
- iii. Wider abutment should be used.
- iv. Retention- and anti-rotation groove should be given over the abutment.
- v. The restoration should have a high precision fit.
- vi. Minimize offset forces on the prosthesis.
- vii. High-strength luting cement should be used.
- viii. The screw-retained prosthesis should be preferred over the cement-retained prosthesis.
- xi. Multiple implants should be splinted together to achieve the adequate retention for the prosthesis.
- x. The prosthesis with minimum cuspal inclination should be used.

Cantilevering of implant prosthesis (AP spread)

The human bone is strong under compressive load but shows lesser strength and gets resorbed under axial load. As the implant does not have any periodontal ligament like the natural tooth, it immediately transfers all the forces to the peri-implant bone. If occlusal forces are more centralized along the body of the implant, the implant transfers these forces to the strong basal bone, but if axial or offset forces are exerted on the implant, it transfers these forces to the ridge crest which may get resorbed

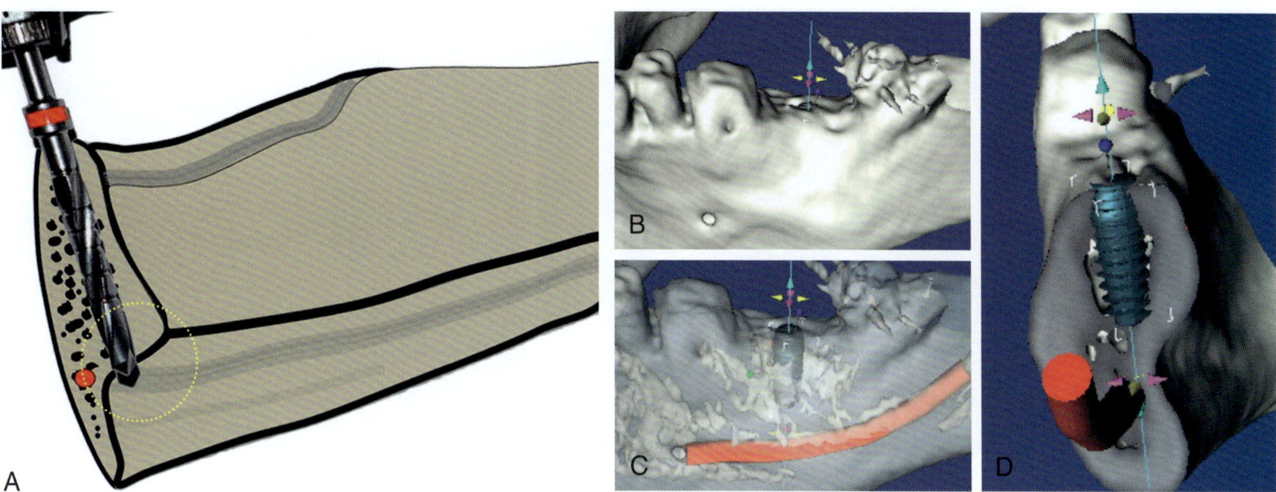

Fig 7.37 (A) Care must be taken to avoid the penetration of the submandibular fossa which is located below the mylohyoid line posterior to the mandibular first molar. Penetration of the lingual plate may be avoided by appropriately directing the pilot drill towards the buccal area and monitoring the area with digital contact while drilling. (B–D) Author recommends CT planning, digital palpation for the location of the lingual undercut, use of short length tapered implant, and tilting of the implant apex a little towards the facial cortical plate to avoid this complication.

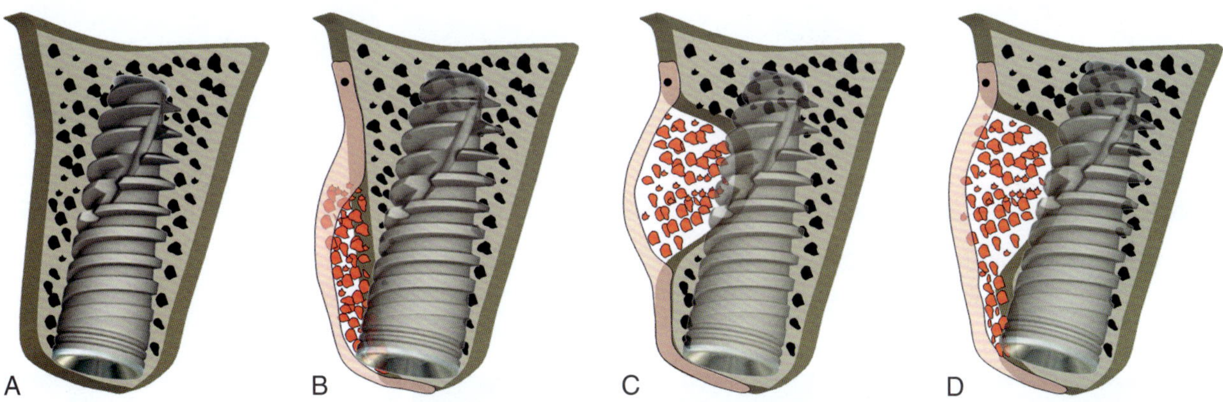

Fig 7.38 (A) Author's classification for the edentulous ridge morphology of anterior maxilla. Adequate facio-palatal ridge width for the insertion of an implant with ideal diameter, without any bone augmentation. (B) Bony ridge deficient at the crestal region requires lateral bone augmentation with or prior to implant placement. (C) Bony ridge with facial concavity at the middle third requires lateral bone augmentation with or prior to implant insertion. (D) Bony ridge with combination of crestal bone deficiency as well as facial concavity needs lateral bone augmentation with or prior to implant insertion.

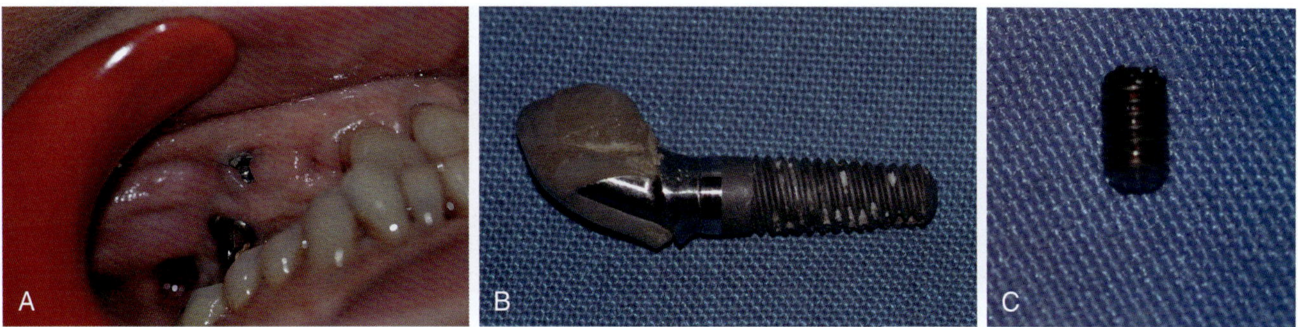

Fig 7.39 (A–C) Implant placement in the laterally resorbed posterior maxilla often leads to large amount of facial cantilevering forces on the implants, which in turn may result in loss of implant, component fracture, crestal bone resorption, etc.

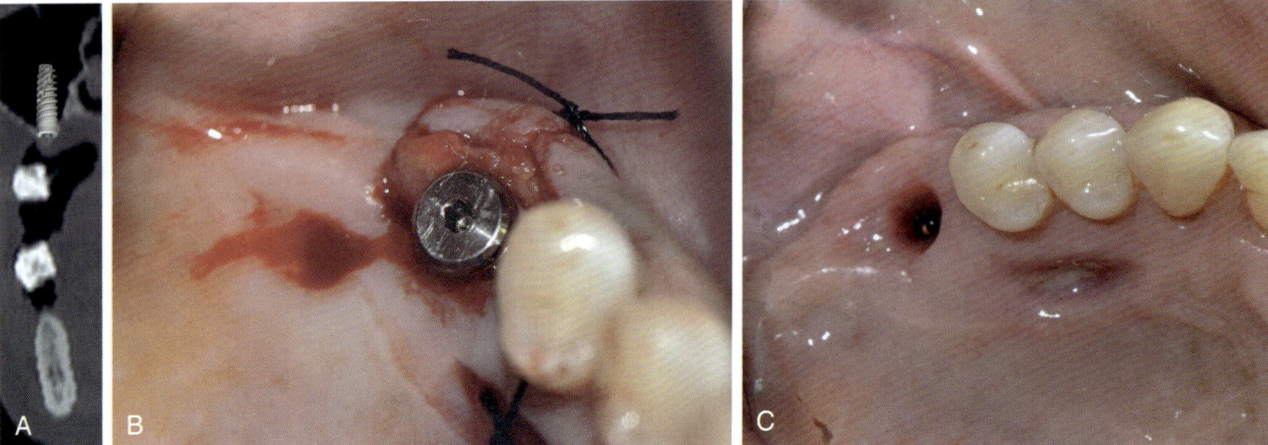

Fig 7.40 (A–C) The long time edentulous posterior maxilla often leads to maxillary sinus pneumatization and lateral ridge resorption towards the palate. Implant placement with only sinus augmentation does not solve problems like facial cantilevering and unaesthetic emergence profile facial to the prosthesis. Lateral bone and soft tissue augmentation procedures should be performed to place the implant at the correct prosthetic position and promote aesthetic soft tissue development facial to the implant prosthesis.

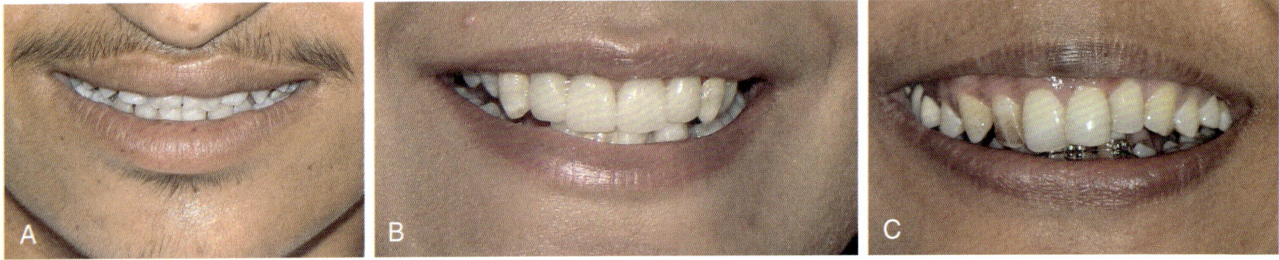

Fig 7.41 (A) Low lip line, (B) medium lip line, (C) high lip line.

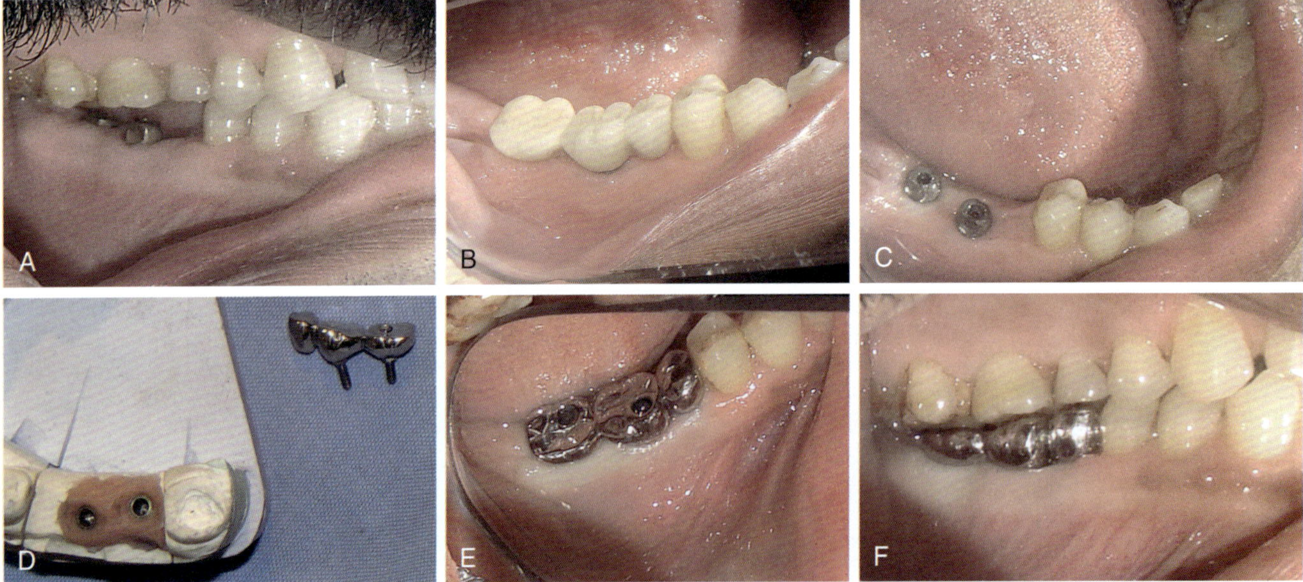

Fig 7.42 (A) Limited crown height space needed reduction of the excessive height of abutments for cement-retained (B) ceramic prosthesis. (C) Because of poor retention, the prosthesis repeatedly gets dislodged in very short spans of time. (D–F) The cement-retained prosthesis is replaced with a screw-retained metal prosthesis to prevent dislodgement and ceramic fracture.

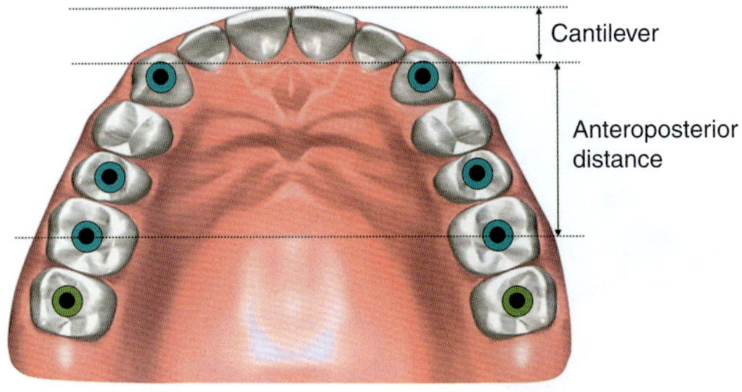

Fig 7.43 The amount of facial cantilevering of full-arch maxillary prosthesis depends on anteroposterior distance between the centres of posterior-most and anterior margin of anterior-most implant. If the facial cantilevering distance is on the higher side either an additional implant should be added on the anterior position or distal to the most posterior implants (shown in green colour).

under axial load. Hence whenever possible, cantilevered/axial/offset forces should be avoided or minimized on the implant prosthesis. The cantilevering of any prosthesis to a limited extent depends on many factors, but the most important are the anteroposterior (AP) distance between the most anterior and the most posterior implant, the dimensions of the implant and bone density.

Based on implant biomechanics, Dr Carl E Misch suggested that the extent of facial or distal cantilevering of a full-arch implant supported maxillary or mandibular prosthesis is directly proportional to the anteroposterior distance in the implant region (Figs 7.43 and 7.44).

Whenever required, the cantilever should extend mesially rather than distally, to reduce the amount of occlusal force on the lever (Fig 7.45A and B). (English CE: Biomechanical concerns with fixed partial dentures involving implants, Implant Dent 1993;2:221–242.)

Maxillomandibular arch relationship

The maxillomandibular arch relationship in the centric occlusion or centric relation position, should be evaluated in both partially as well as completely edentulous patients to avoid or minimize any cantilevered forces over the implant prosthesis. The maxilla is resorbed towards the palate and the mandible widens vertically it gets resorbed, hence inserting implants without evaluating the arch relationship may result in either cross-bite or facial cantilevering on the maxillary implants. For the partially edentulous patients, any improper skeletal position should be corrected orthodontically before implant insertion.

The patient's existing occlusion

The patient's existing occlusal in maximal intercuspation should be closely evaluated for occlusion abnormalities like supra-eruption of opposing tooth, drifting of adjacent teeth, axis inclinations of opposing or adjacent teeth, occlusal forces, and various stress factors (Fig 7.46). Any occlusal discrepancy should ideally be corrected before inserting the implant to achieve the optimal results.

Facial cantilever

As mentioned before, the maxilla resorbs towards the palate and hence reduces in size, in relation to the mandible which enlarges outward as it resorbs. This leads to facial cantilevering on the maxillary implants. Even the normal premaxilla shows facial inclination and hence, when restored with the implant prosthesis it always leads to some amount of facial cantilevering over the implants (Fig 7.47A–C). This cantilevering however, may vary with the maxillary arch form as the squarish maxilla delivers the least and the tapered one the maximum facial cantilevering. The numbers, positions, and angulation of the implants should be planned according to the amount of facial cantilevering. Often, the severely resorbed maxilla needs to be grafted for implant placement at the ideal position to minimize the facial cantilever.

As the maxilla resorbs towards the palate, the placement of the implant in the severely resorbed posterior maxilla often leads to facial cantilevering over the implant prosthesis. Which further get enhanced if such implant restored against the implant prosthesis of resorbed posterior mandible which resorbs facially (Fig 7.48A–D).

Direction of force

As previously mentioned, the jawbone is weaker under axial forces, hence all effort should be made to keep the occlusal forces centralized to the body of the implant. One should evaluate the direction of the occlusal forces if these forces are vertically along the axis of the implant body, less than 15° to the long axis of the implant or more than 15° to the long axis of the implant. With the advancement in implant inventories, the implant which is placed off axis can be restored using different kinds of angled abutments, but this does not avoid the axial forces on the implant body; hence all efforts should be made to place the implant with the correct axis.

Replacement of missing maxillary canine

The replacement of missing maxillary canines with a fixed bridge results in extreme cantilevered forces over the canine pontic during lateral excursive movement of the jaw, specially in patients with canine-guided occlusion; thus whenever the maxillary canine is missing, it should be replaced with implant prostheses. When the teeth adjacent to the missing canine also need replacement, the canine position should always be used as the primary site for implant placement. Whenever cantilevering a multiunit prosthesis in the canine region, it is always prefered to give the cantilever anterior to the canine position, as it offers lower magnitude of occlusal forces (Fig 7.49A–H).

Mandibular flexure

The human mandible distal to the mental foramina flexes towards the midline during opening or protrusive movements, due to internal pterygoid muscle attachment on the ramus. The mandible between the mental foramens is stable, hence whenever possible; the

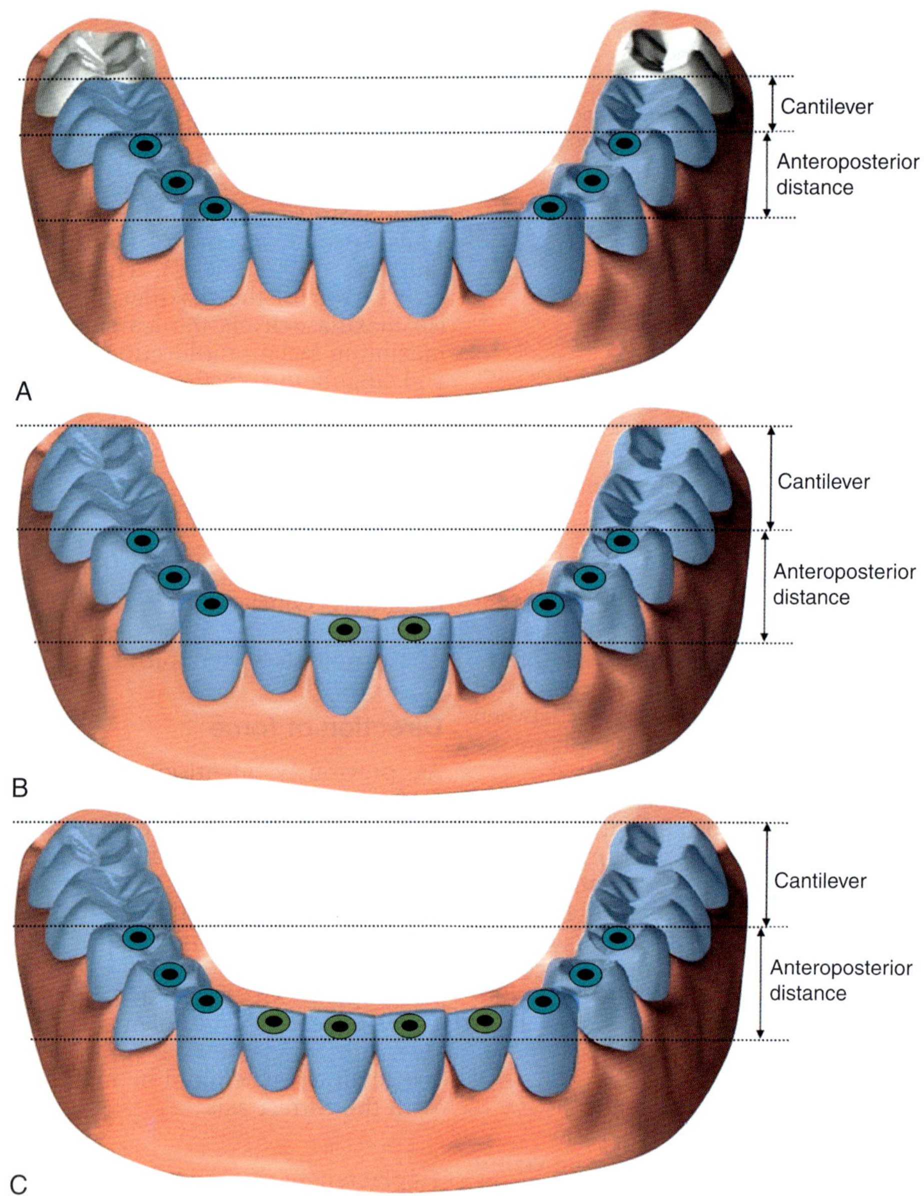

Fig 7.44 (A) If the bone dimensions posterior to the second premolar are inadequate to place an implant, a 12-unit fixed mandibular prosthesis can be given over six implants placed at the canine and premolar positions with the first molars given as the distal cantilever. (B and C) Two to four additional implants should be inserted anterior to the canine positions depending on the dimensions of all the implants used, if a 14-unit fixed prosthesis is planned.

implants placed anterior and posterior to the mental foramina should be restored separately to allow mandibular flexure (Fig 7.50).

Ideal implant numbers and positions to restore edentulous premaxilla with fixed prosthesis

The premaxilla is a common site for the implant prosthesis and this region is considered to be the most difficult to treat in implantology because of high aesthetic demands, compromised bone dimensions, facial cantilevering, etc. Thus using the correct number of implants and placing them at the most appropriate positions is paramount for long-term success and aesthetics. There can be different numbers of implants placed at various positions to support missing maxillary anteriors and this depends on the number of missing teeth, arch form, force factors, etc. (Fig 7.51A–H).

Number and positions of implants to restore edentulous maxilla with fixed prosthesis

The number, sizes and positions of the implants to support a full-arch fixed maxillary prosthesis is critical and largely depend on various factors like arch form, force factors, number of unit prosthesis, facial cantilevering, etc. when the cantilever forces and force factors are minimum, Dr Misch suggested only six implants of ideal sizes placed at the appropriate positions (marked with blue in Fig 7.52), to support a 12-unit maxillary fixed prosthesis. When force

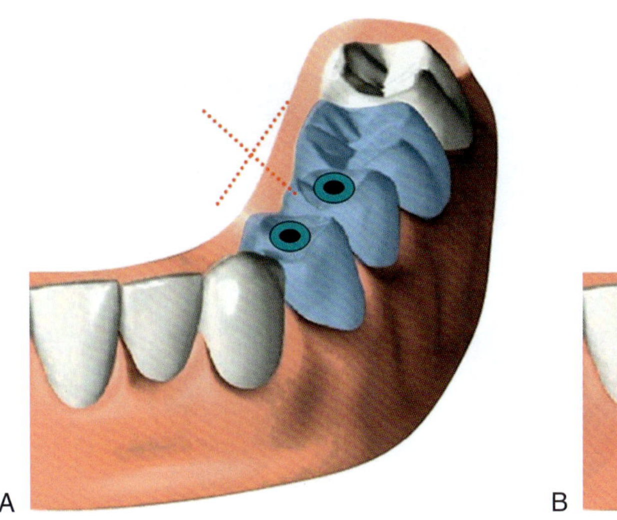

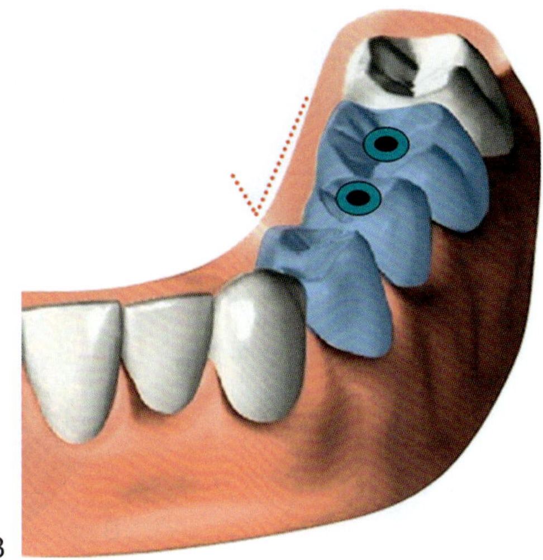

Fig 7.45 (A and B) The cantilever, when needed, should extend mesially rather than distally, to reduce the amount of occlusal force on the lever.

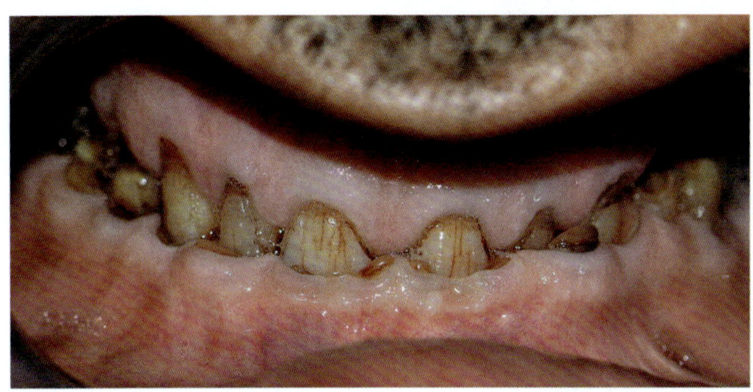

Fig 7.46 Evaluation of patient's existing occlusion is one of the key points to plan the number of implants, their positions and orientations and the kind of future prosthesis.

factors and/or cantilevered forces are moderate to maximum, one or two additional implants are added at the central incisor positions (marked with green in Fig 7.52). Two additional implants should be inserted at the second molar positions, when a 14-unit fixed prosthesis is planned (Fig 7.52).

Number and positions of implants to restore the edentulous mandible, with fixed prosthesis

The number and positions of the implants to support a fixed, implant-supported full-arch mandibular prosthesis depends on various factors like bone availability in posterior mandible, arch form, force factors, number of units in the prosthesis, etc. (Figs 7.53–7.55).

Numbers and positions of implants to restore the edentulous maxilla, with removable prosthesis (implant overdenture)

Fewer implants are required to support a removable prosthesis compared to the fixed prosthesis. The placement of these implants also, does not need to be as specific as in the case of the fixed prosthesis. Usually four implants of adequate sizes placed anterior to the maxillary sinuses are enough to retain a maxillary denture (Fig 7.56A and B).

Numbers and positions of implants to restore edentulous mandible with removal prosthesis (implant overdenture)

Usually the mandible shows high bone density and has no limiting structures in the anterior mandible to prevent placement of long implants. Thus if the ridge form of edentulous mandible is good to excellent, just two implants can give adequate retention to the mandibular overdenture. One should keep in mind, that placing two implants far posterior to the midline may result in forward rocking of the overdenture hence if only two implants are planned, they should be inserted closer to the midline to prevent the forward rocking of the denture. If the ridge form is poor and the patient demands high retention, three to four implants should be inserted (two implants 4 mm anterior to the mental foramina, and one or two implants closer to the midline) to support the mandibular overdenture (Fig 7.57A–D).

Progressive bone loading

When the dentist is planning to insert implants in posterior maxilla, he/she should keep in mind the limiting factors in this region such as poor bone density, higher force factors, pneumatization of sinus, facial cantilevering, etc. Thus various guidelines such as using largest size implant with deeper threads, submerging implant 1 mm apical to the ridge crest, longer time of submerged healing than usual, progressive bone loading, etc. should be followed in this region to deliver an implant prosthesis with long-term success (Fig 7.58A–F).

Fixed orthodontics for ideal implant placement

Any orthodontic treatment required to correct any occlusal discrepancy, create space, distalize the molars, etc. should be completed before implant placement (Fig 7.59A–D).

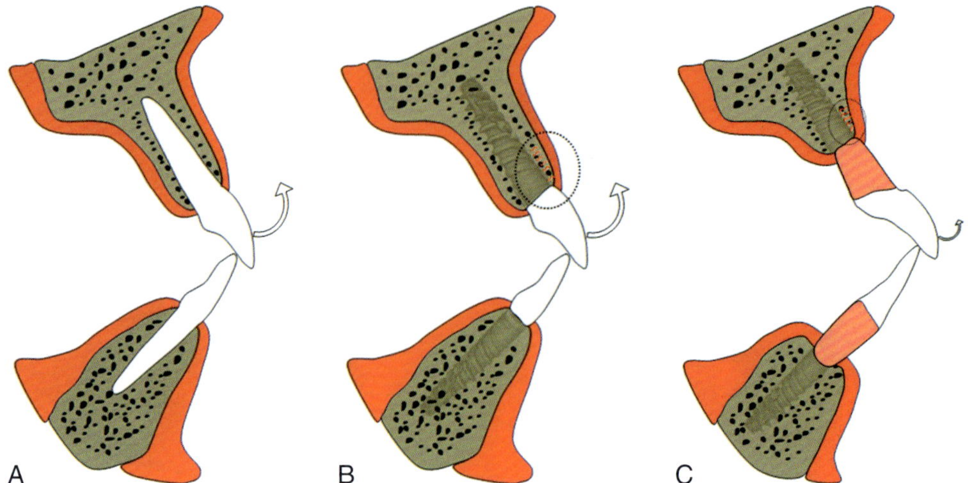

Fig 7.47 (A) The facial cantilevered forces are maximum on the maxillary anteriors, and get further enhanced in patients with bimaxillary protrusion. Whereas the teeth have periodontal ligaments which act as the shock absorber against transverse forces, (B) the implant does not have any such ligament and hence, transfers all such forces to the crestal bone ridge which may lead to the resorption of the thin facial cortical plate. (C) These forces further get enhanced when the premaxilla has resorbed vertically and palatally, and resulted in a long prosthesis with large facial cantilevering, to support the patient's lip from underneath. One should clearly evaluate the faciolingual relation of mandibular anterior teeth to the edentulous premaxilla, to plan for lateral bone augmentation, if required, and placement of implant with the ideal position and angulation to minimize facial cantilevering forces over the thin facial cortical plate.

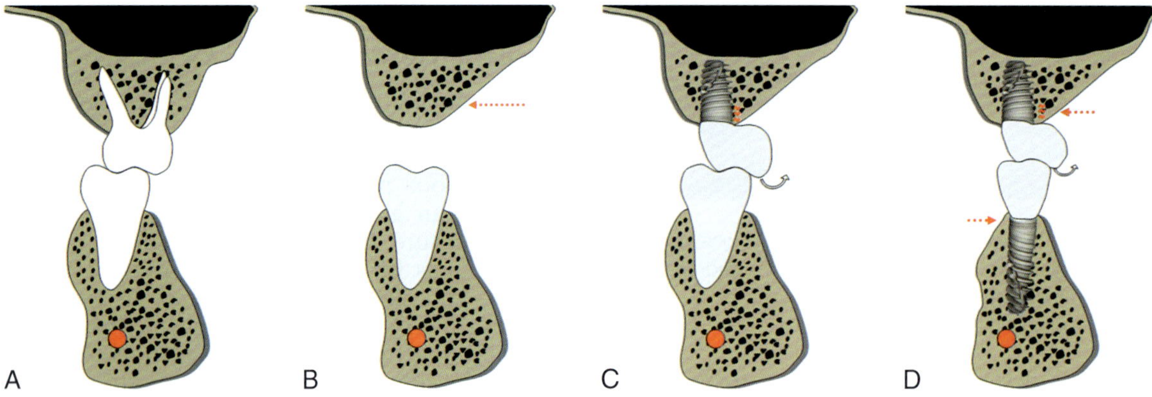

Fig 7.48 (A–C), Placement of the implant in the severely resorbed posterior maxilla often leads to facial cantilevering over the implant prosthesis, as the maxilla resorbs towards the palate which is further enhanced if such an implant is restored against the implant prosthesis of the resorbed posterior mandible, (D) which resorb facially.

Osseous defects

Any present osseous defect should be evaluated and grafted before or at the time of implant placement (Fig 7.60A and B).

Three-dimensional implant positioning in aesthetic region

Implant positioning should be three-dimensionally accurate in the aesthetic region to achieve optimal hard and soft tissue aesthetics. When the adjacent teeth are present with the free gingival collar at the correct position, the implant should be placed in such a way that its platform is finally positioned 2–3 mm apical to the imaginary line connecting the cemento-enamel junction (CEJ) of two adjacent teeth to achieve the adequate emergence profile through the soft tissue. The implant surgeon should also remember that if there is soft tissue recession and root exposure of the adjacent teeth, the implant platform should be placed 2–3 mm above the gingival zenith of adjacent teeth. The implant platform should also be placed 1–1.5 mm palatal to the imaginary line connecting the CEJ of two adjacent teeth (Figs 7.61 and 7.62).

Immediate implant in fresh extraction socket of multi-rooted tooth

When planning to place implant in a fresh extraction socket of a multi-rooted molar, one should place the implant at the ideal position, as placing implant in one of the root socket may result in off axis implant placement and offset forces on the future prosthesis (Fig 7.63A–D).

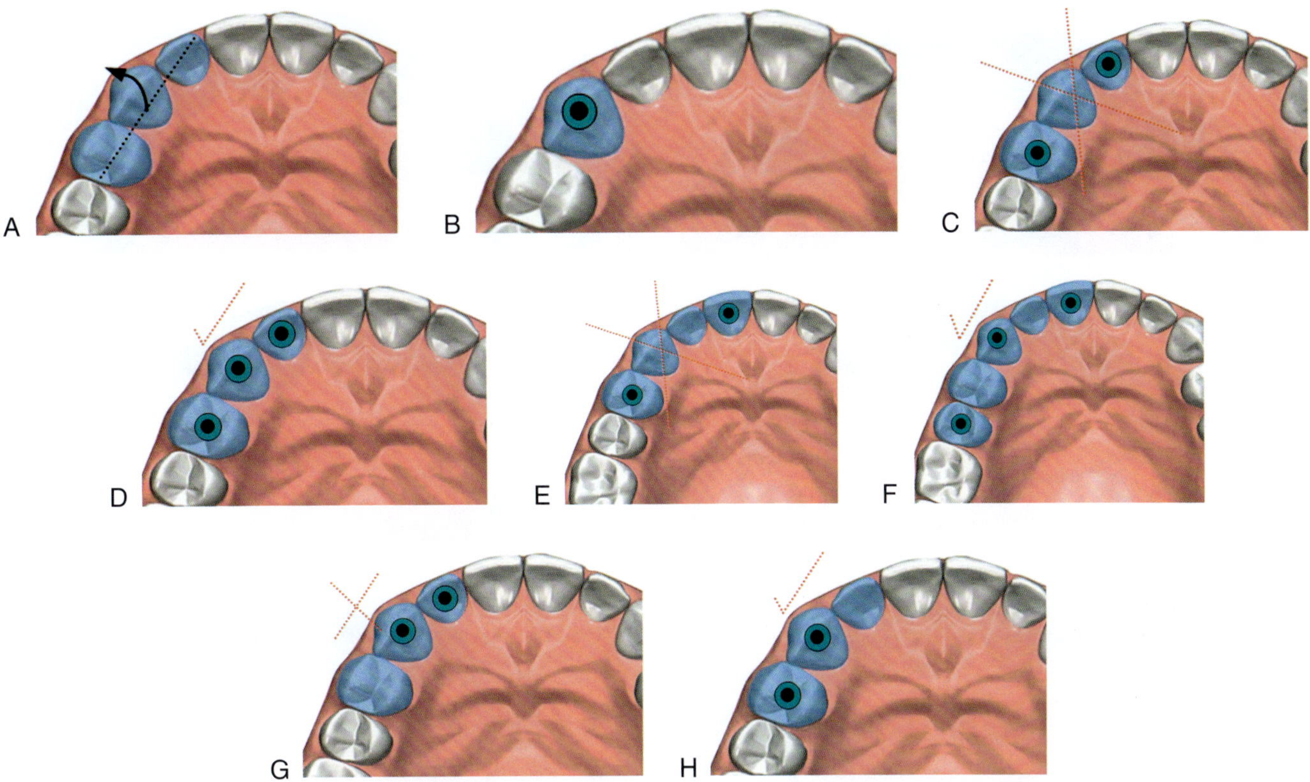

Fig 7.49 (A) The replacement of missing maxillary canine with a fixed bridge results in extreme cantilevered forces over the canine pontic during lateral excursive movement of the jaw, specially in patients with canine-guided occlusion, hence whenever the maxillary canine is missing, should be replaced with (B) implant prosthesis. (C–F) When the teeth adjacent to the missing canine also need replacement, the canine position should not be used for the pontic but the implant should always be placed at the canine position. (G and H) Whenever cantilevering is required in this region, it is preferable to give the cantilever anterior to the canine (less occlusal forces).

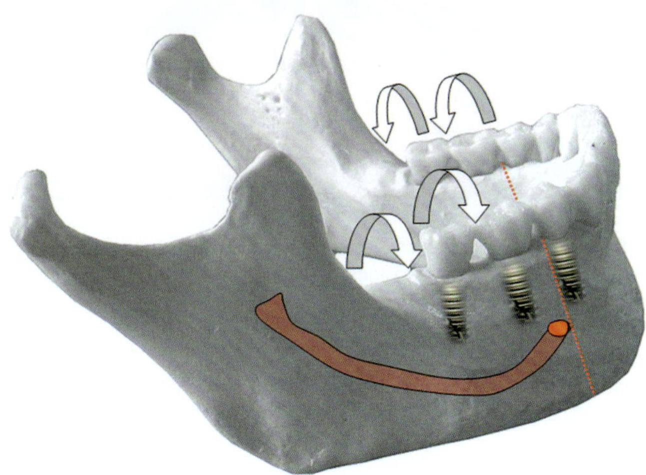

Fig 7.50 The mandible distal to the mental foramina flexes towards the midline during opening or protrusive movements due to internal pterygoid muscle attachment on the ramus. The mandible between the mental foramina is stable; hence whenever possible, the implants placed anterior and posterior to the mental foramina should be restored separately to allow mandibular flexure.

Financial evaluation and management of implant cases

The financial management of implant patients is of great importance for clinicians practicing in countries where patients are not insured for implant treatment. The financial evaluation of the patient seeking the prosthesis is very important and is part of treatment planning. All prosthetic options should always be discussed with patients, with the benefits and drawbacks of the prosthesis in a particular case clearly explained. Considering the high success rate of implant treatment based on literature, documentation and clinical trials of more than 40 years, implants should be the first option given to the patient, if the patient is medically fit for the same. A major disadvantage of the implant is that it needs surgical intervention and is expensive when compared to other prosthetic options. To make the implant treatment affordable and within the reach of the maximum number of patients, the dentist can offer different implant systems with a range of costings. Besides, as the treatment is completed in few months, the dentist may also offer an easy instalment payment option to the patient. The different qualities and costs of implants and prostheses should be discussed separately to the patient, to choose an appropriate option for a particular case. As many implant companies offer warranties on implants and their components, the practicing dentist should also forward these warranties to patients to reduce worries about the success rate and long life of implants. For the denture wearers, the affordable mini implants are the better option to stabilize loose dentures.

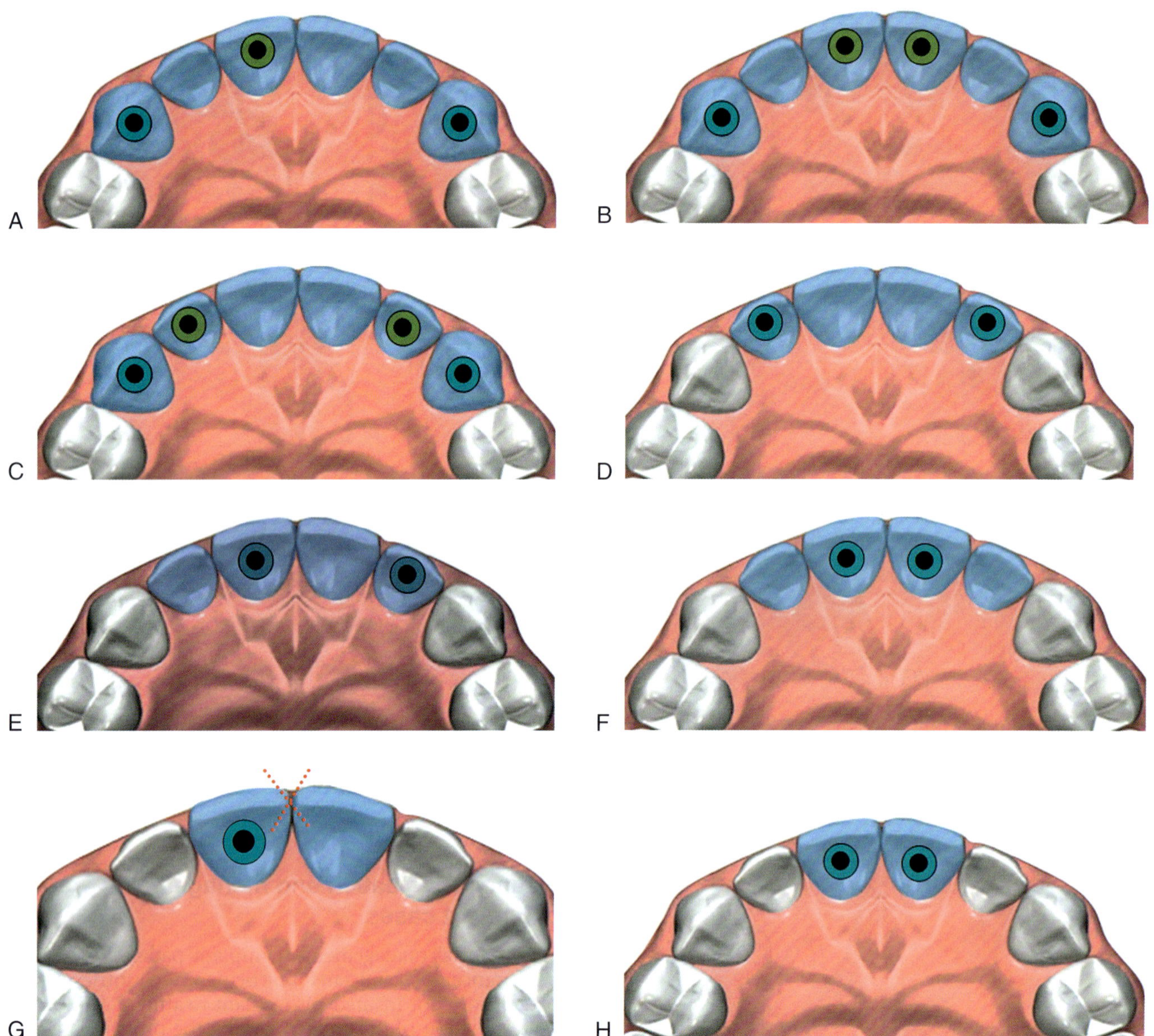

Fig 7.51 (A) When the arch form is squarish and the force factors are minimum, all the maxillary anteriors can be replaced by placing two implants at the canine positions. But if the patient has the oval arch form and the force factors are medium, an additional implant can be inserted at the central incisor position. (B) If the arch form is tapering and subject to maximum force factors, two additional implants should be inserted at the two central incisor positions or (C) at the lateral positions. (D) To replace only missing central and lateral incisors, the two implants should preferably be inserted at the two lateral positions but if the implant placement is not possible at the lateral position because of any bone defect, (E and F) the two implants can be inserted at any central or lateral positions to give the cantilevered prosthesis. (G) If only two central incisors are missing, a cantilevered prosthesis over one implant should be avoided but (H) two implants should be inserted to replace both the incisors.

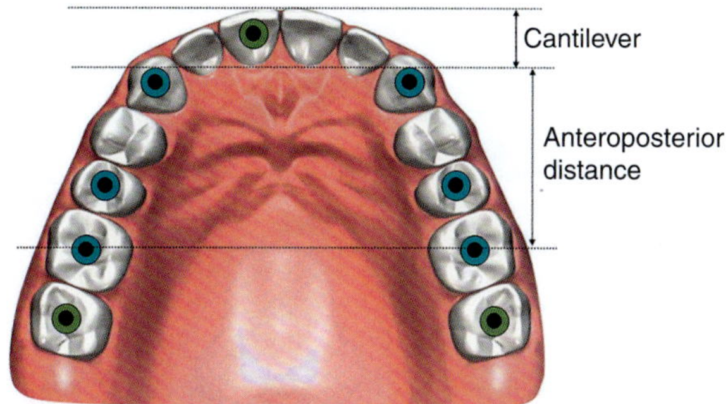

Fig 7.52 When the cantilever forces and force factors are minimum, Dr Misch suggests only six implants of ideal sizes placed at the appropriate positions (marked with blue) to support a 12-unit maxillary fixed prosthesis. When force factors and/or cantilevered forces are moderate to maximum, one or two additional implants are added at the central incisor positions (marked with green). Two additional implants should be inserted at the second molar positions, when a 14-unit fixed prosthesis is planned.

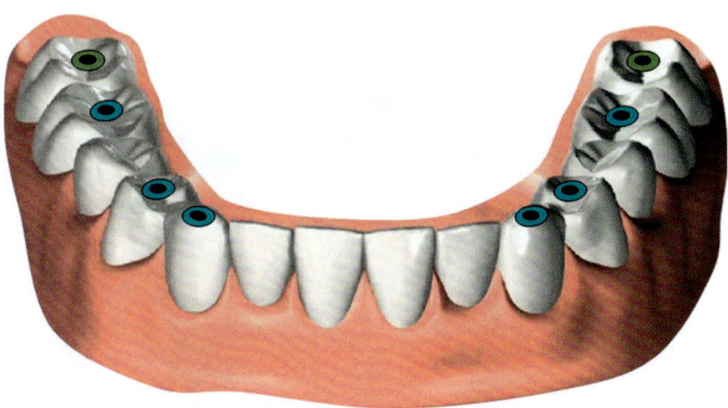

Fig 7.53 When force factors are minimum to moderate, six implants can be placed at the appropriate positions (marked in blue) to support a 12-unit fixed prosthesis. The additional implants should be added at the second molar positions (marked in green) if a 14-unit prosthesis is planned.

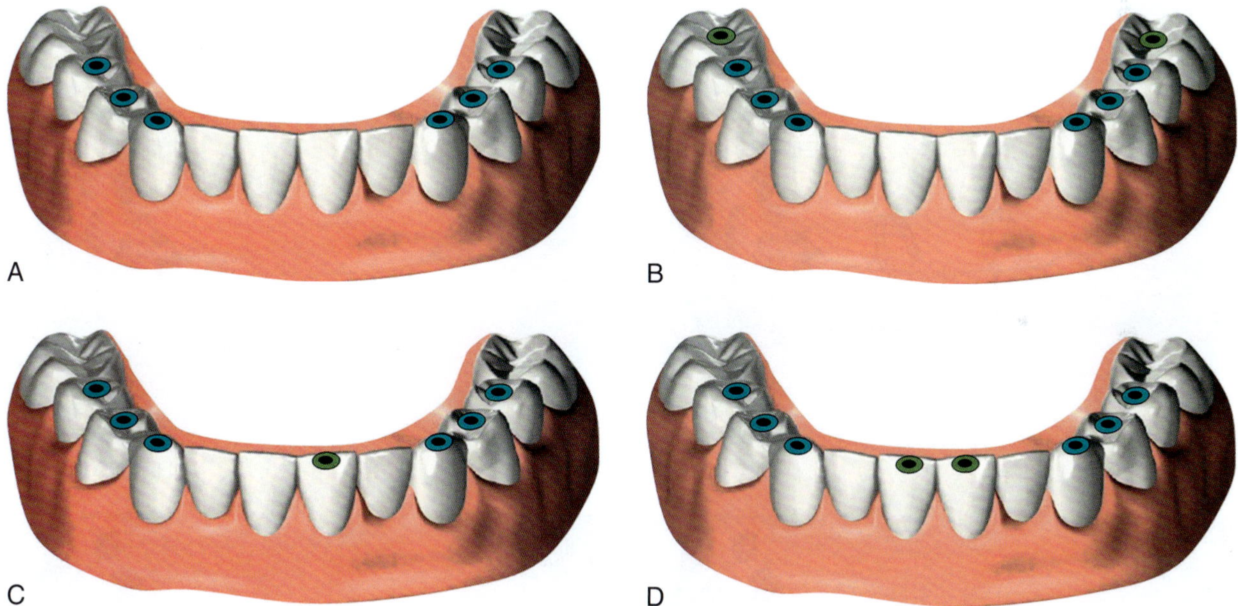

Fig 7.54 (A) If the implant placement at first molar sites is not possible due to insufficient bone dimensions and if the force factors are minimum, a cantilevered prosthesis can be given on six implants for a 12-unit fixed prosthesis. (B) If the force factors are moderate to maximum, and the arch form is square shaped, either two additional implants should be inserted at the molar positions or if not possible, (C and D) one or two implants should be added anterior to the canine positions.

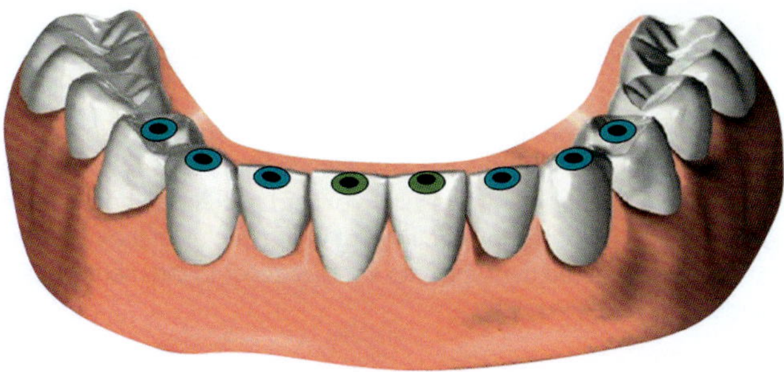

Fig 7.55 If the placement at the second premolar and molar positions is not possible due to inadequate bone volume, a 12-unit cantilevered prosthesis can be given over six to eight implants as shown in the figure.

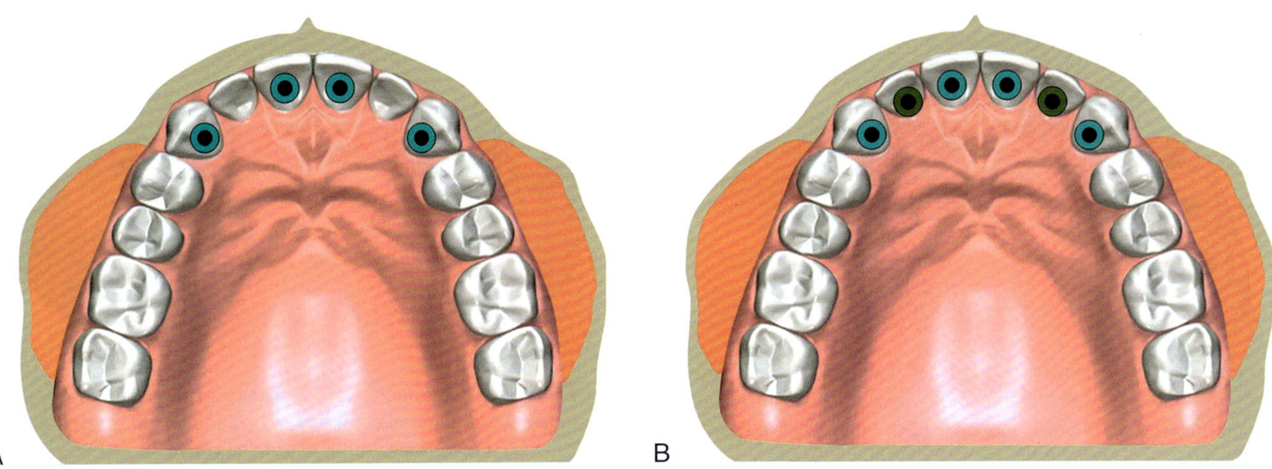

Fig 7.56 Maxillary ridge resorption and pneumatization of the maxillary sinuses often limits the placement of the implants anterior to the anterior wall of the sinus; hence if adequate bone dimensions are available in maxillary anterior region four implants can usually give the adequate retention to a maxillary overdenture. (A) As the maxilla has the medium to low density bone, placement of at least four implants is paramount to retain the maxillary overdenture but if the bone density and the dimensions are not favourable to place regular diameter implants or if the force factors are maximum, (B) two additional implants should be inserted.

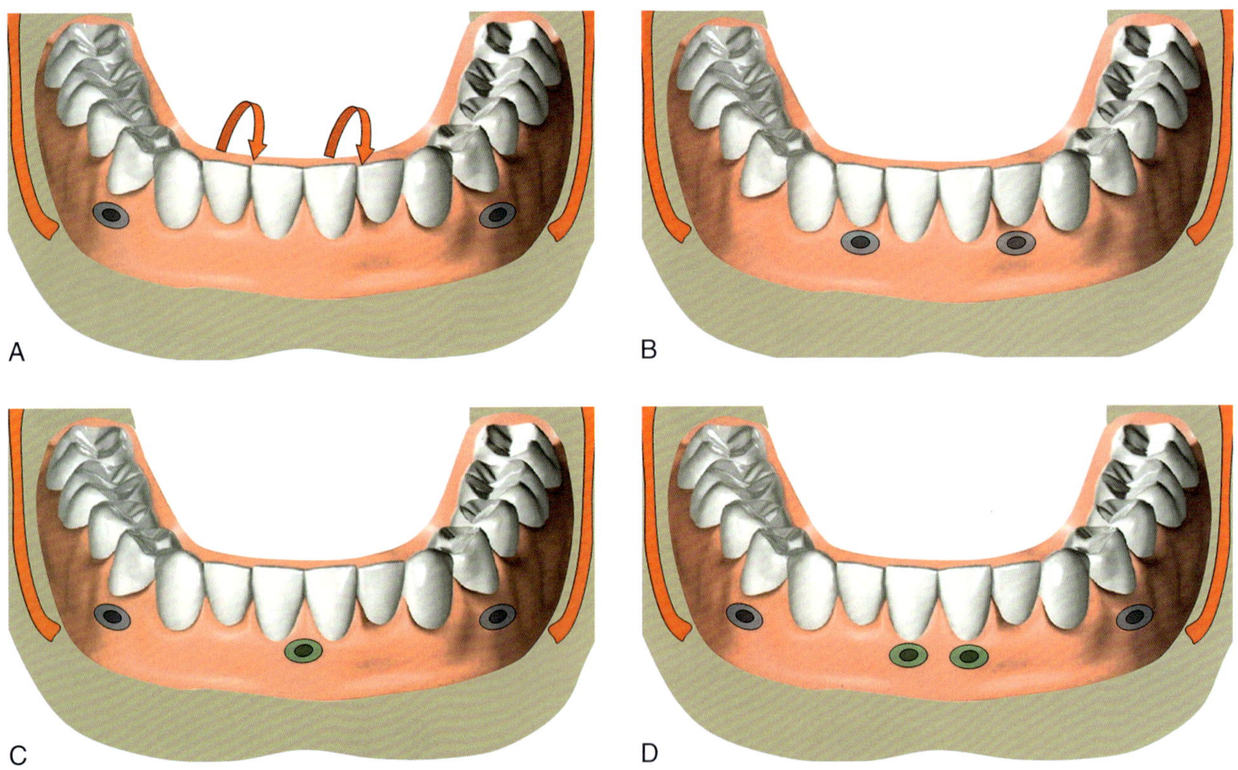

Fig 7.57 Usually the mandible shows high bone density and no limiting structures in the anterior mandible, to place long implants. Thus if the ridge form of edentulous mandible is good to excellent, only two implants can give the adequate retention to the mandibular overdenture. (A) One should keep in mind, placing two implants far posterior to the midline may result in forward rocking of the overdenture hence if only (B) two implants are planned, should be inserted closer to the midline to prevent the forward rocking of the denture if the ridge form is poor and patient is asking for high retention, (C and D) three to four implants should be inserted (two implants 4 mm anterior to the mental foramina, and one or two implants closer to the midline) to support the mandibular overdenture.

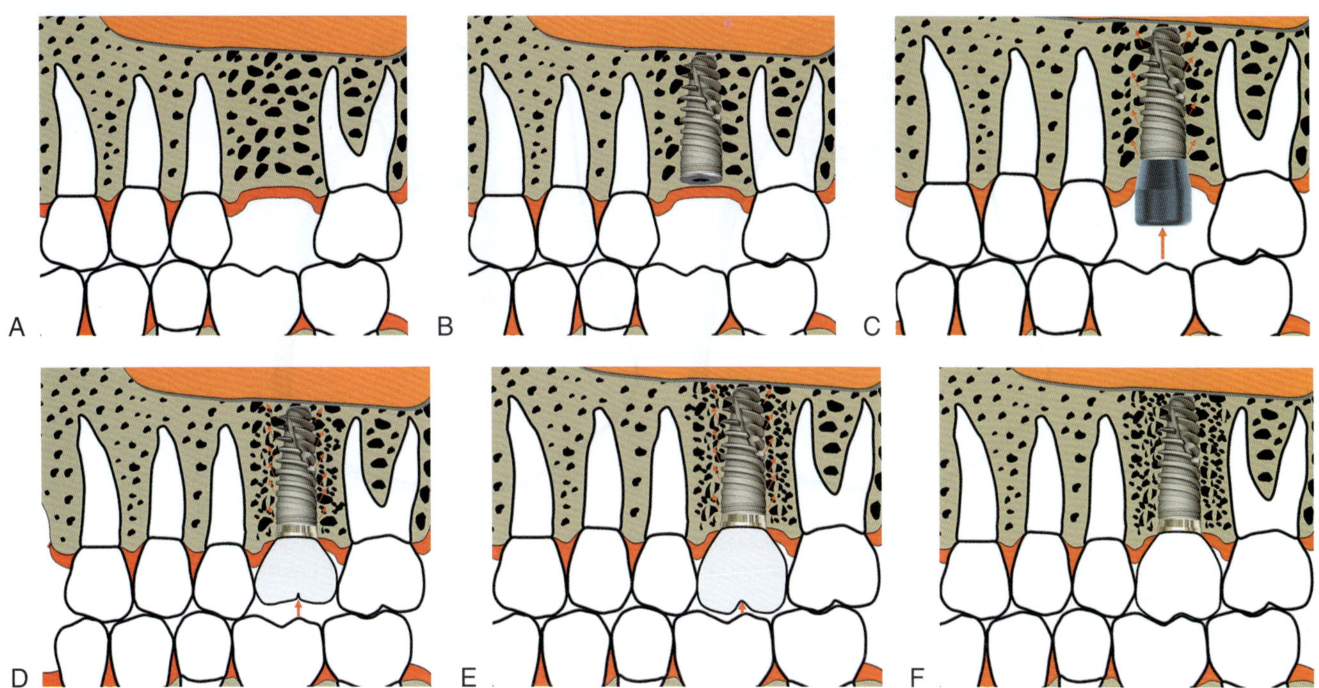

Fig 7.58 (A and B) When implant is inserted into a low density bone (e.g. posterior maxilla), one should plan to submerge the implant 1 mm apical to the ridge crest to avoid premature loading and micromovements during the healing phase. The osseointegrated implant in such bone shows poor amount of trabecular bone attachment to the implant surface (lesser bone implant contact percentage) which does not provide adequate strength to bear the heavy occlusal forces and often result in implant failure after loading. Hence to strengthen the trabecular bone around the osseointegrated implant; the later should progressively be loaded. (C) The osseointegrated implant is uncovered and low profile gingival former is inserted. (D) This gingival former is replaced by a provisional prosthesis which is kept 3–4 mm out of occlusion and patients instructed for not to chew anything very hard. (E) Further, the material is added to the occlusal surface of the provisional prosthesis at two to three weeks intervals. The provisional prosthesis should preferably be fabricated with resilient self-cure acrylic as it acts as the shock absorber and does not immediately transfer the occlusal forces to the implant like the ceramic prosthesis. (F) After the patient has been chewing with the provisional prosthesis for a month, it can be later replaced with the long-term ceramic prosthesis. Progressive loading results in strengthening of the trabecular bone and increased bone density around the implant.

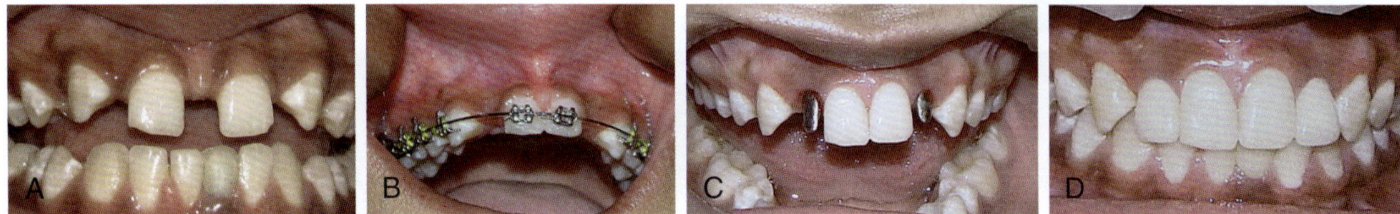

Fig 7.59 (A–D) All the necessary orthodontic treatments should be done, to regain the spaces for implant placement or correct different malpositioning problems, before implant insertion at the appropriate position.

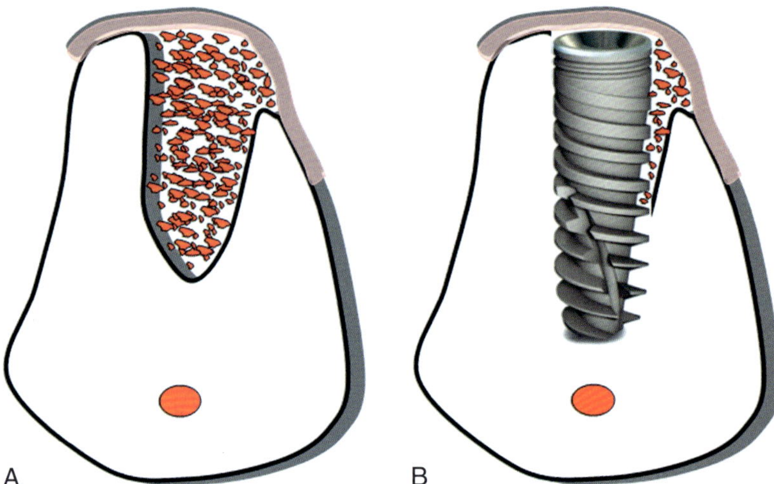

Fig 7.60 Any present osseous defect should be properly evaluated for size and topography with the help of radiograph and dental CT scan. (A) If any defect is present it should be grafted before implant placement or (B) simultaneously with implant placement. Leaving any defect, however small, uncorrected may compromise the life of the implant.

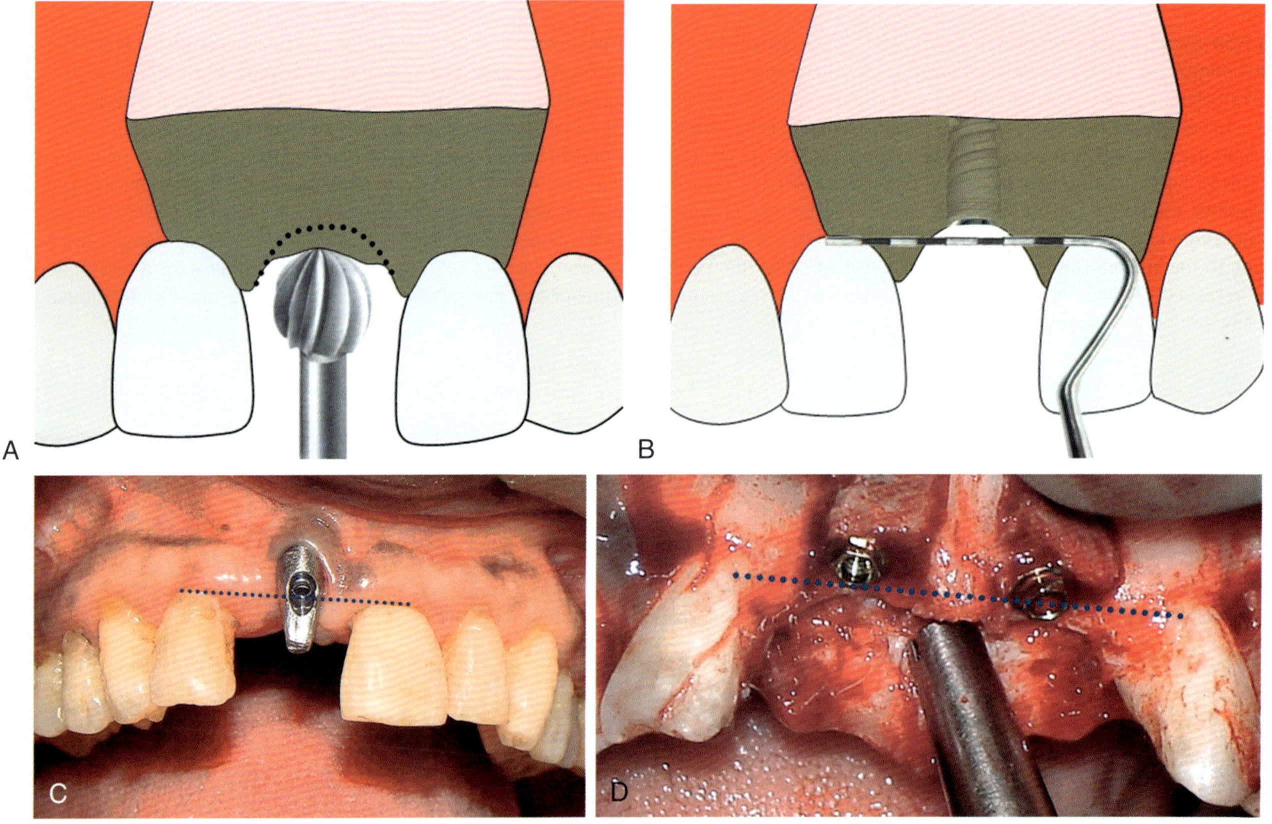

Fig 7.61 (A) When placing an implant in a region with high aesthetics, any irregular bony crest should be ground to create a 'C' shaped osseous topography and (B) the implant is placed 2–3 mm apical to an imaginary line between the CEJ of two adjacent teeth. The implant surgeon should remember, if there is soft tissue recession and root exposure of adjacent teeth, then the implant platform should be placed 2–3 mm above the gingival zenith of adjacent teeth. (C) The incorrectly placed implant. (D) Implants placed correctly 2–3 mm apical to the CEJ of the adjacent teeth.

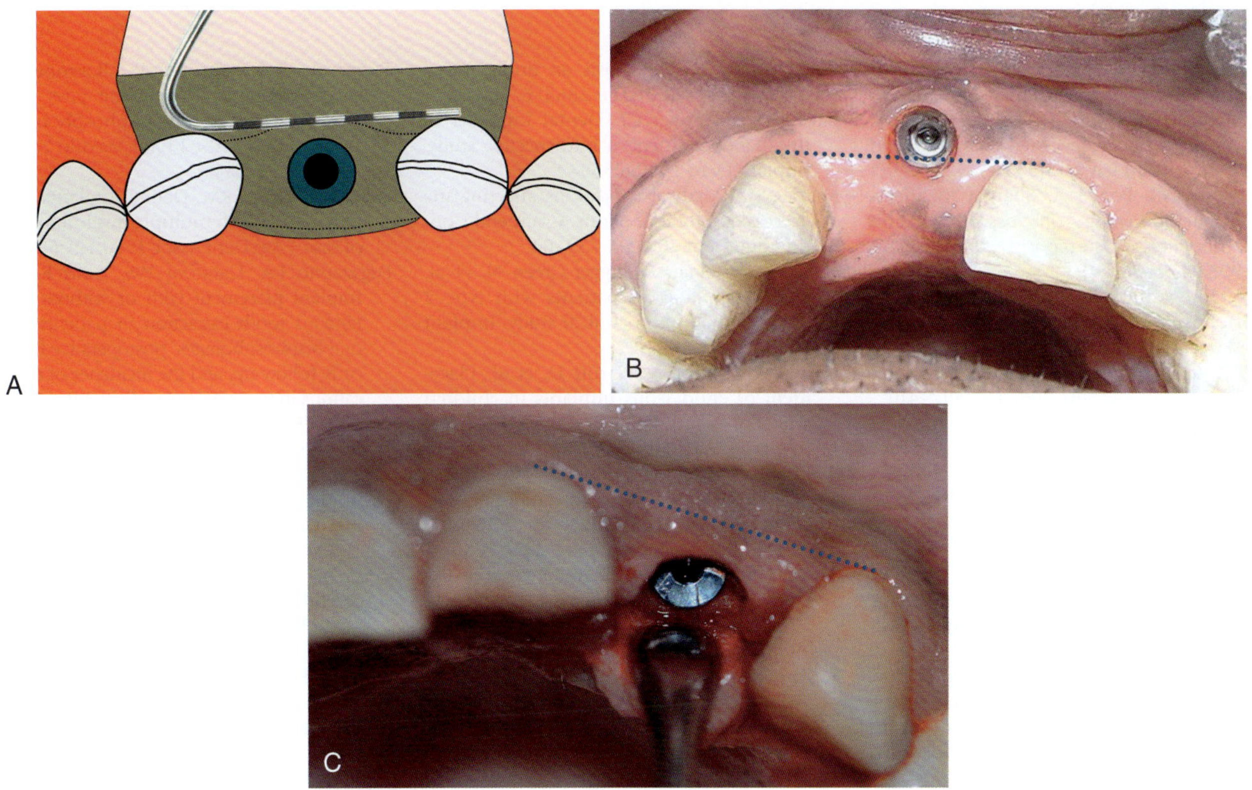

Fig 7.62 (A) The implant should also be placed 1–1.5 mm palatal to the imaginary line between the CEJ of two adjacent teeth. (B) Incorrectly placed implant. (C) Correctly placed implant.

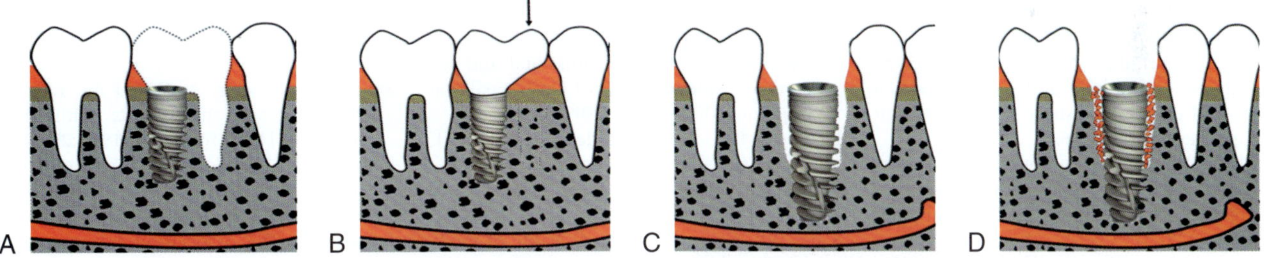

Fig 7.63 (A and B) In the case of immediate implantation in the fresh extraction socket of a molar, if the implant is inserted in any one root socket it may result in a prosthesis with cantilevering effect. (C and D) The implant should be inserted into the inter-radicular region and the peri-implant extraction socket spaces should be grafted using bone substitute (See Chapter 9).

Summary

Patient evaluation and treatment planning play a major role in the success of implant therapy. On first consultation, medical problems such as diabetes, thyroid disorders, hypertension, bone disorders, etc. should be openly discussed with the patient and evaluated to see if the patient is fit for the implant surgery. Thorough clinical examination of the oral cavity and the edentulous ridge site gives an idea about ridge morphology, the soft tissue situation, health of adjacent teeth, force factors, etc. Dental and panoramic radiographs give an idea of the two-dimensional bone available to insert implants, location and path of vital structures such as sinus floor, mandibular canal, etc. The dental CT scan can be very helpful in evaluating bone width, bone density, and accurate three-dimensional bone availability to insert implants of adequate sizes for the best possible future prosthesis. The author suggests fabricating and using a radiographic template for radiographs or dental CT scan of the patient, to closely assess bone density and three-dimensional bone volumes at specific implant sites. Using a surgical guide for implant placement definitely improves accuracy in implant positioning at the correct site and with correct angulation in respect to the future prosthesis. Implant numbers and positions should be thoroughly planned for the full-arch implant-supported prosthesis. The key positions for implant placement, force factors, cantilevers, and ideal implant dimensions for a particular site, vital structures such as mandibular canal, its anterior loop, sinus floor, nasal floor, ridge morphology, any present undercut along the ridge topography, bone density and dimensions, bone angulations, any present osseous defect, the position and angulation of future prosthesis are the factors that the dentist should keep in mind at the time of treatment planning.

Further Reading

Montoya-Carralero JM, Parra-Mino P, Ramírez-Fernández P, et al. Dental implants in patients treated with oral bisphosphonates: a bibliographic review. Med Oral Patol Oral Cir Bucal 2010 Jan 1;15(1):e65–9.

McDonald AR, Pogrel A, Sharma A. Effects of chemotherapy on osseointegration of implant: a case report. J Oral Implant 1998;24:11–3.

Marx RE, Cillo JE Jr, Ulloa JJ. Oral bisphosphonate-induced osteonecrosis: risk factors, prediction of risk using serum CTX testing, prevention, and treatment. J Oral Maxillofac Surg 2007;65:2397–410.

Attard NJ, Zarb GA. A study of dental implants in medically treated hypothyroid patients. Clin Implant Dent Relat Res 2002;4:220–31.

Misch CE. Analysis of medical history pinpoints conditions that contraindicate implants. Dentist 1989;67:23–4.

Wang HL, Weber D, McCauley LK. Effect of long-term oral bisphosphonates on implant wound healing: literature review and a case report. J Periodontol 2007;78:584–94.

American Dental Association Council on Scientific Affairs. Dental management of patients receiving oral bisphosphonate therapy: expert panel recommendations. J Am Dent Assoc 2006;137:1144–50.

Shernoff AF, Colwell JA, Bingham SF. Implants for type 2 diabetic patients: VA implants in diabetes study group. Implant Dent 1994;3:183–5.

Misch E. Contemporary implant dentistry. 3rd ed. Mosby, Inc, an affiliate of Elsevier Inc; 2008, ISBN: 978-81-312-1510-4.

Friberg B, Ekestubbe A, Mellstrom E, et al. Branemark implant and osteoporosis: a clinical exploratory study. Clin Impl Dent Relat Res 2001;3:50–6.

Misch CE. Density of bone: effect on treatment plans, surgical approach, healing and progressive bone loading. Int J Oral Implant 1990;6:23–31.

Corman L, Bolt RJ, editors. Medical evaluation of the pre-operative patient, Med Clin North Am 63:6, 1979.

Raposo V. Simple diagnosis and treatment planning of the implant patient. J Colo Dent Assoc 2001;80:16–7.

Minsk L, Poloson AM. Dental implants outcomes in postmenopausal women undergoing hormone replacement. Compend Contin Educ Dent 1998;19:859–66.

Buser Daniel. Surgical manual of implant dentistry: step by step procedures/Daniel Buser, Jun Y, Cho, Alvin Yeo, p.;cm. ISBN-13:978-0-86715-379-8.

Misch CE, Moore P. Steroids and reduction of pain, edema, and dysfunction in implant dentistry. Int J Oral Implant 1989;6:27–31.

Misch CE. Medical evaluation. In: Misch CE, editor. Contemporary implant dentistry. St Louis: Mosby; 1993.

Chestnut CH. Osteoporosis an undiagnosed disease. JAMA 2001;286:2865–6.

Balshi TJ, Wolfinger GJ. Dental implants in the diabetic patient: a retrospective study. Implant Dent 1999;8:355–9.

Marder MZ. Medical conditions affecting the success of dental implants. Compend Contin Educ Dent 2004;25:739–64.

Peled M, Ardekian L, Tagger-Green N, et al. Dental implants in patients with type 2 diabetes mellitus: a clinical study. Implant Dent 2003;12:116–22.

Kearns G, Sharma A, Perrott D, et al. Placement of endosseous implants in children and adolescents with hereditary ectodermal dysplasia. Oral Surg Oral Med Oral Pathol Oral Radiol Endod 1999;88:5–10.

Blanchaert RH. Implants in the medically challenged patient. Dent Clin N Am 1998;42:1.

Gómez Font R, Martínez García ML, Olmos Martínez JM. Osteochemonecrosis of the jaws due to bisphosphonate treatments. Update. Med Oral Patol Oral Cir Bucal 2008;13:E318–24.

Nevins MI, Karimbux NY, Weber HP, et al. Wound healing around endosseous implants in experimental diabetes. Int J Oral Maxillofac Implants 1998;13:620–9.

Misch CE. Dental implant prosthetics/Carl E. Misch, p.:cm. Includes bibliographical references and index ISBN 0-323-01955-2.

Lambert PM, Morris HF, Ochi S. The influence of smoking on a 3-year clinical success of osseointegrated dental implants. Ann Periodontol 2000;5:79–89.

Sugerman PB, Barber MT. Patient selection for endosseous dental implants: oral and systemic considerations. Int J Oral Maxillofac Implants 2002;17:191–201.

Dempster DW. Bone remodeling. In: Coe FL, Favis MJ, editors. Disorders of bone and mineral metabolism. New York: Raven Press; 1992.

Sabes WR, Green S, Craine C. Value of medical diagnostic screening test for dental patients. J Am Dent Assoc 1970;80:133–6.

Schenkein HA, Gunsolley JC, Koertg TE, et al. Smoking and its effects on early-onset periodontitis. J Am Dent Assoc 1995;126:1107–13.

McCracken M, Lemons JE, Rahemtulla F, et al. Bone response to titanium alloy implants placed in diabetic rats. Int J Oral Maxillofac Implant 2000;15:345–54.

Baim CA. Smoking and implant failure – benefits of a smoking cessation protocol. Int J Oral Maxillofac Implant 1996;11:1667–74.

Marder MZ. Medical conditions affecting the success of dental implants. Compendium 2004;25:739–64.

Visch LL, Van Wass MAJ, Schmitz PIM, et al. A clinical evaluation of implants in irradiated oral cancer patients. J Dent Res 2002;81:856–9.

Ruggiero SL, Mehrotra B, Rosenberg TJ, et al. Osteonecrosis of the jaws associated with the use of bisphosphonates: a review of 63 cases. J Oral Maxillo Fac Surg 2004;62:527–34.

Sager RD, Thesis RM. Dental implants placed in a patient with multiple myeloma. Report of case. J Am Dent Assoc 1990;121:699–701.

Fugazzotto PA, Lightfoot WS, Jaffin R, et al. Implant placement with or without simultaneous tooth extraction in patients taking oral bisphosphonates: postoperative healing, early follow-up, and the incidence of complications in two private practices. J Periodontol 2007;78:1664–9.

Taylor TD, Worthingtom P. Osseointegrated implants rehabilitation of the previously irradiated mandible: results of a limited trial at 3 to 7 years. J Prosthet Dent 1993;69:60–9.

Misch CE. Medical evaluation of the implant candidate. Part I: vital signs and urinalysis. J Oral Implant 1981;9:556–70.

Misch CE. Medical evaluation of the implant candidate. Part II: complete blood count and bleeding disorders. Int J Oral Implant 1982;10:363–70.

Misch CE. Medical evaluation of the implant candidate. Part III: SMA 12/60. J Oral Implant 1981;9:556–70.

Serra MP, Llorca CS, Donat FJ. Oral implants in patients receiving bisphosphonates: a review and update. Med Oral Patol Oral Cir Bucal 2008;13:E755–60.

Chanabaz M. Patient screening and medical evaluation for implant and preprosthetic surgery. J Oral Implatol 1998;24:222–9.

Steiner M, Windchy A, Gould AR. Effects of chemotherapy in patients with dental implants. J Oral Implantol 1995;21:142–7.

Darnell JA, Saunders MJ. Oral manifestations of the diabetic patient. Tex Dent J 1990;107:23–7.

Jeffcoat M. The association between osteoporosis and oral bone loss. J Periodontal 2005;76(Suppl. 11):2125–32.

Statz TA, Guthmiller JM, Humbert LA, et al. Intravenous bisphosphonate-associated osteonecrosis of the jaw. J Periodontol 2007;78:2203–8.

Bain CA, Moy PK. The association between the failure of dental implants and cigarette smoking. Int J Oral Maxillofac Impl 1993;8:609–15.

Granstrom G. Placement of dental implants in irradiated bone: the case of using hyperbaric oxygen. J Oral Maxillofac Surg 2006;64:812–8.

Step by step procedure of implant treatment

8

Ajay Vikram Singh   Amir Gazmawe

CHAPTER CONTENTS HD

Introduction

Once patient evaluation and treatment planning has been completed for a particular implant case and the implant therapy protocol has been finalized, the implant surgeon sets up the operatory for the implant insertion surgery. The implant surgery should not be considered as a normal OPD procedure; it needs a high level of sterility for a predictable success rate. The author recommends that implant dentists should follow all the sterilization parameters that are implemented in hospital operation theatres. It is always better, if possible, to have a special and separate implant unit to perform implant surgical procedures with a high level of sterility. The patient's oral hygiene is one of the key factors for implant success. All periodontal problems must be treated by scaling, curettage, flap surgeries, root planing, polishing, etc. before implant surgery, and the patient should be asked to rinse his/her mouth with 0.12% chlorhexidine for 30 seconds immediately before surgery, to reduce the bacterial count in the oral cavity. The patient should also be encouraged to continue and maintain oral hygiene after surgery also. Implant surgery is an elective surgical procedure and in most cases needs detailed planning and stringent execution, so it should be performed in a calm and comfortable clinical environment.

Setting up the operatory for implant surgery

1. Cleaning, dusting, and mopping of the operatory unit using antimicrobial cleaning agents.
2. The operation theatre should be fumigated using formalin fumigator and the theatre is closed with formalin fumes for 8–12 h (overnight) before implant surgery (Fig 8.1A).
3. Cold sterilize inventories that cannot be autoclaved, e.g. surgical guide (should be dipped into 2% glutaraldehyde for 24 h before implant surgery).
4. The drills and other inventories of the implant surgical kits should be cleaned in an ultrasonic cleaner followed by autoclaving of the fully loaded implant surgical kit wrapped in cloth or in sterilization pouches (Fig 8.1B and C).
5. Instruments and implant motor cord should be autoclaved in pouches.
6. Surgical draping and gauze pieces should be autoclaved.
7. Saline bottles which are to be used during implant osteotomy preparation should be refrigerated.
8. The selected suturing materials (N-W 5002 3-0 ETHICON with cutting edge 3/4 circle needle or non-resorbable, 4-0 vicryl/chromic gut – resorbable) should be ready at hand.
9. The doctor and his assistants should wear sterilized gloves, mask, head cap, and apron (Fig 8.2).
10. Scrub the face of the patient with Betadine/chlorhexidine.
11. Cover the patient's forehead, eyes, and the middle part of the body.
12. Cover all the trays, trolley, radiographic unit, radiographic sensor, etc. with sterilized cloth/wrapping which can be used by surgeon and his assistants during the surgery.

Pre-medication

The patient should be advised to take the following medicines a minimum of 1 h before surgery:

a. Prophylactic antibiotics – amoxicillin 1 g one tab. stat 1 h before surgery. It reduces the chances of post-implantation infection complications. Clindamycin 300 mg can be given to patients who are allergic to penicillin.
b. Analgesic and anti-inflammatory medicine: A combination of aceclofenac, paracetamol and serratiopeptidase (tab. Hifenac-D) should be given to the patient 1 h before surgery. The injectable form of analgesics like diclofenac (inj. Voveran 3 ml IM) or ketorol can be given to the patient who is going to receive multiple implants.
c. Anti-anxiety drugs: alprazolam (tab. Valium 2–5 mg) on the night before and 1 h before surgery, to reduce the anxiety and apprehensions of the patient.
d. Steroid–oral: (tab. Steron forte – 3 tab. stat) or injectable (inj. Dexona IM) form of steroid can be given to patients to reduce the chances of postimplantation swelling.
e. Anti-histaminic (cetrizine): if simultaneous sinus grafting is to be performed with implant insertion.

Anaesthesia

A long-acting anaesthetic, such as bupivacaine (marcaine) 0.5% with epinephrine 1:200,000 should be preferred. Usually the infiltration works well for implant insertion surgery. The nerve block or intravenous sedation can be used for the full-arch implant or implants with other procedures like sinus grafting, nerve transpositioning, etc. (Table 8.1).

Step by step presentation of the single tooth implant

Before making the incision, ask the patient to rinse with 0.12% chlorhexidine (Periogard, Colgate) for 30 s. Several studies have shown that it reduces bacterial count in the oral cavity and complications from post-implantation infection. The implant surgeon can also additionally apply and rub the surgical site with a cotton palate moistened with chlorhexidine.

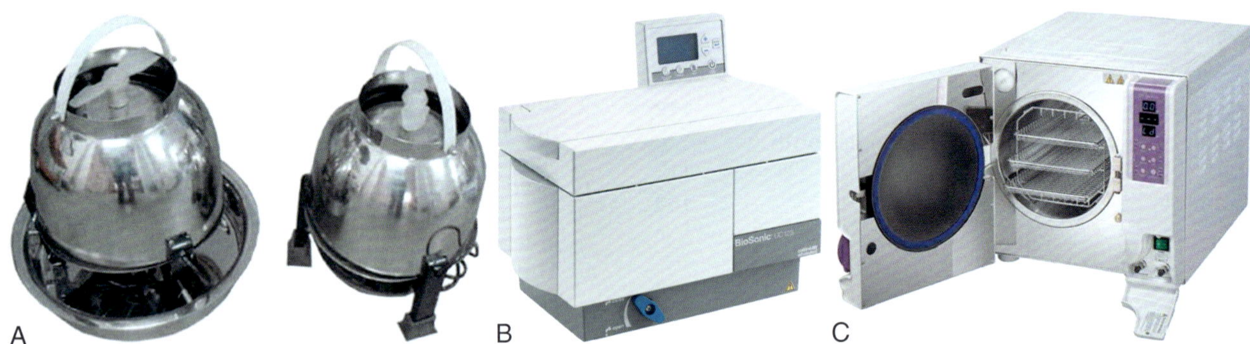

Fig 8.1 (A) Fumigator; (B) Ultrasonic cleaner from Coltene Whaledent, and (C) Front loading autoclave with automatic dry cycle.

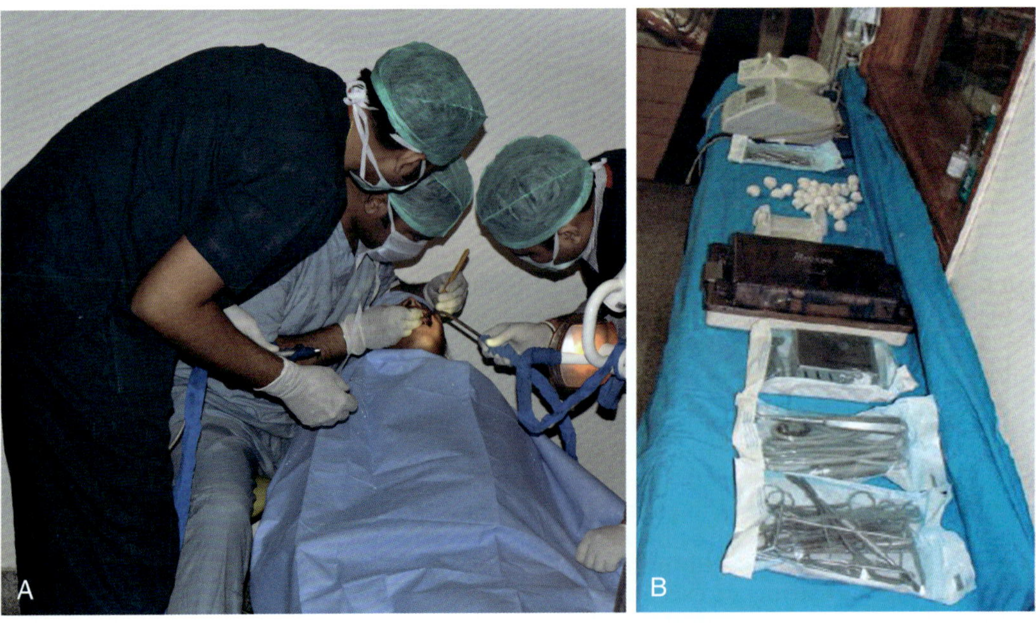

Fig 8.2 (A and B) All sterilization parameters should be followed during implant surgery to avoid any postimplantation infection.

A. **Incision** The type of incision and extent of flap elevation depend on several factors such as the width of the attached keratinized tissue, ridge form, presence of any undercut, any other simultaneous grafting procedure to be done, etc. Usually a mid-crestal incision is given with or without vertical incisions and the flap is elevated to expose the crestal, facial, and lingual parts of the bony ridge (Fig 8.3A and B).

Key points

1. The attached keratinised gingiva at the ridge crest should be evaluated before making the incision.
   a. If the implant site has an adequate buccolingual band of keratinized soft tissue, the incision should be made so as to bisect the keratinized soft tissue band, which results in minimum 2–3 mm keratinized soft tissue on both the labial as well as the lingual side of the implant.
   b. If the implant site has an inadequate keratinized soft tissue band, the incision should be made so as to bisect the thin keratinized soft tissue band and implants are placed and soft tissue grafting should be performed at the stage of re-exposure of the implant.
2. If papillae are intact on the implant site, the papilla preservation incision should be preferred to maintain papillae height and to achieve better soft tissue aesthetics around the future implant prosthesis.

Table 8.1 Different anaesthetic approaches in implant surgery.

INFILTRATIONS	NERVE BLOCK	INTRAVENOUS SEDATION
Single/two/three implants	Several implants placed in one attempt	Full-arch implant placement
Maxillary implants	Mandibular implants	Bilateral sinus lift in one step
Basic implant procedure	Implant placement with other procedures like sinus grafting, ridge splitting, bone grafting, etc.	Nerve transpositioning etc.

B. **Flap elevation** Facial and lingual mucoperiosteal flaps should be elevated to expose the ridge crest as well as the facial and lingual part of the ridge (Fig 8.4A and B)

Key points

1. Both facial as well as lingual flaps are elevated to completely expose the ridge crest and buccal and lingual cortical plates in the case of compromised bone width or ridge with undercuts. This will allow three-dimensional visibility of the bony ridge during implant osteotomy preparation and avoid the chances of inadvertent perforation or dehiscence during drilling.
2. The flaps are elevated to expose the ridge crest and facial cortical plate in case of:
   a. Compromised/limited ridge width or the ridge with facial undercut.
   b. Thin facial and thick palatal cortical plate (e.g. anterior maxilla), which causes the slipping of drills towards the thin facial plate during osteotomy preparation, and may result in dehiscence/perforation through the facial cortical plate. Thus, a direct visualization of the facial cortical plate is paramount during controlled osteotomy preparation.
3. The flaps are minimally elevated to expose the ridge crest in the case of a wide ridge crest with stepped apical widening (e.g. posterior maxilla and posterior mandible). Whereas it has least chances of perforation, unnecessary elevation of the buccal and lingual flaps leads to reduced blood supply to the bone from the periosteum during the initial phase of healing.

C. **Pilot drilling**: After exposing the underlying bony ridge, either a surgical stent is seated on the site or the reference of adjacent teeth is taken to prepare the implant osteotomy, which is three-dimensionally correct for the future prosthesis (Fig 8.5A and B). A sharp pointed lance drill or pilot drill is used to make an initial entry into the bone. Alternatively, a small round bur can be used to mark the implant site and to drill through the high-density crestal bone (Fig 8.5C and D).

Key points

1. If the ridge crest is irregular, it should be flattened using a large round carbide bur before starting pilot drilling.

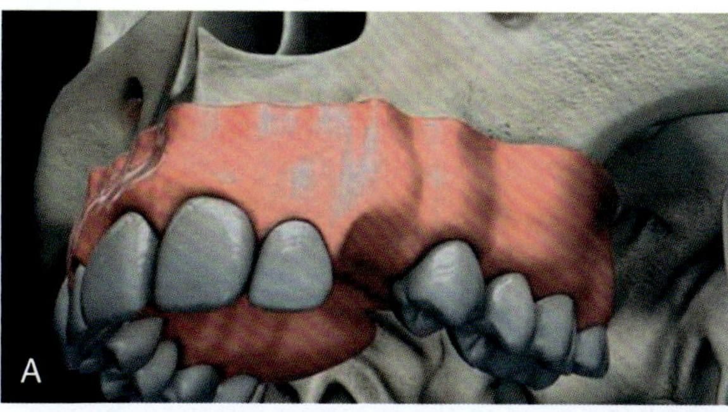

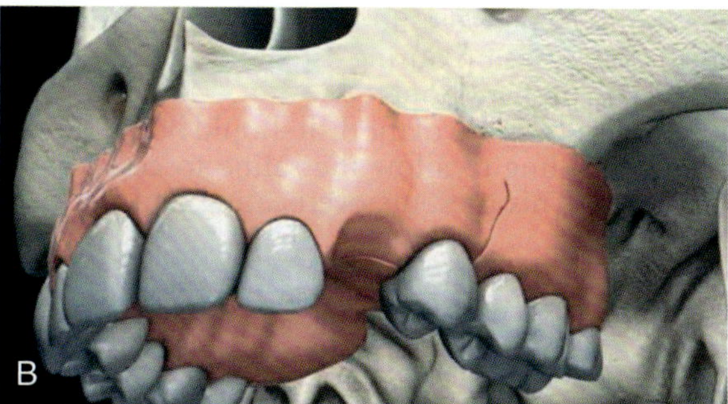

Fig 8.3 (A and B) A mid-crestal incision is given, using 11 or 15 no. blade, which can be further extended with a 12 no. blade in the crevicular area of the adjacent tooth and extended further to the vertical (facial) incision with 11 or 15 no. blade (*Courtesy: Osseolink Implant Company*).

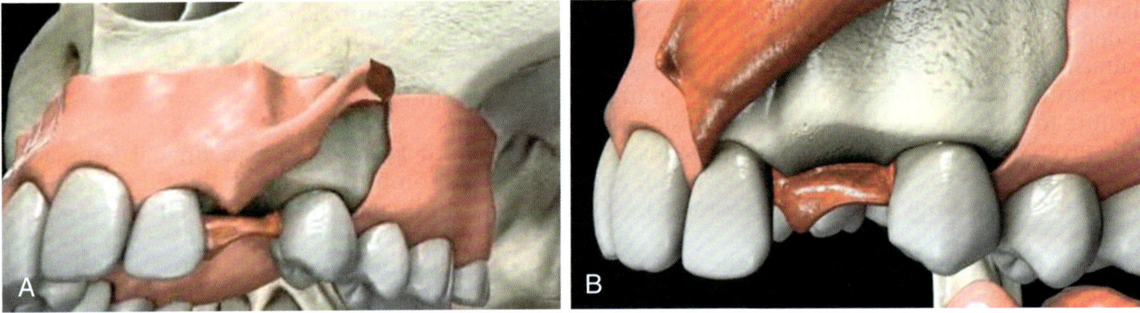

Fig 8.4 (A and B) The facial and lingual mucoperiosteal flaps are elevated to expose the ridge crest as well as the facial and lingual part of the ridge (*Courtesy: Osseolink Implant Company*).

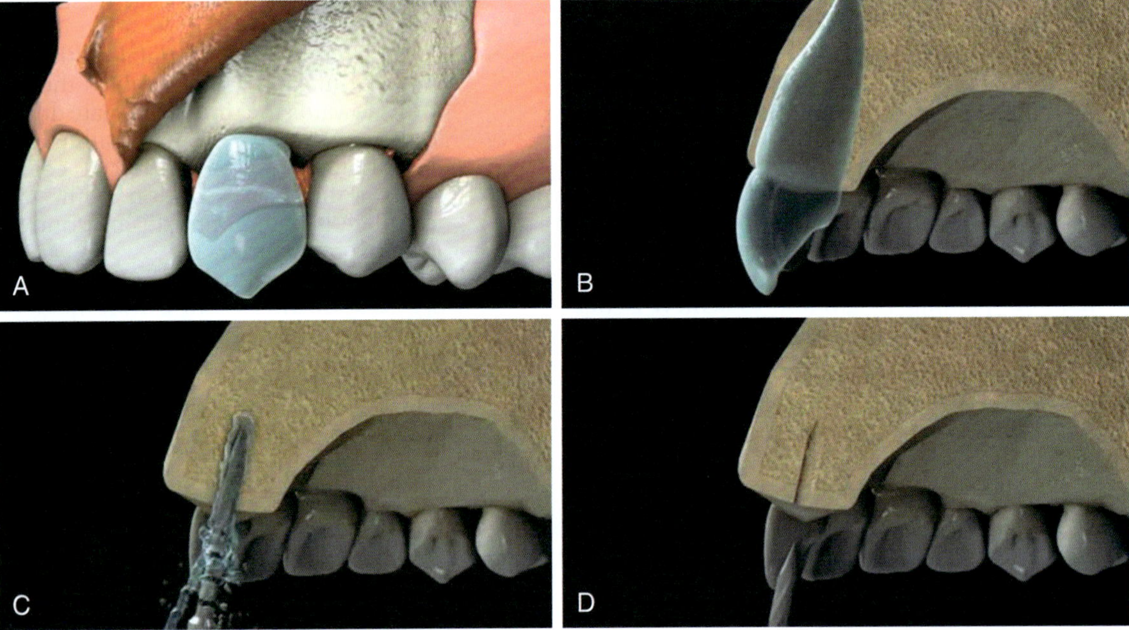

Fig 8.5 (A and B) After exposing the underlying bony ridge, either a surgical stent is seated on the site or the reference of adjacent teeth is taken to prepare the implant osteotomy which is three-dimensionally correct for the future prosthesis. (C and D) A pilot drill which is sharp and pointed is used to mark the position and to drill through the hard cortex to partial depth (*Courtesy: Osseolink Implant Company*).

2. Before using the pilot drill one can also use a small round carbide bur to mark the osteotomy site and to punch through the hard cortex.
3. Drilling (pilot drill to final drill) must be done at speeds of 1200–2500 rpm depending on bone density, under a constant stream of chilled saline. The torque of the implant motor should be adjusted between 30 and 50 Ncm so that the drill does not stop during osteotomy preparation, especially in hard bone.
4. A pumping motion of the drill should be employed during drilling to allow the saline to cool down the bone. This prevents overheating and necrosis of the bone.
5. An intraoral periapical (IOPA) radiograph can be taken at this stage to see the direction of the drill, especially in tight spaces or in the areas of vital structures like the maxillary sinus or mandibular canal. After pilot drilling to partial depth, this drill is inserted into the osteotomy, and a periapical radiograph taken to evaluate the direction of drilling and the availability of the bone dimensions for further osteotomy deepening.

D. **Depth drilling**: The pilot drill or depth drill which usually remain 2 mm of diameter first used to the partial depth and direction of drilling is three-dimensionally evaluated by inserting a parallel pin/force direction indicator in the partially prepared osteotomy. If the direction is correct, the depth drill is further used to the complete depth (Fig 8.6A–D). All the planned osteotomy depth should be attained by pilot drill itself as the rest of the drills are only used to widen the osteotomy. For example, if a 13 mm long implant is planned, depth drill should attain 13 mm depth in the bone before the use of osteotomy-widening drills.

Key points

During or after pilot drilling, if the dentist finds that he/she has drilled in the incorrect direction, he/she can correct the osteotomy direction to some extent by using the special side-cutting Lindemann drill (2 mm diameter)

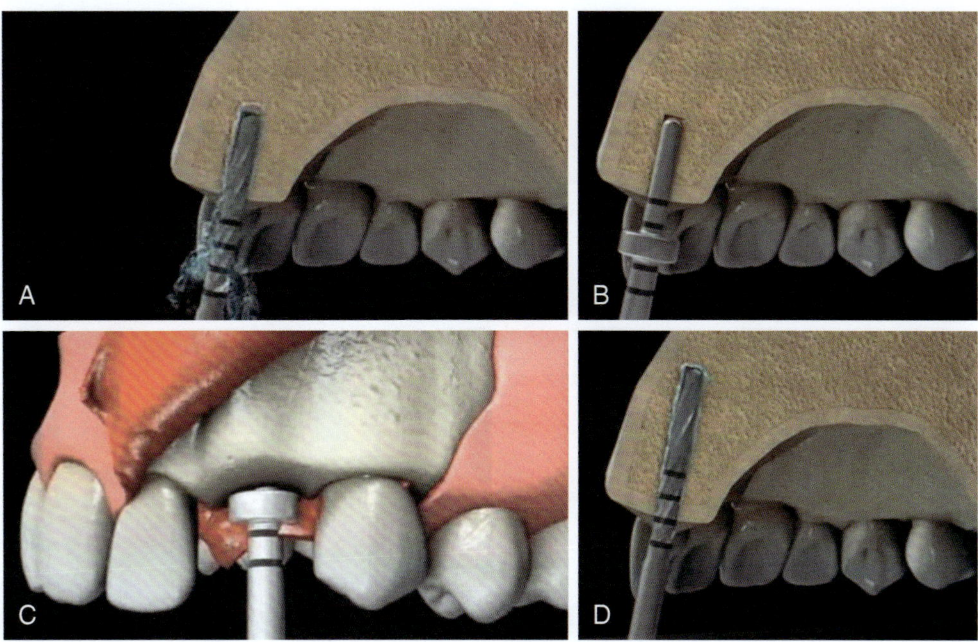

Fig 8.6 (A) Depth drill which is 2 mm in diameter is first used to drill to partial depth and (B and C) direction of drilling is three-dimensionally evaluated by inserting parallel pin/force direction indicator in the partially prepared osteotomy. (D) If the direction is correct, depth drill is further used to the complete depth (depth marks at different lengths on all drills), e.g. for 13 mm long implant, depth drill should attain 13 mm depth in the bone (*Courtesy: Osseolink Implant Company*).

E. **Osteotomy widening:** After pilot drilling to the planned depth, the osteotomy-widening drills are sequentially used to the same depth. A series of different diameter osteotomy-widening drills (e.g. 2.8, 3.2, 3.65, 4.2 mm diameters) are used to the same depth depending on the diameter of the implant (Fig 8.7A–D). Depending on the bone density, the diameter of final drill should be 0.3–0.8 mm less than the diameter of the implant (e.g. if the planned implant diameter is 5 mm, the diameter of final drill must be approximately 4.2 mm in D3/D4 bone and 4.7 mm in D1/D2 bone).

Key points

1. For the implant with non-cutting/nonself-tapping threads, a bone tap or thread former can be used after the final drill and before inserting the implant in high-density (D1 and D2) bone. The bone tap should be used at the speed of 20–30 rpm.
2. Crestal bone drill can be used to submerge the implant platform apical to the ridge crest, if the implant platform is wider than its body. This drill is used at the same speed as the final drill.

F. **Final assessment of prepared osteotomy**: After the final drill, the prepared osteotomy should be checked using a depth probe, for complete depth preparation and also to check any inadvertent perforation that has occurred through the osteotomy walls (Fig 8.8A and B).

Key points

1. Any perforation or thinning of any cortical plate should be finally checked at this stage and if detected, the surgeon should perform bone grafting.
2. The osteotomy site should be irrigated using chilled sterile saline to remove all the residual bone debris which can get collected at the apex and prevent the complete setting of the implant.
3. After irrigating the prepared osteotomy with saline, do not suck the site but let the fresh blood oozing out from within the prepared osteotomy, before inserting the implant. If it is not seen, the surgeon can provoke bleeding by inserting any tool in the prepared osteotomy. For early and predictable osseointegration, the osteotomy should remain filled with fresh blood during implant insertion, for clot formation between the implant surface and osteotomy walls.

G. **Opening the implant packaging**: The implant being highly sterile, remains packed in a sterile vial which is further packed in an outer non-sterile packing. The outer non-sterile covering of the implant vial should be opened by the assistant without touching the inner sterile vial, which contains the implant and cover screw (Fig 8.9A and B). The implant surgeon wearing sterile gloves should open this inner vial to take the implant out from it.

H. **Taking out the implant from its vial and carrying it to the prepared osteotomy**: After the surgeon has opened the inner sterile vial containing implant and cover screw, the implant driver is engaged into the implant connection, the implant is removed from its vial, and carried to the prepared osteotomy without touching its surface (Fig 8.10A–D). An implant mount comes connected into the implant connection in a few systems. This implant mount is used to remove the implant from its vial and to carry it to the osteotomy by hand/hand ratchet adaptor/rotary handpiece adaptor.

I. **Implant insertion**: The implant is carried to the prepared osteotomy and screwed in with clockwise rotations at very slow speed (30–40 rpm) using a rotary handpiece or hand ratchet (Fig 8.11A and B).

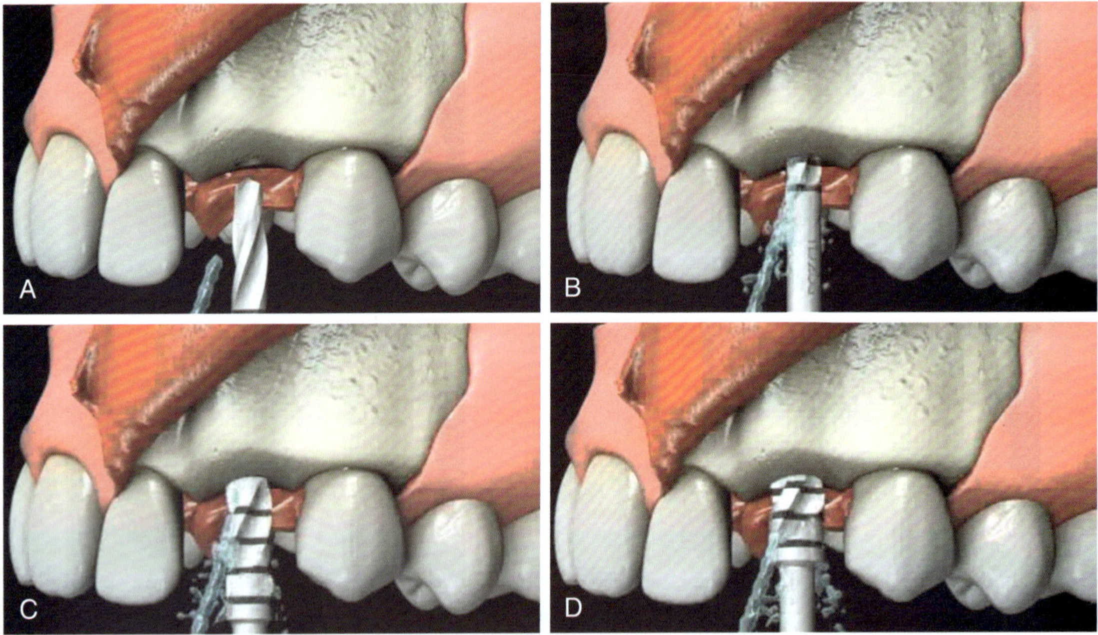

Fig 8.7 (A to D) A series of different diameter osteotomy widening drills (2.8, 3.2, 3.65, 4.2, etc.) are sequentially used to the same depth. Depending on bone density, the finally used drill should have a diameter 0.3–0.8 mm less than the diameter of the implant, e.g. if the implant diameter is 5 mm, the diameter of the final drill must be approximately 4.2 mm in D3/D4 bone and 4.7 mm in D1/D2 bone (*Courtesy: Osseolink Implant Company*).

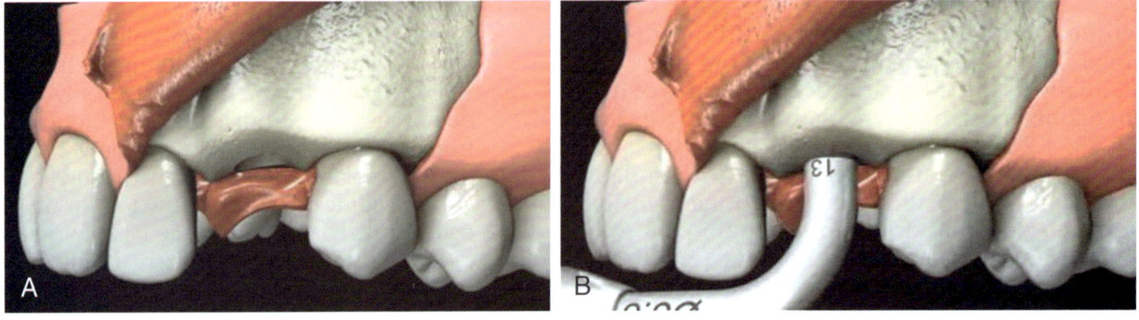

Fig 8.8 (A and B) Depth of completed osteotomy can be checked using a marked depth guide (*Courtesy for diagram's: Osseolink Implant Company*).

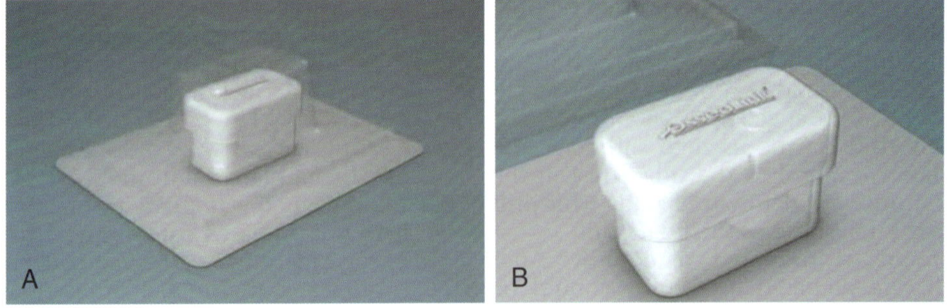

Fig 8.9 (A and B) Implants being highly sterile, remain packed in a sterile vial which further remains packed in an outer non-sterile packing. The outer non-sterile covering of the implant vial should be opened by the assistant without touching the inner sterile vial which contains the implant and cover screw. The implant surgeon wearing sterile gloves should open this inner vial to take the implant out from it (*Courtesy: Osseolink Implant Company*).

Key Points

1. If surgeon feels a little resistance, he/she should stop inserting the implant and wait for a moment. He/she should let the surrounding bone expand and then restart rotating and inserting implant. This can be done several times till all the implant gets completely seated into the osteotomy.
2. If surgeon feels greater resistance he/she should stop inserting the implant, rotate it counter clockwise to unscrew 2–3 threads of the implant

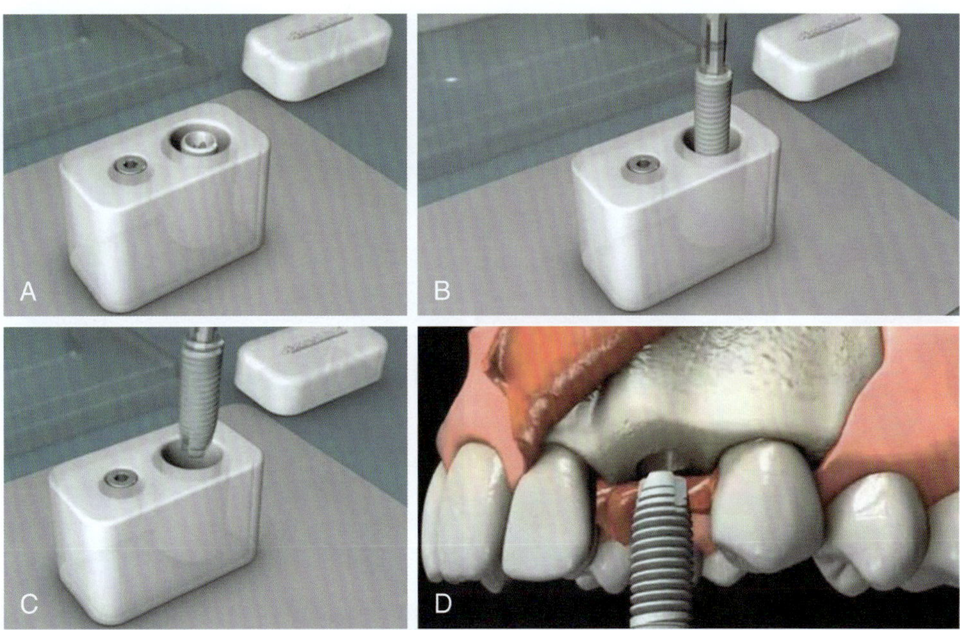

Fig 8.10 (A and B) After opening the inner vial, the implant driver is used to engage the implant hex connection. Make sure that implant driver is secured well into the implant connection to avoid its sudden fall. (C and D) Implant is removed from vial and carried to the prepared osteotomy site with upward position. Implant body surface should not be touched by gloves, any instrument, patient's lip, saliva, etc. to avoid its surface getting contaminated (*Courtesy: Osseolink Implant Company*).

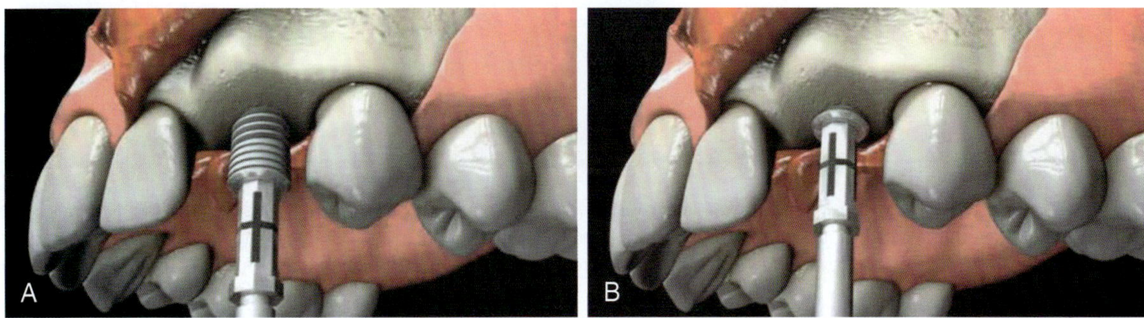

Fig 8.11 (A and B) Secure the implant into the prepared osteotomy and rotate it clockwise at very slow speed (30–40 rpm) using rotary hand piece or hand ratchet (*Courtesy: Osseolink Implant Company*).

to release the pressure on the bone, wait for a moment to let the surrounding bone expand and then restart rotating and inserting the implant. This can be done several times until all the implant gets completely seated into the osteotomy.

3. If implant is not going in by following the above-mentioned two protocols or exerting a greater moment force (more than 40–50 Ncm) on the surrounding bone, then it can cause pressure necrosis of the surrounding bone. Unscrew the implant and remove it from the osteotomy site and transfer it to its sterile vial. Further widen the osteotomy by using the next diameter drill and reinsert the implant.
4. All the implant threads should get submerged into the bone. If any bone defect exists, it can lead to exposure of implant threads. These exposed threads should be covered using bone graft before closing the flap.
5. The complete seating of the implant should present the implant platform flush with the ridge crest in D1, D2, and D3 bone. The implant platform can be submerged 0.5–1 mm apical to the ridge crest in D4 bone, to avoid any premature loading of the implant which may cause micro movement of the implant during its healing phase and may lead to fail to osseointegrate.
6. While inserting the implant in aesthetic regions, the platform of the finally seated implant platform should be 2 mm apical to the cementoenamel junction (CEJ) of adjacent teeth or their gingival zenith, to achieve an acceptable soft tissue emergence around the implant prosthesis. The implant platform should also be placed 2 mm palatal to the imaginary line or straight probe meeting the facial aspects of the CEJ of the two adjacent teeth.

J. **Cover screw insertion and flap suturing**: Following implant insertion, the implant driver is removed from the implant connection, and the cover screw is removed from the implant vial and screwed over the implant connection using a screwdriver. After

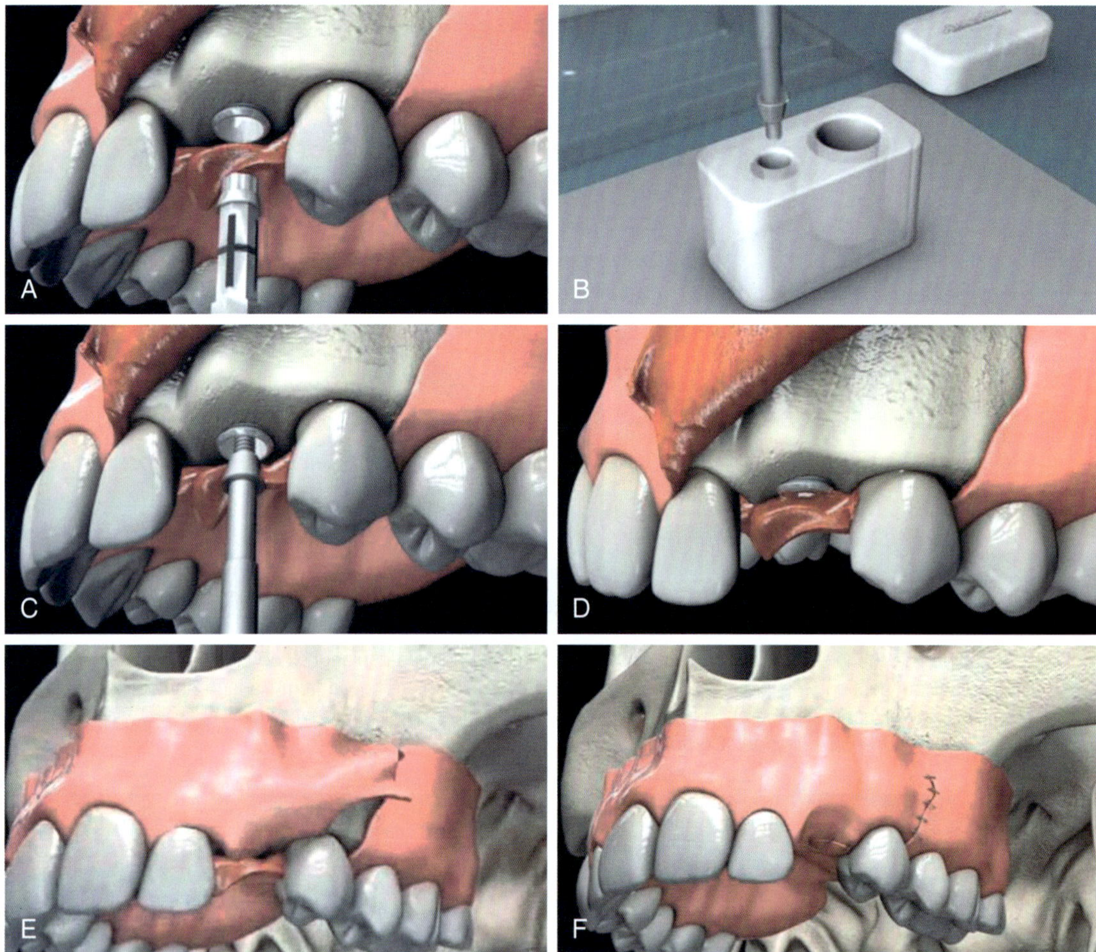

Fig 8.12 Following implant insertion, the implant driver is removed from the implant and implant connection is irrigated with chlorhexidine. The cover screw is removed from the vial using screwdriver and inserted over the implant to cover the implant connection during its (A to D) healing phase. (E and F) After inserting cover screw, the flap is sutured back with tension-free primary closure (*Courtesy: Osseolink Implant Company*).

inserting cover screw, the flap is sutured back with a tension-free primary closure (Fig 8.12A–F).

Key points

1. An antibacterial repellent jelly like Terramycine ointment or Metrohex ointment can be applied over the threads of cover screw before inserting it over the implant, to prevent any microbial growth into the implant connection during its healing phase.
2. The cover screw should not be tightened with great moment force, because this can present problems at removal on uncovery. If it is tightened at a high torque, often the implant itself comes out connected to the cover screw, especially in low-density D4 bone.
3. If the implant surgeon decides on a non-submerged implant healing protocol, a long gingival former can be inserted directly over the implant in spite of using cover screw, and the flap can be sutured around it.
4. Tension-free sutures should be used to avoid the suture line opening because of the tension in the flap.
5. If achieving primary closure becomes difficult, as in cases of implant insertion with simultaneous bone grafting, the flap should be released by making horizontal releasing incisions through the periosteum from underneath the flap. A 3-0/4-0 non-resorbable Ethicon or a resorbable chromic gut suture can be used for the suturing.
6. The sutured tissue surface should be cleaned using chlorhexidine and a light pressure pack of moistened cotton is given. The patient is instructed to keep the mouth closed for 1 h.
7. An ice pack is given to the patient to apply over the facial skin of the surgical site intermittently for 45 min to cool down the bone. The application of a cold pack is beneficial for 48 h after surgery to suppress heat generation and inflammatory oedema, which leads to tension in the soft tissue resulting in suture line opening. Hot fomentations are beneficial after 48 h to diffuse the inflammatory fluid from the site, which reduces soft tissue oedema.
8. If not given before surgery, an intramuscular injection of a potent pain killer like tramadol or diclofenac and a steroid like dexamethasone, can be given after the surgery to reduce the chances of postoperative pain and swelling.
9. Antibacterials like the amoxicillin and clavulanate combination (tab. Augmentin 1 g b.i.d.), analgesics

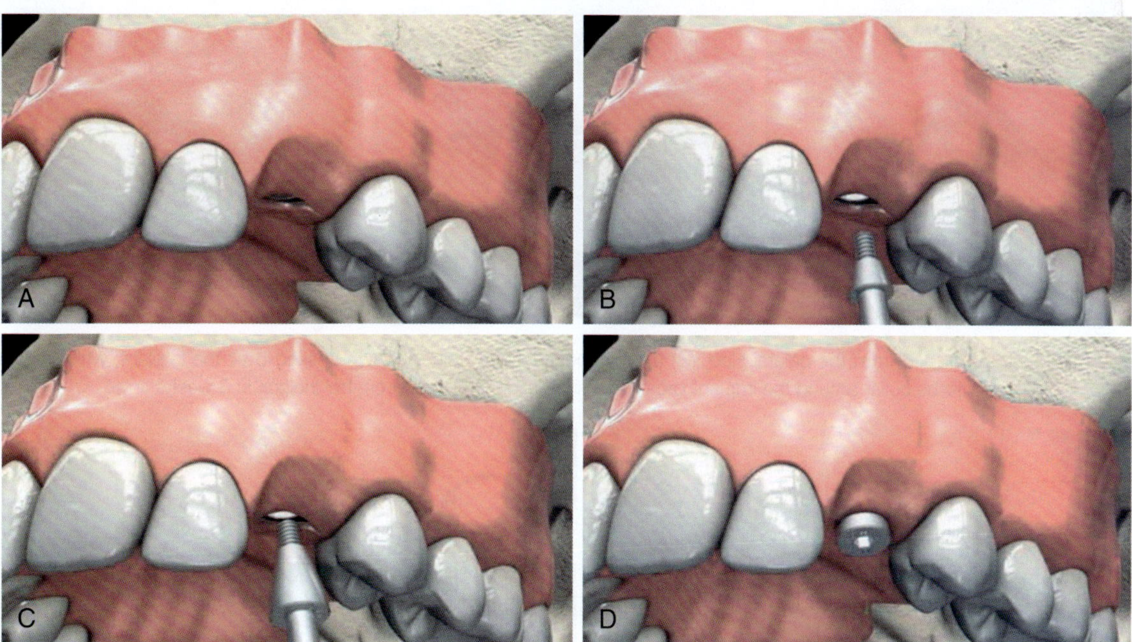

Fig 8.13 (A) After the implant has osseointegrated (3–5 months) with the bone, the cover screw is exposed by giving a small mid-crestal incision or using soft tissue punch. (B) The cover screw is removed using screwdriver and (C and D) a long gingival former is inserted. If required, the flap should be sutured around the gingival former and the site left to heal for 2–3 weeks before making impression (*Courtesy: Osseolink Implant Company*).

like the aceclofenac, paracetamol and serratiopeptidase combination (tab. Hifenac-D, b.i.d.) and multivitamins (cap. Becosule, o.d.) are prescribed for a minimum of 5–7 days.

10. The patient is instructed to take only soft foods for a minimum of 24 h and to avoid any hot and spicy food. The patient should also be instructed to avoid pulling the lip and checking the surgical site, which can result in suture line opening.
11. Patient should be instructed to brush his/her teeth and rinse the mouth 3–4 times a day and after every meal, with 0.12% chlorhexidine (Periogard) to maintain oral hygiene after surgery (after the flap get stabilized).
12. If possible, the patient should be recalled for a follow-up check the day after the surgery.
13. Sutures should be removed after 7–10 days.

K. **Implant uncovery**: Once the implant gets osseointegrated with the bone, the implant is uncovered by making a small crestal incision or using the tissue punch. The cover screw is removed and replaced with a long gingival former/healing abutment/permucosal extension (Fig 8.13A–D).

Key points

1. If adequate width of keratinized soft tissue collar is present on the implant site, the implant can be uncovered by using a soft tissue punch.
2. Gingival formers are available in different heights, thus one with the correct height should be chosen, depending on the soft tissue thickness over the implant.
3. A custom-made gingival former (provisional crown fabricated over a temporary abutment) can also be used to create a 'C' shaped aesthetic soft tissue collar around the future implant prosthesis in an aesthetic region (Fig 8.14A–C).

L. **Making implant impression:** After the soft tissue around the gingival former has healed, the gingival former is removed and an impression post is screwed over the implant. An impression is made in polyether or additional silicon material (Fig 8.15A–D). After removing the impression from mouth, the impression post is removed from the implant and the gingival former is reinserted. The patient is sent back after shade selection and bite registration (Fig 8.15E–H).

Key points

1. The complete seating of the impression post over the implant should be checked with a radiograph before making the impression, because the impression of an incompletely seated impression post can result in incorrect transfer of implant orientation and subsequent inaccurate seating of the final prosthesis.
2. The impression should be made with open tray technique, using a long open tray impression post if the implant is deeply seated in the soft tissue. If the closed tray impression post emerging out of the soft tissue is very short, it may not get properly engaged in the closed tray impression, thus leading to inaccurate transfer of the implant hex position. The open tray posts should also be preferred in multiple implants or full-arch cases, for precision in the fit of the multiunit prosthesis over implants.
3. Screw hole of the impression post should be blocked using wax before making the impression, as it can hinder the reseating of the post into the impression.
4. Usually, the impression post has one long flat side which guides the implant dentist in transferring this post from the implant to the impression with the correct orientation.

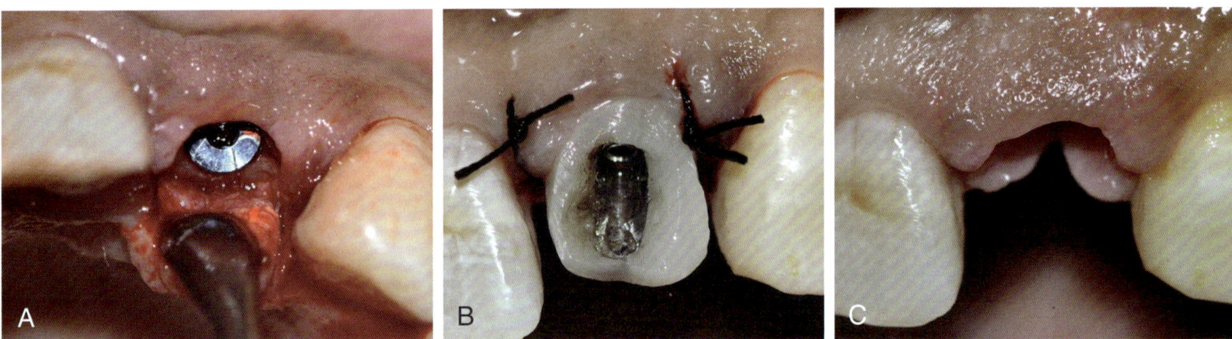

Fig 8.14 (A) The implant is exposed from the palatal side; (B) a provisional screw-retained crown is fixed over the implant, which has created a (C) scalloped 'C' shaped soft tissue collar around the implant prosthesis similar to the adjacent central incisor, in 3 weeks time.

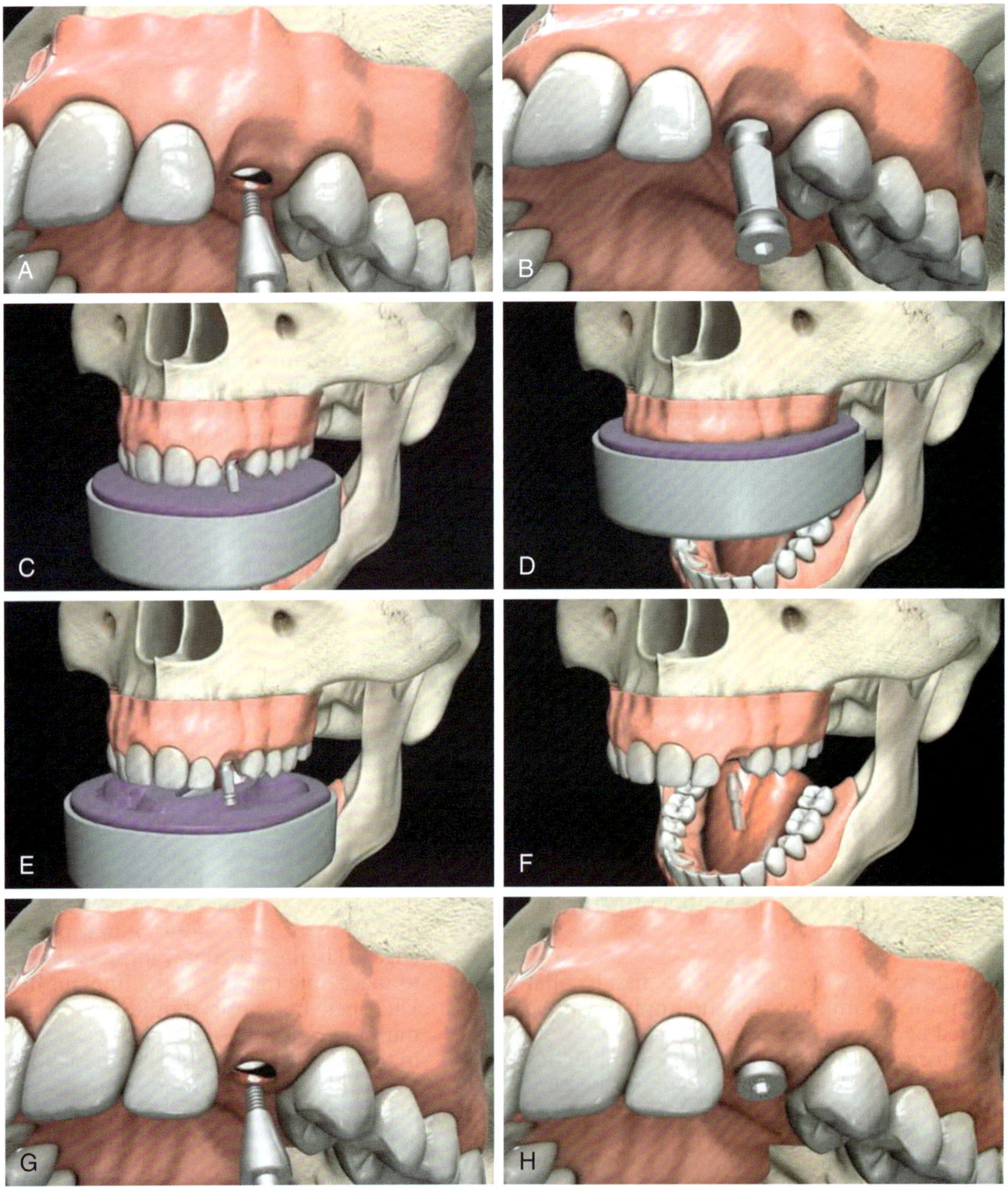

Fig 8.15 (A) After the soft tissue around the gingival former has healed, the gingival former is removed and (B) an impression post is inserted over the implant. (C and D) An impression is made in polyether or additional silicon material. (E) After removing the impression from the mouth, (F) the impression post is removed from the implant and (G and H) gingival former is re-inserted. The patient is sent back after shade selection and bite registration (*Courtesy: Osseolink Implant Company*).

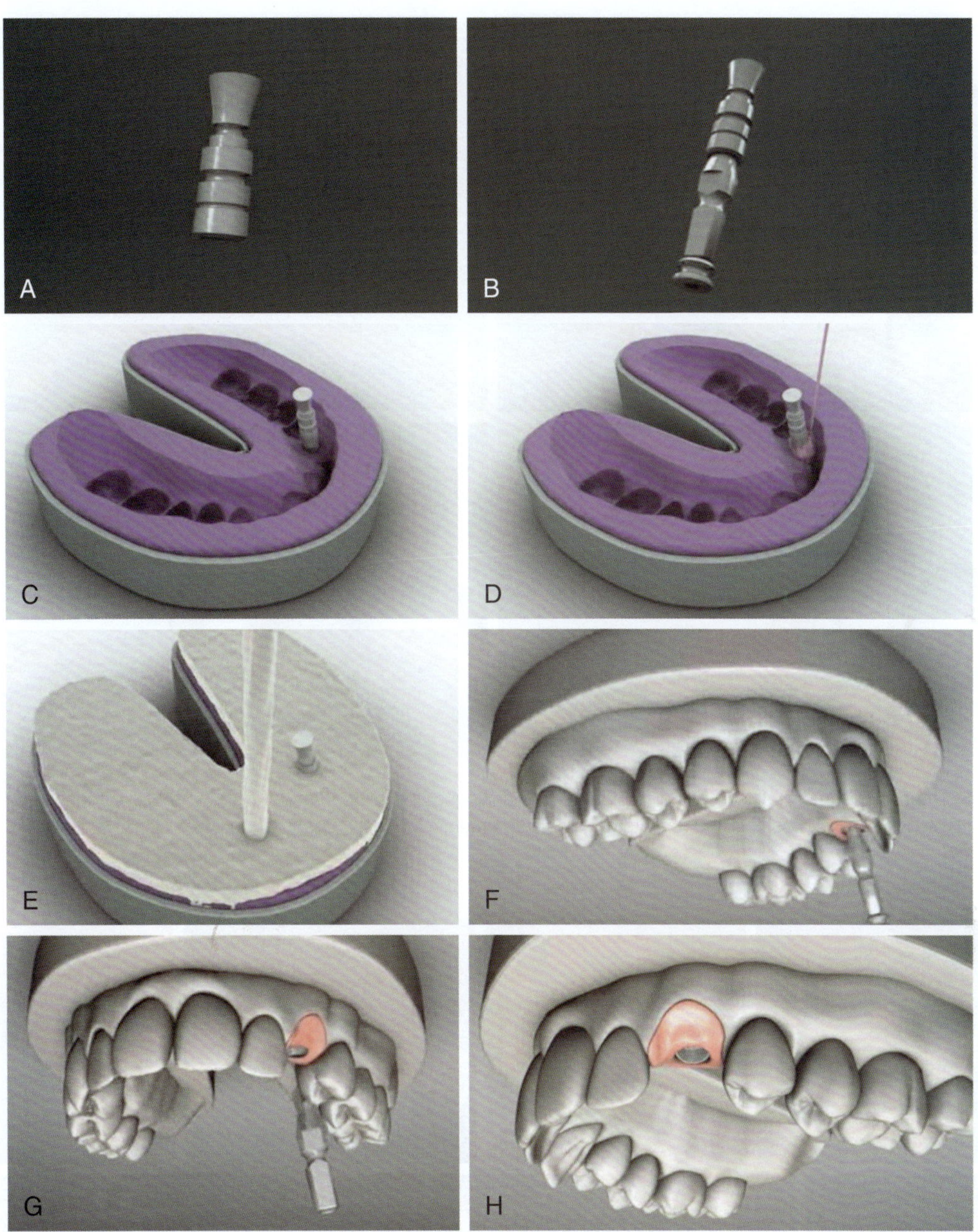

Fig 8.16 The impression post which is removed from the mouth is assembled with the implant analogue that has a different body, but a connection exactly similar to the implant. (A–C) Further, the post assembled with the analogue is re seated into the impression at the same position and with same orientation. (D) The soft tissue replicating material (Multisilk, from Bredent, Germany) is poured around the post-analogue connection followed by pouring of the (E) impression with the high-strength stone plaster. The stone cast is removed from the impression after it has set. (F) The stone cast will contain the analogue inside the stone with the impression post emerging out of it and soft tissue replica around it. (G) The impression post is removed from the analogue. (H) Now the implant connection, position, and orientation is exactly transferred from the mouth to the cast. The soft tissue replica can be removed and reseated as many times as required without any distortion to visualize and to work on analogue abutment connection (*Courtesy: Osseolink Implant Company*).

M. **Pouring the implant impression**: The impression post which is removed from the mouth is assembled with the implant analogue which has different body, but the connection is exactly similar to the implant. Further, the post assembled with the analogue is reseated into the impression at the same position and with same orientation (Fig 8.16A–C). The soft tissue replicating material (Multisilk, from Bredent, Germany) is poured around the post-analogue connection (Fig 8.16D), followed by pouring of the impression with high-strength stone plaster (Fig 8.16E). The stone cast is removed from the impression after it has set. The stone cast will contain the analogue inside the stone with impression post emerging out of it and soft tissue replica around it (Fig 8.16F). The impression post is removed from the analogue (Fig 8.16G). Now the implant connection position and orientation have been transferred exactly from the mouth to the cast (Fig 8.16H). The soft tissue replica can be removed and reseated as many

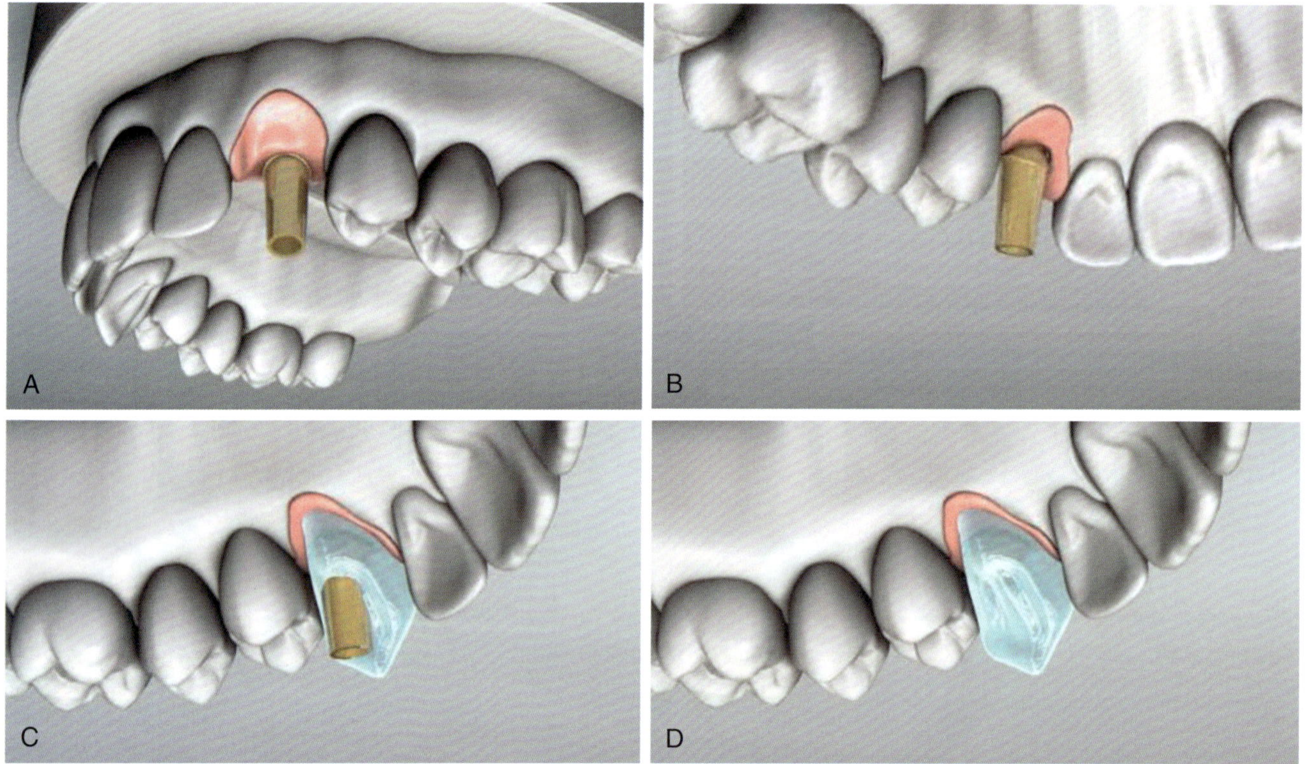

Fig 8.17 (A and B) The final abutment of choice is inserted over the analogue and shaped/milled using carbide/diamond bur for final prosthesis fabrication. (C and D) A desired final prosthesis is fabricated over this abutment (*Courtesy: Osseolink Implant Company*).

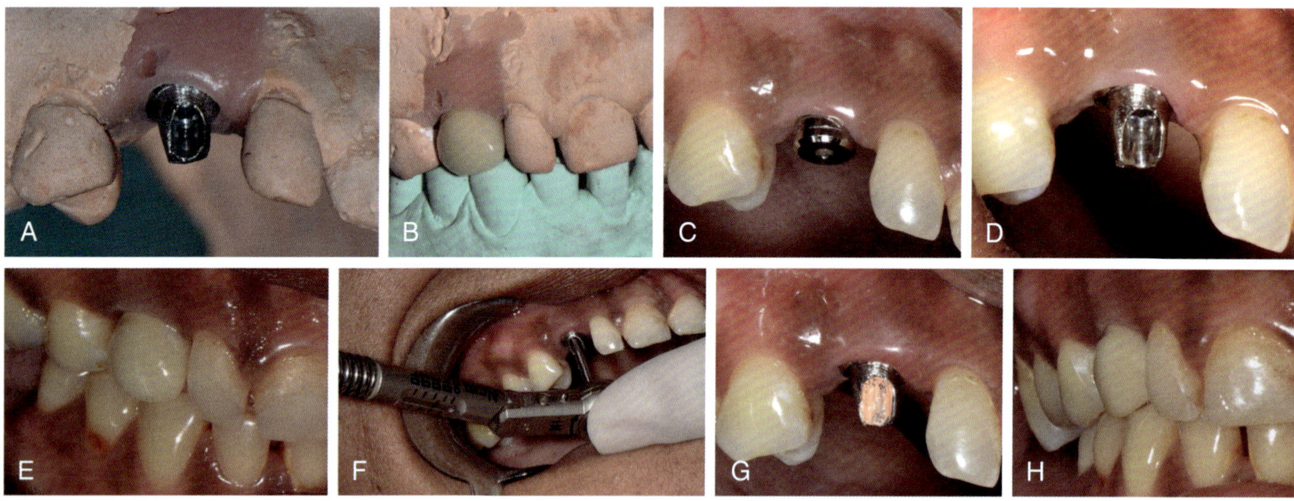

Fig 8.18 Fixing the cement-retained prosthesis. (A) The dentist receives a dental cast from the dental laboratory, which contains an implant analogue connected to metal abutment and (B) the prosthesis over the abutment. (C and D) The gingival former from the patient's mouth is removed and the abutment is transferred from the cast to the implant in patient's mouth with the same orientation. (E) The prosthesis is seated onto the abutment and checked for fitting. (F) After all the required occlusal adjustment has been done, a mechanical screwdriver (torque ratchet) is used to finally tighten the implant abutment connection screw at the moment force of 30–35 Ncm to avoid any future screw-loosening problem under the prosthesis. (H) The screw hole is filled using hot gutta-percha or wax (G) and the prosthesis is fixed using zinc oxide eugenol/zinc phosphate/glass ionomer luting cement (*Courtesy: Osseolink Implant Company*).

times as required, without any distortion to visualize and to work on analogue abutment connection.

N. **Fabrication of the final prosthesis**: The final abutment of choice is screwed over the analogue and shaped/milled using carbide/diamond bur for the fabrication of the final prosthesis. A desired final prosthesis is fabricated over this abutment (Fig 8.17A–D).

Key points

1. At this step, the implant dentist and laboratory technician can decide to fabricate either a cement or screw retained prosthesis of choice. For cement-retained prosthesis fabrication, the technician fixes an appropriate metal abutment over the analogue and shapes it to a desired shape. Further, the technician fabricates the prosthesis over it similar to normal crown fabrication onto the reduced natural tooth abutment. For screw-retained prosthesis fabrication, a plastic castable abutment is fixed onto the analogue, shaped and sent to the dental laboratory. The dental technician makes a wax pattern of the coping over this plastic abutment, removes it from the analogue and after removing its connection screw, he/she casts all together to fabricate a metal coping that can be fixed directly over the analogue using the connection screw. Further, the ceramist builds the ceramic over this casting keeping the patency of fixation screw opening. This screw retained ceramic prosthesis dentist directly fix to the implant in the mouth using connection screw.
2. If the implant placement is not prosthetically guided or if the implant surgeon has intentionally inserted the implant at an angle to the long axis of the prosthesis to insert it in best available bone, one can use an angled abutment to fabricate the prosthesis at the correct axis. The 15–25° angled abutments (metal as well as plastic) are available in most implant systems to correct this prosthetic problem.

O. **Fixing the final prosthesis over the implant**: The dentist receives either the cement-retained or screw-retained prosthesis from the dental laboratory which he/she needs to finally fix onto the implant in the mouth.

1. **Fixing the cement-retained prosthesis**: The dentist receives a dental cast from the dental laboratory, which contains the implant analogue connected to metal abutment and the prosthesis over the abutment. The prosthesis from the abutment is removed and the abutment is marked on the facial side using a permanent ink marker and the same is extended to the cast so that one can correlate the same orientation to the abutment in the patient's mouth. The gingival former from the patient's mouth is removed and the abutment is transferred from the cast to the implant in the patient's mouth with the same orientation. The prosthesis is seated onto the abutment and checked for fitting. One should check the complete seating of the prosthesis with a radiograph. After all the required occlusal adjustment has been done, a mechanical screwdriver (torque ratchet) is used to finally tighten the implant abutment connection screw at the moment force of 30–35 Ncm to avoid any future screw loosening problem under the prosthesis. The screw hole is filled using hot gutta-percha or wax and the prosthesis is fixed using zinc oxide eugenol/zinc phosphate/glass ionomer luting cement (Fig 8.18A–F).
2. **Fixing the screw-retained prosthesis:** The dentist receives from the dental laboratory, the dental cast with implant analogue connected to the prosthesis by a connection screw through a screw hole in the prosthesis. The gingival former is removed from the patient's mouth and the prosthesis is transferred to the implant in the patient's mouth with the correct orientation, and screwed in using the connection screw. The complete seating of the prosthesis is radiographically checked. All the required adjustments are done and a mechanical screwdriver (torque ratchet) is used to finally tighten the connection screw at the moment force 30–35 Ncm. The screw hole is first filled with the hot gutta-percha followed by light cure composite over it to blend its shade to the shade of the prosthesis (Fig 8.19A–H).

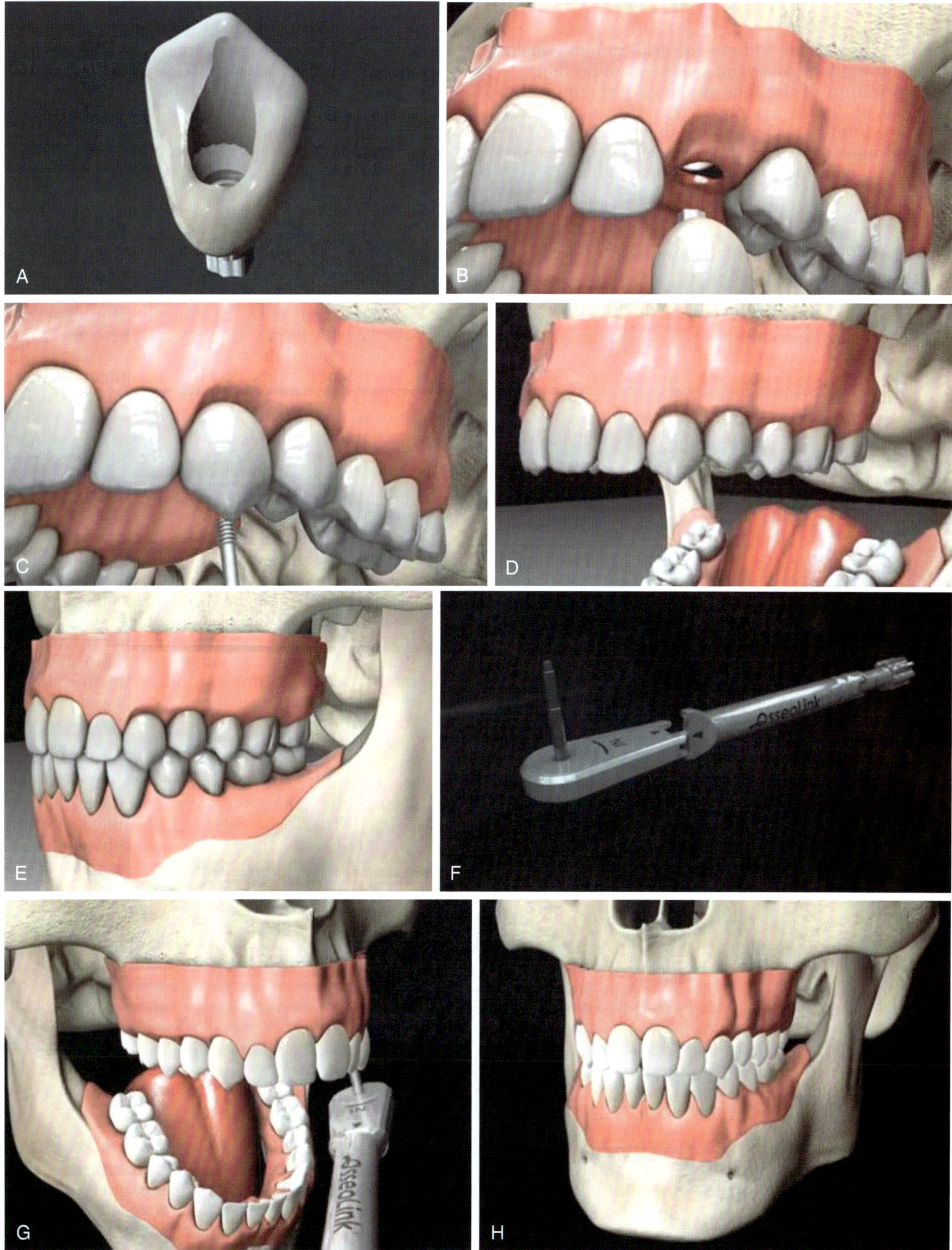

Fig 8.19 Fixing the screw-retained prosthesis. (A) The finally fabricated screw-retained crown. (B–D) Crown is seated over the implant with the correct orientation and fixed using a connection screw which goes through the crown hole to the implant connection. (E) The occlusion is checked and the corrections are made if needed. (F and G) A mechanical torque ratchet is used to finally tighten the connection screw at the moment of 30–35 Ncm for avoiding the screw loosening problem. (H) The screw hole of the crown is filled using gutta-percha and the tooth coloured composite.

CASE REPORT-1

Step by step presentation of implant insertion for the mandibular first molar and its restoration (Figs 8.20–8.33).

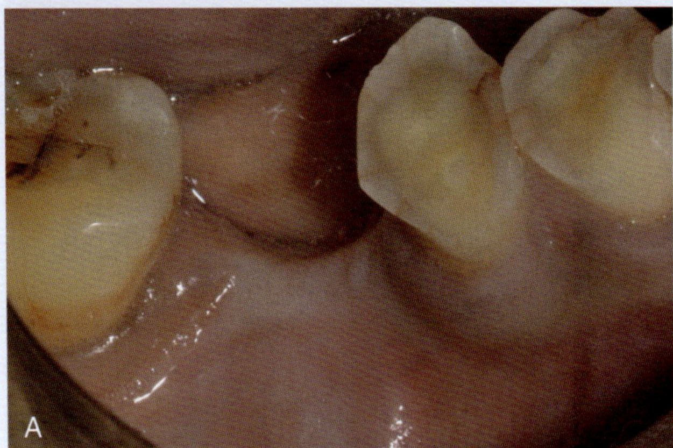

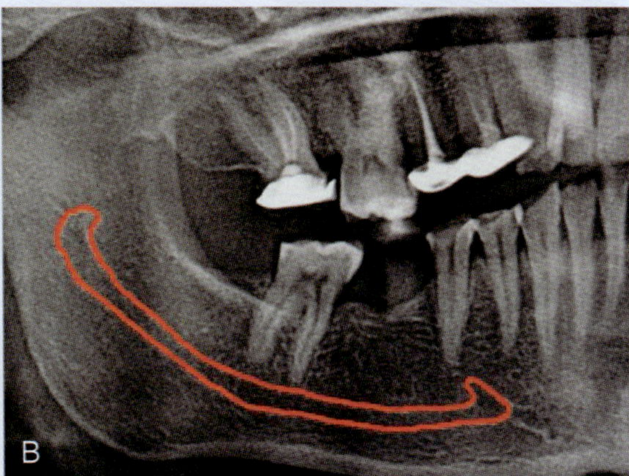

Fig 8.20 (A) Missing right mandibular first molar. (B) Diagnostic radiograph is showing adequate bone height above the mandibular canal to insert adequately long implant.

Continued

CASE REPORT-1—cont'd

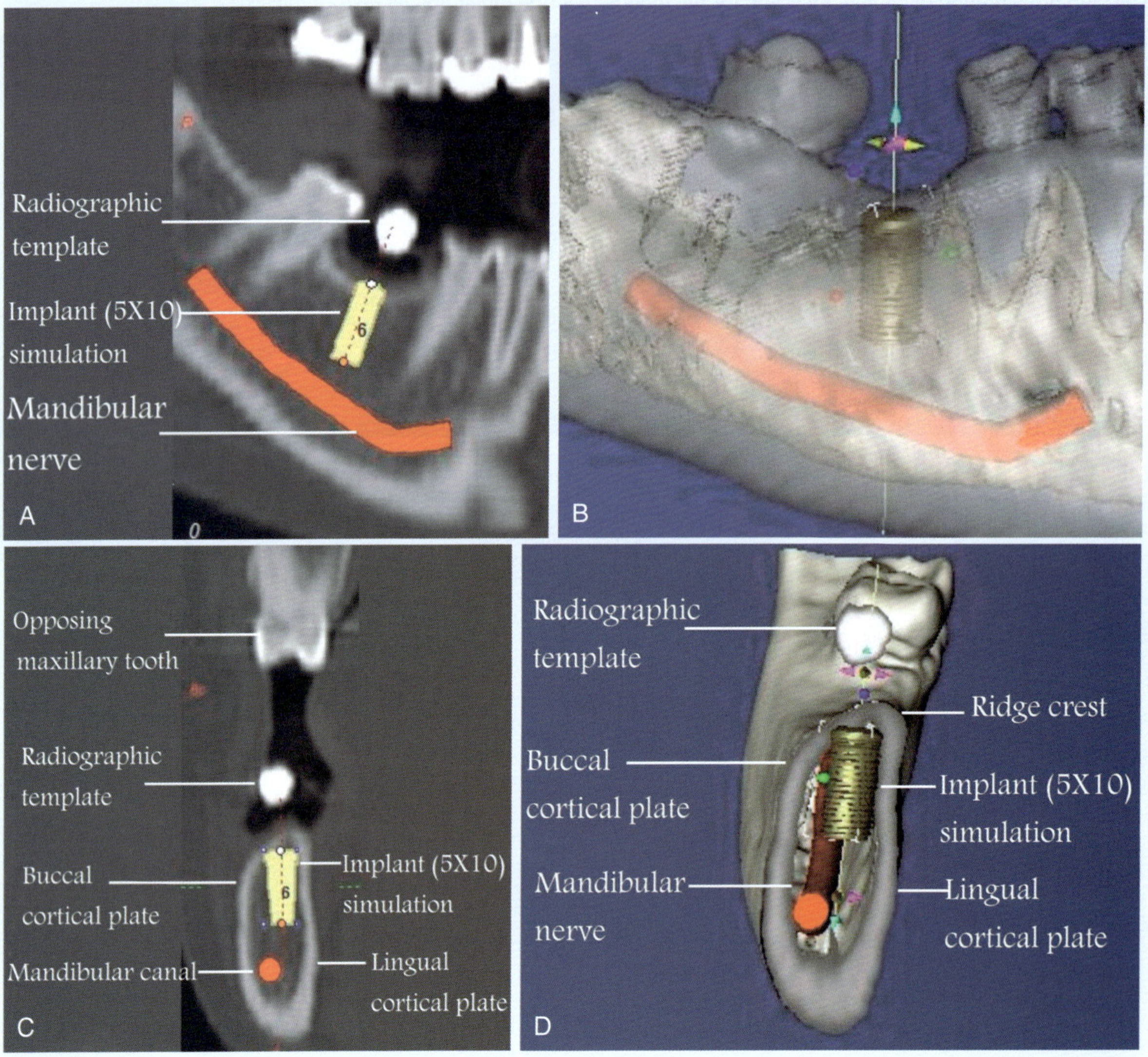

Fig 8.21 (A and B) CT plan shows Implant (5 × 10 mm) simulation. (C and D) Cross-sectional view and section cut of 3D view showing irregular ridge crest, which needs to be flattened to get a flat bone crest for the best possible large diameter implant without any implant thread exposure on the facial aspect of the crest.

CASE REPORT-1—cont'd

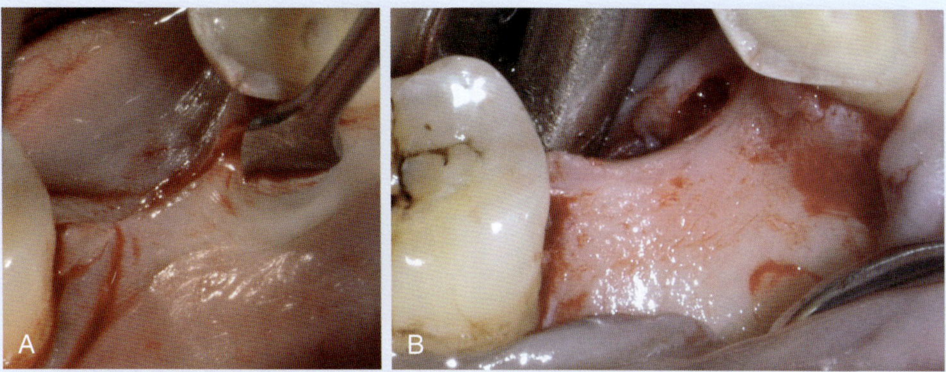

Fig 8.22 (A and B) Mid-crestal and crevicular incisions are made and buccal and lingual mucoperiosteal flaps are elevated to expose the ridge crest.

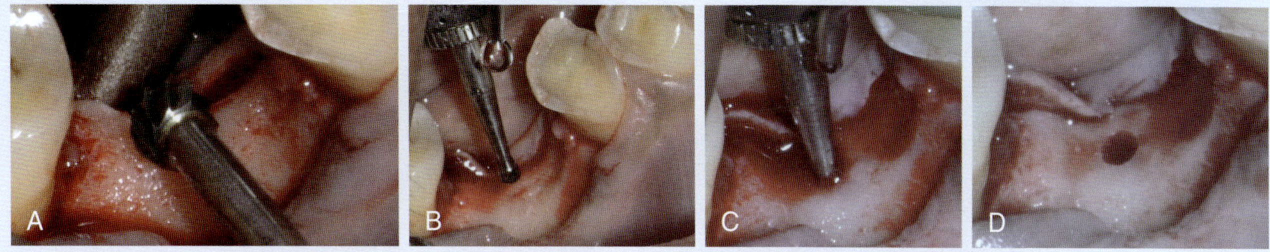

Fig 8.23 (A) The ridge crest is flattened (vertical osteoplasty) using a large round carbide trimmer. A small round carbide bur is used to mark the implant osteotomy site at mesiodistal and buccolingual midpoint of the ridge crest. (B–D) This bur should punch the high density cortical bone to reach to the underlying low density cancellous bone.

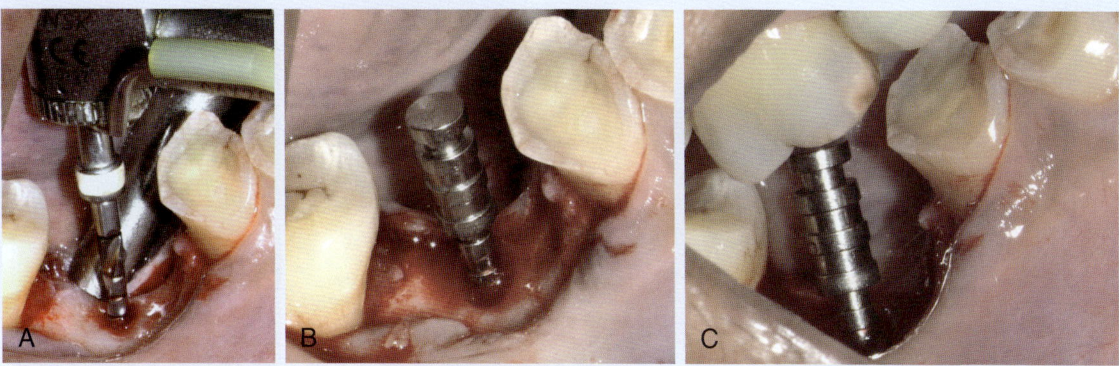

Fig 8.24 Initial osteotomy preparation is done with the pilot drill to a depth of 10 mm. (A) The complete depth should be achieved with this pilot drill as the rest of the drills are osteotomy widening drills. (B and C) The parallel pin/force direction indicator is inserted to check parallelism with the adjacent teeth and also to evaluate the direction of the occlusal forces from opposing tooth over the future implant prosthesis. Any correction, if required, can be done at this stage using the side-cutting Lindemann drill.

Continued

CASE REPORT-1—cont'd

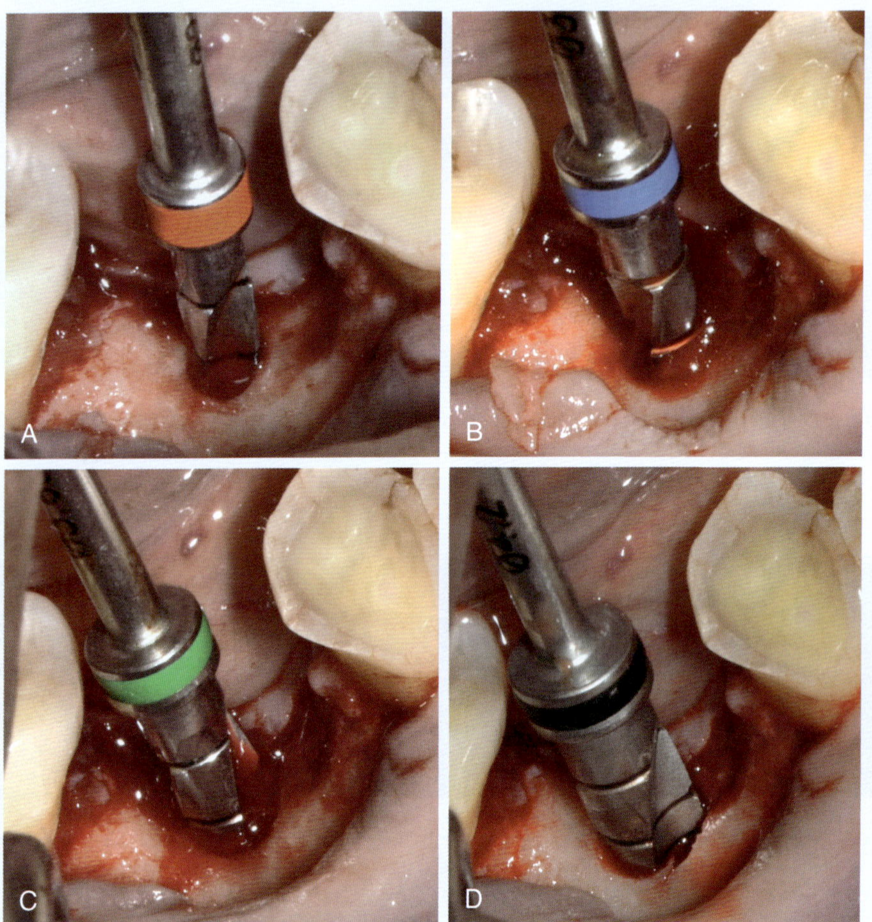

Fig 8.25 (A–D) The rest of the osteotomy-widening drills (2.8, 3.2, 3.65 and 4.2 mm diameter) are sequentially used to widen the osteotomy to the same depth.

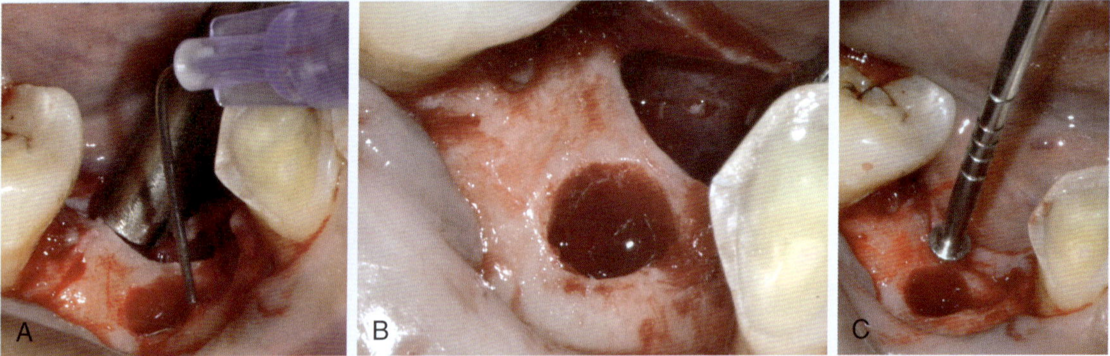

Fig 8.26 (A) The finally prepared osteotomy is irrigated using chilled saline to remove all the bone debris and cool down the bone. The bone debris, if left inside, can be collected at the apex and prevent complete seating of the inserted implant. (B) Finally, prepared osteotomy can be checked using DGI probe for any perforation, and also to induce fresh bleeding. (C) This special instrument can be inserted into the prepared osteotomy and moved up and down along the walls of the osteotomy, to check if any perforation has occurred; its tip gets stuck in the same.

CASE REPORT-1—cont'd

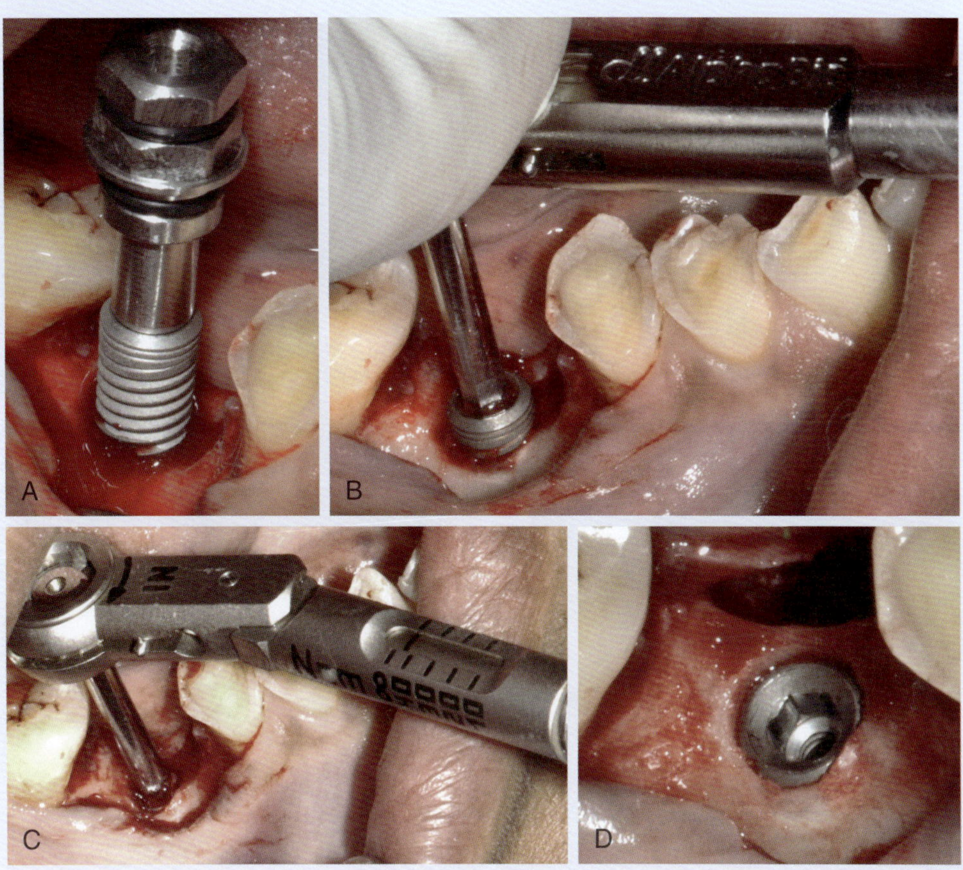

Fig 8.27 (A) Implant is inserted in the prepared osteotomy and (B) screwed in using the hand ratchet till it seats completely. (C) Torque ratchet can be used to evaluate the primary stability of the implant, which is achieved more than 40 Ncm in this case (see the line marks on the ratchet handle). (D) The seated implant with its platform at the level of ridge crest.

Continued

CASE REPORT-1—cont'd

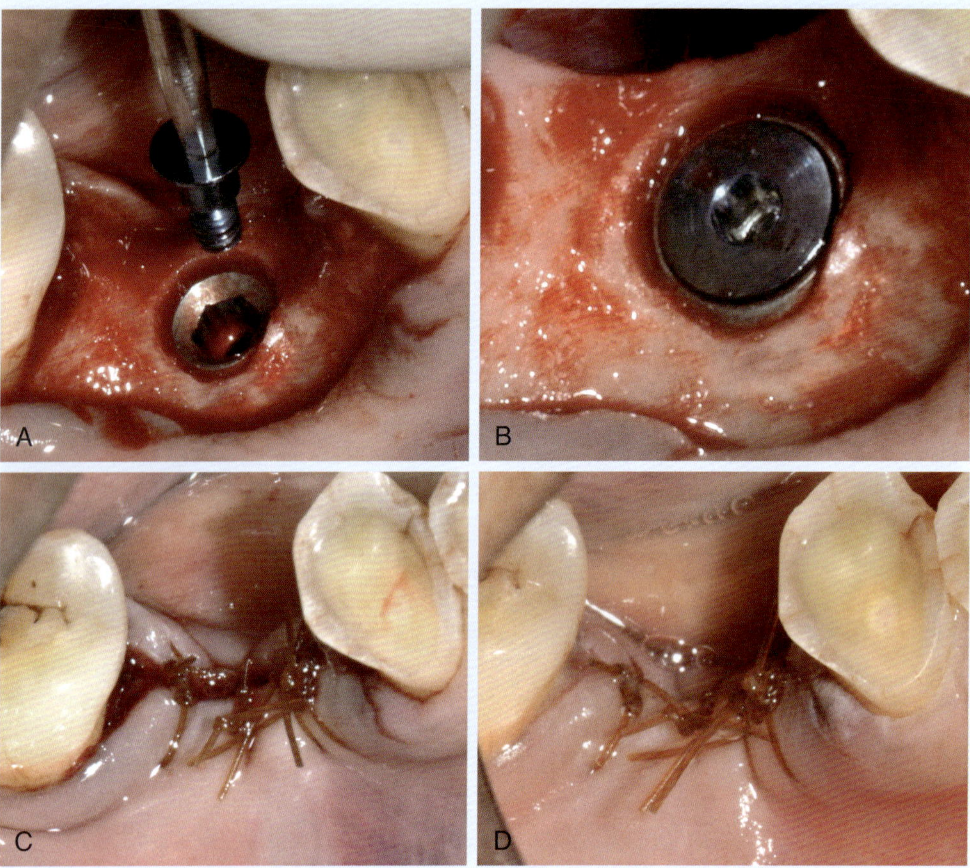

Fig 8.28 (A and B) Cover screw is inserted onto the implant to cover the implant hex connection and (C) the flap is sutured back. (D) Healing of the site on the second day of surgery.

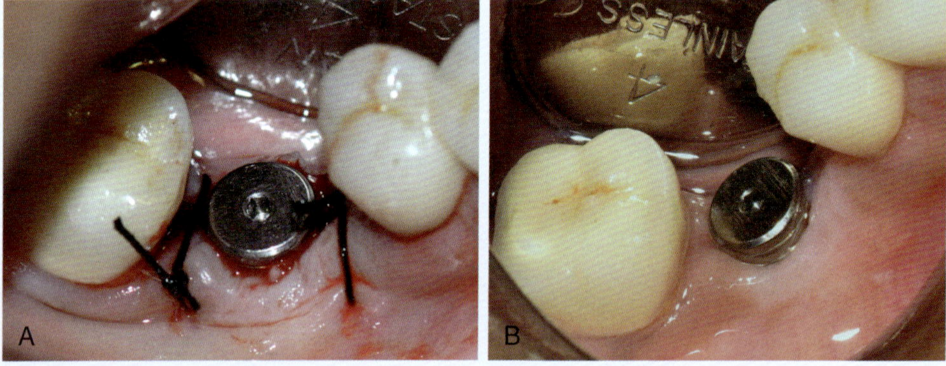

Fig 8.29 The implant is uncovered after it has osseointegrated in 4 months. (A) A mid-crestal incision is given, the cover screw is removed and replaced with the long gingival former, and the flap is sutured back. (B) The soft tissue has adequately healed in 3 weeks after implant uncovery and is ready for the implant impression.

CASE REPORT-1—cont'd

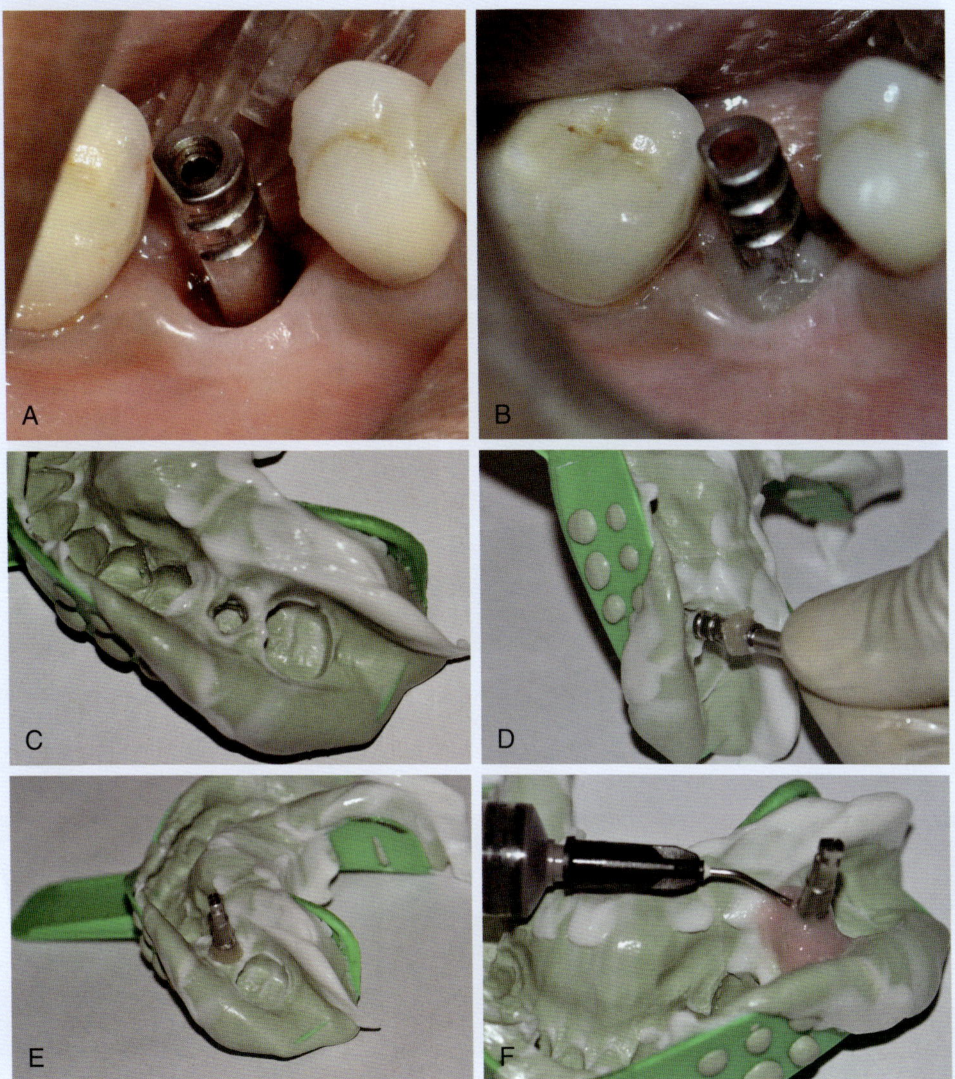

Fig 8.30 (A) The gingival former is removed from the implant and the impression post is inserted. (B) The flow composite is poured and cured into the soft tissue spaces around the impression post for accurately transferring the soft tissue emergence to the working cast. The screw hole of the post is also filled using wax. (C) The closed tray indirect impression of the implant is made, using addition silicon putty and light body, (D and E) the impression post with the composite attached to it, is removed from the implant, assembled with the implant analogue, and transferred to the impression with the same orientation. (F) The soft tissue replicating material (Gi-Mask from Coltene Whaldent) is poured around the post analogue connection.

Continued

CASE REPORT-1—cont'd

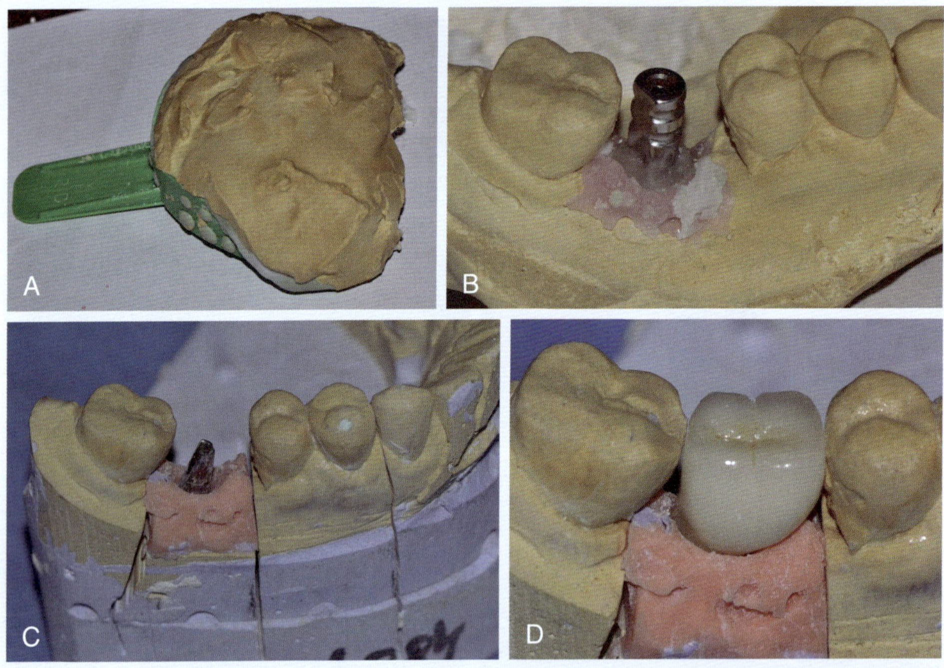

Fig 8.31 (A) The impression is poured using a high strength stone plaster. (B) The stone cast removed from the impression after it has set, shows the impression post connected to the analogue. (C) The impression post is removed and replaced by an appropriate final abutment which is shaped in the dental laboratory. (D) A metal-free zirconium crown is fabricated in the laboratory onto the prepared abutment.

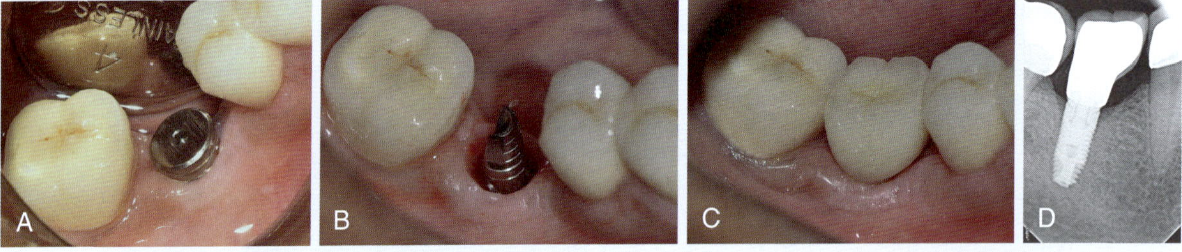

Fig 8.32 (A and B) The gingival former is removed from the implant and replaced with the abutment which is transferred from the cast and fixed to the implant with the same orientation as on the cast. (C) The prosthesis is seated onto the abutment and (D) radiographically checked for its complete and accurate seating onto the abutment.

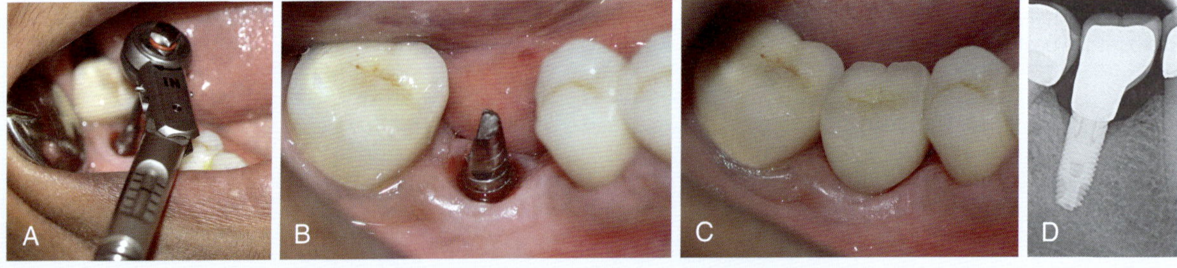

Fig 8.33 (A) The prosthesis is removed and the connection screw of the abutment is finally tightened at the moment of 35 Ncm using torque ratchet. (B) The screw hole of the abutment is filled with the wax. (C) The prosthesis is finally luted onto the abutment using glass ionomer luting cement. (D) A radiograph is taken to check the complete seating of crown and also to check any luting cement in the peri-implant soft tissue. Any cement, if left in the soft tissue pocket, may cause peri-implantitis and crestal bone resorption.

CASE REPORT-2

Flapless (using soft tissue punch) implant insertion for the mandibular first molar and restoration with prepared abutment impression technique (Figs 8.34–8.44).

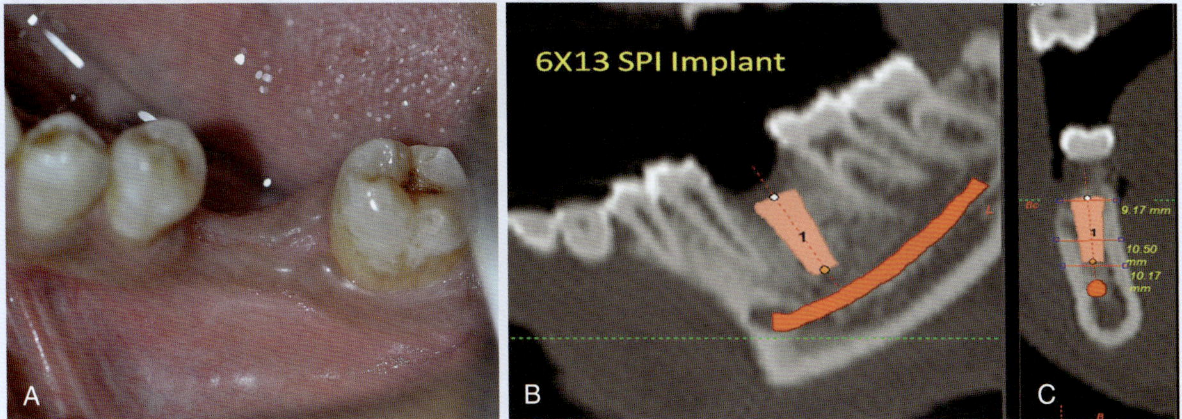

Fig 8.34 (A) Clinical view of missing mandibular first molar shows adequate band of attached keratinized tissue at the ridge crest. (B and C) Three-dimensional CT planning shows adequate amount of bone, without any undercut, available for flapless implant (6 x 13 mm.) insertion.

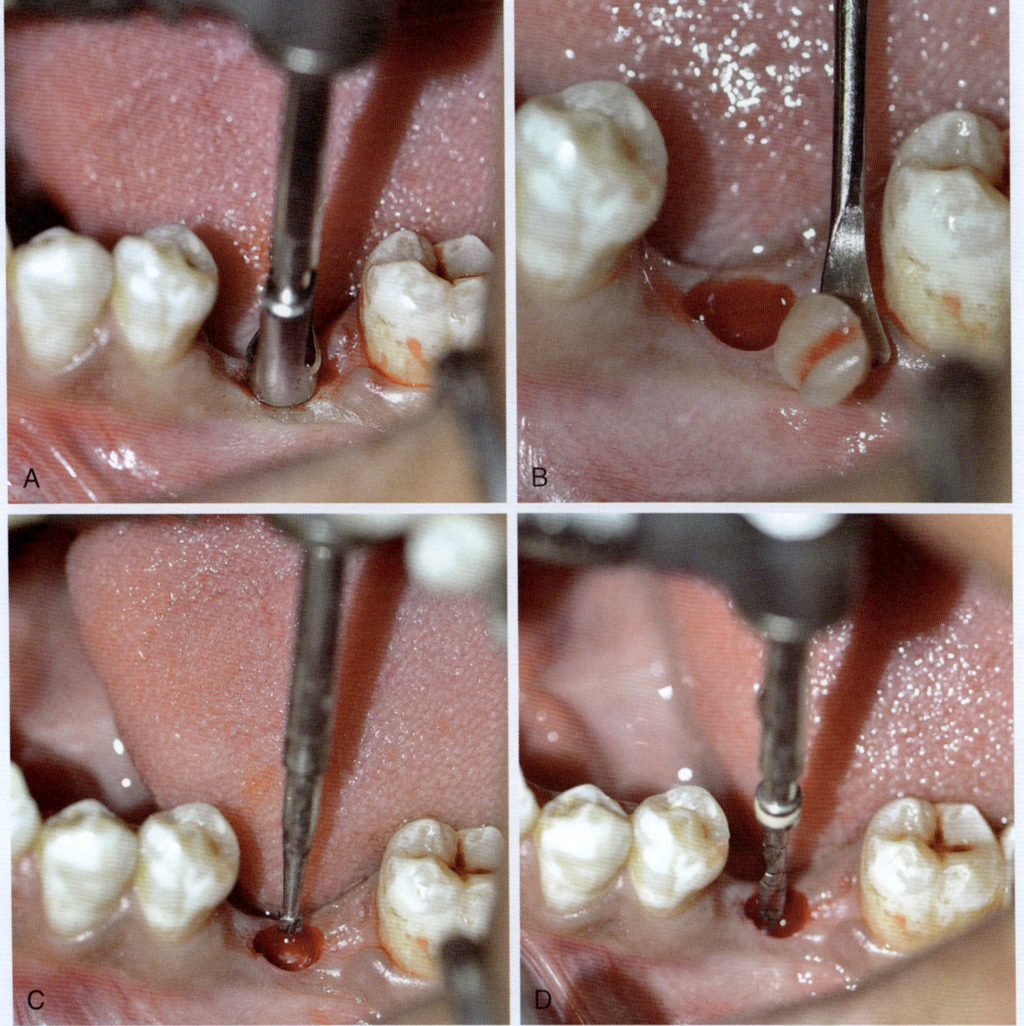

Fig 8.35 (A and B) A tissue punch of 5 mm diameter is used to punch out the soft tissue and (C) a small round carbide bur is used to drill through the ridge crest cortex followed by (D) 2 mm pilot drill to the planned depth.

Continued

CASE REPORT-2—cont'd

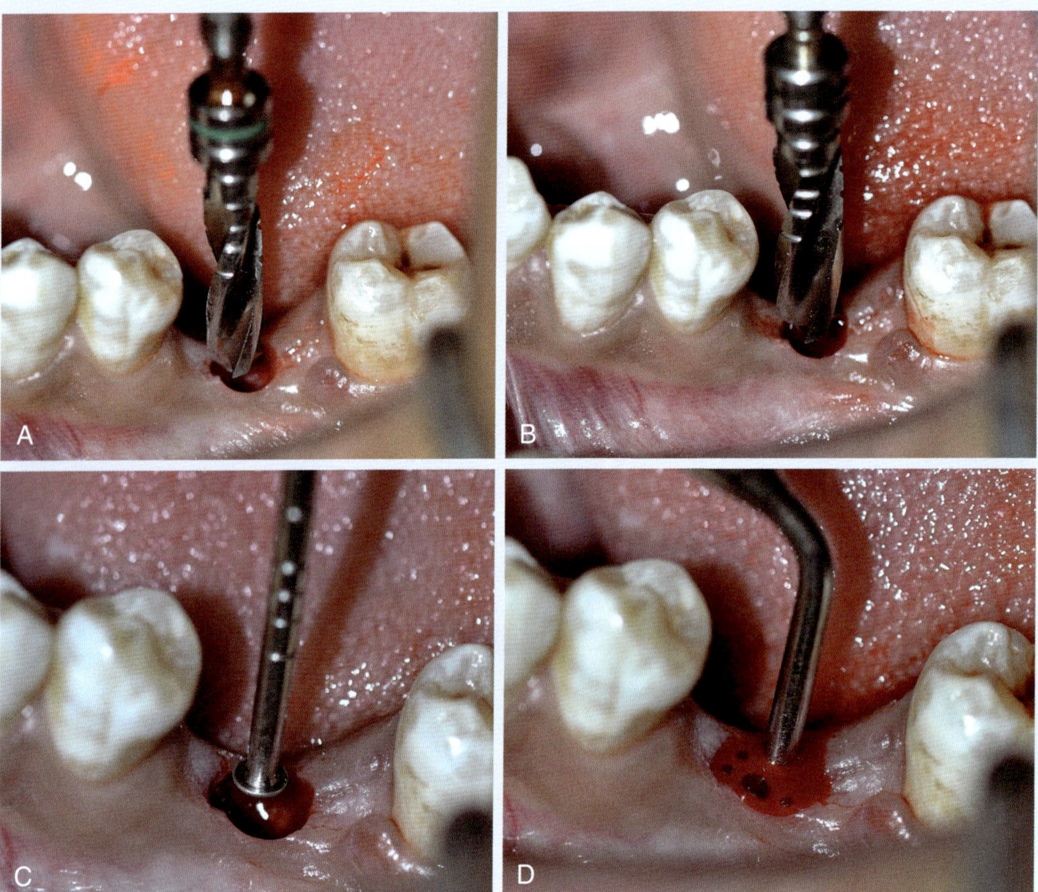

Fig 8.36 (A) The pilot drill should attain the complete depth (13 mm). When inserting implant with flapless technique, the punched out soft tissue height should be measured and added up to the drilling depth because the dentist cannot visualize the bony crest during the drilling, but the soft tissue margin is used as the reference point for the drilling. In this case the soft tissue height is 3 mm; hence, to place 13 mm-long implant, the osteotomy is prepared 16 mm deep from the soft tissue margins. (A and B) All the osteotomy widening drills (φ2.8, φ3.2, φ3.65, φ4.3, φ5.2 mm) are sequentially used to the complete depth. The completed osteotomy is irrigated using chilled saline to cool down the bone and to remove the bony shaving chips (which can prevent the complete seating of the implant) from the osteotomy. (C and D) DGI (defect-specific gingival index) depth probe is inserted to evaluate any perforation and also to provoke fresh bleeding in the osteotomy.

CASE REPORT-2—cont'd

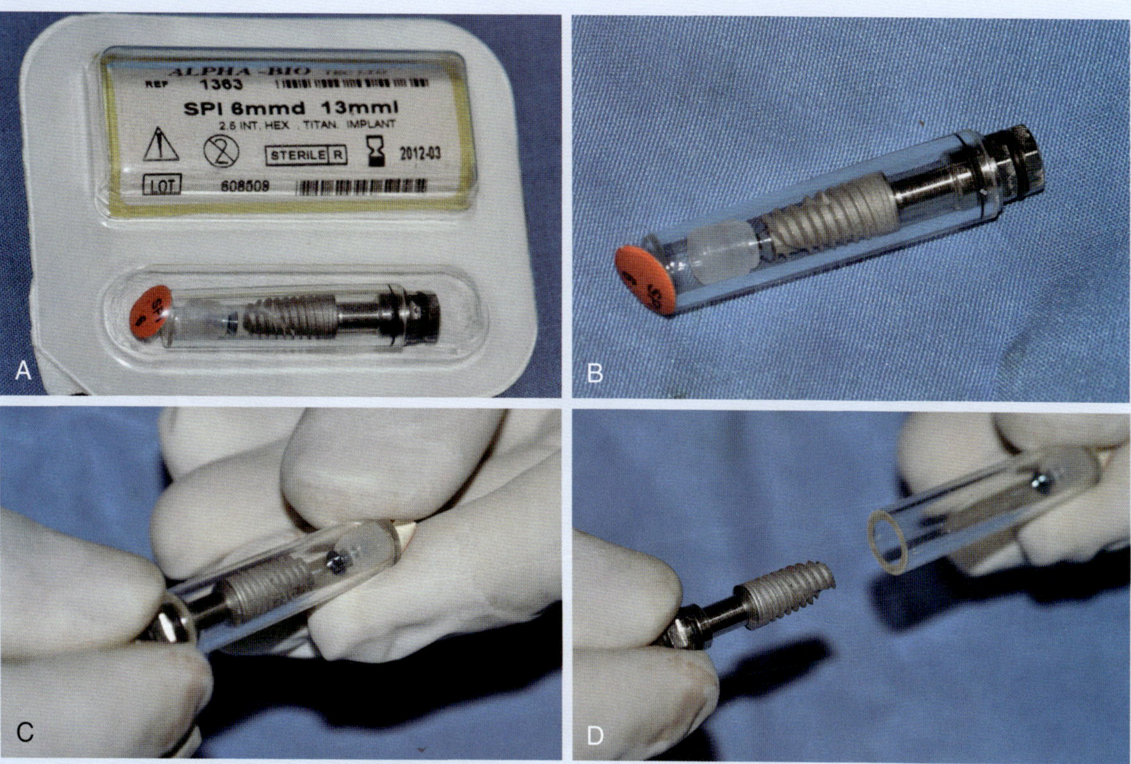

Fig 8.37 (A) Implant packaging, which is unsterile from the outside but has a sterile vial inside and contains implant connected to the mount and one cover screw. (B) The implant packaging is opened and the vial, which contains the implant with mount and cover screw at its base, is removed. (C and D) The implant is removed from the sterile vial by holding the implant mount with gloved hands.

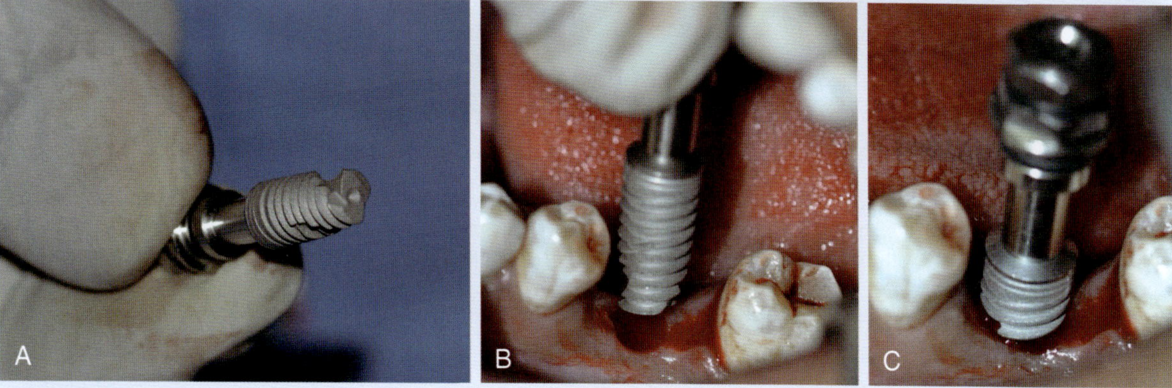

Fig 8.38 The implant surface should not be touched with gloved hands or any instrument which can contaminate its surface. (A) The implant should always be carried to the osteotomy site in the upward position to avoid its sudden detachment from the mount and fall. The osteotomy should remain filled with fresh blood before implant insertion, as this blood carries the different kind of blood cells like platelets and bone morphogenetic proteins (BMPs) from the surrounding bone to the implant surface, which is important for predictable contact osteogenesis. (B and C) The implant is inserted into the osteotomy and threaded with the hand to secure it enough to avoid movement.

Continued

CASE REPORT-2—cont'd

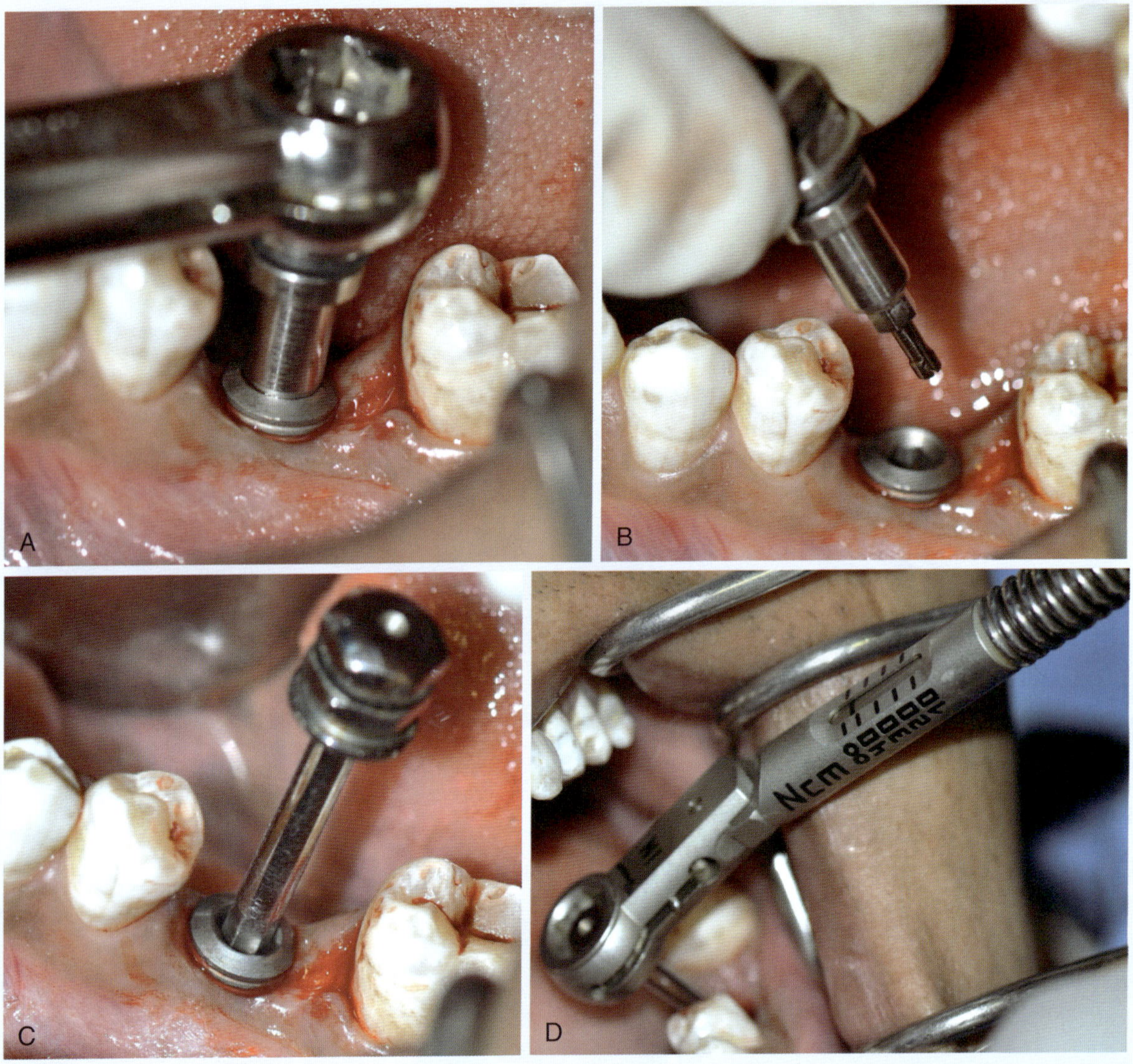

A B C D

Fig 8.39 (A) The implant ratchet is fitted onto the mount head and rotated clockwise to carry the implant further into the osteotomy. If the adjacent teeth start hindering with the short length mount, it can be removed (B) and (C) replaced by a long implant driver. A simple ratchet or a torque ratchet can be used to carry the implant to the complete depth. (D) The torque ratchet shows adequate implant primary stability (40 Ncm) of the implant.

CASE REPORT-2—cont'd

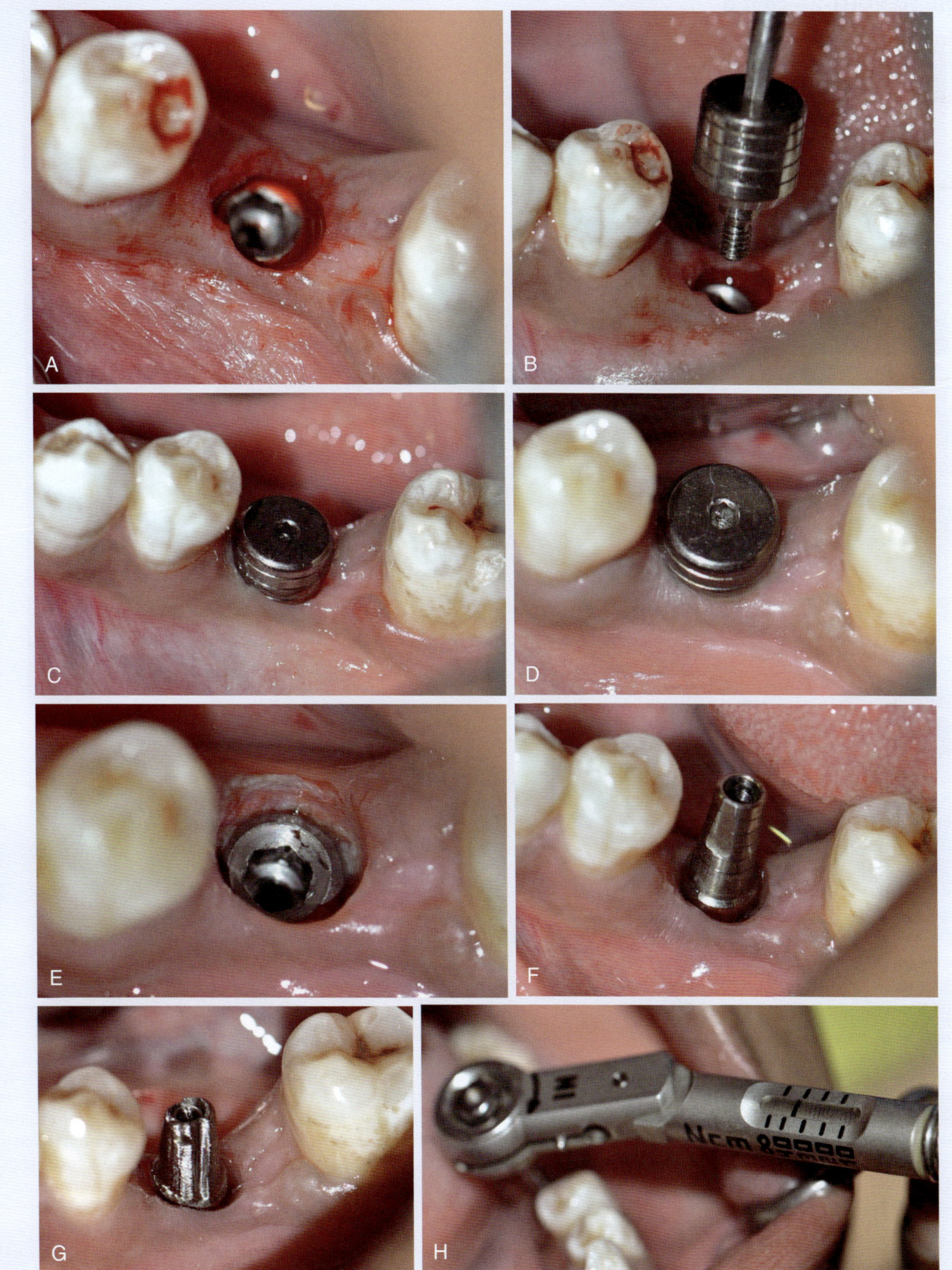

Fig 8.40 (A) Implant at the final position. (B and C) A gingival former inserted to the implant for non-submersed healing. (D) Healing, as seen 2 days after implant insertion. (E) The gingival former is removed after 3 months and (F) a straight abutment is inserted which is prepared in the mouth (G) using carbide burs. (H) The torque ratchet is used to tighten its connection screw at 35 Ncm to avoid any future screw loosening problem.

Continued

CASE REPORT-2—cont'd

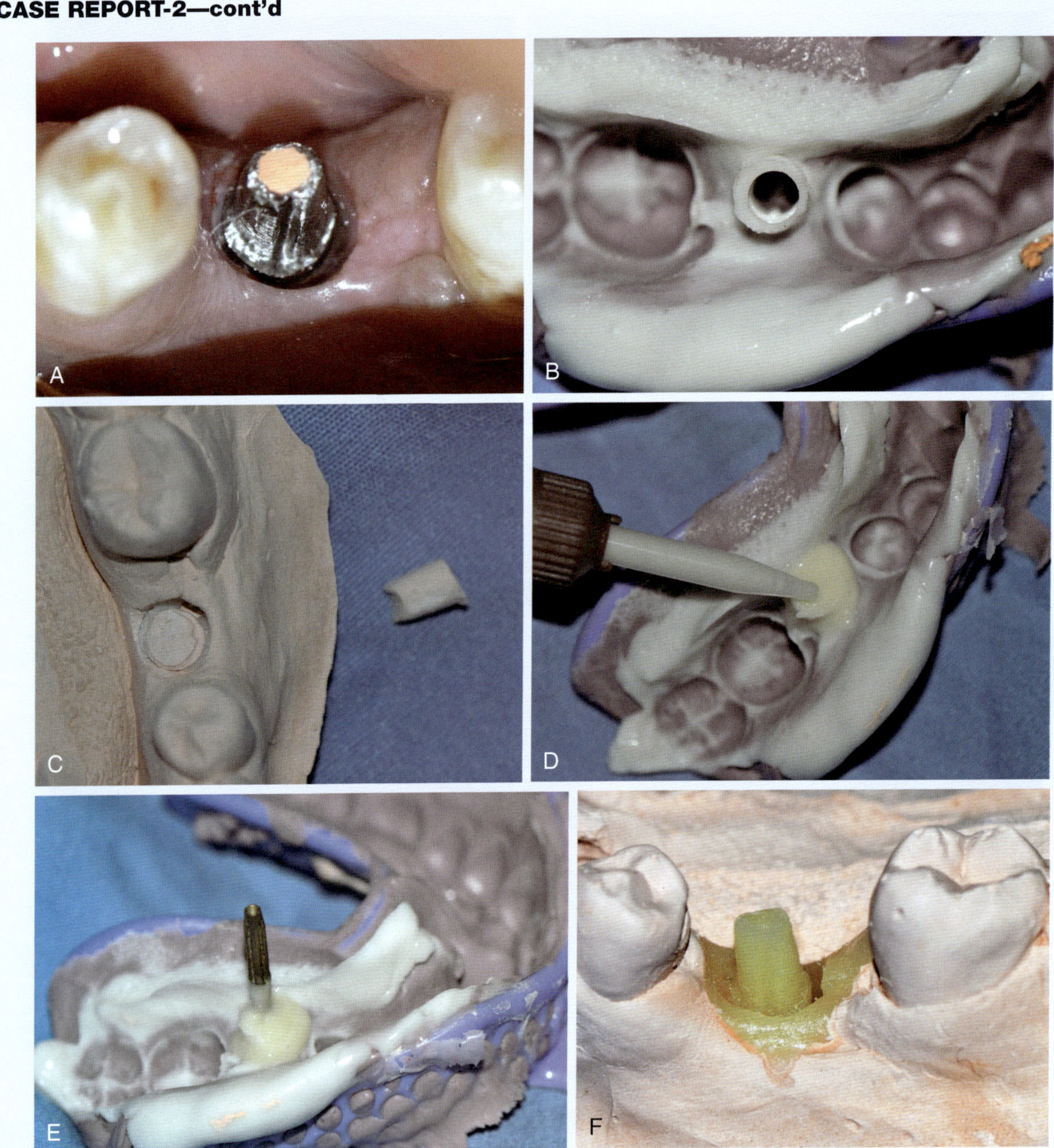

Fig 8.41 (A) The screw hole of the abutment is filled with gutta-percha and (B) the impression is made using additional silicon impression material with direct prepared abutment impression technique. (C) If the impression is poured with stone it may result in the breakage of the thin abutment on removing the cast, so the impression should be poured using a hard material. (D) A dual-cure core build-up material is used to fill the abutment impression and (E) a die pin is inserted to hold it in the stone plaster. The impression is poured with stone plaster. (F) The cast removed shows the abutment of core build-up material. Alternatively, the hard pattern resin material can also be used to pour the abutment area. The crown of choice is fabricated over this abutment in the laboratory.

CASE REPORT-2—cont'd

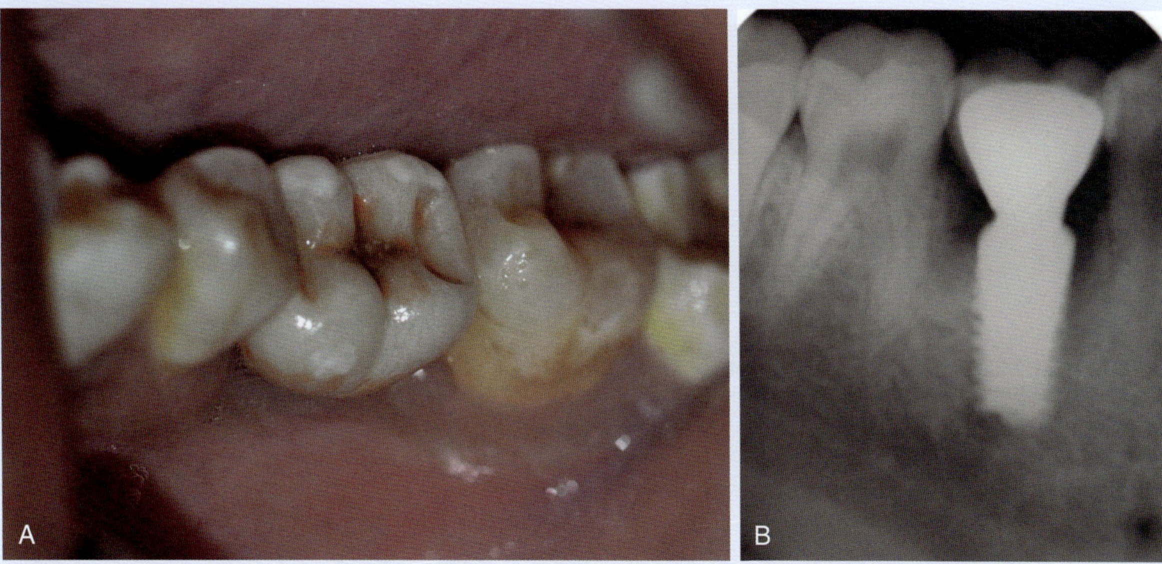

Fig 8.42 (A) The porcelain fused to metal crown is fixed over the implant. (B) Post loading radiograph.

Implant insertion in aesthetic region

The implant therapy in aesthetic region is very challenging to meet the hard and soft tissue aesthetic demands of the patient.

Key Points

1. The implant should be placed at the three-dimensionally correct position and angulation.
2. The implant platform should be placed a minimum of 2 mm above the CEJ of the adjacent tooth to achieve the adequate soft tissue drape and emergence profile. In cases of soft tissue recession from the adjacent teeth, the implant platform should be placed 2–3 mm apical to the gingival zenith (Fig 8.43).
3. Besides placing implant platform 2 mm apical to the CEJ of adjacent teeth or gingival zenith, it should also be placed palatal to the imaginary line connecting the facial aspect of CEJ of two adjacent teeth.
4. The diameter of the implant should be chosen according to the tooth being replaced, to achieve an aesthetic emergence profile of the implant prosthesis. The placement of an implant slightly narrower than the natural tooth root often is indicated to decrease the risk of the lateral perforation of the bone and being too close to the adjacent tooth root.
5. Guided bone and soft tissue regeneration procedure should be performed to repair defects before or at the time of implant therapy.
6. Extensive treatment planning should be done to achieve the optimum aesthetic outcome.
7. The soft tissue should be crafted to achieve the optimal aesthetic outcome at the time of implant uncovering.

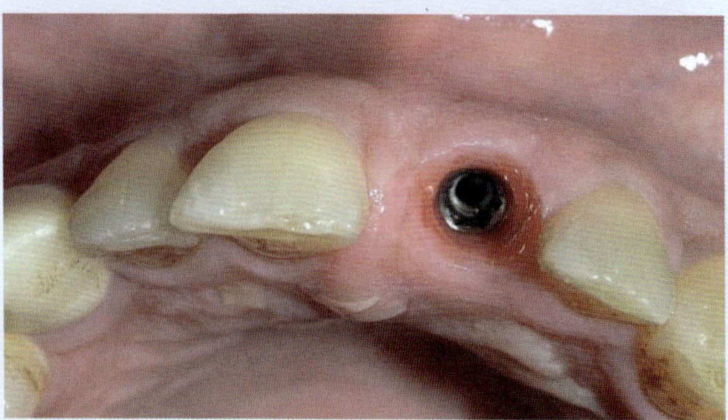

Fig 8.43 In the maxillary aesthetic region, the implant platform should be placed minimum 2 mm above the CEJ of the adjacent tooth, to achieve adequate soft tissue drape and emergence profile. In cases of soft tissue recession from the adjacent teeth, the implant platform should be placed 2–3 mm apical to the gingival zenith. The implant platform should be placed 2 mm apical to the CEJ of adjacent teeth or the gingival zenith, and it should also be placed palatal to the imaginary line connecting the facial aspect of the CEJ of two adjacent teeth.

8. Papillae should be preserved or created.
9. Metal-free zirconium prosthesis should be preferred over porcelain fused to metal prosthesis to achieve high aesthetic results (Fig 8.44A–D).

Continued

CASE REPORT-2—cont'd

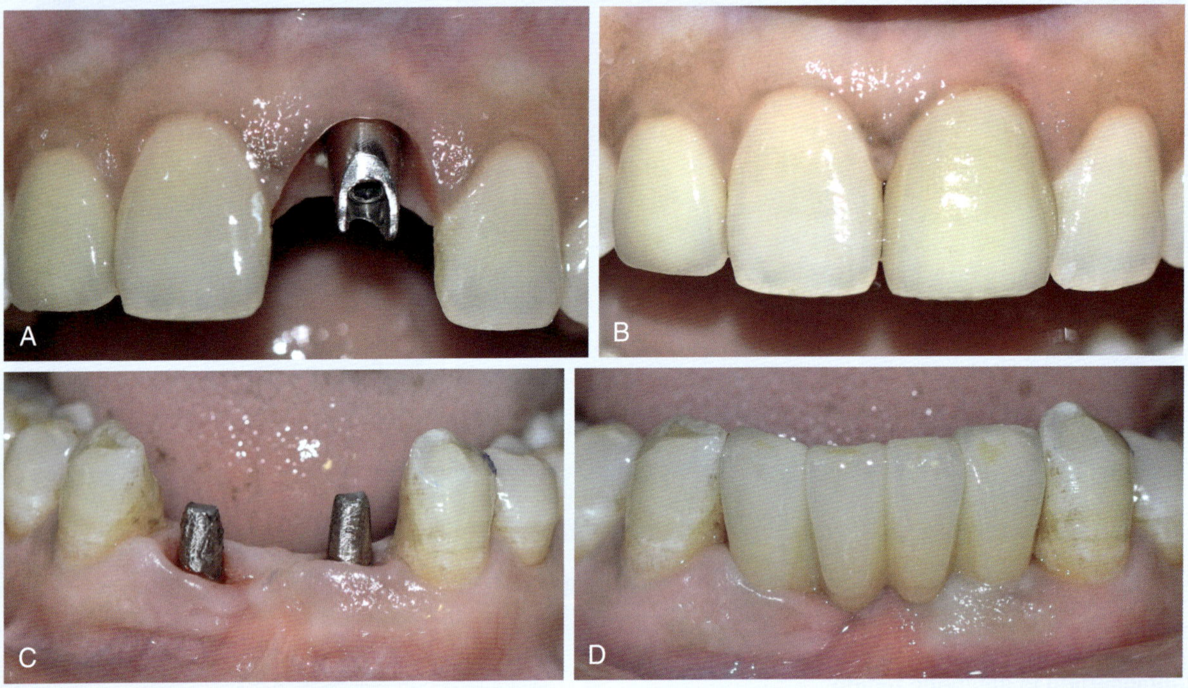

Fig 8.44 (A and B) Implant at maxillary central incisor position is restored using metal-free zirconium crown. (C and D) The two implants at the mandibular anterior position are restored using a zirconium bridge.

CASE REPORT-3

Implants uncovery and soft tissue crafting to create papillae in the maxillary aesthetic region (Figs 8.45–8.53).

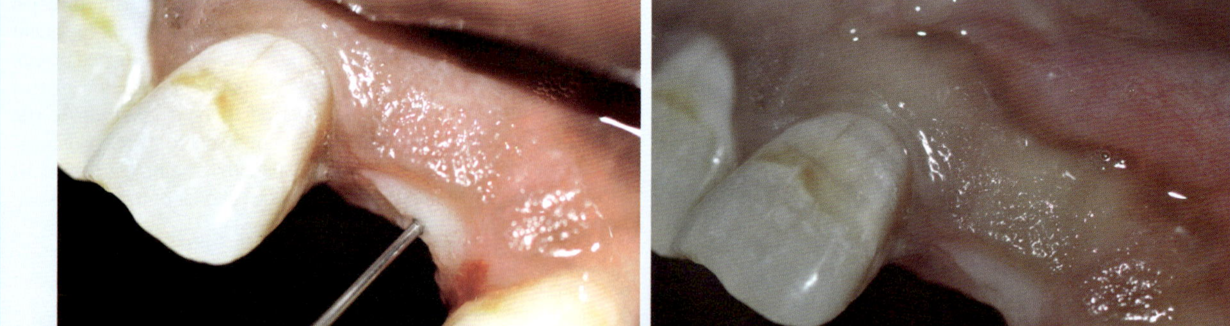

Fig 8.45 (A) A small amount of local anaesthetic is infiltrated directly at the ridge crest for implant uncovery 4 months after implant placement. (B) It causes blanching of the soft tissue. This approach not only anaesthetizes the tissue required to uncover the implant, but also reduces bleeding during uncovery.

CASE REPORT-3—cont'd

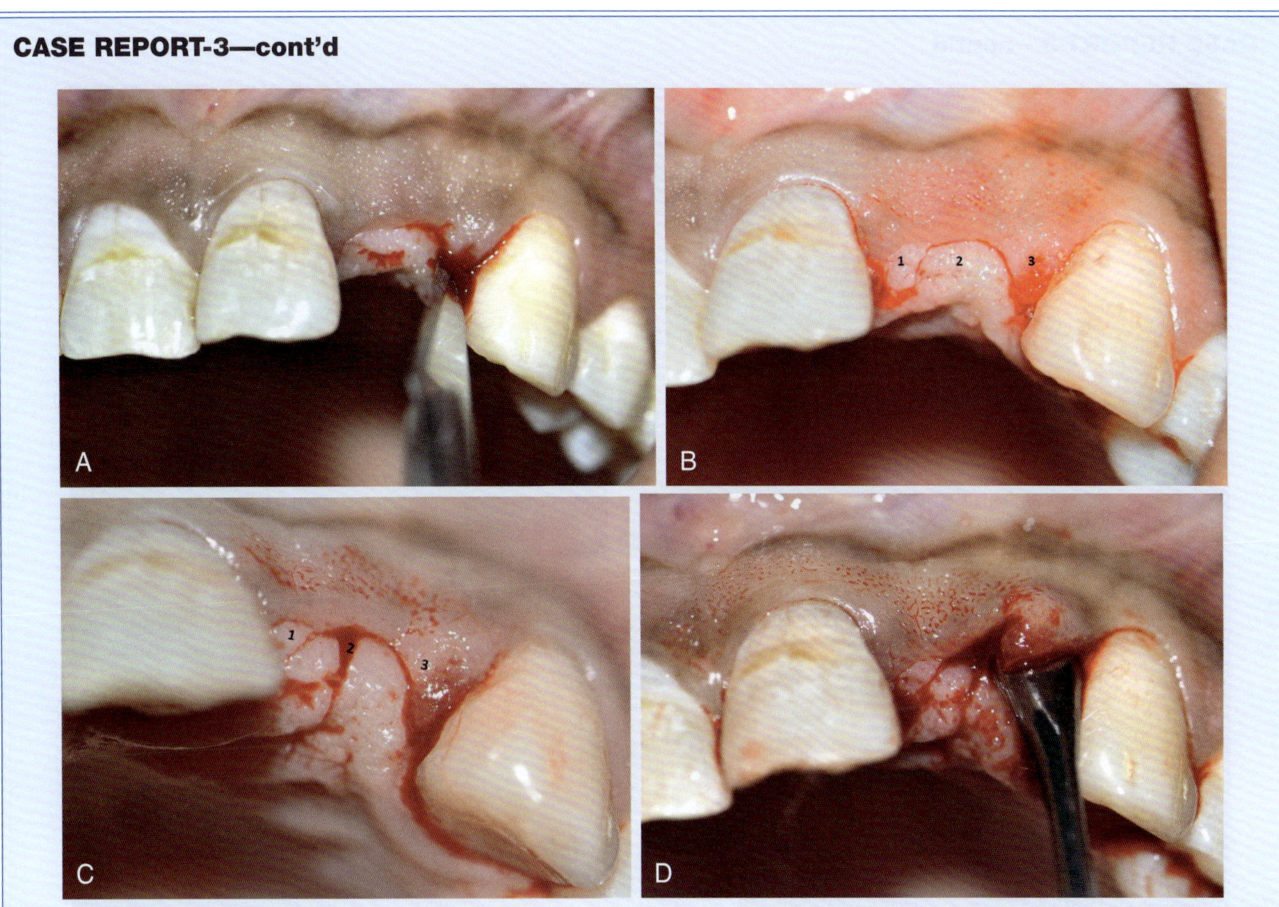

Fig 8.46 (A and B) A three-pronged incision is made (two small buccal and one large palatal). (C) The large palatal finger is bisected in two mesial and distal halves and (D) both the labial fingers are elevated.

Continued

CASE REPORT-3—cont'd

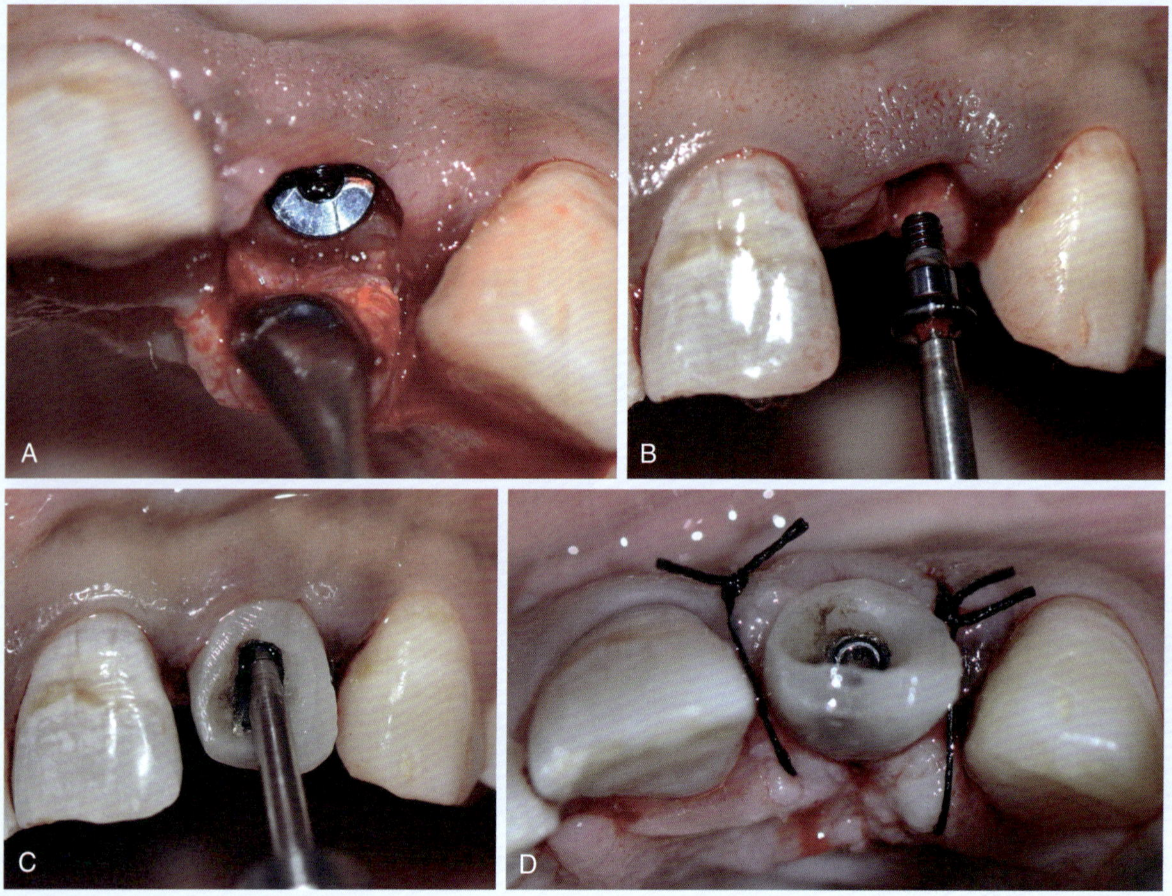

Fig 8.47 (A) The palatal fingers are elevated to uncover the implant and (B) the cover screw is removed. (C) A temporary tooth is fabricated over the aesthetic abutment and fixed to the implant. (D) The split palatal fingers are separated and sutured with the two labial fingers to create both the papillae.

CASE REPORT-3—cont'd

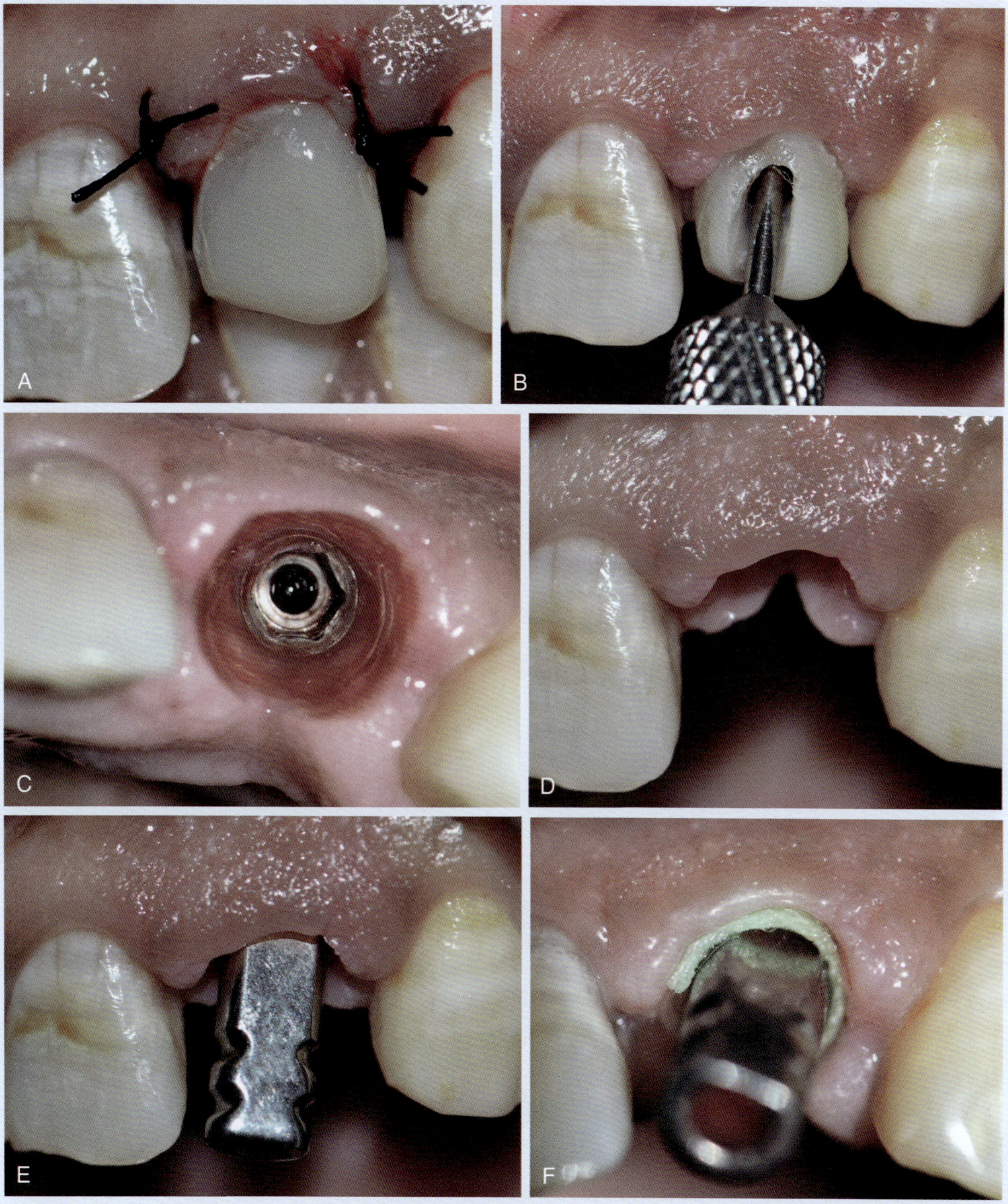

A B C D E F

Fig 8.48 (A) The screw hole is filled with gutta-percha and composite, and left to heal for 3 weeks. (B) The provisional is removed after 3 weeks showing the soft tissue healing with (C) acceptable soft tissue emergence profile. (D) Newly created mesial and distal papillae. (E and F) An impression post is inserted to the implant and its screw hole is sealed with the wax, a gingival retraction cord is used to record the subgingival area in the impression.

Continued

CASE REPORT-3—cont'd

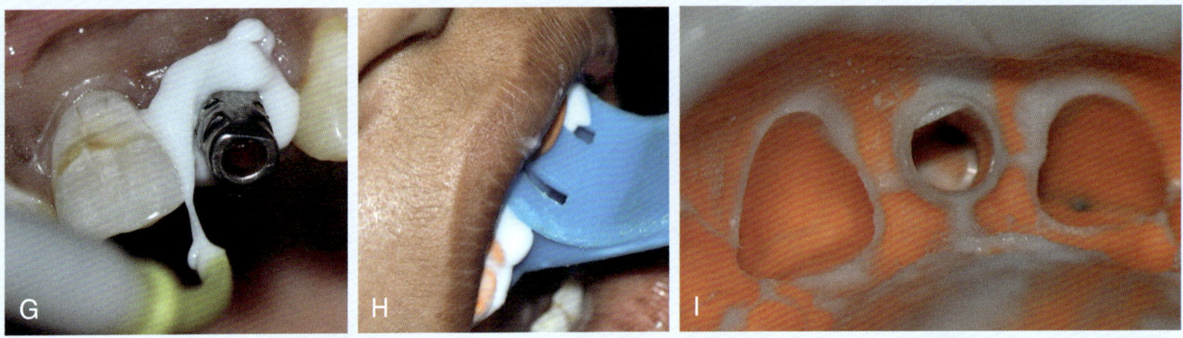

Fig 8.48, cont'd (G–I) An impression is made using additional silicon impression material.

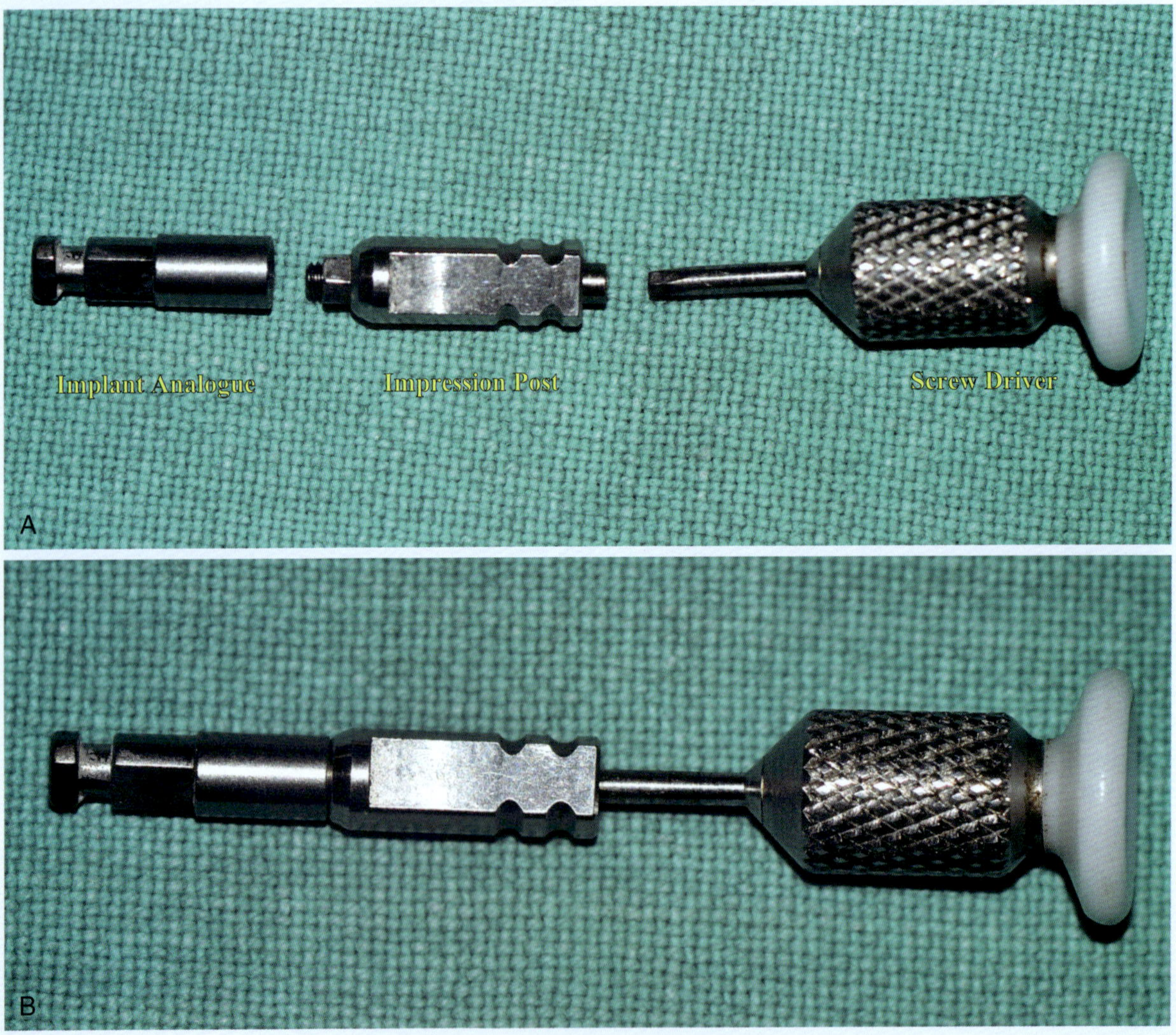

Fig 8.49 (A and B) The impression post is removed from the mouth and assembled with the implant analogue.

CASE REPORT-3—cont'd

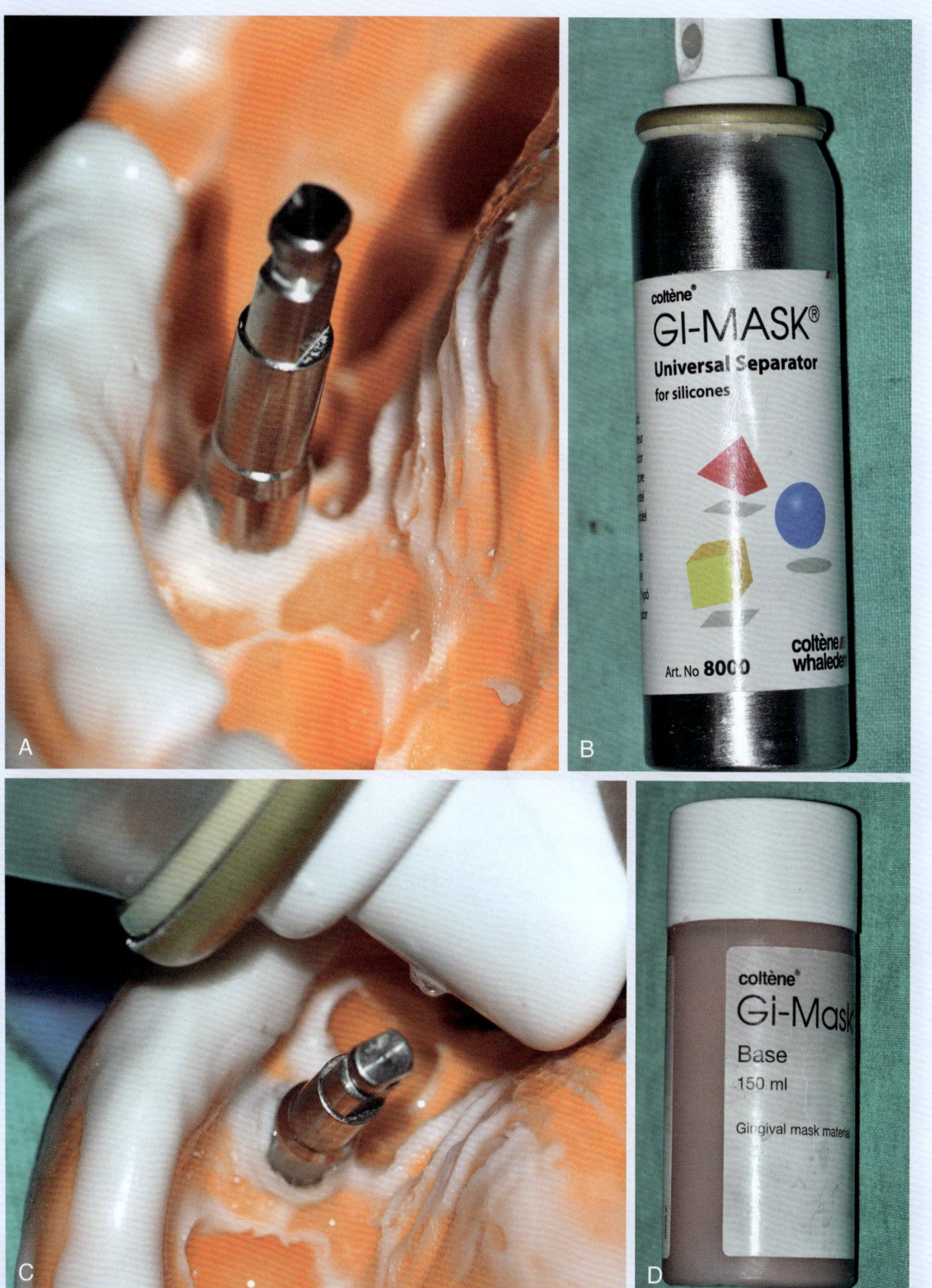

Fig 8.50 (A) The impression post, connected to the analogue, is inserted in the impression with the same orientation as in the mouth (flat surface of the impression post should match the flat surface in the impression). (B and C) A separator is sprayed on the impression and (D–F) Gi-Mask soft tissue replicating material (Coltene Whaledent) is used to pour the impression around the post analogue connection.

Continued

CASE REPORT-3—cont'd

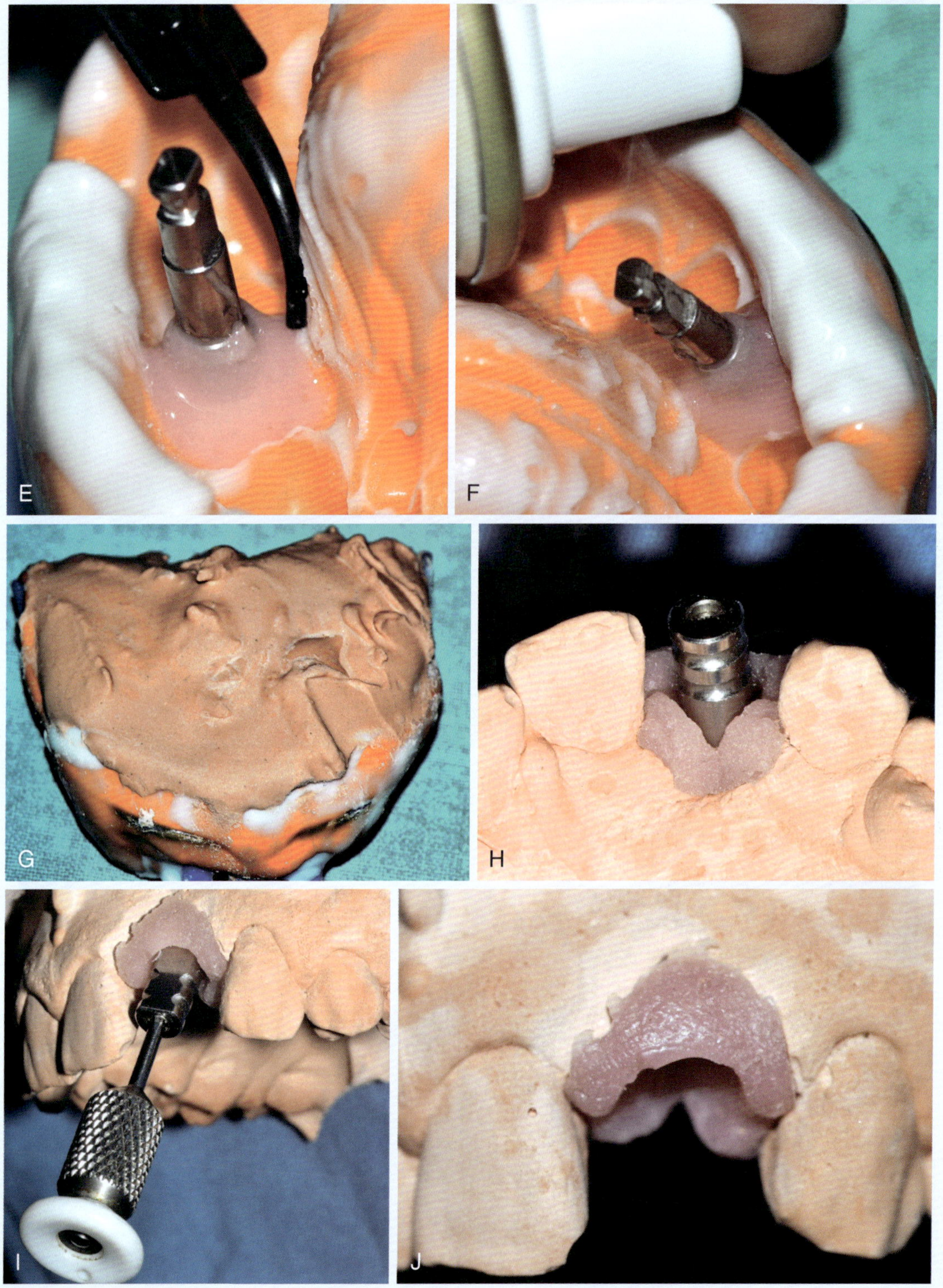

E F G H I J

Fig 8.50, cont'd (G) The impression is poured and stone model is removed after 24 h, showing the impression post connected to the analogue and (H) soft tissue replica around it. (I and J) The impression post is removed from the analogue.

CASE REPORT-3—cont'd

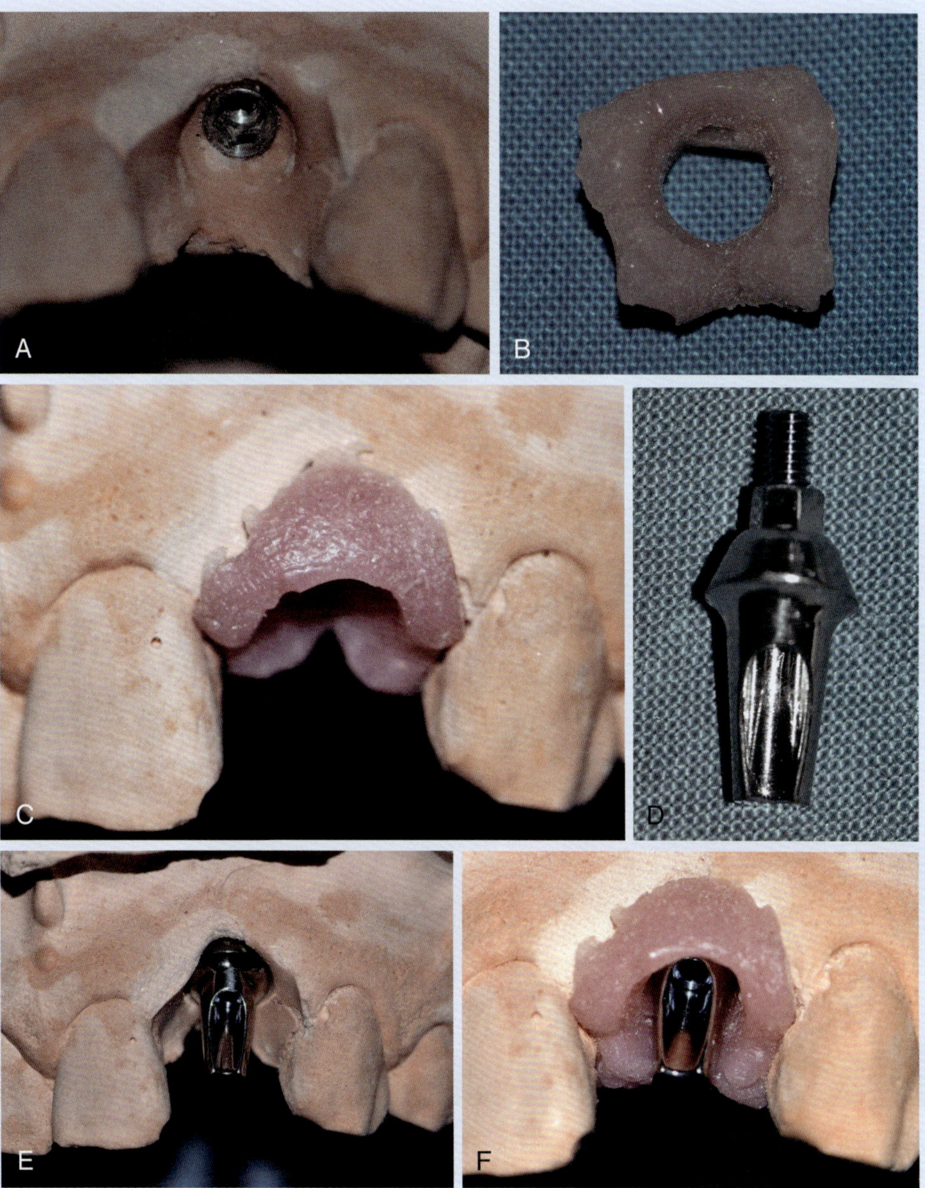

Fig 8.51 (A–C) The soft tissue replica can be removed and re-seated as many times as the clinician or the laboratory technicians needs, to visualize the abutment and analogue connection or the abutment finish line, which is placed subgingival to fabricate the prosthesis with perfect harmony and seal at the finish line. (D–F) An anatomical abutment, which already has the highly polished anatomical finish margins at the cervical region, is connected to the analogue.

Continued

CASE REPORT-3—cont'd

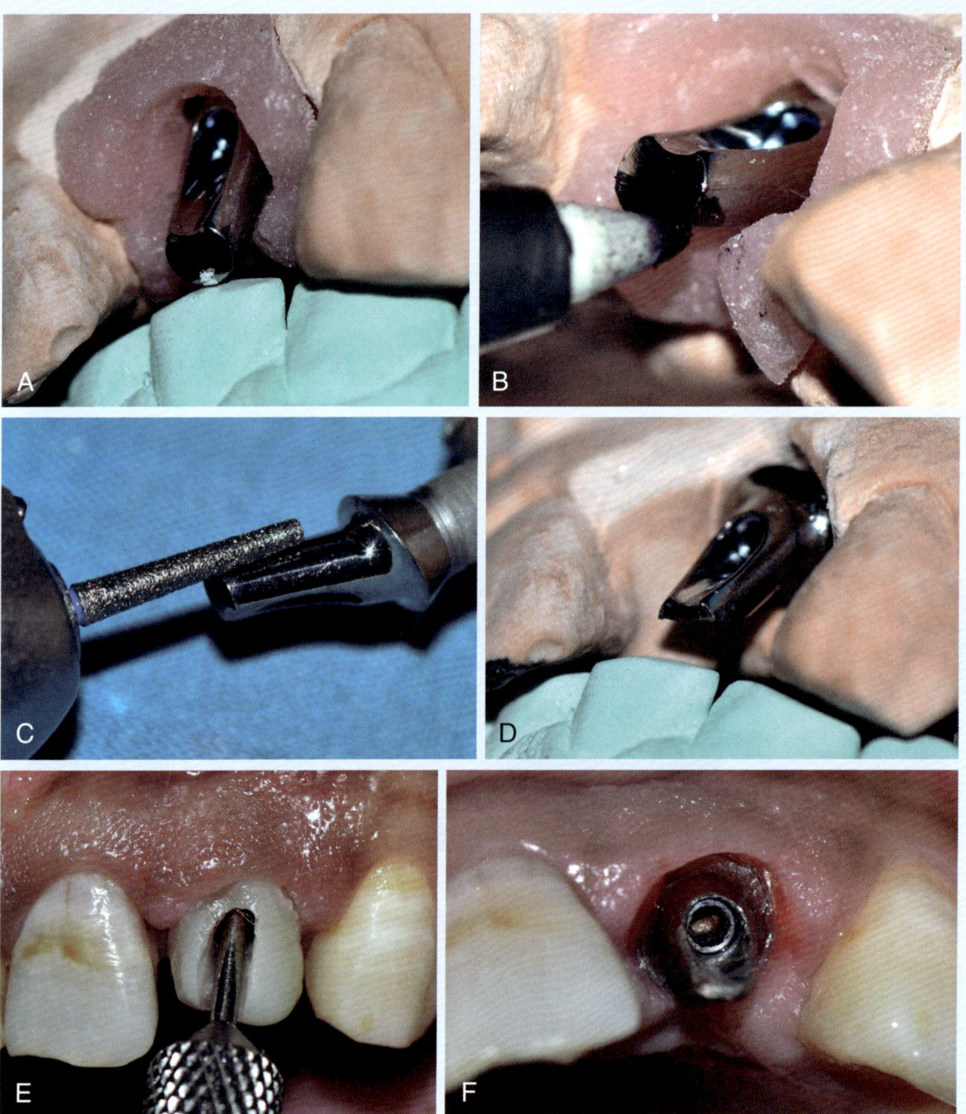

Fig 8.52 (A) The stone casts are articulated, the occlusal clearance is checked, and (B) marked with marker. Now the abutment is removed from the cast and connected to another analogue, and (C) prepared using diamond or carbide bur. Preparing the abutment connected to the cast can result in micromovement of the analogue because of vibration during the abutment preparation/milling. This may lead to inaccurate prosthesis fabrication and problem in seating the same in the mouth. (D) Finally prepared abutment on the model is sent to the laboratory for cement-retained porcelain fused to metal crown fabrication. After the prosthesis is received from the laboratory, the patient is recalled and the provisional prosthesis is removed from the implant. (E and F) The final abutment is transferred to the implant with the correct orientation.

CASE REPORT-3—cont'd

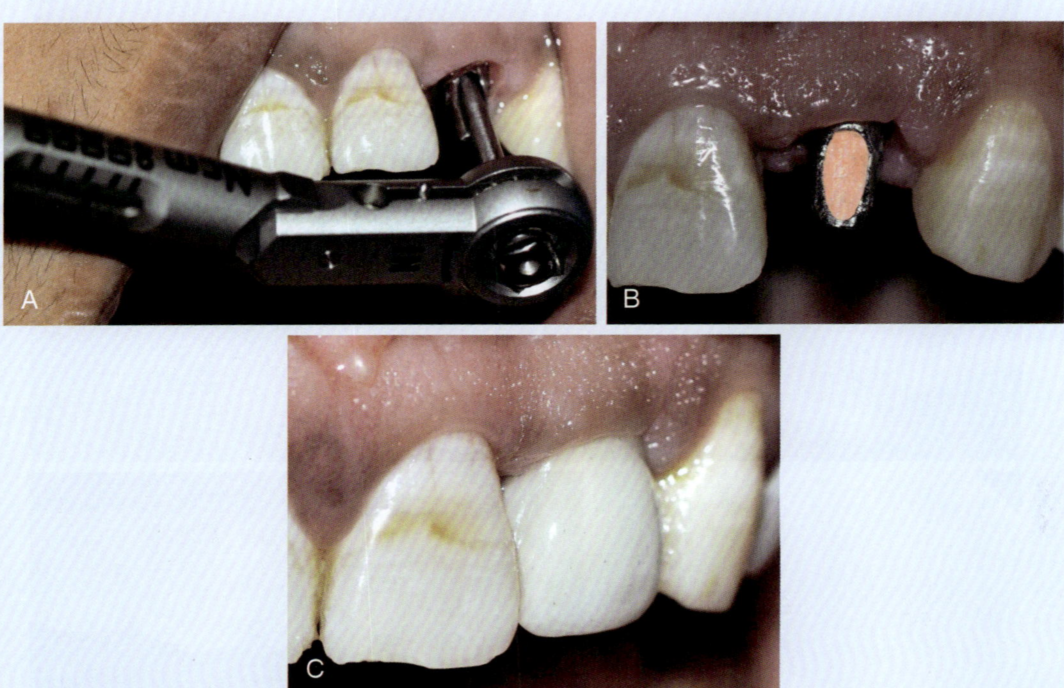

Fig 8.53 (A) The connection screw of the final abutment is tightened using the torque ratchet at 35 Ncm. (B) The screw hole is filled with gutta-percha and (C) the prosthesis is fixed using dual-cure resin cement.

CASE REPORT-4

Single piece implant insertion with immediate restoration in aesthetic region (Figs 8.54–8.61).

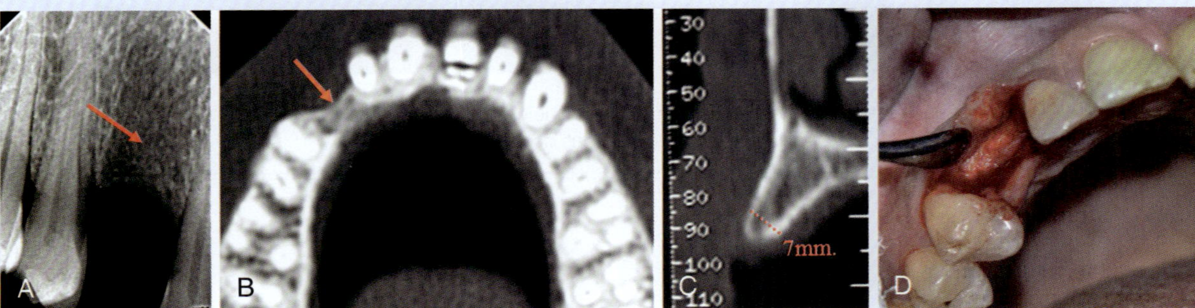

Fig 8.54 (A) Dental radiograph of missing maxillary canine and radiolucency in the crestal half of the ridge indicate thin bone width. (B and C) Axial and cross-sectional views of the dental CT confirm facial concavity in ridge morphology and reduced faciopalatal bone dimensions. (D) Flaps elevated to expose the bony ridge.

Continued

CASE REPORT-4—cont'd

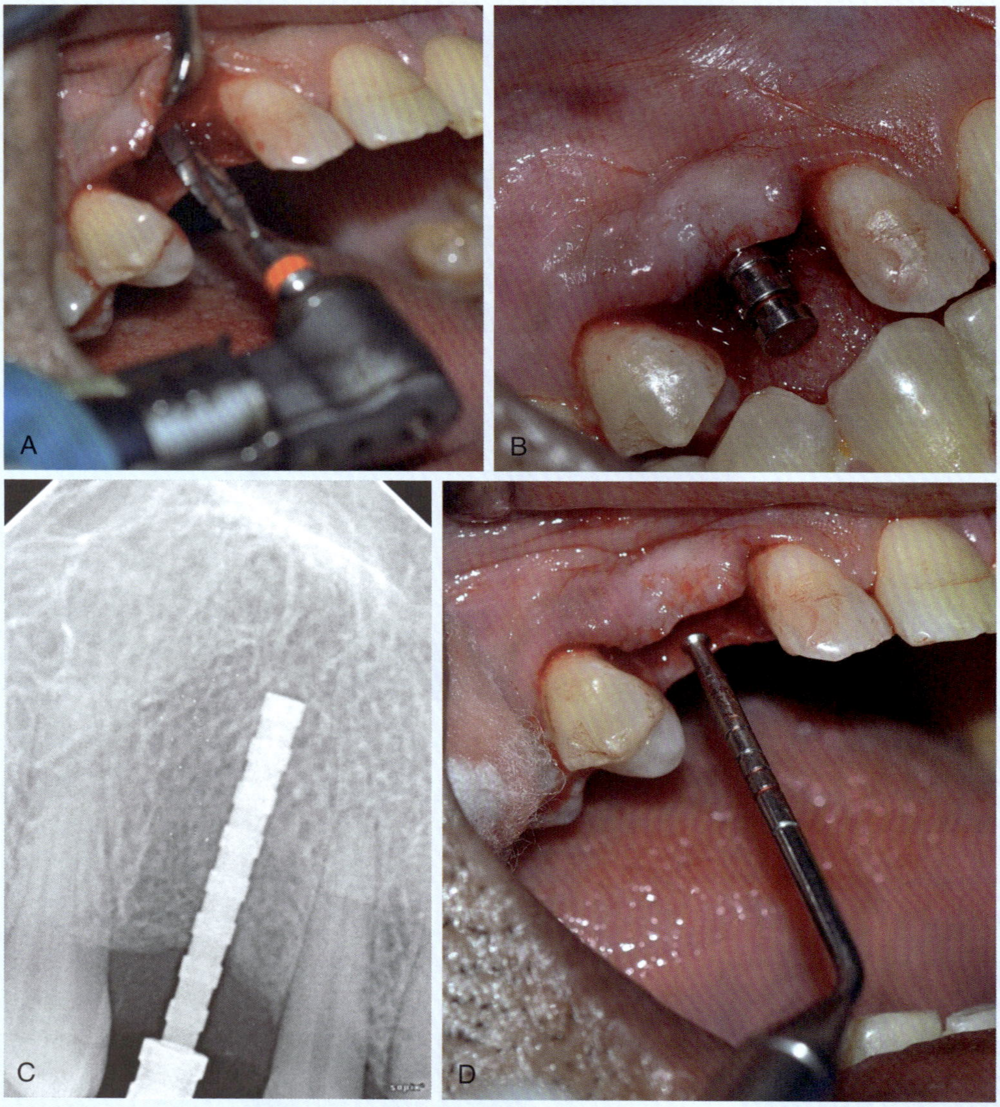

A B C D

Fig 8.55 (A-C) Osteotomy is carefully prepared and its direction and depth is checked by inserting depth pin and taking a radiograph. (D) The finally prepared osteotomy is checked for any inadvertent perforation, if has occurred.

CASE REPORT-4—cont'd

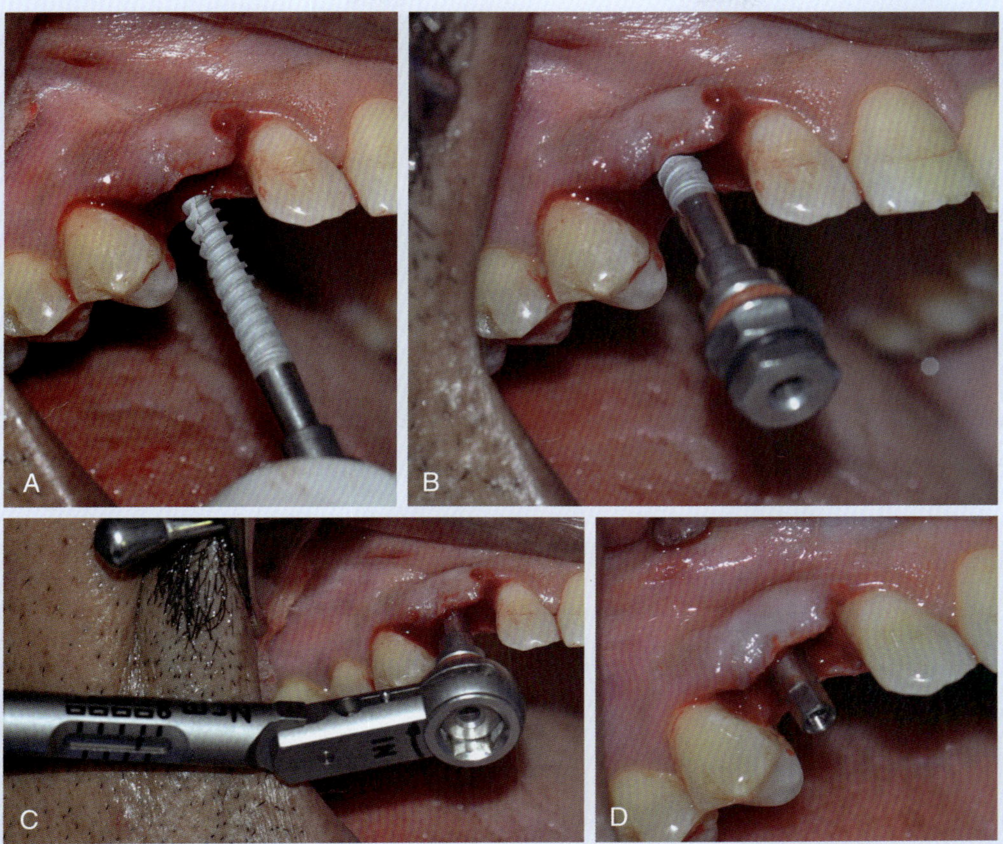

Fig 8.56 (A and B) A narrow diameter, long, one piece implant is inserted, which has attained adequate primary stability (more than 35 Ncm), is measured using (C) torque ratchet. (D) Implant at the final position.

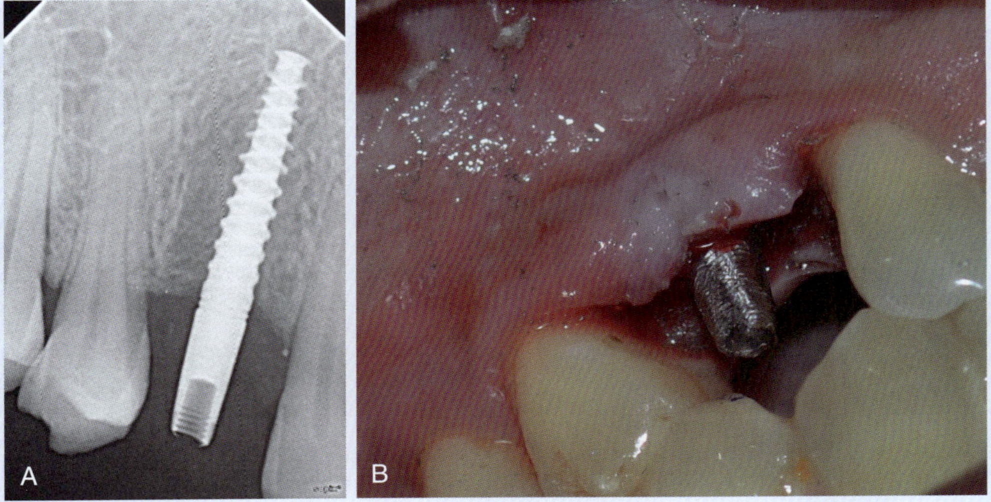

Fig 8.57 (A) Post-implantation radiograph. (B) The implant abutment is prepared using high-speed turbine.

Continued

CASE REPORT-4—cont'd

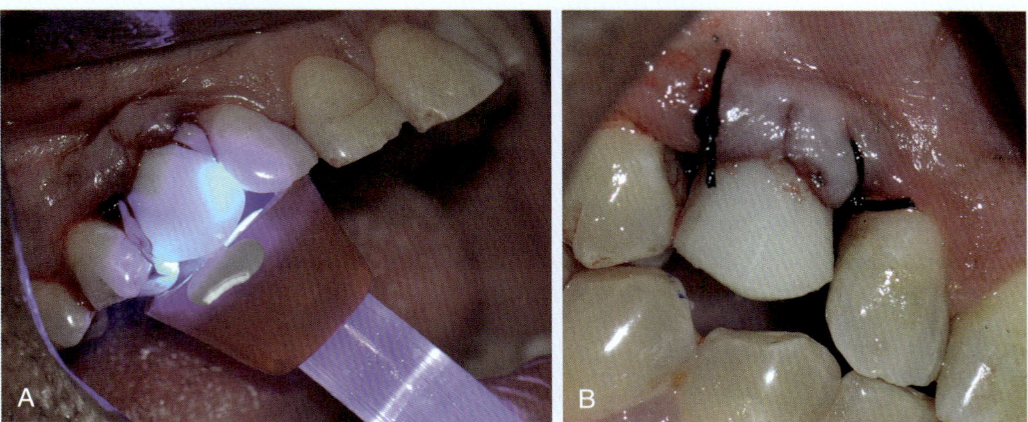

Fig 8.58 (A) An anatomical provisional crown is fabricated in mouth, it is fixed over the implant and (B) the flap is sutured.

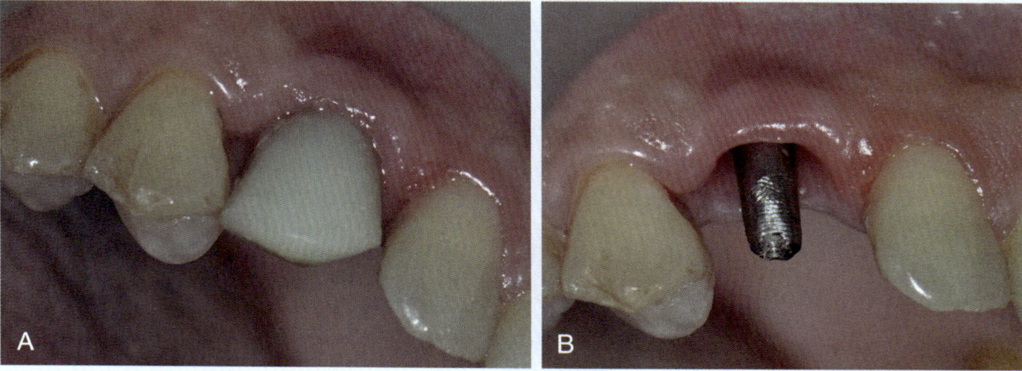

Fig 8.59 (A and B) Healing after 3 weeks has created an aesthetic scalloped soft tissue architecture for the final prosthesis.

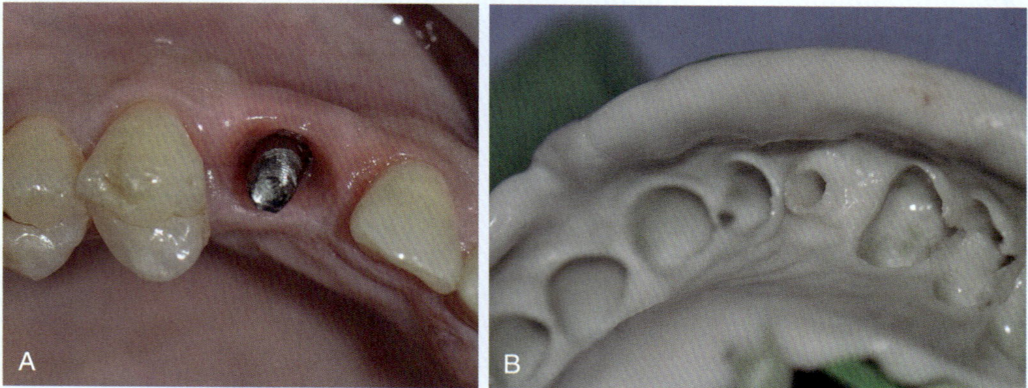

Fig 8.60 (A and B) Impression is made with the prepared abutment technique to accurately record the abutment as well as the soft tissue architecture.

CASE REPORT-4—cont'd

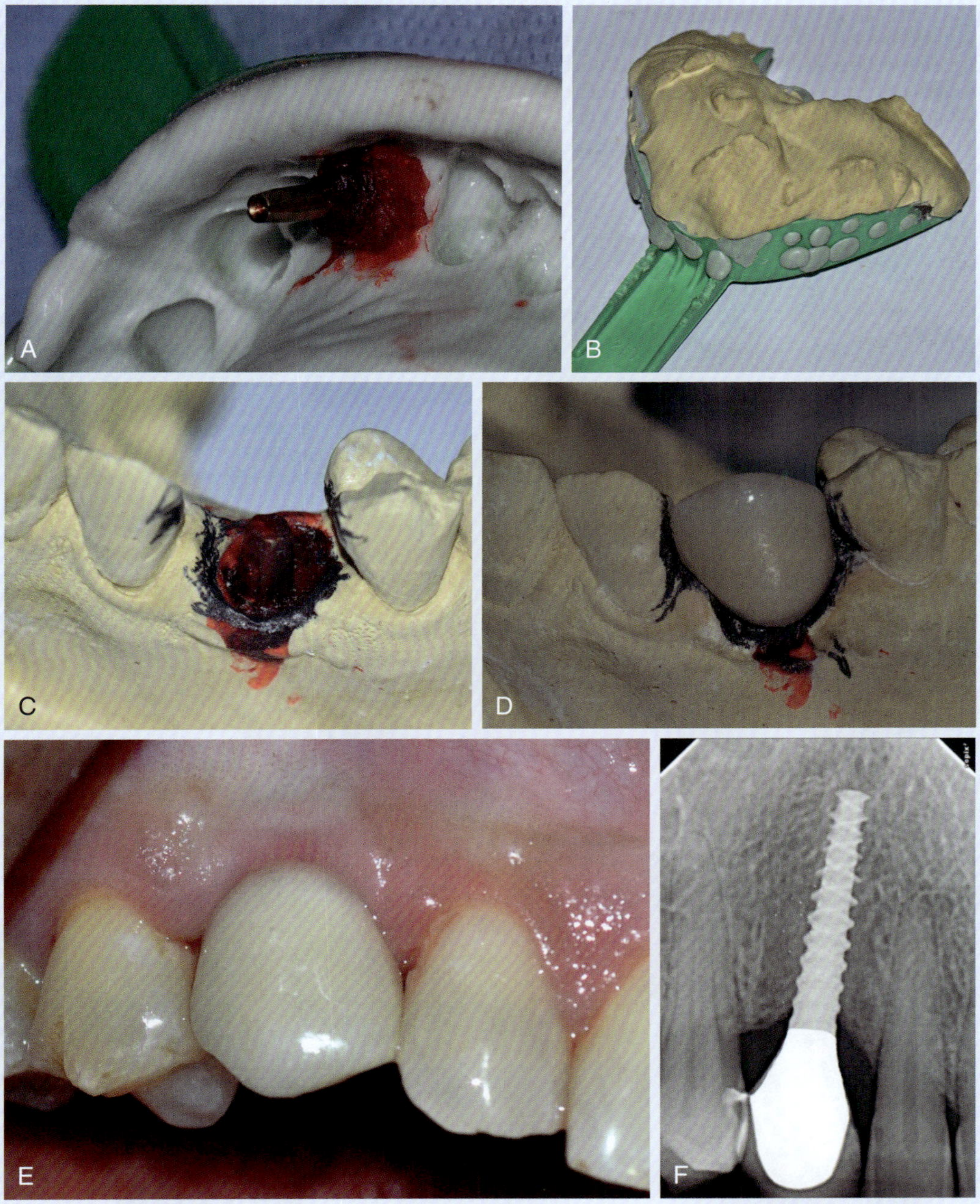

A B C D E F

Fig 8.61 (A) The abutment impression is poured with a high strength pattern resin and a dia pin is inserted. (B) The impression is poured with stone plaster. (C) The impression is removed after 24 h and (D) a metal ceramic crown is fabricated in the laboratory. (E) The prosthesis is fixed over the implant. (F) Post loading radiograph.

Continued

Bone spreading using osteotome: Often patients come with very limited buccopalatal bone dimensions or facial concavities in anterior maxilla with low-density bone where, an implant inserted with normal drilling protocol may result in dehiscence through the thin facial cortical plate. Tatum developed bone spreading to deal with such challenging situations in 1970s. He inserted more than 5000 maxillary anterior implants with this procedure before 1985. Bone spreading not only spreads the narrow ridge faciopalatally but also condenses the soft trabecular bone around the implants, which is normally removed by implant drills (Figure 8.62 a-d). It leads to high primary stability of the implant and more bone implant surface contact area, which is quite important for predictable osseointegration and long-term implant success.

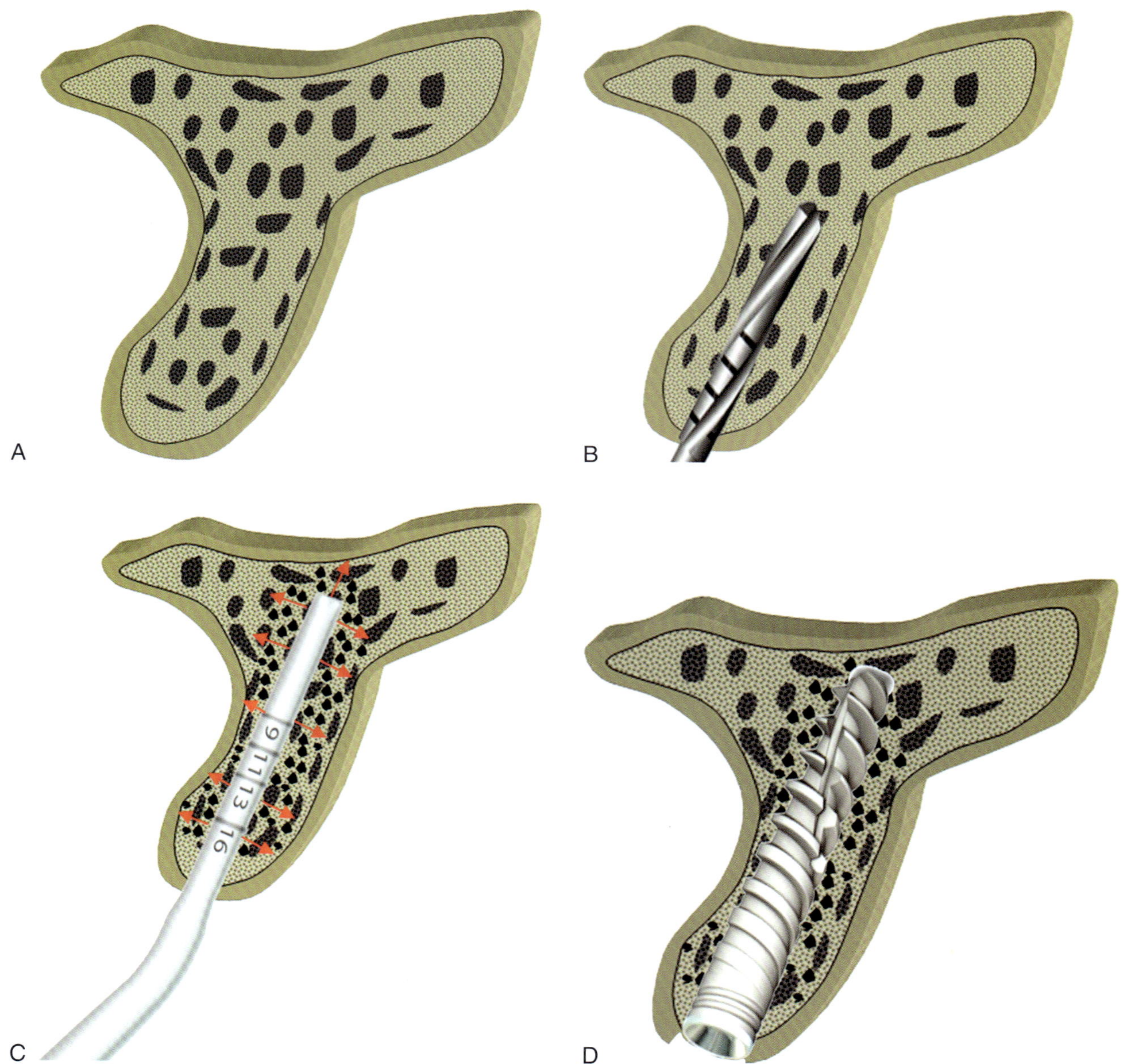

Fig 8.62 (A) Cross-section of edentulous premaxilla with narrow faciopalatal dimensions and low density bone (D3/D4). (B) A pilot drill is used for initial osteotomy preparation followed by use of (C) different sequential diameter osteotomes which spread and condense the surrounding low-density trabecular bone. (D) The implant is inserted in the spreaded and condensed bone with high primary stability and without any dehiscence through the thin labial cortical plate.

CASE REPORT-5

Implant placement in anterior maxilla using bone spreading Osteotomes (Figs. 8.63–8.65).

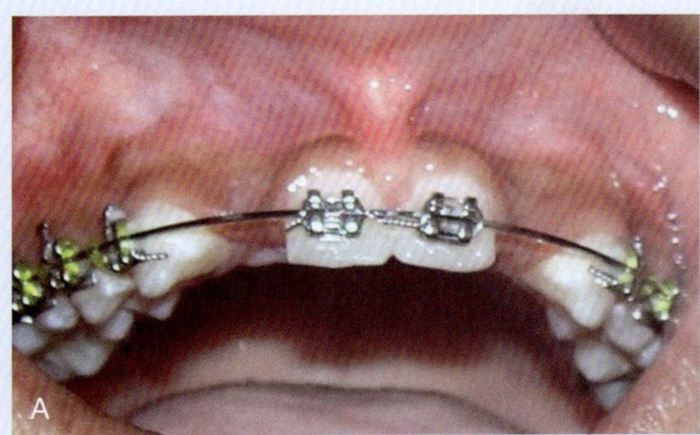

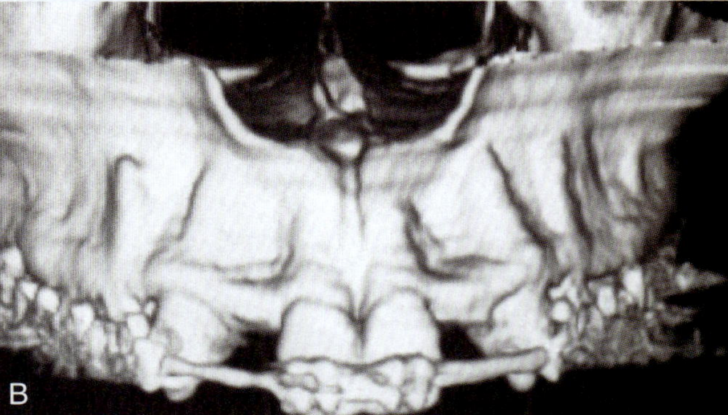

Fig 8.63 (A) Clinical view of the missing maxillary laterals with narrow facio-palatal dimensions and facial concavities, can be seen in the (B) 3D view of the dental CT scan.

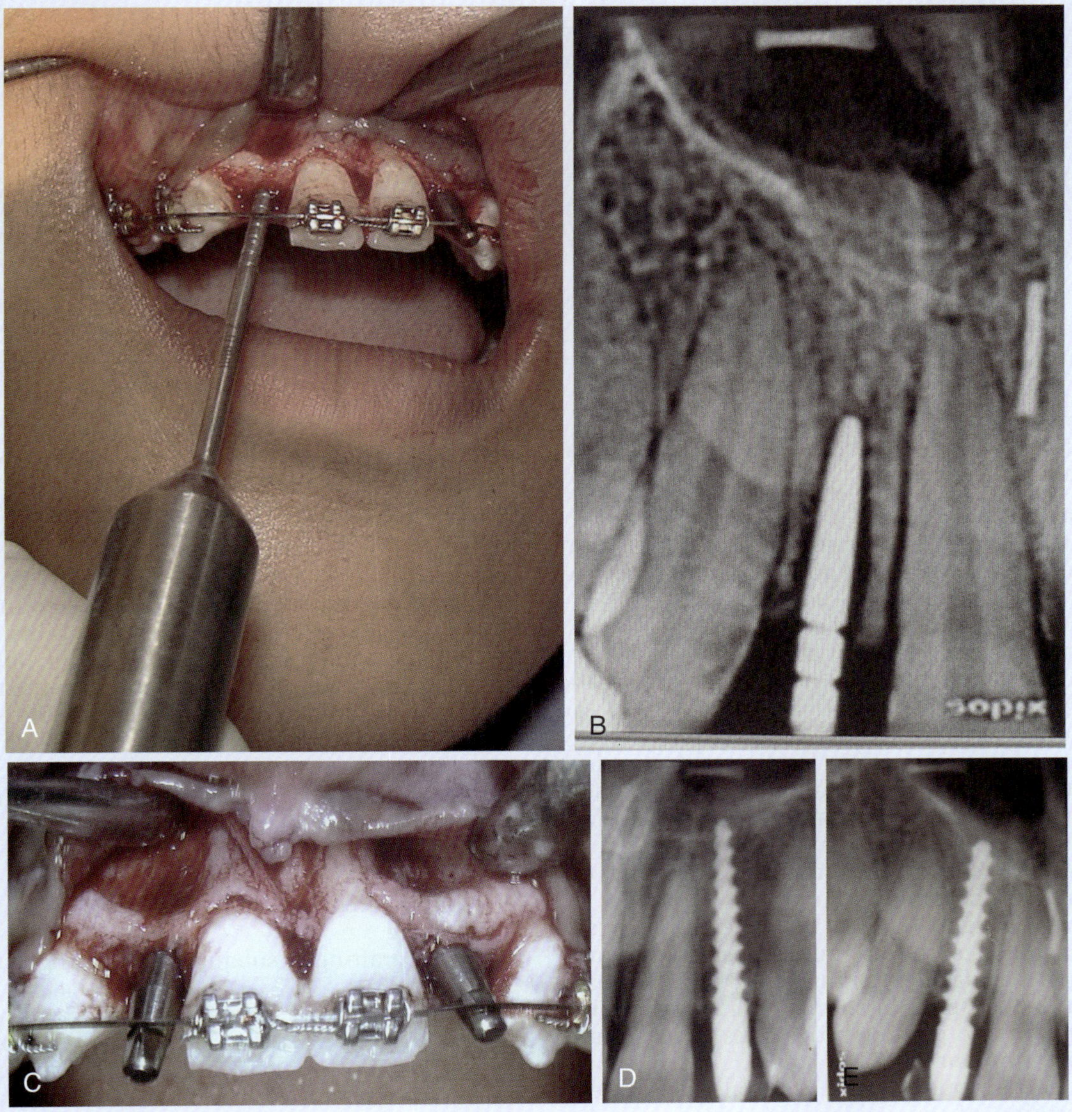

Fig 8.64 (A and B) Osteotome is used to spread and condense the bone. (C) Single piece narrow diameter implants are inserted with high primary stability and without any dehiscence through the facial concavities. (D and E) As can be seen in the radiograph, the apex of the both implants is also stabilized in the high density nasal floor to achieve adequate primary stability as immediate restoration of the implants is planned.

Continued

CASE REPORT-5—cont'd

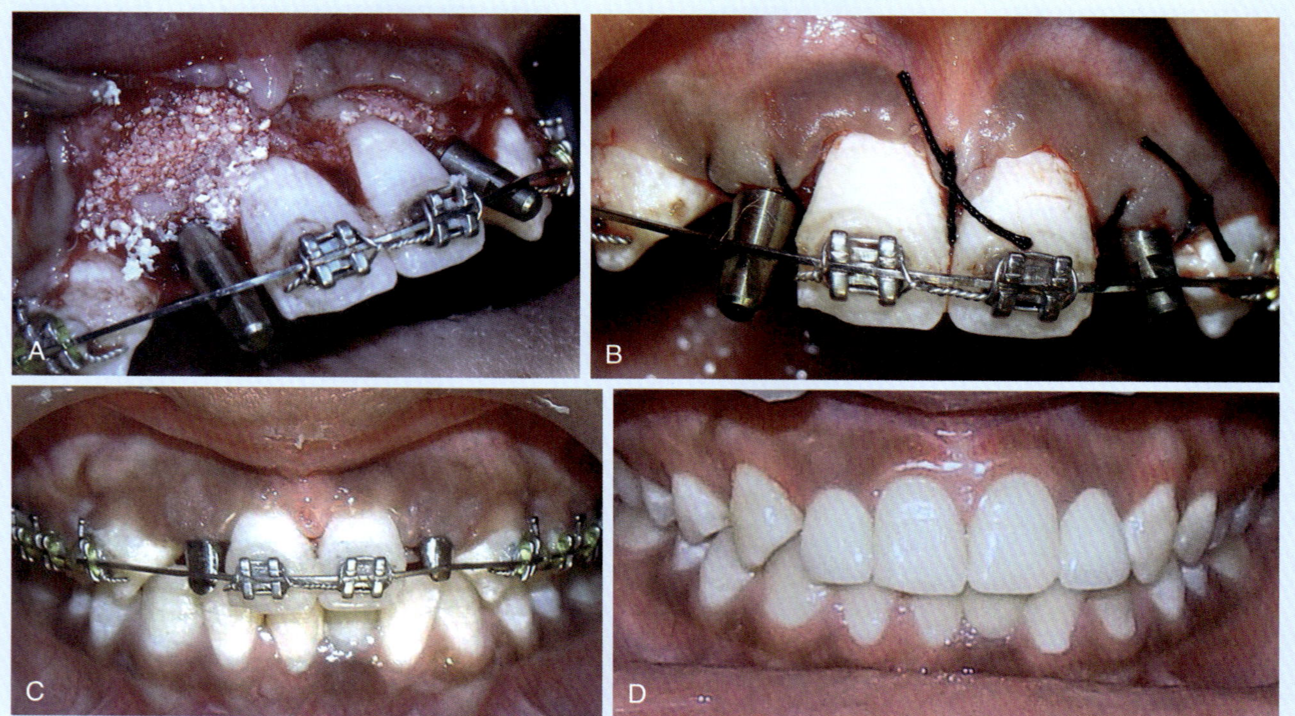

Fig 8.65 (A) The facial concavities are filled with bone graft material (Bio-Oss) to improve the facial tissue aesthetic and (B) the flap is sutured back. (C) Healing after 3 weeks. (D) Implants are restored after required gingivectomy, showing excellent soft tissue aesthetics.

Implant placement in the posterior maxilla

The posterior maxilla often presents a few specific limitations for ideal implant therapy.

Limitations with posterior maxilla

1. Poor bone quality: The posterior maxilla shows poorest bone quality, mostly D3 and D4 bone (Fig 8.66A) which
   a. causes poor initial stability of the implant
   b. delivers poor bone implant contact percentage
   c. causes micromovement of the implant during the healing period leading to failure
   d. takes longer time for the osseointegration
   e. prevents early or immediate loading of the implant
   f. formation of poor bone quality around the osseointegrated implant which can lead to implant failure after loading
   g. requires progressive bone loading to strengthen the peri-implant trabecular bone.
2. Limited bone height: Limited bone height is caused by vertical ridge resorption and expansion (pneumatization) of the maxillary sinus (Fig 8.66B). It leads to either the placement of short implants or requires sinus elevation and grafting procedures to insert adequately long implants.
3. Lateral bone resorption of the residual ridge: Lateral bone resorption of the residual ridge leads to more palatal implant placement and buccal cantilevering of the prosthesis (Fig 8.66C), or requires lateral bone augmentation before implant placement.

Management of reduced bone height is covered in the Chapter 19 'Sinus grafting for dental implants'. The facial cantilevering of the implant prosthesis can be managed by lateral bone augmentation procedures during or before implant placement.

Key Points

1. Lateral bone condensation using osteotomes
2. Achieving higher initial implant stability
3. Using the longest and widest possible implants
4. Submerging implant 1 mm apical to the ridge crest
5. Stabilizing implant apex in the hard cortical sinus floor
6. Using implant with deeper threads with high pitch value
7. Using implant with fast osseointegrating surfaces (HA surface implants from BioHorizons)
8. Avoiding any load on the implant during the healing period
9. Longer healing period of the implant before loading
10. Sinus grafting if subantral bone height is less than 10 mm.
11. Following progressive bone loading protocols:

1. **Bone condensation by using osteotomes:** To increase bone density around the implant, the bone is not removed with normal osteotomy preparation drills; after using the pilot drill a special set of different diameter bone condensers (osteotomes) are used sequentially to laterally condense the low-density cancellous bone (Figs 8.67 and 8.68).

2. **Bone condensation by the implant itself for achieving high primary stability of the implant:** The biggest disadvantage of bone condensation using osteotomes is the psychological trauma to the patient because of tapping with osteotomes. To overcome this problem one can use tapered implants with variable threads design (e.g. Nobel active implants, SPI implant, Taureg implant, etc.) (Figs 8.69 and 8.70).
3. **Using the longest and widest possible implant:** The use of the longest and widest possible implant results in more implant bone contact area and more predictable implant success in the posterior maxilla.
4. **Submerging implant 1 mm apical to the ridge crest:** If the implant platform is submerged 1 mm apical to the ridge crest, the crestal bone takes all the masticatory forces and thus micromovements of the implant during its healing phase can be avoided.
5. **Stabilizing implant apex in the hard cortical sinus floor:** If bone density is very low and the subantral bone height is limited, the sinus floor is fractured upto 1–2 mm, using osteotomes after final osteotomy preparation, so that the longer implant can be placed and its apex can be stabilized in the hard cortical sinus floor to achieve adequate primary stability of the inserted implant. The sinus floor is not augmented in this procedure (Figs 8.71 and 8.72).
6. **Using implant with deeper and more threads:** The deeper threads stabilize the implant in soft cancellous bone and the use of more threads increases the implant bone contact area for better osseointegration.
7. **Using implant with special early osseointegrating surfaces:** According to different studies, a few implant surfaces osseointegrate faster (e.g. Ti-unite surface, SLA surface) than the other surfaces (e.g. sand blasted RBM surfaces). So the implant which has an early osseointegrating nature must be used in low-density bone.
8. **Avoiding any load on the implant during the healing period:** Any soft tissue supported prosthesis should be avoided for at least for 4 months after implant placement.
9. **Longer healing period of the implant before loading:** The lesser the bone volume and density, the longer should be the implant healing period.
10. **Sinus grafting if subantral bone height is less than 10 mm:** To place wider platform implants the sinus floor should be elevated and grafted if the subantral bone height is less than 10 mm, especially if bone width is also compromised.
11. **Following progressive bone loading protocols:** The implant should be progressively loaded in case of D4 type bone, to strengthen the peri-implant trabecular one (see Chapter 7).

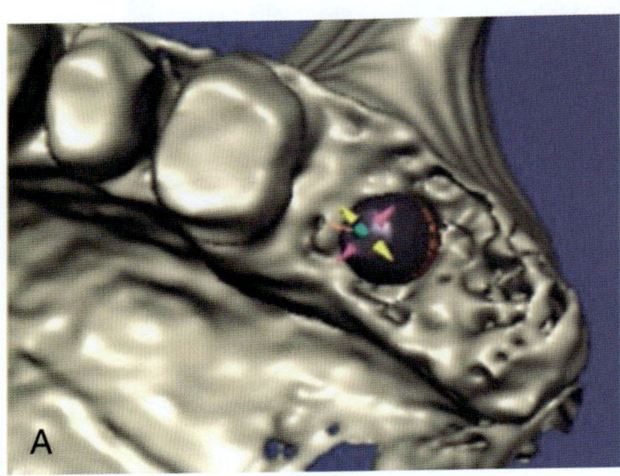

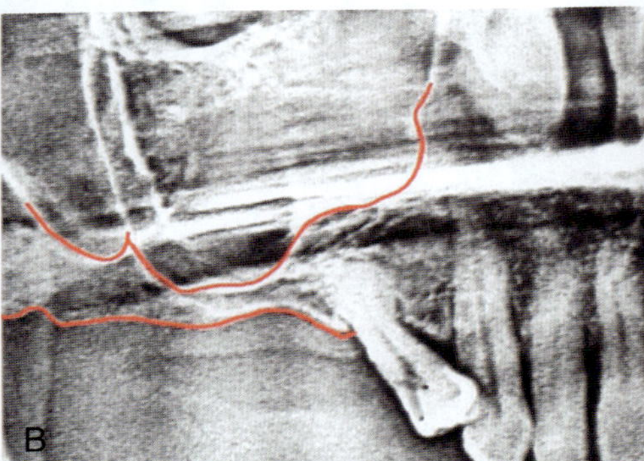

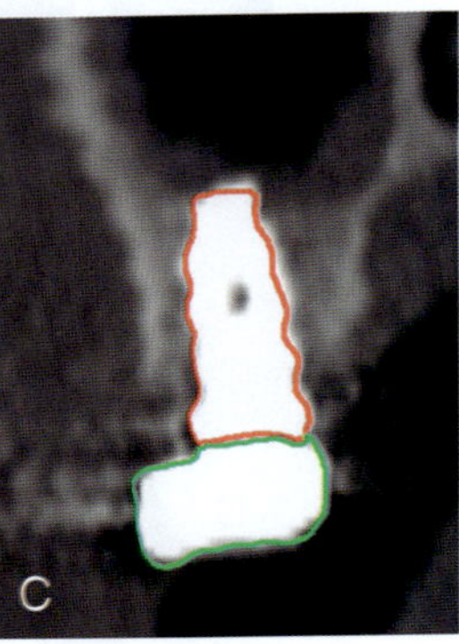

Fig 8.66 (A) DentaScan showing poor bone density in the posterior maxilla, dental radiograph showing limited bone height due to maxillary sinus pneumatization and vertical resorption of the bony ridge. (B) It indicates the need for sinus grafting for implant insertion. (C) Finally restored implant in the posterior maxilla in ideal occlusion with the mandibular natural molar showing facial cantilever due to buccal resorption of the edentulous ridge.

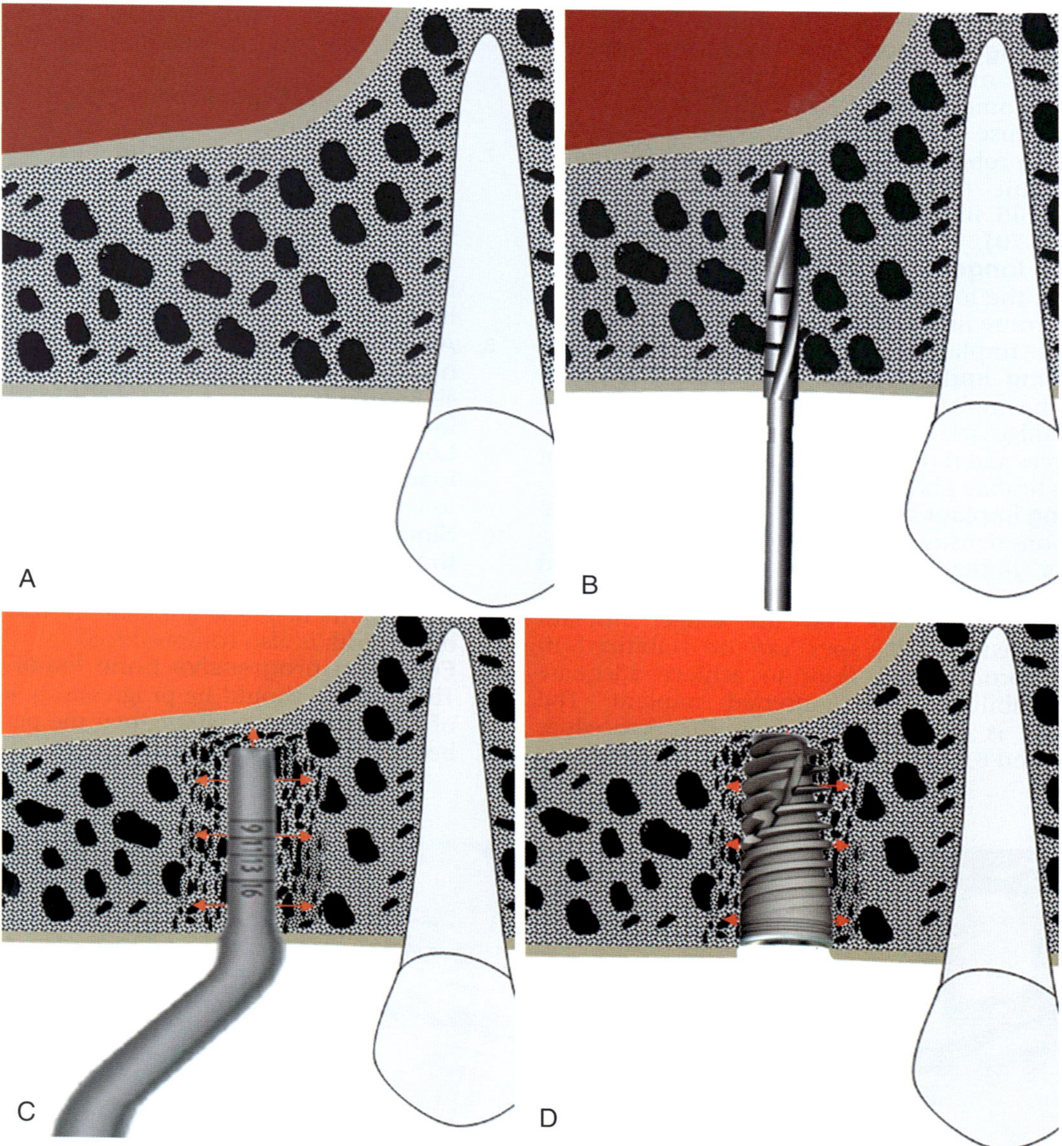

Fig 8.67 (A) Diagrammatic presentation showing low density coarse trabecular bone (D4 bone) in the posterior maxilla. (B) A pilot drill used for initial entry followed by lateral and vertical bone condensation using (C) sequential sized osteotomes and (D) finally implant inserted in the condensed bone. A condensing body implant, wherein the implant itself further condenses the surrounding bone and achieves a high primary stability in low-density bone.

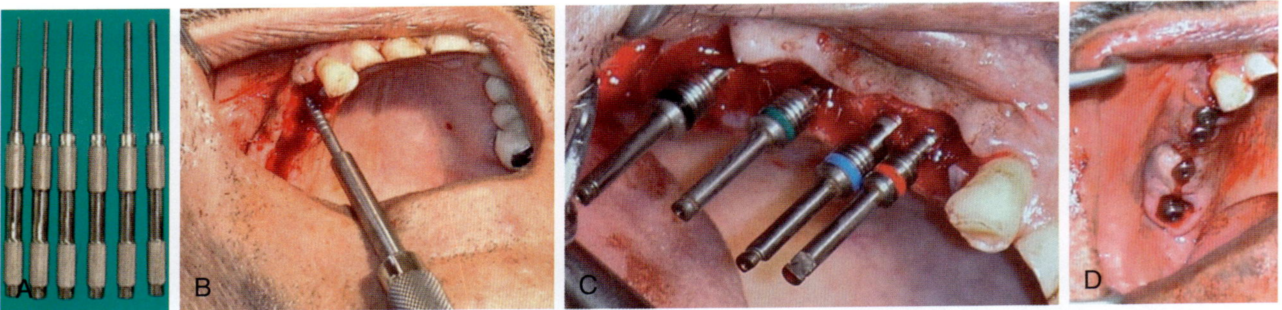

Fig 8.68 (A) Set of different diameter osteotomes. (B) Lateral bone condensation using osteotomes in the posterior maxilla. (C) The finally prepared osteotomy checked for parallelism by inserting final drills. (D) All Implants achieved high primary stability, so gingival formers are inserted over the implants for non-submerged healing.

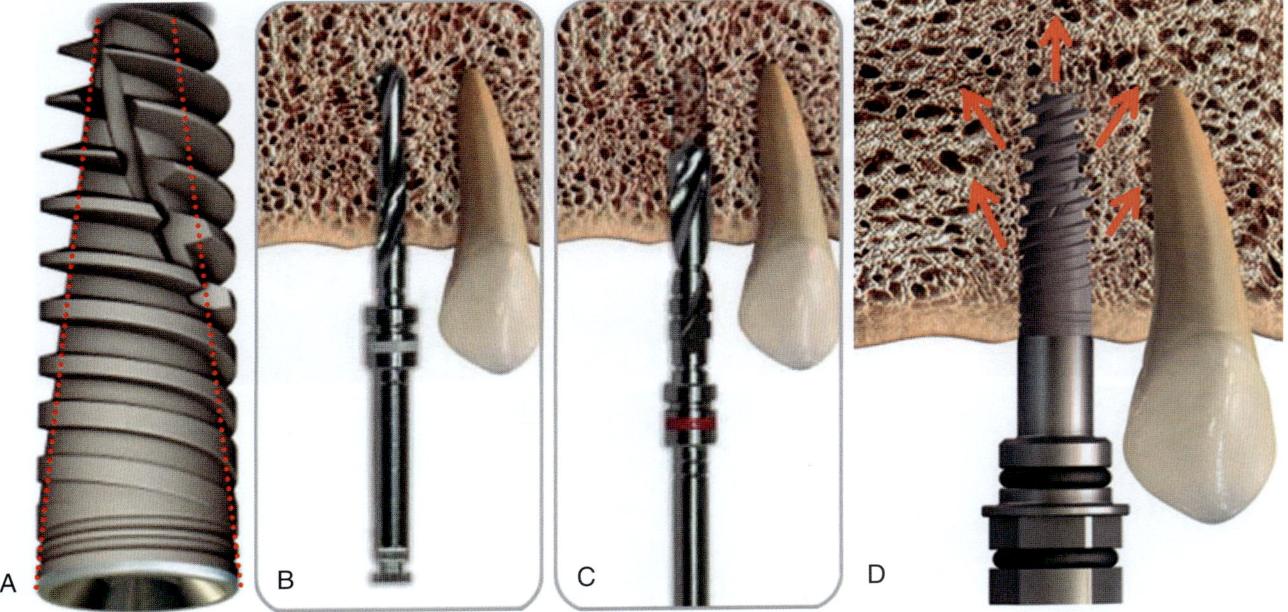

Fig 8.69 (A) SPI implant from Alpha-Bio has a tapered body and variable threads design. It has the implant core diameter much smaller than the thread diameter. The drilling to place this implant in the posterior maxilla is done by limiting the osteotomy preparation with the final drill with diameter matching the core diameter of the implant (e.g. if 5 mm diameter implant is inserted, it has the 2 mm apical diameter, 3.75 mm body diameter, 5 mm diameter just apical to the implant platform and 3.75 mm platform diameter). It has the sharp self-cutting/tapping threads at the apical region which self-prepare the threads into the soft bone to accommodate the wider body threads. It has non-cutting, deeper, self-condensing, square threads at the implant body, which laterally condense the low-density trabecular bone. It has shallow micro rings at the crestal part to avoid stress in the region of high-density crestal bone, which may cause crestal bone resorption. To place the 5 mm. diameter SPI implant, the 2.0 and 2.8 mm diameter drills are used to the complete depth, and 3.2 and 3.65 mm drills are used till the partial depth. These four drills prepare the osteotomy for the core of the implant. (B–D) After using these drills when the implant is inserted, its bone condensing threads laterally condense the soft spongy trabecular bone and achieve adequate primary stability in the low-density posterior maxilla.

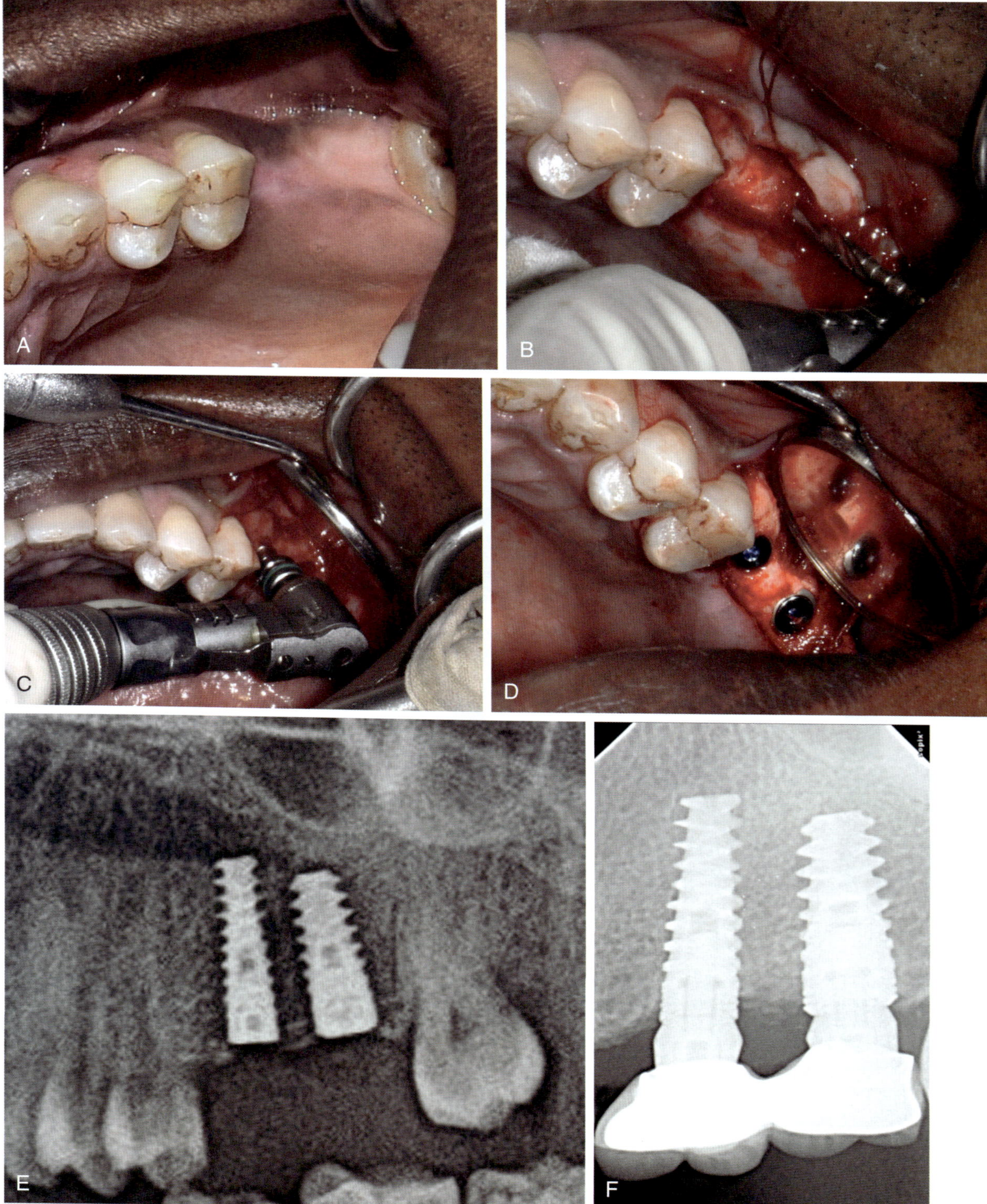

Fig 8.70 (A) Clinical view showing missing 26 and 27 no. teeth with good ridge form, (B) 2.0 mm pilot drill is used for initial osteotomy preparation. (C) The 3.2 and 3.65 mm diameter drills used as the final drills. (D and E) The 4 and 5 mm diameter SPI implants, which achieve high primary stability (more than 35 Ncm), are inserted. (F) Implants are uncovered and restored after 4 months.

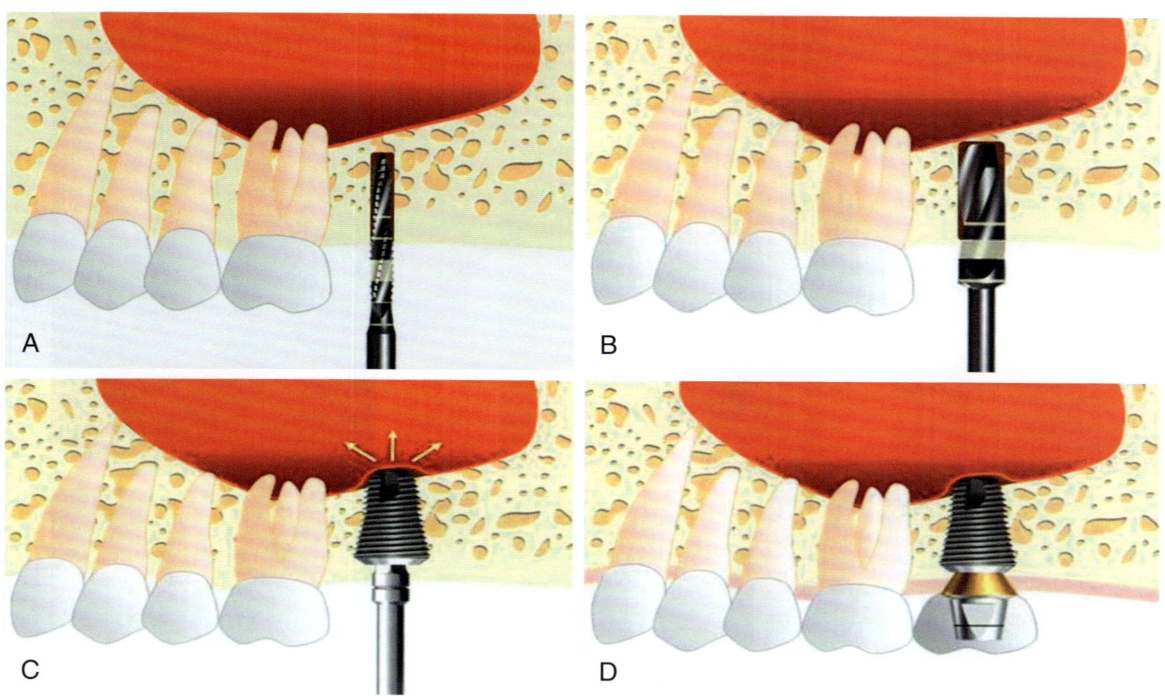

Fig 8.71 (A and B) Implant osteotomy is prepared 1–2 mm short of the sinus floor. (C and D) An adequate size osteotome is used to fracture up the sinus floor and the implant apex is stabilized in the high density sinus floor.

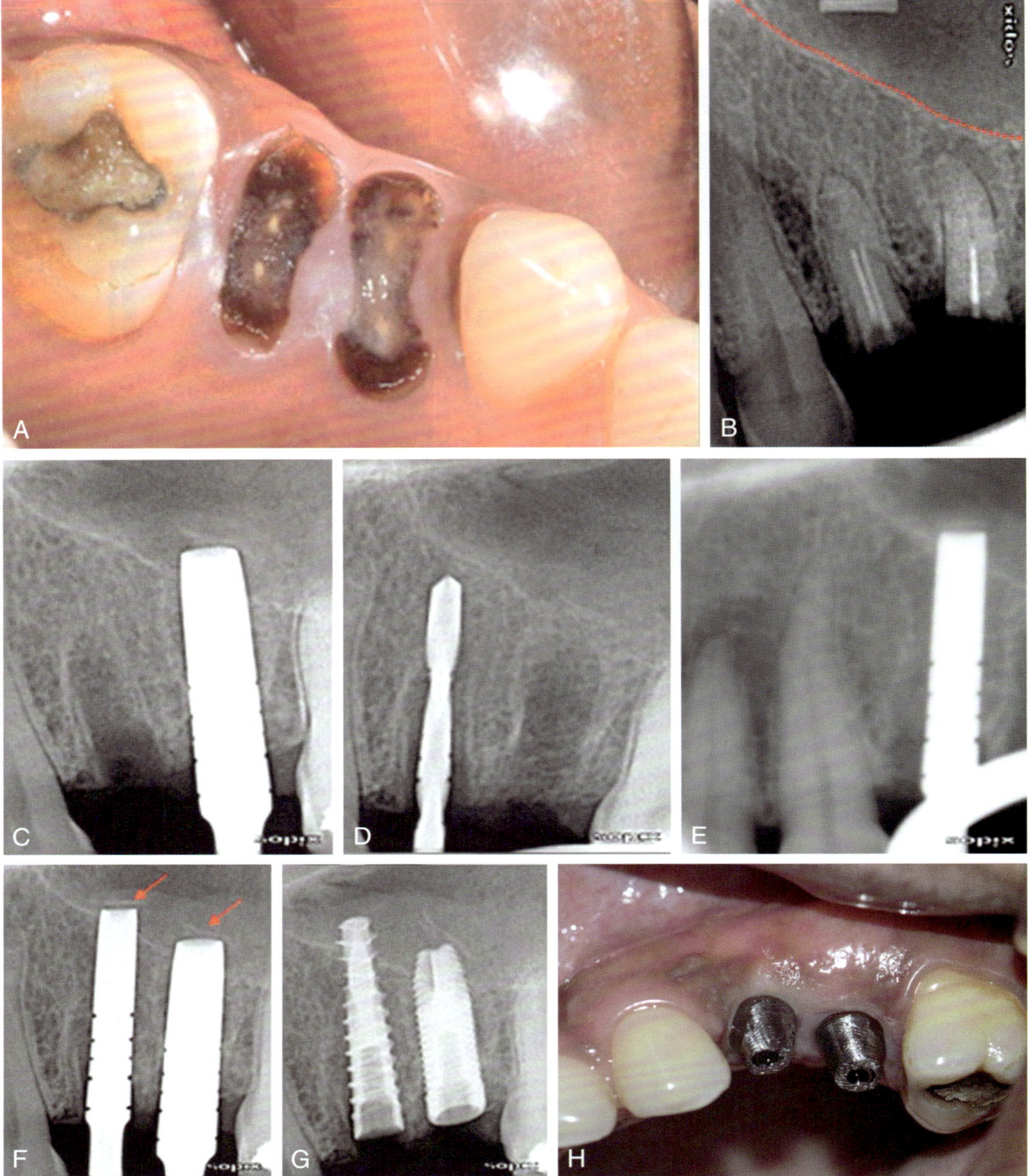

Fig 8.72 (A) Clinical view of the root stumps of left bicuspids, which need to be extracted with immediate implant placement. (B) Dental radiograph shows limited bone height apical to the root stumps (especially in second bicuspid) to engage the immediately inserted implant apex. (C) The root stumps are atraumatically extracted using periotomes and a large 4.2 mm diameter osteotome is inserted into the posterior extraction socket and gently taped to fracture up the hard sinus floor. (D) The implant osteotomy is prepared through the anterior socket 2 mm short of sinus floor. (E) Further, a final drill diameter osteotome is used in a similar fashion to fracture up the sinus floor. (F) Both the osteotomes can be seen in the periapical radiograph reaching beyond the sinus floor with fractured sinus floor bony pieces (red arrows) tenting up the elevated sinus membrane. (G) Both the implants are inserted to engage their apex in the hard sinus floor as well as the ridge crest (bicortical engagement) to achieve high initial implant stability (30–35 Ncm), which is quite necessary for optimal implant success in low-density posterior maxilla. (H and I) Implants are uncovered and restored after 4 months.

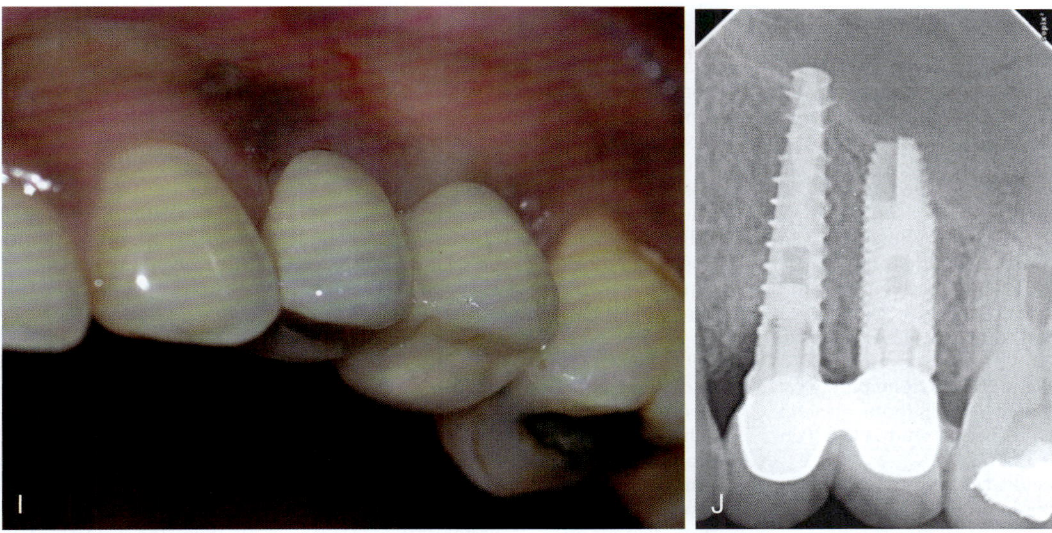

Fig 8.72, cont'd (J) Post loading radiograph shows new bone regeneration at the sinus floor under the elevated membrane. (For interpretations of the references to colour in the Figure legend 8.72F, the reader is referred to the online version of this book.)

Summary

Implant surgery should be performed at a high level of sterility by sterilizing the armamentarium and all implant inventories before surgery. The patient is advised to take prophylactic antibiotics, analgesics, anti-anxiety drugs, and steroid, 1 h before implant insertion surgery. The patient is asked to rinse the mouth with 0.12% chlorhexidine just before making the incision, to reduce the bacterial count in the oral cavity. Usually a mid-crestal incision is made, which can be further extended horizontally or vertically depending on the exposure of the bony ridge required to insert the implant. The mucoperiosteal flap is elevated to expose the bony ridge and osteotomy is prepared for the implant by sequentially using various implant drills to the planned depth and diameter, and the implant is inserted. The implant connection is covered using cover screw and the flap is sutured back. The implant is re-exposed after 3–4 months, once it has osseointegrated with the bone, and the cover screw is replaced with a long transmucosal healing abutment/gingival former for 2–3 weeks. After the soft tissue has healed, the gingival former is removed and the impression of the implant is made by prepared abutment or pick-up technique and is sent to the dental laboratory for the fabrication of cement- or screw-retained prosthesis.

For the prepared abutment impression technique, the gingival former is replaced with an appropriate final abutment which is prepared in the mouth and the impression is made similar to the usual crown and bridge impression technique. The impression is poured and sent to the laboratory for the cement-retained crown fabrication, which is luted over the abutment in the mouth using any appropriate luting cement.

For the pick-up impression technique, the gingival former is removed and replaced with the impression abutment or impression post and impression is made using additional silicon or polyether impression material. The post is removed from the mouth and assembled with the implant analogue. The impression post analogue assembly is inserted in the impression with the same orientation as in the mouth and the impression is poured using high-strength stone. The impression post is removed from the stone cast and the laboratory technician fixes an appropriate final abutment on the cast and fabricates either the cement-retained or screw-retained prosthesis. The dentist fixes this prosthesis on the implant in the patient's mouth.

Further Reading

Norton MR. Multiple single-tooth implant restorations in the posterior jaws: maintenance of marginal bone levels with reference to the implant-abutment micro gap. Int J Oral Maxillofac Implants 2006;21:777–84.

Gotfredsen K. A 5-year prospective study of single-tooth replacements supported by the Astra Tech implant: a pilot study. Clin Implant Dent Relat Res 2004;6:1–8.

Norton M. Biologic and mechanical stability of single-tooth implants: 4- to 7-year follow-up. Clin Implant Dent Relat Res 2001;3:214–20.

Wennström JL, Ekestubbe A, Gröndahl K, et al. Implant-supported single-tooth restorations: a 5-year prospective study. J Clin Periodontol 2005;32:567–74.

Solnit GS, Schneider RL. An alternative to splinting multiple implants: use of the ITI system. J Prosthodont 1998;7:114–91.

Guichet DL, Yoshinobu D, Caputo AA. Effect of splinting and interproximal contact tightness on load transfer by implant restorations. J Prosthet Dent 2002;87:528–35.

Wang TM, Leu LJ, Wang J, et al. Effects of prosthesis materials and prosthesis splinting on peri-implant bone stress around implants in poor-quality bone: a numeric analysis. Int J Oral Maxillofac Implants 2002;17:231–7.

Hansson S. A conical implant-abutment interface at the level of the marginal bone improves the distribution of stresses in the supporting bone. An axis symmetric finite element analysis. Clin Oral Implants Res 2003;14:286–93.

Bozkaya D, Muftu S, Muftu A. Evaluation of load transfer characteristics of five different implants in compact bone at different load levels by finite elements analysis. J Prosthet Dent 2004;92:523–30.

Hansson S. Implant-abutment interface: biomechanical study of flat top versus conical. Clin Implant Dent Relat Res 2000;2:33–41.

Hansson S, Norton M. The relation between surface roughness and interfacial shear strength for bone-anchored implants. A mathematical model. J Biomech 1999;32:829–36.

Palmer RM, Palmer PJ, Smith BJ. A 5-year prospective study of Astra single tooth implants. Clin Oral Implants Res 2000;11:179–82.

Norton MR. The Astra Tech Single-Tooth Implant System: a report on 27 consecutively placed and restored implants. Int J Periodontics Restorative Dent 1997;17:574–83.

Puchades-Roman L, Palmer RM, Palmer PJ, et al. A clinical, radiographic, and microbiologic comparison of Astra Tech and Branemark single tooth implants. Clin Implant Dent Relat Res 2000;2:78–84.

Norton MR. Marginal bone levels at single tooth implants with a conical fixture design. The influence of surface macro and microstructure. Clin Oral Implants Res 1998;9:91–9.

Palmer RM, Smith BJ, Palmer PJ, et al. A prospective study of Astra single tooth implants. Clin Oral Implants Res 1997;8:173–9.

Henry PJ, Laney WR, Jemt T, et al. Osseointegrated implants for single-tooth replacement: a prospective 5-year multicenter study. Int J Oral Maxillofac Implants 1996;11:450–5.

Hwang D, Wang HL. Medical contraindications to implant therapy: part I: absolute contraindications. Implant Dent 2006;15:353–60.

Brägger U. Radiographic parameters for the evaluation of peri-implant tissues. Periodontol 2000 1994;4:87–97.

Albrektsson T, Zarb G, Worthington P, et al. The long-term efficacy of currently used dental implants: a review and proposed criteria of success. Int J Oral Maxillofac Implants 1986;1:11–25.

Markiewicz MR, Raina A, Chuang SK, et al. Full-mouth rehabilitation with single-tooth implant restorations. Overview and report of case. NY State Dent J 2010;76:36–42.

Shin YK, Han CH, Heo SJ, et al. Radiographic evaluation of marginal bone level around implants with different neck designs after 1 year. Int J Oral Maxillofac Implants 2006;21:789–94.

Hansson S. The implant neck: smooth or provided with retention elements. A biomechanical approach. Clin Oral Implants Res 1999;10:394–405.

Scherrer SS, de Rijk WG. The effect of crown length on the fracture resistance of posterior porcelain and glass-ceramic crowns. Int J Prosthodont 1992;5:550–7.

Immediate implant in extraction socket

Ajay Vikram Singh Amir Gazmawe Peter Randelzhofer

CHAPTER CONTENTS HD

Introduction

Based on favourable findings in research and clinical trials, immediate implantation in the fresh extraction socket has become the treatment of choice in implant therapy as it offers many advantages over placing the implant in healed bone. The exact time for placing the implant depends on the structural changes of hard and soft tissue after extraction. Following tooth extraction, the resorption processes of the alveolar bony walls take place. The studies of Araujo et al have shown that the bundle bone is mainly involved in the resorption process, which also results in the loss of buccal bone volume and height. Two-thirds of resorption occurs in the first 3 months post-extraction, and results in a complex clinical situation. The socket grafting or immediate insertion of the implant into fresh extraction sites with simultaneous grafting of peri-implant socket spaces, if needed, prevents this resorption. Immediate implants have proven to be a predictable treatment option. Studies showed a success rate between 93% and 100%. The patient benefits from a less invasive and cost effective procedure resulting in reduced overall treatment time and higher patient comfort. However, immediate implantation requires primary stability and is often accompanied by 'ad hoc' decision making. The possibility of placing an immediate implant depends on the defect anatomy and therefore it is frequently possible to make a decision only at the time of extraction. Cases with thin gingival and high scalloped soft tissue architecture are suitable for the so-called 'open healing' procedure with a wide body-healing abutment placed on top of the implant to support the marginal gingiva. A careful and conservative surgical approach is required to maintain thin papillae and marginal gingiva.

The conventional technique for implant therapy at the site of the diseased tooth which needs replacement, have been discussed in the early Chapters of this book, which encompassed extracting the tooth, waiting 6–8 weeks for the socket to heal, inserting the implant, and further waiting 3–4 months for implant healing and osseointegration. After this procedure, surgical re-entry is necessary to expose the implants and to place a prosthetic abutment. Branemark and co-workers recommended a period of stress-free unloaded healing to ensure the Osseointegration of endosseous implants. High success rates for the two-stage implant protocol have been documented. Valid paradigms have required 3–4 months of healing for tissue integration of the implants following an adequate healing period for the consolidation of the extraction socket. Taking into account the prosthetic treatment also, patients frequently had to wait up to 1 year for a lost tooth to be replaced. In recent years, shorter treatment times from the time of tooth loss to the restoration of teeth with prosthetic appliances on osseointegrated implants have been promoted by many clinicians.

Strategies were developed to substantially shorten the implant treatment time span in extraction and implant insertion cases. There can be various ways of immediate implant insertion in the extraction socket, based on various radiographic and clinical parameters as well as the skilled approach of the implant surgeon, to treat each individual case.

Indications

1. Grossly decayed, nonrestorable, asymptomatic tooth.
2. Traumatic loss of tooth with minimum bone loss.
3. Tooth to be extracted presents no sign of any active infection like pain, swelling, tenderness, purulent discharge, etc.
4. Periodontally compromised tooth without purulent exudate, which needs extraction and replacement.
5. Inability to perform and complete endodontic treatment.
6. Tooth needs immediate implant, shows adequate healthy bone volume apical to the extraction socket to stabilize the implant apex.
7. Tooth needs immediate implant, shows adequate band of thick, stable, and keratinized marginal tissue.
8. Extraction socket is favourable for implant insertion at the correct position and axis for final prosthesis.
9. Extraction socket with small or no osseous defect, where adequate bone–implant surface contact percentage can be achieved and simultaneous bone grafting for the defect is possible with predictable outcome.
10. The dimensions of the socket are favourable for the planned implant dimensions.
11. The adjacent teeth have good periodontal support and present no signs of any active infection.

Contraindications

1. Signs of active infection like pain, swelling, tenderness, purulent discharge etc. related to the tooth planned for extraction.
2. Extraction socket possesses large osseous defect, not favourable for immediate implantation.
3. Inadequate bone volume apical to the extraction socket to stabilize the implant apex.
4. Inadequate band of thick, stable, and keratinized marginal soft tissue around the socket.
5. Extraction socket is unfavourable for implant insertion at the correct position and axis for final prosthesis.
6. The dimensions of the socket are unfavourable for the planned implant dimensions.
7. The adjacent teeth contain active infection or poor periodontal support.

Advantages of immediate implantation in extraction socket

1. Implant can be placed in the same position as the extracted tooth, minimizing the need for angled abutments.
2. Osseointegration is more favourable when implants are placed immediately in the extraction socket.
3. Prevents alveolar ridge atrophy and gingival tissue recession.
4. Nonfunctional restorations can be provided to restore immediate aesthetics, especially in the anterior region.
5. Immediate implantation keeps contaminants away from the socket.
6. More patients opt for implant treatment as there is no waiting time for healing and restoration.
7. Shortens treatment time; treatment is completed in a shorter span of time in comparison to delayed implant insertion.
8. Fewer visits are required.
9. A diminished time period of functional and aesthetic deficiency.

Disadvantages of immediate implantation in extraction socket

1. Not possible in sockets with active infection.
2. Increased risk of infection to the implant.
3. Less initial bone-to-implant contact (BIC) percentage.
4. Grafting required, filling voids and spaces.

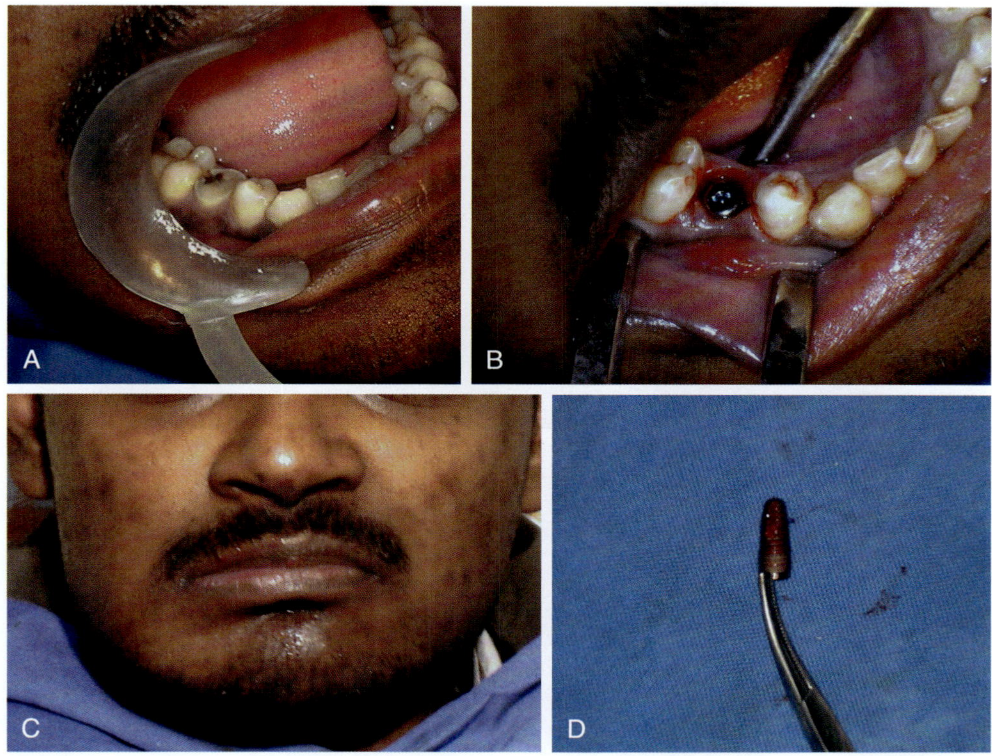

Fig 9.1 (A) Implant placement into an infected socket should be avoided. The tooth number 45 which needs extraction, showed signs of active infection presented with pain on percussion before the extraction. Though, all measures were taken to avoid the infection to the implant, such as prophylactic antibiotics, socket debridement, and flushing the socket with clindamycin before implant insertion, (B) there was infection to the immediately inserted implant, which presented with persistent pain and extraoral swelling even 1 week after (C) the implant placement. (D) When the implant was ultimately removed, the swelling and pain subsided within 24 h with the same antibiotics and analgesics.

5. Difficulty in achieving soft tissue closure.
6. Loss of marginal keratinized soft tissue collar, if flap is released and coronally advanced to achieve primary closure.
7. Micromovement of implant with low primary stability during its healing phase.
8. Technique-sensitive procedure with less control during drilling.
9. Offset implant insertion, if implant is inserted in one of the root sockets of multirooted tooth.
10. Increased cost of the treatment, if grafting materials and collagen barrier membrane are used.

Implant treatment options at the extraction site

Option 1 – extraction and delayed implant insertion in the healed socket

The tooth is extracted and the socket is left to heal for 6–8 weeks before implant insertion with or without simultaneous guided bone regeneration.

Indications

1. Tooth with the active infection (Fig 9.1A–D).
2. Osseous topography of the extraction socket not favourable for immediate implantation.
3. Inadequate bone volume apical to the extraction socket to adequately stabilize the implant.
4. Inadequate band of thick, stable, and keratinized marginal tissue around the extraction socket.

Option 2 – extraction, socket grafting, and delayed implant insertion in healed socket

The tooth is extracted and the socket is grafted using appropriate bone substitute to regenerate the adequate bone dimensions at the extraction site. The grafted socket is left to heal for 4–6 months before implant insertion.

Indications

1. Tooth without any active infection.
2. Osseous topography of the extraction socket is not favourable for immediate implantation (large osseous defect).
3. Inadequate bone volume apical to the extraction socket to adequately stabilize the implant.
4. Inadequate band of thick, stable, and keratinized marginal tissue around the extraction socket.

Option 3 – extraction and immediate implant insertion with submersed healing

Immediate implantation in the extraction socket is performed with or without simultaneous bone grafting and

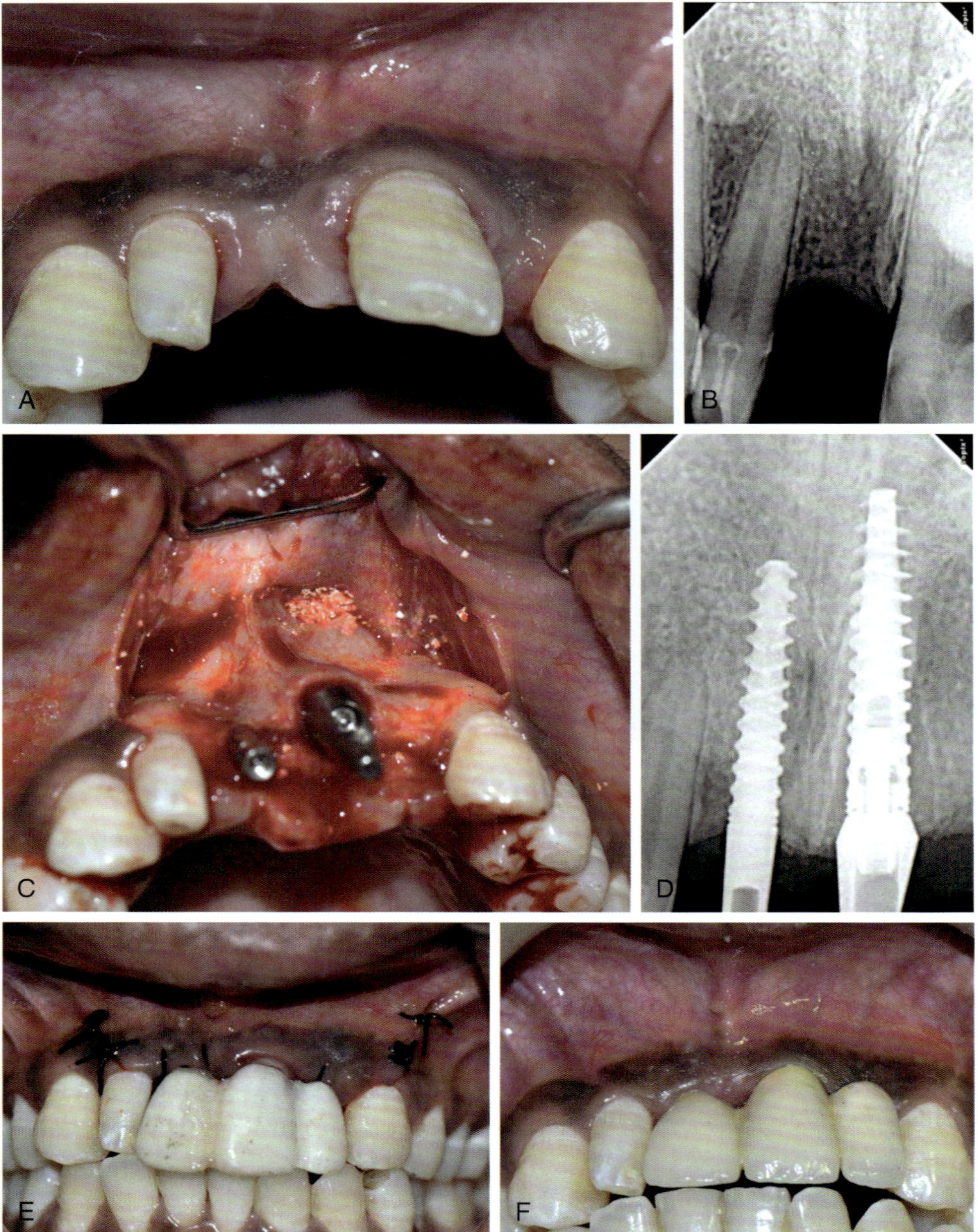

Fig 9.2 (A–D) Teeth are extracted and implants are immediately placed in the sockets of anterior maxilla with apex stabilized in the high density nasal floor to achieve adequate BIC percentage as well as to achieve adequate primary stability of the implants. (E) The inserted implants are immediately restored with a splinted functional prosthesis which is later replaced with the definitive one after the soft tissue (F) healed in 4 weeks.

covered with the soft tissue flap for submerged healing. The site is re-exposed to uncover and restore the implant after 3–4 months.

Indications

1. Tooth without any active infection.
2. Osseous topography of the extraction socket is favourable for immediate implantation with (small osseous defect) or without (no osseous defect) simultaneous bone grafting.
3. Adequate bone volume apical to the extraction socket is present to stabilize the implant.
4. Adequate zone of thick, stable, and keratinized marginal soft tissue around the extraction socket.
5. The inserted implant achieves adequate primary stability (20–25 Ncm).

Option 4 – extraction and immediate implant insertion with non-submersed/open healing

The dental implant is immediately inserted in the extraction socket and a gingival former, emerging out of the soft tissues, is placed on top of the implant and the flap is sutured around it. The site is left to heal for 4 to 6 months before the implant is restored.

Indications

1. Tooth without any active infection.
2. Osseous topography of the extraction socket is favourable for immediate implantation.
3. Adequate bone volume apical to the extraction socket to stabilize the implant.
4. Adequate zone of thick, stable, and keratinized marginal soft tissue around the extraction socket.
5. The coronal advancement of the flap to achieve primary closure may result in shifting of thick, stable, and keratinized marginal soft tissue to the ridge crest.
6. The inserted implant achieves adequate primary stability (30–35 Ncm).

Option 5 – immediate implantation with nonfunctional loading of the implant

The implant is immediately inserted in the extraction socket and a provisional prosthesis is fixed over the implant, and flap is sutured around it. The prosthesis is kept out of occlusion (nonfunctional loading), which is replaced with a definitive prosthesis, in functional occlusion, after 3–4 months.

Indications

1. Tooth in the aesthetic region.
2. Tooth without any active infection.
3. Osseous topography of the extraction socket is favourable for immediate implant insertion.
4. Adequate bone volume apical to the extraction socket to stabilize the implant.
5. Adequate zone of thick, stable, and keratinized marginal soft tissue around the extraction socket.
6. The coronal advancement of the flap to achieve primary closure can result in shifting of thick, stable, and keratinized marginal soft tissue to the ridge crest.
7. The inserted implant achieves adequate primary stability (>35 Ncm).

Option 6 – immediate insertion with functional loading of the implant

The implant inserted in the extraction socket of low stress aesthetic region and achieves higher bone-implant surface percentage and primary stability (more than 35 Ncm). or, multiple implants are immediately inserted in the extraction sockets with high primary stability and a splinted provisional prosthesis, in functional occlusion, is immediately fixed over these implants, which is later replaced with a long-term definitive prosthesis after the soft tissue is healed in 2–3 weeks.

Indications

1. Immediate implant inserted into the extraction socket in the area of low occlusal forces such as aesthetic region and that achieves adequate BIC percentage and primary stability, e.g. long implant in the maxillary anterior tooth socket, stabilized in the high density nasal floor (Fig 9.2A–F), long implant in the mandibular anterior tooth socket stabilized in the high-density basal bone.
2. Multiple diseased teeth without any active infection in the aesthetic region.
3. 'All-on-4'/'All-on-6' implant technique done with immediate implantation.
4. Multiple implants in extraction sockets with immediate full-arch restoration.
5. Immediate implantation with implant overdenture, immediately delivered.
6. Osseous topography of the extraction sockets is favourable for immediate implant insertion.
7. Adequate bone volume apical to the extraction sockets to stabilize the implants.
8. Adequate zone of thick, stable, and keratinized marginal soft tissue around the extraction sockets.
9. The coronal advancement of the flap to achieve primary closure can result in shifting of thick, stable, and keratinized marginal soft tissue to the ridge crest.
10. The inserted implants achieve high primary stability (more than 35 Ncm).

Deciding factors for implant treatment modality in extraction

1. **Osseous topography of extraction socket (bone defect)** – Bone defects can be of different types and sizes as long as the implant is positioned within the bone envelope and interdental bone peaks are present. The mode of implant therapy largely depends on the number of intact bony walls the extraction socket contains (Table 9.1).
    a. **Favourable small to medium osseous defect** These are osseous defects where the implant can immediately be inserted within the bony envelope and the osseous defect can successfully be grafted with predictable outcome (Fig 9.3A).
    b. **Unfavourable small to medium osseous defect** – The osseous defect, where the implant cannot immediately be inserted within the bony envelop and the bony walls do not provide adequate space for guided bone regeneration (Fig 9.3B).
2. **Bone dimensions (height and width)** – Treatment modality largely depends on the three-dimensional bone dimensions of the socket and the available bone volume apical to the socket to engage the widest and longest possible implant with adequate initial stability and BIC percentage. As a general rule, a minimum 3–5 mm of bone height apical to the extraction socket, should be available to adequately engage the implant apex (Fig 9.4A–C). One should also remember that, if any noninfected periapical lesion related to extracted tooth is present, the implant should further be engaged 3–5 mm apical to that radiolucent lesion (Fig 9.5A and B).
3. **Bone density** – The density of the bony walls of the socket as well as of the bone apical to the socket also plays a key role in achieving the adequate primary stability of the implant. An implant inserted in the extraction socket achieves less BIC percentage when compared to the implant inserted in the healed socket/bone. Further, if the bone density in the socket area is low, achieving adequate primary stability of the implant can be a challenge for the surgeon, and can lead to micromovements of the implant during its healing phase and subsequent failure. To overcome this complication, the implant surgeon should follow

the following guidelines when inserting the implant in the extraction socket in the areas of low-density bone:

a. Placing widest and longest possible implant to achieve maximum area of contact between the bone and implant surface.
b. Using an implant with deeper threads and with high pitch value to engage maximum bone and achieve adequate primary stability.
c. Bone condensing using osteotomes.
d. Submerging the implant platform 1–2 mm apical to the bone crest to avoid micromovement under occlusal forces.
e. Bicortical engagement of the implant.
f. Using implant with the fast osseointegrating surfaces (e.g. SLA surface, anodized surface, etc.).

4. **Occlusal forces** The implants inserted in the extraction sockets of maxillary and mandibular anterior regions usually can immediately be restored with nonfunctional loading to fulfil the aesthetic demands of the patient, as the occlusal forces in this region are very low, compared to the posterior segments. The immediate restoration/loading of the single implant should be avoided in the posterior segment.
5. **Primary stability of dental implant** The mode of implant therapy in the extraction socket largely depends on the primary stability of the implant inserted in the fresh extraction socket.
   a. **Primary stability less than 25 Ncm** – The implant should be submerged for closed healing to avoid micromovement during the phase of osseointegration.
   b. **Primary stability between 25 and 35 Ncm** – Open or nonsubmerged healing protocol with immediately placed healing abutment/gingival former on top of implant can be preferred.
   c. **Primary stability more than 35 Ncm:** The implant can immediately be restored with the nonfunctional (out of occlusion) loading in the aesthetic region.
6. Region
   a. **Aesthetic region** – Immediate restoration of aesthetics may be the treatment of choice in the aesthetic region. If the post-implantation situation is favourable for open healing and immediate restoration (nonfunctional), a provisional prosthesis can immediately be placed over the implant; but if implant dentist decides to go for closed healing protocol for the inserted implant, he/she can chose a resin-bonded or soft tissue-supported provisional prosthesis to restore the patient's aesthetic during the submerged healing of the implant.
   b. **Nonaesthetic region** – Immediate restoration, even nonfunctional, of the implant inserted in extraction socket of nonaesthetic region should be avoided to avoid any micromovement of the implant during the phase of its osseointegration. This author recommends closed (submerged) healing protocol in posterior nonaesthetic regions. The open healing protocol (transgingival healing)

Table 9.1 Types of osseous topography of the extraction socket and implant placement modalities

OSSEOUS TOPOGRAPHY OF SOCKET	TREATMENT MODALITY
1. Socket with five bony walls	Immediate implantation with simultaneous grafting of peri-implant socket spaces, if required, using any resorbable graft material.
2. Socket with four bony walls	Immediate implantation with simultaneous grafting of peri-implant socket spaces and lost bony wall using autogenous bone or any resorbable graft material covered with a barrier membrane.
3. Socket with three bony walls	Immediate implantation with simultaneous grafting of peri-implant socket spaces and lost bony walls using autogenous bone mixed with any resorbable graft material covered with a barrier membrane supported by the tent screw from underneath for space maintenance.
4. Socket with two bony walls	Option 1. Socket grafting using autogenous bone mixed with resorbable graft material covered with barrier membrane supported by the tent screw from underneath for space maintenance. Implant placement after 4–6 months in healed bone. Option 2. Block grafting and delayed implant placement in the healed bone after 4–6 months.
5. Socket with one bony wall	Block grafting and delayed implant placement in the healed bone after 4–6 months.

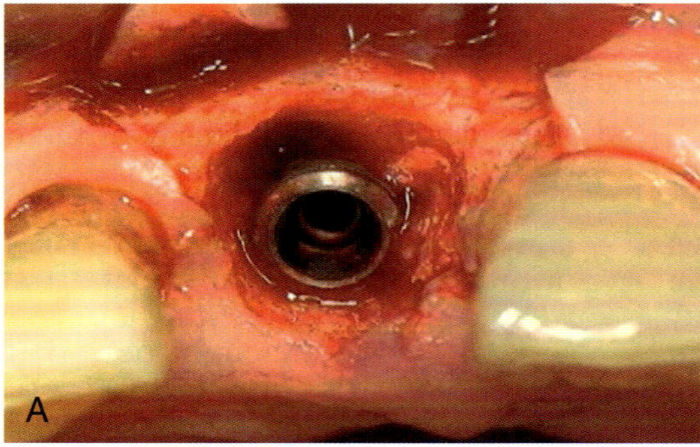

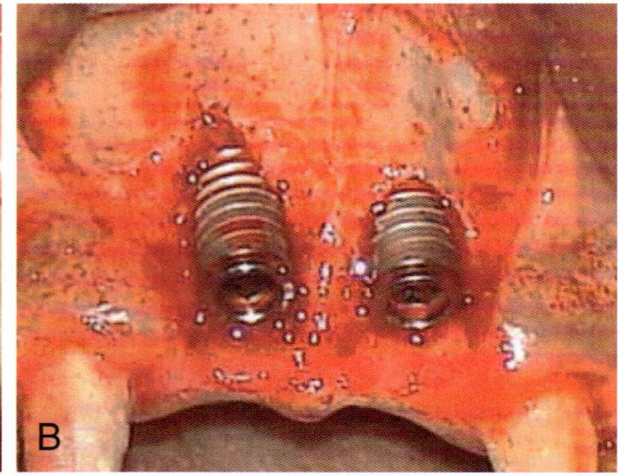

Fig 9.3 (A) Favourable osseous defect and (B) unfavourable osseous defect.

by immediate placement of a healing abutment on top of the implant is only preferred if:

i. Osseous topography of the post-extraction socket is favourable.
ii. Achieving primary closure of the soft tissue is difficult.
iii. Bone density of the area is favourable (posterior mandibular region).
iv. Primary stability of the implant is more than 30 Ncm.

7. Situation of soft tissues

A. **Biotype**

a. **Thick biotype** – Thick soft tissue biotypes are more resistant to recessions and infection and are hence considered to be the best for any kind of implant insertion modality in the extraction socket

b. **Thin biotype** – Thin biotype is less resistant to recession and peri-implant infections (peri-implantitis); hence restoration of this biotype should be done before choosing the open or closed implant healing protocols. The author suggests connective tissue grafting to change thin biotype to thick biotype at the stage of uncovery of the implant or before prosthetic procedures.

B. **Soft tissue collar**

a. **Keratinized** – One should plan to achieve minimum 3–4 mm thick, stable, and keratinized marginal soft tissue collar around the implant

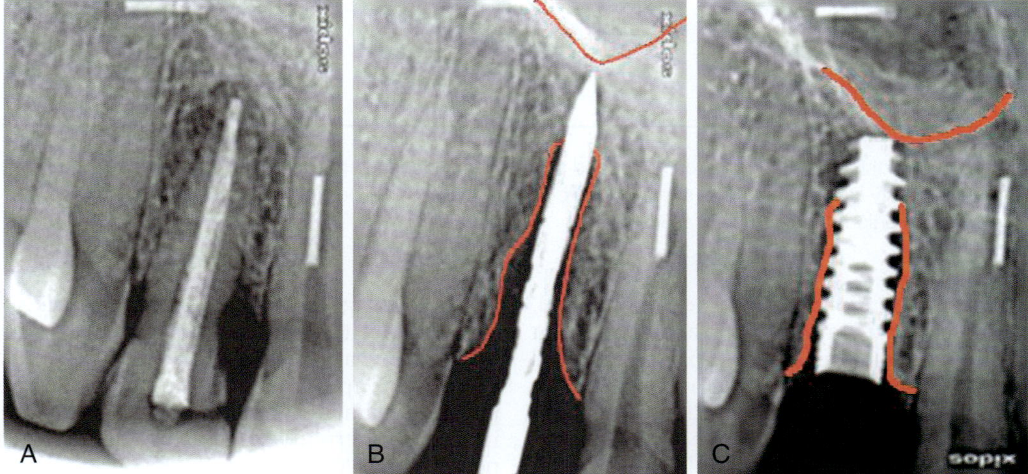

Fig 9.4 (A–C) The apex of the implant should be engaged into 3–5 mm healthy bone apical to the extraction socket to achieve adequate primary stability.

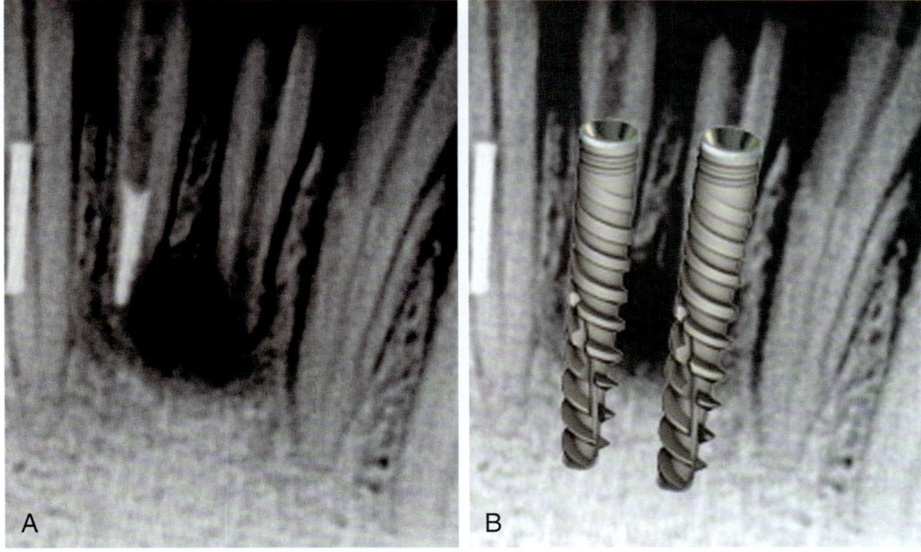

Fig 9.5 (A and B) If any noninfected periapical cyst/radiolucency related to the extracted tooth is present, the implant should further be engaged 3–5 mm apical to the radiolucent area.

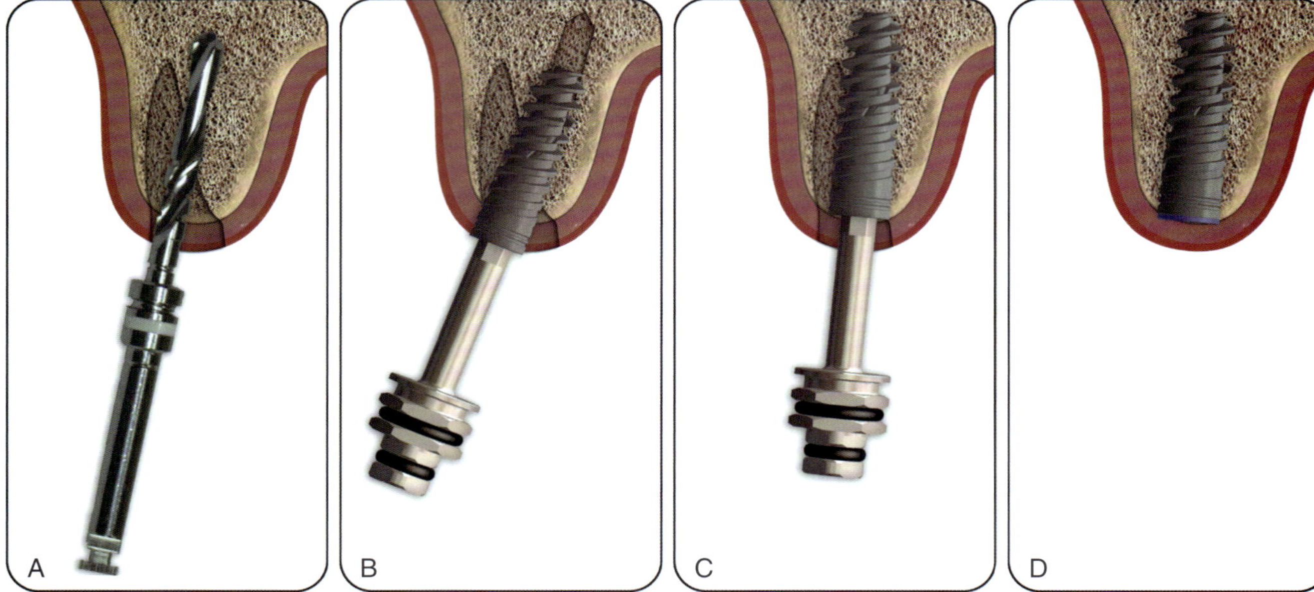

Fig 9.6 The implant with deeper threads with high pitch value, and sharp cutting blades at the apex should be preferred in immediate implantation cases to achieve adequate primary stability. (A–D) The sharp cutting blades at the implant apex also help in directing the implant to the correct three-dimensional positions during insertion *(Courtesy: Alpha-Bio, Israel).*

prosthesis as it is more resistant to muscle pull, recession, and peri-implantitis. If a large amount of keratinized soft tissue collar is present around the socket, the implant surgeon can choose immediate implant insertion and healing with any protocol depending on other parameters.

b. **Nonkeratinized** – If a thin, mobile, and non keratinized marginal soft tissue collar is preset around the socket, the extraction and delayed implant insertion in the healed socket should be preferred as it generates a thick keratinized soft tissue over the healed socket, which can be displaced facial to the implant inserted in the healed socket. If the surgeon prefers to immediately insert the implant into the fresh extraction socket, he/she should perform the soft tissue grafting with the implant insertion or at the time of implant uncovery, to regenerate a thick, stable, and keratinized marginal soft tissue collar around the final prosthesis.

C. **Interdental papilla**

a. **Intact papilla** – The implant should be inserted immediately and a provisional prosthesis should be placed to support the papilla. If the implant cannot be immediately restored, an anatomical provisional prosthesis bonded to the adjacent teeth must be given to support the intact papillae.

b. **Compromised or missing papilla** – The implant can be inserted with the submerged technique. The papillae, if lost can be re-formed with the finger tip incision technique at the time of implant uncovery.

D. **Primary closure of soft tissue after extraction and implant insertion**

a. **Possible**

b. **Problematic.**

If achieving the primary closure of the soft tissue looks difficult and the clinical situation of the inserted implant is not favourable for nonsubmerged healing, one can harvest a thick epithelialized connective tissue graft from the patient's palate and suture over the inserted submerged implant. Alternatively, the implant surgeon can use the nonresorbable cytoplast barrier membrane to cover the socket opening. This membrane can be left exposed in the oral cavity and immobilized by figure of eight sutures.

8. **Implant selection**

a. **Tapered implant** – For immediate implant placement in an extraction, initial fixation is very important because the contact area between fixture and bone is inevitably small. Therefore, a tapered implant which has excellent initial fixation is more favourable than the parallel body implants (Fig 9.6A–D).

b. **The implant with self-tapping/self-cutting, deeper threads at the apex**, is preferred for immediate implantation cases as it achieves high initial anchorage/stability in the small amount of healthy bone present apical to the extraction socket.

c. **Wide implants** – The implant is selected with a diameter capable of minimizing the gap between the implant surface and socket walls. The reason why a wide diameter is recommended is that it is favourable for initial fixation and does not require guided bone generation. Wide-diameter tapered implants that decrease in size in the apical portion obdurate the socket, eliminating the need for membranes or guided bone regeneration. The staggered decreasing apical diameters prevent perforations of the concavity through the labial plate

d. **Back tapered coronal design (platform shifting)** – Implants like NobelActive (from Nobel Biocare),

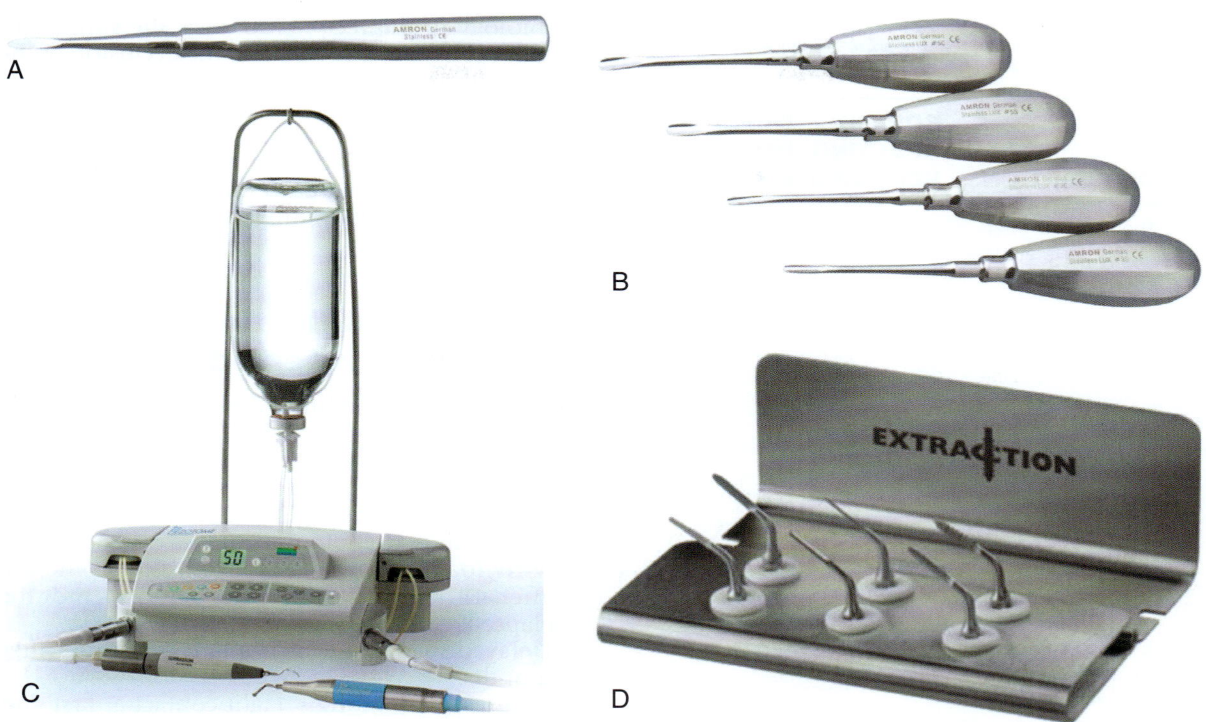

Fig 9.7 Use of (A) periotomes, (B) luxators is highly recommended for atraumatic extraction of the tooth planned for immediate implantation. (C) The piezotome with (D) its special extraction kit offers several advantages for atraumatic extraction of the tooth planned for immediate implantation *(Courtesy: Amron Instrument Company, and Setlec, France).*

which has the reverse coronal thread design are preferred for immediate implant in the extraction socket, as it avoids the pressure against the thin bony crest margins of the extraction socket, which may result in crestal bone resorption. It allows a stress-free environment at the crestal region for clot formation and the regeneration of a good amount of hard and soft tissue around its reverse coronal part. This not only prevents crestal bone resorption but also permits the formation of thick soft tissue at the crest resulting in high soft tissue aesthetic around the final prosthesis.

   e. **Implant surface** – The implants with TiUnite (Nobel Biocare) or SLA surface should be preferred, as several studies have shown these surfaces to have the property of early and enhanced osseointegration, thereby increasing the predictability of treatment in immediate implant cases.

9. **Oral hygiene** – Oral hygiene of the patient should be improved before implant insertion in the extraction socket by scaling, root planing, etc. For such cases, the closed healing protocol should be preferred to avoid any postimplantation infection.
10. **Aesthetic and functional demands of the patient** – If conditions are favourable, the immediate implant should be preferred in the aesthetic region. It can be immediately restored (nonfunctional) to fulfil the aesthetic demands of the patient. If the implant does not achieve adequate primary stability (more than 35 Ncm) it can be left with submerged healing, and a fixed prosthesis bonded to the adjacent teeth can be given for the aesthetic purposes.
11. **Number of implants**
    a. **Single-tooth replacement**
    b. **Multiple teeth replacement** – In the case of multiple implants, if immediate functional or nonfunctional restoration is planned, then all the implants should be splinted together using a rigid prosthesis to minimize the micromovements of the implants during function.

Special armamentarium required for immediate implantation in the extraction socket

The implant surgeon should have the armamentarium for atraumatic extraction to preserve the hard and soft tissue architecture of the socket for ideal implant placement. The implant surgeon needs to have the set of periotomes and luxators for atraumatic extraction (Fig 9.7A and B). The special extraction kit of the piezotome, offers several advantages for atraumatic extraction (Fig 9.7C and D).

Grafting the peri-implant socket spaces (jumping distance of osseointegration)

Following tooth extraction, however, a socket often presents dimensions that may be considerably greater than the diameter of a conventional implant. Hence,

Table 9.2 Extraction socket seal classification by Krauser and Hahn

GRADE	DESCRIPTION	BONE GRAFTING REQUIRED	IMMEDIATE IMPLANT INDICATED
Grade 1	The socket is completely obliterated by the implant	No	Yes
Grade 2a	An ovoid or triangular void between the implant and the socket wall without any vertical bone loss	Yes	Yes
Grade 2b	It is the same as grade 2a but with a much larger void	Yes	No Unless primary stability achieved
Grade 3	The buccal bone of the extraction socket is lost prior or during the extraction-only horizontal bone loss	Yes	No Unless primary stability achieved
Grade 4	Horizontal as well as vertical bone loss of the socket observed around the implant	Yes	No

following implant installation a gap may occur in the marginal part of the recipient site. There are many schools of thought on whether to graft or not to graft these spaces, but as the various studies and clinical trials have shown, any space between implant surfaces and the socket wall which is more than 2 mm may lead to the soft tissue ingrowths, and hence need to be grafted. But if the space is less than 2 mm, the bone will grow to fill the space. This distance is called the 'jumping distance of osseointegration'.

Extraction socket seal classification – Unlike sockets which are oval and tapered along their length, implants are round. Due to this geometric discrepancy the implant may not completely fill the extraction socket. Krauser and Hahn classified and graded the implant socket on the extent to which an implant occupies the space created by extraction (Table 9.2).

Immediate or early loading of the implant inserted in a fresh extraction socket

Based on past studies and clinical trials, the implant inserted in the fresh extraction socket can immediately be restored with functional or nonfunctional loading, especially in the area of high aesthetic concern (maxillary and mandibular anteriors) and lower occlusal stress. Immediate loading of implants requires an understanding of the biology of the recipient tissues, the surgical trauma, the wound-healing process, and the occlusion of the prosthetic reconstruction.

Wound-healing studies have demonstrated osteocoating after 1–2 weeks following the insertion of implant with an osteophilic surface. Implant loading after 2 weeks may therefore turn into a feasible protocol. Certainly, early loading after 6 weeks has become routine.

Loading classification for the immediately inserted implant

1. **Conventional loading** – The implant is loaded after 3 – 6 months of subgingival healing.
2. **Immediate restoration** – The implant is restored out of occlusion, within 48 h of insertion.
3. **Immediate loading** – The implant is restored in occlusion, within 48 h of insertion.
4. **Early loading** – The implant is restored in occlusion, after 48 h of insertion and before 4 months have elapsed.
5. **Delayed loading** – The implant is restored after 3 – 6 months.
6. **Progressive loading** – Light contact at first and gradual loading to full occlusion.

Criteria for successful loading in the aesthetic zone

1. Good primary stability – torque >35 Ncm (Chiapasco, 2003)
2. No excessive micromovement – <100 μ (Brunski, 1999)
3. Implant length – minimal, 10 mm (Wang, 2006)
4. Bone density type – high-density bone (D1 or D2)
5. Bicortical anchorage of implant (Glauser, 2003).

Risk factors for immediate implantation and functional loading[1]

1. Parafunction – Bruxism
2. Low quality bone (Type D4)
3. Infected implantation sites
4. Large osseous defect.

Consensus conference on immediate loading[2]

1. Implant length: >10 mm
2. Implant diameter: >3.3 mm
3. Implant design: Screw form/tapered
4. Implant surface: Rough titanium surface
5. Occlusal scheme: No occlusal or lateral forces.

[1]Tarnow DP, et al. Int J Oral Maxillofac Implants 1997;12:319–324. Aparicio C Clin Implant Dent Relat Res 2003;5:57–60.
[2]Wang, Ormianer, Palti, Perel, Trisi, Sammartino, Implant Dent 2006.

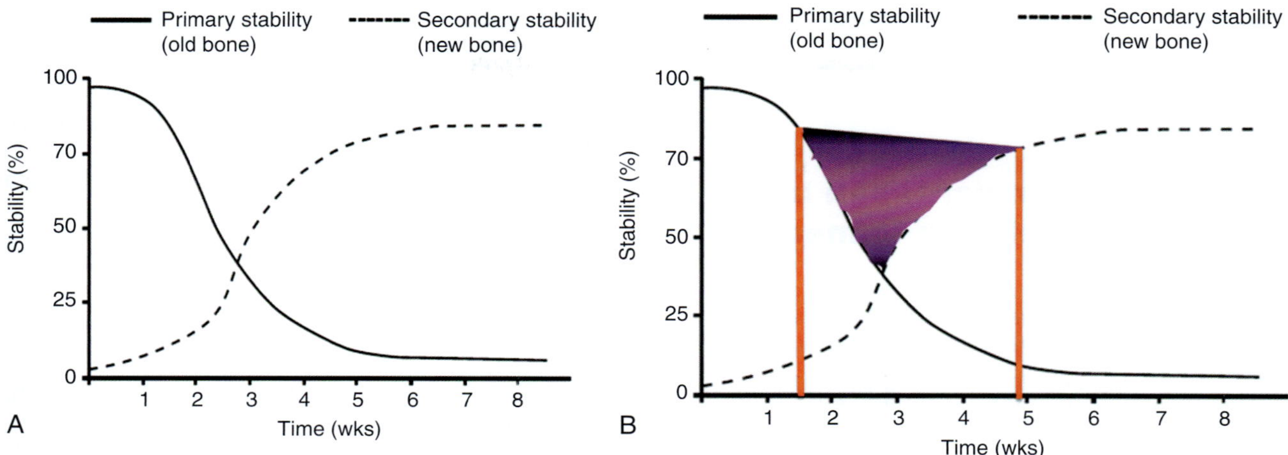

Fig 9.8 (A and B) The implant's primary and secondary stability curves as well as their transition period when the implant remains at higher risk of micromovement and fails to osseointegrate. *Source:* Raghavendra et al. Int J Oral Maxillofac Implants 2005;20:425–431.

Primary and secondary implant stability

Osseointegration requires bone apposition on the implant surface, without any micromovement. During implant insertion, any stability that the, implant achieves is completely mechanical and is called the primary stability of the implant. Further, during the biological processes of osseointegration of the implant, the surrounding bone physiologically changes in the multiple phases of bone resorption and new bone apposition over the implant surface. During the healing period, however, the biological processes of osseointegration change to a mixture of mechanical and biological stability (secondary stability). Any micromovement of the implant during this phase may lead to the failure of implant osseointegration with the bone. The primary or mechanical stability changes to the secondary or biological stability, once the osseointegration of the implant is completed. Based on different studies this process may, however, take 4 to 6 months (Fig 9.8A and B).

Importance of primary stability for immediately loading the implants

The concept of primary stability is of paramount importance for the survival of immediately loaded implants. Cameron and co-workers attempted to define the conditions under which porous metal will bond to bone, with respect to implant movement. Pilliar and co-workers stated that micromovement above 150 µm should be considered excessive and therefore, deleterious to osseointegration. Brunski stated that "micromotion can be deleterious at the bone-implant interface, especially if it occurs soon after implantation." According to Brunski, micromovement of more than 100 µm should be avoided, as it will cause the wound to undergo fibrous repair rather than bone apposition. Preventing excessive micromovement during function, may facilitate the integration of implants with the surrounding bone. The question of how to avoid or prevent excessive micromovement during function remains. The more pronounced the primary stability, the longer will be the period of mechanical stability, during which the implant will be osseointegrated. The idea is to preserve primary stability during 'functional loading' long enough to attain biological stability.

Achieving primary stability

1. The most important factor is the bone at the implant site, which must present adequate density (Dl or D2 bone) and volume to place the implant with desired dimensions and with adequate initial stability.
2. Splinting of the multiple implants by a multiunit joint bridge so that micromovement of implants during the healing period can be prevented.
3. Use of stepped tapper screw implants design with deeper self-tapping threads.
4. Stabilizing implant apex in high density nasal floor, sinus floor or basal bone.
5. Lateral bone condensation.

Optimized surgical preparation of the implant bed includes a tapered screw implant that is wider than the prepared implant bed, inserted and fastened to a torque of minimum 35 Ncm (Fig 9.9).

Optimized implant form and surface to achieve good primary stability

1. Tapered shape
2. Wide screw with sharp and deep thread edges
3. Implant surface resembling the surrounding bone morphologically, with sandblasted acid-etched implant surface to maximize osseous contact during early integration. Bone healing is accelerated to achieve earlier osseointegration, resulting in faster secondary stability for successful loading. It has been documented that if a 20-Ncm counter clockwise torque does not loosen the implants at placement, the splinted multi-implant

restoration may be loaded immediately. If a 50-Ncm counterclockwise torque does not loosen the implant, a functional single-tooth restoration may be placed immediately.

Advantages of implantation in the extraction socket with immediate loading

1. Crestal bone maintenance – Reports indicate that by delaying implant loading a significant amount of crestal bone is lost.
2. Osseointegration is more favourable after immediate implant placement following an extraction.

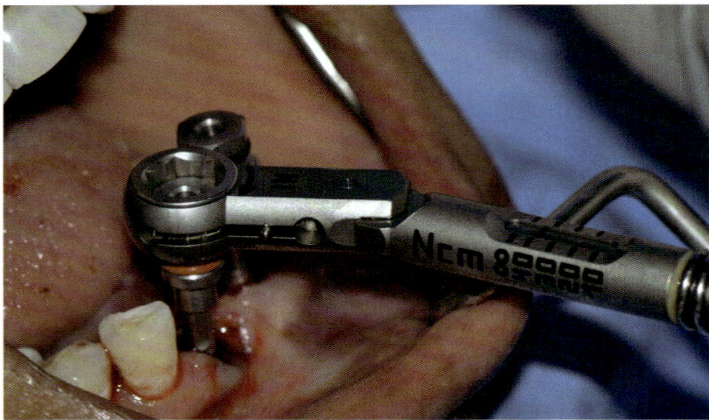

Fig 9.9 Demonstrates the application of a torque on the inserted implant exceeding 35 Ncm.

3. Single-piece implants may be used (no risk of loosening abutments, low cost).
4. For implants in periodontally involved areas, immediate placement and loading enhances bone maintenance without adversely affecting osseointegration.
5. Fewer office visits are required
6. Shorter treatment time to complete the implant therapy.
7. Lower cost to patients.
8. No removable interim denture is required.
9. Increased acceptance of treatment by patients.
10. Fewer surgical procedures.
11. Preservation of gingival aesthetics (Fig 9.10).
12. Less chair time needed for dentists.

The protocol for successful osseointegration has been based on the concept of delayed loading for over 20 years, but this concept is increasingly being questioned. After reviewing available literature, the author concludes that there is sufficient evidence to show that, when placed in bone of adequate quality and volume, screw-type implants can be loaded immediately if splinted together by a rigid bar at least in the areas of less occlusal load and high aesthetic demand.

Advantages of single-piece implants

1. No re-entry (second surgical) procedure is required
2. No risk of abutment loosening
3. No need for cover screws or healing abutments (economy)
4. During insertion, the visible abutments guide operators to parallelism with adjacent implants and teeth.

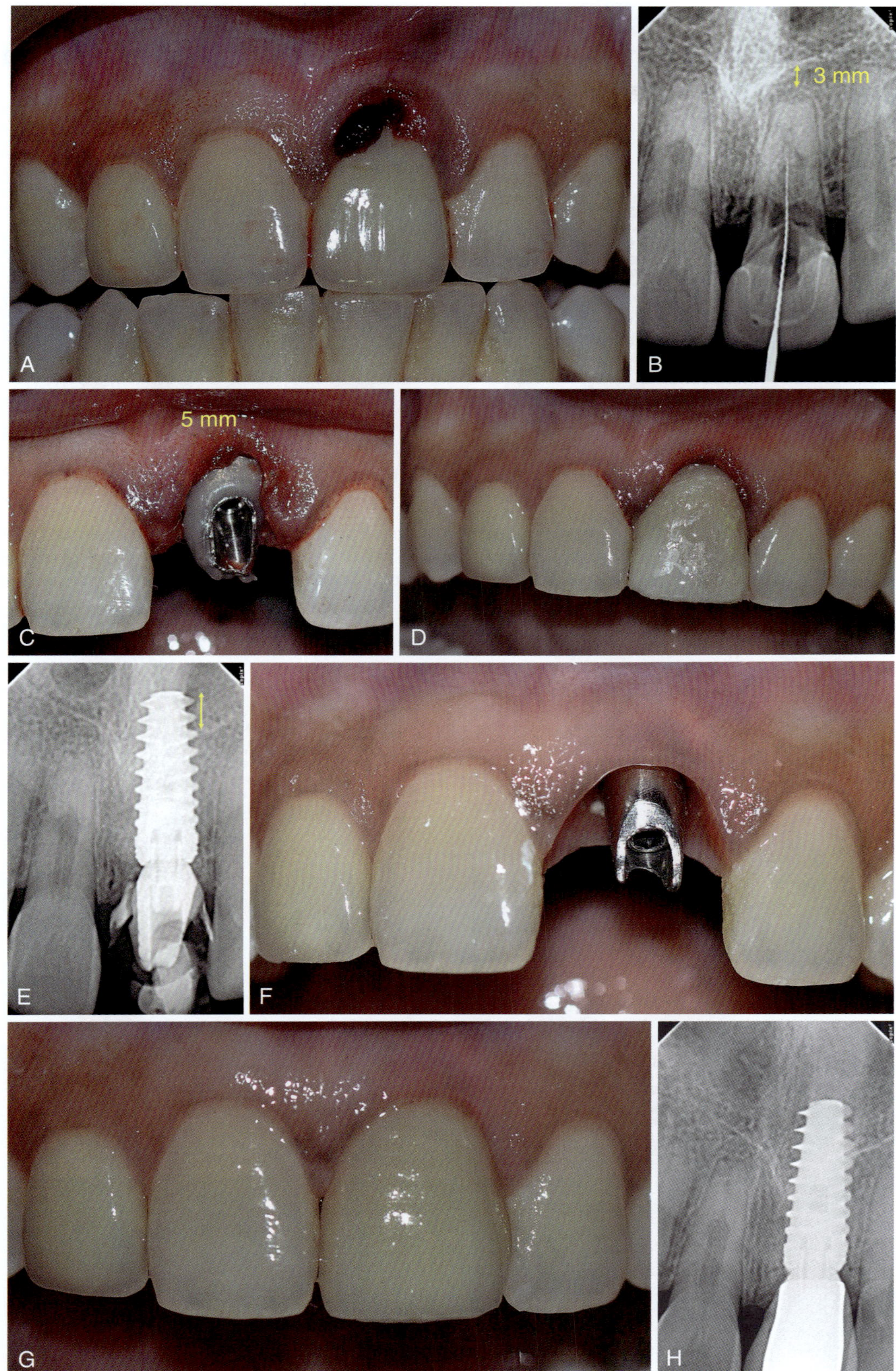

Fig 9.10 Tooth number 21 presented with root caries and calcified canal and therefore needed extraction and replacement. (A and B) The immediate implant in extraction socket with immediate restoration was planned to support the soft tissue architecture of the socket and for immediate aesthetic rehabilitation of the patient, but radiographs showed only 3 mm of bone apical to the socket. Thus a wider diameter long tapered implant was placed and adequately stabilized along the socket walls and into the nasal floor. (C and D) The implant was restored immediately after the placement. (E) The post-implantation radiograph shows the implant apex stabilized into the nasal floor. (F–H) After the soft tissue healed, the implant was restored using metal-free zirconium crown. The implant has been in function without any crestal bone resorption for more than 2 years.

Immediate implantation in the extraction socket of anterior maxilla – a step by step diagrammatic presentation (Figs 9.11–9.13)

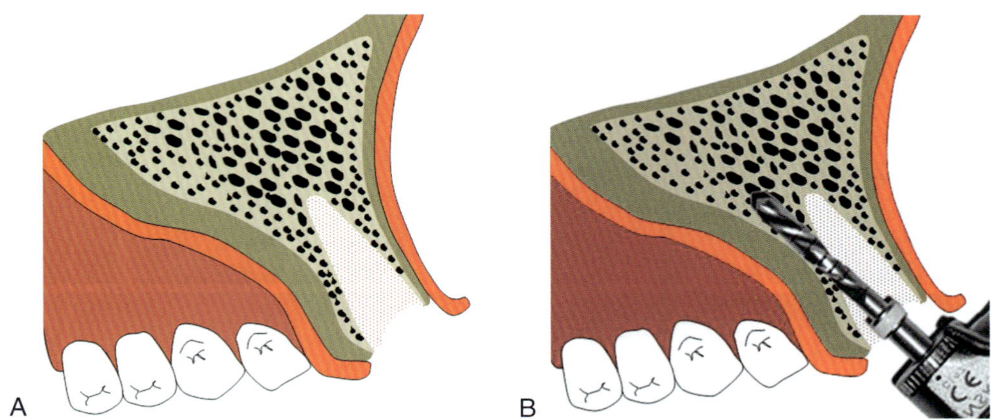

Fig 9.11 (A) The extraction socket of the premaxillary region often shows a thin facial cortical plate, which is prone to perforation/dehiscence during implant osteotomy preparation because the drill tends to slip away from the hard palatal cortical bone towards the thin facial plate. (B) To overcome this problem the osteotomy preparation should be started with the drilling slightly towards the hard palatal cortex using a pilot drill, which should reach minimum 4–5 mm deep apical to the extraction socket.

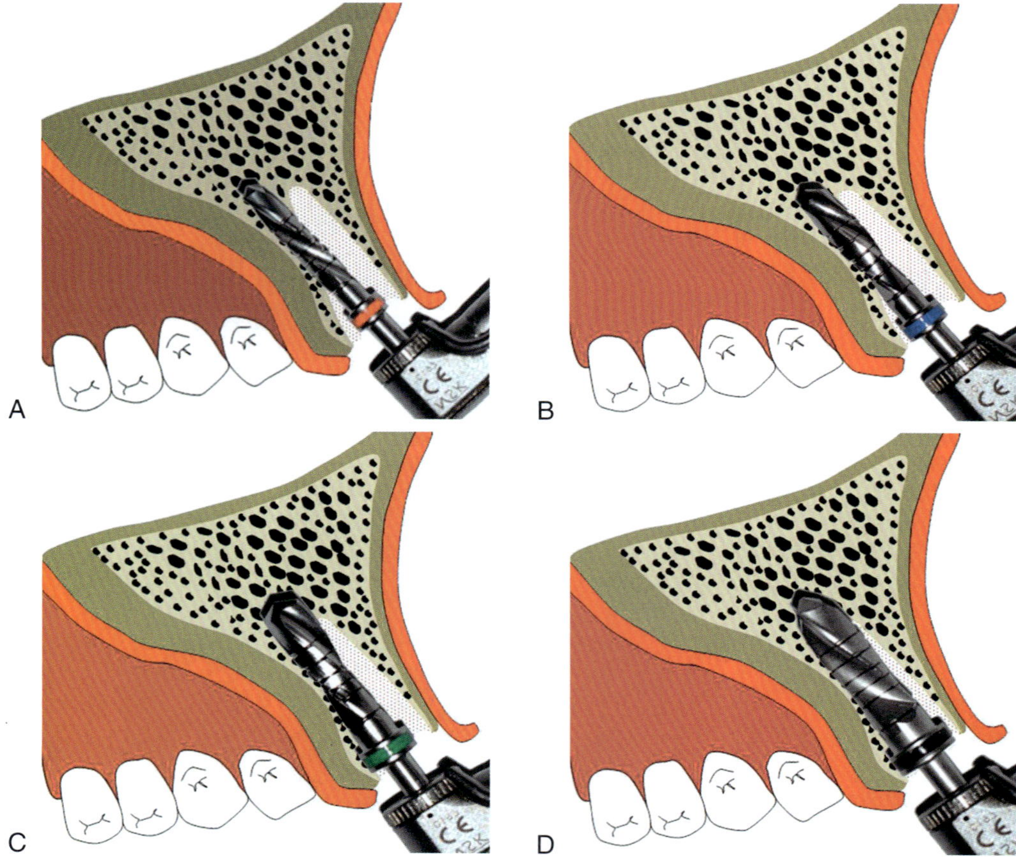

Fig 9.12 (A–D) All the osteotomy widening drills are used to the same direction and depth, keeping away from the thin facial plate. During drilling, the three-dimensional orientation of the final implant position should also be visualized.

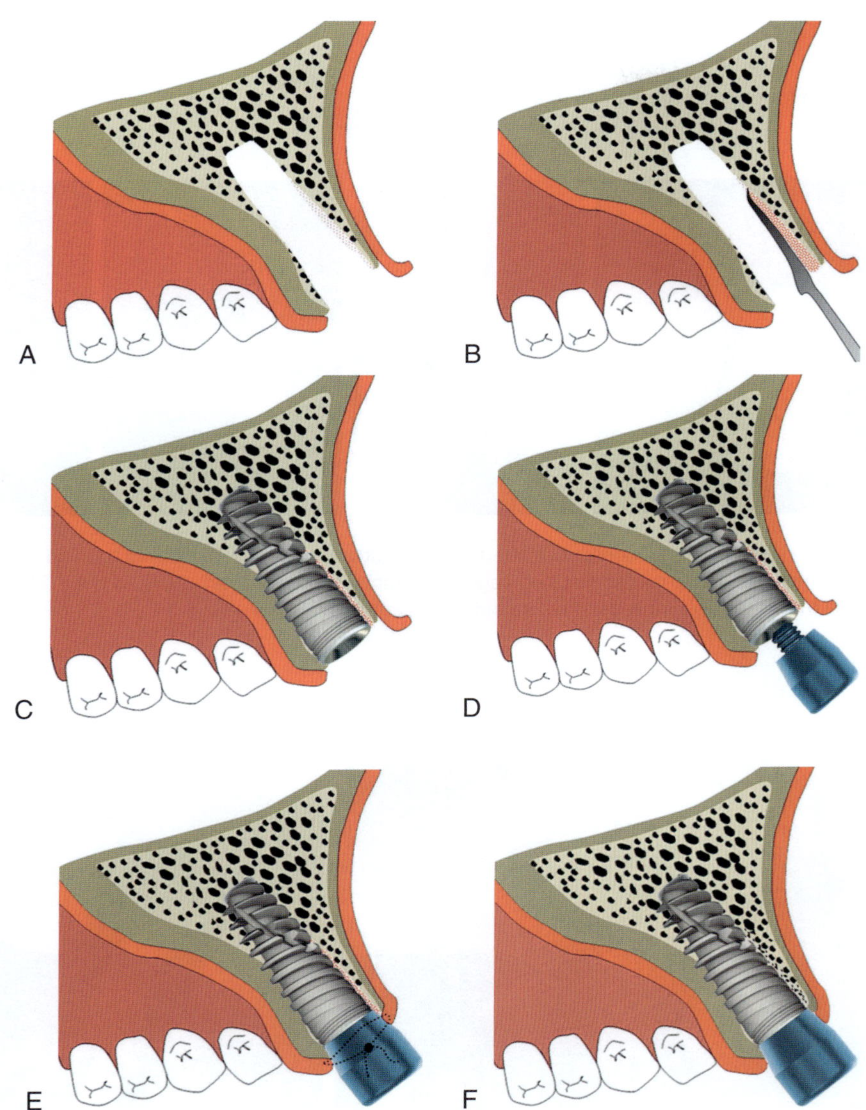

Fig 9.13 (A) Once the osteotomy has been prepared, either the autogenous bone, collected from the drills, or (B) the bone substitute is used to reinforce the thin facial plate. (C) This is followed by implant placement at the correct position and axis. (D and E) If implant has achieved adequate primary stability, a transmucosal abutment (gingival former) is inserted on top of implant and soft tissue, if required, is sutured around the same. (F) The grafting against the thin facial plate ultimately resulted in regeneration of thick bone facial to the implant collar, which is more resistant to resorption under functional load.

CASE REPORT-1

Immediate implant with open (nonsubmerged) healing (Figs 9.14–9.19).

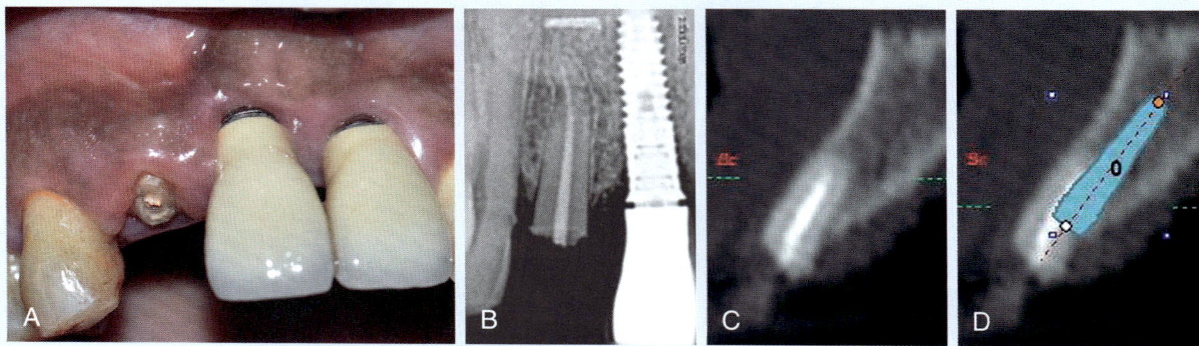

Fig 9.14 (A) Fractured and nonrestorable endodontically treated maxillary lateral incisor. (B–D) Radiograph and CT cross-sectional images showing adequate bone volume apical to the root socket to engage a long tapered screw implant. As seen in the CT cross-sections a very thin bone is present facial to the tooth root, hence needs to be grafted for its long-term survival.

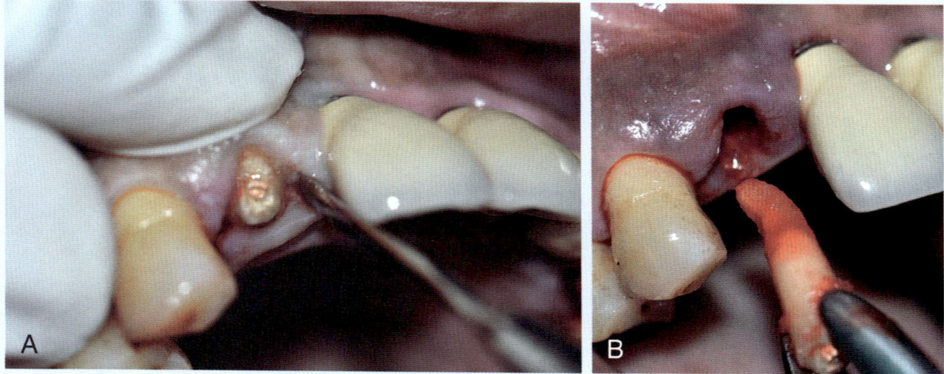

Fig 9.15 (A and B) The root is atraumatically extracted using periotomes to preserve the hard and soft tissue architecture of the socket.

CASE REPORT-1—cont'd

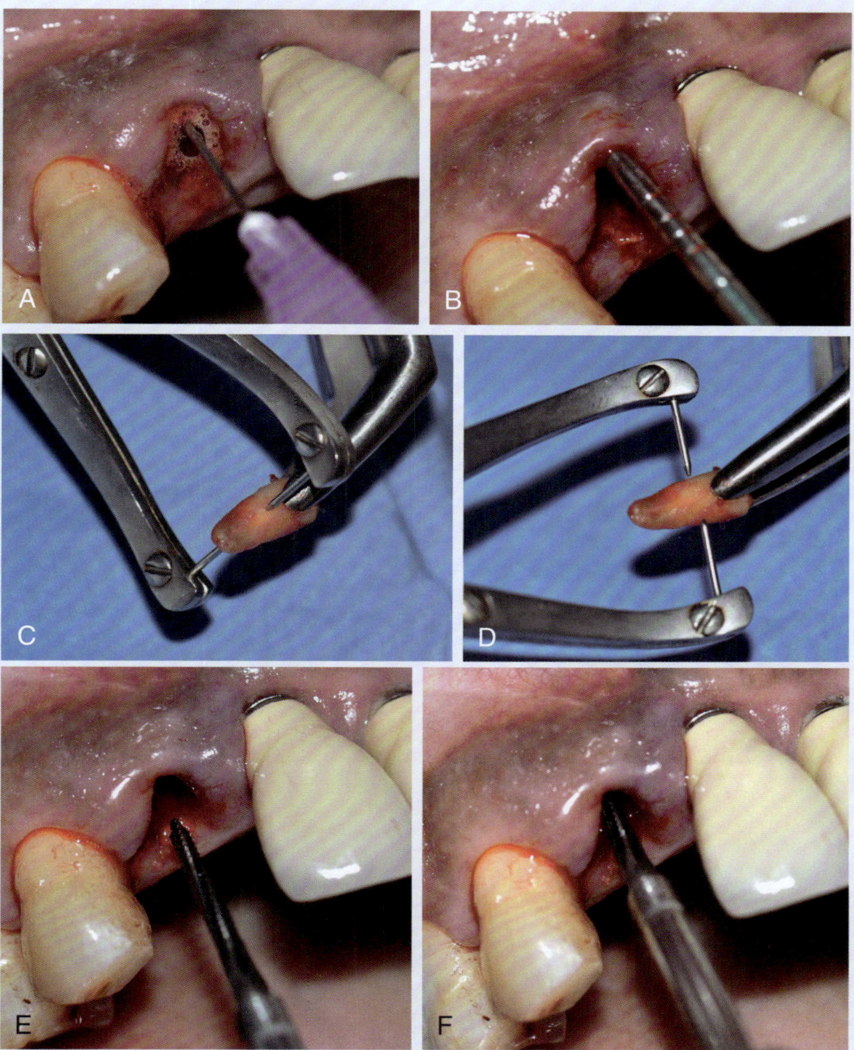

Fig 9.16 (A) The socket is first irrigated using antibiotic (injection clindamycin 600 mg) to kill the residual pathogens, if present. (B) The bony crest of the facial plate is palpated to measure the soft tissue height, so that the implant platform can be finally positioned at the level or 1 mm apical to the crest. (C and D) The root dimensions can be measured to select the implant of appropriate diameter and length. (E and F) A sharp, pointed side cutting Lindemann drill is used for controlled initial osteotomy preparation towards the hard palatal cortex.

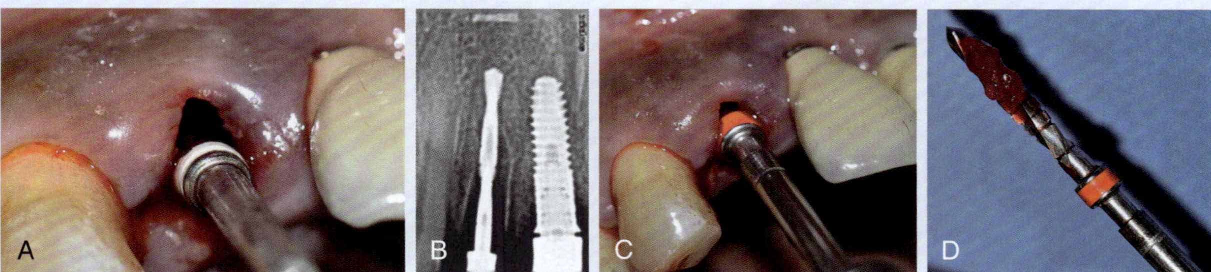

Fig 9.17 (A) The pilot drill is used to the same direction, avoiding the thin labial cortex, to reach the complete depth. (B) A radiograph is taken, with pilot drill inserted in the prepared osteotomy, to evaluate the correct direction and depth. (C) Further, the osteotomy widening drills are used to widen the osteotomy at slow speed and (D) the bone scraping which comes out with the drill is collected.

Continued

CASE REPORT-1—cont'd

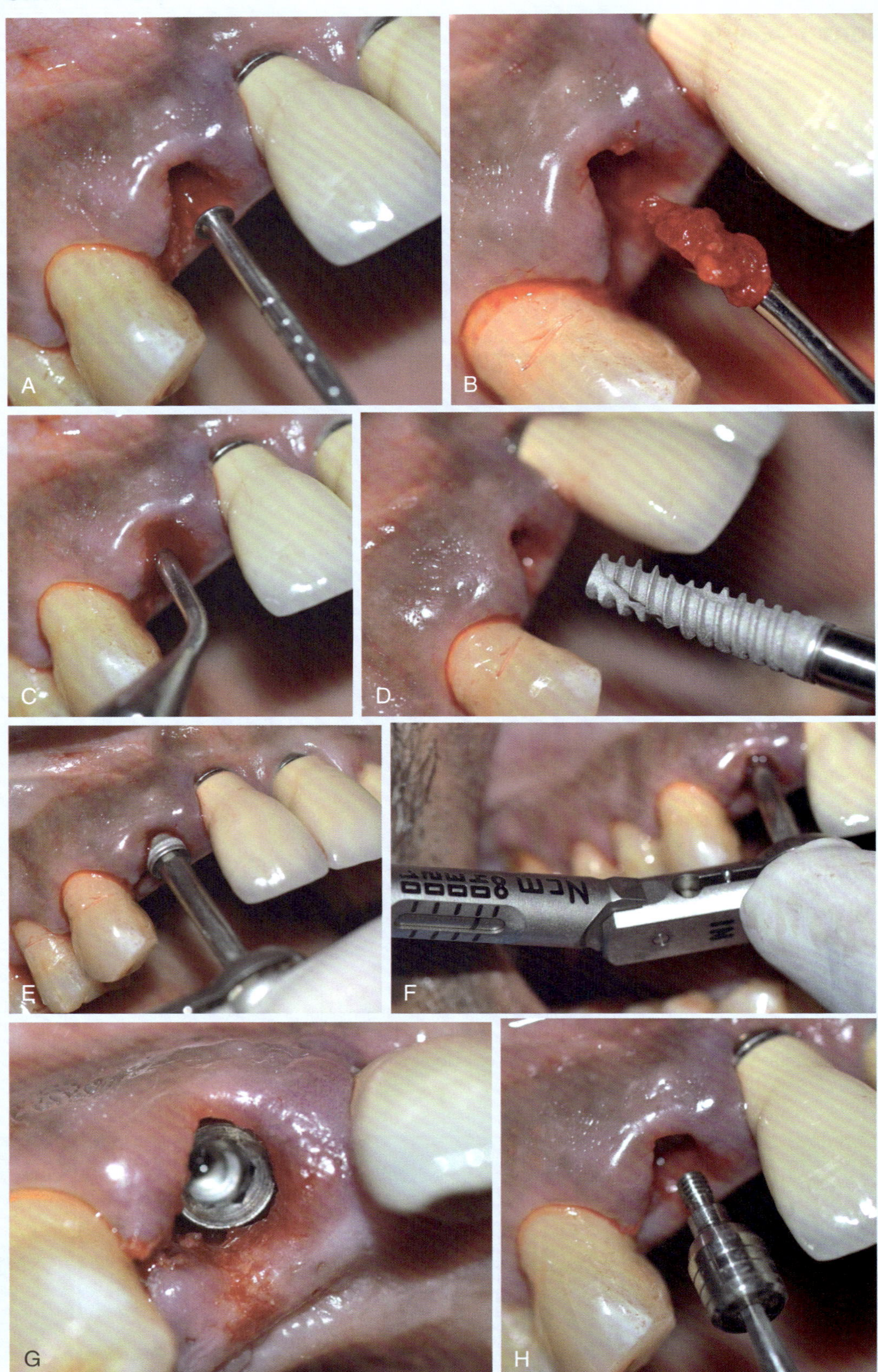

Fig 9.18 (A) The DGI depth probe is used to check any dehiscence/perforation, if has occurred and (B and C) autogenous bone is grafted to reinforce the thin labial plate. (D and E) A tapered screw-shaped implant (4.2 x 16 mm) is inserted. (F) The mechanical ratchet shows primary stability of the implant at more than 40 Ncm. (G–H) Once the implant is completely seated, a gingival former is inserted for its transgingival healing.

CASE REPORT-1—cont'd

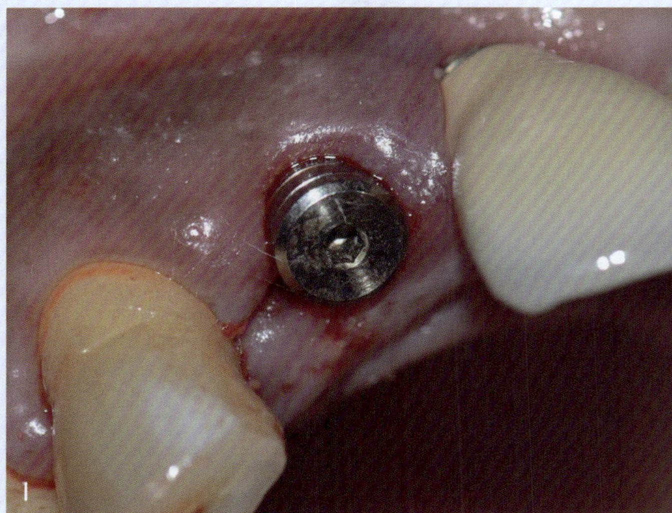

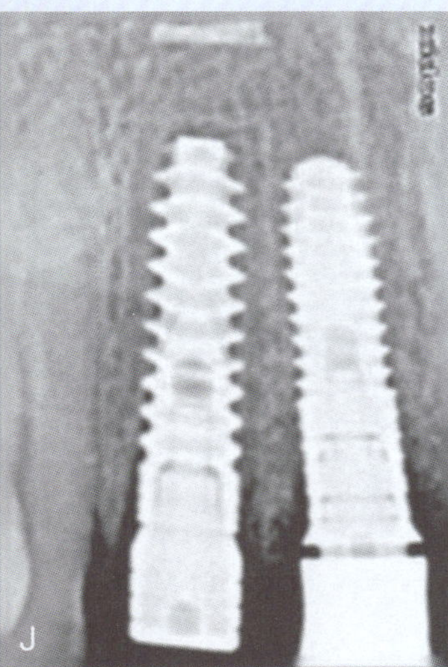

Fig 9.18, cont'd (I and J) Post-implantation clinical view and radiograph.

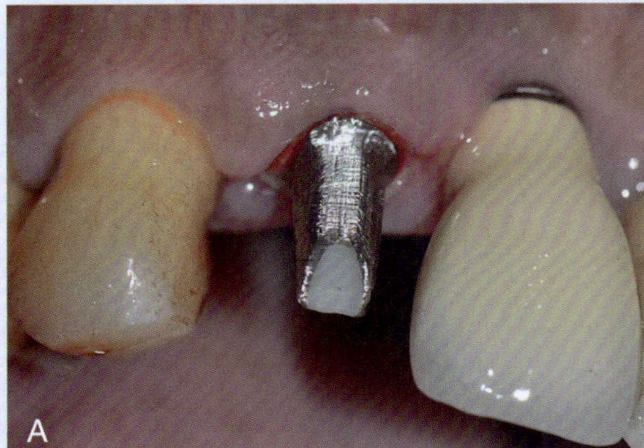

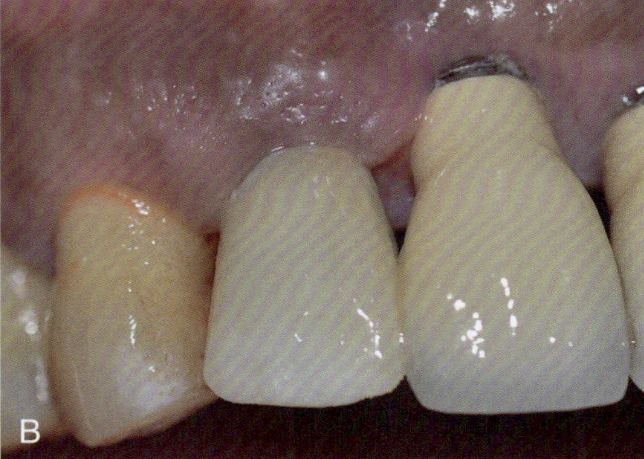

Fig 9.19 (A and B) The final abutment is inserted and implant is restored after 4 months.

CASE REPORT-2

Immediate implantation with bone grafting of large osseous defect *(Courtesy: Dr Peter Randelzhofer and Dr Gert de Lange)* (Figs 9.20–9.22).

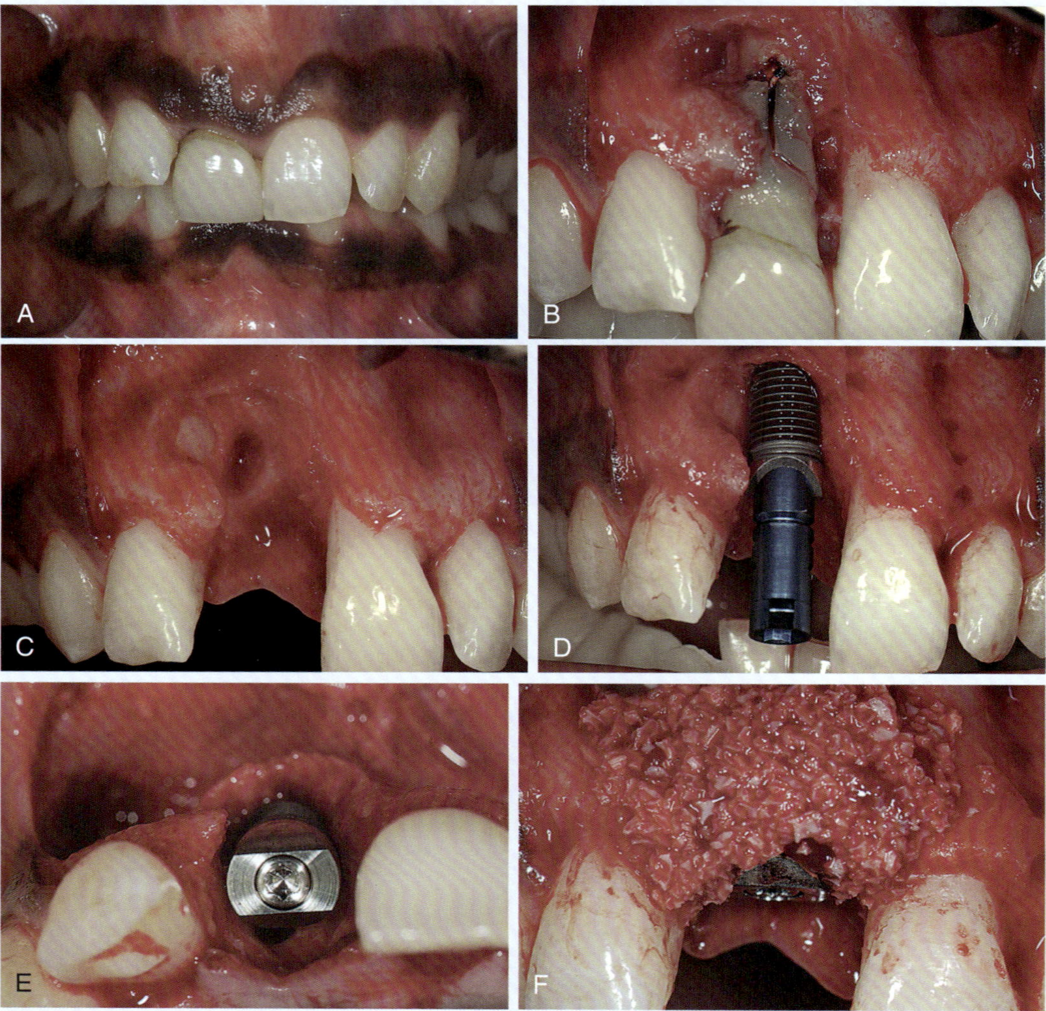

Fig 9.20 (A) Tooth number 11 with poor prognosis due to vertical root fracture. (B) The vertical bone defect affects two-thirds of the buccal bone plate. (C) An extensive bone deficit becomes visible after tooth extraction. (D and E) Implant is inserted within the bony envelope and at the correct prosthetic position. Due to the pronounced bone defect a closed healing approach is chosen. Autologous bone chips are harvested using a trephine drill from the retromolar area and are placed onto the implant surface. Geistlich Bio-Oss® is mixed with blood and applied onto the bone chips to prevent primary resorption of the autologous bone. (F) The regenerated hard tissue will provide the basis for stable soft tissue architecture.

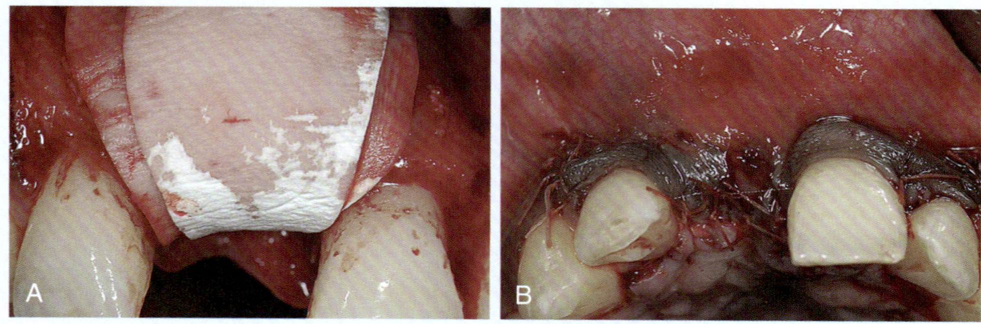

Fig 9.21 The augmented area is covered with the Geistlich Bio-Gide® membrane. (A) The membrane is placed in the double layer technique to provide stable protection for bone regeneration. For additional soft tissue augmentation a connective tissue graft from the palate is sutured to the flap. In order to guarantee a tension-free closure the flap is mobilized by a split flap technique. (B) Primary wound closure is achieved with resorbable vicryl sutures 6.0/5.0.

CASE REPORT-2—cont'd

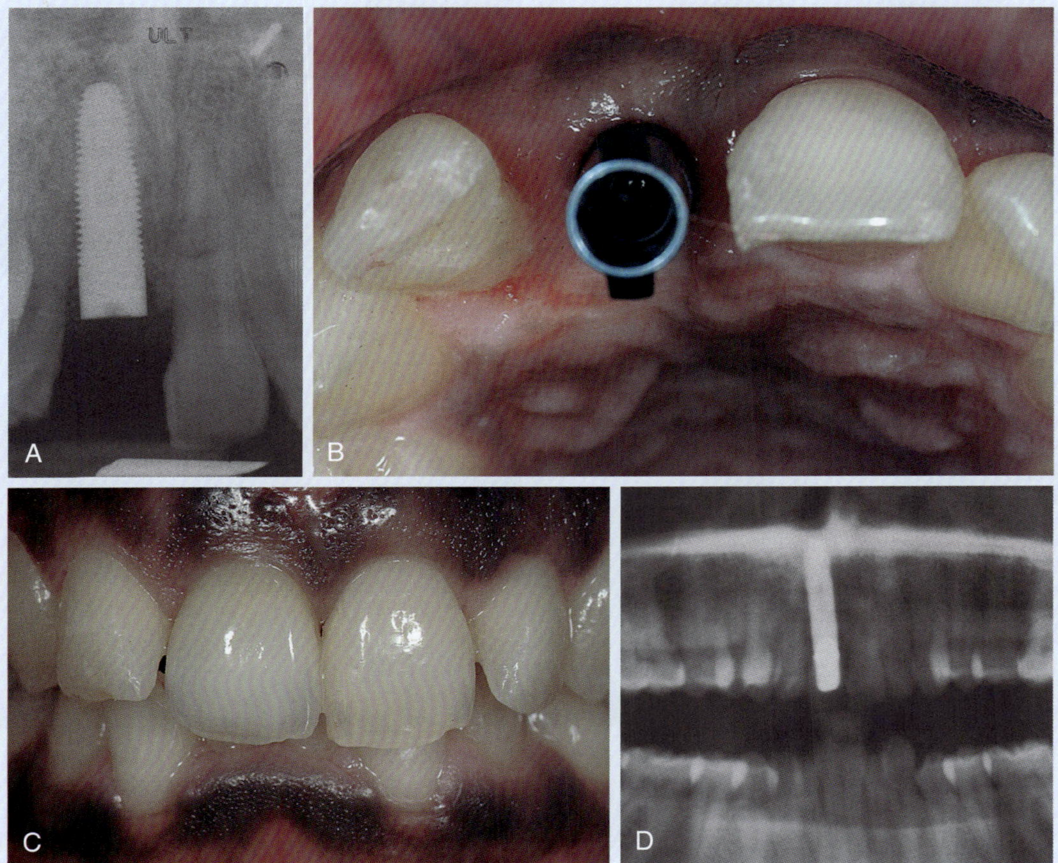

Fig 9.22 (A) Post-implantation radiograph. (B) Implant is uncovered after 4 months of submerged healing and (C) restored using metal-free zirconia prosthesis with excellent aesthetic outcome; (D) post loading radiograph.

CASE REPORT-3

Immediate implant with bone grafting of a small osseous defect and immediate restoration *(Courtesy: Dentium Co., Ltd/Well Dental Clinic)* (Figs 9.23–9.33).

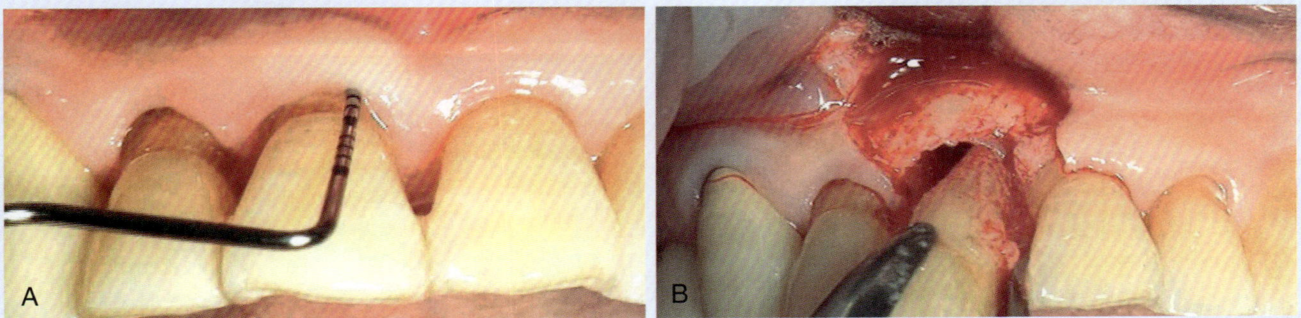

Fig 9.23 (A) The right central incisor, which shows mobility, needs extraction and immediate implant insertion. (B) The facial flap is elevated to expose the labial osseous defect and tooth is atraumatically extracted.

CASE REPORT-3—cont'd

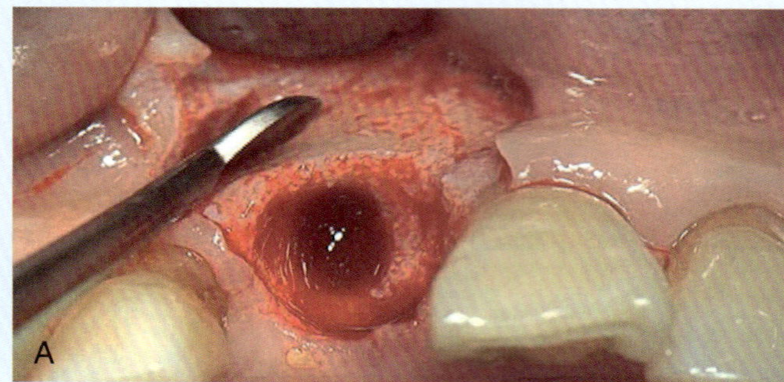

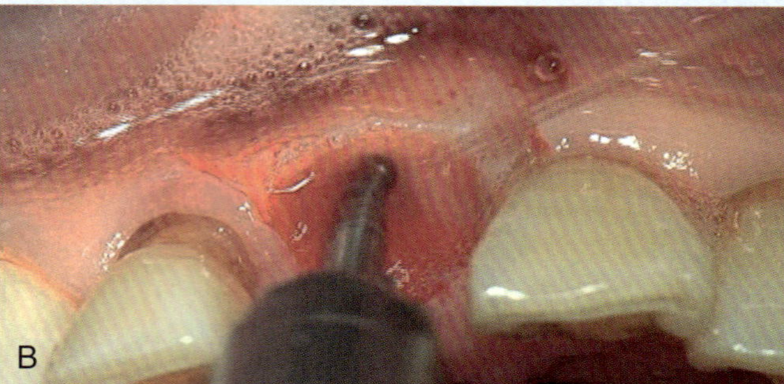

Fig 9.24 (A) All the granulation tissue, which if left behind can cause infection to the implant, is curetted out from the socket. (B) Grinding of fibro-osseous tissue was done using round carbide bur. It removes all the dead fibro-osseous tissues covering the inner lining of the socket walls; it also induces the fresh bleeding from the underlying bone which nourishes the bone graft to regenerate a predictable amount and quality of new bone in the defective area.

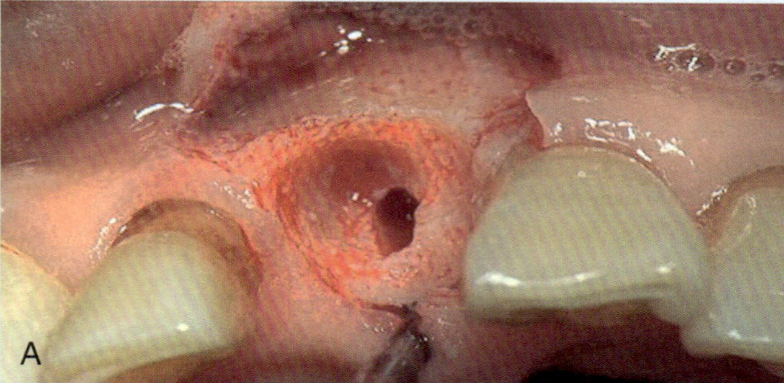

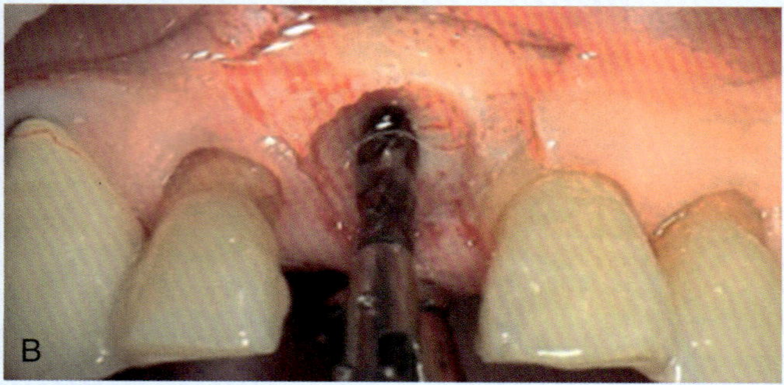

Fig 9.25 (A) The osteotomy preparation site is marked using a small round carbide bur. It avoided the chances of offset osteotomy preparation with pilot drill. (B) Lindemann first drill/pilot drill used to deepen the osteotomy to the predetermined depth. Lindemann drills have the side cutting advantage over the normal pilot drill, so one can change the drill orientation/direction during drilling to achieve better control during initial implant osteotomy preparation. Drilling done at 1000 rpm using 35–45 Ncm torque with continuous chilled saline irrigation. The adjacent central incisor was used as the reference to prepare the osteotomy with the correct direction so that the finally inserted implant comes along the correct three-dimensional position for the final prosthesis.

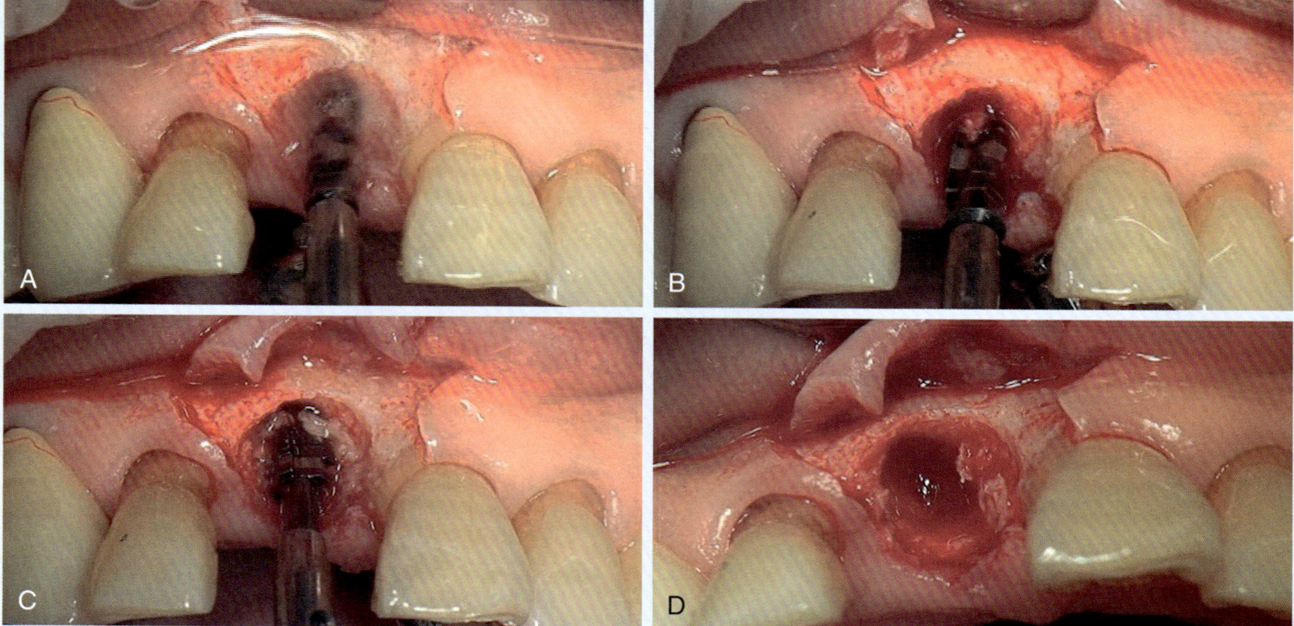

Fig 9.26 (A and B) The rest of the osteotomy widening drills are used to widen the osteotomy (C). A 4.3-mm diameter countersink drill was used to the partial depth at the speed of 20 rpm and 30–45 Ncm torque. This drill is used to submerge the implant platform apical to the bone crest. (D) Finally prepared osteotomy.

CASE REPORT-3—cont'd

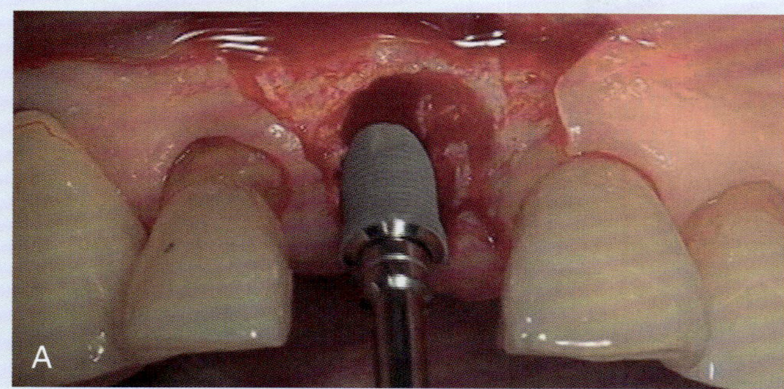

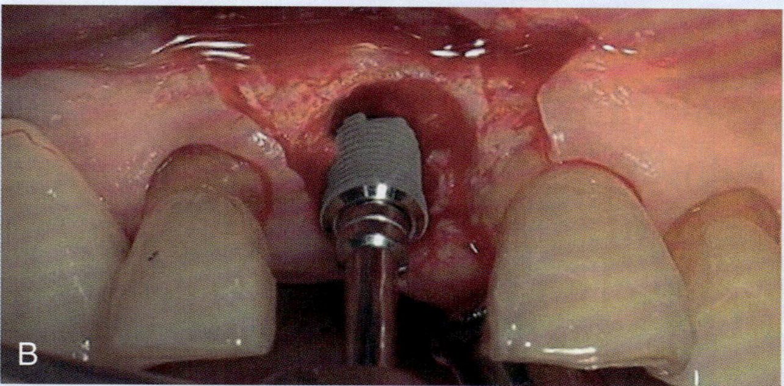

Fig 9.27 (A and B) A superline 4.5 mm diameter and 10 mm long implant fixture inserted in the prepared osteotomy at the rotational speed of 20 rpm and 30–45 Ncm torque.

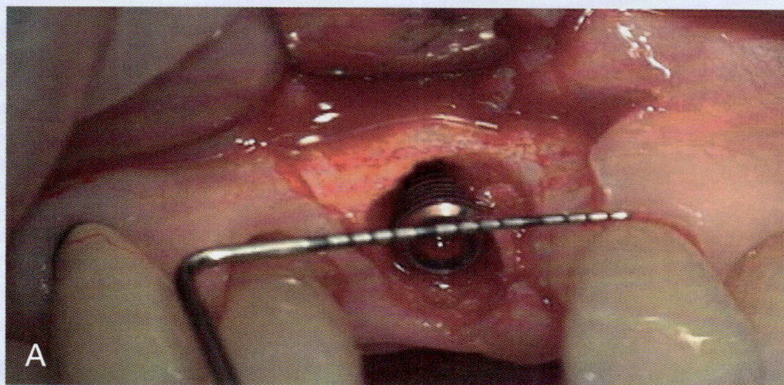

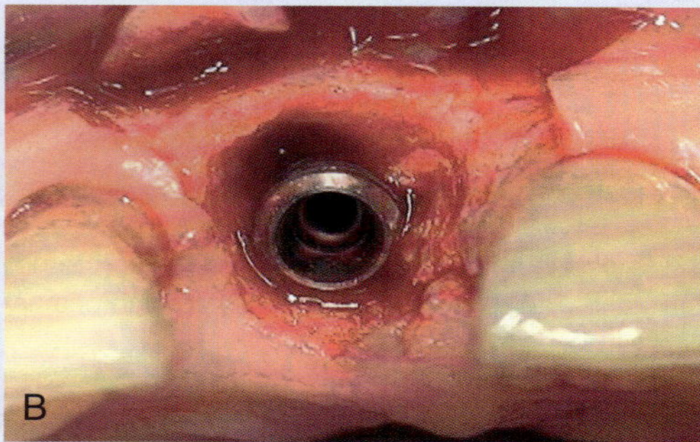

Fig 9.28 (A) Three-dimensional position of the implant is checked. Implant is placed closer to the palatal cortical plate to provide room for bone grafting and thick amount of new bone regeneration facial to the implant head. The implant platform should be placed 2–3 mm apical to the cementoenamel junction of the adjacent natural tooth. (B) The labial defect, which needs to be grafted, can be seen after final implant insertion.

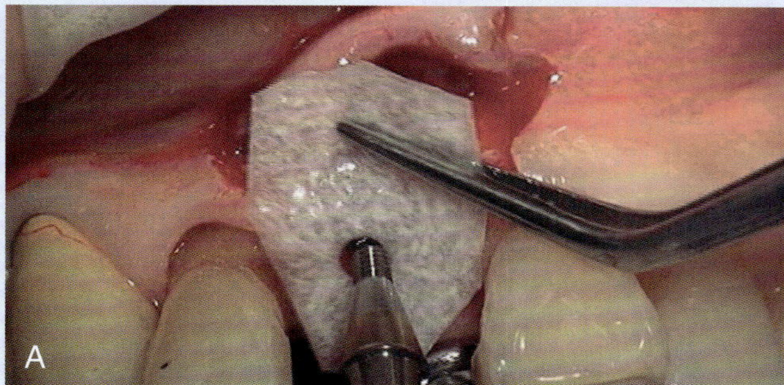

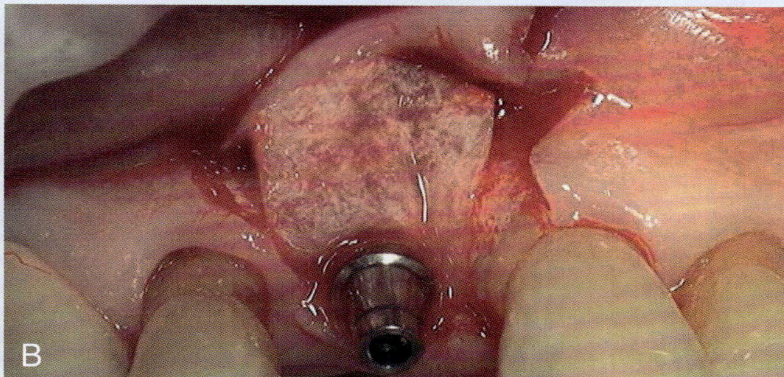

Fig 9.29 (A and B) A collagen barrier membrane shaped to size, punched to make a hole and engaged with the implant using combi abutment.

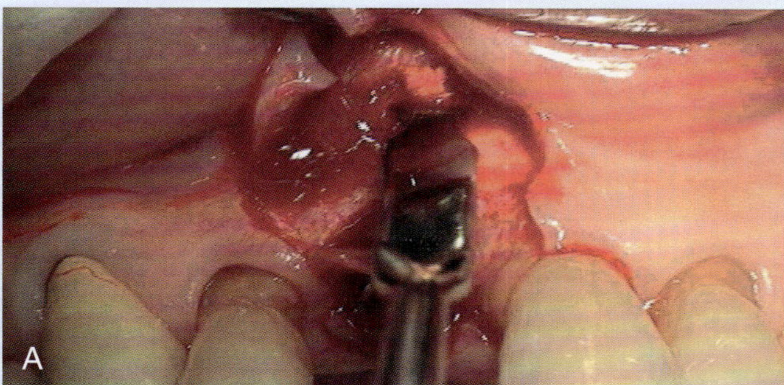

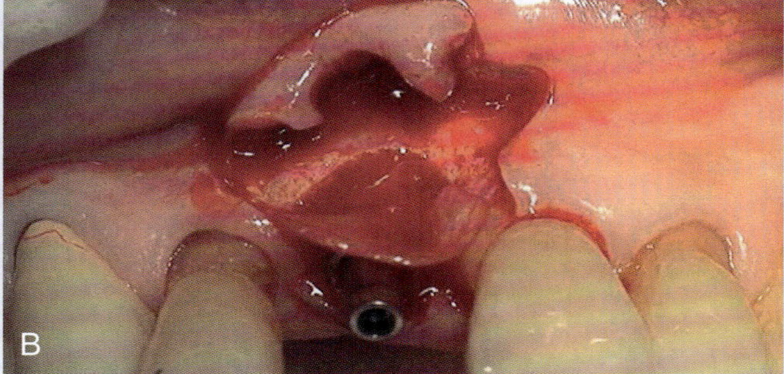

Fig 9.30 (A) Small amount of autogenous bone is harvested from the subnasal region using sharp chisel and (B) placed as the base layer in the osseous defect.

Continued

CASE REPORT-3—cont'd

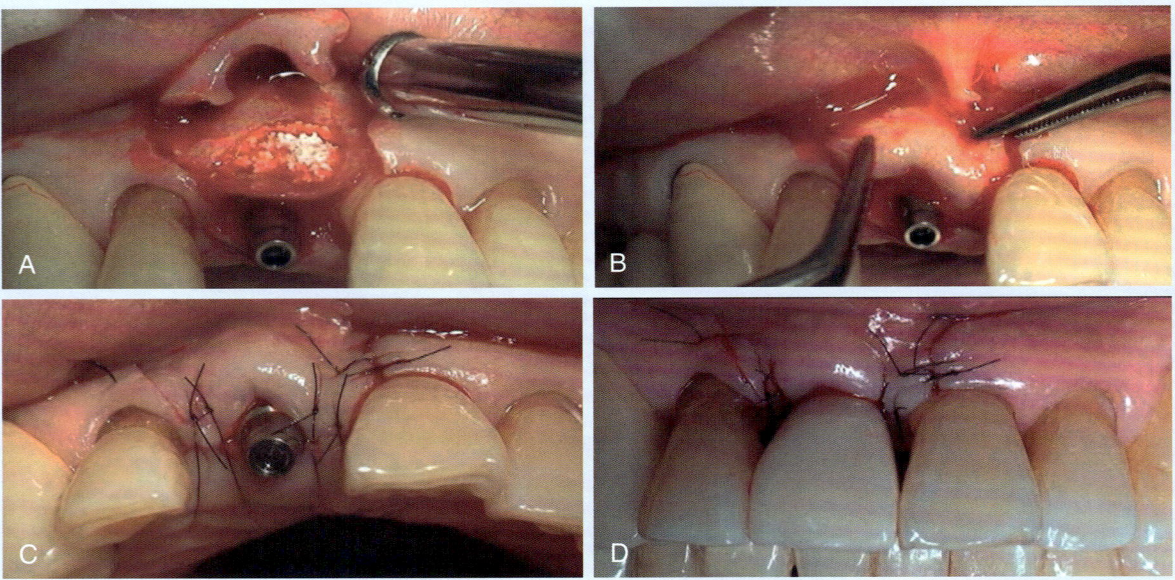

Fig 9.31 (A) The defect is further grafted using osteon bone graft on top of autogenous bone. Grafted site is covered with barrier collage membrane (B) and (C) flap is sutured back. (D) As high primary stability of the implant is achieved; the implant is immediately restored using a provisional prosthesis.

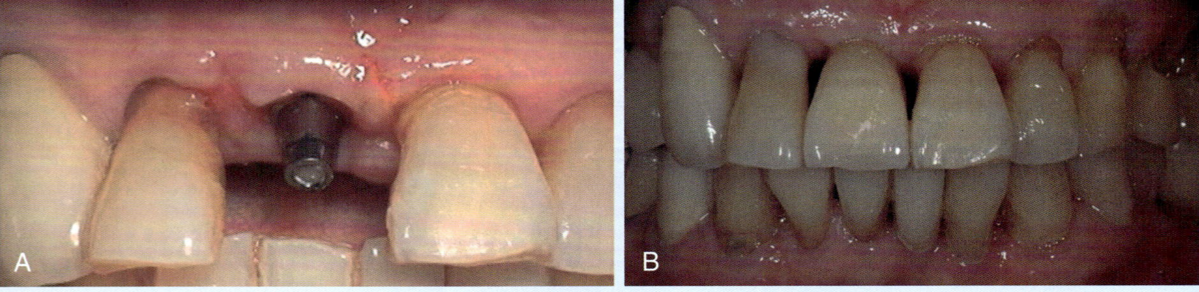

Fig 9.32 (A) The provisional prosthesis is removed after 3 weeks and (B) the implant is restored using a metal-free zirconium prosthesis with an acceptable aesthetic outcome.

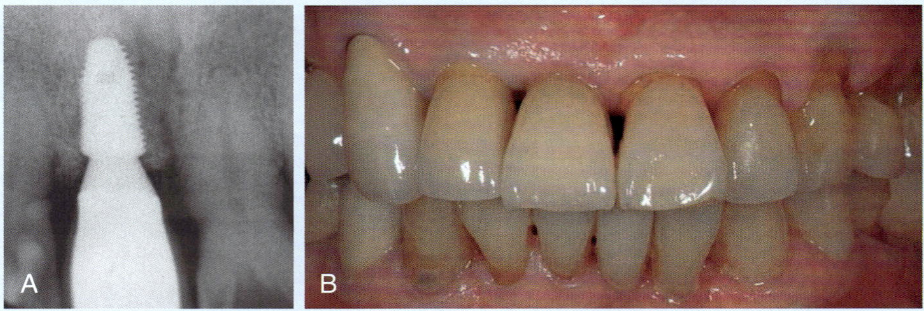

Fig 9.33 (A) Post-implant loading radiograph and clinical view at 11 months follow-up. (B) The soft tissue is seen to have adapted well around the implant prosthesis.

CASE REPORT-4

Immediate implantation with grafting of dehiscence occurred during osteotomy preparation (Fig 9.34 A-H).

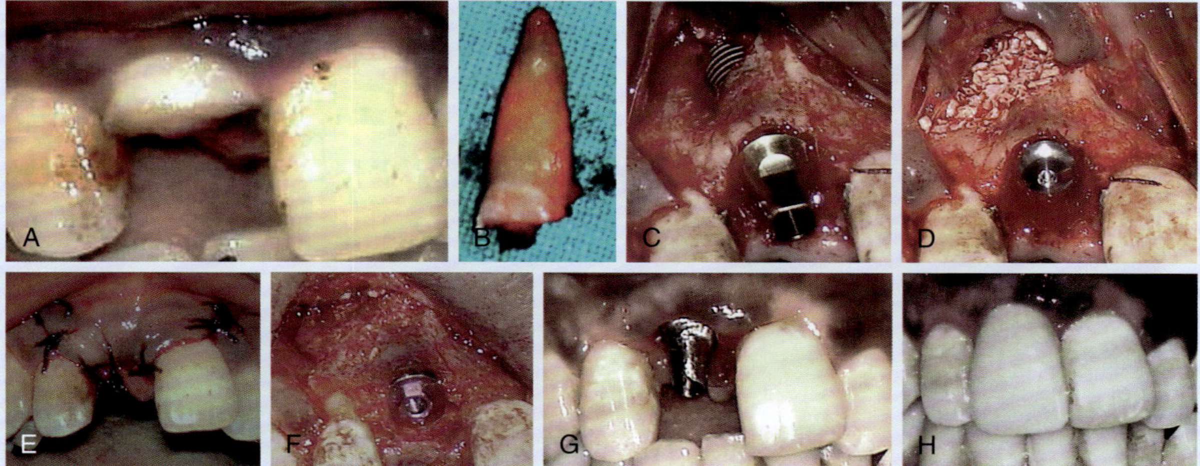

Fig 9.34 (A and B) Accidentally fractured tooth is extracted and implant is inserted. (C) A dehiscence through the labial cortex is visible which is grafted using (D) Bio-Oss particulate graft and (E) the flap is sutured back with primary closure. (F) The implant is uncovered after 4 months showing new bone regeneration at the dehiscence area. (G and H) Implant is restored using ceramic prosthesis.

CASE REPORT-5

Immediate implant with immediate restoration in the maxillary anterior socket (Figs 9.35–9.38).

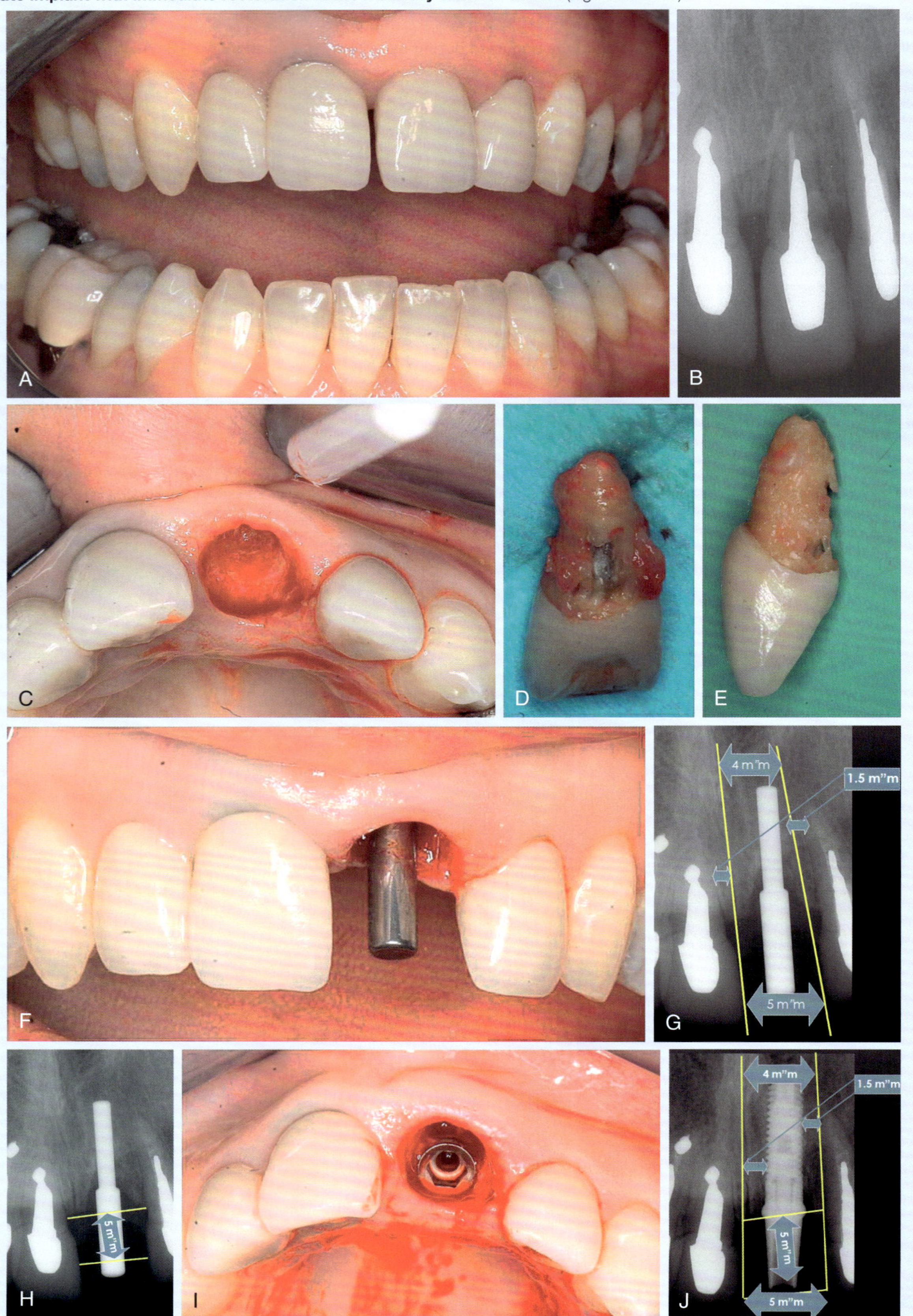

Fig 9.35 (A and B) Tooth number 21 showing root resorption, is atraumatically (C-E) extracted. (F-H) The osteotomy is prepared with correct direction and angulation, evaluated with radiographs, and (I and J) the implant is inserted at the three-dimensionally correct position.

CASE REPORT-5—cont'd

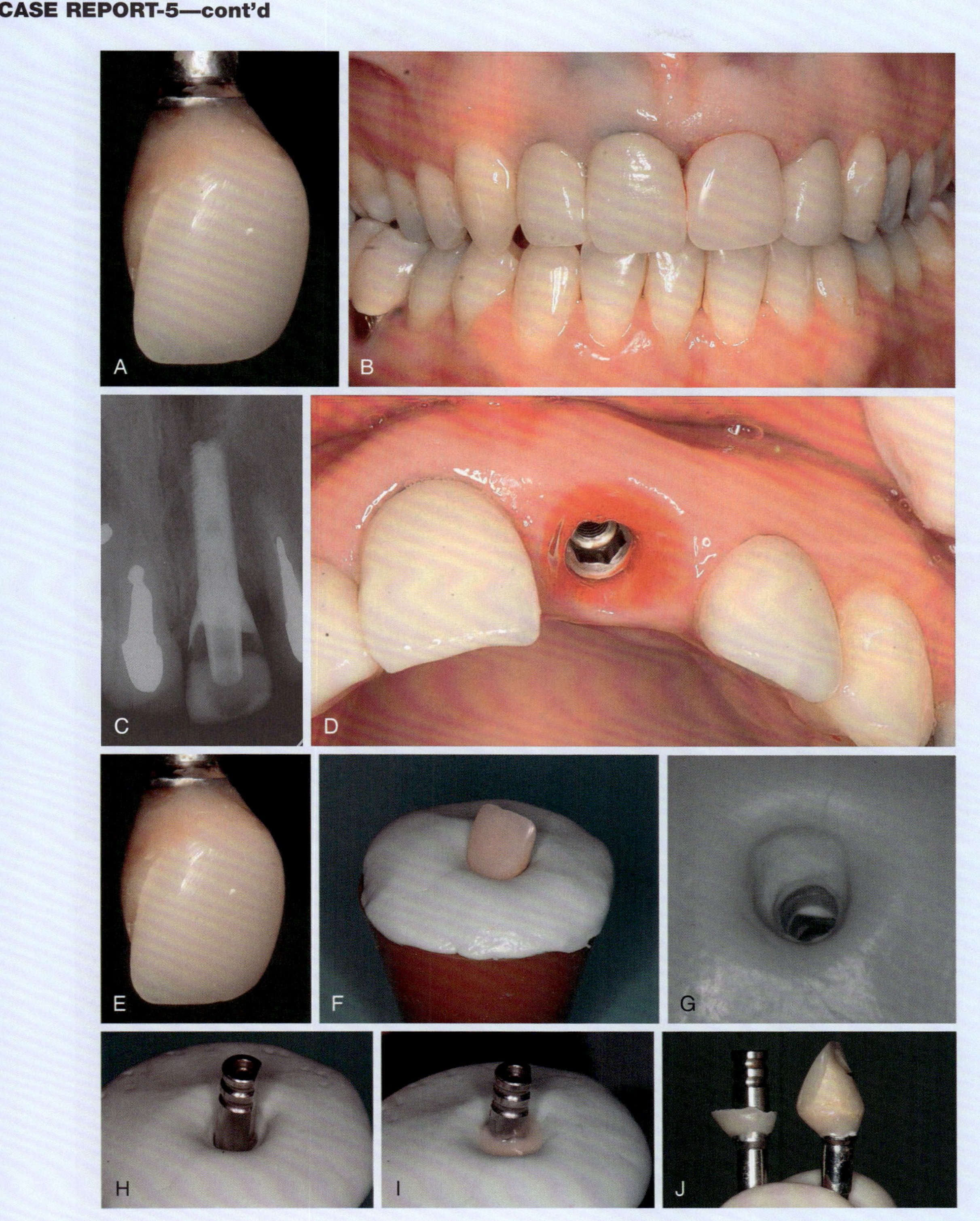

Fig 9.36 (A–C) A provisional crown, similar in form to the extracted tooth, is fabricated and fixed to the implant to support the soft tissue architecture. (D) Removal of the provisional crown, after 4 months, shows the formation of aesthetic emergence profile of the healed soft tissue. Now transferring this soft tissue profile to the working cast is paramount to fabricate the definitive crown with appropriate aesthetic emergence in the cervical region. (E–G) The provisional crown with abutment is assembled with the implant analogue and a putty impression was made. (H) Now the analogue is removed, assembled with impression abutment, and again seated in the impression. (I and J) The cavity around the impression abutment is filled with flowable composite to replicate the cervical emergence of the provisional crown.

Continued

CASE REPORT-5—cont'd

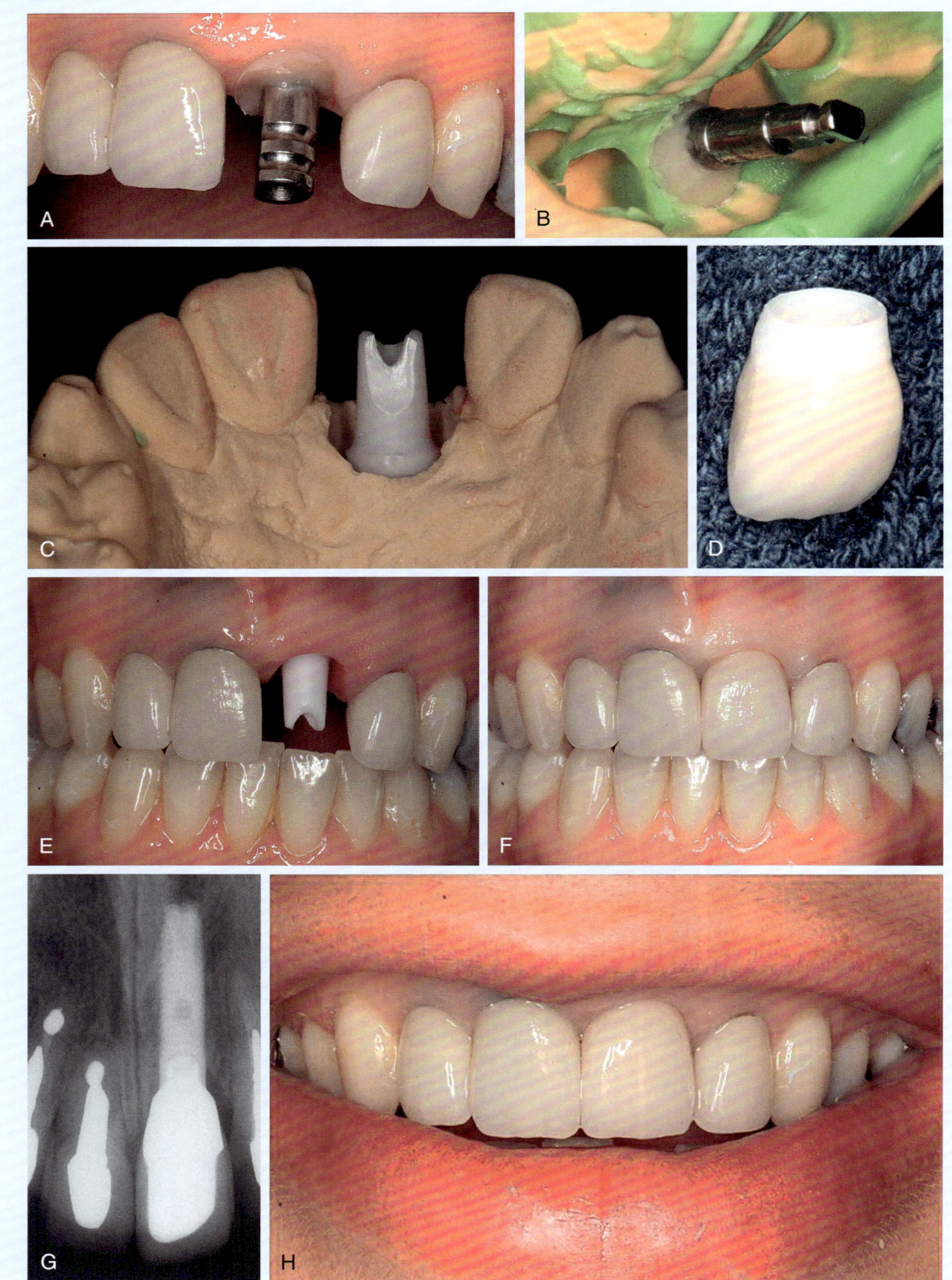

Fig 9.37 (A and B) Impression abutment with bonded composite is fixed to the implant with the correct orientation and an impression is made. (C) It has transferred the soft tissue emergence accurately to the working cast. (D–F) A zirconium crown fabricated and fixed in the mouth shows that a high aesthetic outcome has been achieved. (G and H) Follow-up radiograph and clinical picture show stable hard and soft tissue around the implant and prosthesis.

CASE REPORT-5—cont'd

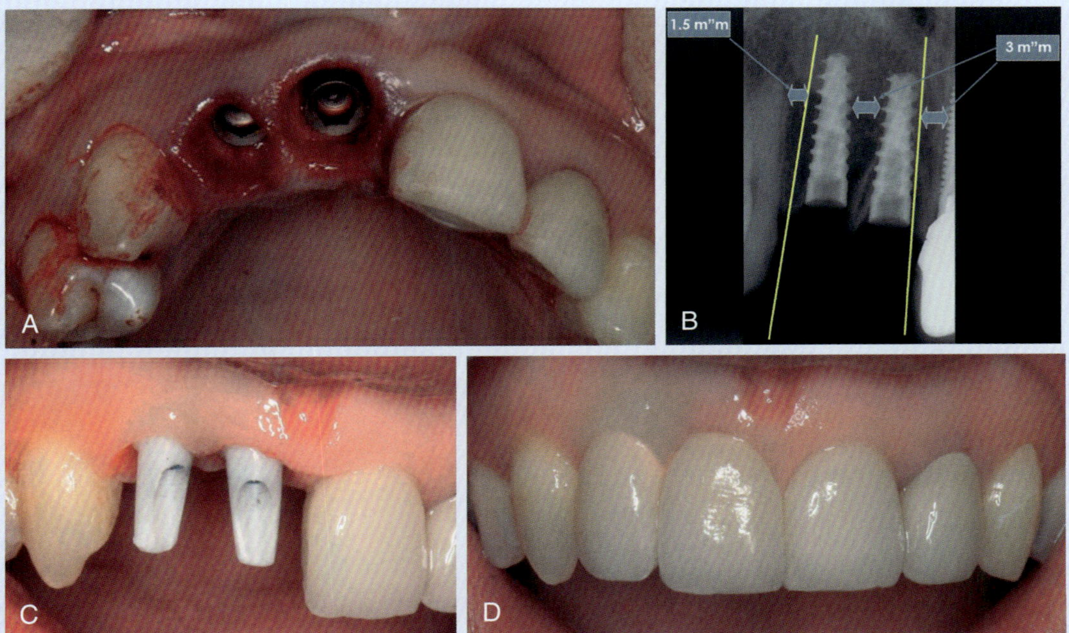

Fig 9.38 (A and B) After a couple of months, tooth numbers 11 and 12 got fractured hence replaced with immediate implant in a similar way. (C and D) Implants are restored using zirconia crowns over zirconium abutments.

CASE REPORT-6

Immediate implant preparation using osteotome with immediate loading of inserted implant (Figs 9.39–9.41).

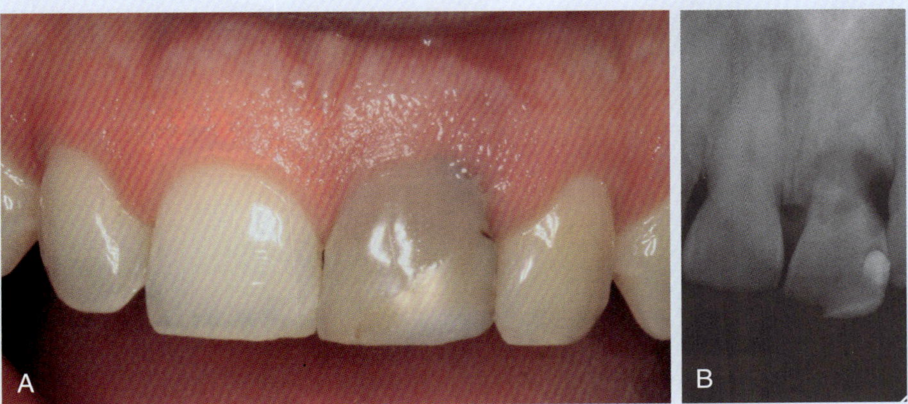

Fig 9.39 (A and B) Tooth number 21 showing severe root resorption.

Continued

CASE REPORT-6—cont'd

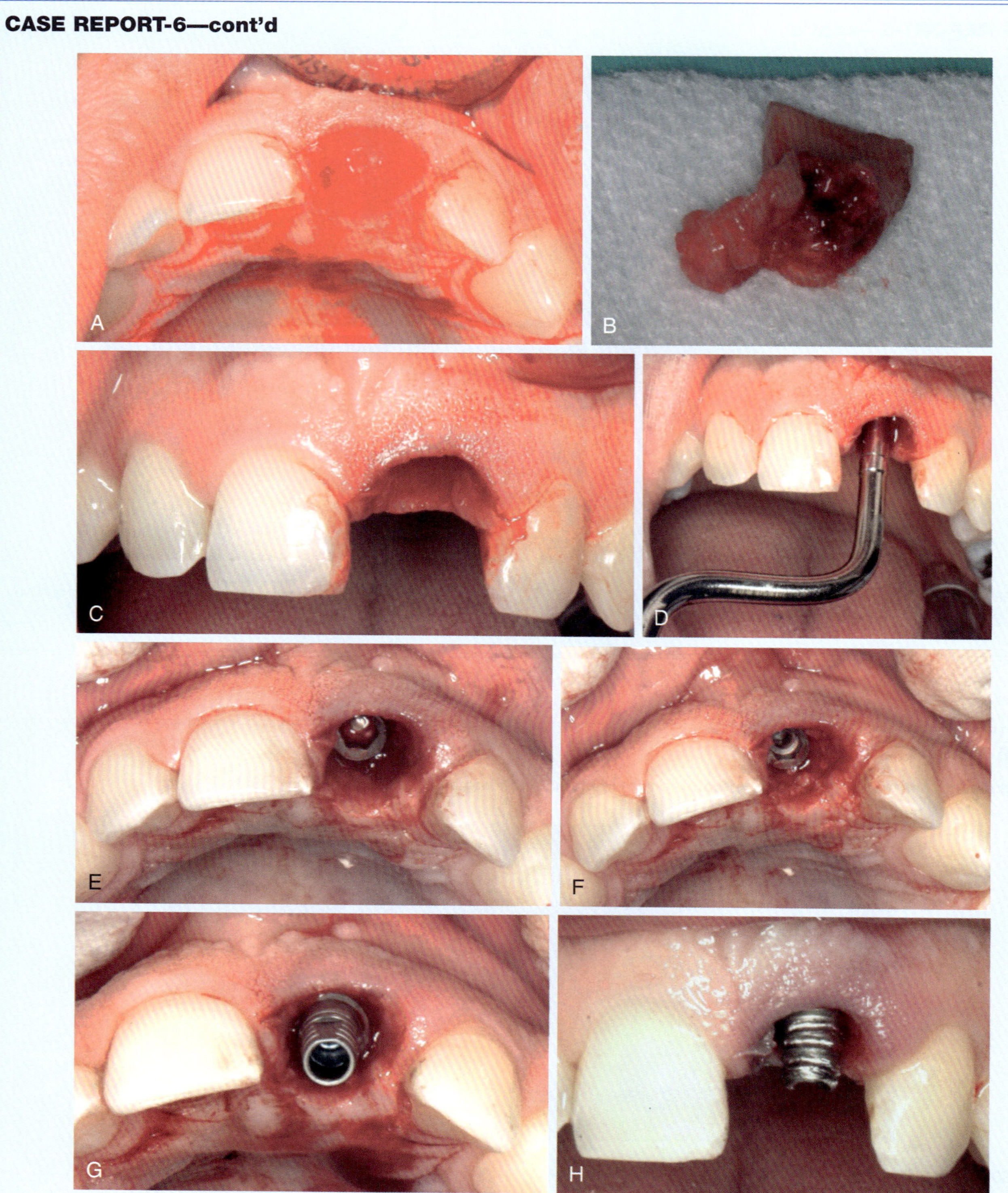

Fig 9.40 (A–C) Tooth is extracted and (D) implant osteotomy is prepared using bone condensing osteotomes. (E) The implant is inserted at the correct prosthetic position. (F) The peri-implant socket spaces are packed using bone graft and (G) abutment is inserted. (H) Abutment is reduced and retention grooves are prepared over abutment surface.

CASE REPORT-6—cont'd

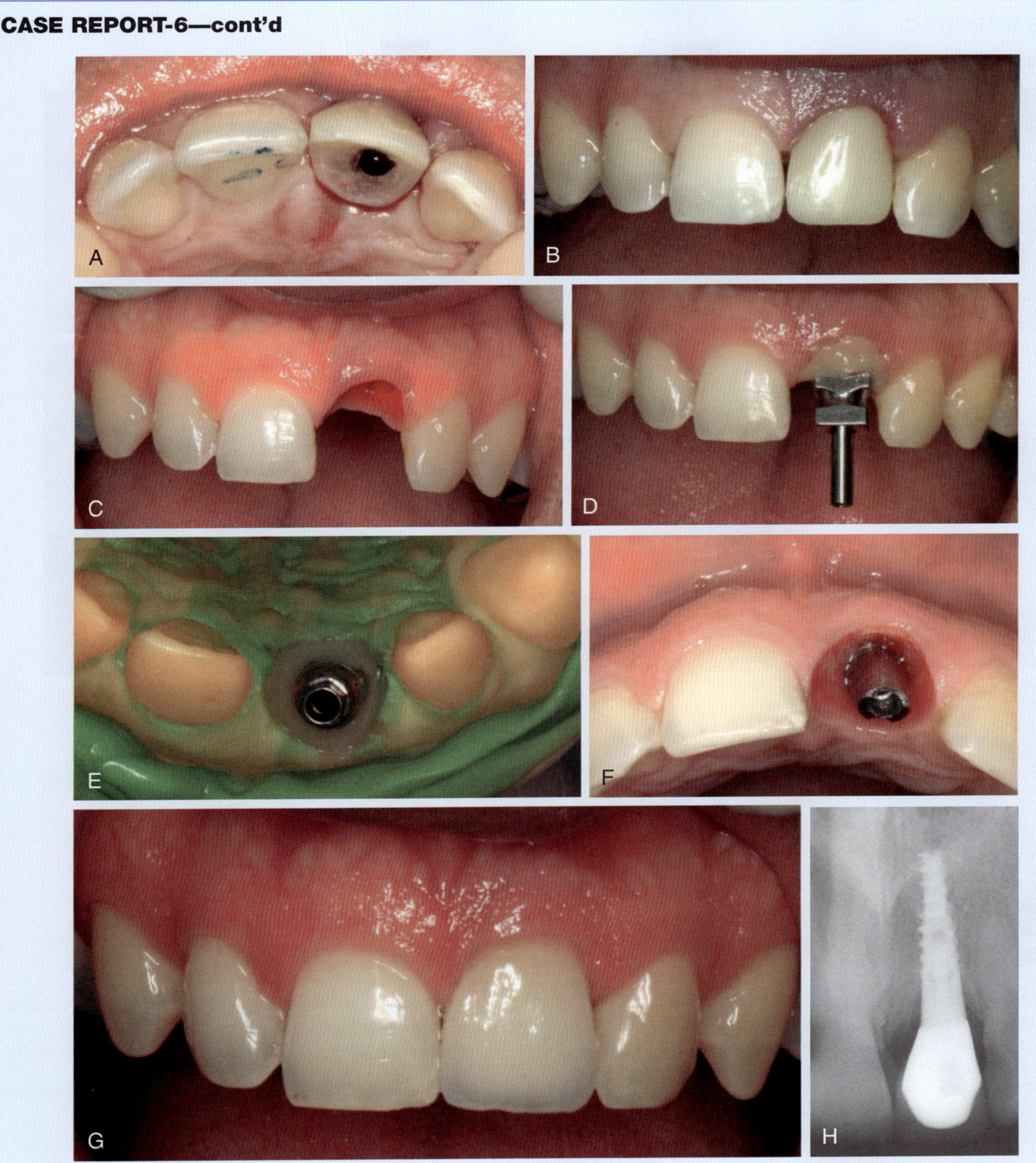

Fig 9.41 (A and B) A screw-retained provisional crown is fabricated and fixed over the implant. (C) Scalloped soft tissue healing can be seen when the provisional crown is removed after 4 months. (D and E) Impression is made with the soft tissue emergence transfer technique, and (F and G) the implant is restored using metal-free zirconium crown. (H) Post loading radiograph.

CASE REPORT-7

Immediate implantation with delayed loading (Figs 9.42–9.44).

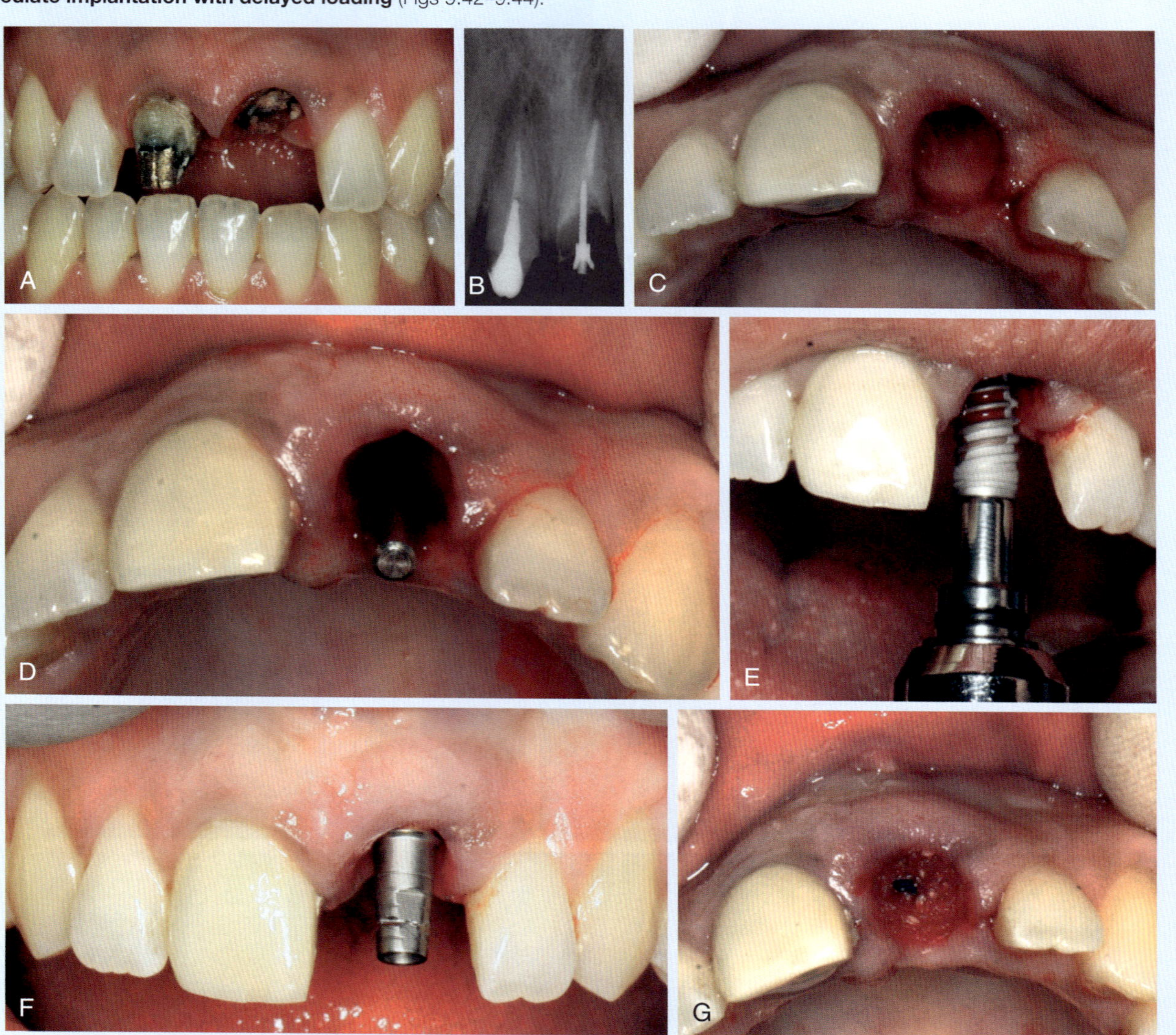

Fig 9.42 (A–C) Fractured tooth, number 21, is atraumatically extracted. (D–F) Implant osteotomy is prepared and the implant is inserted at the correct prosthetic position. Implant could not achieve adequate primary stability and BIC percentage because of large peri-implant socket spaces; therefore, the abutment is removed and the decision is taken to leave the implant for submerged healing. (G) The peri-implant socket spaces are filled using synthetic bone graft material.

CASE REPORT-7—cont'd

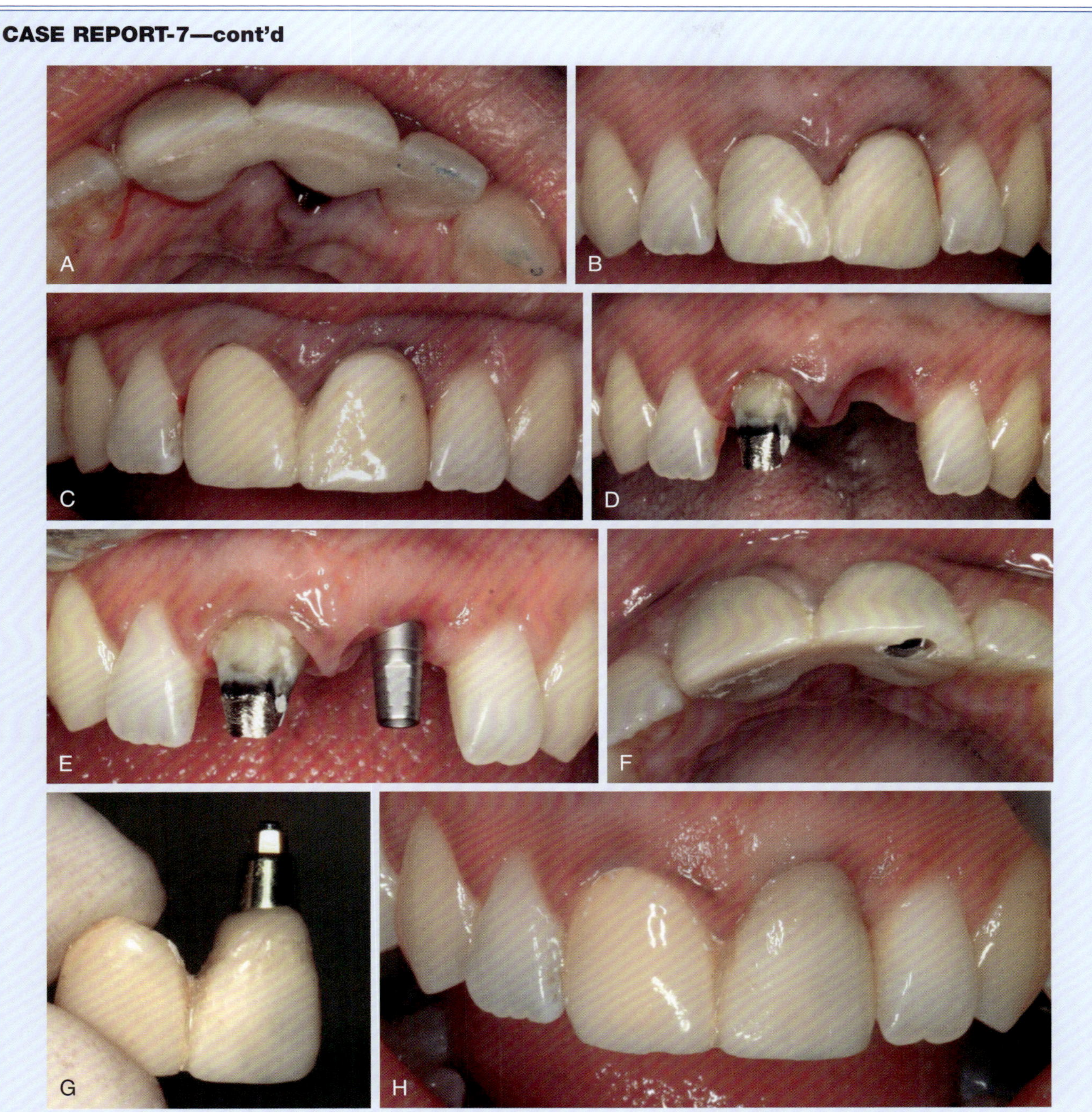

Fig 9.43 (A and B) A provisional prosthesis with an aesthetic shape is fixed over the adjacent tooth which not only supports the soft tissue but also prevents the loss of the graft from the socket. (C and D) Healing after 4 months showed the formation of nicely scalloped soft tissue at the cervical region. (E) Implant is uncovered using tissue punch, and (F–H) implant is restored with an anatomic provisional crown.

Continued

CASE REPORT-7—cont'd

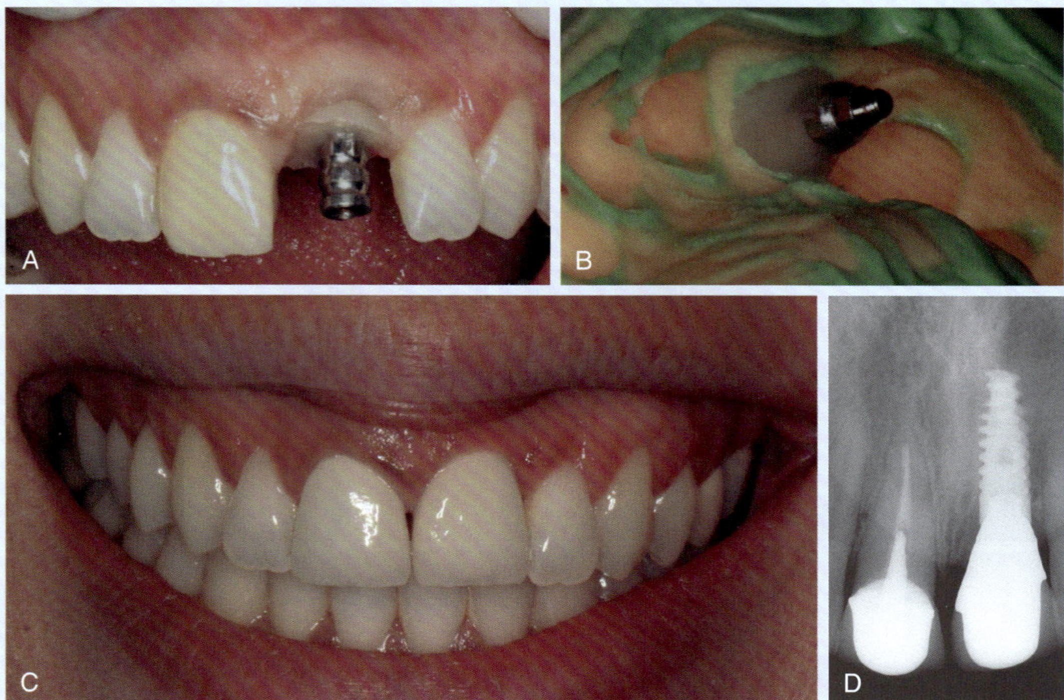

Fig 9.44 (A and B) Once the soft tissue got healed, the impression was made with 'soft tissue emergence transfer technique'. (C and D) Implant as well as adjacent tooth are restored using metal-free zirconia crowns.

CASE REPORT-8

Immediate implantation in maxillary premolar socket (Figs 9.45–9.48).

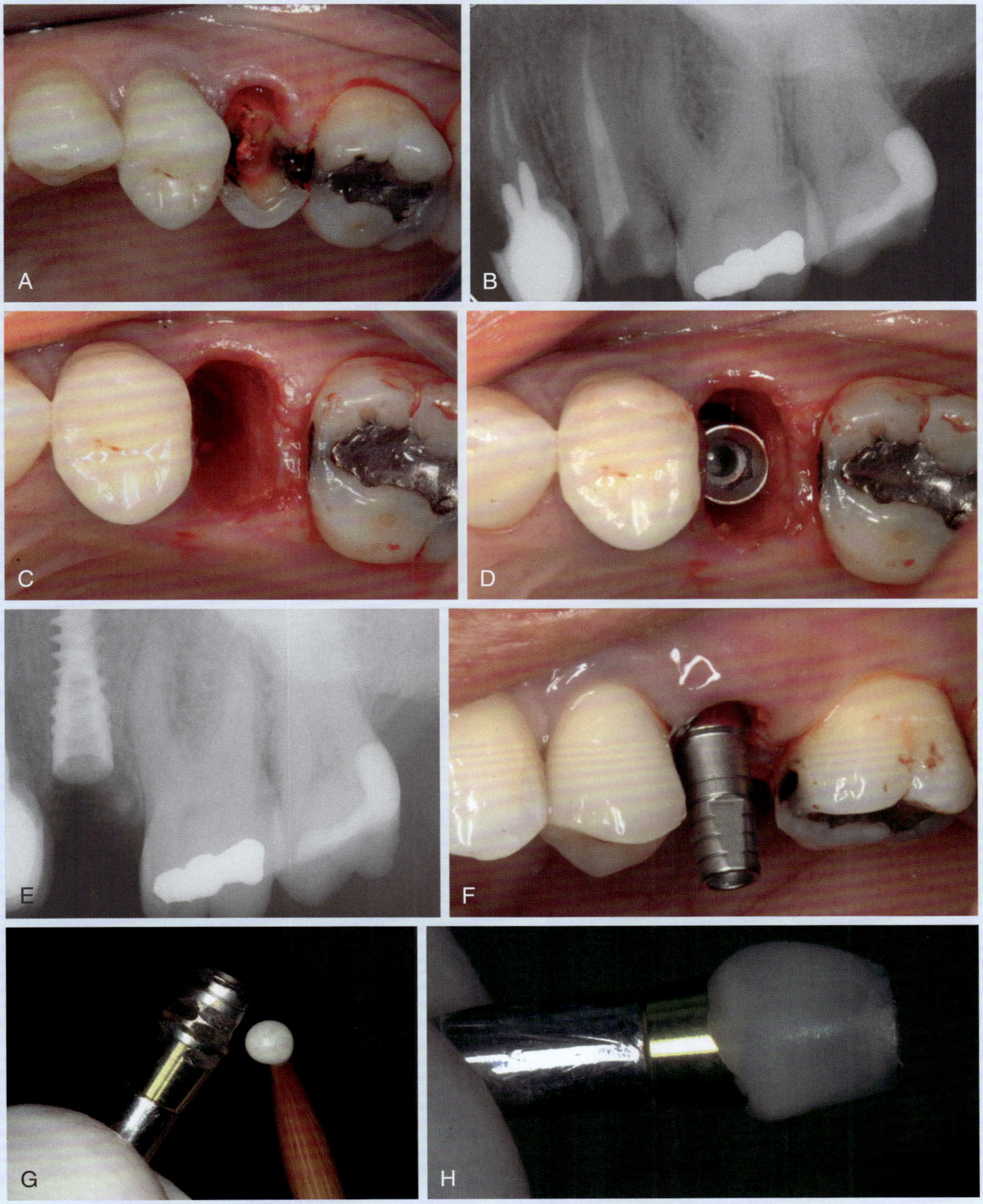

Fig 9.45 (A and B) Fractured tooth number 25 is extracted and (C–E) implant is inserted at the correct position with good primary stability. (F) Abutment is inserted, prepared, removed, and (G) assembled with analogue. (H) Self-cure resin is built up over the abutment.

Continued

CASE REPORT-8—cont'd

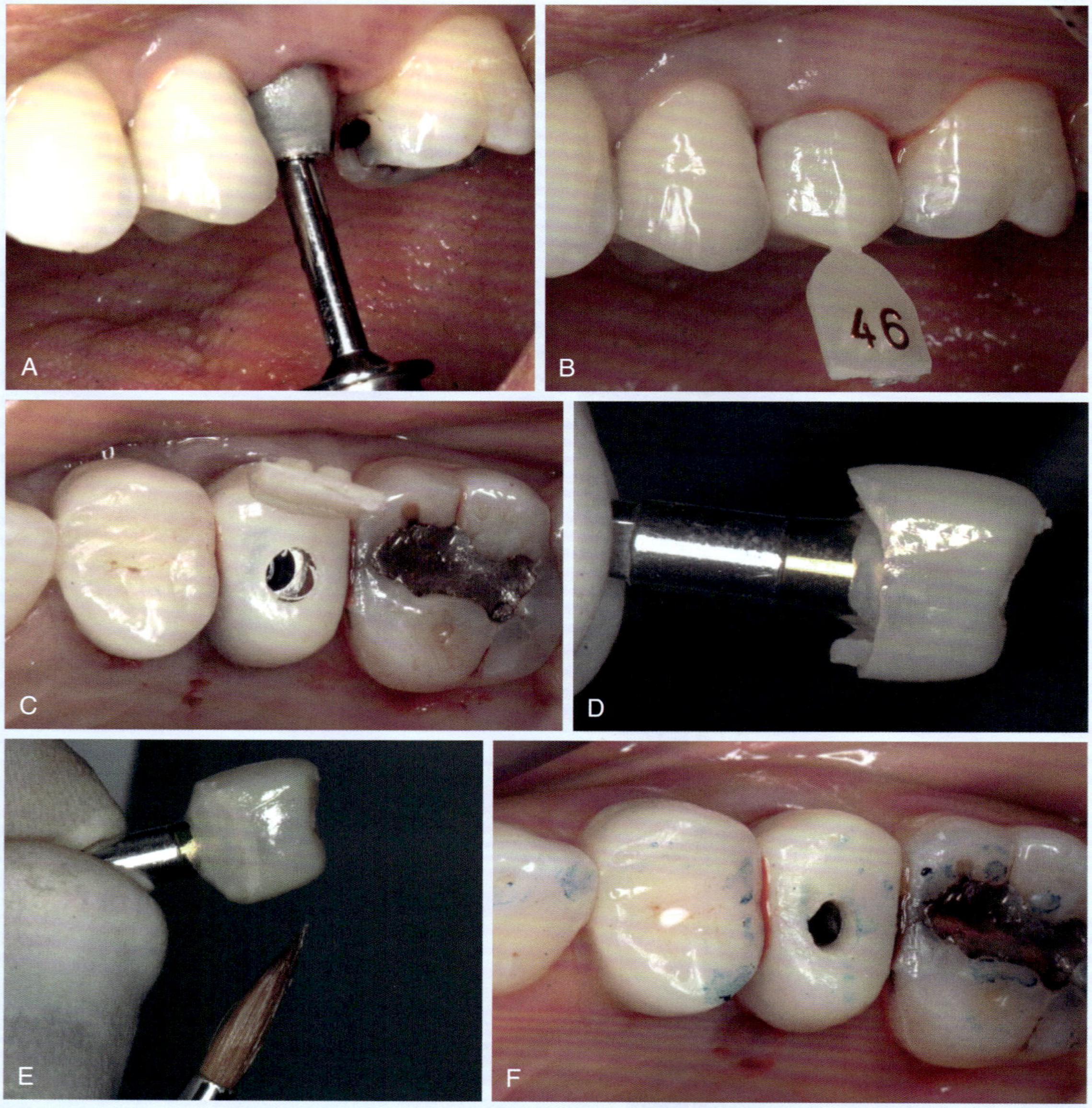

Fig 9.46 (A) Abutment is again screwed to the implant and (B) a poly crown is used to fabricate a provisional crown. (C) An entry to the screw hole is prepared and (D) abutment with attached crown is unscrewed from the implant and assembled to the analogue. (E) The self-cure resin is further added in the cervical area to form an aesthetic soft tissue emergence profile. (F) The crown is screwed to the implant.

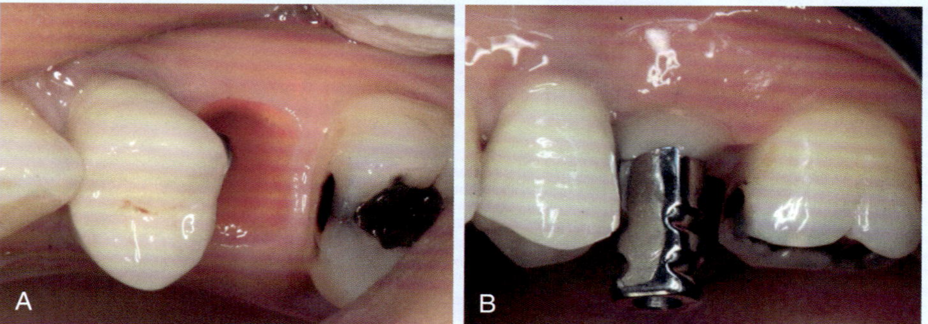

Fig 9.47 (A) Healing after 4 months shows formation of an excellent anatomical emergence profile of soft tissue. (B) An impression abutment with flowable composite in place.

CASE REPORT-8—cont'd

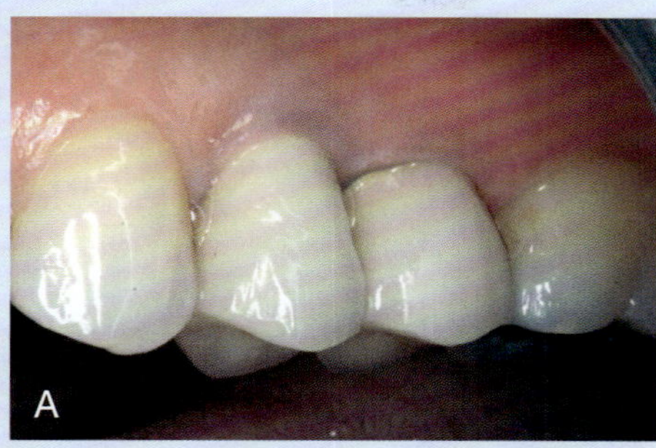

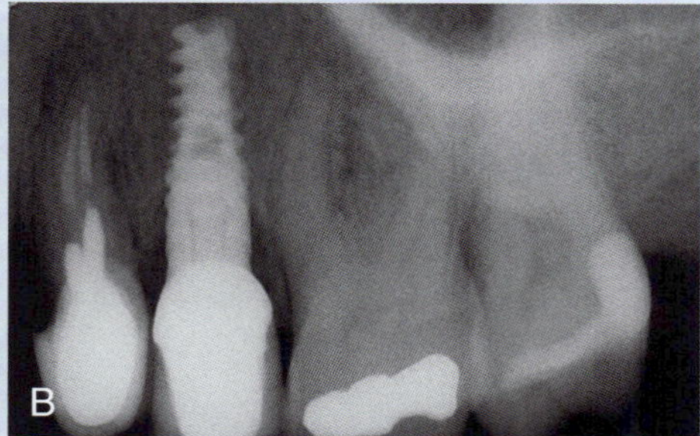

Fig 9.48 (A) Implant is restored using metal-free zirconium crown. (B) Post losing radiograph.

Immediate implants in mandibular anterior extraction sockets

The periodontal breakdown with excessive mobility of mandibular incisors is one of the most common problems that patients come in with, in day-to-day general dental practise. Stabilizing such teeth, which show more than 50% of vertical bone loss is not a definitive treatment, hence such teeth should be extracted and replaced with implant supported prostheses. The bone in the mandibular anterior region is usually found adequate in height and density to insert long implants with good primary stability, and hence, usually can be immediately restored to fulfil the aesthetic and functional demands of the patient. There are many advantages in this region, which facilitate immediate implantation with immediate loading:

1. No anatomical structures which can hinder placement of implants.
2. Longest (16–18 mm long) implants can be inserted to achieve a high initial stability.
3. Long implant can be stabilized in high density basal bone.
4. Less number of the implants can be inserted to support a multiple unit bridge, 4–6 unit bridge over two implants.
5. The cost of the treatment can be reduced by placing longer and fewer implants.
6. Since the bone is very dense in this region the implants achieve very high initial stability, and hence can immediately be loaded.
7. Most of the patients opt for this treatment as they get fast and fixed replacement for their mobile teeth.

CASE REPORT-9

Immediate implant with immediate loading in the mandibular anterior region (Figs 9.49–9.56).

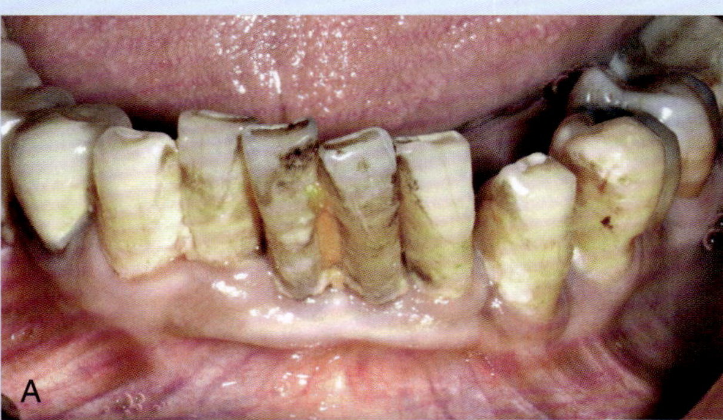

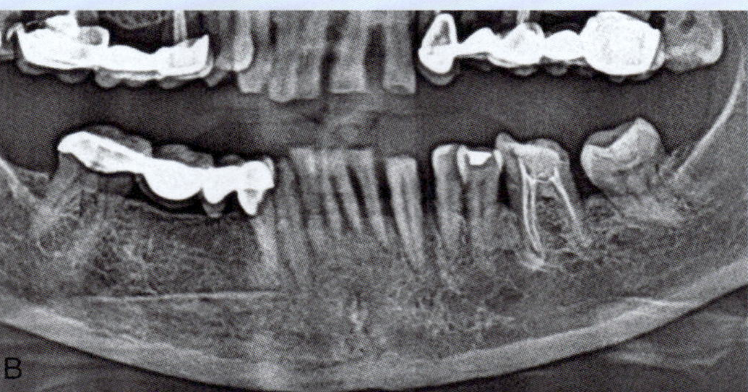

Fig 9.49 (A) A 50-year-old female patient clinically presented all mandibular incisors, left canine and first premolar with grade 3 mobility. (B) Panoramic radiograph shows severe vertical bone loss around the roots of the mobile teeth.

Continued

CASE REPORT-9—cont'd

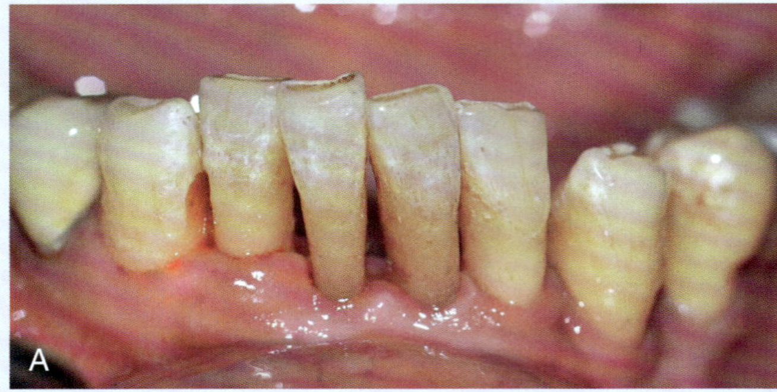
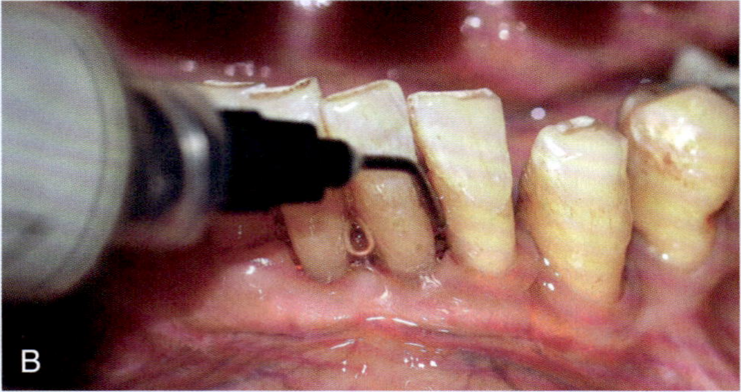

Fig 9.50 (A) Scaling and root planing is done and (B) citric acid injected in the periodontal pockets to kill the pathogens and to improve soft tissue healing. Patient is advised to rinse the mouth many times in the day with the 0.12% chlorhexidine solution and local application of Metrohex ointment. Prophylactic antibiotics (amoxicillin 1 g + metronidazole 500 mg) was prescribed for 24 h before implant surgery.

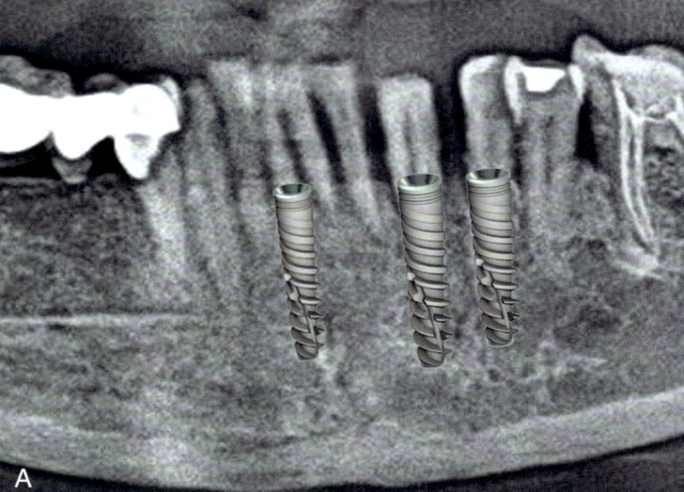
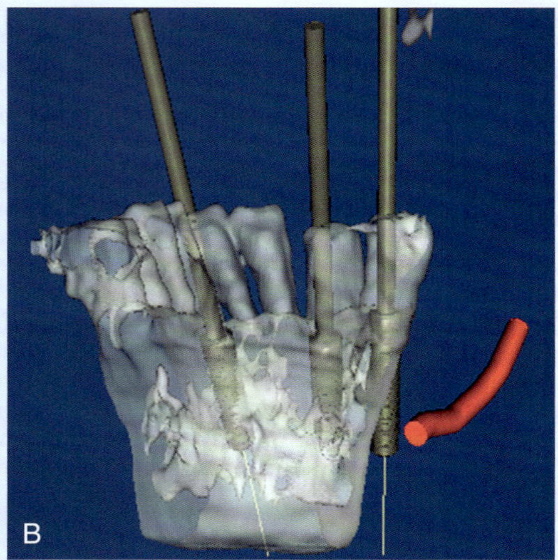

Fig 9.51 (A and B) Three implants (3.3 × 16 mm) were planned with radiographs and dental CT images for immediate insertion in extraction sockets.

CASE REPORT-9—cont'd

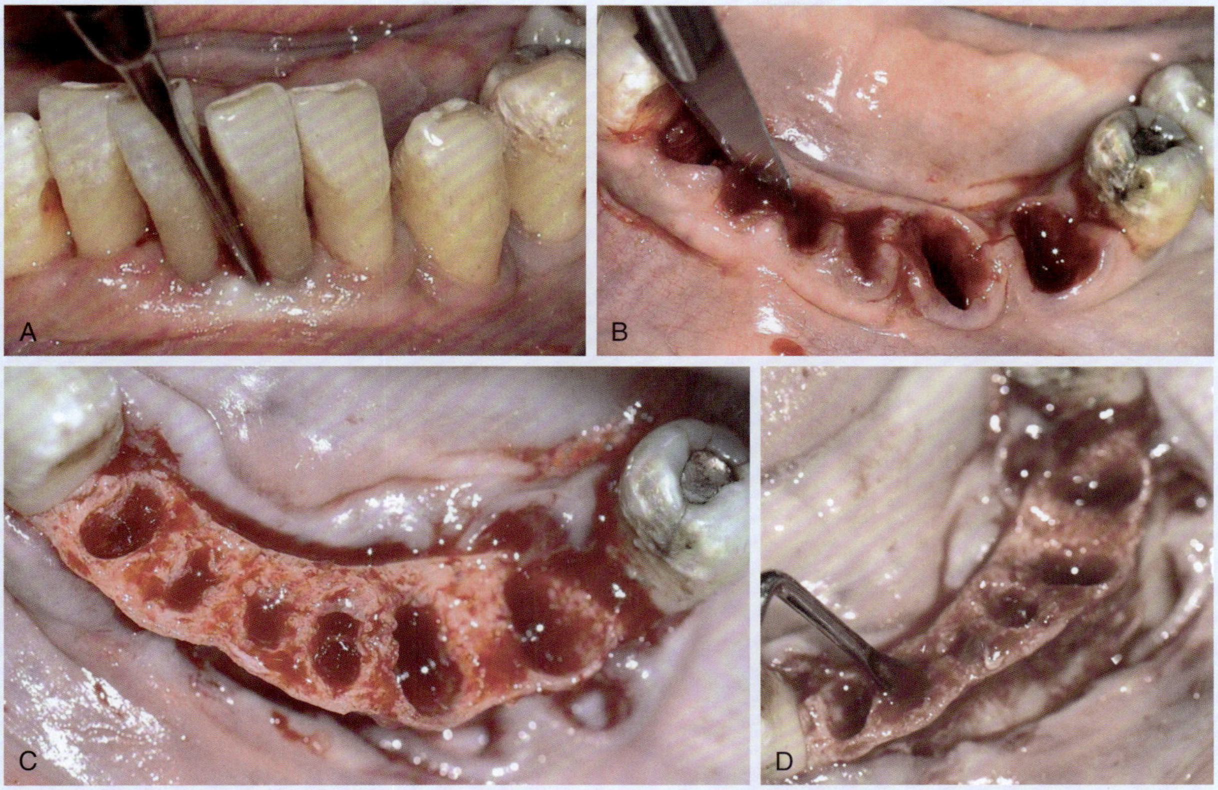

A B C D

Fig 9.52 (A and B) The patient is recalled on the next day and all the mobile teeth are extracted atraumatically using a set of periotomes. (C) A midline incision is given and mucoperiosteal flaps are elevated to expose the bony sockets. (D) All the granulation tissue present in the sockets is curetted out because if left behind, it can infect the implants.

Continued

CASE REPORT-9—cont'd

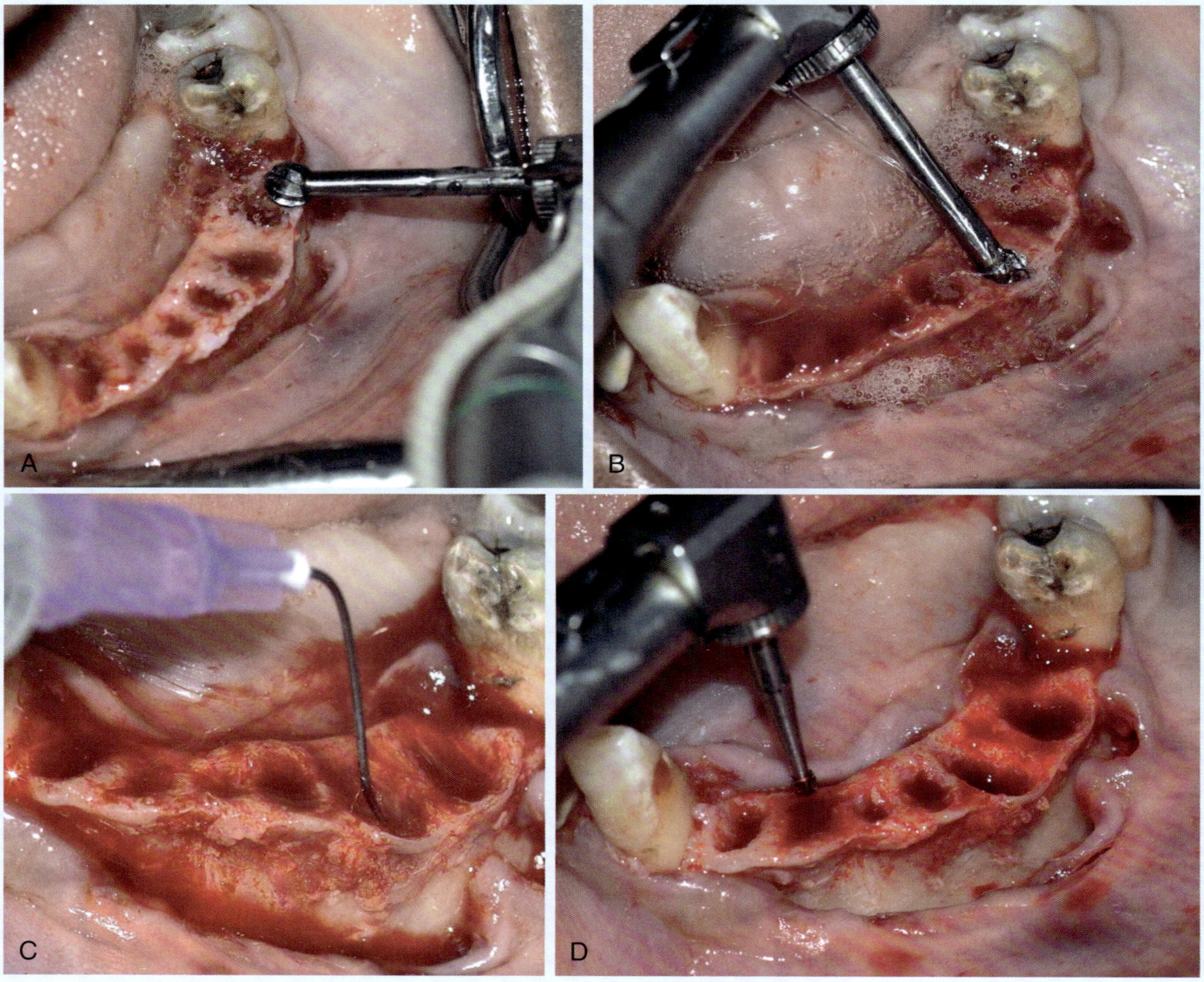

Fig 9.53 (A and B) A large round carbide bur can further be used to remove the fibrosseous tissue from the socket. All the infected granulation tissue should be removed from the socket as it can be transported deep into the prepared osteotomy and can infect the inserted implant. (C) Further, the extraction sockets are irrigated with clindamycin (Dalacin C injection 600 mg) to kill the residual pathogens. The antibiotic is left filled in the socket for at least 30 s to kill the pathogens. (D) A small round carbide bur is used to start the implant osteotomy because, unlike the pilot drill, it avoids slipping towards the thin and week labial cortical plate to cause dehiscence.

CASE REPORT-9—cont'd

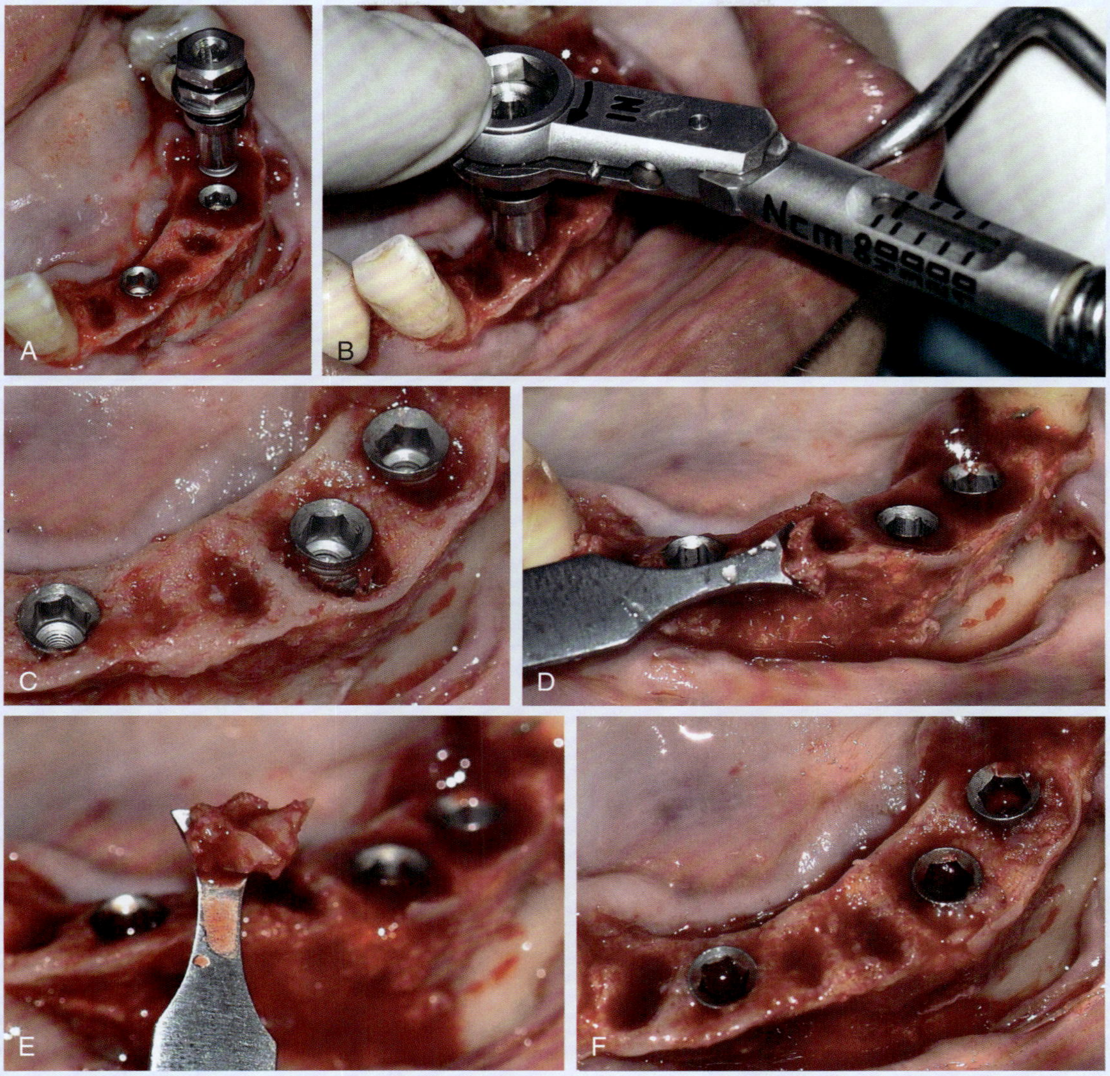

Fig 9.54 (A) The osteotomy is prepared and three screw-type tapered implants (3.3 × 16 mm) are inserted. (B) All three implants achieved the high primary stability. (C) Two implants show large peri-implant socket spaces, (D–F) a small amount of autogenous bone was harvested from the adjacent socket wall and the spaces grafted.

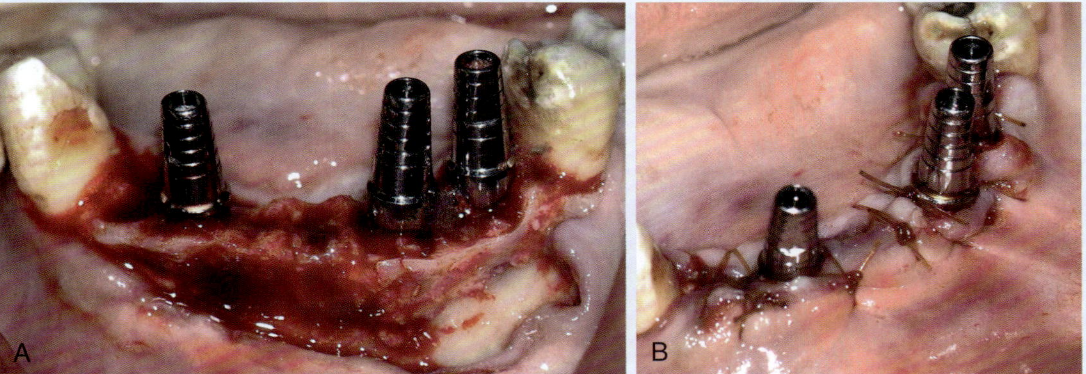

Fig 9.55 (A) The appropriate abutments are inserted on top of implants and (B) the flap is sutured back around the abutments.

CASE REPORT-9—cont'd

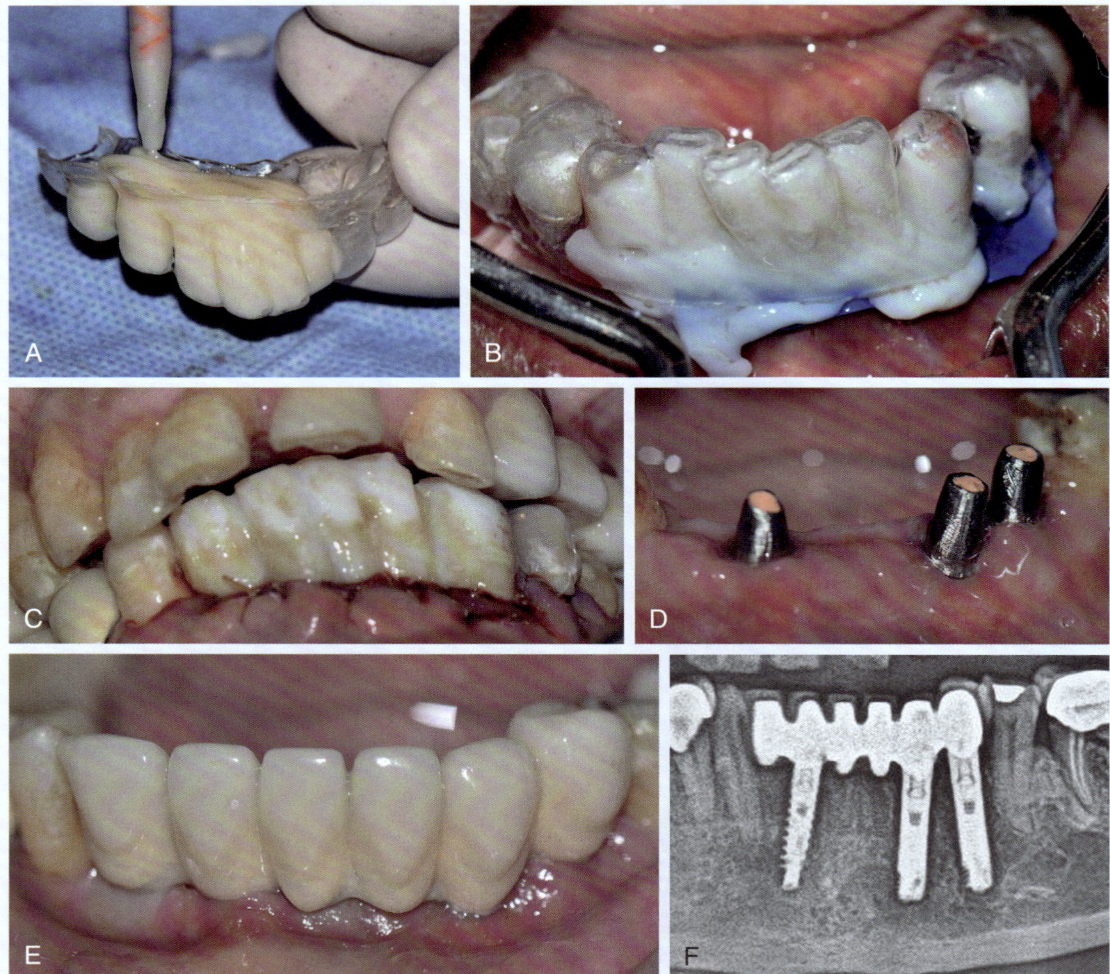

Fig 9.56 (A) The prefabricated mould is filled with the Protemp provisional fabrication material, and (B) seated in the patient's mouth at the correct position. (C) The provisional bridge finished, polished, stained, and used as the provisional restoration for 3 weeks until the soft tissue get healed. (D) The provisional bridge is removed after 3 weeks and finally milled abutments are inserted and (E) implants restored with ceramic bridge. (F) Post loading radiograph. The implants are in function since more than 3 years without any noticeable crestal bone loss.

CASE REPORT-10

Immediate insertion of narrow diameter single body implants with immediate loading (Figs 9.57 and 9.58).

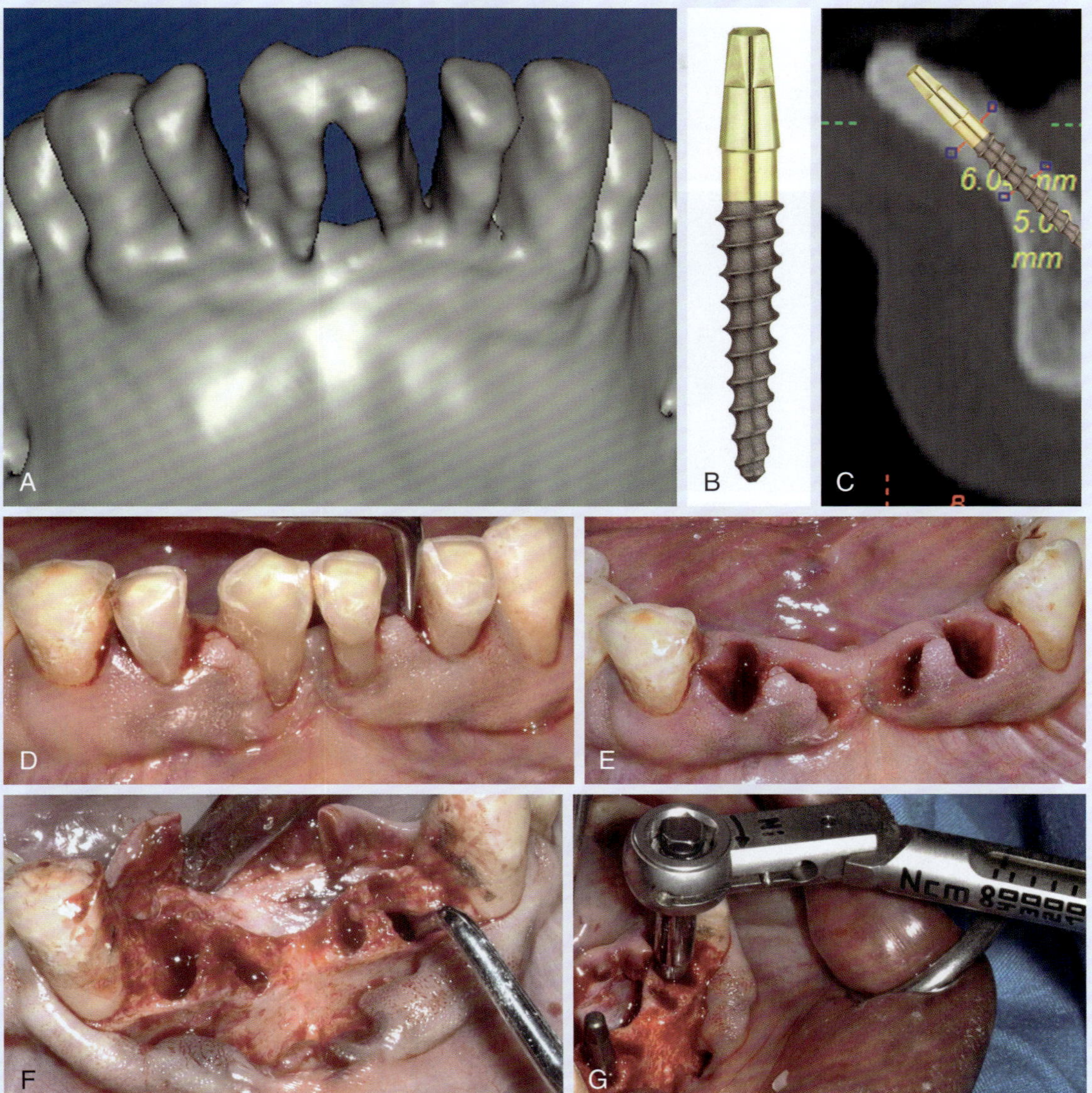

Fig 9.57 (A) The 3D view of the mandible shows the vertical bone loss with mandibular incisors. (B and C) As seen in CT cross-sectional image, the buccolingual bone width is only 5–6 mm, thus narrow diameter (3 × 15 mm) one-piece implants (ARRP) are planned for insertion at the laterals positions to support a four-unit bridge. (D and E) Teeth are atraumatically extracted out using periotomes. (F) The mucoperiosteal flaps are elevated to expose the bony sockets and all the granulation tissue is currated out. (G) The implant osteotomies are prepared using 2 mm diameter pilot drill and two arrow press implants are inserted at the lateral positions with good primary stability as shown with the torque ratchet.

Continued

CASE REPORT-10—cont'd

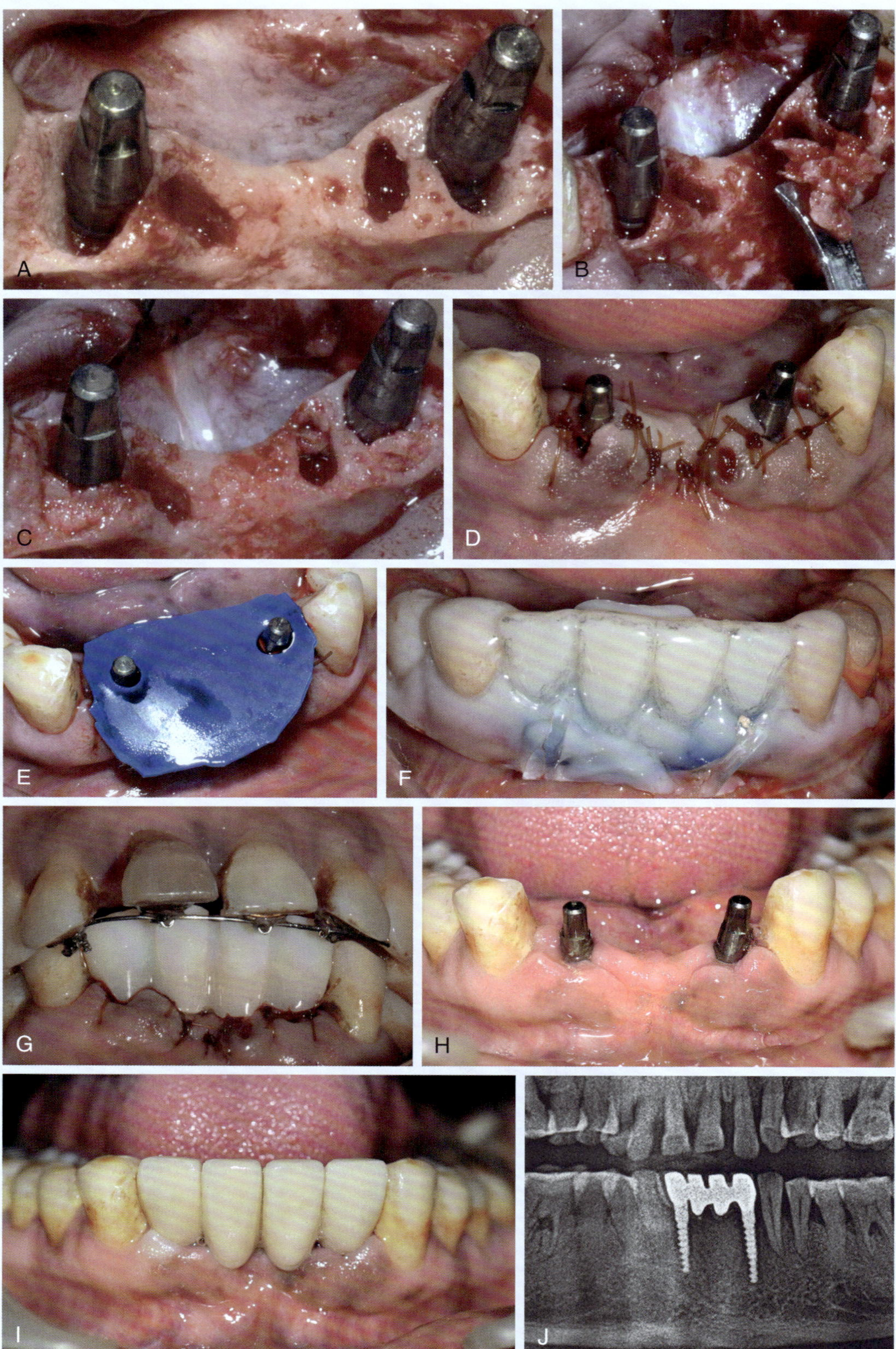

Fig 9.58 (A) Both the inserted implants show the large peri-implant socket spaces, which need to be grafted for predictable osseointegration and to avoid soft tissue ingrowth in the socket spaces. (B and C) A small amount of autogenous bone was harvested from the adjacent socket wall and the socket spaces are filled using this bone. (D) The flap is sutured around the implant abutments and implants are immediately restored with the joined provisional prosthesis fabricated using Protemp. (E–G) A piece of rubber dam should be used to cover the sutured flap surface to prevent any Protemp material flowing into the suture line and getting entangled with the sutures. (H and I) The provisional prosthesis is removed after 3 weeks and replaced with the final ceramic prosthesis. (J) Post loading radiograph. The implants are in function since more than 2 years without any noticeable crestal bone loss.

CASE REPORT-11

Flapless immediate implantation with immediate loading (Figs 9.59–9.61).

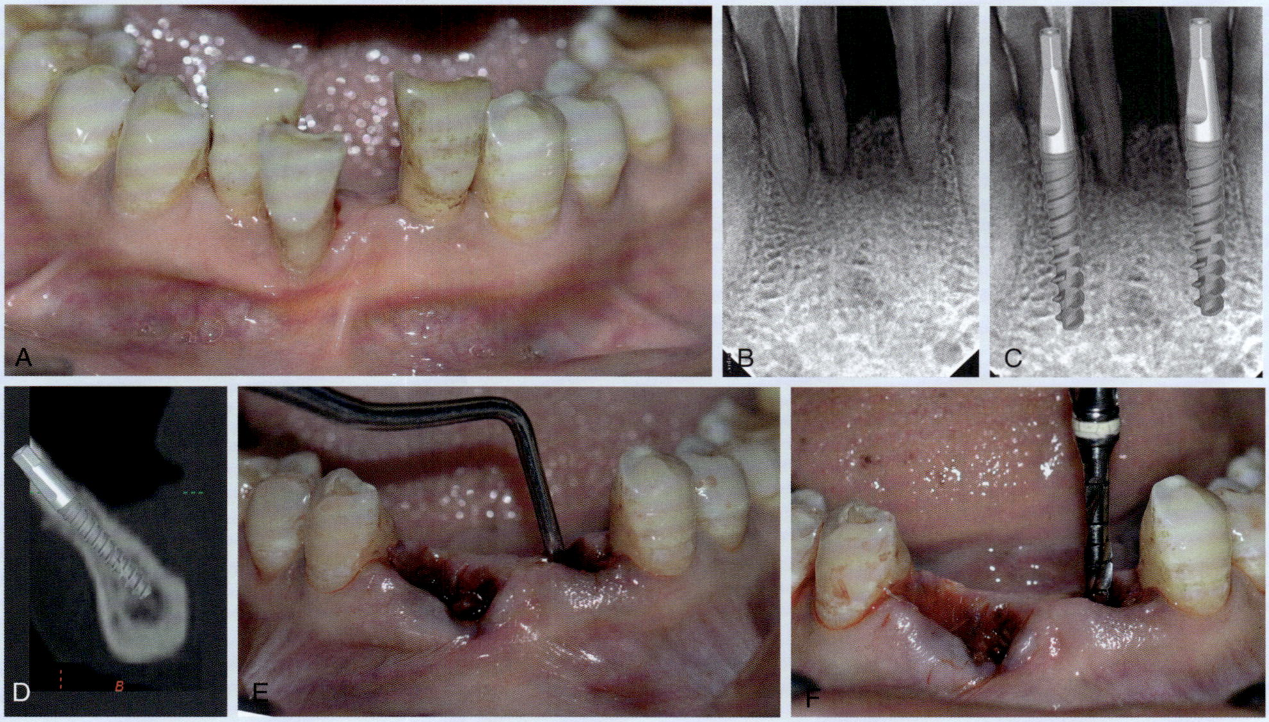

Fig 9.59 (A and B) Mandibular incisors, which need replacement because of severe vertical bone loss and mobility. (C) Two single-body implants (3 × 15 mm) are planned to support a four-unit ceramic prosthesis. (D) The CT cross-sectional scans showed no severe undercuts in the ridge morphology or any osseous defect, thus flapless implant placement is planned. (E) Teeth are atraumatically extracted, all the granulation tissue is curetted out and sockets are disinfected using parenteral form of clindamycin. (F) The implant osteotomies are prepared at the correct predetermined axis.

Continued

CASE REPORT-11—cont'd

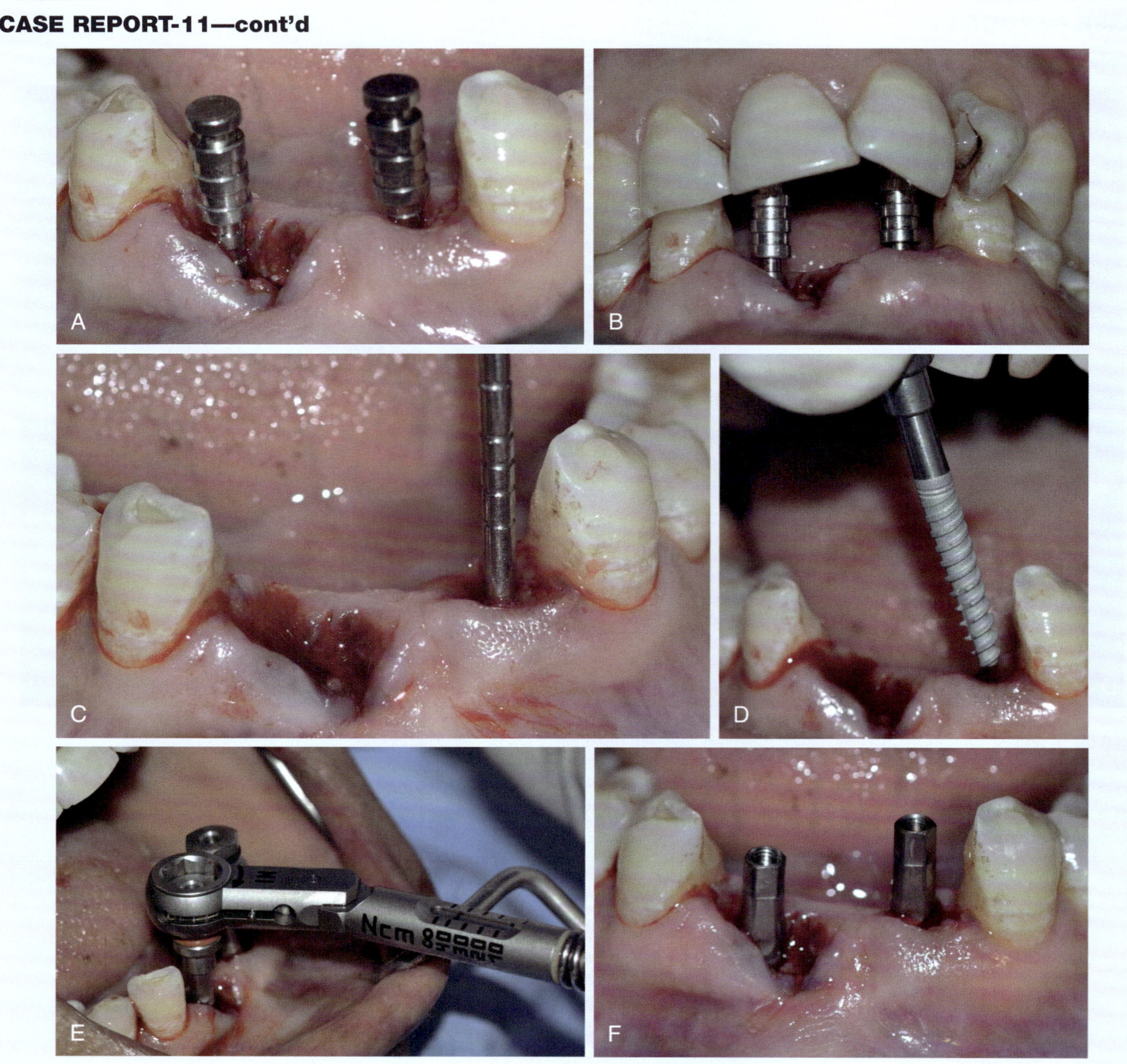

Fig 9.60 (A) The guiding pins are inserted in the prepared osteotomy to check the parallelism as well as the (B) occlusal direction. (C) The osteotomy is also checked for any perforation using a depth probe. (D – F) Two long single-body implants (3 × 15 mm), which achieved primary stability more than 35 Ncm, are inserted.

CASE REPORT-11—cont'd

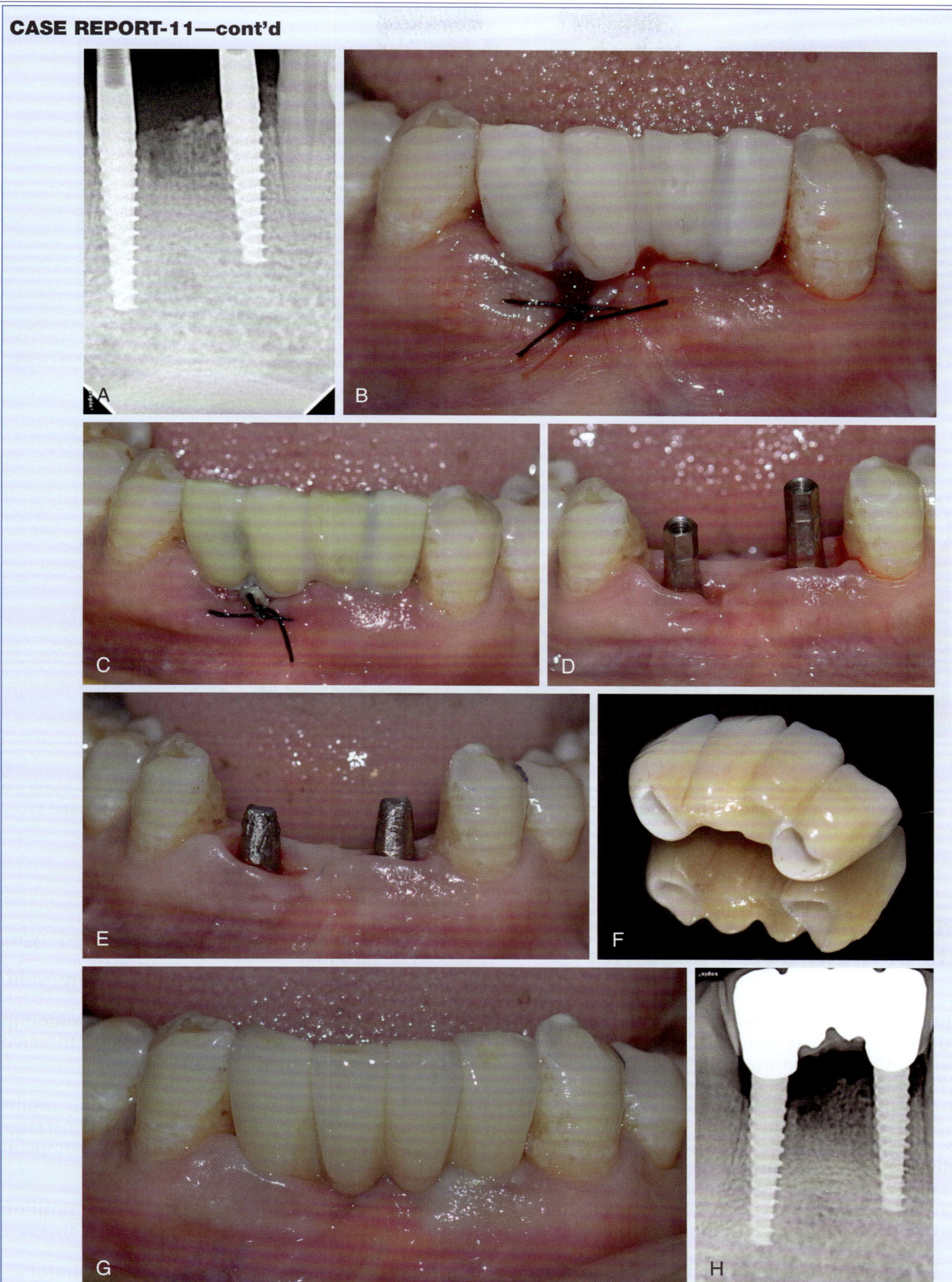

Fig 9.61 (A) Post-implantation radiograph. (B) Implants are immediately restored in functional occlusion. (C and D) Provisional prosthesis is removed from the implants, once soft tissue gets healed in 3 weeks. (E) The abutments are prepared in the patient's mouth, (F–H) impression is made with prepared abutment technique and implants are finally restored using definitive zirconium prosthesis.

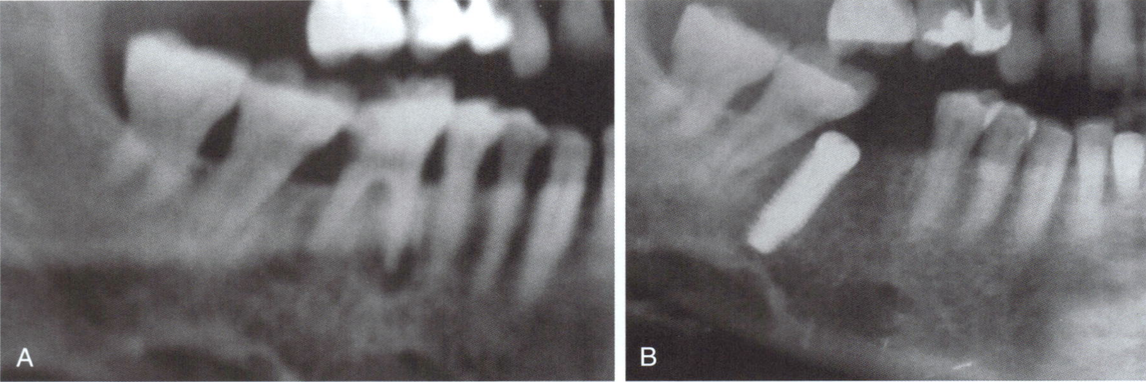

Fig 9.62 (A and B) If one of the root sockets of a multirooted molar is chosen for implant insertion, it may lead to large offset forces on the implant, once restored in function.

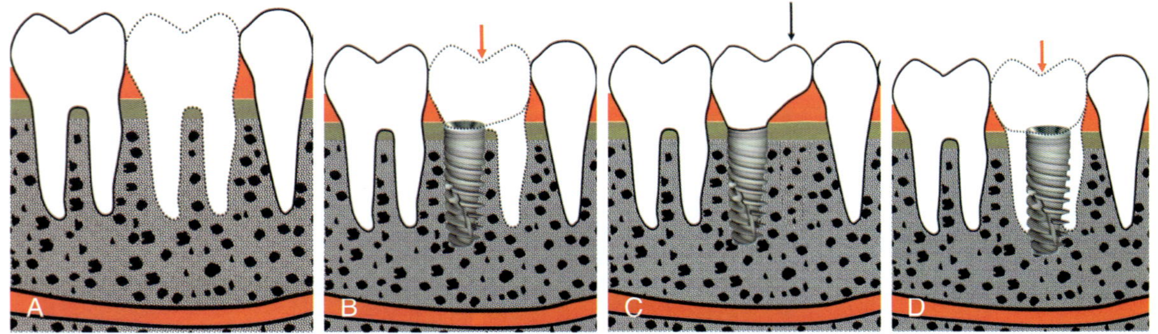

Fig 9.63 (A) Post-extraction socket of the mandibular molar poses two root sockets, and (B and C) if the implant is inserted in one of the extraction sockets, it may result in offset (cantilevered) forces on the implant once it finally restored in function. (D) Ideally, the implant should be inserted at the midpoint of mesiodistal dimensions between two adjacent teeth but are often inserted at the interradicular septal region, to avoid the offset forces on the implant prosthesis.

Immediate implants in extraction sockets of multirooted posterior teeth

As described earlier in this chapter, the high success rate of immediate implants in extraction sockets has been documented. Although immediate implantation has been successful in the anterior region or in a single-rooted extraction socket, fewer articles describe attempts to place an implant in the posterior multirooted sockets. The main reason is the topography of the resultant extraction socket, which is two-rooted in mandibular and 3-rooted in the maxillary molar area. When planning immediate implant in the extraction socket of a multirooted tooth, the implant surgeon may choose one of the two protocols:

Protocol 1 – Implant insertion in any one of the root sockets. The choice of the root socket depends on a few anatomical and radiographic features of the particular root socket. The following socket types should be preferred:

a. Socket with more intact osseous topography (minimum or no wall defects)
b. Socket more close to the mesiodistal midpoint between two adjacent teeth; it avoids cantilevered forces on the inserted implant.

The disadvantage of this protocol is that it may results in off-axis implant placement, which may result in a large amount of cantilevered forces on the inserted implant (Figs 9.62 and 9.63).

Protocol 2 – The implant insertion at the ideal position (into inter-radicular septal region) (Fig 9.63D).

Step by step diagrammatic presentation of immediate implant in multirooted tooth socket (Figs 9.64 and 9.65).

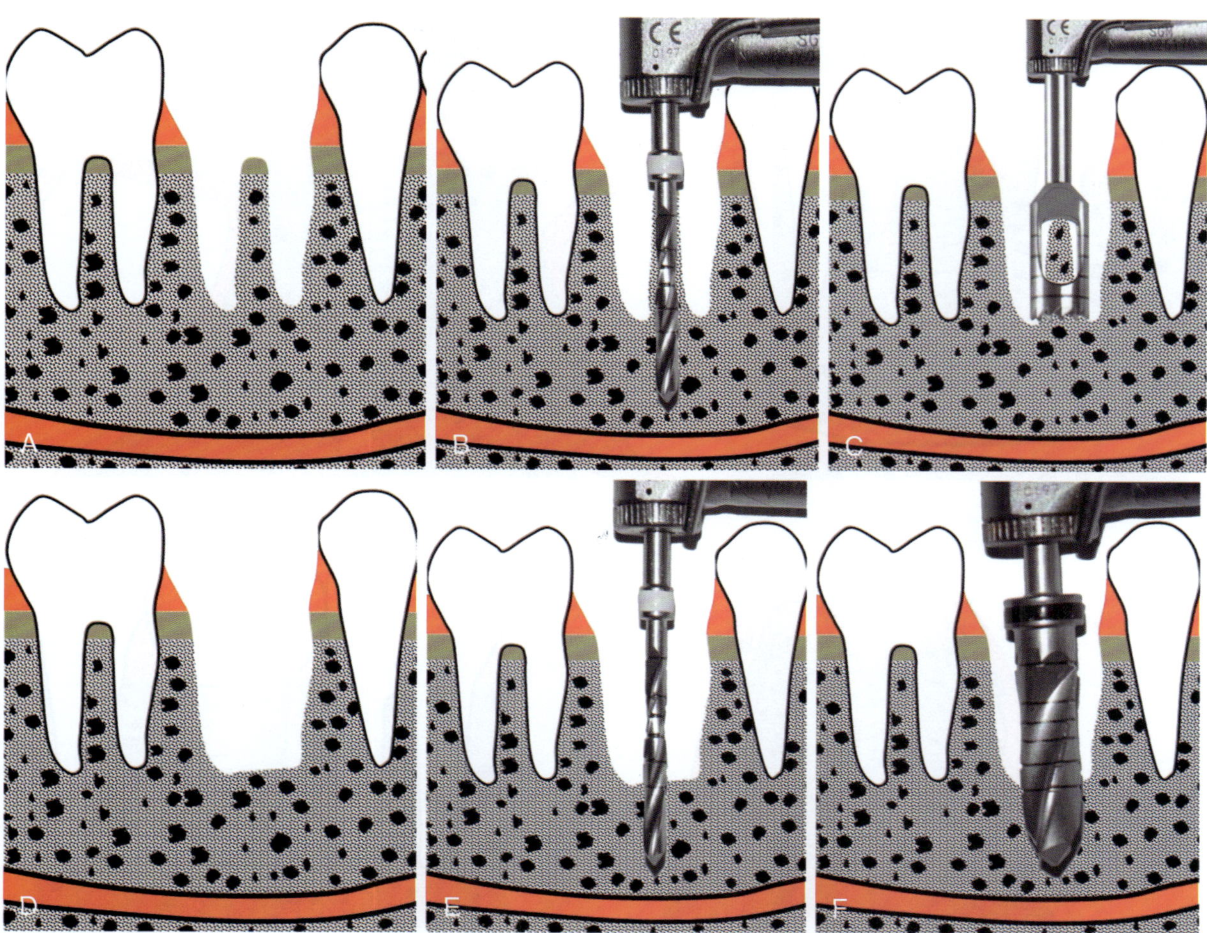

Fig 9.64 (A) Atraumatic extraction of multirooted tooth is done and (B) the osteotomy preparation begins using a sharp pointed drill in the region of the interradicular septa. (C and D) Alternatively, one can use a trephine drill to prepare the implant osteotomy and to remove interradicular septa which can be used to graft the post-implantation peri-implant socket spaces. (E and F) Further, the osteotomy is prepared 3–5 mm apical to the extraction socket using all implant drills to engage the implant apex in the healthy dense bone and to achieve adequate primary stability of the implant .

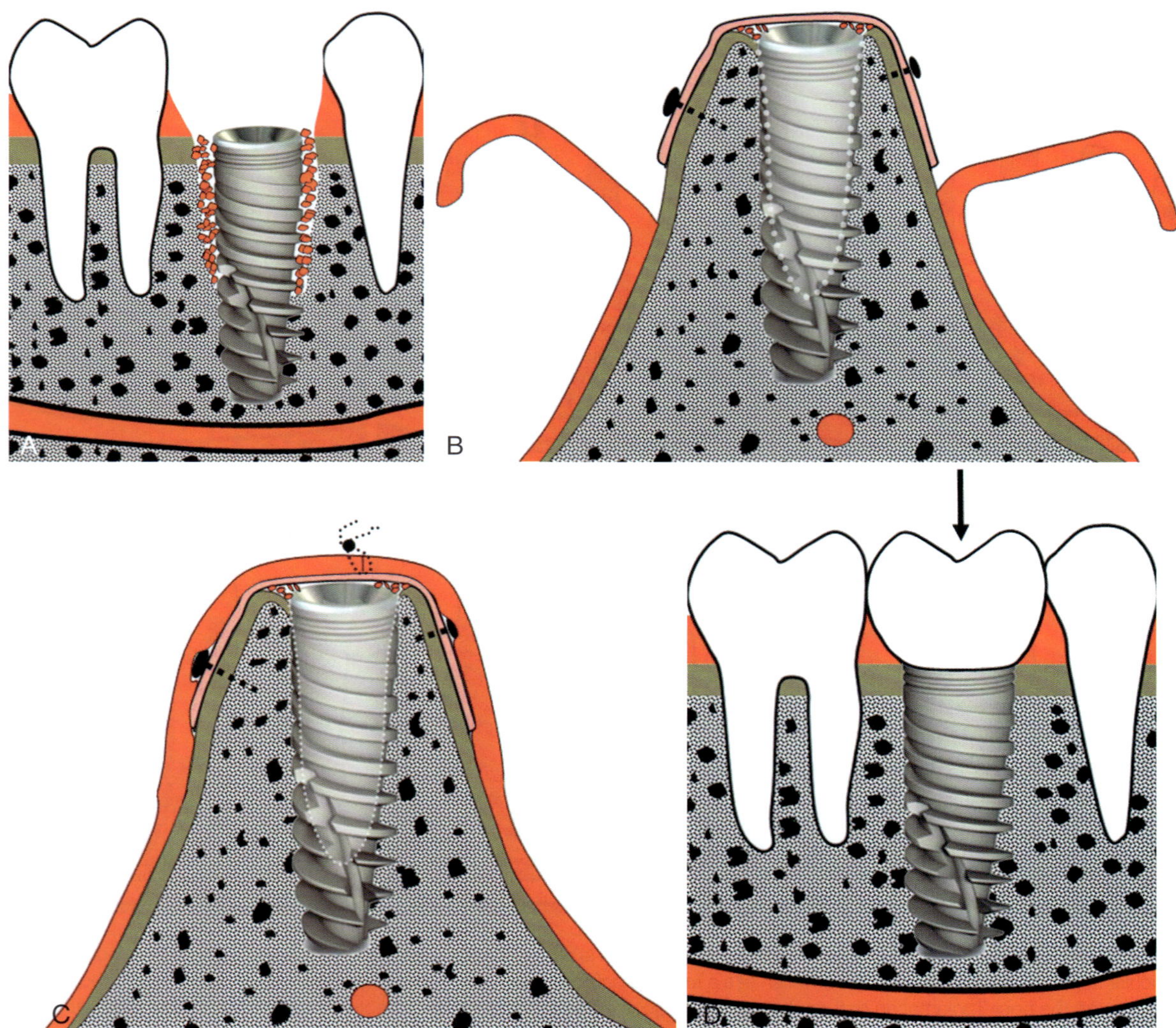

Fig 9.65 (A) The implant is inserted into the septal region and the peri-implant socket spaces are grafted using autogenous bone alone or mixed with bone substitute. (B) For large grafted spaces, a barrier membrane should be used to cover the socket and (C) the flap is sutured back for submerged implant healing, for a minimum of 4 months. (D) Implant is uncovered after 4 months and restored with an ideal prosthesis which has the entire occlusal load along the implant axis.

CASE REPORT-12

Immediate implant in the mandibular molar socket with peri-implant socket space grafting and use of nonresorbable cytoplast TXT membrane (Figs 9.66–9.70).

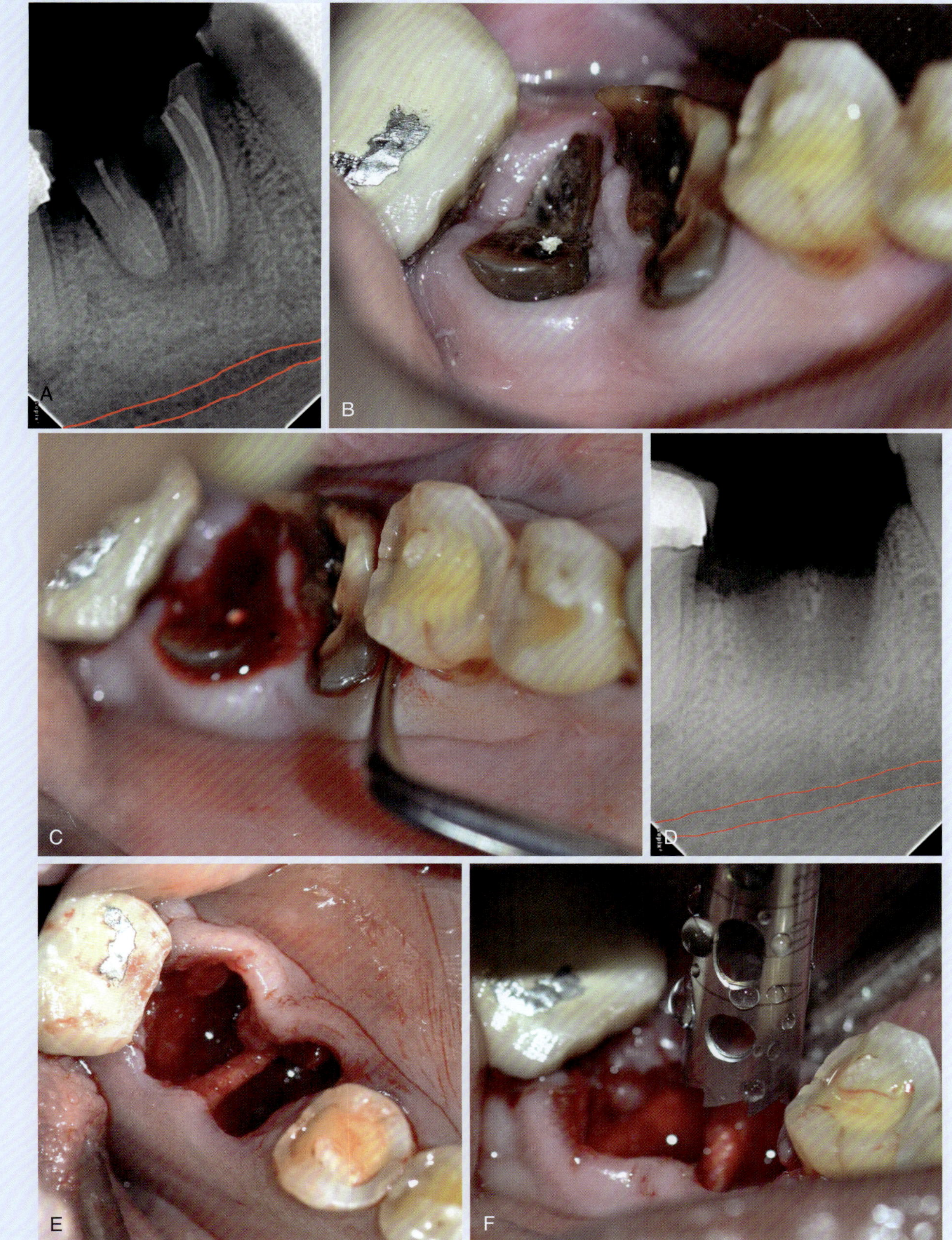

Fig 9.66 (A and B) Nonrestorable root stumps of the mandibular molar which need extraction and replacement with implant prosthesis. (C and D) Both roots are extracted atraumatically using a set of periotomes and luxators. (E) The interradicular bony septa is removed using a (F) large trephine drill.

CASE REPORT-12—cont'd

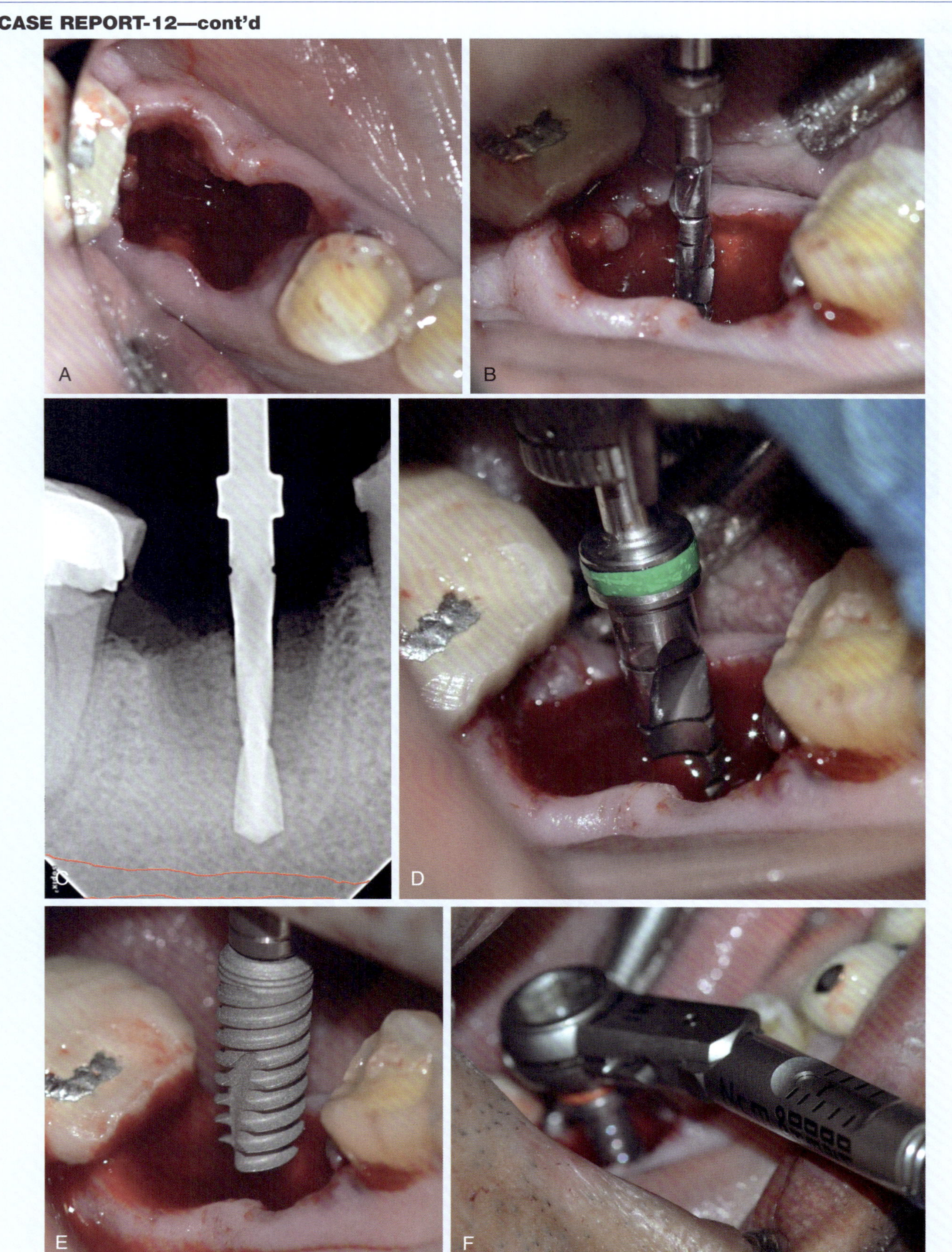

Fig 9.67 (A) Once the septum has been harvested, (B) a pilot drill is used to prepare the osteotomy into the mesiodistal midpoint of two adjacent teeth. (C) The radiograph is showing the pilot drill reaching 5 mm apical to the extraction socket and 2 mm short of the mandibular canal. (D) The rest of the osteotomy widening drills are used to the same depth, and (E) a self-taping screw-type implant (5 x 13 mm.) with deeper threads at the apex is inserted. (F) The inserted implant has achieved primary stability more than 35 Ncm as evaluated using mechanical torque ratchet.

CASE REPORT-12—cont'd

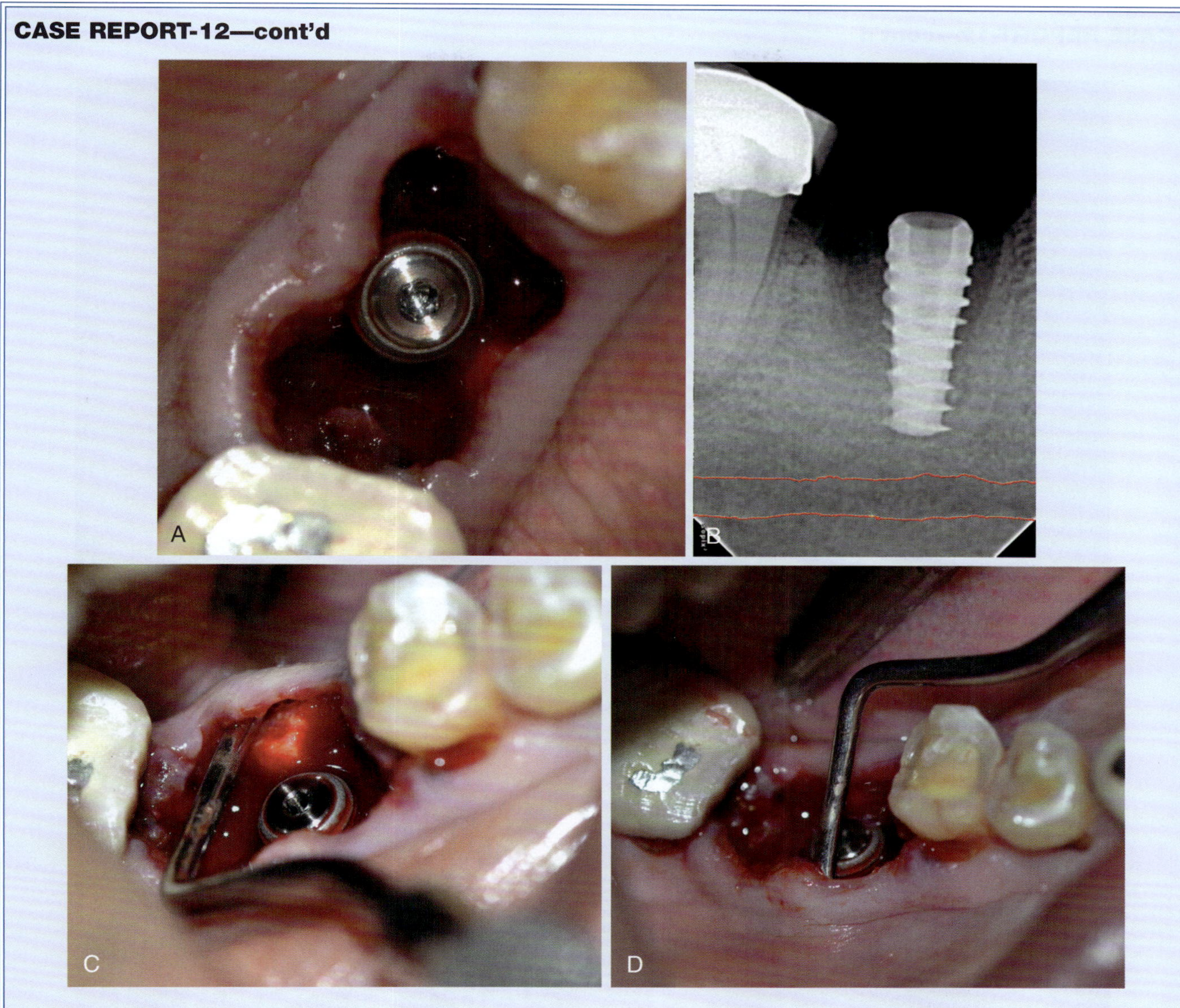

Fig 9.68 (A and B) Once the implant has been installed at the final position, (C and D) the lingual and buccal soft tissue periosteum is minimally elevated to create the buccal and lingual subperiosteal pouches.

Continued

CASE REPORT-12—cont'd

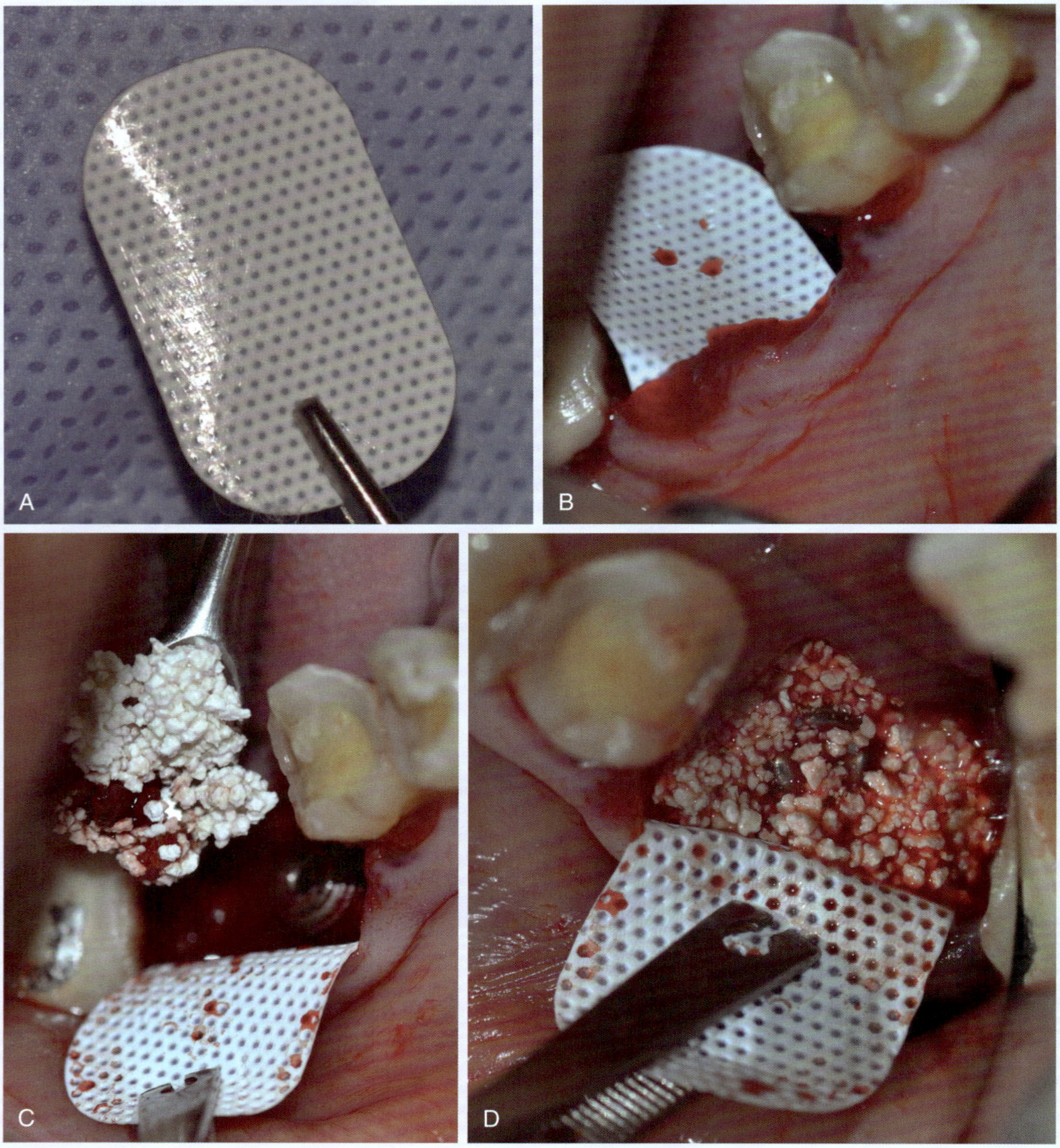

A B C D

Fig 9.69 (A and B) One end of a nonresorbable cytoplast TXT membrane is inserted in the buccal pouch and (C and D) the peri-implant socket spaces are loosely filled using a mixture of autogenous bone and hydroxyapatite graft.

CASE REPORT-12—cont'd

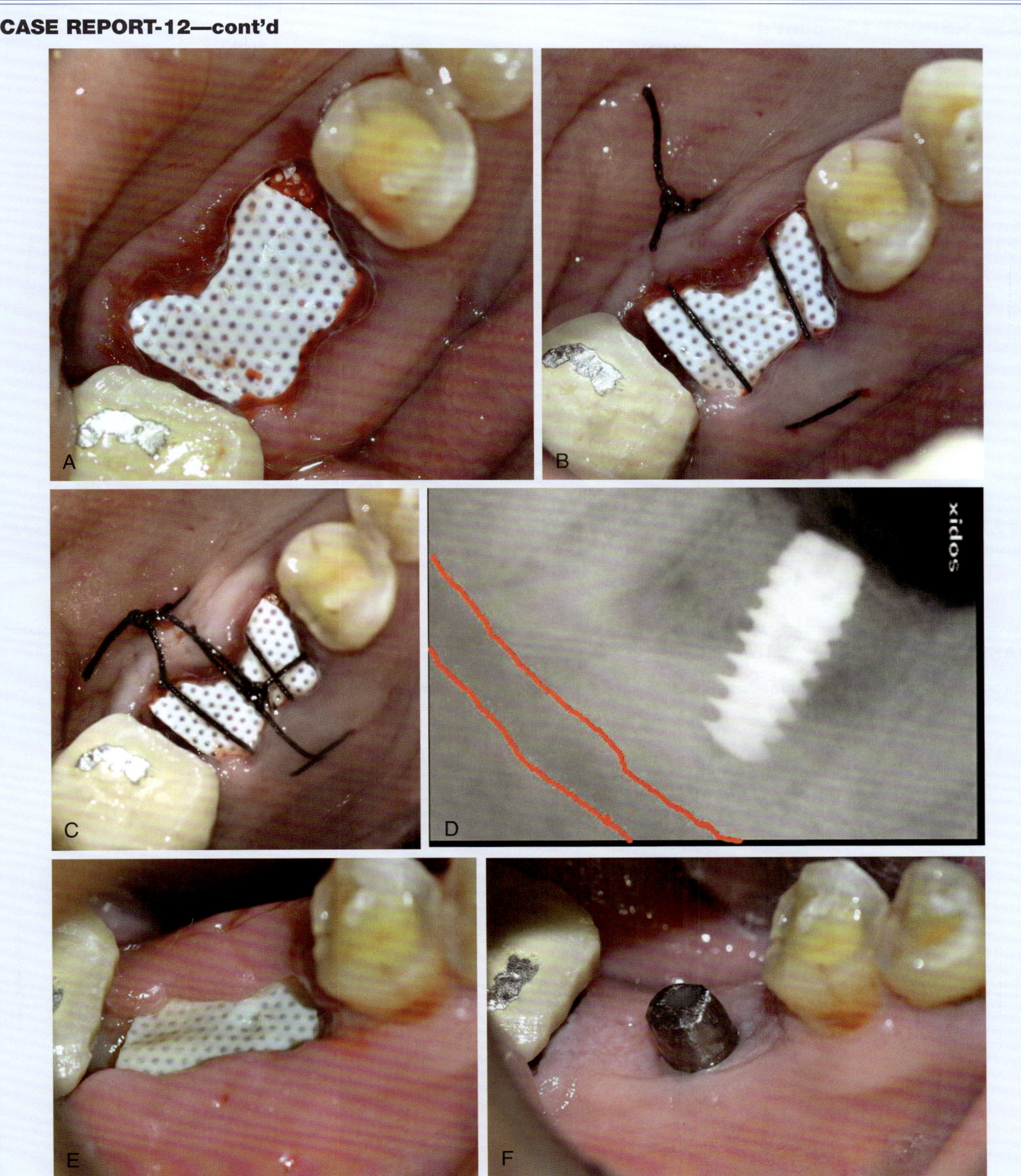

Fig 9.70 (A) The other end of the membrane covering the graft is inserted in the lingual pouch and (B) membrane is immobilized using sutures. (C) Another suture is given at approximate buccal and lingual soft tissue margins. (D) The post-implantation radiograph showing the implant inserted at the ideal location and grafted socket spaces. (E) The sutures are removed after 1 week. The membrane is removed after 3 weeks using an explorer. (F) The implant is uncovered after 4 months using a tissue punch.

Continued

CASE REPORT-12—cont'd

Fig 9.70, cont'd (G) implant is restored using a metal ceramic crown. (H) Post loading radiograph. This implant is in function since one year without any noticeable crestal bone loss.

CASE REPORT-13

Extraction of deciduous and immediate implantation at the mandibular molar site (Figs 9.71 and 9.72).

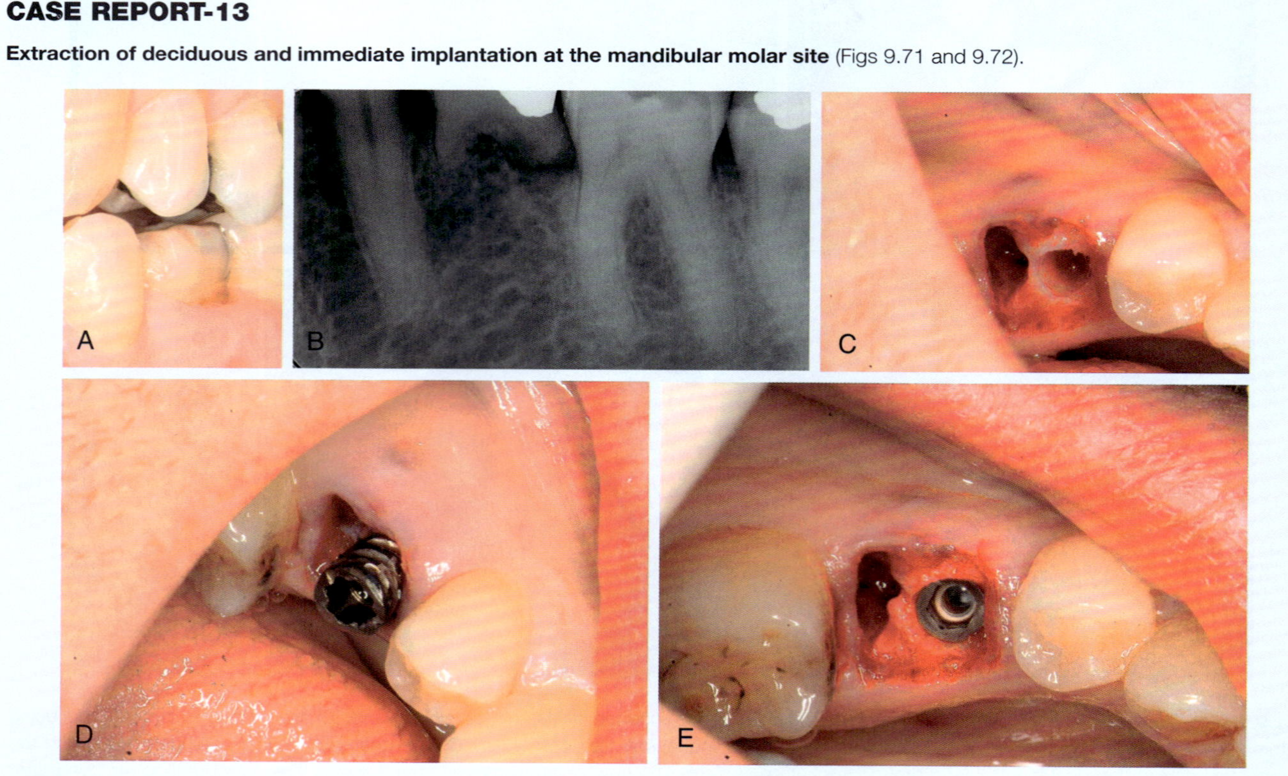

Fig 9.71 (A–C) Over-retained deciduous molar is extracted and (D) an implant is inserted at the correct position. (E) An abutment, with prepared retention grooves, is inserted over the implant.

CASE REPORT-13—cont'd

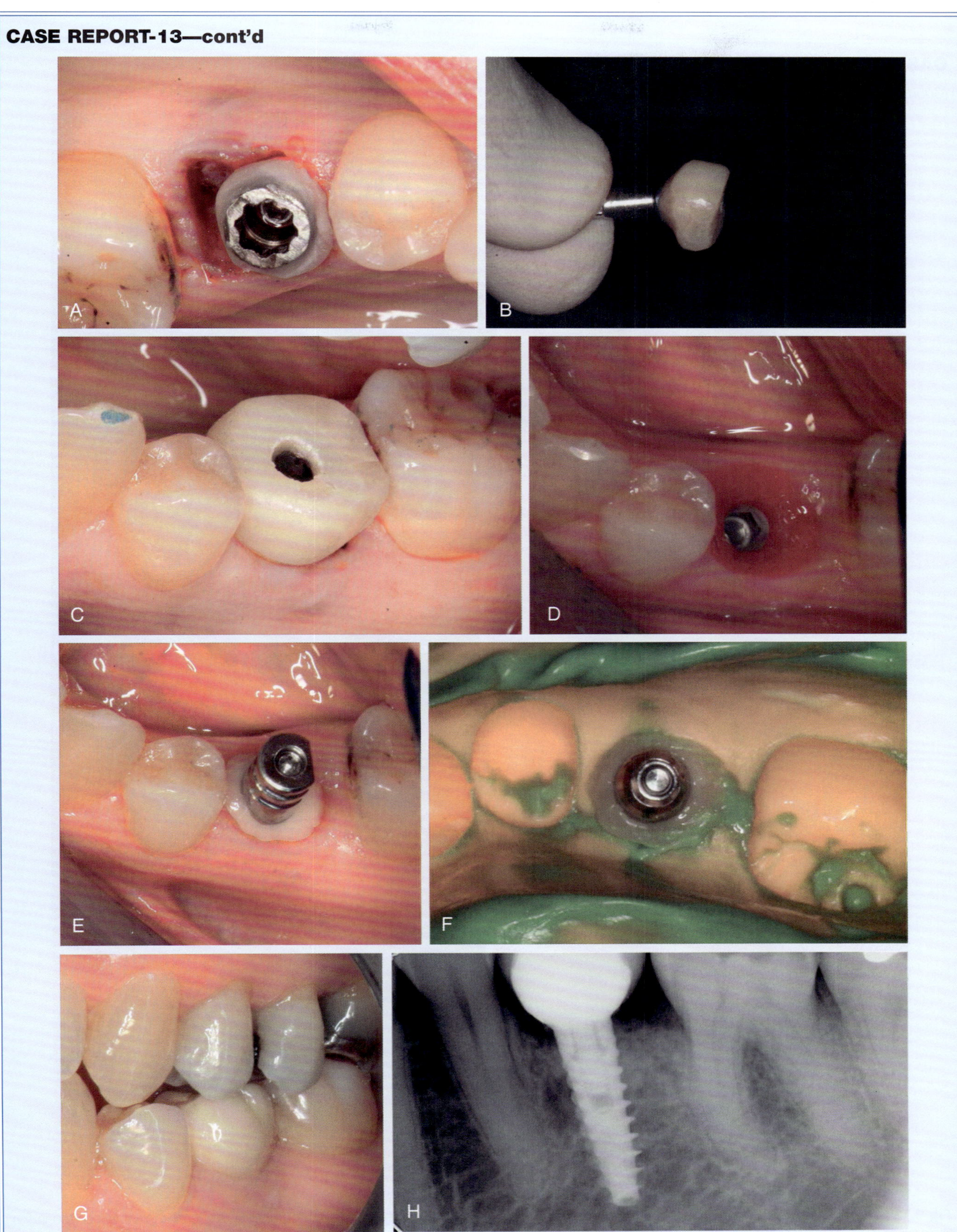

Fig 9.72 (A and B) The self-cure resin is built up over the abutment and (C) a provisional crown is fixed onto the implant, which has created (D) the scalloped soft tissue emergence in 4 months of implant healing. (E and F) An impression is made with soft tissue emergence transfer technique and (G) the implant is restored with high aesthetics. (H) Post loading radiograph.

CASE REPORT-14

(Courtesy: Dentium Co. Ltd, Well Dental Clinic, Seoul, Korea) (Fig 9.73A–H).

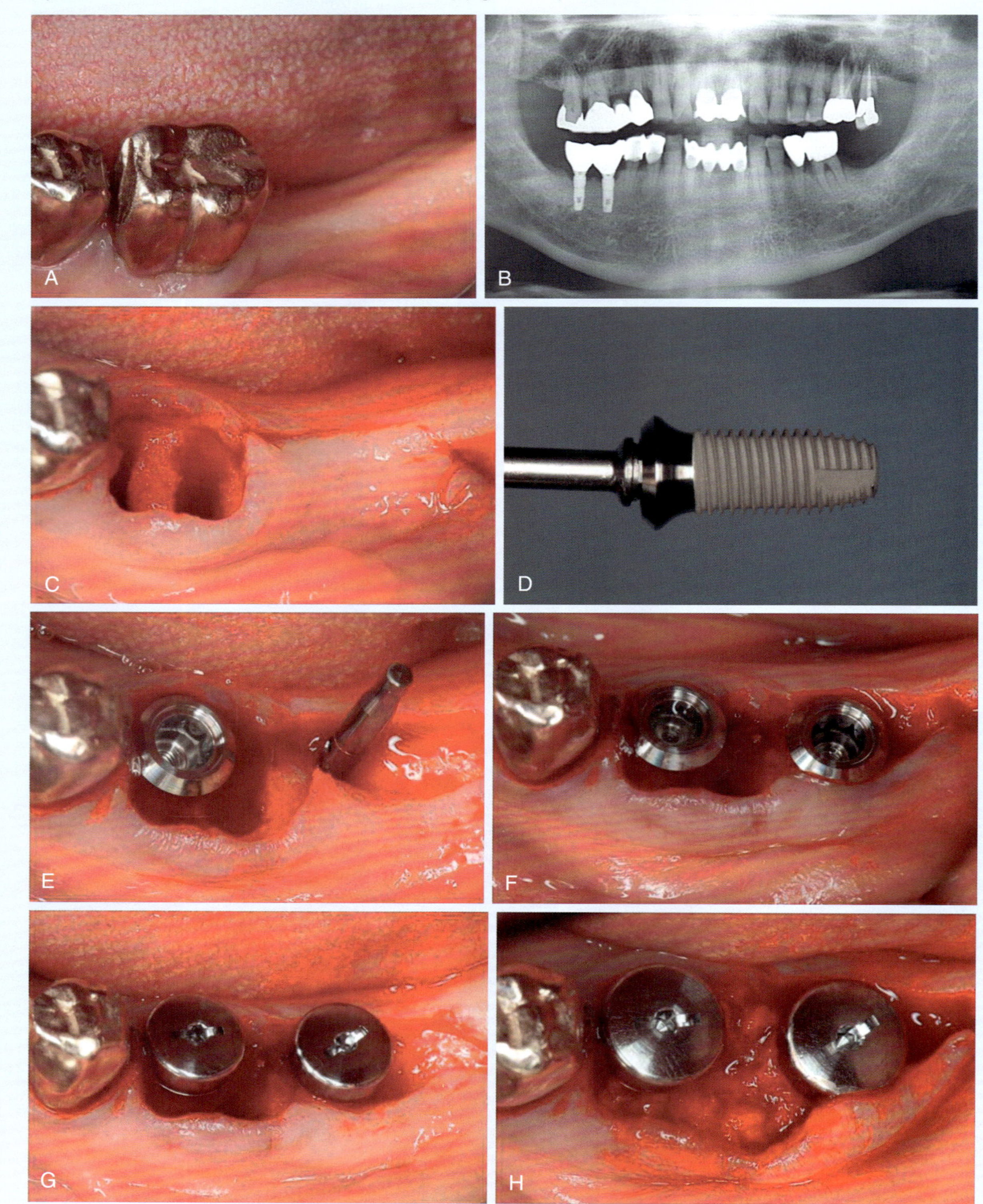

Fig 9.73 (A–C) Mandibular first molar which needs extraction, is atraumatically extracted and (D and E) a wide diameter implant is inserted in the mesial root socket. (F and G) Another implant is inserted distal to the distal root socket to give a two-unit fixed prosthesis. (H) The socket spaces are grafted using autogenous bone graft.

CASE REPORT-14—cont'd

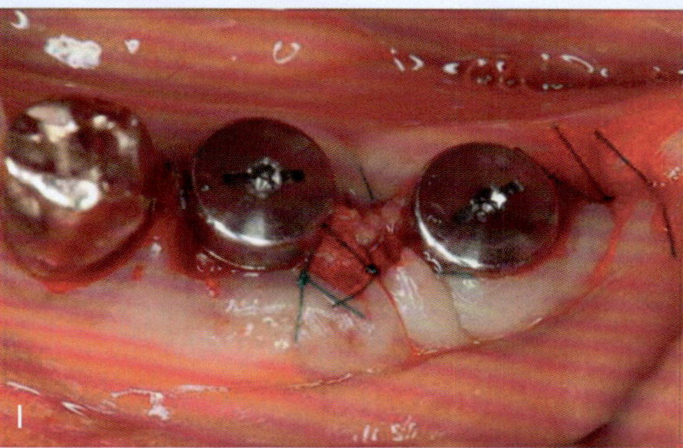

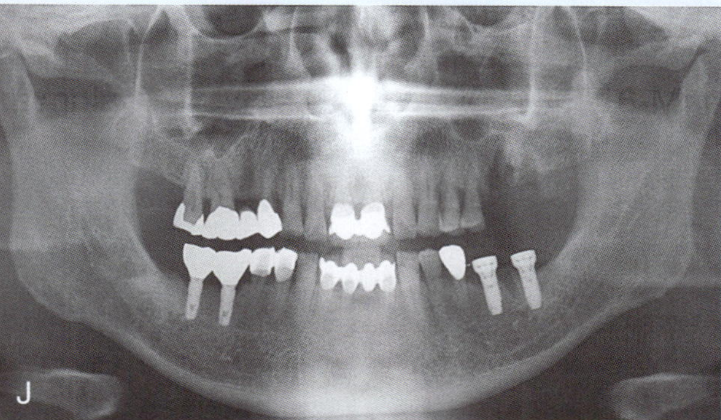

Fig 9.73, cont'd (I) The flap is sutured back for trans gingival healing of the implants. (J) Post-implantation radiograph. But leaving the bone graft exposed to the oral environment often leads to some complications like loss of graft or infection. The author recommends that the graft should be covered either using a barrier membrane or a provisional crown fixed over the implant that completely seals the grafted area.

CASE REPORT-15

Immediate implant into extraction sockets of mandibular molars and use of epithelialized connective tissue graft to achieve soft tissue closure. *(Courtesy: Jun Shimada, Japan)* (Figs 9.74 and 9.75).

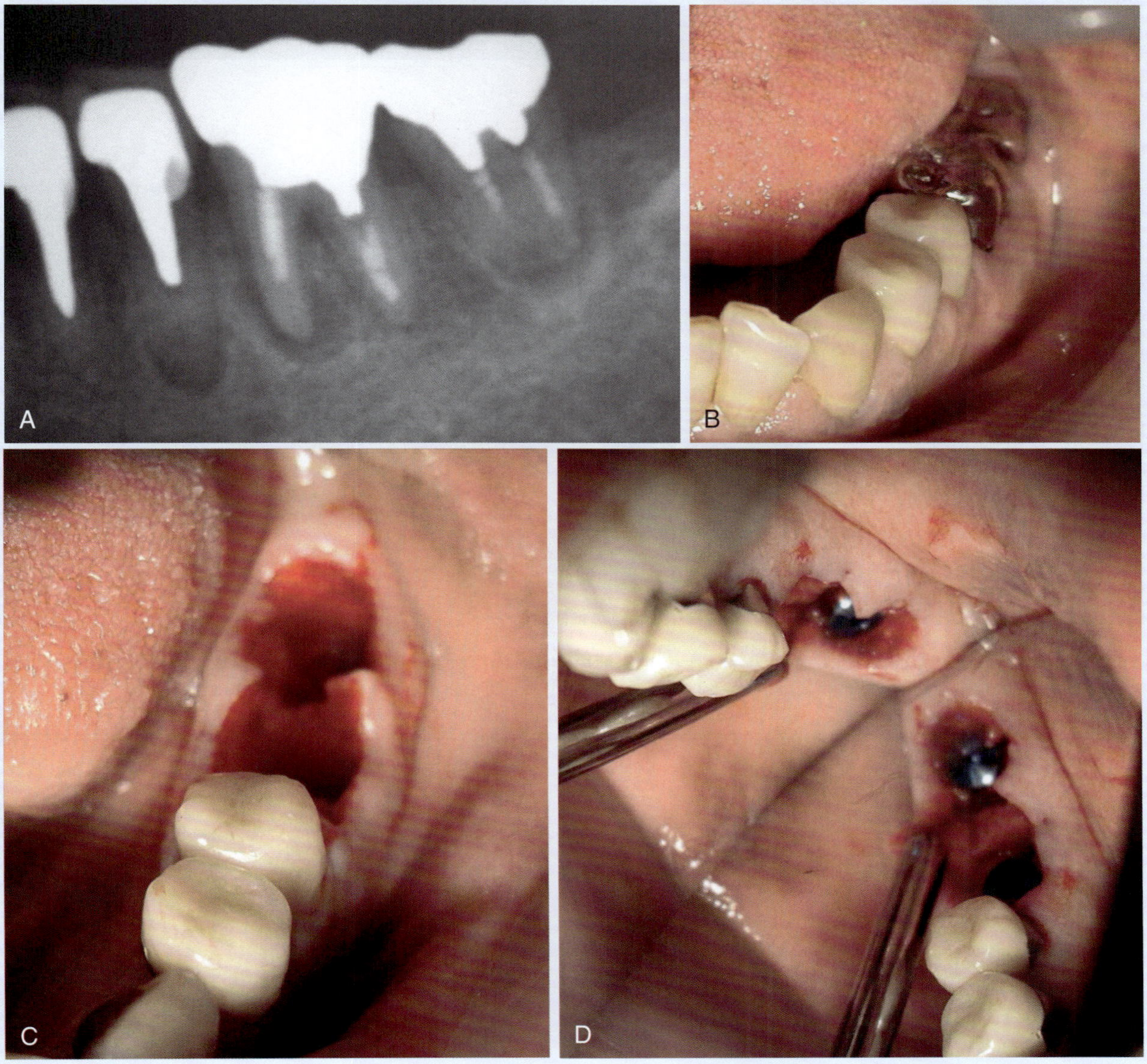

Fig 9.74 (A–C) Two mandibular molars which need extraction, atraumatically extracted preserving hard and soft tissue architecture of the socket. (D) Two implants inserted at the ideal positions into both the sockets.

CASE REPORT-15—cont'd

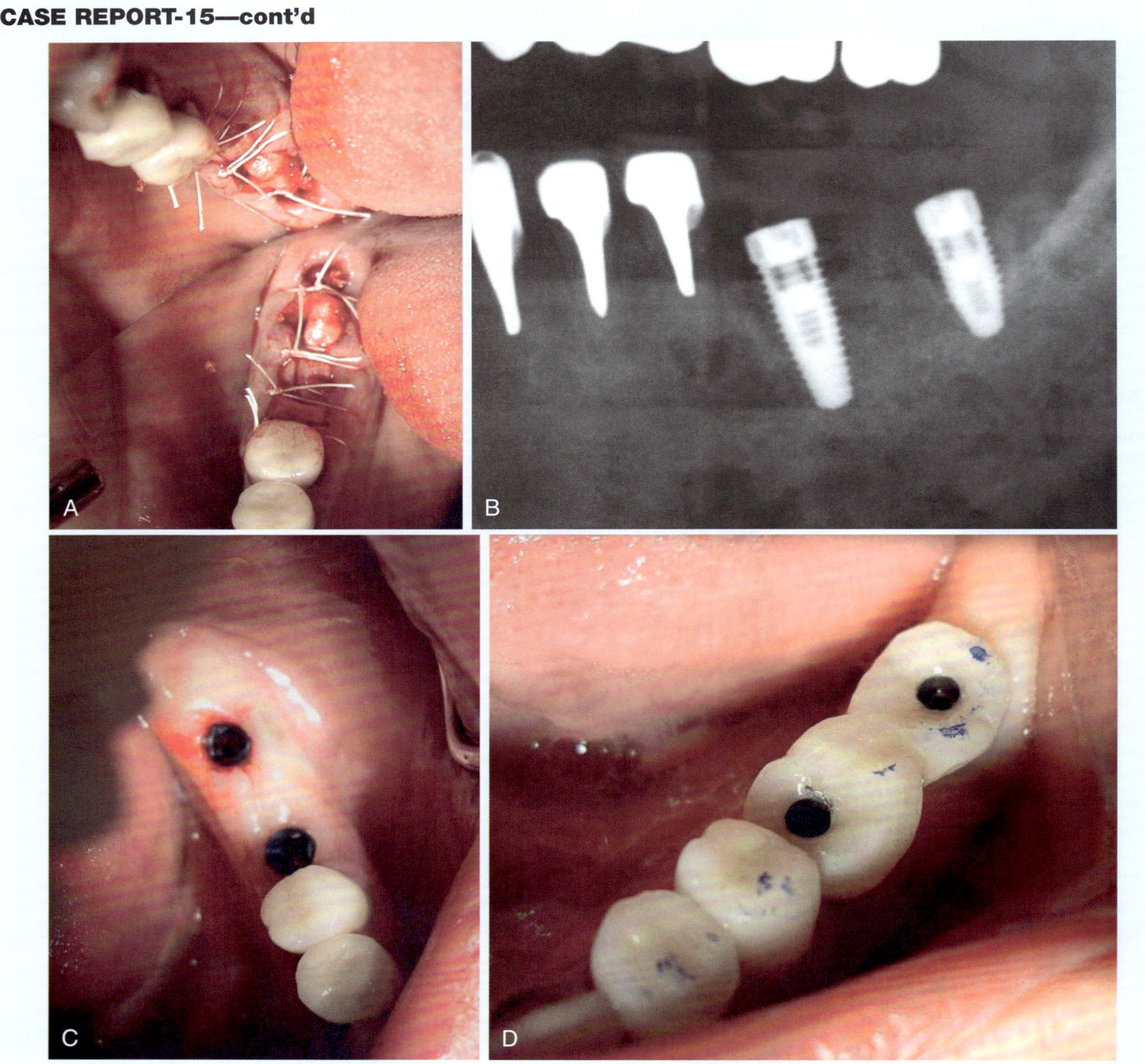

Fig 9.75 (A) A thick epithelialized connective tissue graft is harvested from the patient's palate and sutured to cover the socket. (B) Post-implantation radiograph. (C) Implants are uncovered after 4 months using a tissue punch and (D) restored using screw-retained prosthesis.

Socket lifting in maxillary posterior region

CASE REPORT-16

Achieving adequate primary stability is a challenge in immediate implantation in the socket of the posterior maxilla because of the poor density of the bone. Lateral bone condensation and stabilizing the implant apex in the high-density sinus floor can provide the adequate primary stability in such cases (Fig 9.76A–J).

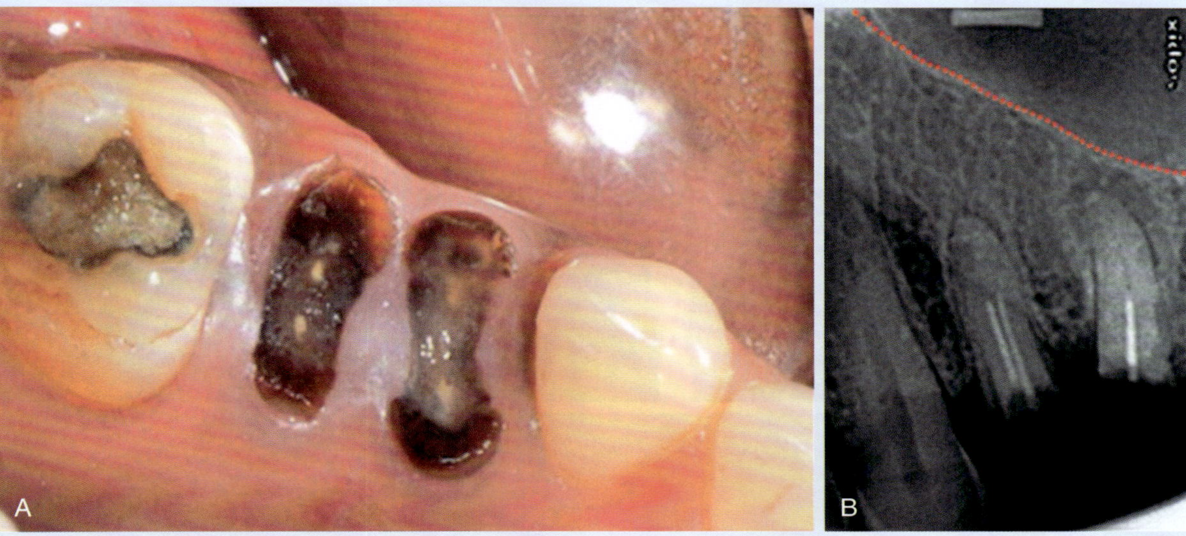

Fig 9.76 (A) Clinical view of the root stumps of left bicuspids which need to be extracted with immediate implant placement. (B) Dental radiograph shows limited bone height apical to the root stumps (especially in the second bicuspid) to engage the immediately inserted implant apex.

Continued

CASE REPORT-16—cont'd

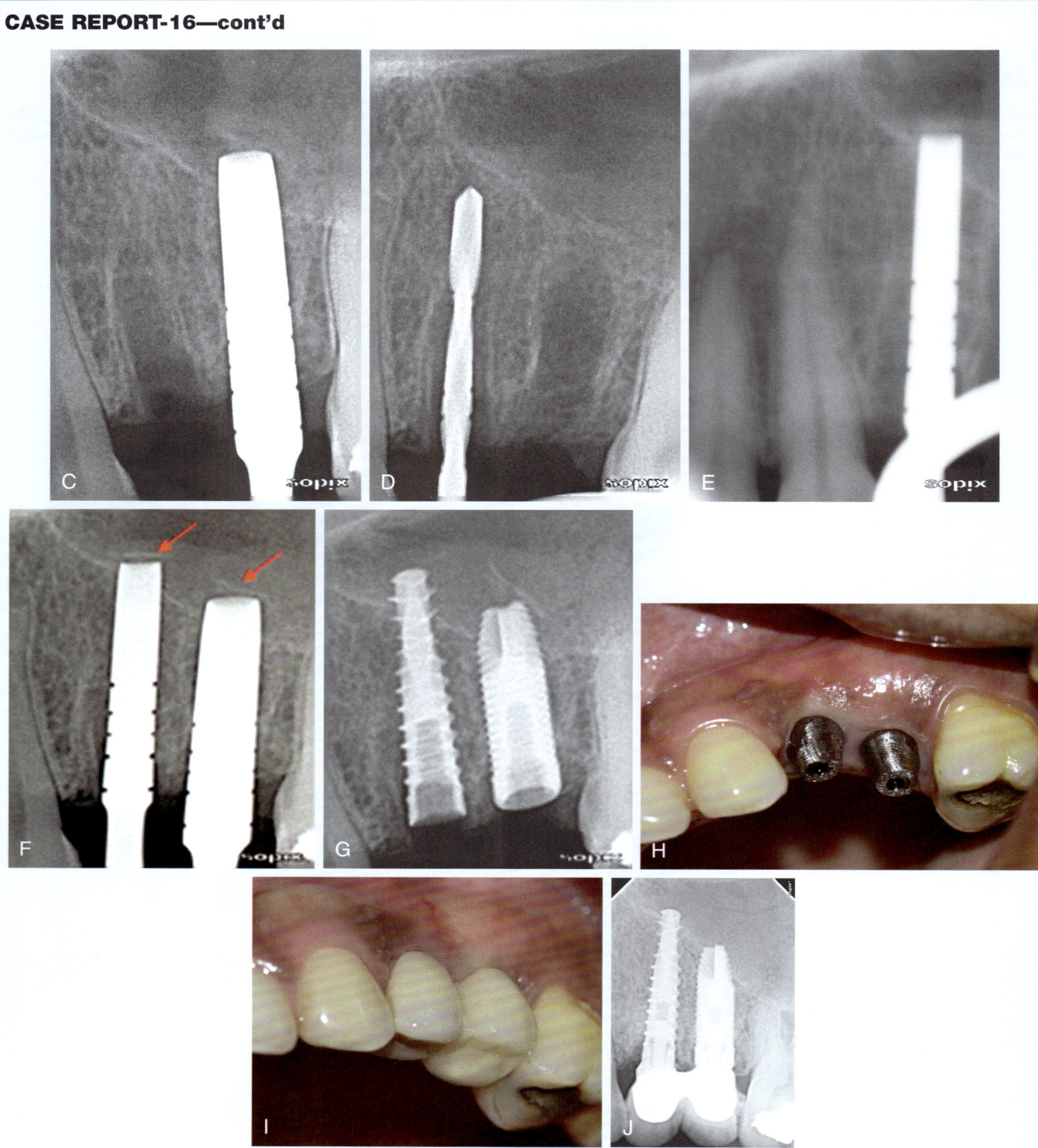

Fig 9.76, cont'd (C) The root stumps are atraumatically extracted using periotomes and a 4.2 diameter osteotome is inserted into the posterior extraction socket and gently taped to fracture up the hard sinus floor. (D) The implant osteotomy is prepared through the anterior socket just 2 mm short of the sinus floor. (E) Further, a final drill diameter osteotome is used in similar fashion to fracture up the sinus floor. (F) Both the osteotomes can be seen in the radiograph reaching beyond the sinus floor with fractured sinus floor bony pieces (red arrows) tenting up the elevated sinus membrane. (G) Both the implants are inserted to engage their apex in the hard sinus floor as well as the ridge crest (bicortical engagement) to achieve adequate initial implant stability (30–35 Ncm), which is quite necessary for optimal implant success in the low-density posterior maxilla. (H and I) Implants are uncovered and restored after 4 months. (J) Post loading radiograph 6 months after implant insertion shows new bone regeneration in the elevated sinus. Even though no bone graft material was used to fill the elevated sinus floor, the reason for new bone formation is that the implant apex kept tenting the elevated membrane and provided the space for new bone growth.

Summary

Backed with scientific literature and clinical trials, immediate implantation in the extraction socket has now been established as a proven implant technique. Usually immediate implants should be performed in single-rooted sockets, as placing the implant in the extraction socket of a multirooted tooth often results in multiple problems like lower percentage of bone–implant surface contact, inadequate primary stability of the implant, difficulty in achieving primary closure of the flap, off-axis implant placement, loss of graft, infection, etc. In addition, a large amount of graft is often required to fill the peri-implant sockets as well as a collagen membrane to cover it, which increases the cost of the procedure. Immediate implant in the aesthetic region offers several advantages over conventional implant placement in healed socket. Immediate implantation cases should be thoroughly planned with study models, radiographs, and dental CT images, to place the implant at the correct position in the socket without perforating any socket wall. The tooth needs to be extracted with the minimum trauma and should preserve the existing bony and soft tissue architectures of the socket. The implant surgeon should use good quality periotomes and luxators for this purpose. The socket for immediate implantation should not contain any active infection as it can transport pathogens to the bone and later can infect the inserted implant; all the granulation tissue should be curetted out and the socket should be disinfected using clindamycin or tetracycline to kill residual pathogens before the start of drilling. Osteotomy preparation for immediate implant in some sockets is more difficult than in healed bone, as the implant drills often slip towards the low-density, thin, cortical plate of the socket, which may lead to perforations. Efforts should be made to stabilize the implant in the healthy bone present apical to the socket. The longest and widest possible implant, which leaves minimum peri-implant socket spaces without compromising the resultant thickness of the peri-implant socket walls, should be placed. Several studies have shown good results in the immediate implant with immediate loading in the anterior region, if the force factors are minimum and the implant has achieved primary stability more than 35 Ncm. The author has substantial experience in immediate implantation with immediate loading in the maxillary and mandibular anterior region. In his view, if multiple implants are being inserted, they should be splinted together using a joint provisional prosthesis. The peri-implant socket spaces, if they are more than 2 mm wide, should be grafted and either a barrier membrane or an anatomical crown prosthesis should be fixed on top of implant to cover the graft. The immediate implant should be avoided in sockets with large osseous defects.

Further Reading

Araujo MG, Lindhe J. Dimensional ridge alterations following tooth extraction: an experimental study in the dog. J Clin Periodontol 2005;32:212–8.

Schropp L, Wenzel A, Kostopoulos L. Impact of conventional tomography on prediction of the appropriate implant size. Oral Surg Oral Med Oral Pathol Oral Radiol Endod 2001;92:458–63.

Kan JY, Rungcharassaeng K. Immediate implant placement and provisionalization of maxillary anterior single implants: a surgical and prosthodontic rationale, pract periodont. Asthet Dent 2000;12:817–24.

Schropp L, Wenzel A, Kostopoulos L, et al. Bone healing and soft tissue contour changes following single-tooth extraction: a clinical and radiographic 12-month prospective study. Int J Periodontics Restorative Dent 2003;23:313–23.

Araujo MG, Sukekava F, Wennström JL, et al. Ridge alterations following implant placement in fresh extraction sockets: an experimental study in the dog. J Clin Periodontol 2005;32:645–52.

Gomez-Roman G, Kruppembacher M, Weber H, et al. Immediate post extraction implant placement with root analog stepped implants: surgical procedure and statistical out come after 6 years. Int J Oral Maxillofac Implants 2001;16:503–13.

Maiorana C, Beretta M, Salina S, et al. Reduction of autogenous bone graft resorption by means of Bio-Oss coverage: a prospective study. Int J Periodontics Restorative Dent 2005;25:19–25.

Schwartz-Arad D, Chaushu G. Placement of implants into fresh extraction sites: 4 to 7 years retrospective evaluation of 95 implants. J Periodontol 1997;68:1110–6.

Brazilay I. Immediate implants, their current status. Int J Prosthodont 1993;6:169.

Schlegel KA, Fichtner G, Schultze-Mosgau S, et al. Histological findings in sinus augmentation with autogenous bone chips versus a bovine bone substitute. Int J Oral Maxillofac Implants 2003;18:53–8.

Becker W, Dahlin C, Becker BE, et al. The use of e-PTFE barrier membranes for bone promotion around titanium implants placed into extraction sockets: a prospective multicenter study. Int J Oral Maxillofac Implants 1994;9:31–40.

Tehemar S, Hanes P, Sharawy M. Enhancement of osseointegration of implants placed into extraction sockets of healthy and periodontally diseased teeth by using graft material, an ePTFE membrane or a combination. Clin Implant Dent Relat Res 2003;5:193–211.

Rosenquist B, Granthe B. Immediate placement of implants into extraction sockets: implant survival. Int J Oral Maxillofac Implants 1996;11:205–9.

Tarnow DP, Eskow RM. Preservation of implant aesthetics, soft tissue and restorative considerations. J Esthet Dent 1996;8:12–9.

Lang NP, Brägger U, Hämmerle CH, et al. Immediate transmucosal implants using the principle of guided tissue regeneration. I. Rationale, clinical procedures and 30-month results. Clin Oral Implants Res 1994;5:154–63.

Schwartz-Arad D, Chaushu G. Immediate implant placement: a procedure without incisions. J Periodontol 1998;69:743–50.

Brägger U, Hämmerle CH, Lang NP. Immediate transmucosal implants using the principle of guided tissue regeneration (II). A cross-sectional study comparing the clinical outcome 1 year after immediate to standard implant placement. Clin Oral Implants Res 1996;7:268–76.

Botticelli D, Berglundh T, Lindhe J. Hard-tissue alteration following immediate implant placement in extraction sites. J Clin Periodontal 2004;31:820–8.

Schwartz-Arad D, Chaushu G. The ways and wherefores of immediate placement of implants into fresh extraction sites: a literature review. J Periodontol 1997; 68(10):915–23.

Van Steenberghe D, Callens A, Geers L, et al. The clinical use of deproteinized bovine bone mineral on bone regeneration in conjunction with immediate implant installation. Clin Oral Implants Res 2000;11:210–6.

Lang NP, Tonetti MS, Suvan JE, et al. Immediate implant placement with transmucosal healing in areas of esthetics priority: a multicenter randomised controlled clinical trial. I. Surgical outcomes. Clin Oral Implants Res 2007;18:188–96.

Hämmerle CH, Lang NP. Single stage surgery combining transmucosal implant placement with guided bone regeneration and bioresorbable materials. Clin Oral Implants Res 2001;12:9–18.

Glauser R, Sennerby L Meredith N, et al. Resonance frequency analysis of implants subjected to immediate or early functional occlusal loading. Successful vs. failing implants. Clin. Oral Impl. Res 2004;15: 428–34.

Meyer U, Wiesmann HP, Fillies T, et al. Early tissue reaction at the interface of immediately loaded dental implants. Int J Oral Maxillofac Implants 2003;18(4):489–99.

Schropp L, Wenzel A, Kostopoculos L, et al. Bone healing and soft tissue contour changes following single tooth extraction: a clinical and radiograph 12-month prospective study. Int J Periodontics Restorative Dent 2003;23:313–23.

Esposito MA, Koukoulopoulou A, Coulthard P, et al. Interventions for replacing missing teeth: dental implants in fresh extraction sockets (immediate, immediate-delayed and delayed implants). Cochrane Database Syst Rev 2006;4:CD005968.

Immediate implantation in fresh extraction sockets. A controlled clinical and his-tological study in man. J Periodontol 2001;72(11):1560–71.

Ericsson I, Randow K, Nilner K. Peterson: early functional loading of Branemark dental implants: 5-year clinical follow-up study. Clin Implant Dent Relat Res 2000;2(2):70–7.

Immediate load implant system, Tokyo: Quintes. Int Oral Maxillofac Implants May science 1998.

Ferrara A, G'Alli C, Mauro G, et al. Immediate provisional restoration of post extraction implants for maxillary single tooth replacement. Periodontics Restorative Dent 2006;26:371–7.

De Smet E, Jaecques S, Vandamme K, et al. Positive effect of early loading on implant stability in the bi-cortical guinea-pig model. Clin Oral Implants Res 2005; 16(4):402–7.

Balshi T, Wolfinger G. Immediate functional loading of implants. Implant Dent 2002;10:231.

Schwartz Ard D, Laviv A, Lavin L. Survival of immediately provisionalized dental implants placed immediately into fresh extraction sockets. J Periodontol 2007;78:219–23.

Misch CE, Wang HL. The procedures, limitations and indications for small diameter implants and a case report. Oral Health 2004;94:16–26.

Schwartz D, et al. The clinical effectiveness of implants placed immediately into fresh extraction sites of molar teeth. J Periodontol 2000;71:839–44.

Paolantonio M, Dolci M, Scarano A, et al. Immediate versus non-immediate implantation for full-arch fixed reconstruction following extraction of all residual teeth: a retrospective comparative study. J Periodontol 2000;71(6):923–8.

Roynesdal AK, Ambjornsen E, Haanaes HR. A comparison of 3 different endosseous nonsubmerged implants in edentulous mandibles: a clinical report. Int J Oral Maxillofac Implants 1999;14(4):543–8.

Becker W, Dahlin C, Becker BE, et al. The use of e-PTFE barrier membranes for promotion around titanium implants placed into extraction sockets, a prospective multicenter study. Int J Oral Maxillofac Implants 1994;9:31–40.

Saadoun AP, Landsberg CT. Treatment classification and sequencing for post extraction implant therapy: a review. Pract Perio Rest Dent 1997;9:933–41.

Ganeles J, Rosenberg MM, Holt RL, et al. Immediate loading of implants with fixed restorations in the completely edentulous mandible: report of 27 patients from a private practice. Int J Oral Maxillofac Implants 2001;16(3):418–26.

Brunski JB. Biomechanical factors affecting the bone-dental implant interface. Clin Mater 1992;10(3):153–201.

Ogiso N, Tabata T, Lee RR, et al. Delay method of implantation enhances implant binding, a comparison with the conventional method. Int J Oral Maxillofac Implants 1995;10:415–20.

Schropp L, Isisor F, Kostopoulos L, et al. Interproximal papilla levels following early versus delayed placement of single-tooth implants: a controlled clinical trial. Int J Oral Maxillofac Implants 2005;20:753–61.

Pilliar RM, Lee JM, Maniatopoulos C. Observations on the effect of movement on bone ingrowth into porous-surfaced implants. Clin Orthop Relat Res 1986;208:108–13.

Implant overdentures

10

Ajay Vikram Singh   Saâd Zemmouri

CHAPTER CONTENTS HD

Introduction

The prosthetic management of the completely edentulous patient has long been a major challenge in dentistry. The conventional edentulous ridge supported dentures, in use over centuries, has been the traditional standard of care for these patients. However, most patients do not achieve satisfactory comfort with conventional dentures; hence, the implant-retained overdenture can be one of the ultimate options for these patients. After losing teeth, the ridge gets slowly resorbed as the normal course of disuse atrophy, which further gets enhanced by using the tissue supported dentures for several years. The worst cases are the patients who lose their teeth because of advanced periodontitis; their periodontal bone gets vertically resorbed because of periodontitis, leaving compromised ridge height inadequate to retain ridge-supported dentures. The implant retained overdentures improve chewing efficiency, comfort, and overall maxillofacial prosthesis of the patient. Besides, the placement of implants anchors the jaw bone and prevents the further bone loss. Depending on the bone volume available for implant placement, arch form, bone density, and force factors, two to four implants are inserted to retain the mandibular denture, whereas four to six implants are required to retain the maxillary denture (Fig 10.1A–E).

Prosthetic options for completely edentulous patients

1. Conventional ridge-supported dentures
2. Implant-retained overdentures
3. Implant-supported full arch fixed prosthesis.

Problems associated with conventional dentures

1. Inadequate retention and stability
2. Inability to chew and eat
3. Soft tissue abrasions
4. Continuous bone loss
5. Large size prosthesis with long flanges and palate extension
6. Phonetic problem
7. Longer period required to get used for the dentures
8. Teeth setting in the neutral zone causes altered maxillofacial prosthesis.

Indications for implant overdenture

1. Inadequate bone volume to insert the number of implants required for full arch fixed prosthesis
2. When the relation between the two arches makes the achievement of a fixed prosthesis difficult
3. Palatal/ridge defect which makes conventional denture fabrication difficult
4. Highly resorbed ridge, inadequate to retain the conventional denture
5. Phonetic problems caused by difficult control of the saliva movement between the prosthesis and the maxillary gum
6. High aesthetic expectations.

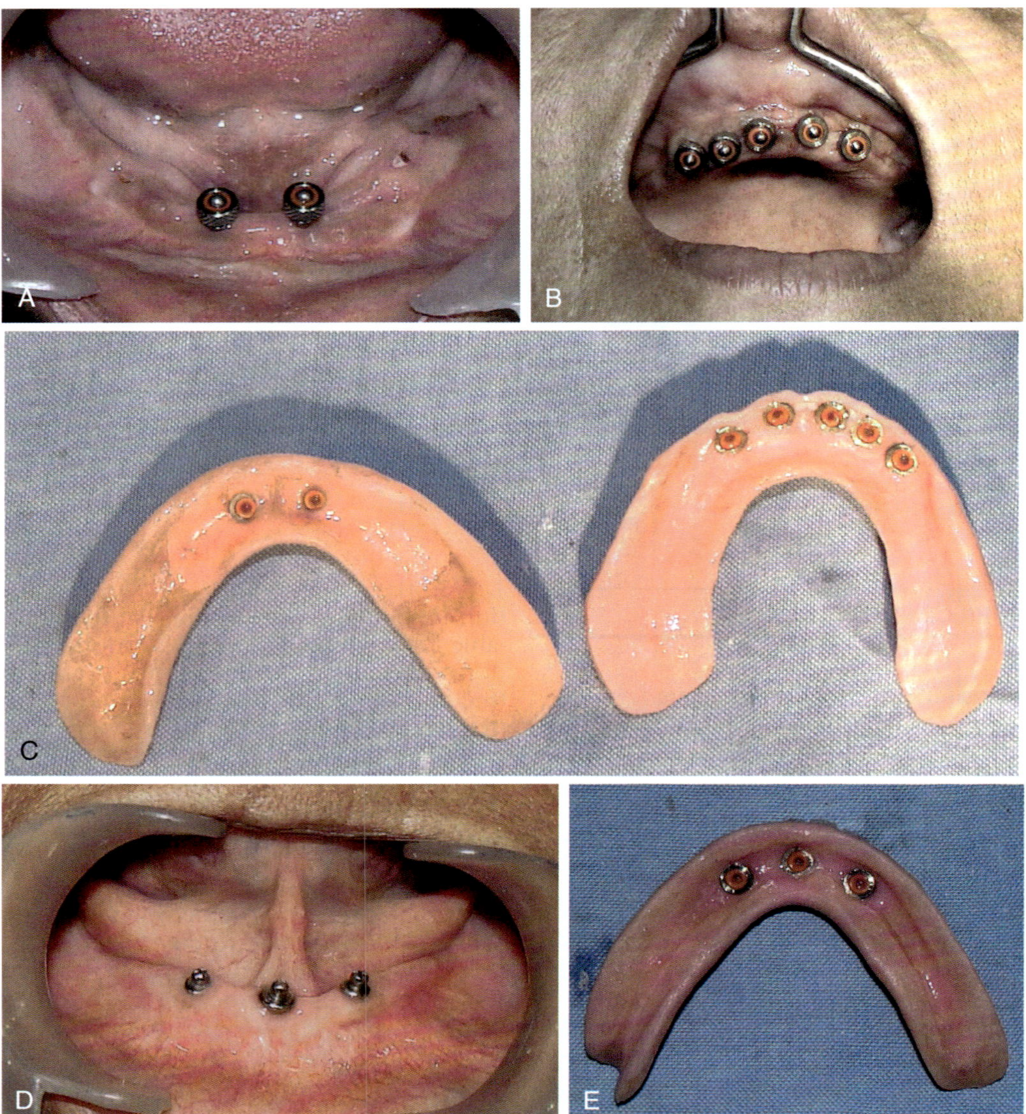

Fig 10.1 (A–E) Depending on the ridge form and bone available to insert the longest and widest possible implants, a minimum of 2–4 implants are required to retain the mandibular overdenture, whereas a minimum of 4–6 implants are required to retain the maxillary overdenture. The low-density bone and presence of facial cantilevering are the reasons to place more number of implants for the maxillary overdenture. If two implants are planned for the mandibular overdenture, both implants should be inserted closer to the midline, to avoid anteroposterior rocking of the denture.

7. Limited financial budget for the prosthesis
8. Medically compromised patients for whom the placement of a large number of implants, grafting procedures, etc. are not possible
9. Patients with complaints of low retention of their old conventional dentures
10. Patients with a history of poor oral hygiene maintenance.

Advantages of the implant overdenture over the ridge supported denture

1. Implants prevent further bone loss
2. Improved denture retention, support and stability
3. Reduced denture size eliminates palate extension and deep flanges of the denture
4. Decreased soft tissue abrasions
5. Improved chewing efficiency
6. Improved occlusion – original centric occlusion can be reproduced
7. Improved maxillofacial appearance as the implant-retained prosthesis can better support the lip and cheek muscles
8. Improved retention and removal of palatal extension improves speech.

Advantages of the implant overdenture over the fixed implant prosthesis

1. Fewer implants are required for overdenture
2. Less specific implant placement
3. Grafting procedures (e.g. sinus grafting, vertical bone augmentation, etc.) can be avoided

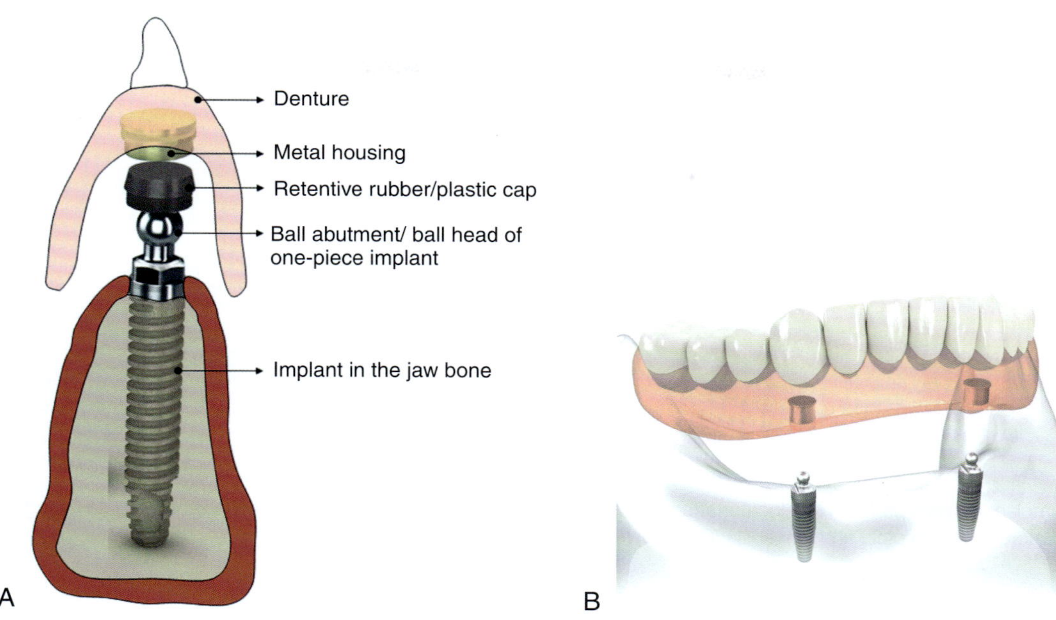

Fig 10.2 Either a single-body, ball head implant or a two-piece implant with ball abutment is inserted into the jaw bone. A retentive rubber or plastic cap is inserted in the metal housing before placement over the ball abutment. When the denture filled with self-cure acrylic is seated over the metal housing, the latter comes out embedded in the tissue surface of the denture. (A and B) When this denture with the female part (metal housing with retentive cap inside) is seated over the male part of the implant (ball abutment), it provides adequate retention to the removable implant overdenture *(Courtesy: Nobel Biocare).*

4. Improved maxillofacial aesthetics with labial flanges, soft tissue drape, and prefabricated denture teeth
5. Lower cost to the patient
6. Easy oral hygiene maintenance
7. Easy repair
8. Reduced stress on the implants as the prosthesis can be removed at night.

Disadvantages of the implant overdenture

1. Patient's psychological feeling against wearing a removable prosthesis.
2. Needs regular maintenance like denture relining, change of retentive components, new prosthesis after few years etc.
3. Continuous posterior bone loss.
4. Denture movement where only two implants are used for denture retention.
5. More interarch space is required to compensate the denture base and the implant superstructure.
6. Food impaction under the prosthesis.
7. Soft tissue abrasions in the posterior region.

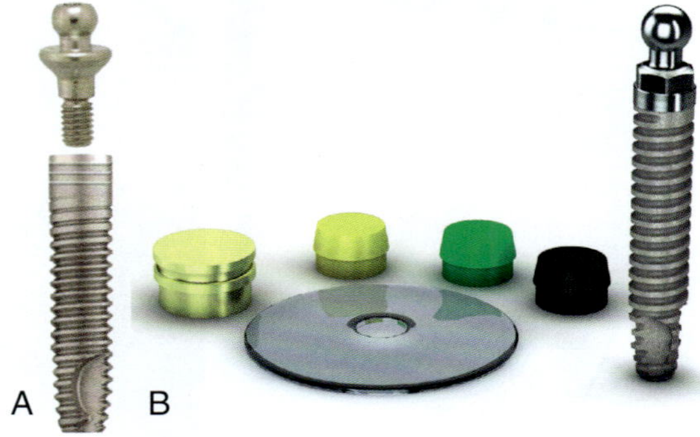

Fig 10.3 (A) Either a ball abutment is screwed onto the two-piece implant or (B) a single-body ball abutment implant is used for overdenture cases. Different kinds of plastic/rubber caps ranging from hard to soft consistency (colour coded) can be used under the metal housing, depending on the degree of retention required for the denture. Ideally, if immediately loaded, one should use the soft low retention cap, and it should be replaced with a medium to hard one, after the implants have osseointegrated with the bone *(Courtesy: Biohorizons Implant Systems Inc).*

Components required

Several kinds of prosthetic components are placed over implants as well as into the tissue surface of the denture. These components may vary in shape, size, design from one implant system to the other, with the type of retention device the dentist delivers to his/her patient, e.g. ball and socket, locator abutment, bar header clip type, etc. (Figs 10.2–10.4).

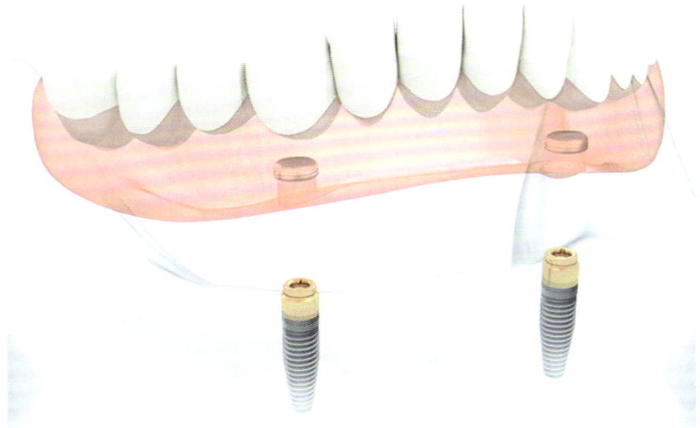

Fig 10.4 Many implant dentists prefer to use locator attachments over the 'O' ring or cap attachment because of many advantages like need of less interarch space, more precision of fit, and longer life *(Courtesy: Nobel Biocare).*

CASE REPORT

Ball abutment and cap retained mandibular overdenture (step by step presentation) (Figs 10.5–10.9).

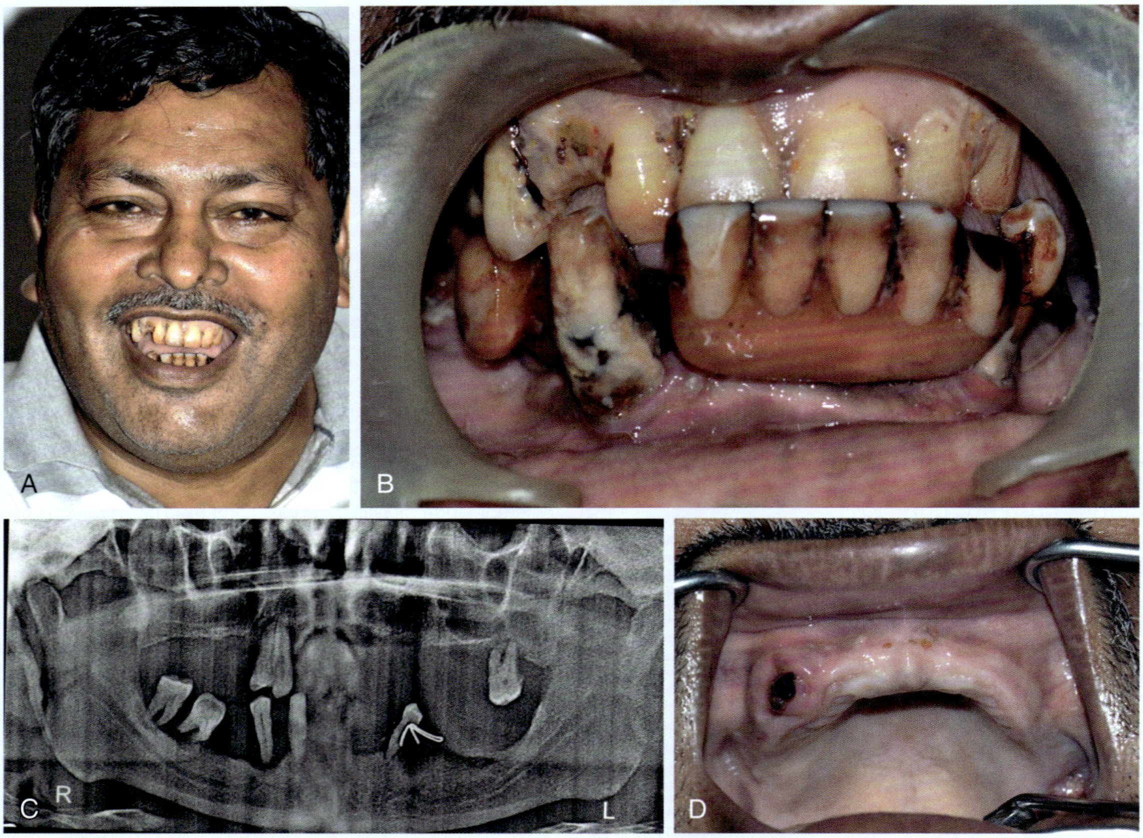

Fig 10.5 (A and B) Patient with faulty dentures and periodontally compromised teeth. (C) Radiograph shows the need for extraction of all teeth and replacement with the full mouth prosthesis. (D) The maxillary ridge after the extractions, showing a good ridge form to retain a soft tissue supported denture.

CASE REPORT—cont'd

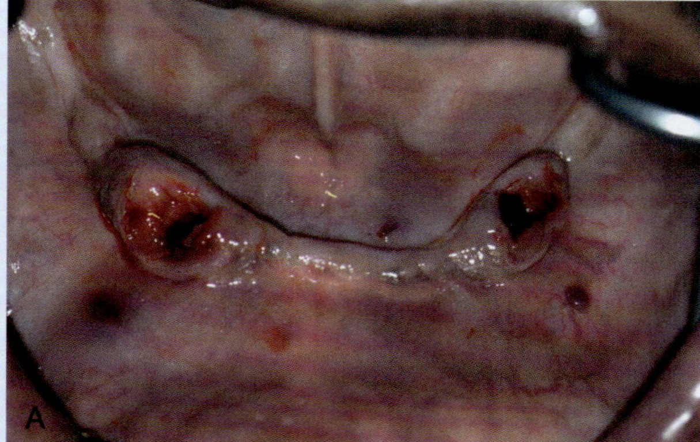

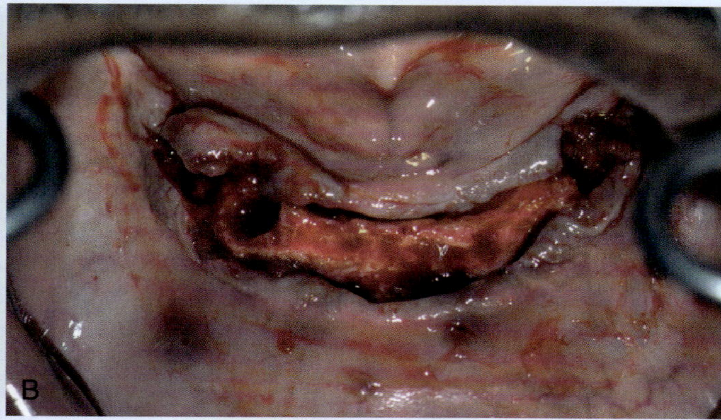

Fig 10.6 (A) Lower ridge is very poor in form, hence implant supported overdenture is planned. (B) Mid-crestal incision is given and the flap is elevated to expose the bony ridge.

CASE REPORT—cont'd

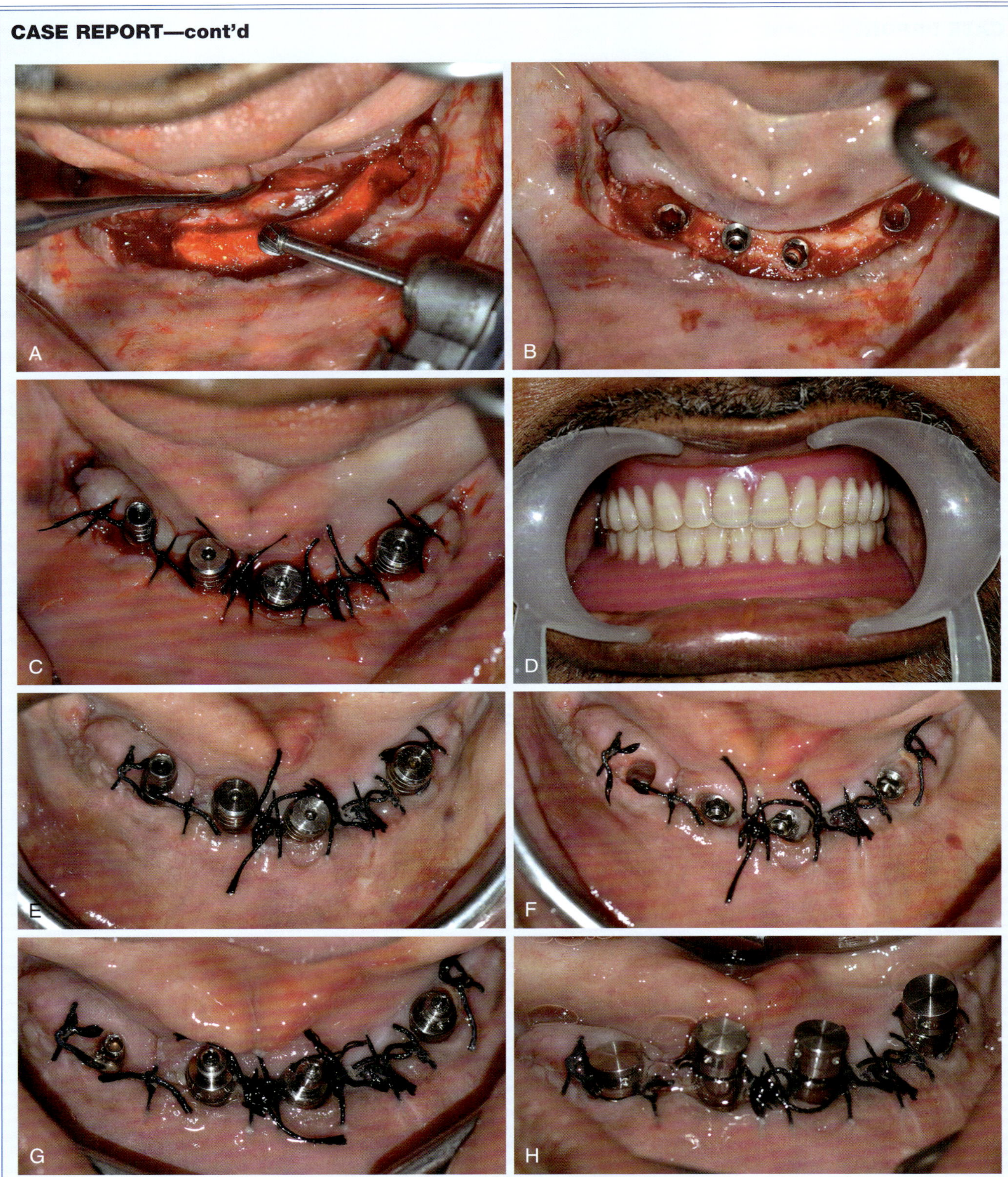

Fig 10.7 (A) Osteoplasty, using the large round carbide bur, is done to flatten the ridge crest and (B) four implants are inserted between two mental foramina. (C) Transgingival healing abutments are inserted and flaps are sutured back. (D) A complete denture is fabricated for the patient. (E–G) The transgingival abutments are removed after 3 days and replaced with ball abutments. (H) The metal housings carrying retentive plastic caps fitted inside, are seated on top of the ball abutments.

CASE REPORT—cont'd

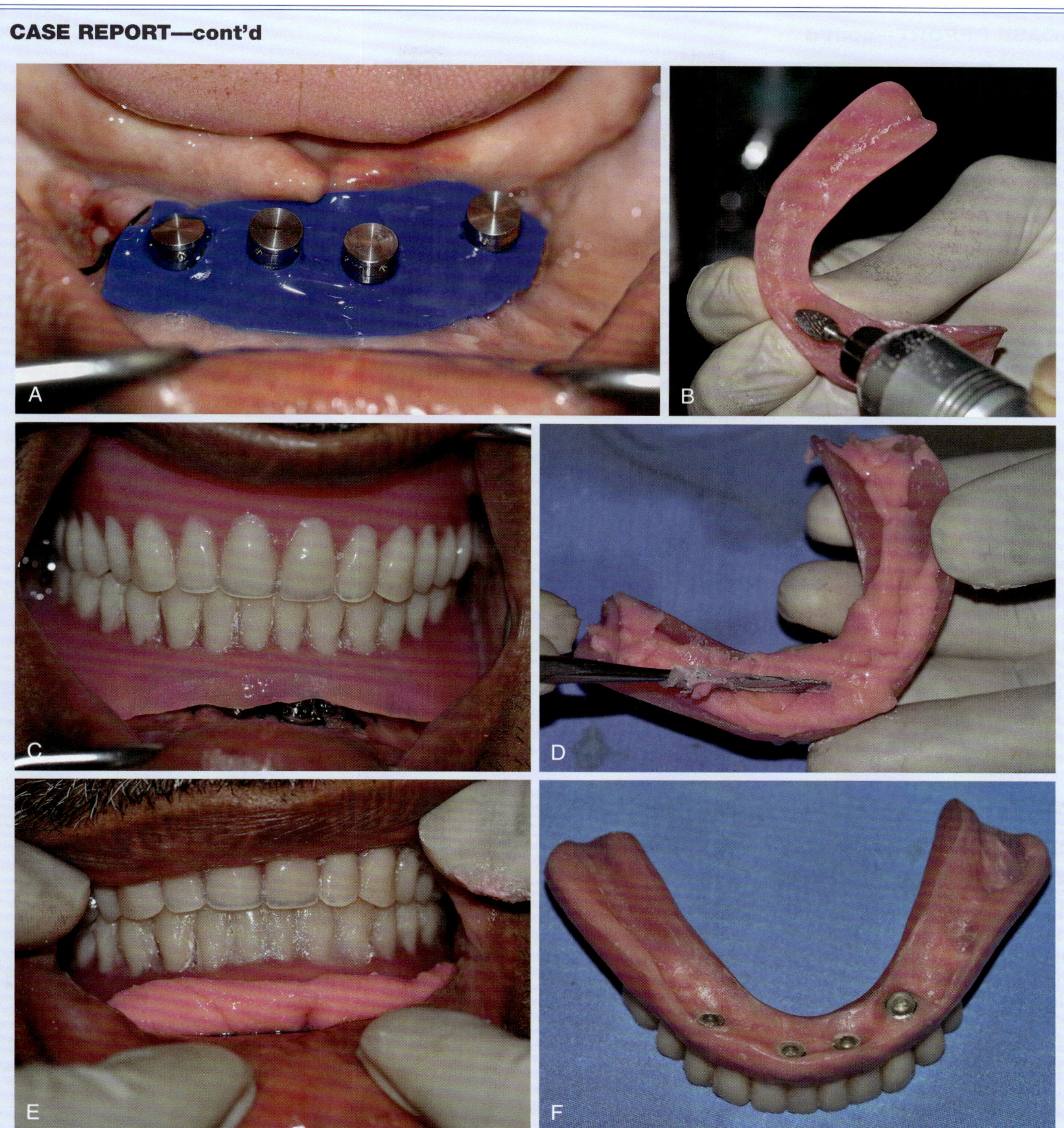

Fig 10.8 (A) A piece of rubber dam is used to cover the sutures and block the undercuts under the metal housing. It prevents the flow of the acrylic and its locking into the undercut areas. (B and C) The tissue surface of the lower denture is reduced and the denture is tried in the patient's mouth for complete and passive seating over the metal housing. The tissue surface of the denture is reduced to create minimum 2 mm space all around, between the metal housing and the denture surface, for the self-cure acrylic. (D and E) The tissue surface of the denture is filled with self-cure acrylic and the denture is seated in the patient's mouth in the correct occlusion. The denture surface, except its tissue surface, should be coated with petroleum jelly before it is filled with self-cure acrylic to avoid unnecessary adhesion of acrylic over the denture flanges and teeth. (F) After the acrylic has set, the denture carrying the metal housings embedded in the tissue surface, is removed from the mouth.

CASE REPORT—cont'd

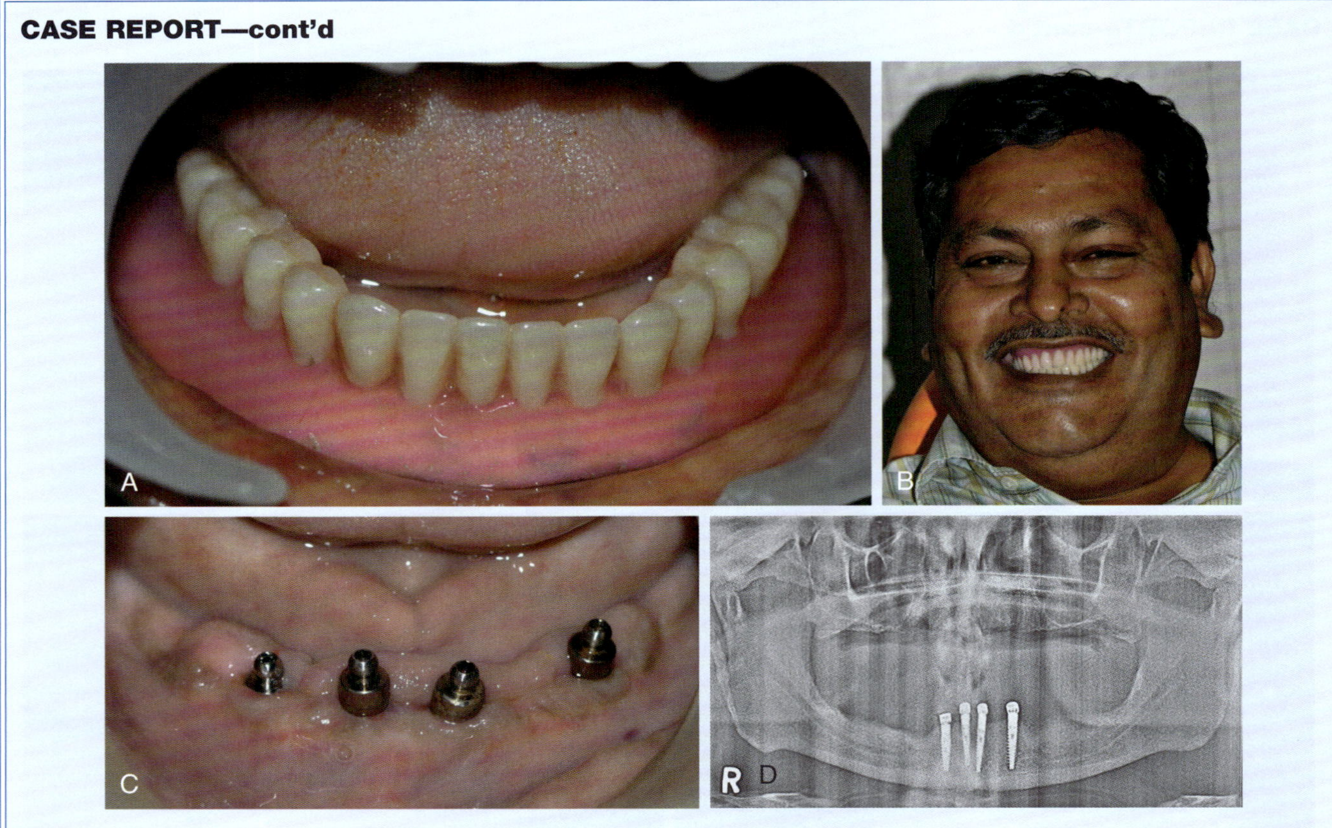

Fig 10.9 (A and B) The denture is finished, polished, and seated over the implants in the patient's mouth. (C) Soft tissue healing after 1 week. (D) Post loading radiograph.

Decision making for immediate, early, or delayed implant loading in overdenture cases

The immediate or delayed stabilization of the denture over the implant depends on various factors such as bone density, bone volume, number of implants required to support the denture, implant sizes, soft tissue type, force factors, and the primary stability of the inserted implant (Table 10.1). Implants are usually inserted in the anterior segment of the maxillary and/or mandibular ridge, to retain the dentures where density of the bone is usually found to be adequate in volume, with no structures limiting the placement of the longest possible implants. Moreover, favourable bone density is also usually found to adequately stabilize the implants in these segments, especially in the anterior mandible. Thus in most cases, the denture can be immediately or early stabilized over these implants using ball abutments and metal housings. For immediate loading, efforts should be made to insert the longest possible implants and stabilize them in basal bone/nasal floor to achieve adequate initial stability (more than 35 Ncm). However, if adequate stability cannot be achieved (less than 35 Ncm) for any implant, the implant should be loaded only after it has osseointegrated with the bone in 2 to 3 months (Fig 10.10A–F). For cases, where adequately long implants cannot be placed and a predictable amount of primary stability

Table 10.1 Various deciding factors for immediate or delayed loading in overdenture cases

DECIDING FACTORS	IMMEDIATE STABILIZING DENTURE	DELAYED LOADING OF IMPLANTS (AFTER 3–4 MONTHS)
Bone density	High (Type I or Type II)	Low (Type III or Type IV)
Bone volume	Adequate to place long implants	Inadequate to place long implants
Soft tissue	Adequate band of keratinized tissue at the ridge crest	Inadequate band of keratinized tissue at the ridge crest, which needs soft tissue grafting at implant's uncovery stage
No. of implants	Adequate	Fewer implants for cost effective treatment
Primary stability of implants	More than 35 Ncm	Less than 35 Ncm

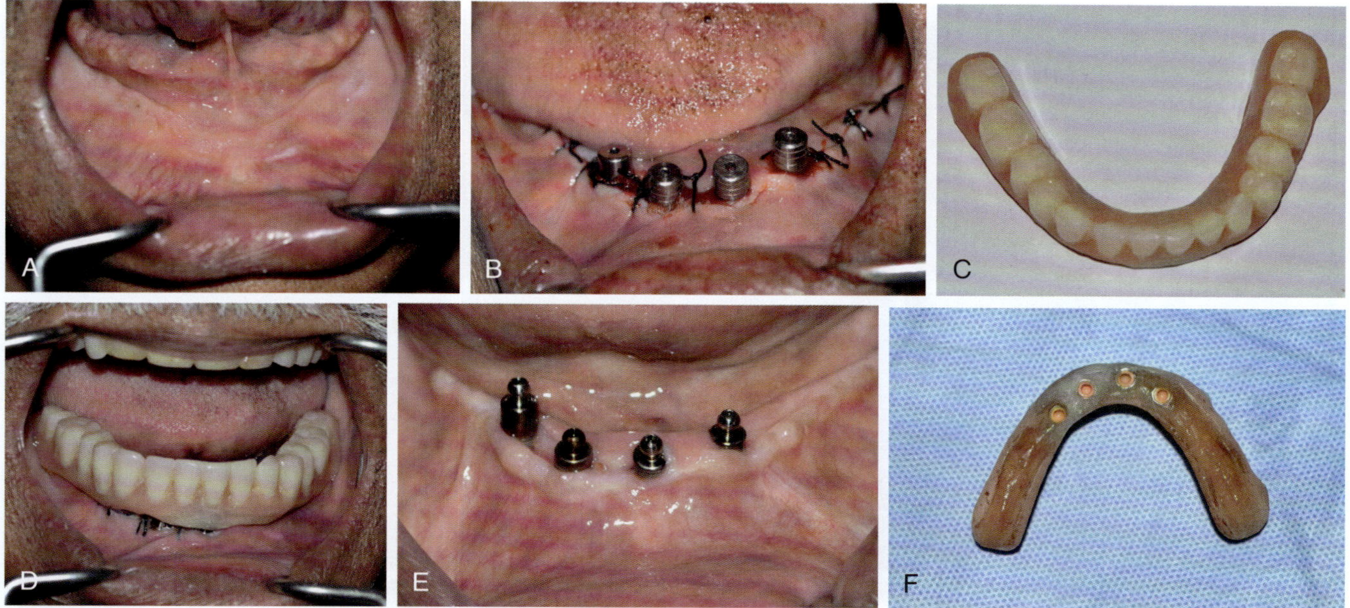

Fig 10.10 (A) The patient who had been wearing ridge-supported dentures for more than 10 years, presented with complaint of poor retention of the mandibular denture because of continued vertical ridge resorption in the course of time. Four implants were inserted in the anterior mandible but most of the implants achieved primary stability between 25 and 30 Ncm. (B) The implants were left for open healing with long healing abutments. (C and D) The denture was re-lined in mouth over these abutments and stabilized, as the immediate placement of the ball and socket connection causes a large amount of pulling forces on the implants during denture removal, which may result in implant failure. (E) After the implants were osseointegrated with the bone, the healing abutments were replaced with ball abutments and (F) the retention housings were placed into the tissue surface of the denture.

cannot be achieved, the conventional two-stage protocol should be followed. In such cases the implants are left for subgingival healing for 3 to 4 months and then uncovered, and the implant is stabilized over implants (Fig 10.11A–L).

Bar-retained overdenture

Many dentists prefer to fabricate a metal bar which is screwed over the implants, with either header clips or locator attachments used to retain the denture onto the bar (Fig 10.12A and B). When compared to the ball or locator attachments, bar-retained dentures offer better retention and support to the patient; but fabrication of a bar which can be passively seated over the implants and the placement of header clips into the tissue surface of denture needs good laboratory support and multiple sittings with the patient (Figs 10.12 and 10.13).

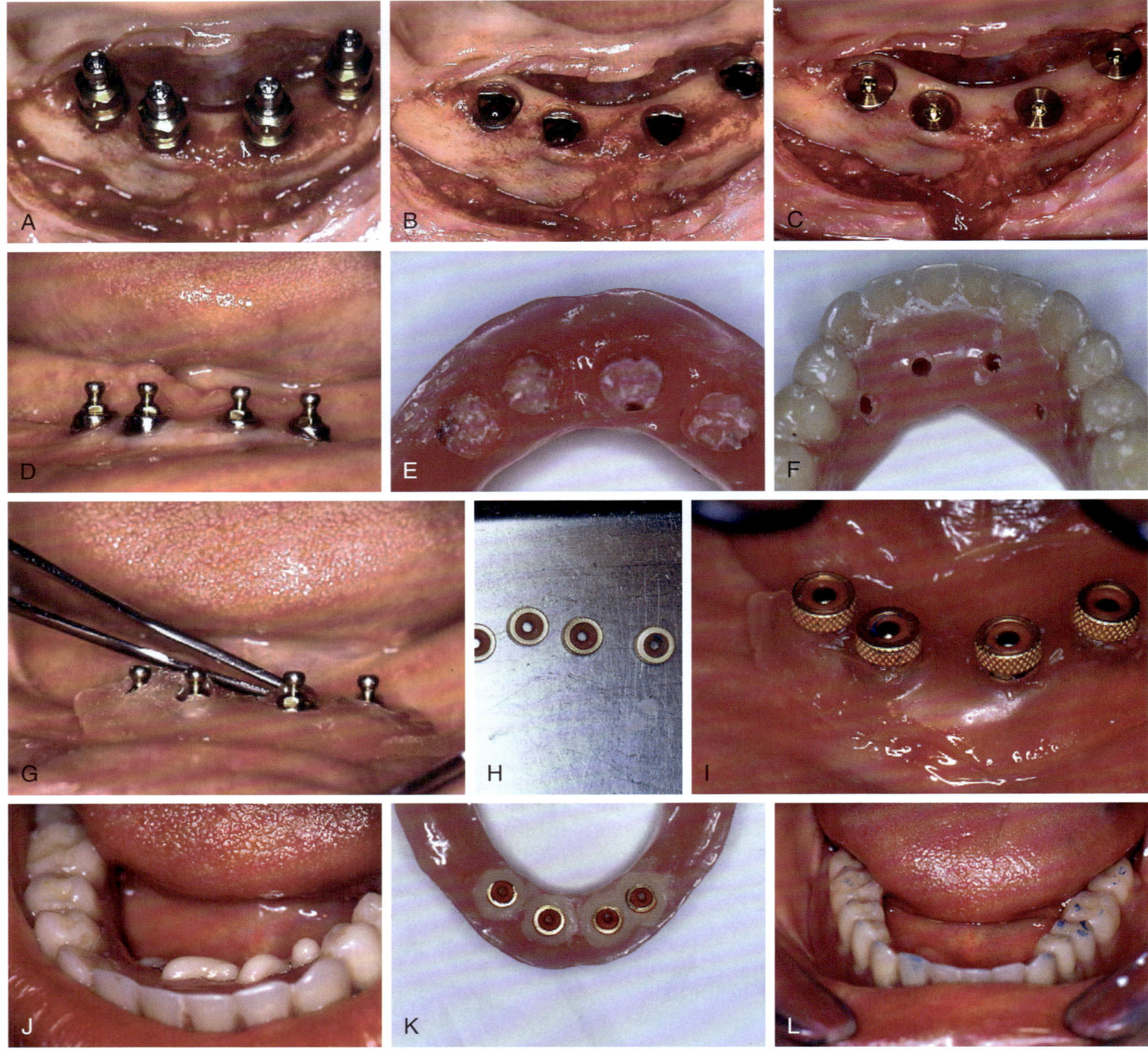

Fig 10.11 (A–C) Four implants are inserted in the anterior mandible with submerged healing for 3 months. (D) Implants are uncovered and ball abutments are inserted. (E and F) Tissue surface of the denture is prepared. (G) The undercuts of the ball abutments are blocked using modelling wax. (H and I) The appropriate 'O' rings are selected and seated onto the ball abutments. (J) The self-cure acrylic is filled into the prepared tissue surface and denture is seated over the 'O' rings in the correct occlusion. (K) Denture is removed after the resin has set, showing the 'O' rings in the denture. (L) Denture is finished, polished, and seated in the patient's mouth.

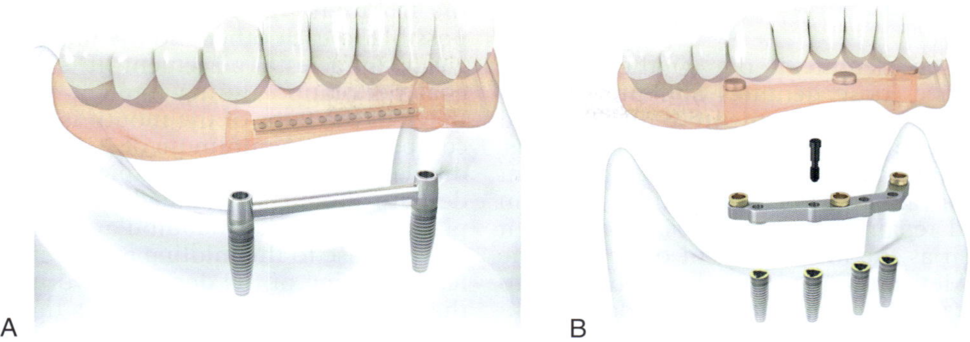

Fig 10.12 (A and B) Many dentists prefer to fabricate a metal bar which is screwed over the implants and either header clips or locator attachments are used to retain the denture onto the bar. When compared to the ball or locator attachments, bar-retained dentures offer better retention and support to the patient *(Courtesy: Nobel Biocare).*

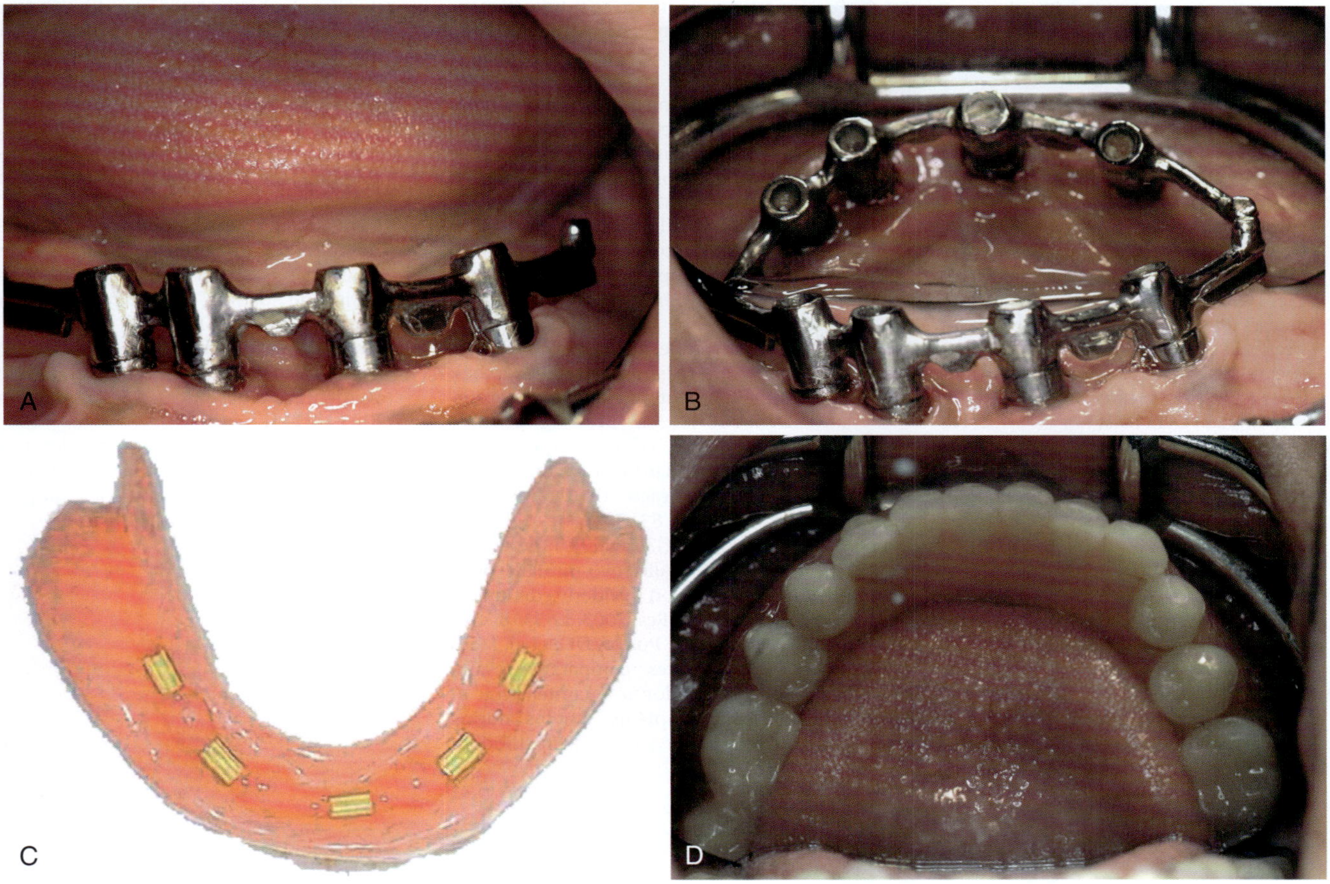

Fig 10.13 (A and B) A cast metal bar is seated and screwed over the implants. (C) The header clips are placed into the tissue surface of the denture in the dental laboratory, (D) which gets locked over the bar to retain the denture.

Summary

Implant-retained overdenture is one of the preferred options to stabilize loose dentures and prevent further bone loss. The implant overdenture offers several advantages over the implant supported fixed prosthesis, such as lower treatment cost, fewer and specific implant placement, less invasive surgery, no grafting, ease in maintenance and repair of the prosthesis, etc. Thus it should be chosen as the first treatment option for the old age patient. Meticulous planning should be done to insert the longest possible implants, to provide immediate and long-term stability for the dentures. A simple, uncomplicated one-stage surgical protocol is considered the technique of choice, with implants as parallel as possible to each other and the implant platforms being given supracrestal placement. It is critical to avoid lingual perforation during implant placement. Haemorrhage of the floor of the mouth is a potentially serious complication. A minimum of 2–4 implants for the mandibular denture and 4–6 implants to support maxillary denture should be planned. If only two implants are placed to support a mandibular denture, they should be placed close to the midline to prevent the anterior posterior rocking of the denture. Two implants (ideally in the canine or lateral position) is the minimal implant standard of care in the edentulous anterior mandible to retain an overdenture.

Further Reading

Carpentieri, JR, Tarnow, DP. The mandibular two-implant overdenture first-choice standard of care for the edentulous dentaure patient. Pract Proced Aesthet Dent. 2003 Nov-Dec;15(10):750–2.

Phillips K, Wong KM. Space requirements for implant-retained bar-and-clip overdentures. Compend Contin Educ Dent 2001;22:516–8; pp. 520, 522.

Zitzmann NU, Marinello CP. Treatment outcomes of fixed or removable implant-supported prostheses in the edentulous maxilla. Part I: patients' assessments. J Prosthet Dent 2000;83:424–33.

Branemark PI, et al. Branemark Novum: a new treatment concept for the rehabilitation of the edentulous mandible – preliminary results from a prospective clinical follow – up study. Clin Implant Dent Relat Res 1999;1:2–16.

Mericske-Stern R. Prosthodontic management of maxillary and mandibular overdentures. In: Feine JS, Carlsson GE, editors. Implant overdentures: the standard of care for edentulous patients. Chicago, IL: Quintessence Pub. Co.; 2003. pp. 83–98.

Branemark PI, Zarb GA, Albrektsson T. Tissue-integrated prostheses: osseointegration in clinical dentistry. Chicago, IL: Quintessence; 1985.

Awad MA, Lund JP, Shapiro SH, et al. Oral health status and treatment satisfaction with mandibular implant overdentures and conventional dentures: a randomized clinical trial in a senior population. Int J Prosthodont 2003;16:390–6.

Balsi TJ, Wolfinger GJ. Immediate loading of Branemark implants in edentulous mandibles: a preliminary report. Implant Dent 1997;6:83–8.

Quirynen M, Alsaadi G, Pauwels M, et al. Microbiological and clinical outcomes and patient satisfaction for two treatment options in the edentulous lower jaw after 10 years of function. Clin Oral Implants Res. 2005;16:277–87.

Zitzmann NU, Marinello CP. A review of clinical and technical considerations for fixed and removable implant prostheses in the edentulous mandible. Int J Prosthodont 2002;15:65–72.

Grunder U. Immediate functional loading of immediate implants in edentulous arches: two year results. Int J Periodontics Restorative. Dent 2001;21:545–51.

Feine JS, Carlsson GE, editors. Implant overdentures: the standard of care for edentulous patients. Chicago, IL: Quintessence Pub. Co.; 2003. pp. 83–98.

Morais JA, Heydecke G, Pawliuk J, et al. The effects of mandibular two-implant overdentures on nutrition in elderly edentulous individuals. J Dent Res. 2003;82:53–8.

Watson GK, Payne AG, Purton DG, et al. Mandibular overdentures: comparative evaluation of prosthodontic maintenance of three different implants systems during the first year of service. Int J Prosthodont 2002;15:259–66.

Krennmair G, Weinlander M, Krainhofner M, et al. Implant-supported mandibular overdentures retained with ball or telescopic crown attachments: a 3-year prospective study. Int J Prosthodont 2006;19:164–70.

Jemt T, Chai J, Harnett J, et al. A 5-year prospective multicenter follow-up report on overdentures supported by osseointegrated implants. Int J Oral Maxillofac Implants 1996;11:291–8.

Cooper L, et al. Immediate mandibular rehabilitation with endosseous implants: simultaneous extraction, implant placement, and loading. Int J Oral Maxillofac Implants 2002;17:517–25.

Gulizio MP, Agar JR, Kelly JR, et al. Effect of implant angulation upon retention of overdenture attachments. J Prosthodont 2005;14:3–11.

Shor A, Goto Y, Shor K. Mandibular two-implant-retained overdenture: prosthetic design and fabrication protocol. Compend Contin Educ Dent 2007;28:80–8.

Implant impressions and prosthetics

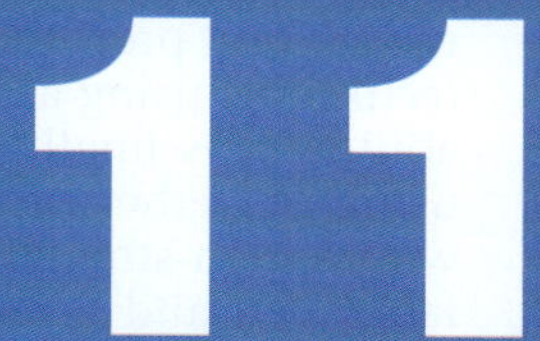

Ajay Vikram Singh

CHAPTER CONTENTS HD

Introduction

An accurate impression of the implant as well as the surrounding hard and soft tissue structures is known to be the backbone to deliver a desired implant prosthesis with an accurate fit and in harmony with the marginal soft tissues. Studies have shown that most implant practitioners do not give enough attention to implant impressions, and often the impressions sent to the dental laboratories show visible errors, which may result in multiple problems with implant restoration, such as nonpassive fit, incomplete seating, tight contact, improper retention, and an unharmonious prosthesis with marginal soft tissues.

More accurate transfer is required in the indirect impression technique (pick up technique) as any change in transferring the position and orientation of the post from the mouth to the impression and later on in the working cast, may end up with various prosthetic fabrication and fixing problems. With advancements in implant prosthetics, several types of implant prosthetic options are being offered, which require various types of implant and abutment level impressions to deliver a prosthesis with high accuracy. As described in earlier chapters, the implant differs from the natural tooth in not having any periodontal ligament; hence, any nonpassive prosthesis fitted over the implant does not shift the implant from its position like the natural tooth to relieve stress, but the stress gets transferred to the crestal bone with the implant and may result in crestal bone resorption. The type of impression selected, depends on the type of prosthesis the dentist has planned to use to restore the implant.

Many types of implant restorations are being done and the selection of a particular prosthesis largely depends on factors, such as the number of implants supporting the prosthesis, their insertion angulations and parallelism in respect to each other, soft tissue depth, available crown height space, the desired aesthetics, the position of the connection screw, the weight of the desired prosthesis, its profile, retrievability of the prosthesis, ease of repair, the prosthetic components available in the implant system and stress factors. Fabrication of implant restorations requires accurate impression transfer, good laboratory support, and effective communication between the restoring dentist and the laboratory technician.

There are many impression procedures for implant restoration and each has its own indications and advantages. The dentist should have a knowledge of how the impression for a particular implant should be made, in order to deliver a planned prosthesis with a high level of precision.

Impression materials

The impression of the implant should be made using rubber based impression materials as dimensional accuracy is required in the impression, to achieve predictable results in the fit and for precision in the implant prosthesis. Considering all the advantages, the following materials are preferred to make implant impressions:

1. **Polyether**: Being hydrophilic in nature, this is the material of choice for the implant impression, to accurately record and transfer the implant position and orientation from the patient's mouth to the working cast. The only disadvantage with this material is that it cannot be stored for a long time because the dimensions of this material start changing after few days, which may lead to inaccuracy of the prosthesis in precision of fit.
2. **Polyvinylsiloxane** (addition silicon): This is a material which is widely used to make implant impressions because of its dimensional accuracy, stability, and long storage life without any distortion in dimensions.

Implant impression procedures

There are many ways to make implant impressions and a particular method is chosen based on the requirements of the particular implant case.

1. **Direct/prepared abutment impression technique**: In the prepared abutment technique, the final abutment is fixed on top of the implant in the patient's mouth and prepared with a normal crown and bridge technique, using a diamond or carbide bur. Once the abutment is finally prepared, an impression is made using polyether or addition silicon material, poured with a high-strength stone material. The prosthesis is fabricated and cemented in the mouth by following crown and bridge technique steps.

   Indications
   a. Single-body/one-piece implant.
   b. Implant in nonaesthetic posterior region.
   c. Cement-retained prosthesis where high precision is not a concern.
2. **Indirect/pick-up impression technique**: This is the most common impression technique in implant practised and practised in most dental implant cases, as it precisely and accurately transfers the implant position and orientation from the patient's mouth to the working cast. The impression should be recorded using a rigid impression material expressed around the impression components as well as in the tray. This impression can be made using either an open tray or closed tray technique.
   a. **Closed tray technique**: An impression material with soft to medium consistency (less rigid) should be used in the closed tray technique, for ease of removal from the mouth without any tearing of the impression around the impression posts. The gingival former is removed from the implant in the patient's mouth and a closed tray impression transfer abutment is inserted onto the implant using a connection screw. The accurate and complete seating of the impression abutment on the implant should be checked with a radiograph. An impression of this impression abutment using polyether or addition silicon material is made. After successfully recording the impression, the impression abutment is removed from the implant and assembled with an appropriate implant analogue. The impression abutment–analogue assembly is reinserted at the corresponding location in the impression, making sure that the impression transfer abutment is inserted with the same orientation as in the mouth. The impression is sent to the dental laboratory to fabricate the working model. It is recommended to pour a soft tissue replicating material (Multisil from Bredent, Germany) around the implant analogue because it facilitates the removal of the impression abutment after the stone die is poured and provides ease of working to the laboratory technician, to the level of implant abutment connection.
   b. **Open tray technique**: The open tray technique transfers the implant position and orientation more precisely and accurately than the closed technique and thus should be followed when a higher level of accuracy is required. It is required to be followed when castable implant components ,which need a high level of precision to accurately seat the finally cast prosthesis onto the implants in the mouth, are used. This technique should also be followed in cases of multiple implants inserted at different angulations, as the closed tray technique may tear the impression in such cases on removal from the mouth. The open tray technique is also helpful if the implants are seated very deep in the soft tissue, as this causes the emergence of a very short part of the closed tray impression abutment out of the thick soft tissue, which hardly gets engaged firmly in the impression.

   Indications
   i. Multiple number of implants which are not parallel to each other.
   ii. Full arch implant supported fixed prosthesis.
   iii. Abutment level impressions of multiple to full arch implant case.
   iv. Joint screw-retained prosthesis over multiple implants.
   v. Deep seated implants.

Implant versus abutment level impression

In most implant cases implant level impressions are made where the impression abutments are inserted to the implant, and after recording open or closed tray pick-up impression, these impression abutments are removed from the implant and assembled with the implant analogue. The abutment level impression technique is practised in cases of screw-retained multiple unit to full arch joint implant prosthesis. In this technique, the gingival formers/healing abutments are removed from the implants and replaced with the appropriate abutments which are called 'abutment for screw.' At one side this abutment for screw is screwed to the implant in the mouth and on top of it another abutment or the prosthesis is fixed using the connection screw. Thus after these abutments for screw are inserted on top of implants, the impression posts are screwed over these abutments and an abutment level impression with closed or open technique is made. After successfully recording the impression, the impression posts are assembled with the 'abutment analogue' and the impression is poured in the usual fashion. The restoration is then fabricated over the abutment analogues on the working model and fixed over the abutments for screw in the patient's mouth.

A. Steps for the fabrication of a cement-retained prosthesis with the direct/prepared abutment technique:
   Step 1: One piece implant in the mouth or gingival former is removed and the final abutment is fixed over the two-piece implant.
   Step 2: The implant abutment is prepared in the mouth using carbide or diamond burs in the usual fashion, as in the natural tooth preparation with high speed turbine.
   Step 3: The impression of this prepared abutment is made using silicon material similar to the usual crown and bridge cases.

Step 4: The impression is poured, using a high strength stone, to make a working cast.

Step 5: The prosthesis is fabricated similar to the crown and bridge in the laboratory, and is fixed over the implant abutment using appropriate luting cement, following the principles of normal crown and bridge technique (Figs 11.1–11.4).

B. Steps for the fabrication of a cement-retained prosthesis with the closed tray implant level impression technique:

Step 1: The gingival former is removed from the implant and a closed tray impression post is inserted on top of the implant. The impression is made using silicon impression material (polyether or addition silicon).

Step 2: The impression post is removed from the mouth and assembled with an appropriate implant analogue. The post assembled with the analogue is inserted into the impression at the correct position and with correct orientation.

Step 3: The impression is poured using high strength stone plaster, after the pouring of gingival mask around the post–analogue connection. Working cast is removed after it has hardened.

Step 4: The impression post is removed from the analogue leaving the analogue in the stone cast. An appropriate final metal abutment is selected and screwed over the analogue, using the connection screw.

Step 5: The final abutment is prepared and the desired prosthesis (porcelain-fused-to-metal [PFM] or metal free zirconium) is fabricated over it.

Step 6: The abutment is transferred to the implant in the patient's mouth with the same orientation as on the cast. The connection screw is finally tightened at the moment of 30–35 Ncm using mechanical driver and the screw hole of the abutment is

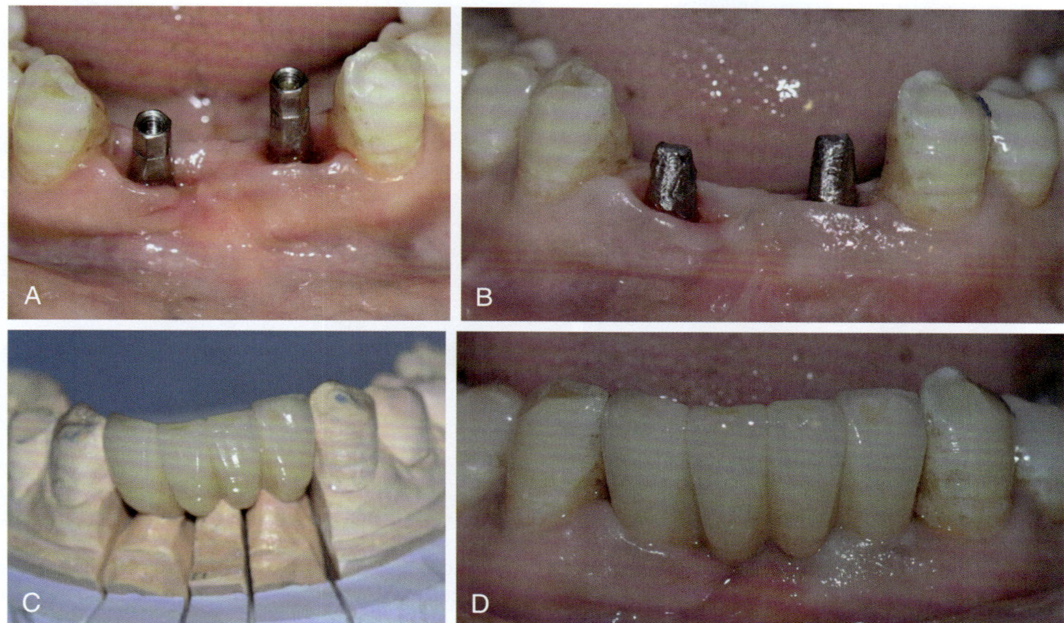

Fig 11.1 (A and B) Abutments of single-piece implants are prepared in the mouth. (C) Impression is made with the prepared abutment technique and sent to the dental laboratory where the technician poured the impression using high strength stone and fabricated the four-unit ceramic bridge prosthesis. (D) The prosthesis is fixed over the implants using dual cure resin cement.

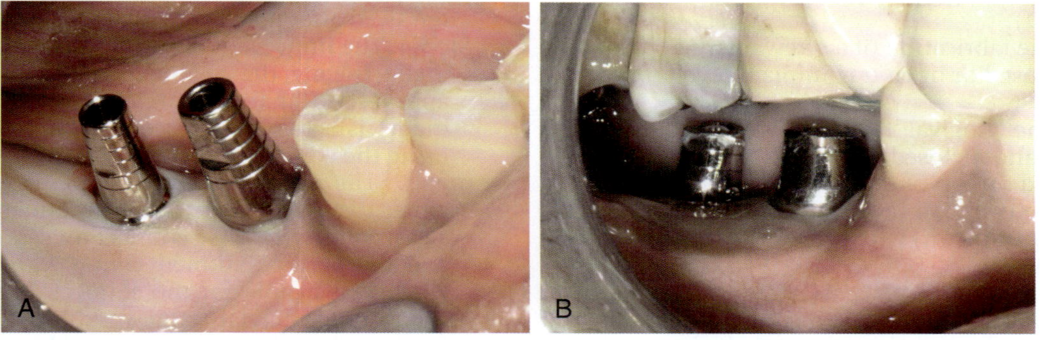

Fig 11.2 (A) The healing abutments are removed and replaced with the appropriate final abutment over the two-piece implants. (B) The abutments are prepared in the mouth using high speed turbine with carbide/diamond burs.

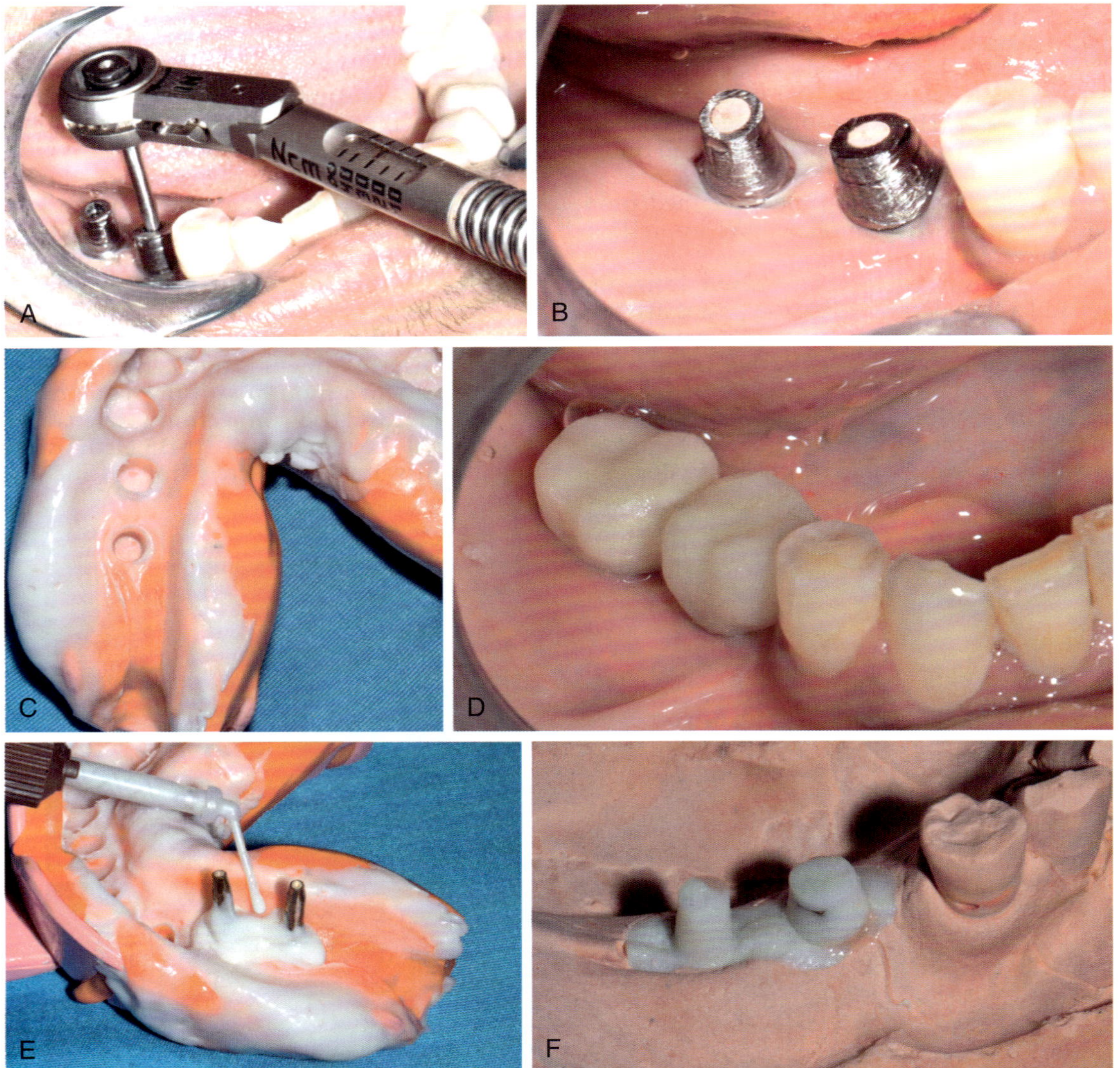

Fig 11.3 (A) The connection screw is finally tightened, using a mechanical torque ratchet, at 35 Ncm (B) the screw holes are filled using gutta-percha and (C) impression is made in silicon material. (D) A provisional prosthesis in function is fixed over the abutments which also avoids oral soft tissue abrasions with the abutment. (E) The abutment region of the impression is poured using the high strength core build-up material or pattern resin with dia pins inserted into it. (F) The impression is further poured with dia stone and a working cast is prepared.

sealed using retrievable material such as gutta-percha or wax. The prosthesis is fixed over the abutment using appropriate luting cement. (Figs 11.5–11.9).

c. Steps for the fabrication of a screw retained prosthesis with the closed or open tray implant level impression technique

Step 1: The gingival former is removed from the implant and a closed or open tray impression post is inserted on top of the implant. The impression is made using silicon impression material (polyether or addition silicon) with open or closed impression technique.

Step 2: The impression post is assembled with an appropriate implant analogue. The post assembled with the analogue is inserted into the impression at the correct position and with correct orientation, if closed tray technique is used.

Step 3: The impression is poured using high strength stone plaster, after pouring the gingival mask around the post–analogue connection. The working cast is removed after it has hardened.

Step 4: The impression post is removed from the analogue leaving the analogue in the stone cast. An appropriate final castable abutment (plastic abutment) is selected and screwed over the analogue, using the connection screw.

Step 5: The plastic abutment is prepared and a wax pattern is built up onto this abutment to fabricate a cast framework. The connection screw is removed and the plastic abutment along with wax pattern, which has a hole for the connection screw, is cast to fabricate a metal framework, just like the metal framework of the PFM crown and bridge prosthesis.

Step 6: The try-in of the metal framework is done in the patient's mouth to check its accurate and passive

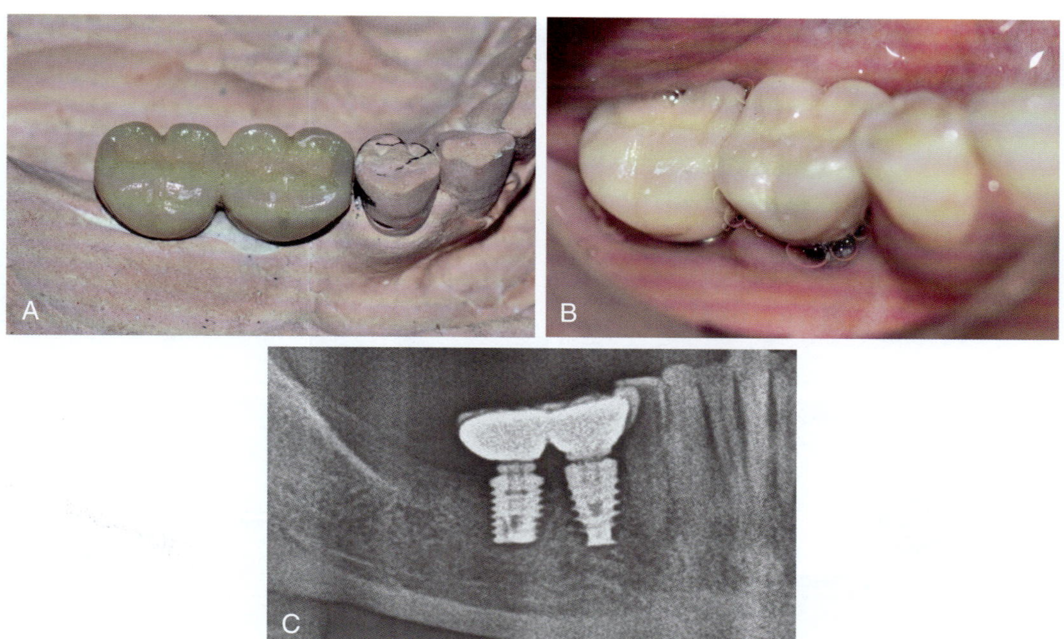

Fig 11.4 (A) A PFM prosthesis is fabricated over the cast, (B) which is transferred and fixed over the implant abutments in the mouth following normal crown and bridge technique. (C) Post loading radiograph.

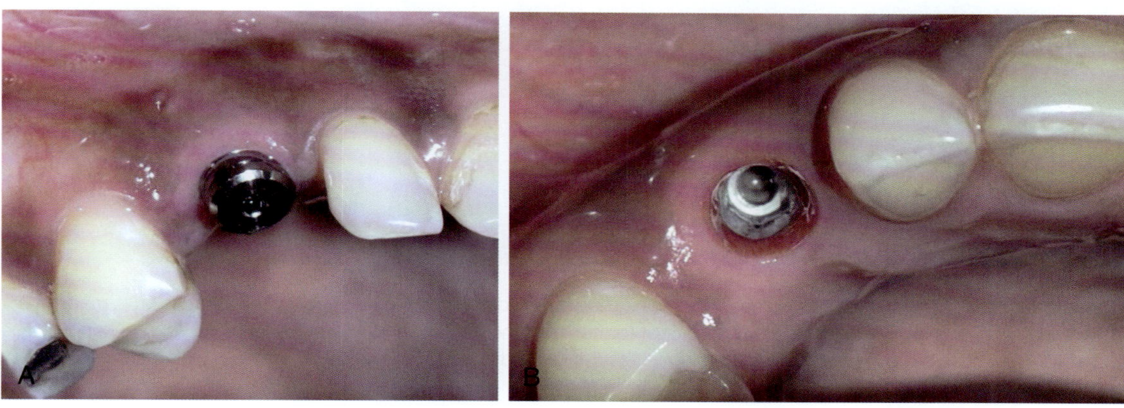

Fig 11.5 (A and B) Gingival former (healing abutment) is removed from the implant.

seating over the implant. To fabricate the final prosthesis, the ceramic build-up (for the PFM prosthesis) or an acrylic denture curing (for the hybrid prosthesis) is done over this framework, preserving the patency of the connection screw holes.

Step 7: The final prosthesis is fixed in the patient's mouth over the implants using connection screws, and the screw holes of the prosthesis are filled first with gutta-percha and then with a composite of a blending shade (Figs 11.10–11.16)

D. Steps for the fabrication of a screw-retained prosthesis with the closed or open tray abutment level impression technique:

Step 1: The gingival formers are removed from the implants and replaced with the abutments for screw. Alternatively the abutments for screw are placed on top of implants immediately after implant insertion or uncovery.

Step 2: Either closed or open tray impression posts are placed on top of these abutments. The impression is made using silicon impression material (polyether or addition silicon) with open or closed impression technique.

Step 3: The impression posts are assembled with abutment analogues. The posts are assembled with the abutment for screw analogues and inserted into the impression at the correct position and with correct orientation, if the closed tray technique is practised.

Step 4: The impression is poured using high strength stone plaster, after the pouring of the gingival mask around the post–analogue connections. The working cast is removed after it has hardened.

Step 5: The impression posts are removed from the analogue leaving the analogues in the stone cast. The appropriate final castable abutments (plastic

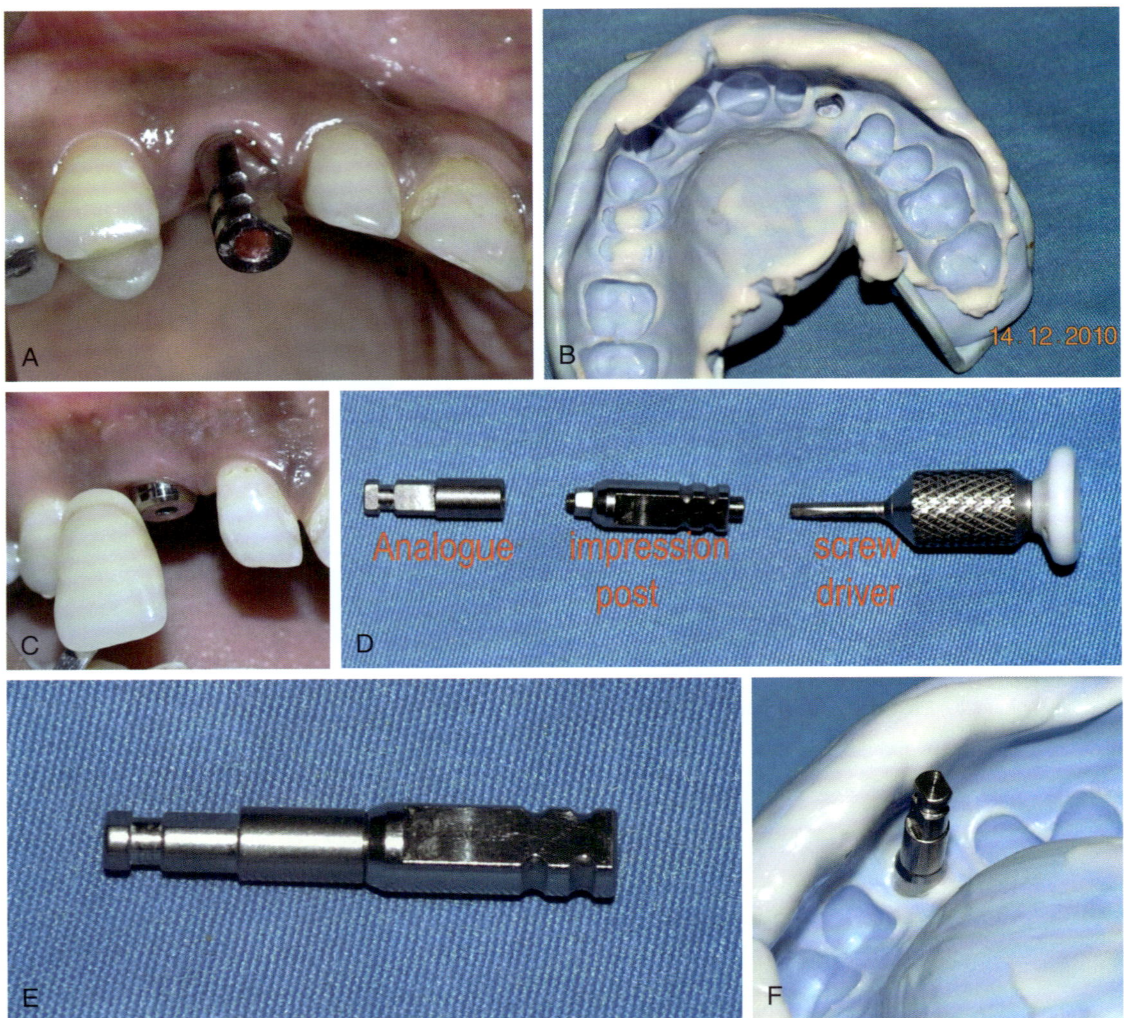

Fig 11.6 (A) The impression post for closed tray impression technique is inserted over the implant and (B) the impression is made in addition silicon material. (C) The impression post is again replaced with gingival former over the implant and shade selection is done. (D and E) The impression post is assembled with an appropriate implant analogue using a screwdriver and (F) inserted into the impression with the same orientation as in the mouth.

abutments) are selected and screwed over the abutment analogues using the connection screw.

Step 6: The plastic abutments are prepared and a wax pattern is built up onto these abutments to fabricate a cast framework. The connection screws are removed and the plastic abutments along with the wax pattern, which has a hole for the connection screw, are cast to fabricate a metal framework, just like the metal framework of the PFM crown and bridge prosthesis.

Step 7: The try-in of the metal framework is done in the patient's mouth to check its accurate and passive seating over the implants. To fabricate the final prosthesis, the ceramic build-up (for the PFM prosthesis) or an acrylic denture curing (for the hybrid prosthesis) is done over this framework, preserving the patency of the connection screw holes.

Step 8: The final prosthesis is fixed in the patient's mouth over the implants using connection screws and the screw holes of the prosthesis are filled first with gutta-percha and then using a composite of a blending shade (Figs 11.17–11.21).

E. Steps for stabilizing dentures over implants (ball and socket type):

1. **Direct technique**

Step 1: The gingival formers are removed from the implants and replaced with ball abutments. Alternatively the ball abutments are inserted over the implants immediately after the implant insertion or at the stage of implant uncovery.

Step 2: The 'O' rings with retention rubbers within or metal housings with plastic housings within are seated on top of the ball abutments. The tissue surface of the patient's denture is prepared in such a way that it can be passively seated over the ridge with a minimum 2 mm space all around the 'O' rings or metal housings for the acrylic.

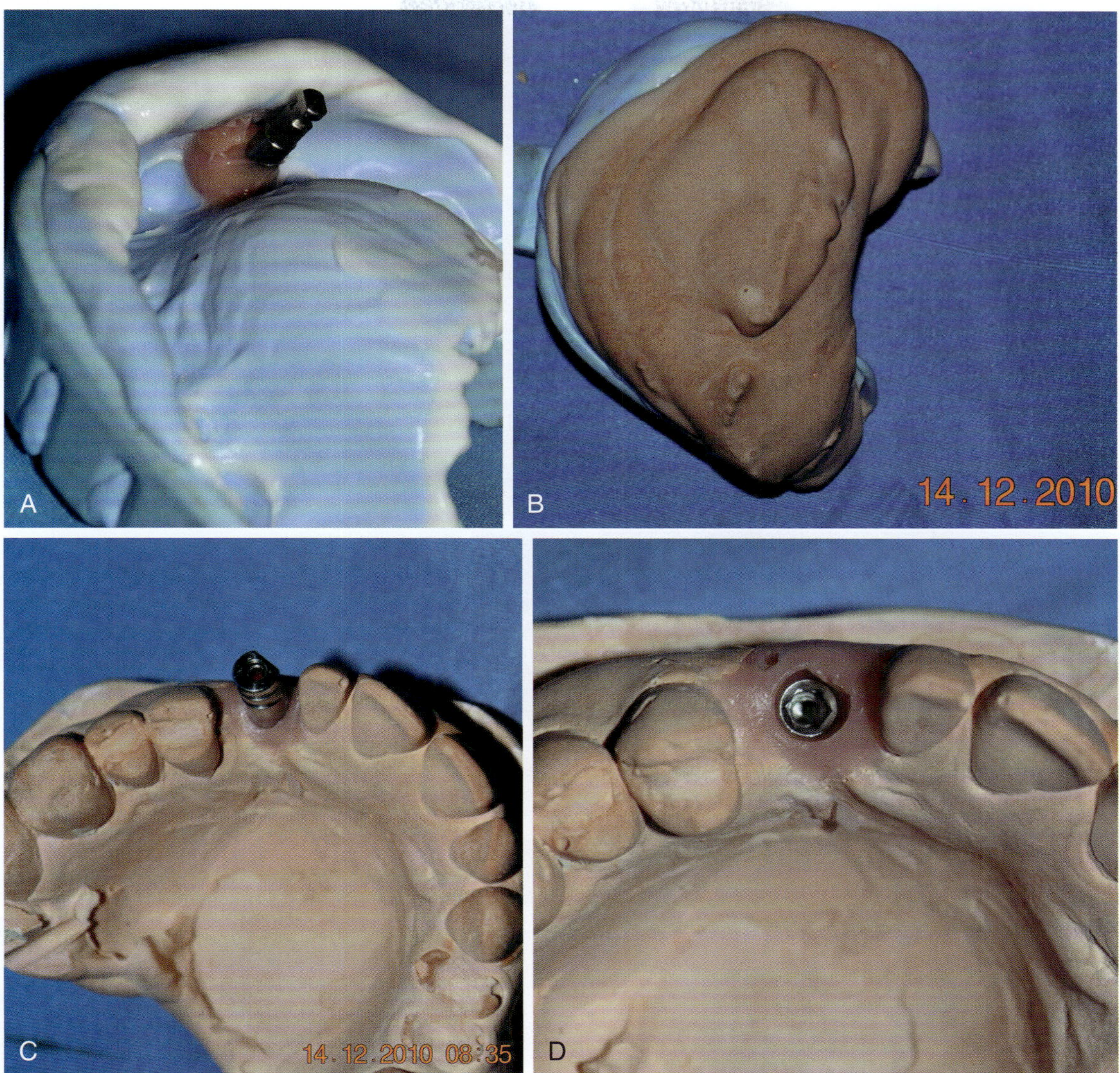

Fig 11.7 (A) A soft tissue masking material (Gi-Mask, Coltene Whaledent or Multisil, Bredent) is poured around the impression post to the level of post–analogue connection. (B) The impression is poured further using the stone. (C and D) The impression post, which accurately has transferred the position and orientation of implant connection from the patient's mouth to the working cast, is removed from the analogue.

Step 3: Self-cure acrylic is filled into the prepared tissue surface of the denture and the denture is seated over the metal housings in the correct occlusion.

Step 4: After the acrylic has set, the denture is removed from the mouth carrying the metal housings within the tissue surface of the denture.

Step 5: The denture is finished, polished, and seated in the mouth. The relative housings get locked over the ball abutments and provide adequate retention to the denture. (Figs 11.22–11.25).

2. **Indirect technique**: In the indirect technique for implant overdenture, the impression of the implants is made with open or closed impression technique using impression posts and sent to the laboratory. In the laboratory, the technician assembles the posts with analogues and pours the impression using high strength stone plaster. The technician places the ball abutments and metal housings over the model and reduces the denture surface. Then he/she fixes the metal housing in the tissue surface of the denture using cold or heat cure resin and sends the denture with the metal housings within, back to the clinician. The dentist transfers the ball abutments from the model to the implants with the similar orientation and at similar positions. The denture is seated over the abutments in the patient's mouth.

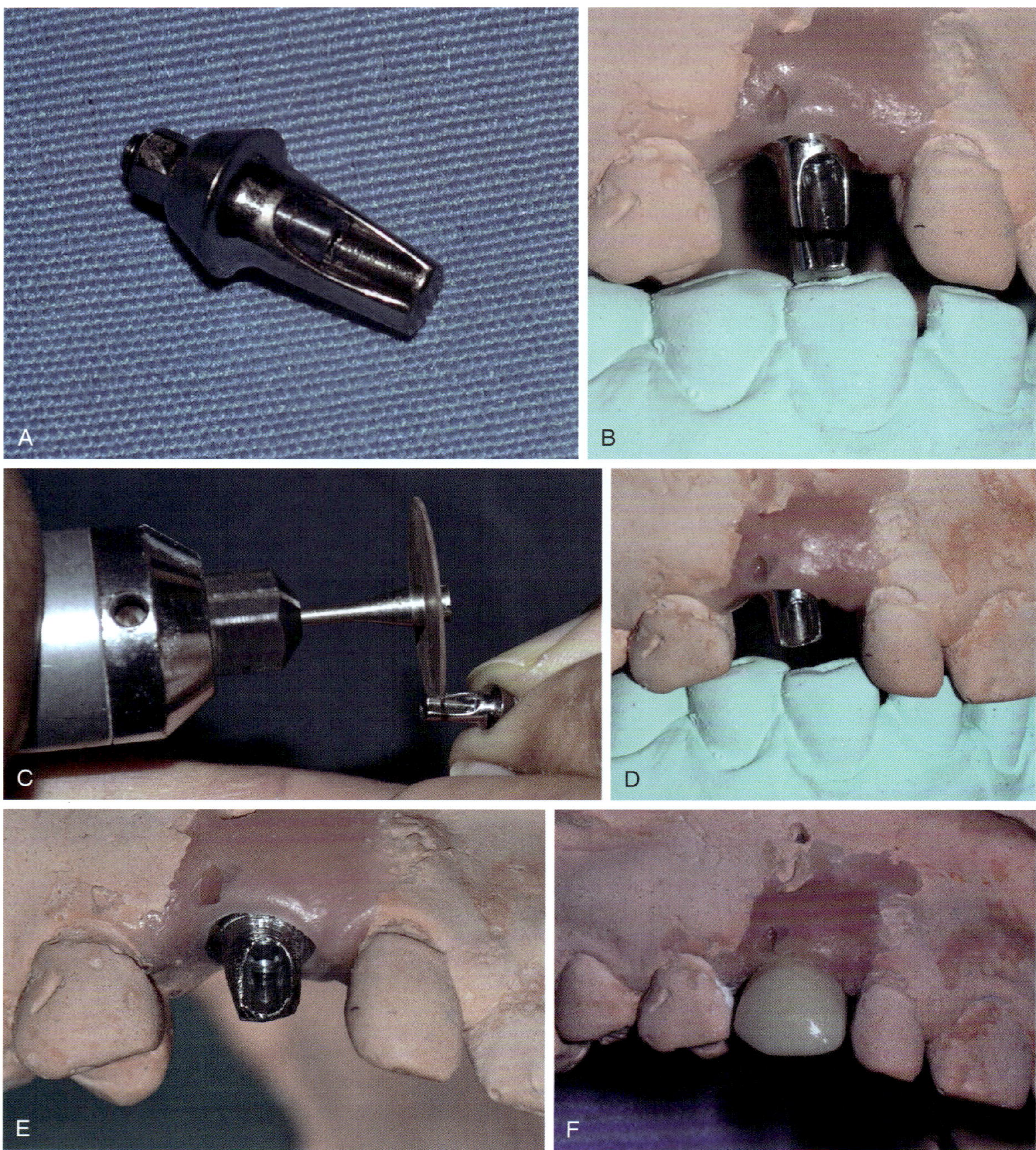

Fig 11.8 (A) An appropriate final abutment is selected and (B) fixed over the analogue. (C and D) The height of the abutment is marked and reduced. (E) The abutment is further prepared like a normal crown abutment preparation. For the abutment cutting and preparation, it should be removed from the analogue and assembled with another analogue because vibration can loosen the analogue within the stone cast. (F) A ceramic prosthesis is fabricated over the abutment.

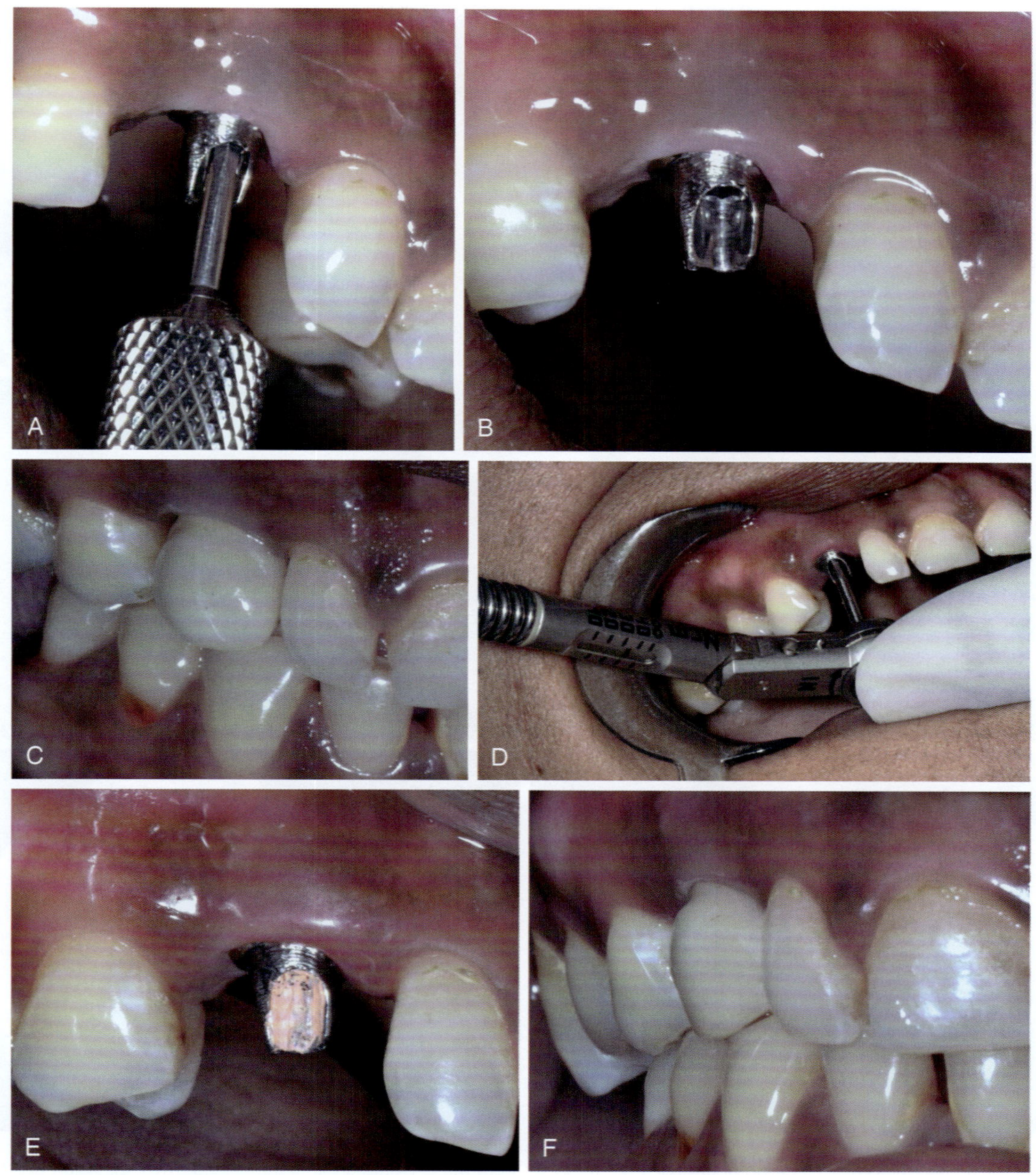

Fig 11.9 (A and B) The abutment is transferred to the implant with correct orientation and (C) the try-in of the prosthesis is done to check for its fitting. All the required occlusal adjustments are done. (D) The connection screw is finally tightened at 35 Ncm using a torque ratchet. (E) The screw hole is filled using warm gutta-percha and (F) the prosthesis is fixed over the abutment using glass ionomer luting cement.

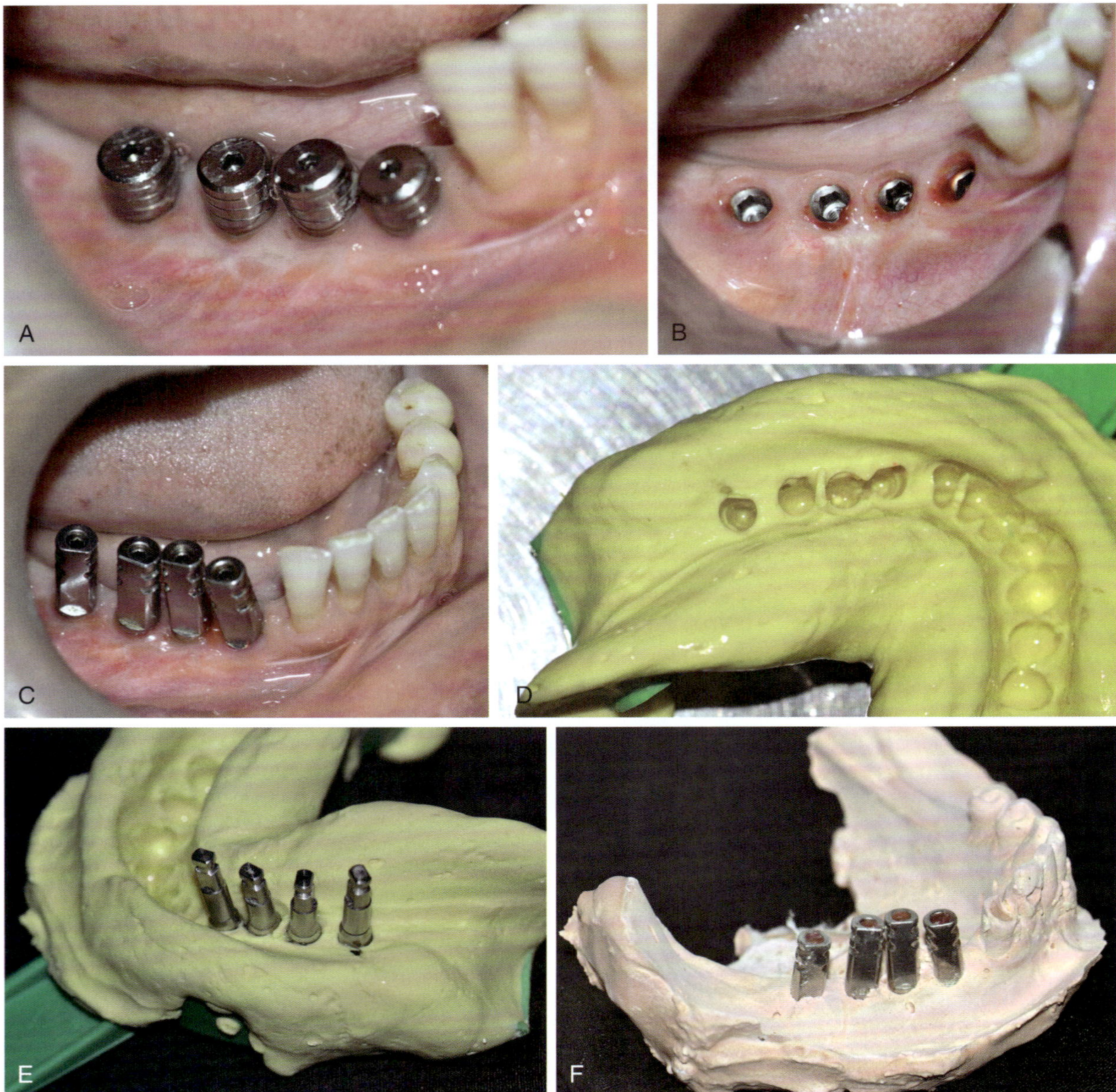

Fig 11.10 (A and B) Gingival formers (healing abutments) are removed from the implants and (C) the closed tray impression posts are inserted. (D) A closed tray impression is made and (E) the posts assembled with implant analogues are inserted into the impression with correct position and (F) orientation to prepare a stone cast.

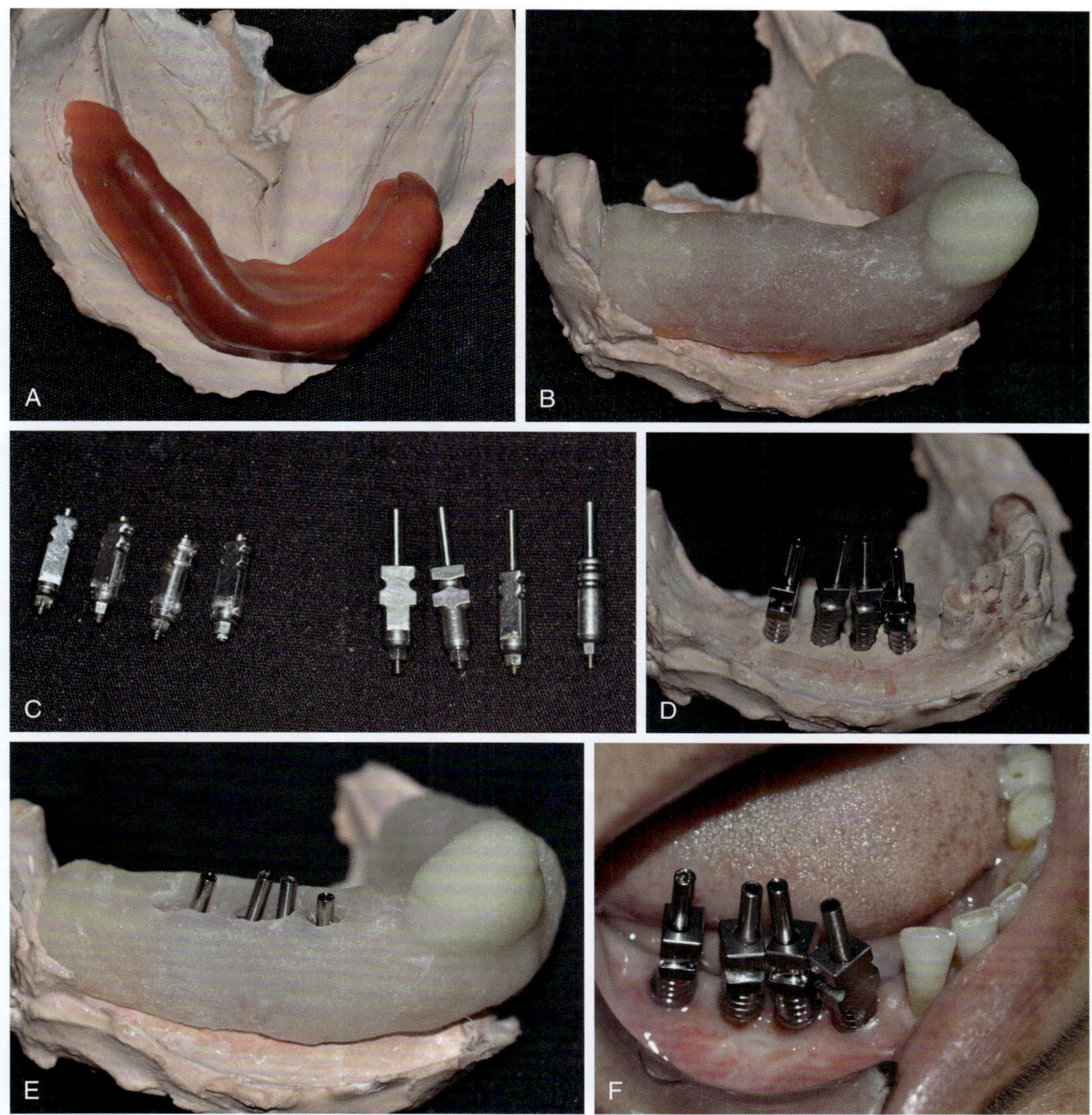

Fig 11.11 (A) Wax is used as the spacer and to block the undercuts, and (B) a special tray is fabricated over the cast. (C and D) The closed tray impression posts are removed from the cast and replaced with the open tray impression posts. (E) The spacer is removed from the special tray and holes are prepared over the implant sites, so that the long connection screws of the impression posts emerge out and above the impression tray. (F) The open tray impression posts are inserted over the implants in the patient's mouth.

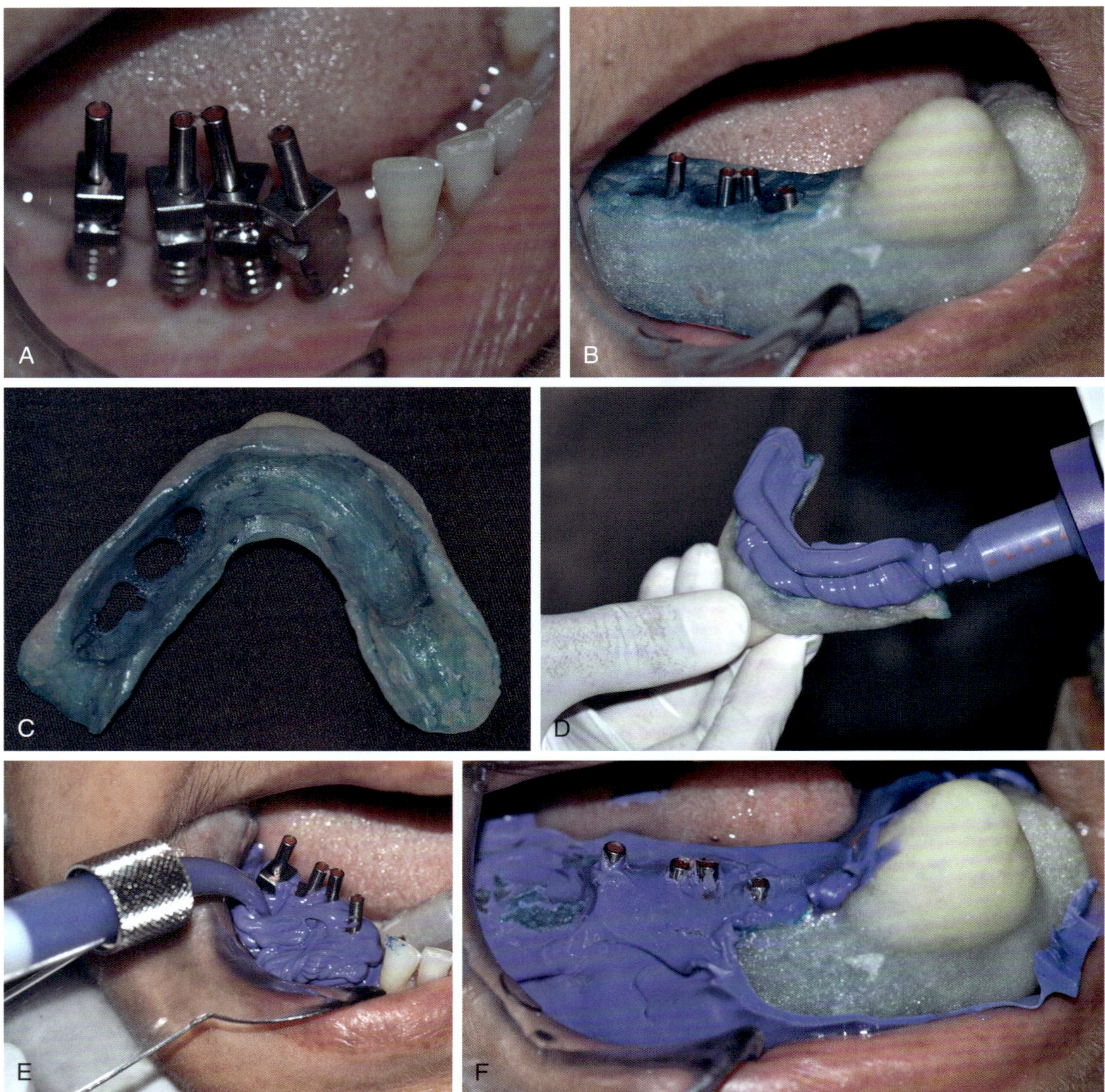

Fig 11.12 (A) The screw holes are blocked using wax and (B) try-in, for complete and passive seating of the special tray, is done. (C) A tray adhesive should be used on the inner surface and edges of the tray. (D–F) The impression is made using polyether (3M ESPE, Impregum Penta) impression material with the post screws emerging out and above the impression.

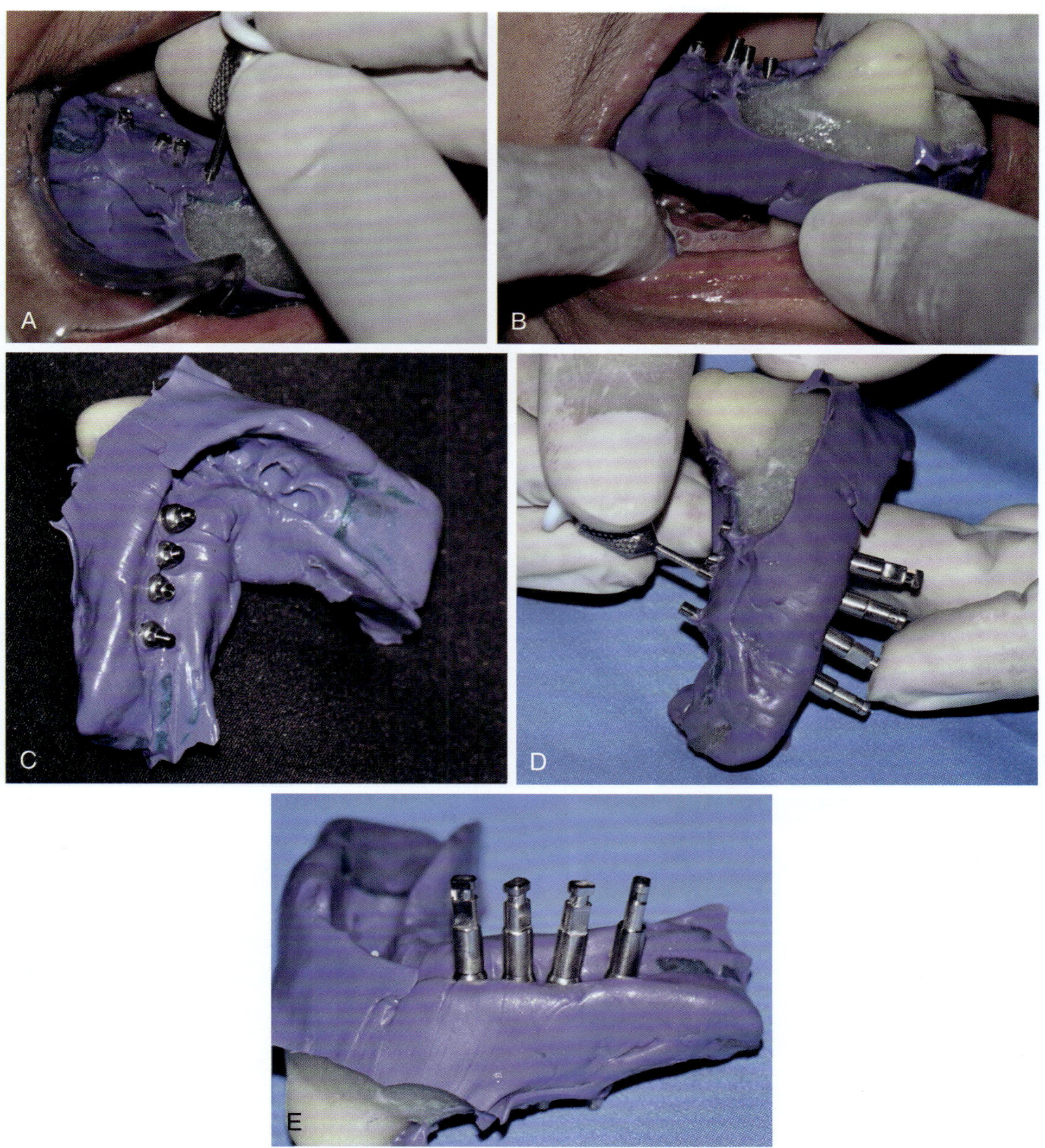

Fig 11.13 (A) All the connection screws should be unscrewed from the implants, (B) before removing the impression from the patient's mouth. (C) On removing the impression from the patient's mouth, the open tray posts come out firmly engaged within the impression. (D and E) The analogues are assembled with the posts and connection screws are tightened.

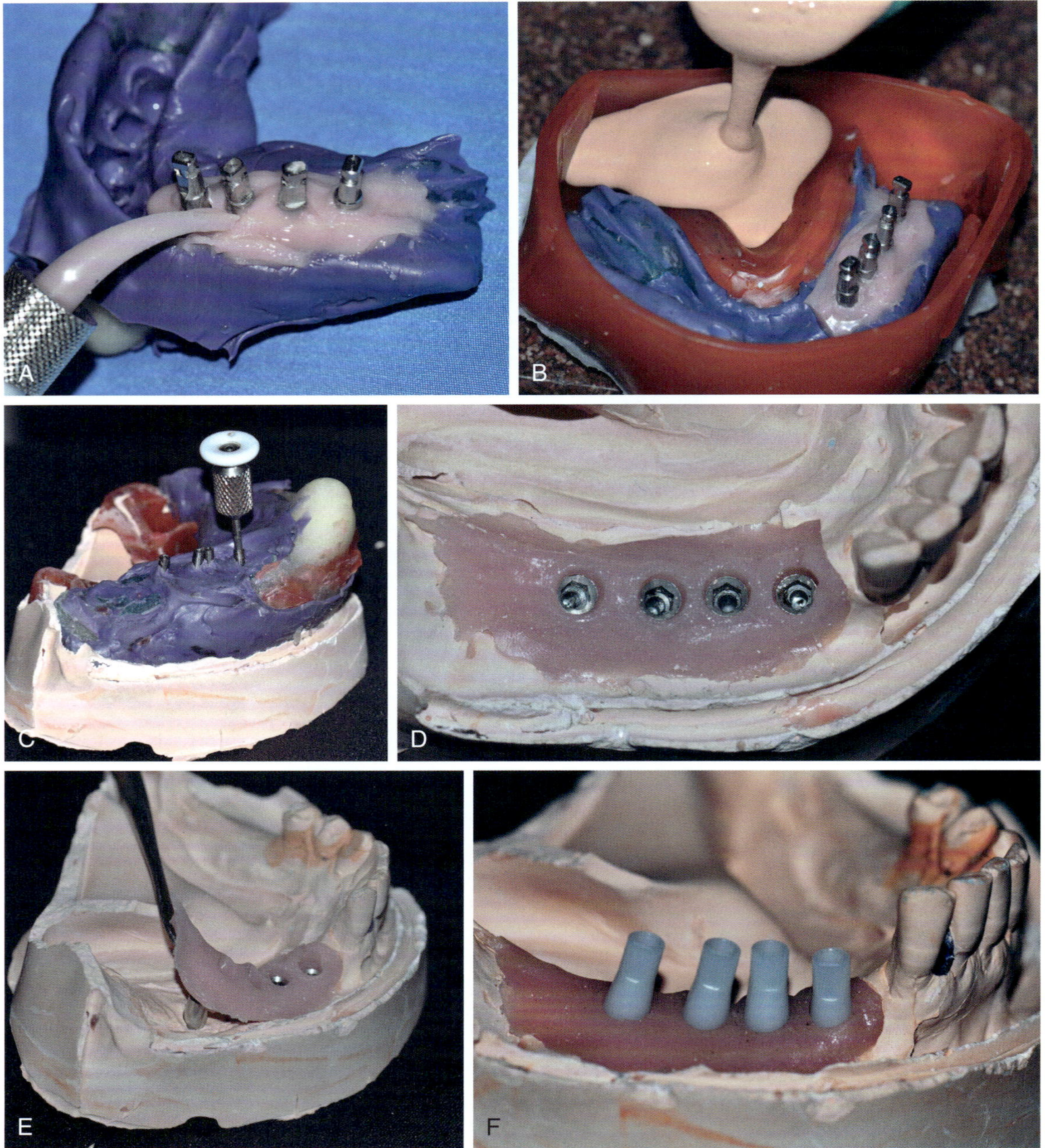

Fig 11.14 (A) First, a soft tissue replicating material (Multisil Mask, Bredent, Germany) should be poured around the post analogue connections in the impression (B) followed by the pouring of the impression using high strength stone material. (C and D) Again the post screws should be unscrewed from the analogues before removing the impression from the cast. (E) Use of soft tissue replicating material has the advantages of easy removal of the posts from the analogues without cast material fracture, easy visualization and working at the analogue platform by the laboratory technician as this material can be removed and replaced as many time as required without any distortion. (F) The appropriate castable plastic abutments are inserted over the analogues and fixed using titanium connection screws.

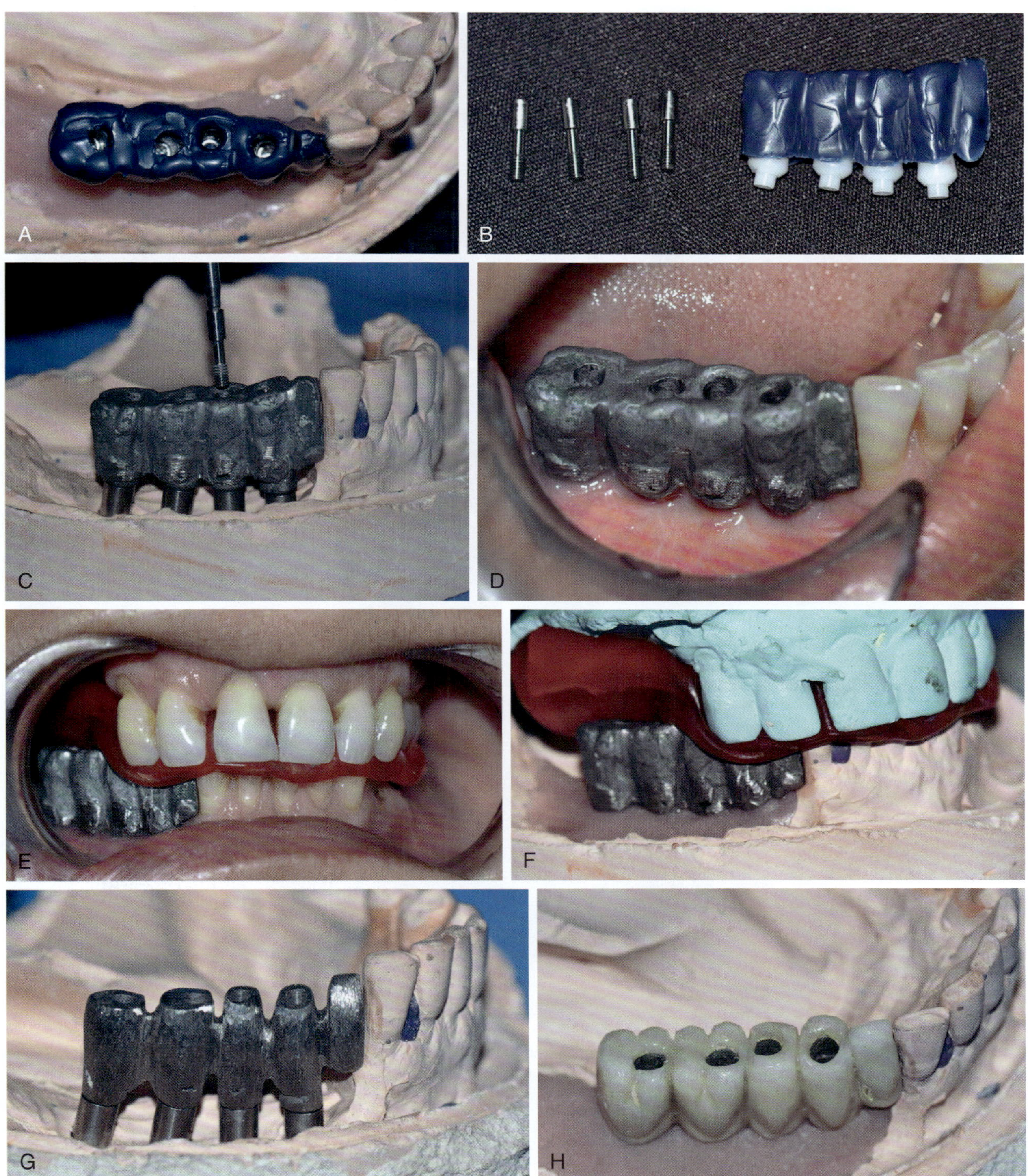

Fig 11.15 (A) The wax pattern is prepared over the abutments and (B) the abutments along with the pattern are removed from the cast. The connection screws are removed from the pattern and the pattern along with castable abutments are cast to a metal framework preserving the holes for the connection screws. (C and D) The complete and passive seating of metal framework is checked over the model as well as in the patient's mouth. The radiograph should be taken to make sure the cast framework is completely seated over the implants. (E and F) The bite registration is done and transferred to the cast to articulate the models in the correct centric position. (G) The required shaping and finishing of the metal framework is done and (H) the ceramic build-up is done over it, preserving the screw holes.

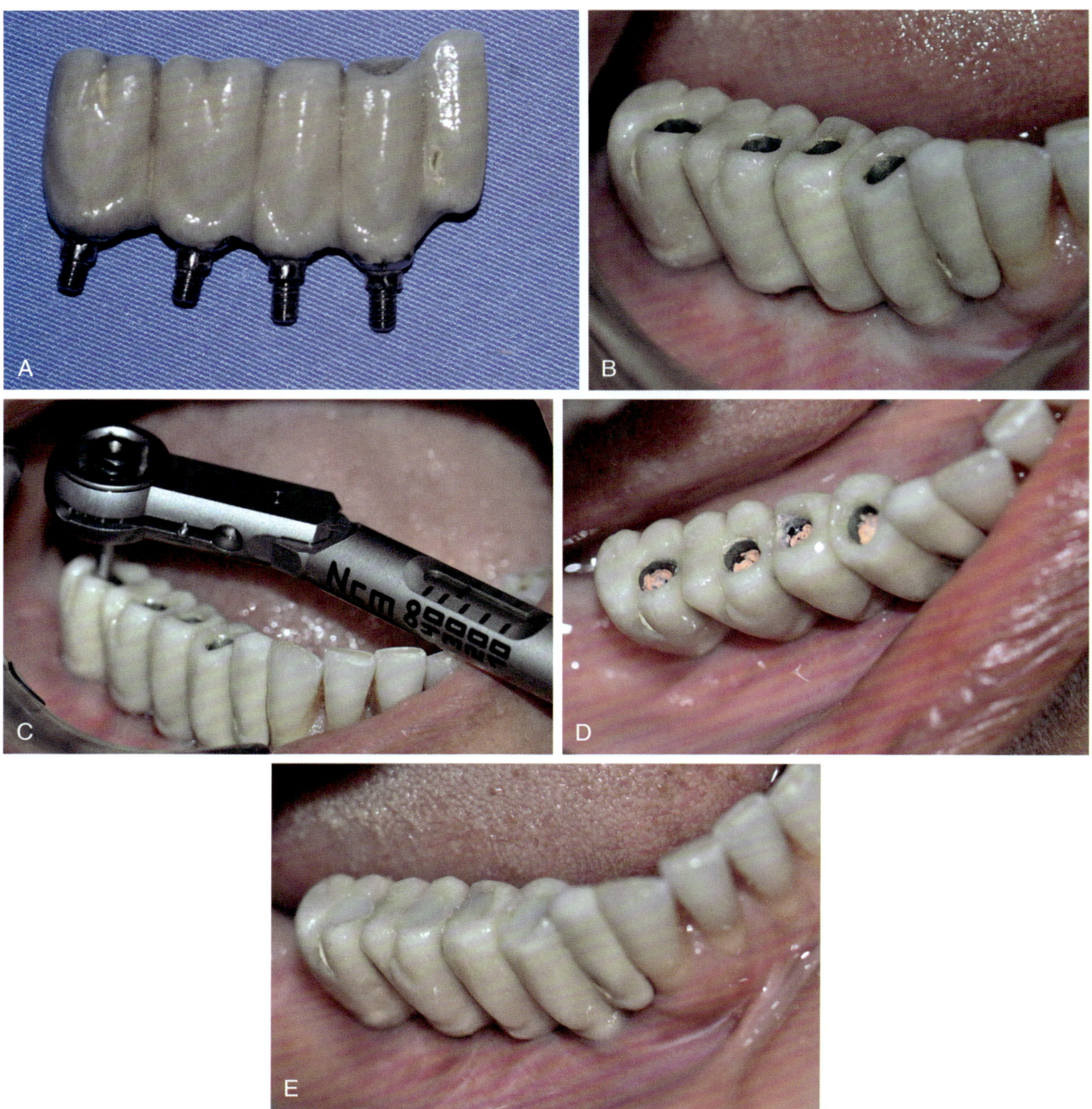

Fig 11.16 (A) The prosthesis is removed from the cast and (B) transferred to the implants in the patient's mouth. (C) The connection screws are finally tightened at 35 Ncm using a torque ratchet. (D) The screw holes are first filled with gutta-percha (E) followed by light cure composite resin.

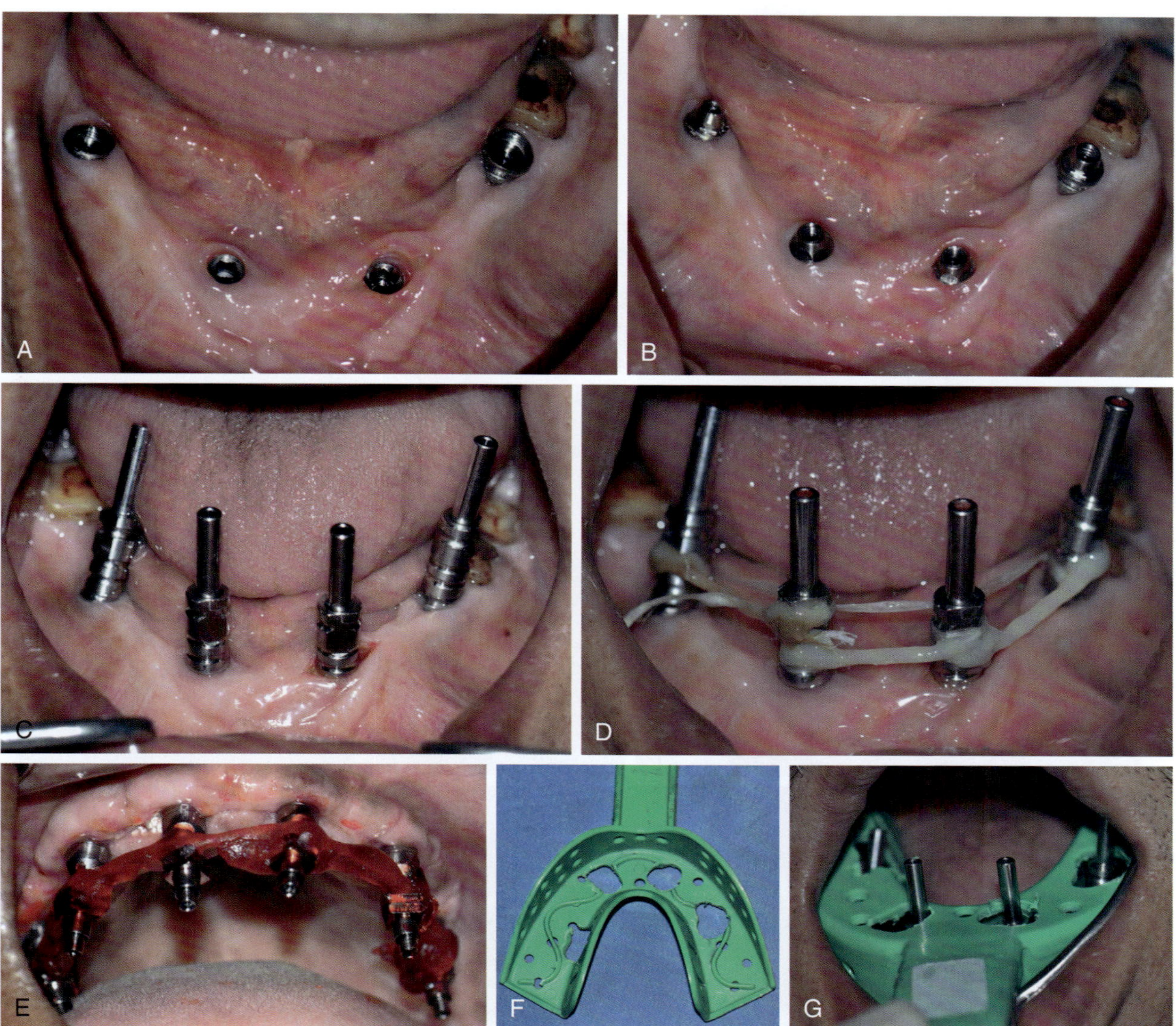

Fig 11.17 (A and B) Healing abutments are removed from the implants and 'abutments for screw' are inserted over the implants. (C) The open tray impression posts are placed on top of the abutments for screw. (D) Before making the impression, the impression posts should be splinted together using a light cure flow composite, self-cure acrylic, or (E) pattern resin to avoid any movement of the posts within the impression. The holes are prepared through a custom tray at the impression posts site and the tray is tried in the patient's mouth for passive seating. (F and G) The long fixation screws of the posts emerge out and above the impression tray.

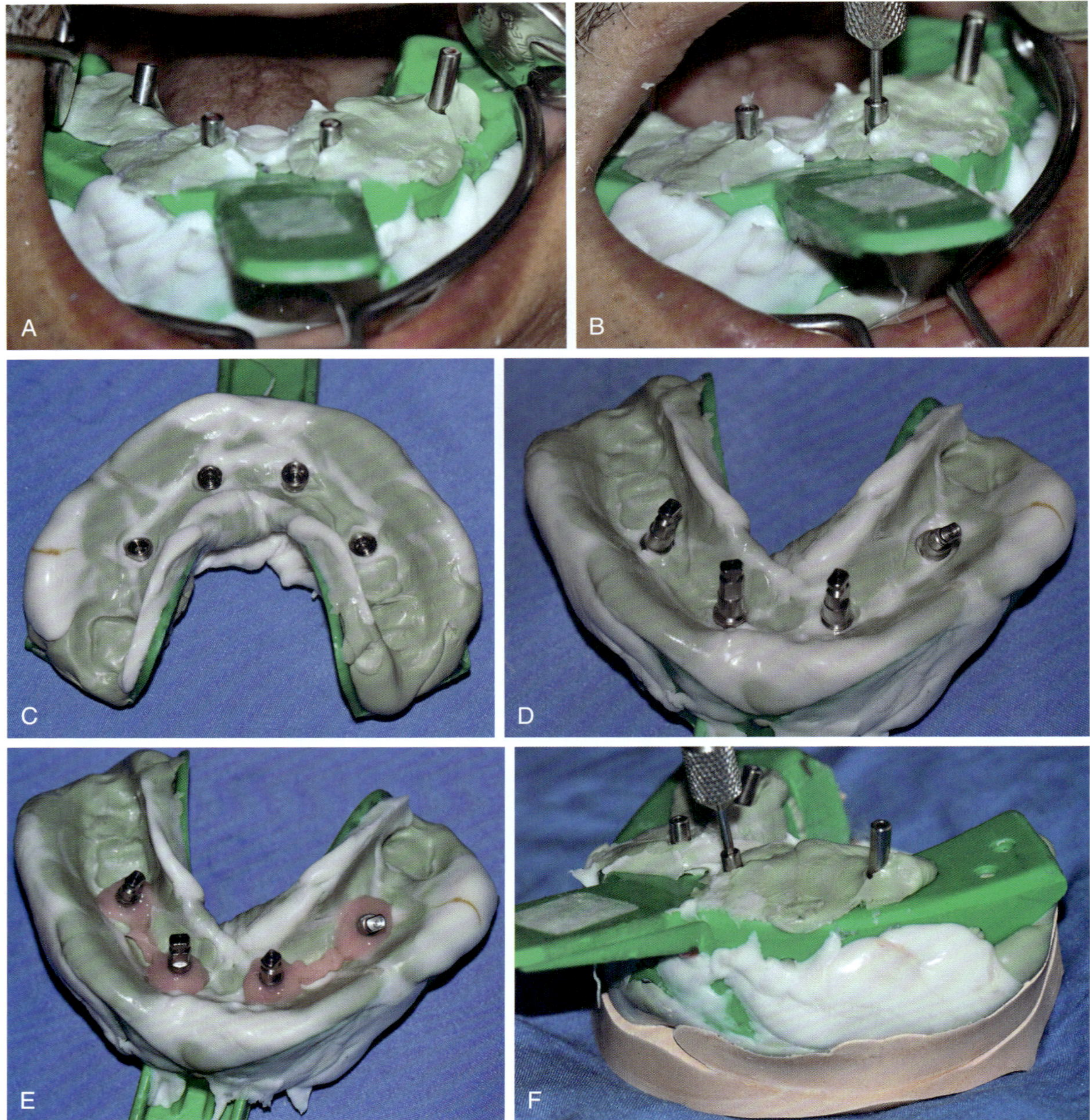

Fig 11.18 (A) The impression is made using addition silicon material with the long connection screws of the impression posts emerging out and above the impression. (B) The fixation screws should be unscrewed from the abutments for screw before removing the impression from the patient's mouth. (C and D) The impression posts, which come out within the impression are assembled with the abutment for screw analogues. (E) The soft tissue replicating material is poured around the post–analogue connections before impression is poured using the stone. (F) The fixation screws should be unscrewed from the analogues before removing the impression from the working cast.

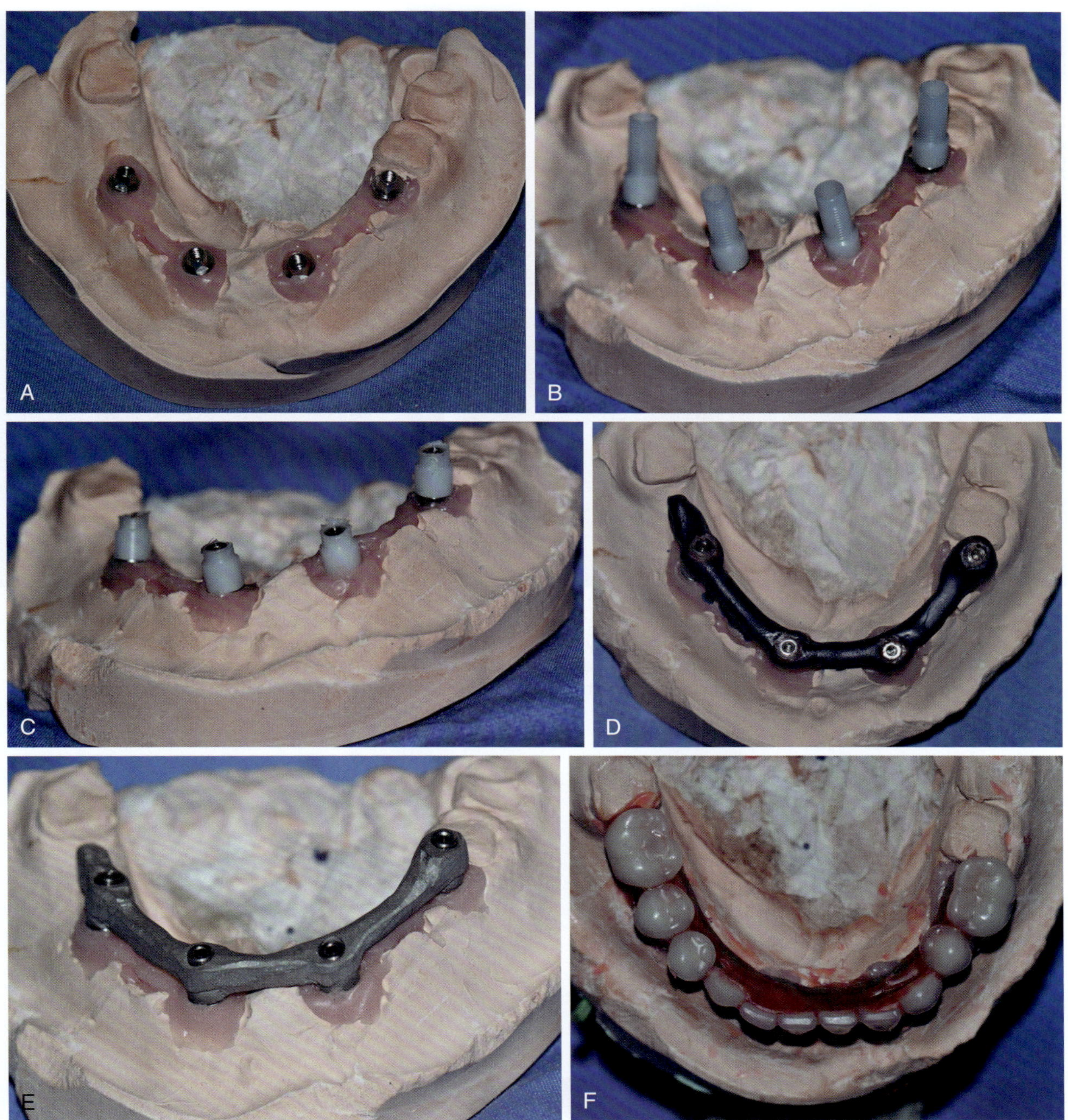

Fig 11.19 (A and B) The castable plastic abutments are screwed on top of abutment analogues on the working cast and (C) reduced to the planned height. (D) The wax pattern is prepared onto the castable abutments and (E) cast to fabricate a cast metal framework. (F) The teeth set-up is done over the cast framework to fabricate a screw-retained hybrid prosthesis.

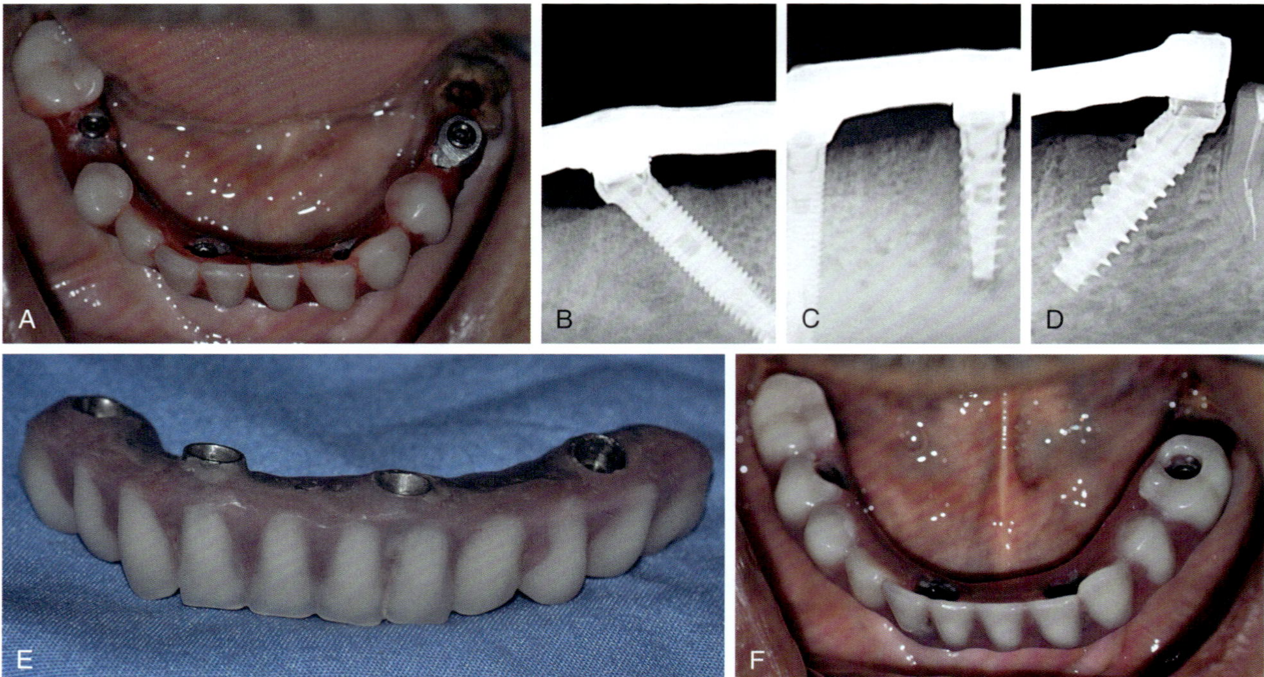

Fig 11.20 (A) The try-in of the framework along with teeth set up is done in the patient's mouth to check accurate and passive seating over the abutments for screw. The teeth from the wax can be removed during try-in at the sites where the teeth come over the screw holes. (B–D) Radiographs are taken to evaluate the complete seating of the framework onto the abutments for screw. (E) The teeth set-up is acrylized over the metal framework to finally fabricate the hybrid prosthesis. (F) The prosthesis is fixed in the mouth over the abutments for screws, using the connection screws.

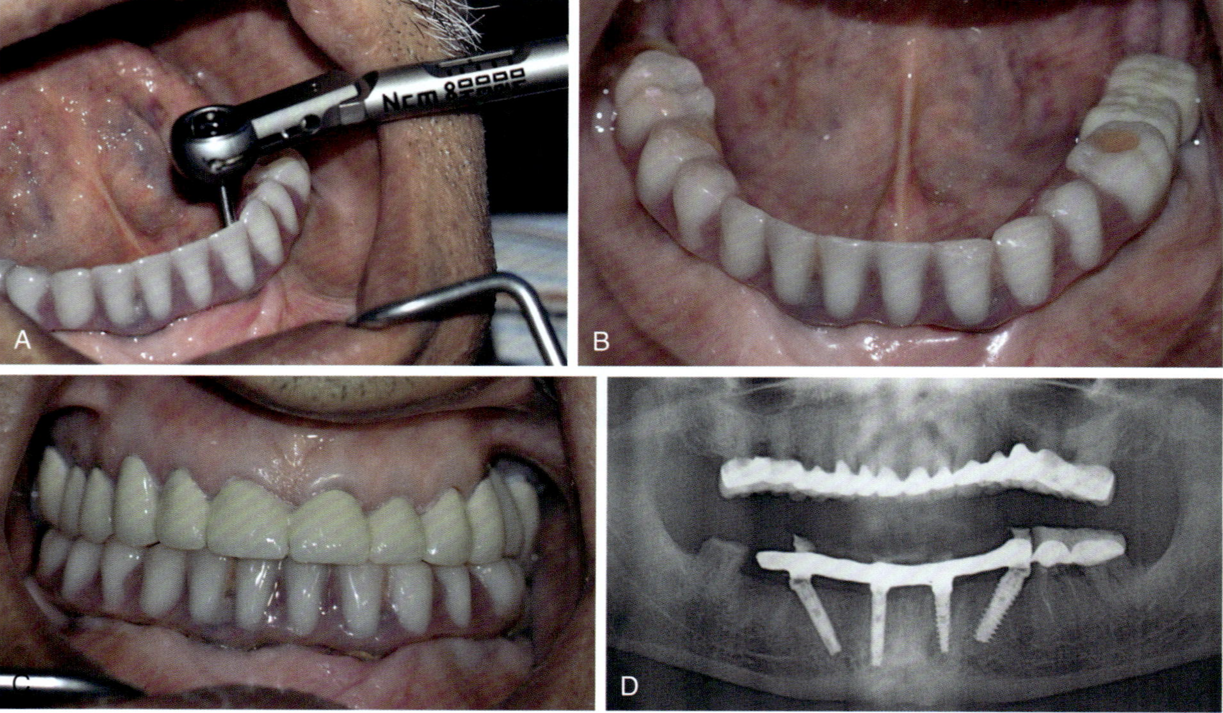

Fig 11.21 (A) The torque ratchet is used to finally tighten the connection screws at 30 Ncm and (B) screws holes are filled using gutta-percha followed by the light cure composite. (C) Prosthesis in occlusion. (D) Post loading radiograph.

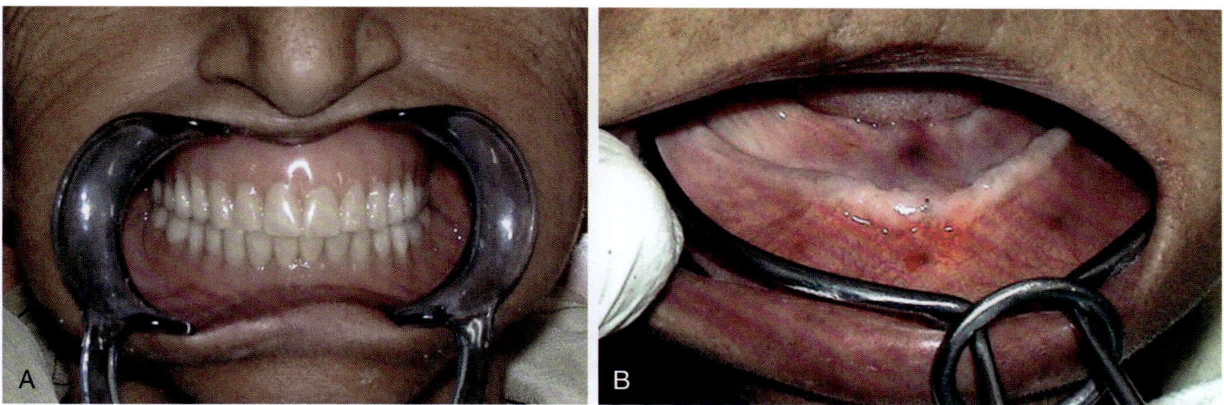

Fig 11.22 (A) The patient with maxillary and mandibular ridge supported dentures presented complaining of poor retention of the mandibular denture. (B) Poor mandibular ridge height, caused by vertical ridge resorption, can be seen.

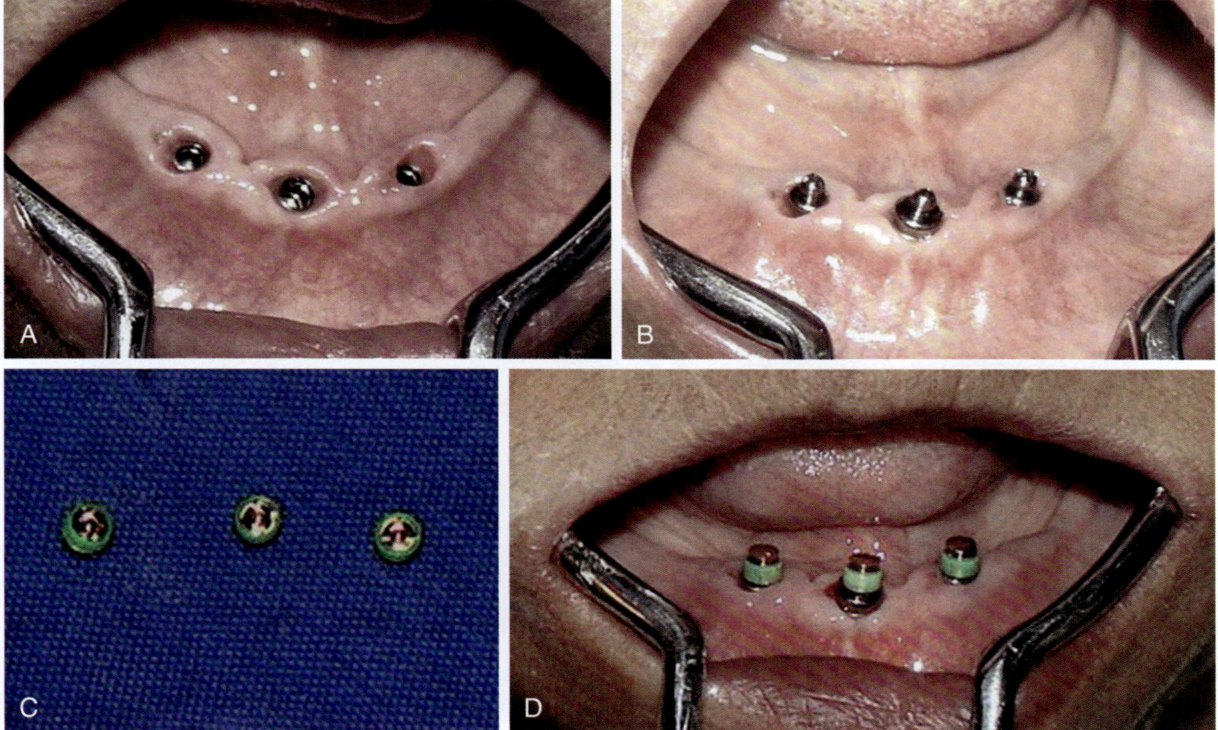

Fig 11.23 (A) Three implants are inserted in the anterior mandible to provide adequate retention to the same denture. (B) Ball abutments are inserted on top of the implants as the male part and (C and D) metal housings are placed onto the ball abutments as the female part.

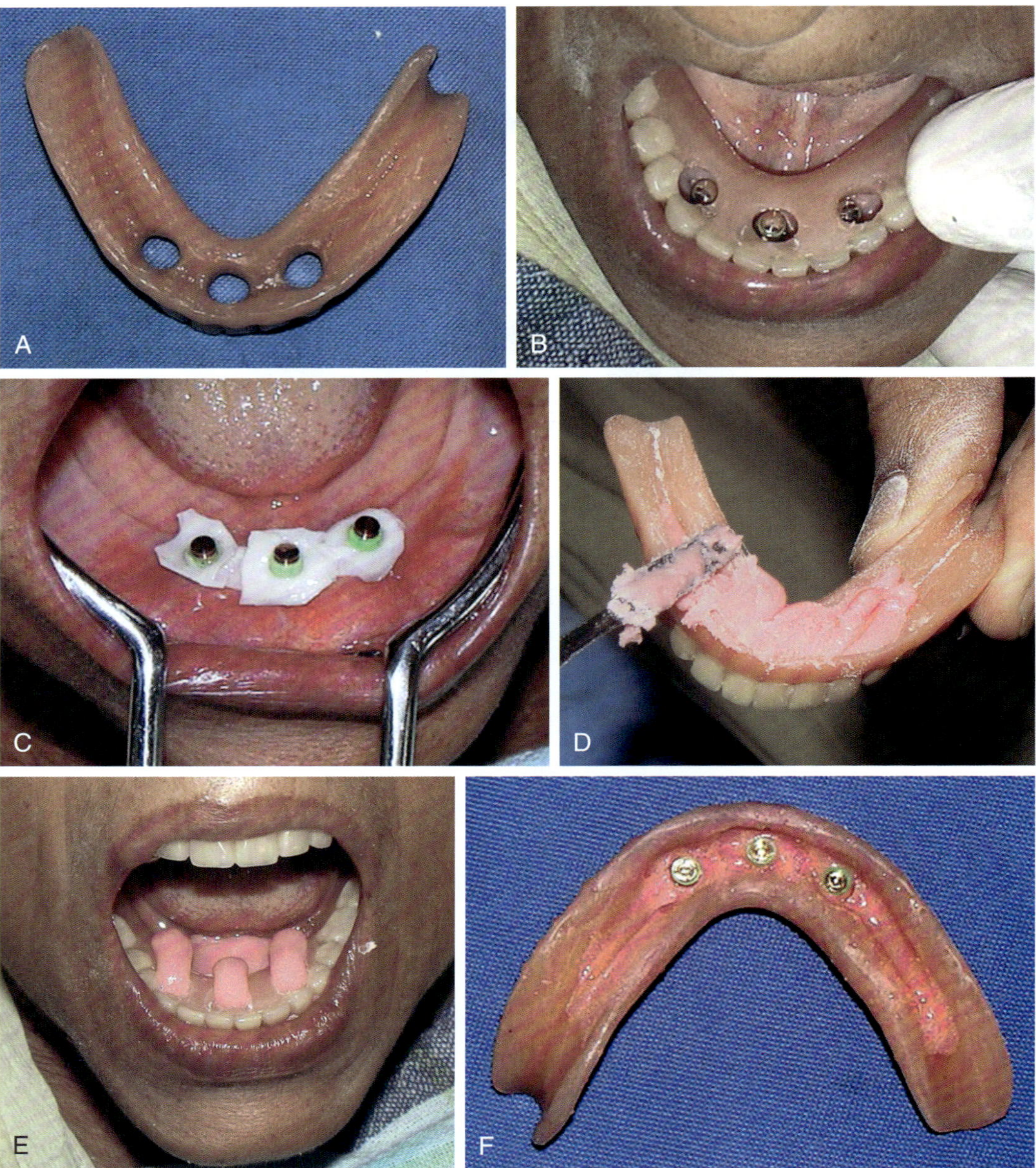

Fig 11.24 (A) The holes are prepared through the tissue surface of the denture, at the implant sites and (B) denture try-in is done for passive seating over the ridge with the metal housing in place. Sufficient space (minimum 2 mm) should be provided in the denture all around the metal housings, to adequately retain the housings in the self-cure resin. (C) The undercuts underneath the metal housings are blocked using a rubber dam sheath or thick glove sheath to prevent the self-cure resin flowing down and getting locked in the undercuts. (D) The self-cure resin is mixed and filled into the tissue surface of the denture. (E) The denture is seated over the metal housings in the patient's mouth and the patient is asked to close the dentures in occlusion. (F) The denture is removed after the self-cure resin has set, with the metal housings coming out from within the denture.

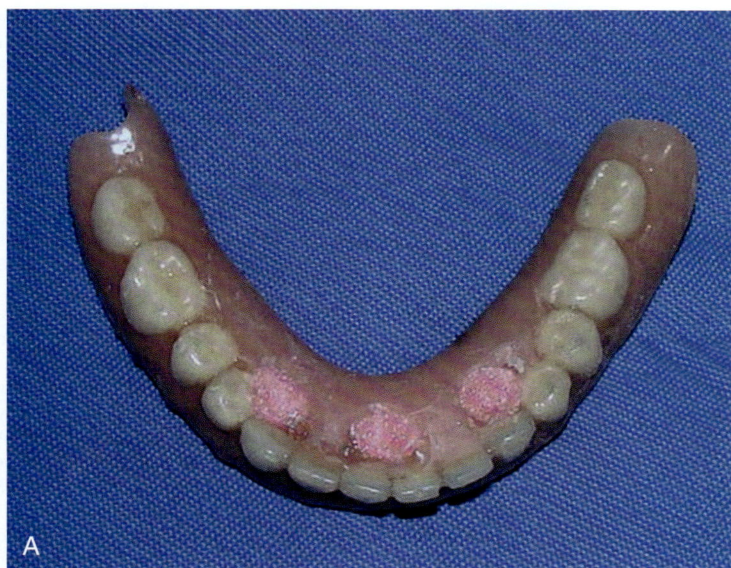

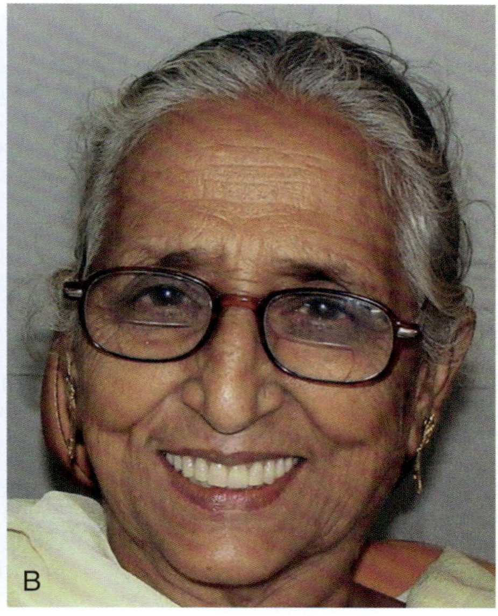

Fig 11.25 (A and B) The denture is finished, polished, and seated in the patient's mouth with high degree of retention from the implants.

Summary

Choosing the appropriate method of impression transfer and performing it with the highest possible accuracy and precision is paramount for fabricating an implant prosthesis with high level of precision in fit and desired accuracy. An appropriate impression material should be used to make the implant impressions, polyether and addition silicon are the materials of choice for making implant impressions. The prepared abutment technique can be practised where a high level of precision is not a concern or in the cases of one-piece implants. The open tray impression transfer technique should be preferred over the closed tray method in cases of multiple implants, full arch cases, deep seated implants, and screw-retained, multiple unit/full arch prosthesis because the open tray technique transfer the implant platform, connection positions, and orientation more accurately. For the open tray impression of multiple implants, the impression posts should be splinted together using pattern resin to avoid any possible movement of the posts within the impression, in respect to each other. Abutment level impressions should be preferred in cases of multiunit or full arch, screw-retained implant prosthesis. The tray adhesive should always be used to minimize the separation of the impression from the tray. The implant impressions should always be checked by the clinician for any errors and discrepancies before it is sent to the laboratory. Besides making accurate impression, choosing a laboratory which has expertise in fabricating the implant prosthesis, and using the correct prosthetic implant components are mandatory to obtain the desired prosthetic results. The overdenture cases can be done with the direct technique but it should be done with the indirect technique if a high level of retention of the metal housing is desired in the denture base.

Further Reading

Conrad HJ, Pesun IJ, DeLong R, et al. Accuracy of two impression techniques with angulated implants. J Prosthet Dent 2007;97:349–56.

Assunção WG, Cardoso A, Gomes EA, et al. Accuracy of impression techniques for implants. Part 1 – influence of transfer copings surface abrasion. J Prosthodont 2008;17:641–7.

Kohavi D. Complications in the tissue integrated prostheses components: clinical and mechanical evaluation. J Oral Rehabil 1993;20:413–22.

Assuncao WG, Filho HG, Zaniquelli O. Evaluation of transfer impressions for osseointegrated implants at various angulations. Implant Dent 2004;13:358–66.

Inturregui JA, Aquilino SA, Ryther JS, et al. Evaluation of three impression techniques for osseointegrated oral implants. J Prosthet Dent 1993;69:503–9.

Wee AG. Comparison of impression materials for direct multi-implant impressions. J Prosthet Dent 2000;83:323–31.

Liou AD, Nicholls JI, Yuodelis RA, et al. Accuracy of replacing three tapered transfer impression copings in two elastomeric impression materials. Int J Prosthodont 1993;6:377–83.

Carr AB. Comparison of impression techniques for a five-implant mandibular model. Int J Oral Maxillofac Implants 1991;6:448–55.

Cabral LM, Guedes CG. Comparative analysis of 4 impression techniques for implants. Implant Dent 2007;16:187–94.

Choi JH, Lim YJ, Yim SH, et al. Evaluation of the accuracy of implant-level impression techniques for internal-connection implant prostheses in parallel and divergent models. Int J Oral Maxillofac Implants 2007;22:761–8.

Daoudi MF, Setchell DJ, Searson LJ. A laboratory investigation of the accuracy of two impression techniques for single-tooth implants. Int J Prosthodont 2001;14:152–8.

Burawi G, Houston F, Byrne D, et al. A comparison of the dimensional accuracy of the splinted and unsplinted impression techniques for the Bone-Lock implants system. J Prosthet Dent 1997;77:68–75.

Hsu CC, Millstein PL, Stein RS. A comparative analysis of the accuracy of implant transfer techniques. J Prosthet Dent 1993;69:588–93.

Naconecy MM, Teixeira ER, Shinkai RS, et al. Evaluation of the accuracy of 3 transfer techniques for implant- supported prostheses with multiple abutments. Int J Oral Maxillofac Implants 2004;19:192–8.

Daoudi MF, Setchell DJ, Searson LJ. An evaluation of three implant level impression techniques for single tooth implant. Eur J Prosthodont Restor Dent 2004;12:9–14.

Carr AB. Comparison of impression techniques for a two-implant 15-degree divergent model. Int J Oral Maxillofac Implants 1992;7:468–75.

Nissan J, Ghelfan O. The press-fit implant impression coping technique. J Prosthet Dent 2009;101:413–4.

Lorenzoni M, Pertl C, Penkner K, et al. Comparison of the transfer precision of three different impression materials in combination with transfer caps for the Frialit-2 system. J Oral Rehabil 2000;27:629–38.

Wenz HJ, Hertrampf K. Accuracy of impressions and casts using different implant impression techniques in a multi-implant system with an internal hex connection. Int J Oral Maxillofac Implants 2008;23:39–47.

Carr AB, Master J. The accuracy of implant verification casts compared with casts produced from a rigid transfer coping technique. J Prosthodont 1996;5:248–52.

Barrett MG, de Rijk WG, Burgess JO. The accuracy of six impression techniques for osseointegrated implants. J Prosthodont 1993;2:75–82.

Vigolo P, Fonzi F, Majzoub Z, et al. An evaluation of impression techniques for multiple internal connection implant prostheses. J Prosthet Dent 2004;92:470–6.

Vigolo P, Majzoub Z, Cordioli G. In vitro comparison of master cast accuracy for single-tooth implant replacement. J Prosthet Dent 2000;83:562–6.

Del'Acqua MA, Arioli-Filho JN, Compagnoni MA, et al. Accuracy of impression and pouring techniques for an implant supported prosthesis. Int J Oral Maxillofac Implants 2008;23:226–36.

Wee AG, Aquilino SA, Schneider RL. Strategies to achieve fit in implant prosthodontics: a review of the literature. Int J Prosthodont 1999;12:167–78.

Kim S, Nicholls JI, Han CH, et al. Displacement of implant components from impressions to definitive casts. Int J Oral Maxillofac Implants 2006;21:747–55.

Assif D, Marshak B, Schmidt A. Accuracy of implant impression techniques. Int J Oral Maxillofac Implants 1996;11:216–22.

Lee H, Ercoli C, Funkenbusch PD, et al. Effect of subgingival depth of implant placement on the dimensional accuracy of the implant impression: an in vitro study. J Prosthet Dent 2008;99:107–13.

Vigolo P, Majzoub Z, Cordioli G. Evaluation of the accuracy of three techniques used for multiple implant abutment impressions. J Prosthet Dent 2003;89:186–92.

Assif D, Nissan J, Varsano I, et al. Accuracy of implant impression splinted techniques: effect of splinting material. Int J Oral Maxillofac Implants 1999;14:885–8.

Lee H, So JS, Hochstedler JL, et al. The accuracy of implant impressions: A systematic review. J Prosthet Dent 2008;100:285–91.

Herbst D, Nel JC, Driessen CH, et al. Evaluation of impression accuracy for osseointegrated implant supported superstructures. J Prosthet Dent 2000;83:555–61.

Jemt T, Lindén B, Lekholm U. Failures and complications in 127 consecutively placed fixed partial prostheses supported by Branemark implants: from prosthetic treatment to first annual checkup. Int J Oral Maxillofac Implants 1992;7:40–4.

Assif D, Fenton A, Zarb GA, et al. Comparative accuracy of implant impression procedures. Int J Periodontics Restorative Dent 1992;12:113–21.

Spector MR, Donovan TE, Nicholls JI. An evaluation of impression techniques for osseointegrated implants. J Prosthet Dent 1990;63:444–7.

Vigolo P, Fonzi F, Majzoub Z, et al. Master cast accuracy in single-tooth implant replacement cases: an in vitro comparison. A technical note. Int J Oral Maxillofac Implants 2005;20:455–60.

Dental implants for periodontally compromised patients

12

Frédéric Joachim Issam Joachim-Samaha Jacques Charon

CHAPTER CONTENTS HD

Introduction

An increasing number of patients are benefiting from implants placed to replace missing teeth that were lost due to periodontal diseases. A logical and fundamental question arises as to whether a history of periodontitis affects implant outcomes.

Implantologists, before starting any implant therapy on patients suffering from periodontal diseases, should ask themselves:

1. What are periodontal diseases?
2. Do peri-implant diseases exist?
3. Is periodontitis a risk factor outcome for implant treatment?
4. Does a specific protocol exist for implant therapy for patients suffering from periodontal diseases?

The aim of this chapter is to answer these questions and to evaluate the effect of untreated periodontitis on implant outcomes.

A complete protocol to maximize success, will also be described. Finally, in order to illustrate this chapter, clinical cases treated in a private practise will be presented.

Infectious periodontal diseases

Periodontal diseases are complex infections that occur in susceptible hosts and are caused by biofilms that form on tooth surfaces. These biofilms comprise microorganisms that are components of normal oral microbiota. However, the host-response determines whether loss of attachment, as determined by probing and radiographs, will or will not occur (Figs 12.1 and 12.2).

It is clearly established that without effective treatment, periodontal diseases cause loss of attachment or even loss of the teeth in severe cases. The prevalence of the most severe advanced periodontitis has been found in 10–15% of randomized populations.

However, periodontally compromised teeth, if well-maintained and treated at regular intervals, show very high survival at 10 years (92–93%). So, it is clear that periodontal therapy is still a very good up-to-date and economical solution, especially when epidemiological studies showed that the survival of oral implants after 10 years, varies between 82% and 94%.

Nevertheless, for the 7–10% of teeth lost during periodontal treatment, implant therapy seems to be a good alternative to fixed bridges or removable dentures.

Definition, aetiology and clinical features of peri-implant diseases

Peri-implant diseases or peri-implantitis are essentially infectious diseases responsible for the majority of implants lost [11]. They are the result of an imbalance between bacterial load and host defence but the main aetiological factor is a special biofilm.

Many studies showed that bacterial flora related to periodontitis and peri-implantitis are quite similar. Therefore, when the periodontium of natural teeth is infected, there is a high risk of similar bacterial infection around the implant. This is called translocation and in these circumstances, peri-implant disease may appear.

Peri-implant diseases may affect the peri-implant mucosa only (i.e. peri-implant mucositis) or also involve the supporting bone (i.e. peri-implantitis). When peri-implantitis is diagnosed too late, complete loss of osseointegration

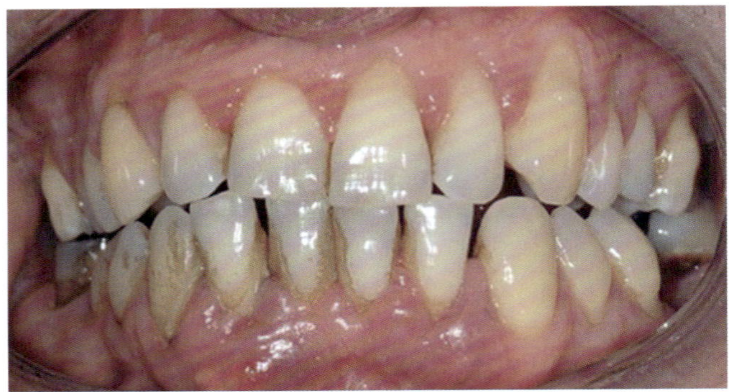

Fig 12.1 Front clinical view of a 36-year-old male patient suffering from aggressive periodontitis. Note the severe inflammation with gingival recessions, bleeding, abscesses, and migrations. This patient was also suffering from halitosis, pain and finally, mobilities of the lower front teeth.

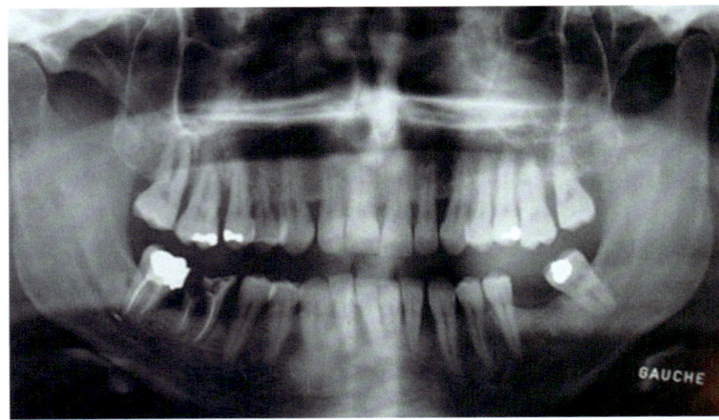

Fig 12.2 Panoramic radiograph of the same patient showing severe loss of attachment from 50% to 80%.

CASE REPORT

Showing 28 years follow-up periodontal treatment results on a patient with aggressive periodontitis (Figs 12.3–12.6).

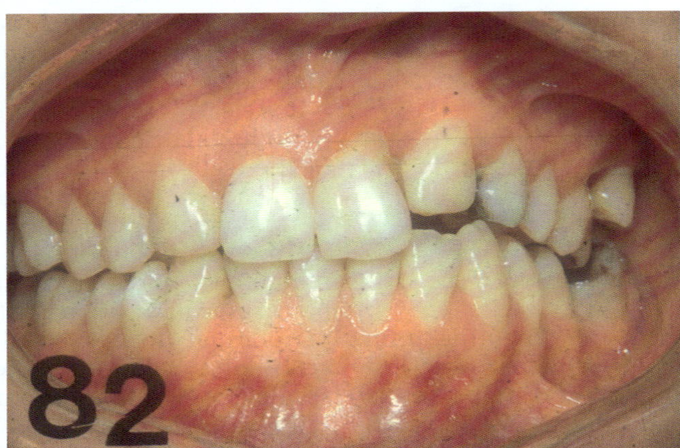

Fig 12.3 Front clinical view of a female who was 26 years old in 1982. This patient suffered from an aggressive form of periodontitis. She was treated for 1 year to stabilize her disease. Then, she had orthodontic treatment associated with upper front splinting. Finally, she underwent maintenance procedure once in a year.

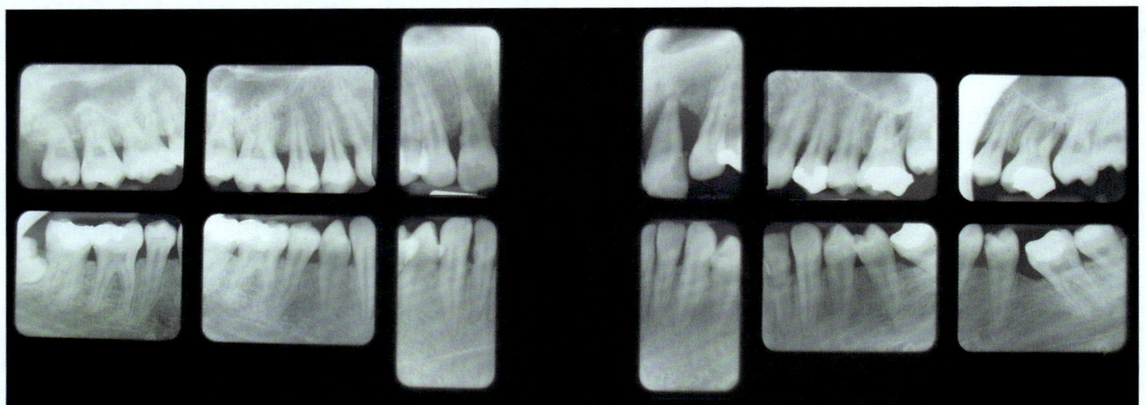

Fig 12.4 'Long-cone' radiographs of 1982. The radiographs confirmed the aggressive state of the periodontitis.

CASE REPORT—cont'd

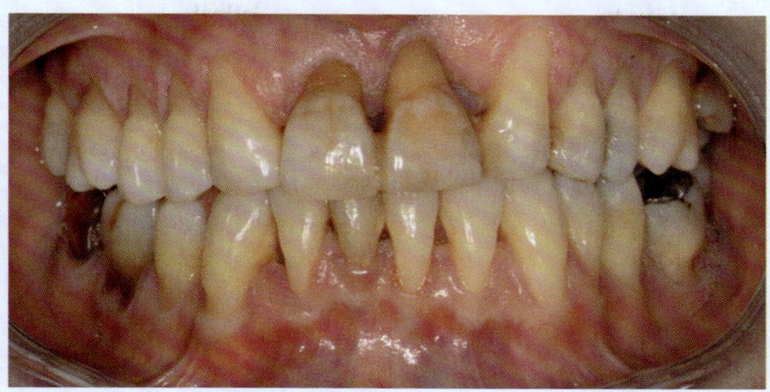

Fig 12.5 Front clinical view on December 2010. This patient comes every year for a recall session. She is 54 years old and she follows her maintenance protocol very carefully. Her cooperation is perfect. She has no functional complaint and is very happy that she has been able to keep her teeth.

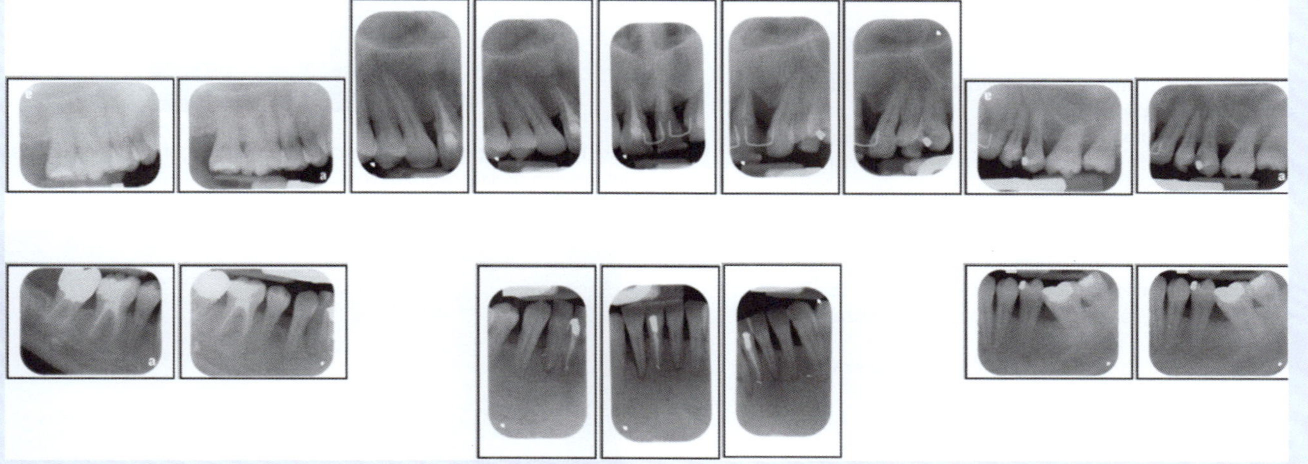

Fig 12.6 'Long-cone' radiographs of 2010.There have been 28 years of follow-up since the first appointment (Fig 12.4).

occurs, followed by the removal of the implant (Figs 12.7 and 12.8).

A high number of implant losses are observed when implant therapy is undertaken on patients suffering from untreated or poorly maintained periodontal disease [5,10]. Many similarities with periodontal diseases have been observed with regard to epidemiology, aetiology, risk factors, clinical features, pathogenesis, and progress in peri-implantitis. Therefore, the most efficient weapon against peri-implantitis and for its prevention, is to avoid all periodontal infection before implant therapy.

Risk factors of peri-implant diseases

Patients suffering from periodontal diseases are at high risk to develop peri-implantitis when periodontitis is not treated. This risk is increased when the patient is a smoker.

As with periodontal diseases, several risk factors may increase the speed and the severity of the peri-implantitis

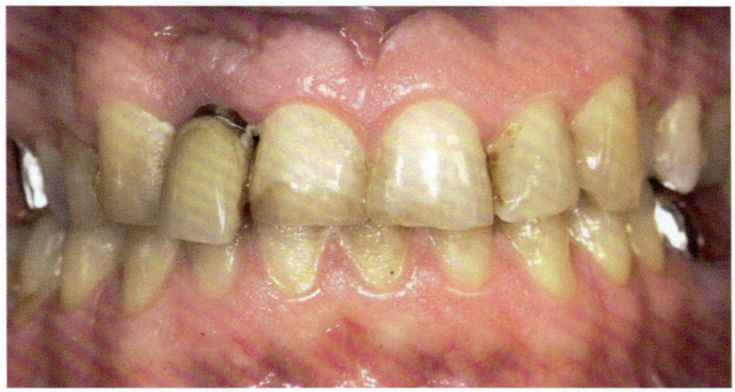

Fig 12.7 Complete loss of osseointegration in the upper lateral right incisor. Migration and mobility were observed and the implant had to be removed. Please note that for personal reasons, there was no maintenance protocol for this patient for a period of 14 years.

[5,12]. Several of the risk factors are well established whereas others need to be proved. They can be classified as follows:

1. The established risk factors are:
   a. Poor oral hygiene
   b. History of periodontitis
   c. Cigarette smoking
2. Possible risk factors that still need to be proved because of limited evidence:
   a. Diabetes
   b. Alcohol consumption (more than 10 mg/day)
3. Conflicting and limited evidence of risk factors that need to be proved:
   a. Genetic traits
   b. Height of keratinized mucosa
   c. Implant surface.

CASE REPORT

Showing the protocol to be followed in periodontally compromised patients.

A rigorous protocol has to be followed in periodontally compromised patients who need implant therapy. When this protocol is followed by the patient and the implantologist, it is possible to reach a high success level close to those obtained with healthy periodontal patients.

The step by step protocol for perioimplant patient therapy is:

- Aetiological periodontal diagnosis and prognosis
- Clinical, bacteriological and radiological stabilization of the periodontitis
- Clinical, radiological, prosthetic and surgical examinations
- Implant surgery
- Prosthesis
- Periodontal and prosthetic maintenance.

The following case illustrates the above. The patient suffers from severe periodontitis. There have been 28 years of periodontal and 5 years of implant follow-up.

Mr Michel And, 38 years old, heavy smoker (40 cigarettes per day), with a stressful job, came to our practise on the 25th of May 1983 with periodontal complaints. According to his age and the clinical, radiological and bacteriological examinations, he was diagnosed as suffering from a general aggressive periodontitis (Figs 12.9 and 12.10).

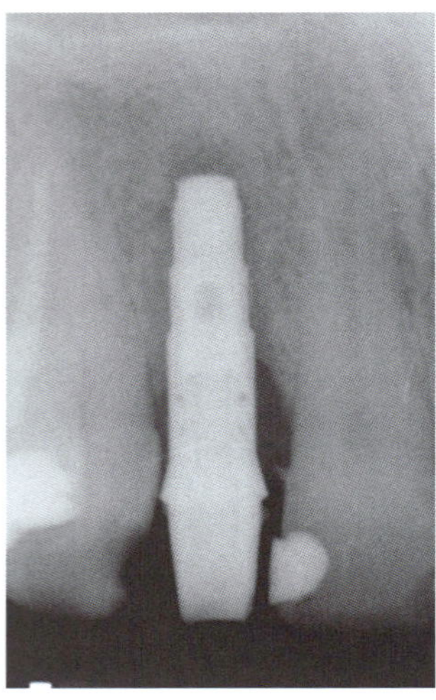

Fig 12.8 Radiograph of the implant showing a complete loss of osseo-integration and its migration out of the bone.

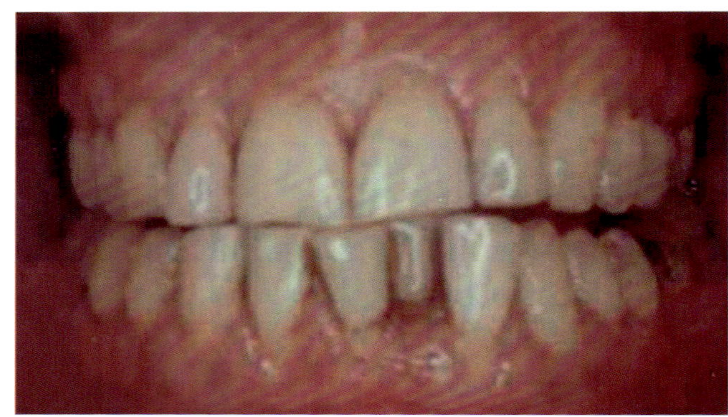

Fig 12.9 Clinical front view during the first appointment. The patient was 38 years old.

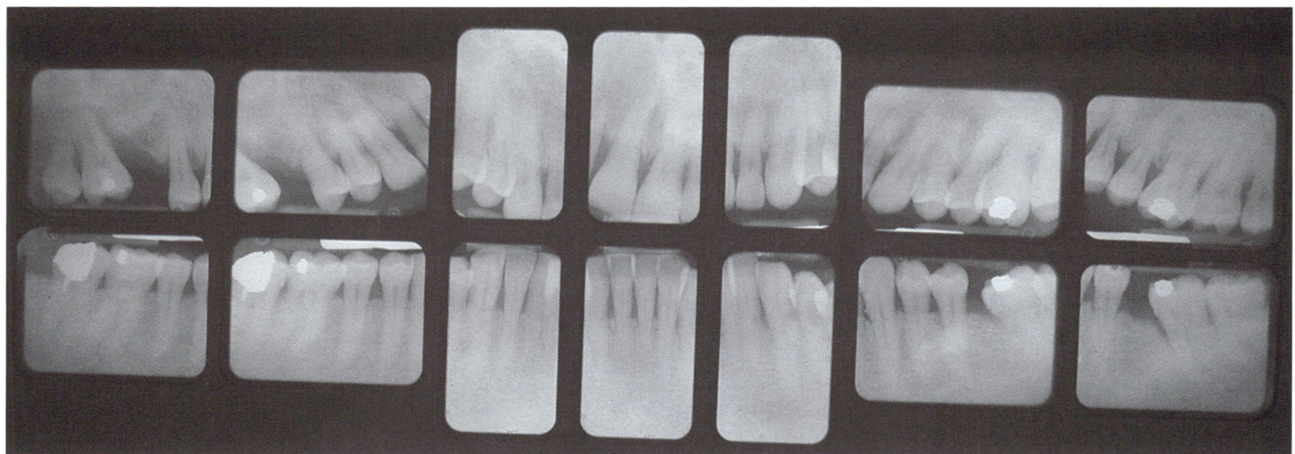

Fig 12.10 'Long-cone' radiographs taken during the first appointment. Note that loss of attachment varied between 20% and 70%.

The periodontal treatment was undertaken until clinical, radiological and bacteriological stabilization of the disease was obtained. The patient was then placed on a twice a year maintenance protocol.

However, due to private and professional reasons, the patient did not come to the maintenance visits between 1986 and 1993. A that time, an upper right tooth was spontaneously lost. Clinical, bacteriological and radiological examinations showed increasing periodontal loss of attachment (Fig 12.11).

A new periodontal treatment had to be undergone again. The conditions to get long-term success were clearly explained to the patient. An upper partial denture was made to facilitate the chewing.

The periodontitis was stabilized. The cooperation of the patient has been excellent since that time (Figs 12.12 and 12.13).

At the 2005 recall session, the patient, who had quit smoking, decided to remove the upper denture and to replace it by implant therapy. An implant protocol was decided on, and the teeth numbers 12, 14, 27, and 28 were extracted because of poor prognosis (Fig 12.14). A new upper denture was inserted during the time of implant osseointegration (Fig 12.15). The implants were inserted at the same time as a sinus bone graft surgery.

Because of the severity of the periodontitis and the size of the prosthetic reconstruction, the patient was seen twice a year in recall appointments. The patient is now 66 years old and expresses his gratitude. Twenty-six years after the first appointment, a better function and an acceptable aesthetic were obtained (Figs 12.16 and 12.17). The implantology was undertaken under good conditions and the patient understood that long-term success depended on his behaviour being modified to prevent the recurrent periodontal infections observed between 1986 and 1993.

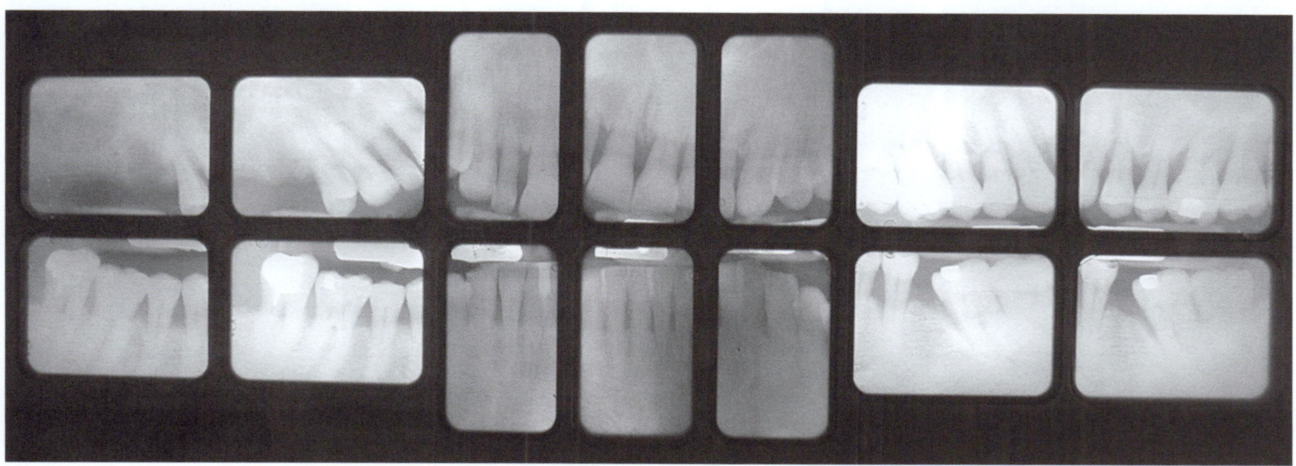

Fig 12.11 'Long-cone' radiographs shot in 1993 showing the loss of the upper right molars and the increased loss of attachment, essentially at the upper arch.

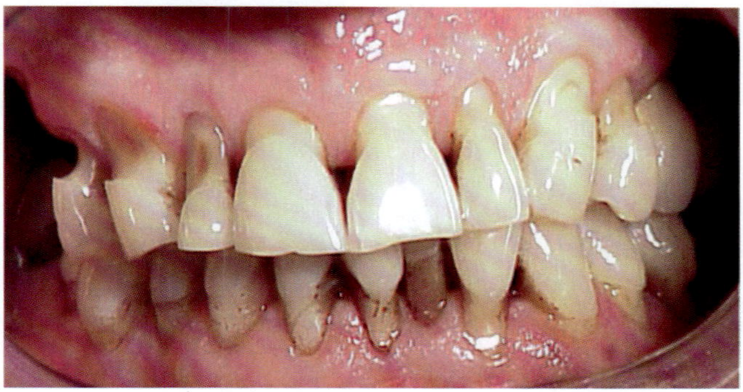

Fig 12.12 Clinical front view during 2000, 17 years after the first appointment.

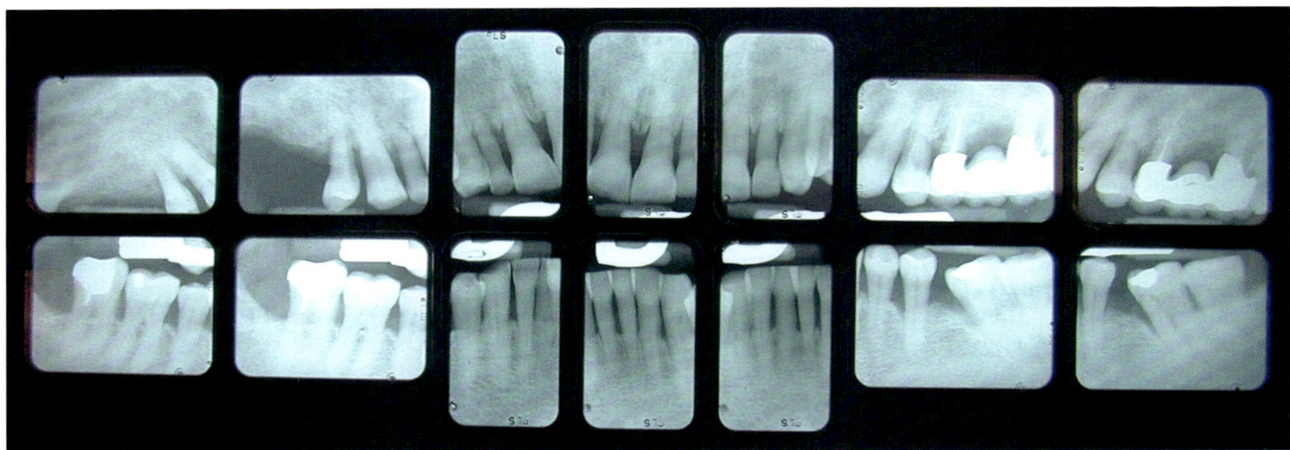

Fig 12.13 'Long-cone' radiographs shot in 2000 showing stabilization of the lesions. The upper first left molar had to be removed.

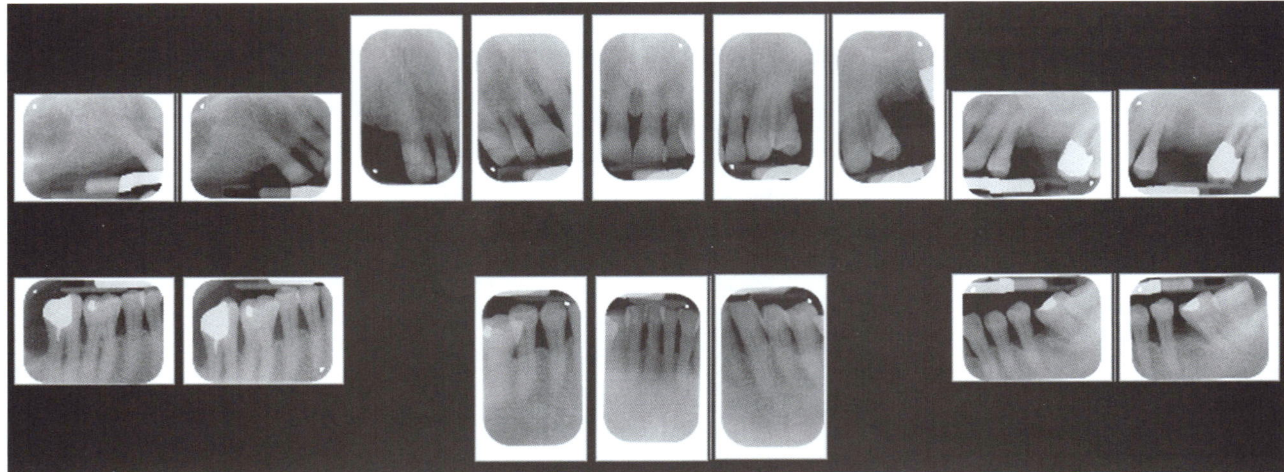

Fig 12.14 'Long-cone' radiographs taken before implant therapy in 2005.

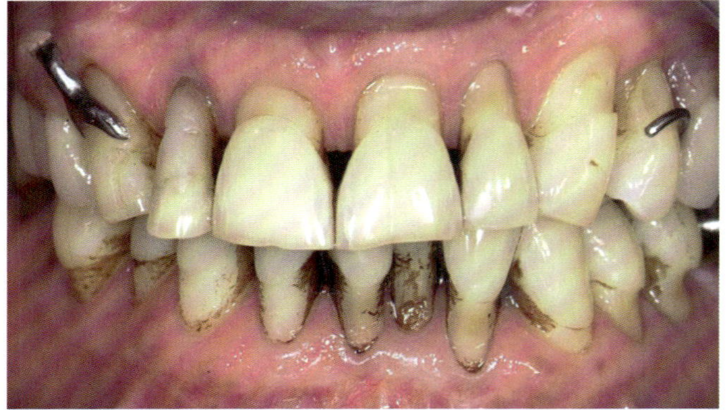

Fig 12.15 Front clinical view in 2005, showing the healthy periodontium and the upper denture.

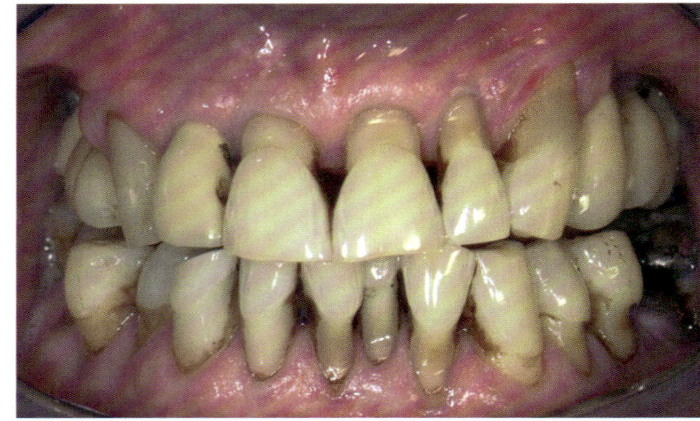

Fig 12.16 Front clinical view taken during a recall session in 2010. Please note ulceration due to strong brushing.

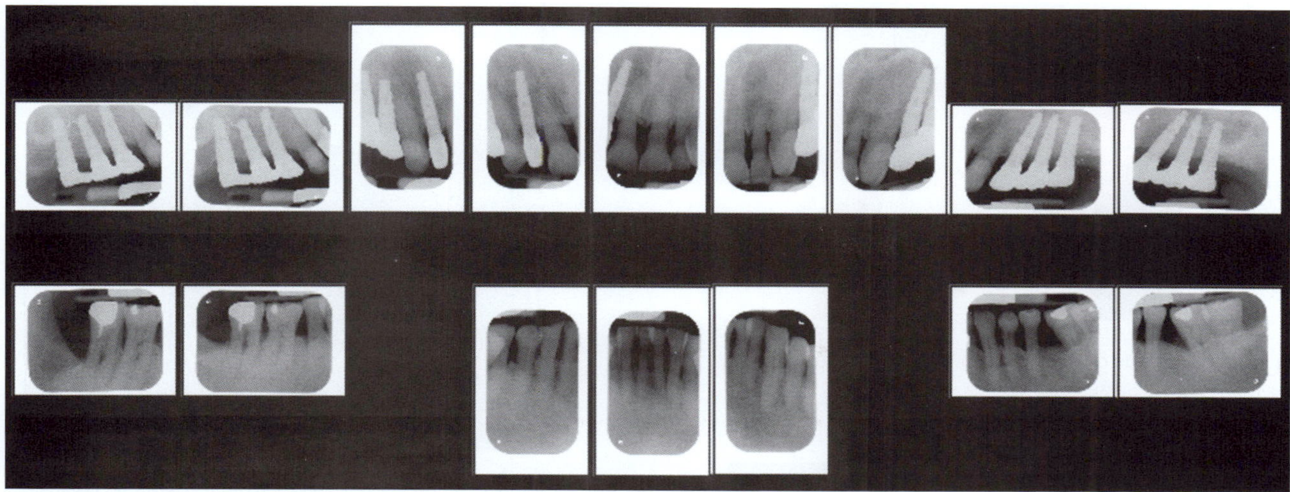

Fig 12.17 'Long-cone' radiographs taken during the recall session in 2010.

Clinical cases

CASE REPORT-1

Retaining partially removable prosthesis on a patient with chronic adult periodontitis (follow-up: 19 years-periodontitis/ 9 years-implantology) (Figs 12.18–12.21).

In 1991, Mrs Pierrette Der, 54 years old, came to the practise in order to treat her adult chronic periodontitis. After her periodontal treatment, she was on maintenance treatment once a year. In 2001, the maxillary right bridge had to be removed due to the fracture of the root of the second premolar. As the patient did not accept the sinus bone graft, it was decided to realize a removable denture. In order to reduce its size, avoid an unaesthetic clasp and increase its stabilization, an implant with a retainer was inserted and replaced the tooth number 15. The patient is now 73 years old and still very happy with this solution. The long-term success was possible because of her very good compliance with the periodontal maintenance protocol.

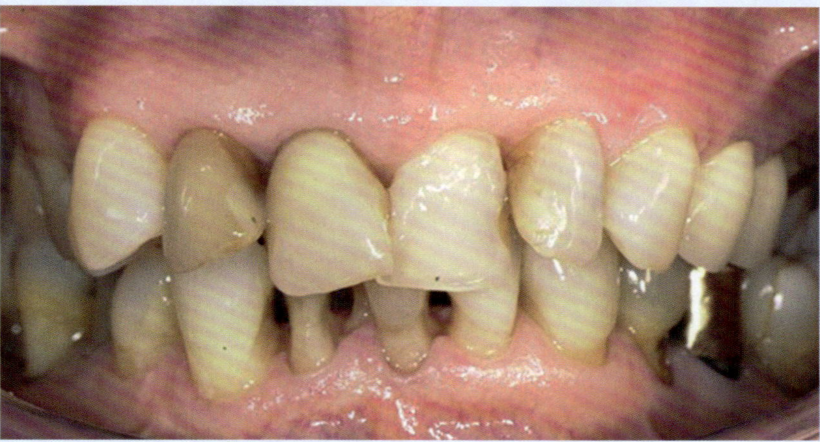

Fig 12.18 Clinical front view observed during a 2010 recall session. The periodontitis is still stable and the implant has been in function for 9 years.

Continued

CASE REPORT-1—cont'd

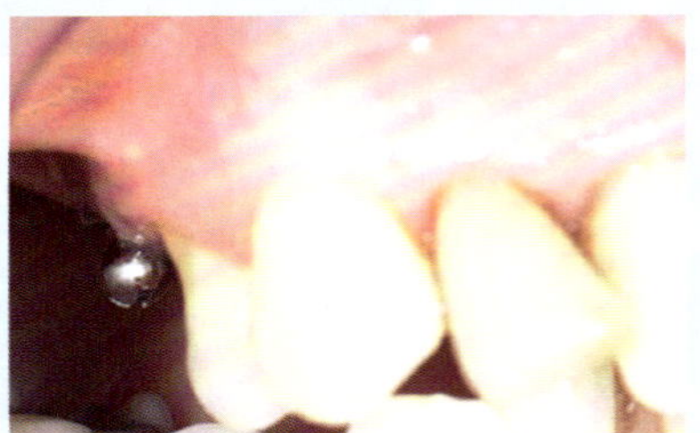

Fig 12.19 Right side clinical view showing the retainer.

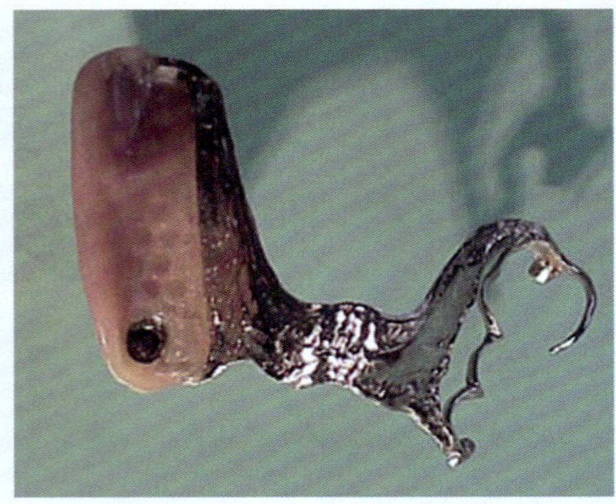

Fig 12.20 View of the upper denture. Note the reduced palatal surface of the denture.

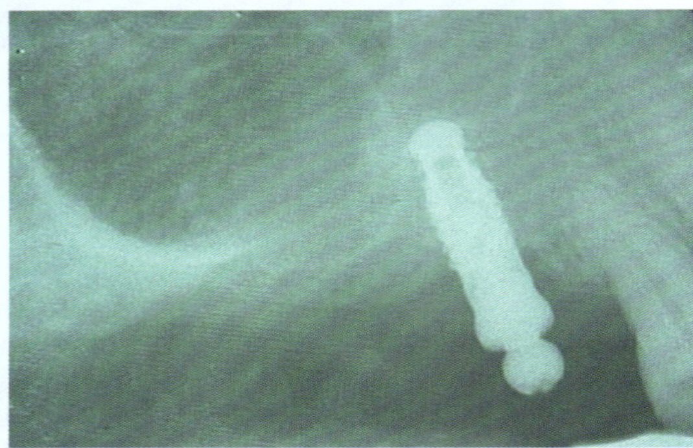

Fig 12.21 Radiographs of the implant after 10 functional years.

CASE REPORT-2

Lower front edentulism on patient with chronic adult periodontitis: fixed prosthesis on implants (follow-up: 17 years-periodontitis/16 years-implantology) (Figs 12.22–12.26).

Mrs Colette Thi, 57 years old, consulted for the first time on the 20th of October 1993. She complained of periodontal disease. A diagnosis of adult chronic periodontitis was established and treatment was initiated. At the end of the treatment (April 1994) she wanted to replace the lower denture with a fixed prosthesis. Two implants were placed at teeth numbers 41 and 32 and a ceramic bridge was realized. At the last recall session, the patient was 74 years old and her plaque control, which allowed the success of the periodontal/implant treatments, was still excellent.

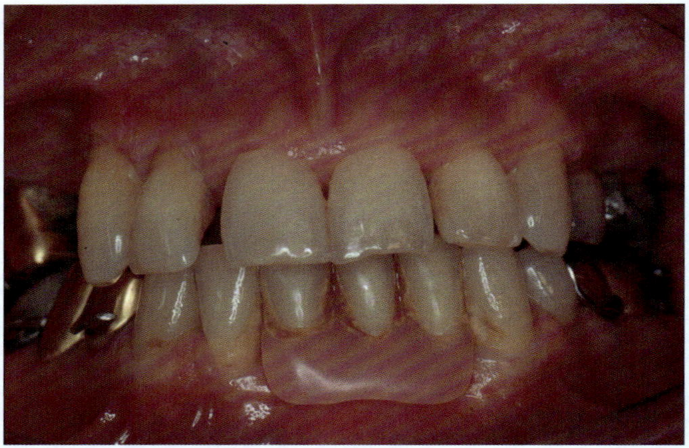

Fig 12.22 Clinical front view in 1994 at the end of the periodontal treatment. Please note the very good oral hygiene.

CASE REPORT-2—cont'd

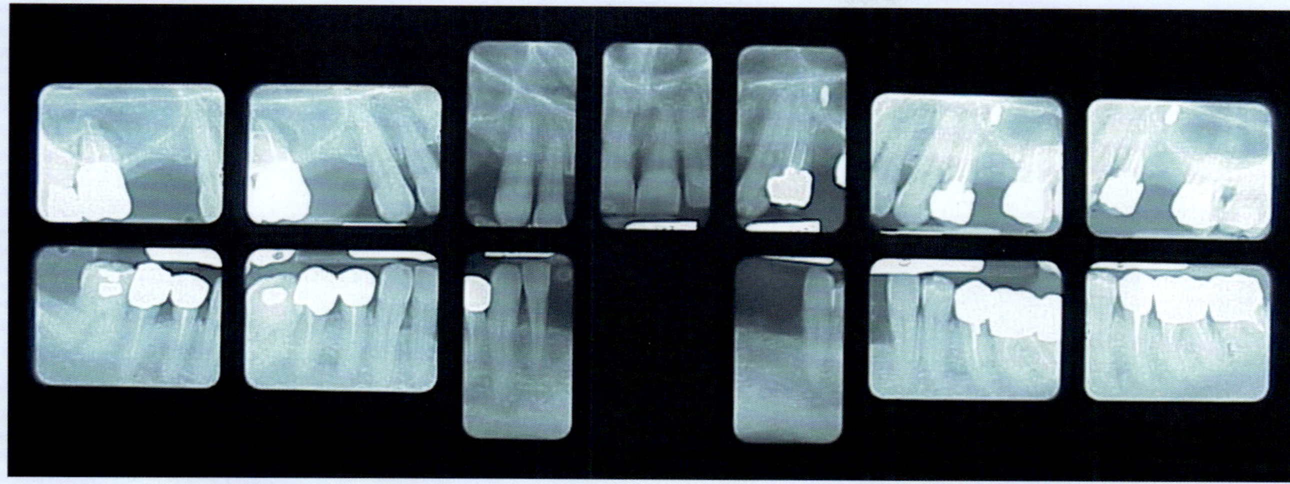

Fig 12.23 'Long-cone' radiographs taken at the end of the periodontal treatment in 1994.

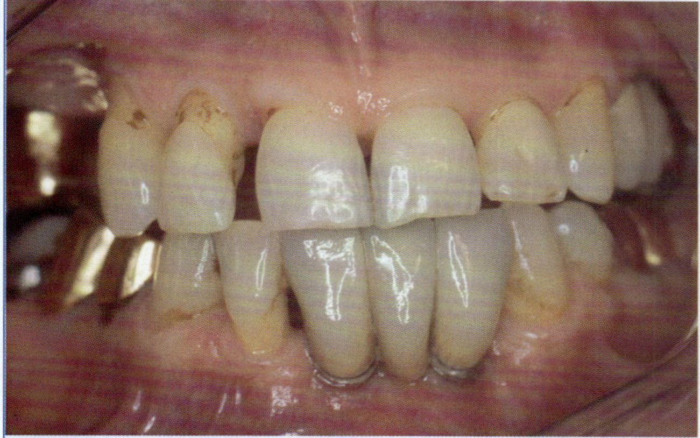

Fig 12.24 Clinical front view at the first postimplant recall in 1995.

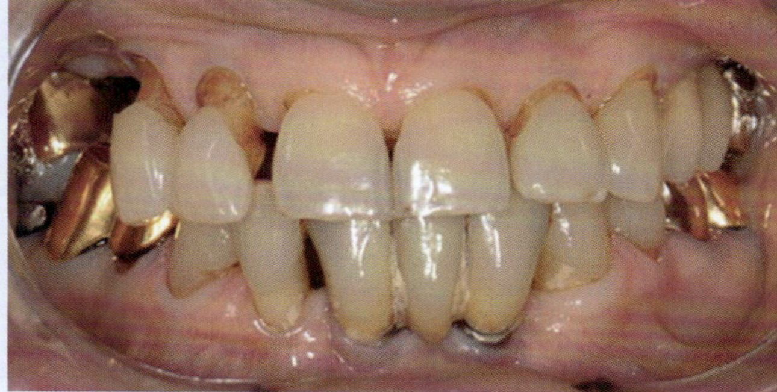

Fig 12.25 Clinical front view in 2010. The patient is now 74 years old and the situation still excellent. There is no inflammation.

Continued

CASE REPORT-2—cont'd

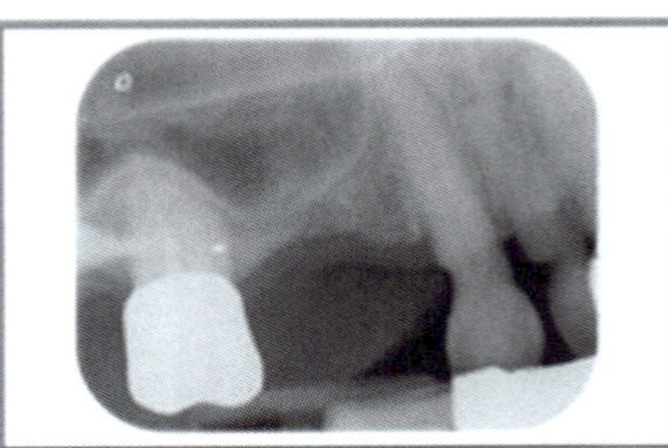
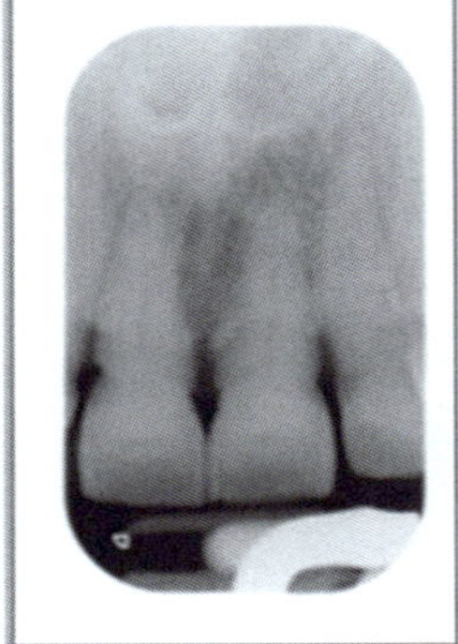
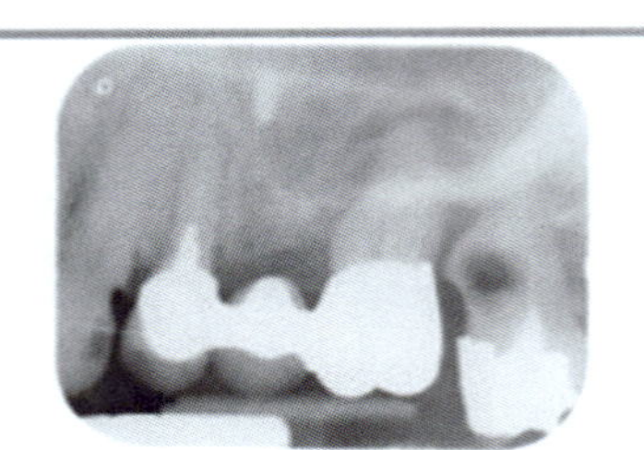
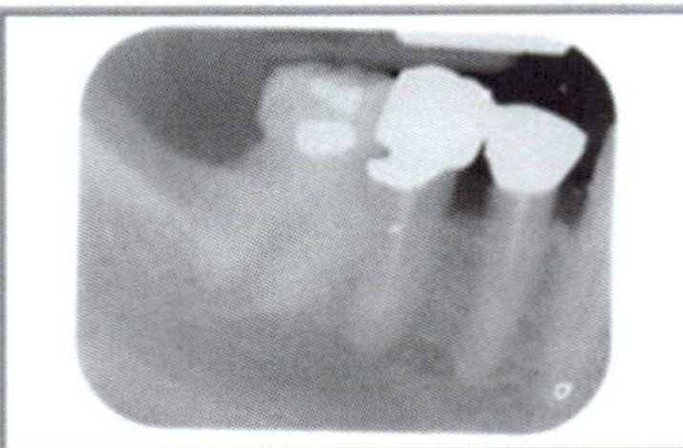
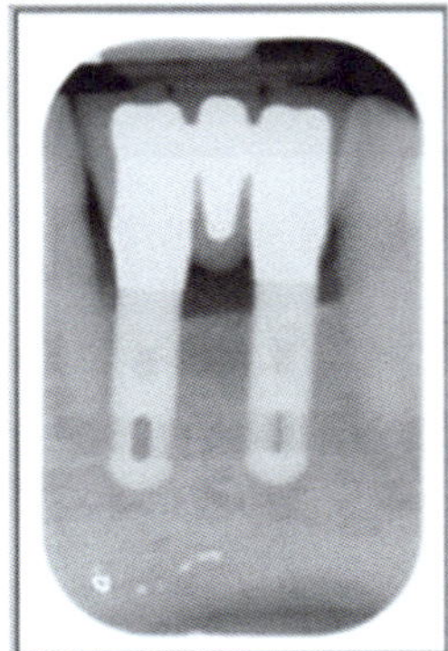
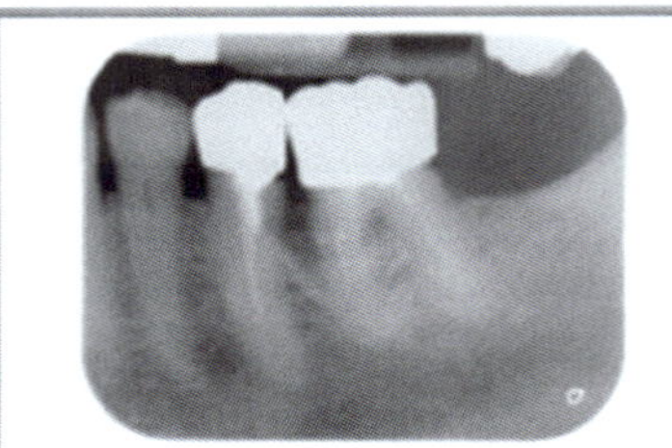

Fig 12.26 'Long-cone' radiographs taken at the 2010 recall session.

CASE REPORT-3

Lower left edentulism on a patient with chronic adult periodontitis: fixed prosthesis on implants (follow-up: 7 years-periodontitis/5 years-implantology) (Figs 12.27–12.30).

In September 2003, Mrs Martine Dut, 50 years old, came to the practise because she was suffering from periodontitis and wanted to avoid dentures. The periodontal treatment was successful and was terminated in November 2004. However, in 2005, teeth numbers 35 and 36 were pulled out because of root fractures. Three implants and ceramic crowns were put inserted to replace the teeth numbers 35, 36 and 37. The patient is now seen once a year on maintenance protocol.

Fig 12.27 Clinical front view in 2010 during a recall appointment. Please note the very good plaque control.

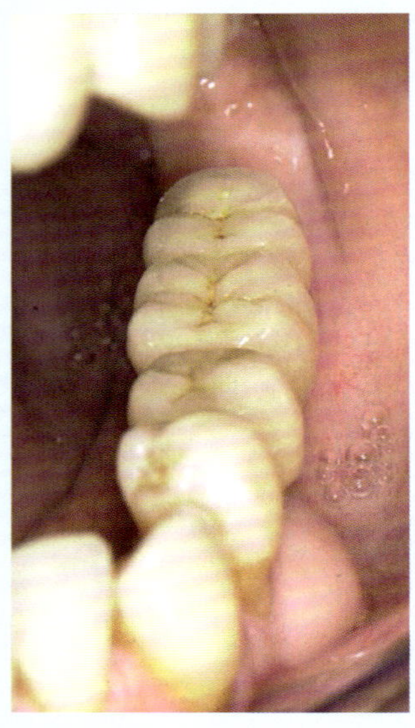

Fig 12.28 Upper view of the bridge.

CASE REPORT-3—cont'd

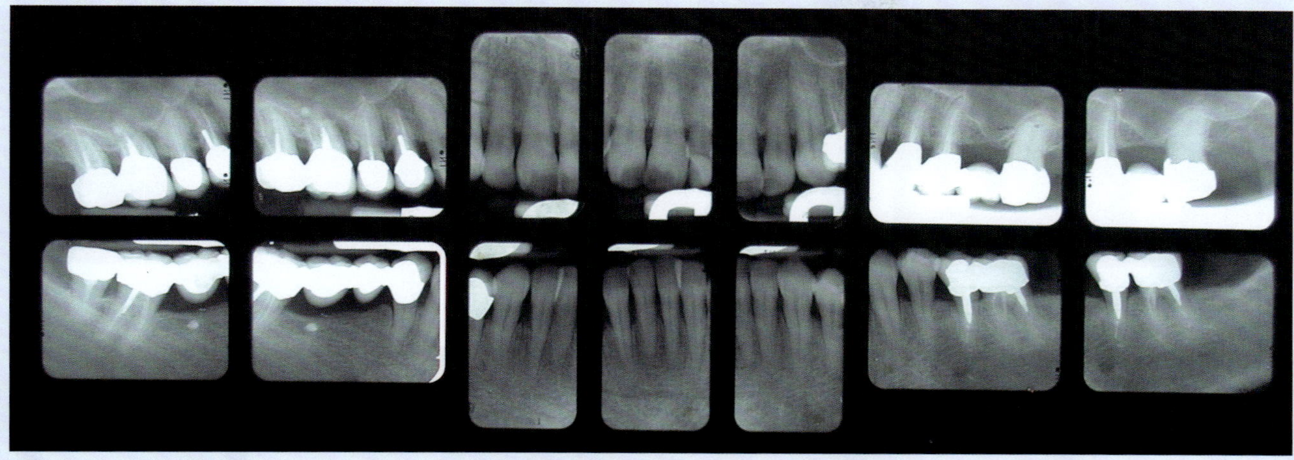

Fig 12.29 'Long-cone' radiographs taken at the end of the periodontal treatment in 2004.

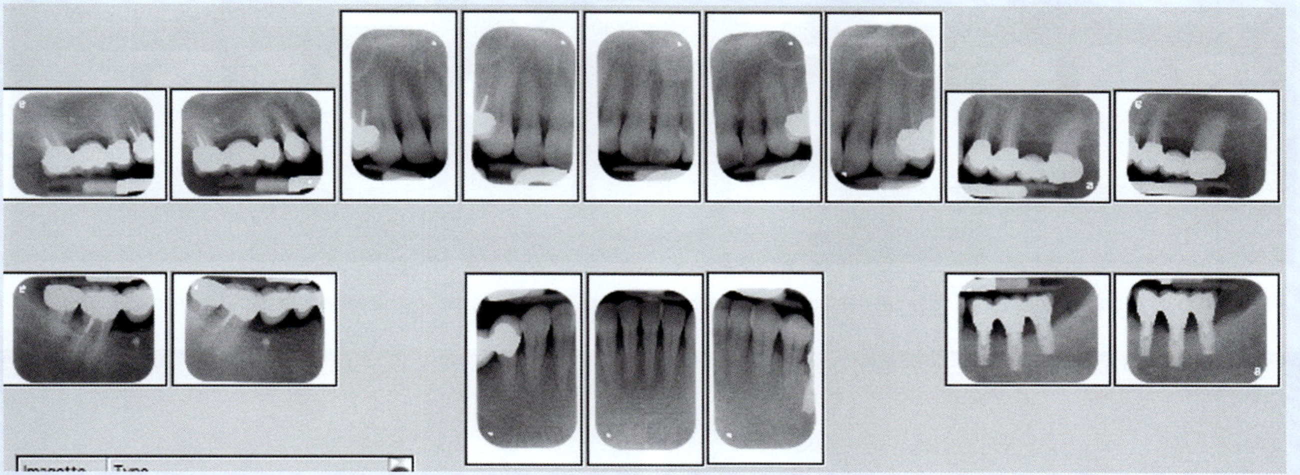

Fig 12.30 'Long-cone' radiographs taken at the last recall session in November 2010.

CASE REPORT-4

Maxillary edentulism on patient with severe periodontitis: fixed prosthesis on implants without sinus lift bone graft (follow-up: 10 years-periodontitis/6 years-implantology) (Figs 12.31–12.35).

Mrs Anne-Marie Bast, 51 years old, was seen for the first time in January 2000 because of significant mobilities of the upper left and right posterior bridges. Severe caries and endodontic cysts were diagnosed along with severe adult chronic periodontitis. Periodontal treatment was undertaken up to January 2002. Due to severe caries, teeth numbers 17, 16, 15, 23, 24, 25, 26, 27, 36, 38 and 48 were extracted. In June 2002, implant therapy was decided on, but the patient refused sinus and mandibular bone grafts. The oral prosthetic rehabilitation was limited to the second premolars. The prosthetic therapy took place only in January 2004, because during 2003 the patient had surgery and chemotherapy to treat breast cancer. Since that period, she followed a very careful maintenance protocol once a year. The therapeutic solution restricted to the short arches has not been bothering the patient in respect of aesthetic and masticatory functions. It confirmed findings in literature that the masticatory function could be established and maintained in subjects receiving fixed dental prosthesis with severely reduced but healthy periodontal tissue support.

Continued

CASE REPORT-4—cont'd

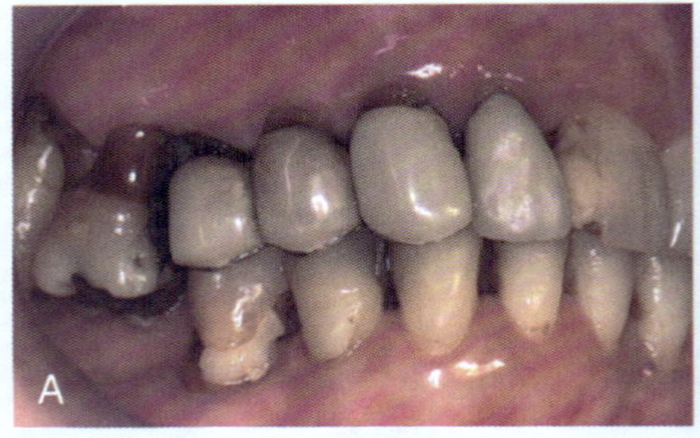

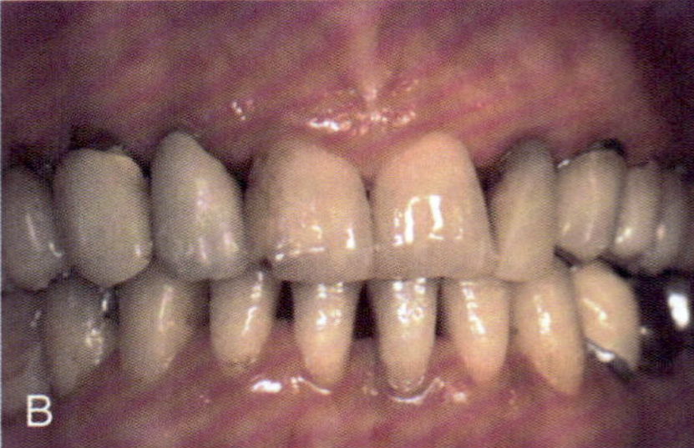

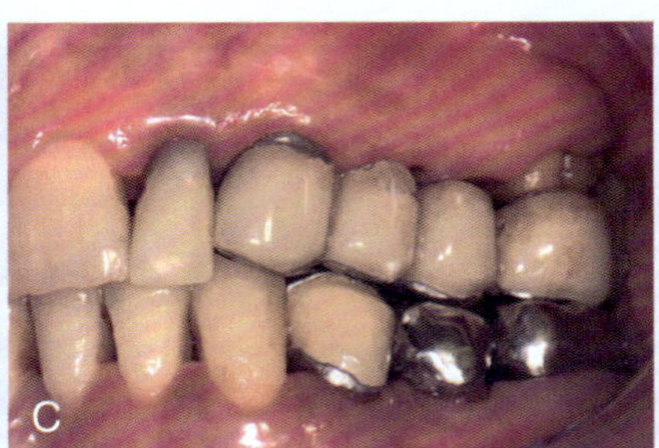

Fig 12.31 (A–C) Clinical views taken at the first appointment (January 2000).

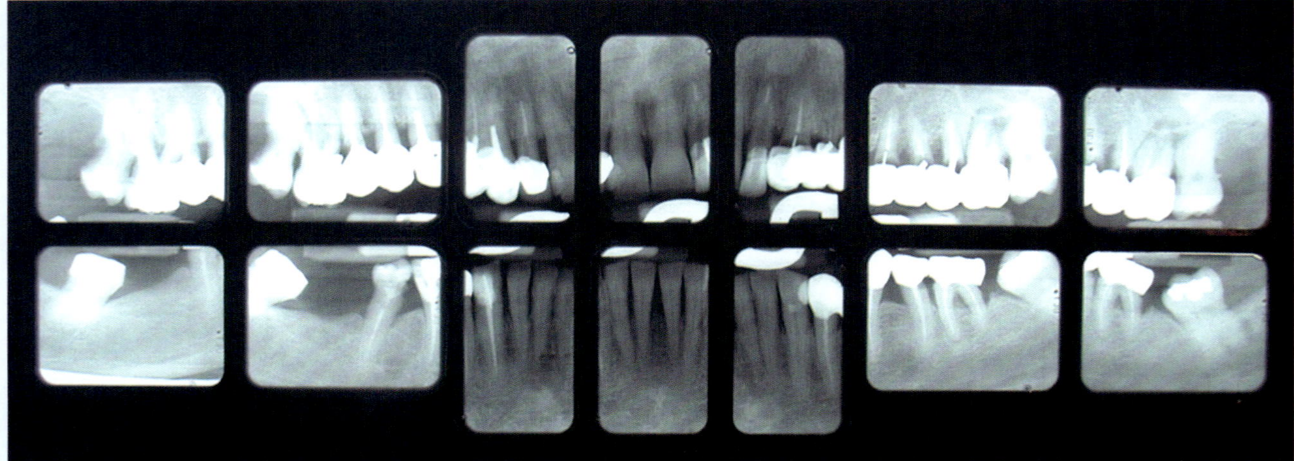

Fig 12.32 'Long-cone' radiographs taken at the first appointment in January 2000. Note the loss of attachment and numerous caries.

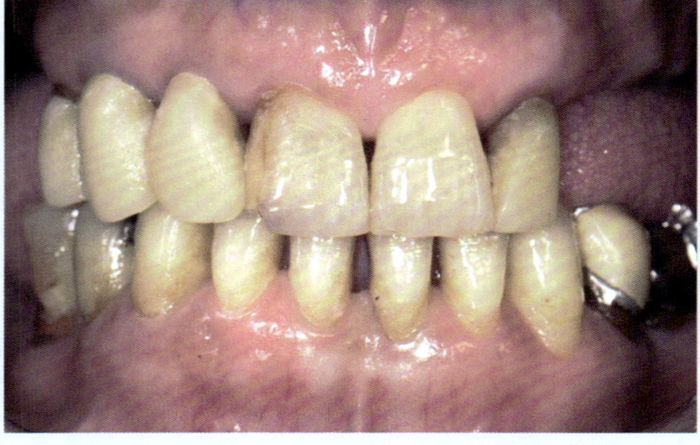

Fig 12.33 Clinical front view after periodontal treatment and extraction of teeth, but before implant surgery (January 2002).

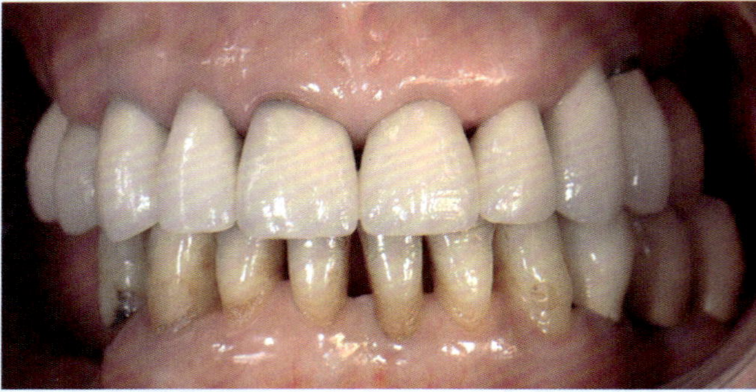

Fig 12.34 Clinical front view during a recall session at the end of 2010. Note the perfect oral hygiene.

CASE REPORT-4—cont'd

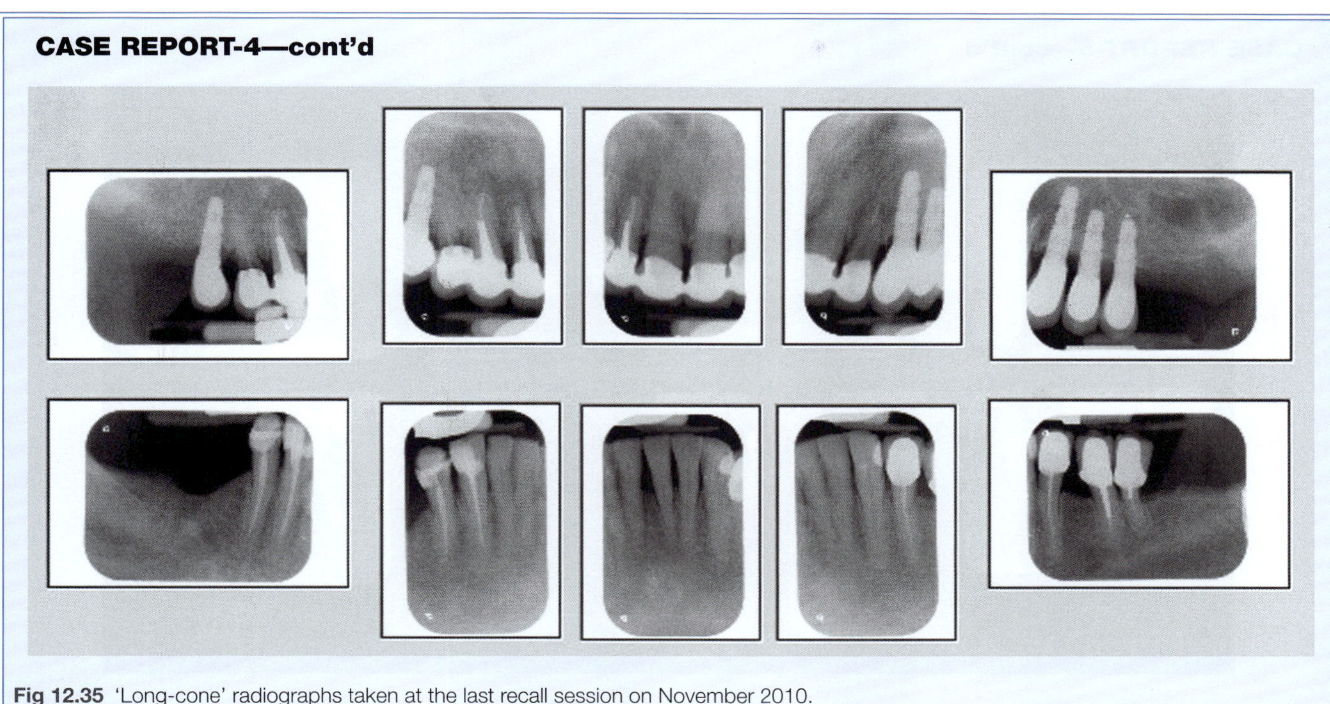

Fig 12.35 'Long-cone' radiographs taken at the last recall session on November 2010.

CASE REPORT-5

Lateral left maxillary edentulism on a patient with severe periodontitis: fixed prosthesis on implants after orthodontic treatment but without sinus bone graft augmentation (follow-up: 12 years-periodontitis/8 years-implantology) (Figs 12.36–12.39).

On 1999, Mrs Francoise Lec, 54 years old, suffered from severe periodontitis with 50–90% loss of attachment. Her major complaints were mobility and loss of aesthetics due to migration. When the periodontitis was stabilized, a 2-year orthodontic treatment was undertaken and it ended in 2003, after which it was decided to splint the front upper and lower teeth to avoid recurrence of migration. It was also decided to remove the tooth number 24 and put two implants in situation numbers 24 and 25 (the patient did not want to go through a sinus lift procedure). The crowns were settled at the end of 2003. Since then, the patient is seen once a year on a routine periodontal and implant maintenance protocol. As in case report-4, this short left arch therapeutic solution has made the patient happy in respect of aesthetic and masticatory functions. However, it is very important to realize that long-term success depends on the compliance of the patient.

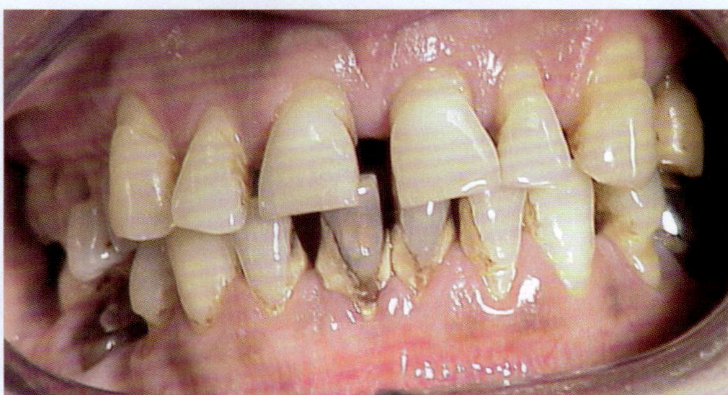

Fig 12.36 Clinical front view during the first appointment in November 1999.

Continued

CASE REPORT-5—cont'd

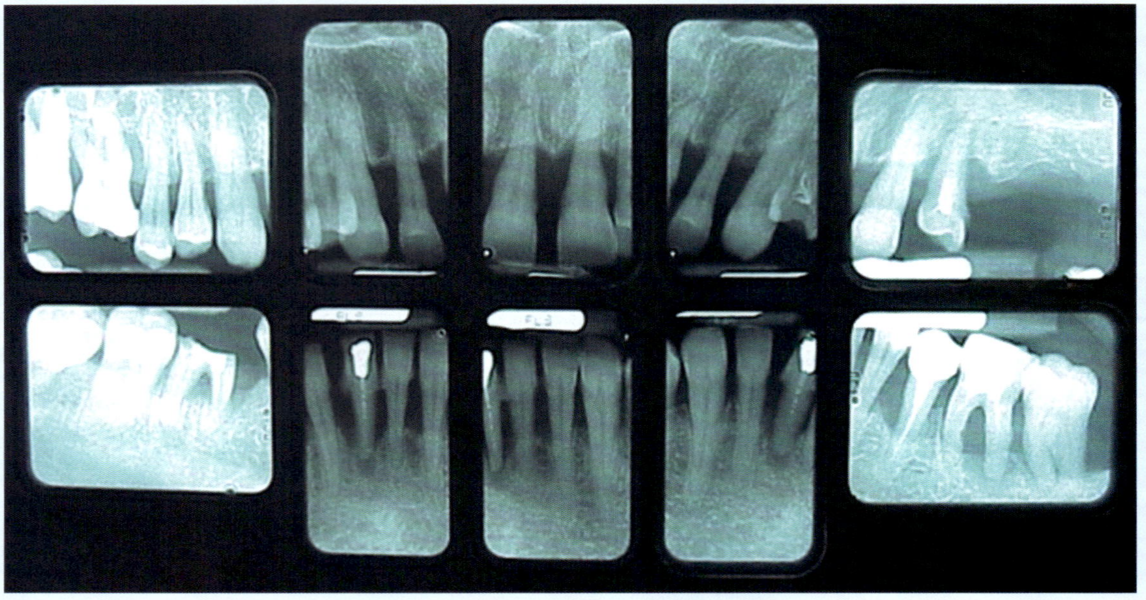

Fig 12.37 'Long-cone' radiographs taken at the first appointment. Note the severe loss of attachment.

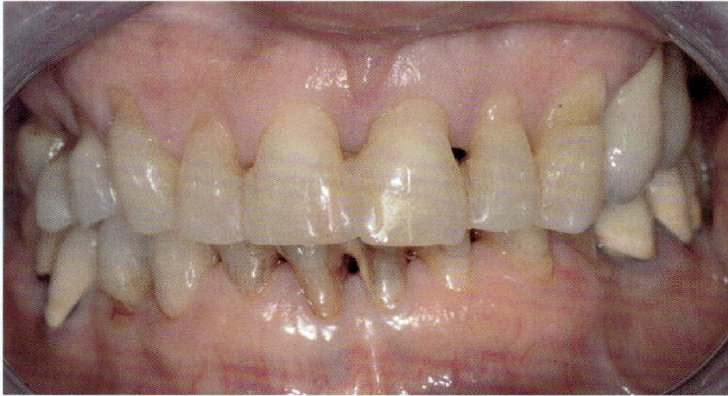

Fig 12.38 Clinical front view during the last recall session on January 2011. Note the lack of inflammation even after 12 years of periodontal follow-up.

CASE REPORT-5—cont'd

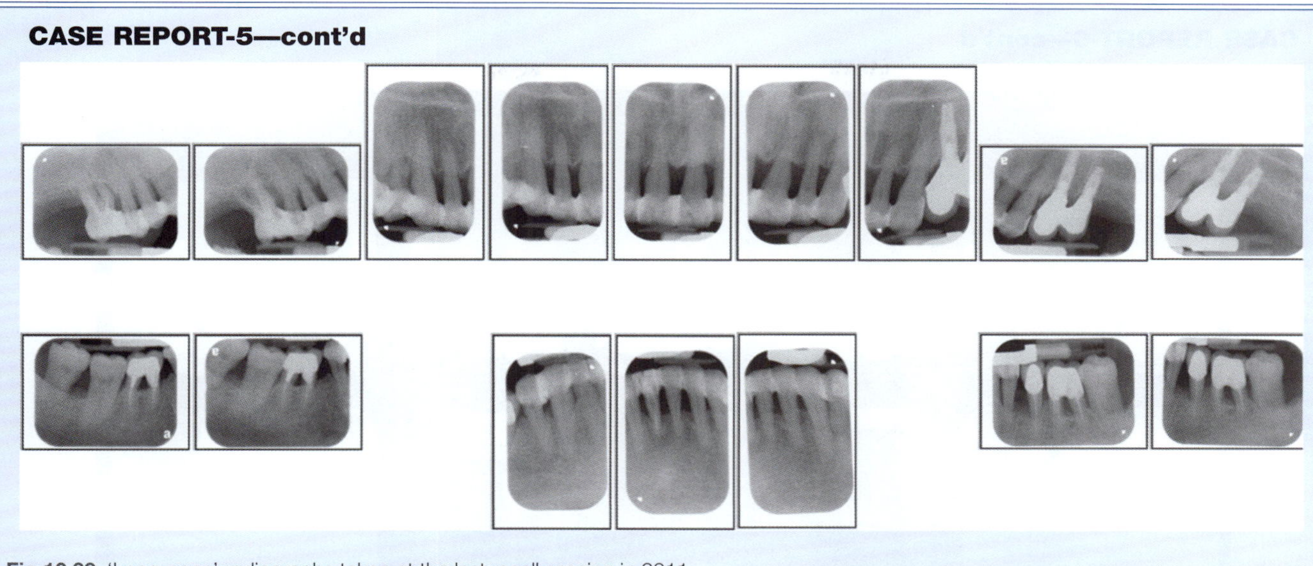

Fig 12.39 'Long-cone' radiographs taken at the last recall session in 2011.

CASE REPORT-6

Full mouth rehabilitation: full bridge on implants after bone grafts on the upper jaw and full bridge on periodontal compromised treated teeth on the lower jaw (follow-up: 13 years-periodontitis/9 years-implantology) (Figs 12.40–12.44).

Mrs Michèle Den, 45 years old on September 1997, consulted the practise because she was suffering from severe mobility of an upper bridge associated with pain and abscesses. Subterminal loss of attachment on the upper jaw and moderate loss of attachment on the lower jaw, were observed. Therefore, it was decided to realize a full upper arch bridge associated with autograft bone augmentation procedures in the horizontal and vertical dimensions (sinus floor elevation procedures included). Before the graft procedures, all endodontic and periodontal infections were eliminated. The periodontal treatment at the lower jaw was successful.

On January 2001, the patient was periodontally, prosthetically and psychologically ready to receive the grafts. The implants were inserted in September 2001 and fixed dentures were put in at the end of the year. Since this period, the patient has been under a routine maintenance follow-up once a ear.

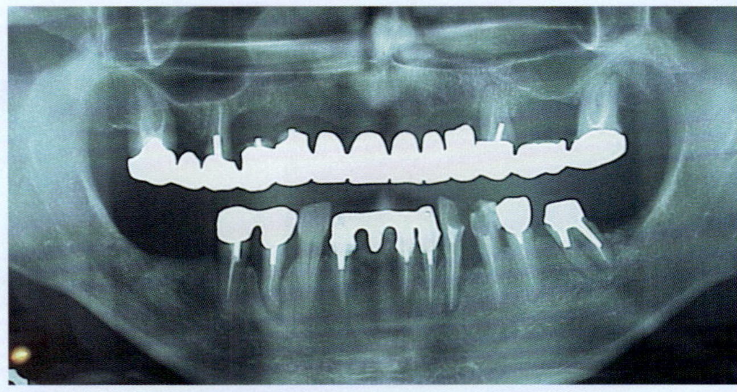

Fig 12.41 Panoramic radiograph taken just before the full upper arch bone augmentation grafts (2001).

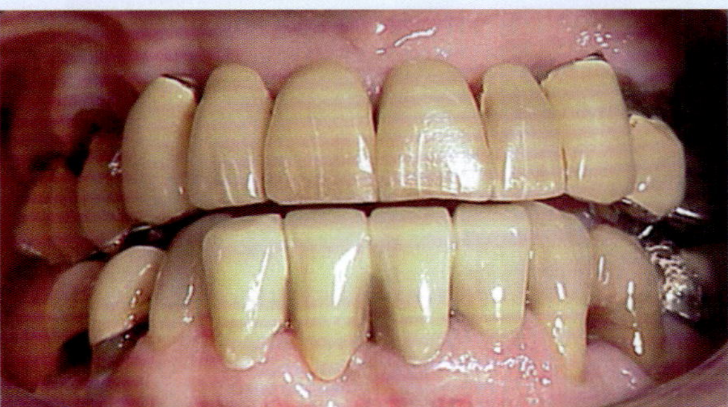

Fig 12.40 Clinical view before graft surgeries (2001). The mobile full bridge of 1997 was used to avoid (as long as possible) a full removable denture.

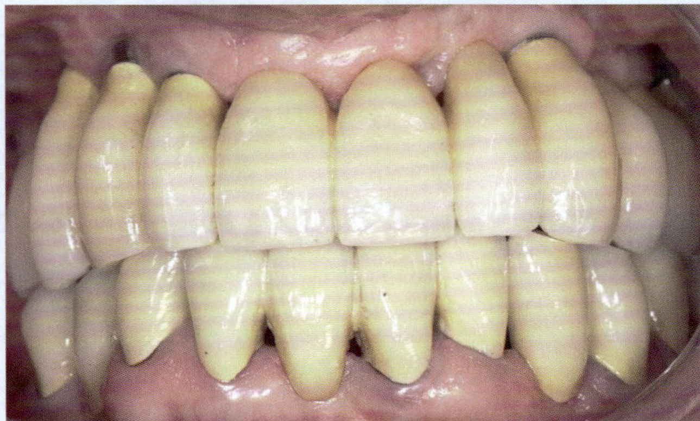

Fig 12.42 Clinical view (September 2010), 13 years after the first periodontal appointment and 9 years after the grafts and implant surgeries. Note the excellent dental plaque control and the lack of inflammation. These two conditions are the major features of long-term success.

Continued

CASE REPORT-6—cont'd

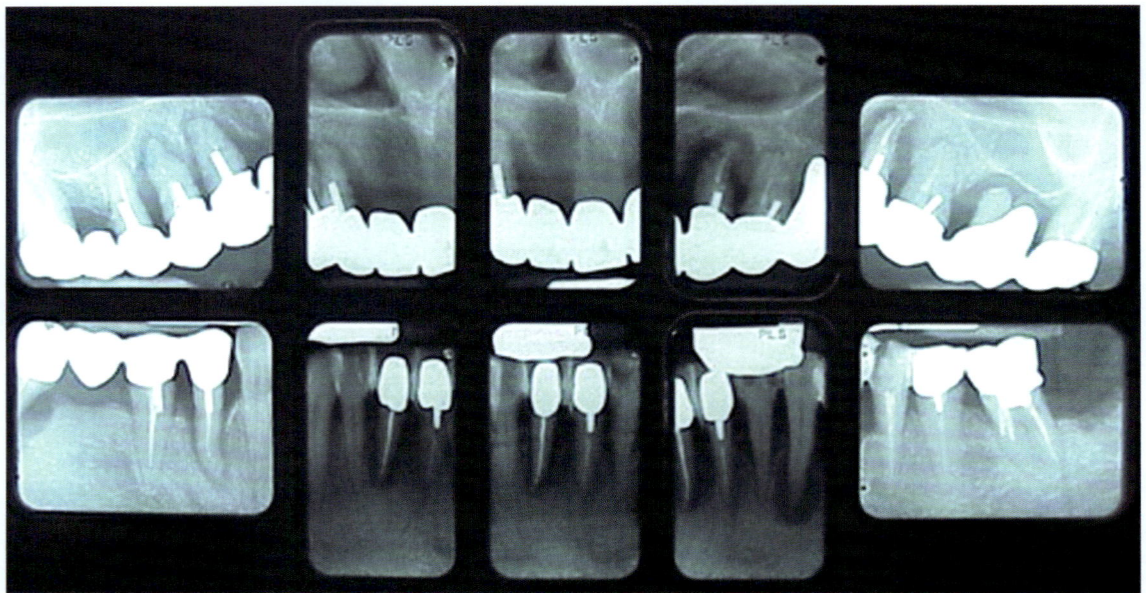

Fig 12.43 'Long-cone' radiographs at the first appointment (1977). Note the severe loss of attachment (often, even more than 100%).

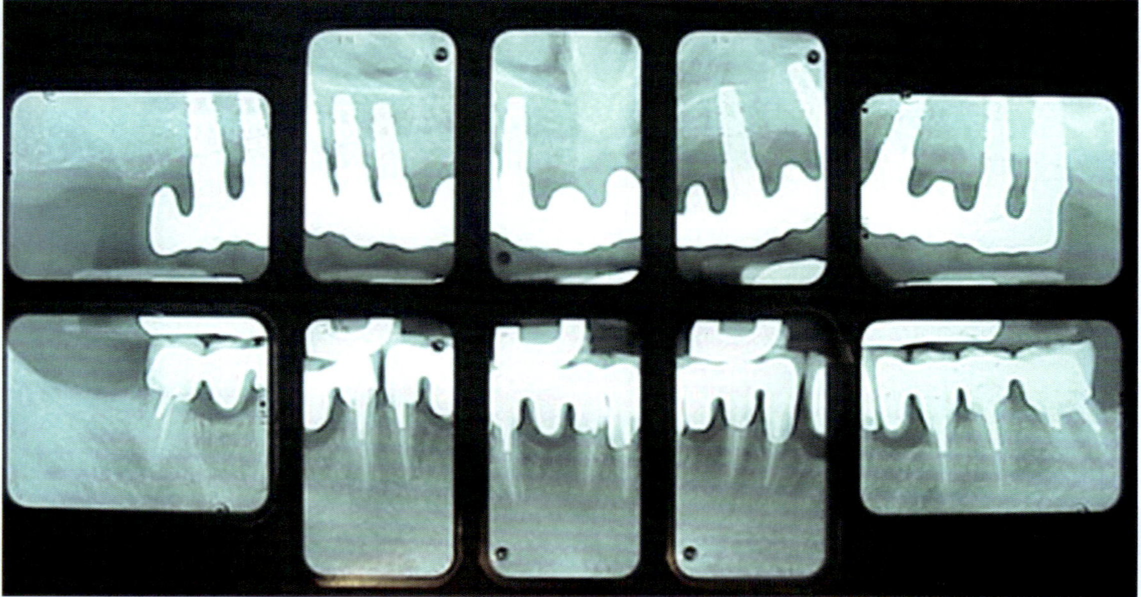

Fig 12.44 'Long-cone' radiographs taken in 2010. Note the good osseointegration of the implants and the stabilization of the loss of attachment of the lower jaw.

Summary

The success of a more or less complex implant treatment for a patient suffering from periodontal disease depends on the patient's compliance to a rigorous protocol. This protocol goes from the periodontal diagnosis up to different therapeutics including periodontal treatment, implant surgery, prosthetic treatment and finally, periodontal and prosthetic maintenance. Good maintenance is one of the key factors of long-term success.

According to the human and financial investment involved in these heavy treatments, it is necessary to offer patients the best and most up-to-date concepts, the most recent scientific, fundamental, and clinical knowledge, recognized techniques, and materials capable of assuring a high rate of long-term success.

Further Reading

Armitage GC, Cullinan M. Comparison of the clinical features of chronic and aggressive periodontitis. Periodontol 2000, 2010;53:12–27.

Aspe P, Ellen RP, Overall CM, et al. Microbiota and crevicular fluid collagenase activity in the osseointegrated dental implant sulcus: a comparison of sites in edentulous and partially edentulous patients. J Periodontal Res 1989;24:96–105.

De Bruyn H, Collaert B. The effect of smoking on early implant failure. Clin Oral Implants Res 1994;5:260–4.

Gatti C, Chiapasco M, Esposito M. Outcome of dental implants in partially edentulous patients with and without a history of periodontitis: a 5-year interim analysis of a cohort study. European J Oral Implantol 2008;1:45–51.

Heitz-Mayfield LJA. Peri-implants diseases: diagnosis and risk indicators. J Clin Periodontol 2008;35(Suppl. 8):292–304.

Hinode D, Tanabe S-I, Yokoyama M, et al. Influence of smoking on osseointegrated implant failure: a meta-analysis. Clin Oral Impl Res 2006;17:473–8.

Holm-Pedersen P, Lang NP, Müller F. What are the longevities of teeth and oral implants? Clin Oral Impl Res 2007;18(Suppl. 3):15–9.

Joachim F, Dujardin S. Implantologie et parodontopathies: quelles décisions thérapeutiques en 2009? Le fil Dentaire 2009;39:26–8.

Karoussis IK, Salvi GE, Heitz-Mayfield LJ, et al. Long-term implant prognosis in patients with and without a history of chronic periodontitis: a 10-year prospective cohort study of the ITI dental implant system. Clin Oral Impl Res 2003;14:329–39.

Koka S, Razzoog ME, Bloem TJ, et al. Microbial colonization of dental implants in partially endentulous subjects. J Prosth Dent 1993;70:141–4.

Lang NP. Implants and teeth in harmony with biology. Wiley-Blackwell Dentistry News 2008;1:3.

Lindhe J, Meyle J. Peri-implant diseases: consensus report of the sixth European workshop in periodontology. J Clin Periodontol 2008;35(Suppl. 8):282–5.

Loe H, Anerud A, Boysen H, et al. Natural history of periodontal disease in man rapid, moderate and no loss of attachment in Srilankan laborers 14 to 46 years of age. J Clin Periodontol 1986;13:431–40.

Lulic M, Brägger U, Lang NP, et al. Ante's (1926) law revisited: a systemic review on survival rates and complications of fixed dental prostheses (FDPs) on severely reduced periodontal tissue support. Clin Oral Impl Res 2007;18(Suppl. 3):63–72.

Mombelli A, Marxer M, Gaberthuel T, et al. The microbiota of osseointegrated implants in patients with a history of periodontal disease. J Clin Periodontol 1995;22:124–30.

Papapanou PN, Wennstrom JL, Sellen A, et al. Periodontal treatment needs assessed by the use of clinical and radiographic criteria. Community Dent Oral Epidemiol 1990;18:113–9.

Quirynen M, Teughels W. Microbiological compromised patients and impact on oral implants. Periodontol 2000, 2003;33:119–28.

Rams TE, Roberts H, Feik D, et al. Subgingival bacteriology of periodontally healthy and diseased human implants. IADR Abstract 267. J Dent Res 1984;63:200.

Schou S, Holmstrup P, Worthington HV, et al. Outcome of implant therapy in patient with patient in previous tooth loss due to periodontitis. Clin Oral Impl Res 2006;17(Suppl. 2):104–23.

Silverstein LH. The microbiota of peri-implant region in health and disease. Impl Dent 1994;3:170–4.

Zitzmann NU, Berglundh T. Definition and prevalence of peri-implant disease. J Clin Periodontol 2008;35(Suppl. 8):286–91.

Basics of bone grafting and graft materials 13

Ajay Vikram Singh Sunita Singh

CHAPTER CONTENTS HD

Introduction

"Bone grafting is a surgical procedure replacing missing bone in order to repair bone defects."

Bone usually has the ability to regenerate completely but requires a very small defect space or some sort of scaffold called 'bone graft' to do so. Most bone grafts are expected to get reabsorbed and replaced as the natural bone heals over a few months' time.

Bone grafting is the process of surgically placing autogenous bone or bone substitutes to repair bone defects or to regenerate desired bone volume for successful placement of an implant of adequate size and at the desired axis. In many instances, a desired implant site in the maxilla or the mandible does not offer enough bone volume or quantity to accommodate a root form implant of desired dimensions or in the proper place, which is ideal for the future prosthesis. This is usually a result of bone resorption that has taken place following loss of one or more teeth or trauma. As described in previous chapters, the bone gets resorbed at a variable pace after tooth loss, due to disuse atrophy, if it has not been replaced with implant restoration. Approximately, two-thirds of the resorption occur in the first 3 months post extraction, which results in a more complex clinical situation. Socket grafting or immediate implant into extraction socket with simultaneous grafting of peri-implant socket spaces, if needed, prevents this resorption.

Many dentists do not give much attention to this problem, and they leave the site either edentulous for a long time or replace the lost tooth with fixed bridges or removable dentures, which causes loss of bone dimensions, necessitating bone grafting before or at the time of implant insertion. Bone grafting procedures usually try to re-establish bone dimension, which has been lost due to resorption.

Either the patient's own bone (autogenous) in different physical forms or bone substitutes with or without autogenous bone, are used to regenerate new bone in and over the bone defect or deficient ridge area.

For successful implant placement, an adequate volume and quality of bone is essential at the site of the implant insertion. However, many patients seeking implant-supported restoration are deficient in bone volume, and hence, bone grafting has become an integral part of day-to-day implant surgery.

In about 40% of all implantations, clinicians use various regenerative procedures to build up the desired quantity and quality of bone and soft tissue. The use of bone substitutes and barrier membranes is now a standard therapeutic approach in implantology.

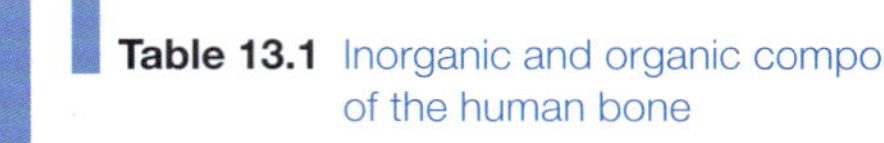

Table 13.1 Inorganic and organic components of the human bone

INORGANIC PHASE (wt%)	ORGANIC PHASE (wt%)
Hydroxyapatite ~60	Collagen ~20
Carbonate ~4	Water ~9
Citrate ~0.9	Noncollagenous proteins ~3 (osteocalcin, osteonectin, osteopontin, thrombospondin, morphogenetic proteins, sialoprotein, serum proteins)
Sodium ~0.7	
Magnesium ~0.5	
Other: Cl^-, F^-, K^+, Sr^{2+}, Pb^{2+}, Zn^{2+}, Cu^{2+}, Fe^{2+}	Other traces: polysaccharides, lipids, cytokines. Primary bone cells: osteoblasts, osteocytes, osteoclasts

Biological mechanism of bone formation at the grafted site

Osteoconduction

Osteoconduction occurs when the bone graft material serves as a scaffold for new bone growth that is perpetuated by the native bone. Osteoblasts from the margin of the defect that is being grafted utilize the bone graft material as a framework upon which to spread and generate new bone. At the very least, a bone graft material should be osteoconductive.

Osteoinduction

Osteoinduction involves the stimulation of osteoprogenitor cells to differentiate into osteoblasts that then begin new bone formation. The most widely studied type of osteoinductive cell mediators are bone morphogenetic proteins (BMPs). A bone graft material that is osteoconductive and osteoinductive does not only serve as a scaffold for currently existing osteoblasts but also triggers the formation of new osteoblasts, theoretically promoting faster integration of the graft.

Osteopromotion

Osteopromotion involves the enhancement of osteoinduction without the possession of osteoinductive properties. For example, enamel matrix derivatives have been shown to enhance the osteoinductive effect of demineralized freeze-dried bone allograft (DFDBA), but they will not stimulate de novo bone growth alone.

Osteogenesis

Osteogenesis occurs when vital osteoblasts originating from the bone graft material contribute to new bone growth along with bone growth generated via the other two mechanisms (osteoconduction and osteoinduction).

Composition of natural bone

Hydroxyapatite and collagen form the major part of the human bone while water, minerals and proteins remain minor elements (Table 13.1).

Types of bone grafts

The autogenous bone remains the gold standard for bone augmentation procedures but the need of another surgical site to harvest the bone, inadequate bone volume availability, donor site morbidity, etc. are problems attendant to the use of autogenous bone. To overcome these problems, bone substitutes alone or mixed with autogenous bone have very successfully been used in intraoral bone augmentation procedures. Various types of bone grafts, which are used in bone augmentation procedures are described here.

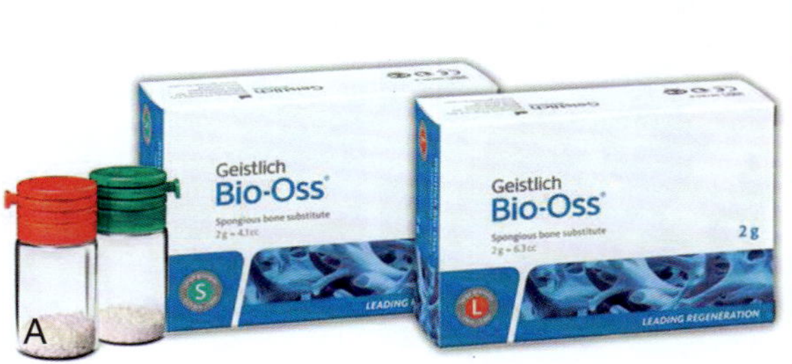

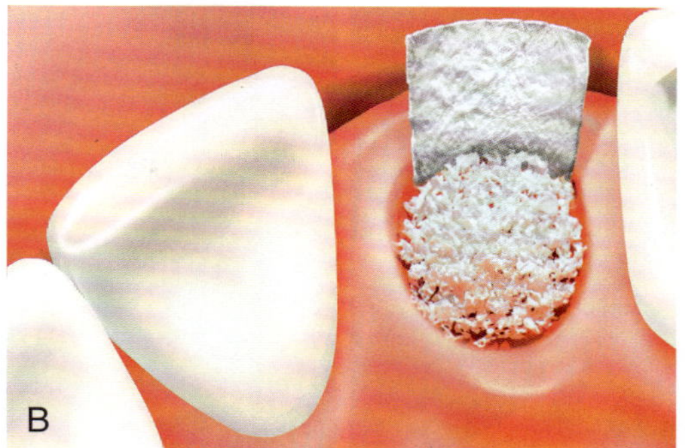

Fig 13.1 Bio-Oss is a natural, osteoconductive bone substitute that promotes bone growth in periodontal and maxillofacial osseous defects. It consists of the mineral portion of bovine bone. (A and B) Bio-Oss provides the body with a matrix for bone cell migration and is integrated into the natural physiologic remodelling process *(Courtesy: Geistlich Biomaterials).*

Autologous/autogenous bone graft/autograft

The bone graft, which is harvested from the patient's own body and immediately used to graft the osseous/ridge defect is called the autogenous bone graft. Autogenous bone remains the 'gold standard' for bone augmentation procedures, as it forms the bone by all three mechanisms of bone formation (osteoconduction, osteoinduction, and osteogenesis). Moreover, the use of autogenous bone as the graft also reduces the cost of the procedure. The drawbacks of using autogenous bone are the need for another intraoral or extraoral site to harvest the bone graft, donor site morbidity, increased time of surgery, and the need for a skilled surgeon to harvest the graft of desired volume, dimension, and quality.

Donor sites

Various intraoral as well as extraoral sites have been used as donor sites to harvest autogenous bone, depending on the volume and quality of bone graft required.

1. Intraoral sources – mandibular symphysis, mandibular ramus/buccal shelf, maxillary tuberosity, etc.
2. Extraoral sources – iliac crest, tibia, etc.

Advantages

1. Less risk of the graft rejection because the graft is originated from the patient's own body.
2. It has all three new bone regeneration properties – osteoconductive, osteoinductive and osteogenic.
3. Reduced cost of the procedure.

Disadvantages

1. An additional surgical site is required to harvest autograft, in effect adding another potential location for postoperative pain and complications.
2. Donor site morbidity.
3. Skilled approach is required to harvest the graft of desired volume and dimensions.
4. Increased time of surgery.
5. Resorbs faster, if used alone in an area of low oxygen like the maxillary sinus.

Bone graft substitutes

Various bone substitutes are available to be used for bone grafting. These bone substitutes remain biocompatible and show the histomorphological similarities more or less, to the human bone. Use of bone substitutes offers several advantages like increase in the graft volume when mixed with the autogenous bone, provision of a bioactive and bioinert scaffold for new bone regeneration, reduced time of grafting procedure, etc. These bone substitutes can either be used mixed with autogenous bone (composite graft) or used alone to regenerate new bone dimensions in many bone augmentation cases. Based on their source they can be classified as:

1. Allograft
2. Xenograft
3. Synthetic bone graft/alloplastic graft.

Allograft

The bone graft which is harvested from cadavers, processed in bone banks to make it usable in the human body is called allograft (e.g. Grafton).

Types of bone allograft

1. Fresh or fresh-frozen bone
2. Freeze-dried bone allograft (FDBA)
3. Demineralized freeze-dried bone allograft (DFDBA).

Xenografts

The bone which is harvested from the animals (bovine source), processed in bone banks to make it usable in the human body is called xenograft.

Thus, these bone substitutes have their origin from a species other than human, such as bovine (e.g. Bio-Oss).

Review of literature on xenograft (Bio-Oss)

Bio-Oss: an ideal osteoconductive material for use in dental implant surgery

Bio-Oss natural bone mineral offers predictable results which have been proven through years of clinical experience and extensively documented in published scientific literature (Fig 13.1A and B).

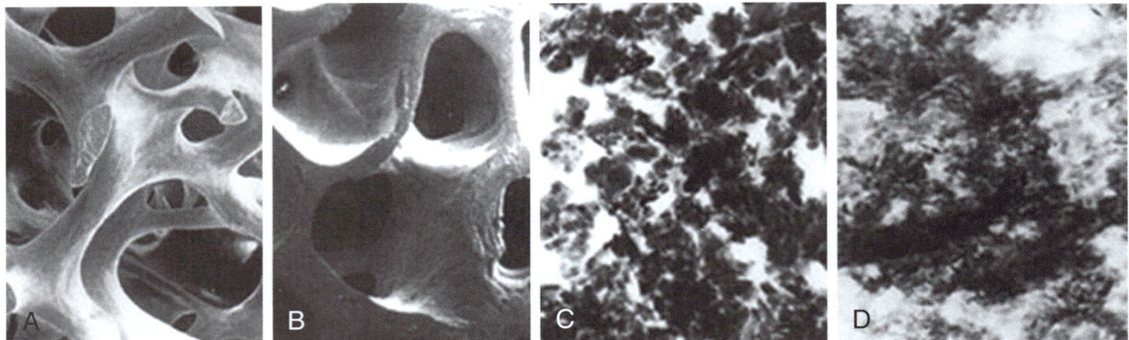

Fig 13.2 Cancellous structure of Bio-Oss. (A) Structure of autogenous bone. (B) Small and compact nanocrystals of Bio-Oss similar to human bone (TEM 100,000×). (C) Human bone – (D) small and compact natural apatite crystals (TEM 100,000×).

Bio-Oss: morphology like the human bone

Geistlich Bio-Oss® is a natural bone substitute material obtained from the mineral portion of bovine bone. The reason for the good bone regeneration seen with Geistlich Bio-Oss® is its close resemblance to human bone. Bio-Oss was developed as an ideal bone substitute that would replicate the structure of autogenous bone. Each step in the development of Bio-Oss was conducted with this goal in mind, resulting in a matrix that is very similar in physical and chemical composition to human bone (Fig 13.2A–D). The trabecular architecture and fine crystalline structure of the natural bone in Bio-Oss are preserved through a patented manufacturing process, resulting in an exceptional osteoconductive matrix.

Process of natural bone regeneration with Bio-Oss

When Bio-Oss is grafted at the osseous defect, it provides a bioinert and bioactive scaffold, into which new blood vessels grow from the peripheral host bone and osteoblasts migrate into the graft and form a new bone at the graft site. The graft gets slowly replaced by new bone via resorption and substitution during remodelling phase of bone (Fig 13.3).

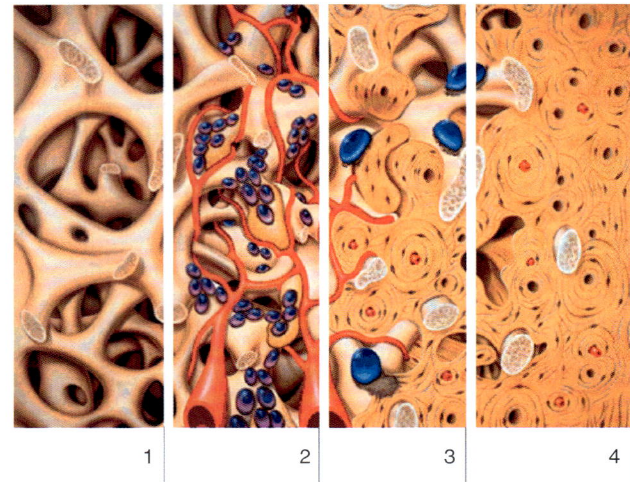

Fig 13.3 Clot stabilization facilitated by Bio-Oss interconnecting macro- and micropores (1). Revascularization (red), migration of osteoblasts (purple) and in-growth of woven bone (yellow) is enhanced by Bio-Oss scaffolding (2). Lamellar bone (dark yellow) and Bio-Oss (light yellow) are successfully integrated after approximately 6 months. Bio-Oss is included in the natural physiologic remodelling process (osteoclasts – blue) (3). Finally remodelled new bone formation at the site grafted with the Bio-Oss (4).

Advantages of Bio-Oss

1. Superior handling characteristics made possible by the large hydrophilic inner surface area similar to human bone.
2. Promotes revascularization and clot stabilization, due to its interconnecting macropores and micropores.
3. Facilitates bone formation by providing an exceptional osteoconductive scaffolding, which results from the retention of the natural porous architecture and trabeculation of human cancellous bone.
4. Effective space maintenance, and when integrated, provides mechanical strength and stiffness due to retention of the natural mineral content.
5. Optimal integration with the patient's own bone aided by a chemical composition analogous to human bone with fewer hydroxyl and more carbonate groups than most synthetic materials.
6. Bio-Oss is integrated during the natural remodelling process of the human bone and slowly resorbed due to small crystallite size, which is comparable to human bone.
7. Effective bone regeneration that has been clinically and scientifically proven for more than 15 years.
8. Bio-Oss prevents newly formed bone from rapid resorption and leads to a long-term preservation of bone volume.

Disadvantages of Bio-Oss

The only disadvantage of Bio-Oss is its slow substitution rate, as the material may appear as pebbles or gel upon re-entry to the grafted site.

Synthetic bone graft/alloplastic graft

The bone grafts which are created from the synthetic source (ceramics) such as calcium phosphates (e.g. hydroxyapatite and tricalcium phosphate), bioglass,

Table 13.2 Mechanisms of bone formation by various types of bone grafts

GRAFT TYPE	OSTEOCONDUCTIVE	OSTEOINDUCTIVE	OSTEOGENETIC
Alloplast	+	–	–
Xenograft	+	–	–
Mineralized allograft	+	±	–
Demineralized allograft	+	+	–
Autograft	+	+	+

and calcium sulphate are called alloplastic or synthetic bone grafts.

Alloplastic grafts are often made of hydroxyapatite or other naturally occurring and biocompatible substances with mechanical properties similar to those of bone. Hydroxyapatite is a synthetic bone graft, which is the most commonly used among other synthetic grafts due to its osteoconduction property, hardness, and acceptability by bone. Hydroxyapatite (HA), if used in combination with tricalcium phosphate (TCP), gives both osteoconduction and resorbability, and thus is being widely used in bone regeneration procedures (OSTEON graft).

Rationale for the use of bone graft substitutes

1. Expands autogenous bone graft volume to graft the large defects.
2. Provides scaffold for osteoconduction.
3. Participates in phase II remodelling.
4. Physical support for guided bone regeneration (GBR) procedures.

Graft quality for successful osteoconduction

1. The graft must provide a bioinert or bioactive scaffold at the ectopic site for new bone formation with the process of osteoconduction.
2. The material should be porous and hydrophilic to favour tissue growth and bony deposition.
3. It should be slowly replaced by new bone via resorption and substitution during the remodelling phase of bone.
4. The scaffold should have a microtopography similar to bone.

Mechanism of bone regeneration by various types of grafts

As described earlier in this chapter, bone formation at the grafted site occurs by three mechanisms – osteoconduction, osteoinduction, and osteogenesis. Various types of grafts play different roles in bone formation depending on their source. The alloplastic or synthetic grafts and xenografts show only osteoconductive properties and only provide a bioinert and bioactive scaffold onto which the blood vessels and osteoblasts migrate from the host bone, to form the new bone. The allograft shows the osteoconductive and also a variable degree of osteoinductive properties. Thus, besides providing a scaffold at the ectopic site, it may also induce the host bone into the procedure of bone formation at the grafted site. Besides showing more enhanced properties of osteoinductivity and osteoconductivity, the demineralization of allografts results in the graft becoming a little osteogenic. The autograft therefore forms bone by all three mechanisms – osteoconduction, osteoinduction, and osteogenesis. Besides providing a scaffold and inducing the host bone into bone formation like the allografts, the autograft also contains the vital cells to begin new bone formation at the graft site before bone formation occurs by the other two mechanisms (Table 13.2).

Growth factors

Growth factor enhanced grafts are produced using recombinant DNA technology. They consist of either human growth factors or morphogens (BMPs in conjunction with a carrier medium, such as collagen). The implant surgeon can also extract the growth factors such as platelet-rich plasma (PRP), Plasma rich in growth factors (PRGF), or platelet rich-fibrin (PRF) from the patient's venous blood just before surgery and mix in the graft to enhance its bone regeneration properties (Fig 13.4A and B).

Composite graft

A composite graft consists of a mixture of autogenous cancellous marrow and a slow-substitution rate bone graft substitute, in a specified ratio.

Two-phase theory of osteogenesis

The new bone formation at the grafted site occurs in two phases when an osteogenic graft (autograft) is used.

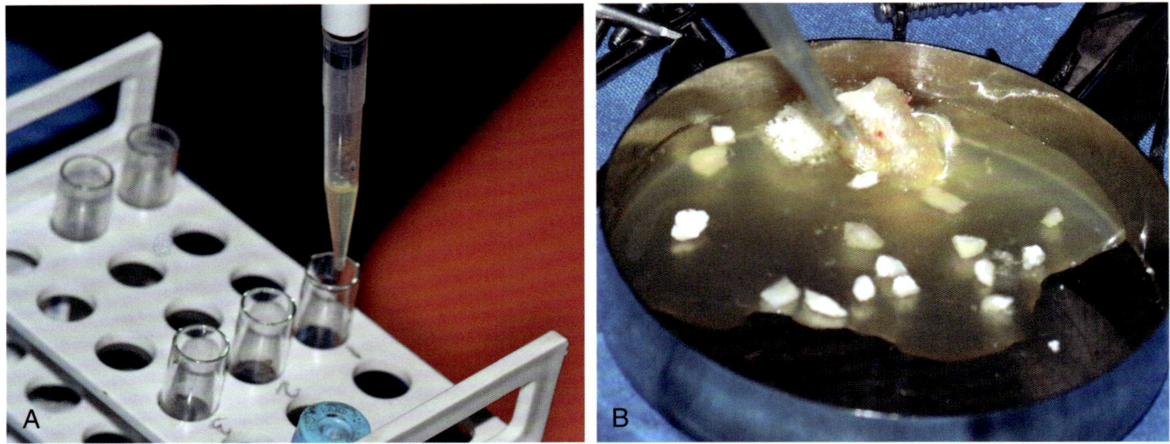

Fig 13.4 (A) Plasma rich in growth factors (PRGF) is separated from the venous blood. (B) PRGF being mixed with the bone substitute.

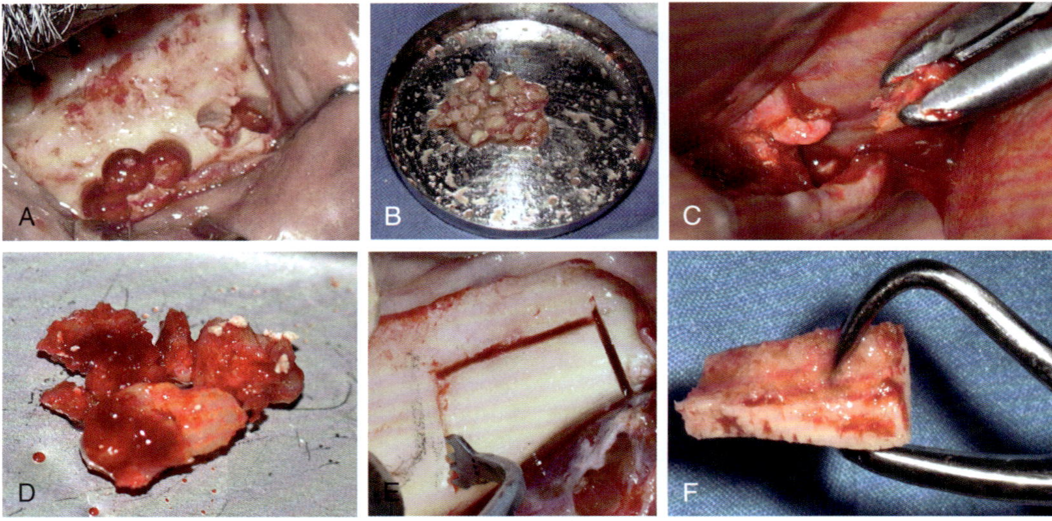

Fig 13.5 Figures showing autogenous bone in various physical forms – autogenous cortical bone harvested from the mandibular symphysis using trephines (A) and (B) crushed to be used as particulate cortical chips. (C and D) The cancellous bone harvested from the maxillary tuberosity and used as a particulate autograft. (E and F) The cortical block graft harvested from the mandibular buccal shelf.

Phase I

Volume yield from graft depends upon the concentration of viable cells transplanted from the donor through the process of osteogenesis. The autogenous cancellous marrow grafts are known to be the 'Gold Standard' for phase I osteogenesis. They are the most useful and predictable grafts because they transfer the viable osteoblast and osteoprogenitor cells to support phase I bone graft healing.

Phase II

Osteoinduction and osteoconduction of osteocompetent cells from the recipient site responsible for graft incorporation, remodelling and replacement according to local stress and strain factors mediated by site specific signalling.

The two-phase theory can be simplified as the autogenous graft transfers the viable osteoblasts and osteoprogenitor cells, which initiate new bone formation at the graft site (phase I osteogenesis), and later on the osteocompetent cells from the recipient site, which get incorporated into the graft, cause remodelling and replacement of the graft with new bone by the process of osteoinduction and osteoconduction (phase II osteogenesis).

Physical forms of grafts

Different types of grafts can be available or harvested in various physical forms and clinically used according to the requirements of the particular case of bone augmentation. The autogenous bone can be harvested and used in various forms like bone blocks (only cortical or corticocancellous), strips, and particulate graft (only cortical chips, corticocancellous, or only cancellous) (Fig 13.5A–F). The different bone substitutes can also be commercially available in various physical forms such as particulate form, putty/gel form, cortical

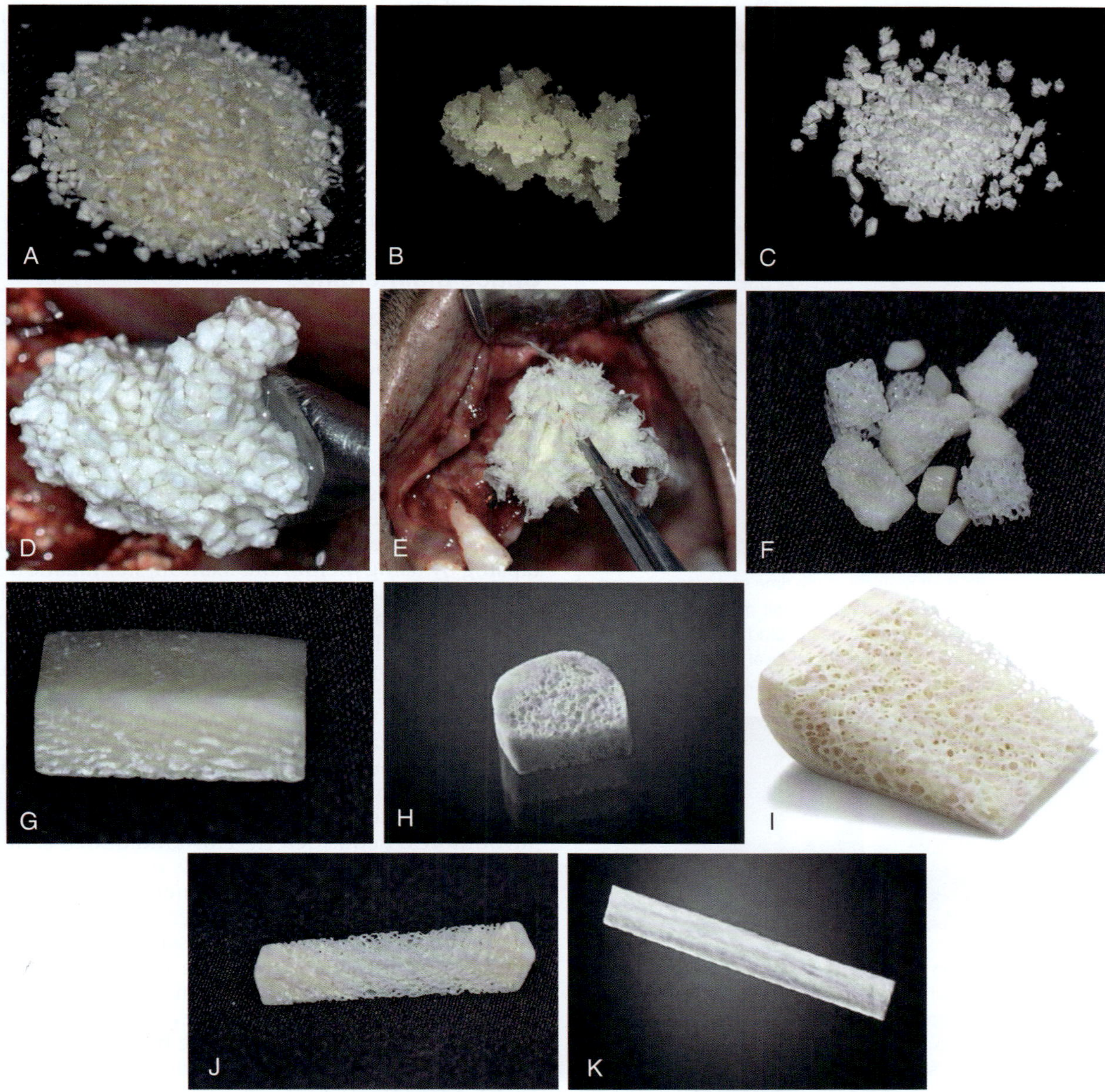

Fig 13.6 (A) Figures showing bone substitutes in various physical forms – particulate form of mineralized and (B) demineralized bone allograft. (C) Particulated xenograft, (D) particulated form of HA + β-Tcp mixture, (E) demineralized allograft in putty form, (F) allograft in the form of corticocancellous chips, (G) cortical block allograft, (H) cancellous block allograft, (I) corticocancellous block allograft *(Courtesy: Zimmer Dental)*, (J) cancellous strip allograft, (K) cortical strip allograft.

chips, strips, and cortical or corticocancellous block form (Fig 13.6A–K).

Keys for successful bone grafting

Surgical asepsis/absence of infection

Infected sites should never be selected for bone grafting until all the infection has been removed and the site has healed with no sign of any active infection like pain, swelling, and purulent discharge. Bacterial infection reduces the pH level at the infected site, which causes solution-mediated rapid resorption of grafted material. There should be no clinical or radiographic findings of any active infection at the site chosen to graft (recipient site) or harvest (donor site) bone graft material. The grafted site should also be prevented from receiving any infection after the procedure because of poor oral hygiene, suture line opening, or membrane or graft exposure to the oral environment, etc. Antibiotics can be added to alloplastic material and autograft. Although tetracycline is often used in periodontal bone grafting to improve collagen formation, it chelates calcium and arrests the bone formation process. Instead, parenteral penicillin, cephalosporin, or clindamycin should be mixed into the graft material, because these antibiotics do not affect the process of bone

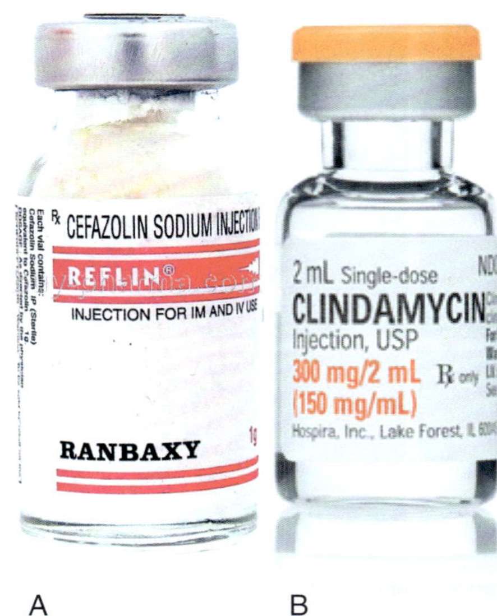

Fig 13.7 (A) A parenteral form of cefazolin sodium (Reflin) or (B) clindamycin can be mixed with graft material at the time of grafting procedure. These antibiotics can also be added to the graft material when the site has been contaminated and has become infected in the early phase of the healing process. This provides increased level of antibiotic concentration at the site, even though vascularization is incomplete.

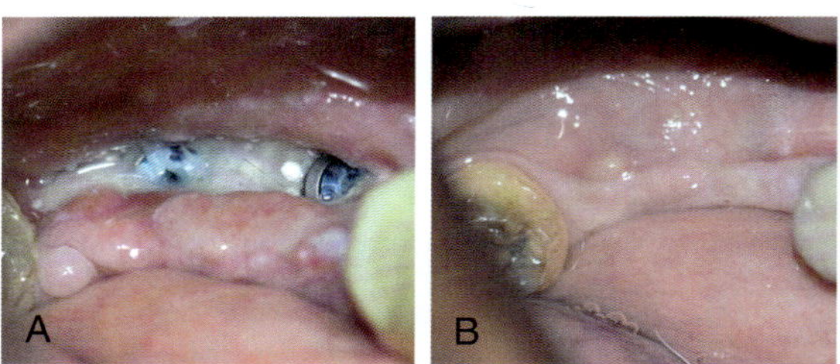

Fig 13.8 Suture line opening can result in loss of graft, soft tissue ingression, and infection to the graft. To prevent the exposed graft getting contaminated/infected, the site can be irrigated with parenteral antibiotics (e.g. cefazolin or clindamycin) two to three times a day till the site gets healed with secondary intension (A and B). This provides increased level of antibiotic concentration at the site, even though vascularization is incomplete.

regeneration (Fig 13.7A and B). Suture line opening can result in loss of graft, soft tissue ingression, and infection to the graft. To prevent the exposed graft getting contaminated/infected, the site can be irrigated with parenteral antibiotics (e.g. cefazolin or clindamycin) two to three times a day till the site gets healed with secondary intension (Fig 13.8A and B). This provides an increased level of antibiotic concentration at the site, even though vascularization is incomplete.

Space maintenance

Space maintenance at the bone graft site is paramount to the bone formation process. The space of the graft site refers to the anatomical site and contour of the desired augmentation, and maintenance refers to the fact that the space must exist long enough for bone to fill the desired region. The barrier membrane which is used to cover the graft often collapses in the grafted space, which leads to the loss/resorption of a partial volume of the graft and results in under contoured new bone formation. The barrier membrane can be prevented from collapsing by using membrane fixation/stabilization screws ('membrane tacks') but better contour can be achieved by using a fixation screw which is elevated above the host bone level to the height/width of the desired bone volume to support the barrier membrane from underneath; this screw is called 'tent screw.' Tent screws, titanium mesh or titanium-reinforced membrane and graft materials beneath the membrane have been advocated to maintain the desired space during the bone grafting process. The osseous defect, which itself can provide adequate space for new bone regeneration is called 'favourable osseous defect.' This kind of defect does not need any tent screw but the walls of the osseous defect itself keep tenting the barrier membrane to maintain the space for new bone regeneration (Fig 13.9A–F). The osseous defect with the missing walls which cannot provide the adequate space by itself for the new bone regeneration is called an 'unfavourable bone defect'. This kind of osseous defect needs the use of the tent screw to keep tenting up the barrier membrane, to maintain adequate space for bone regeneration (Figs 13.10–13.12).

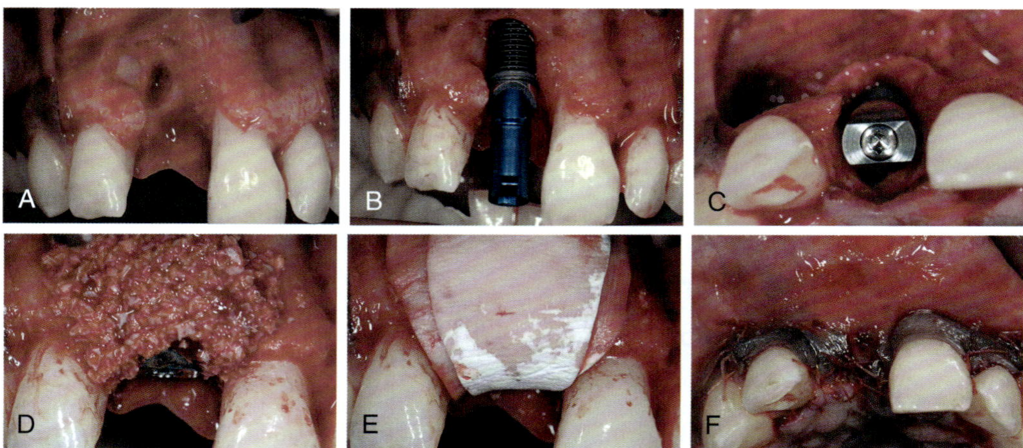

Fig 13.9 The favourable osseous defect, where implant placement has been possible within the osseous envelope of the defect. (A–F) The walls of the defect have provided adequate space maintenance for the graft by tenting up the membrane from underneath *(Courtesy: Dr Peter Randelzhofer, DDS, private practice, Germany)*.

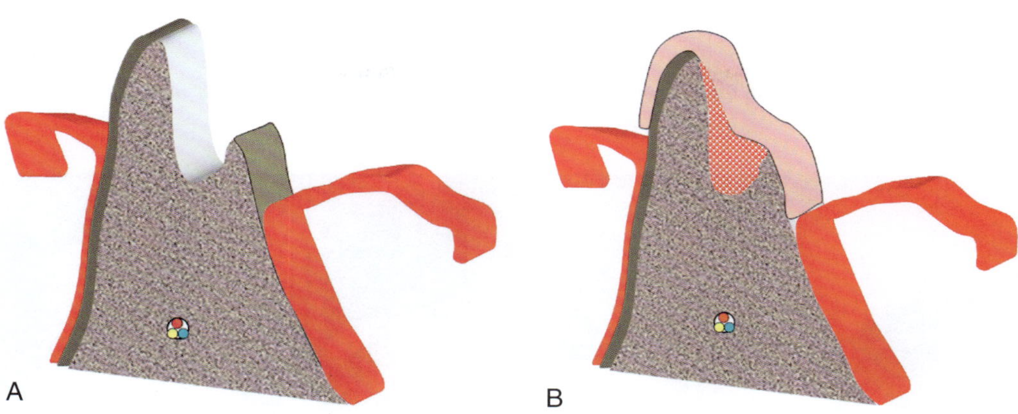

Fig 13.10 An unfavourable bone defect is grafted using particulate bone graft covered with barrier membrane. (A and B) The barrier membrane collapsed in the defect, resulting in compromised space for new bone formation of desired volume and contour.

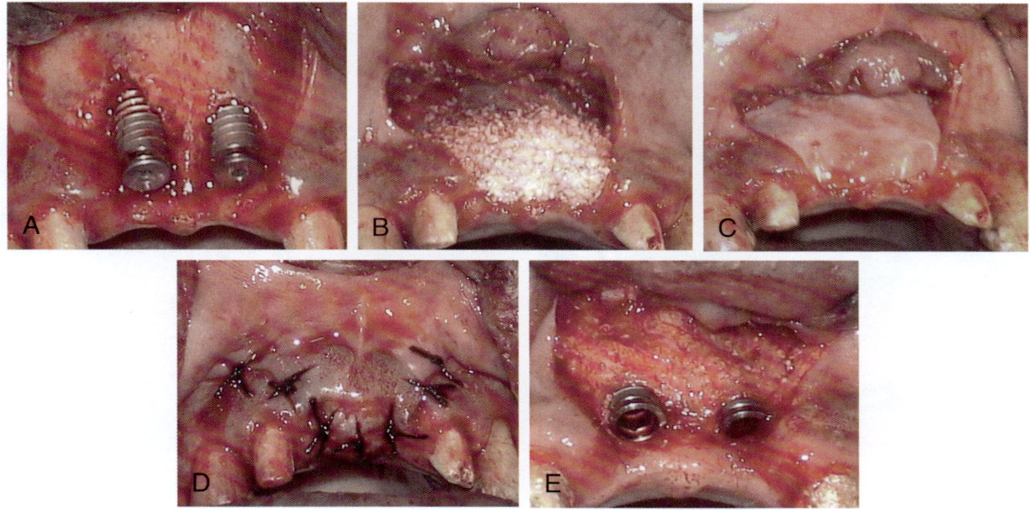

Fig 13.11 Unfavourable osseous defects, where implants could not be placed within the bony envelope. (A–E) Even the defects have been adequately grafted and covered with barrier membrane; the uncovering of the implants shows inadequate amount of bone formation because of inadequate space maintenance and loss of graft.

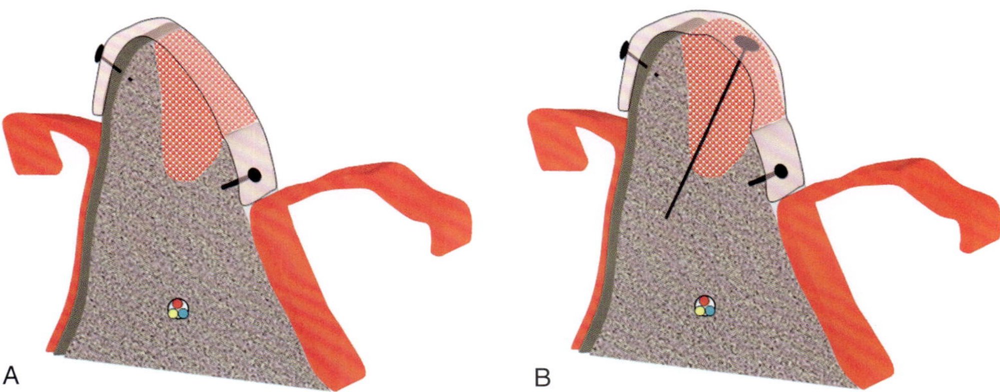

Fig 13.12 (A) The barrier membrane, which is stabilized using fixation screws (membrane tacks) to prevent the membrane from collapsing. (B) Using a long tent screw, which supports the membrane from underneath, results in better space maintenance for the graft and new bone formation of the desired volume and contour.

CASE REPORT

Lateral and vertical bone augmentation in the posterior mandible using tent screws *(Courtesy: Dr Jun Shimada, Japan)* (Figs 13.13–13.15).

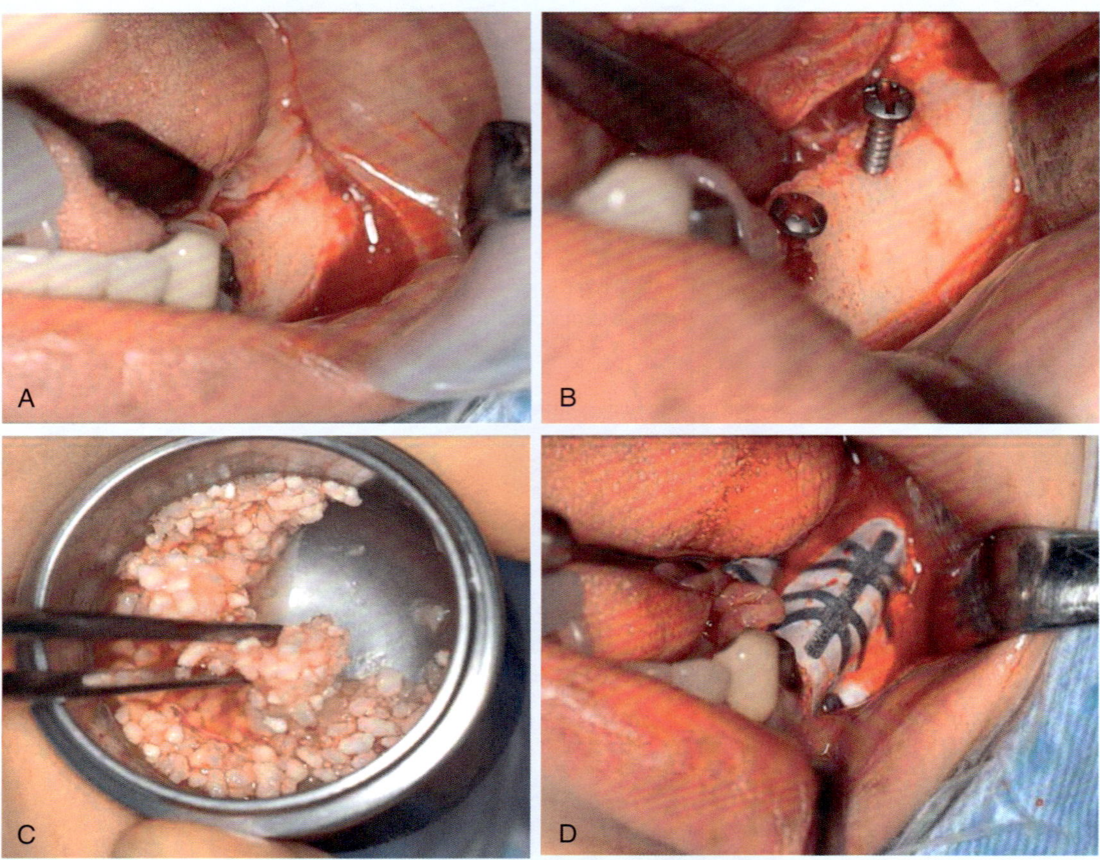

Fig 13.13 (A) The edentulous posterior mandibular ridge shows vertical as well as horizontal bone deficiency. (B) Two tent screws are fixed to the host site keeping them well emerged out of the bony surface. (C) A particulated allograft mixed with platelet-rich plasma (PRP) is used to augment the deficient area to the desired dimensions and covered with titanium-reinforced nonresorbable TXT membrane, which is supported by the (D) elevated tent screws from underneath.

CASE REPORT—cont'd

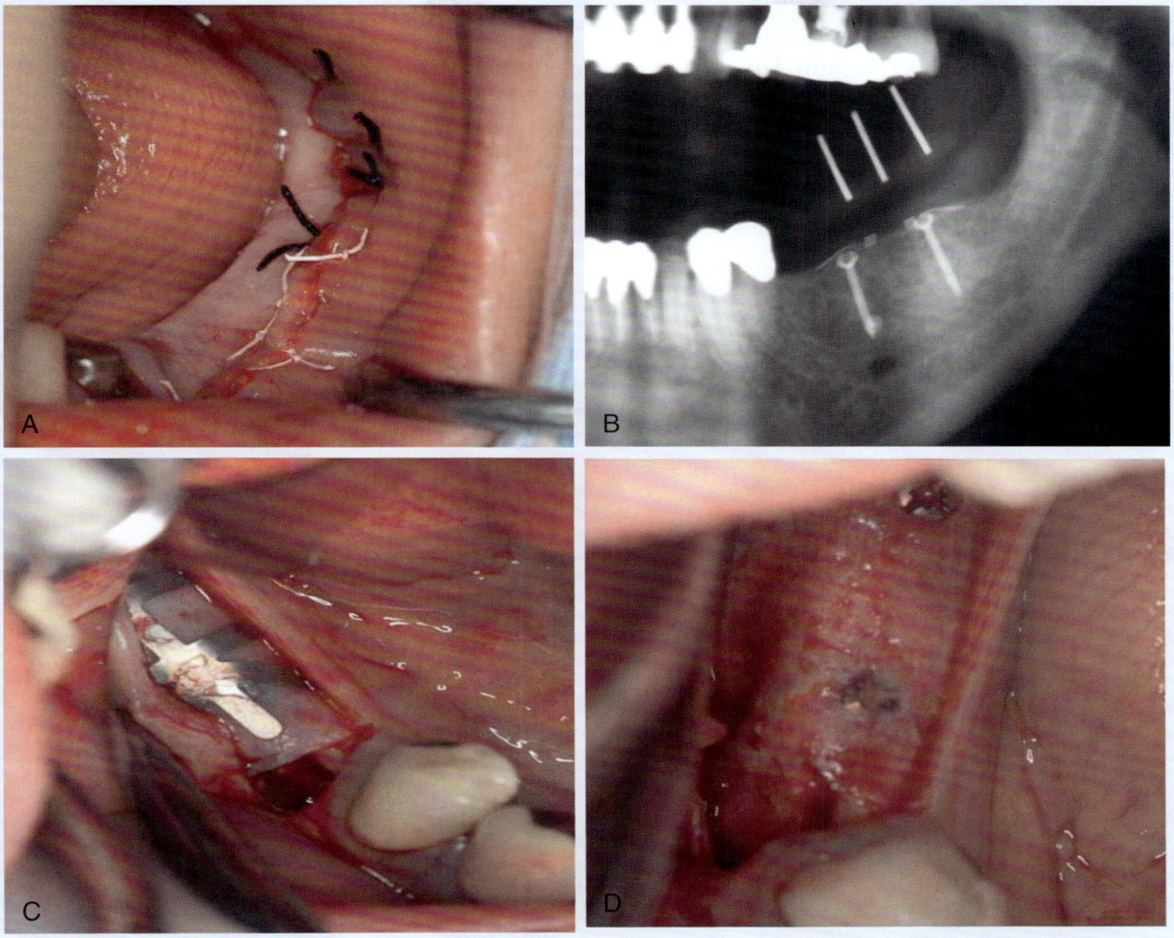

Fig 13.14 (A) The periosteum is released and sutured to achieve a watertight primary closure. (B) Postgrafting radiograph. (C) The site is uncovered after 4 months of healing period and the TXT membrane is removed. (D) The grafted site shows a remarkable amount of new bone regeneration.

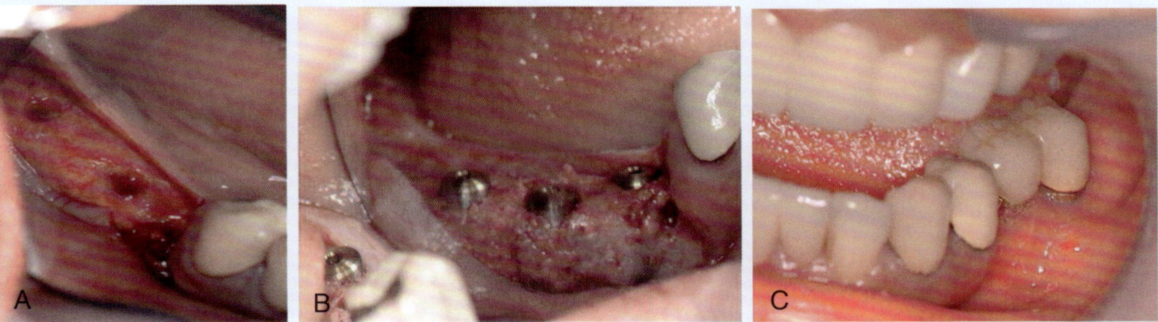

Fig 13.15 (A) The tent screws are removed and (B) implants of adequate sizes are inserted. (C) Clinical view after implants have been restored in function.

Soft tissue closure

The primary closure of the soft tissue is mandatory for the success of the grafting procedure, as it prevents the loss of graft from the site and prevents infection. However, if primary closure is not achieved (e.g. socket grafting), a non-resorbable cytoplast TXT membrane can be used to cover the grafted site to prevent any microbial invasion into the graft or loss of graft material. The primary soft tissue closure ensures healing by primary intension and requires minimal soft tissue collagen formation and soft tissue remodelling. It also minimizes postoperative discomfort to the patient. Often, it becomes difficult to achieve a primary closure over the grafted site because the volume underneath the flap increases after bone grafting. In such cases, primary closure can be achieved by releasing

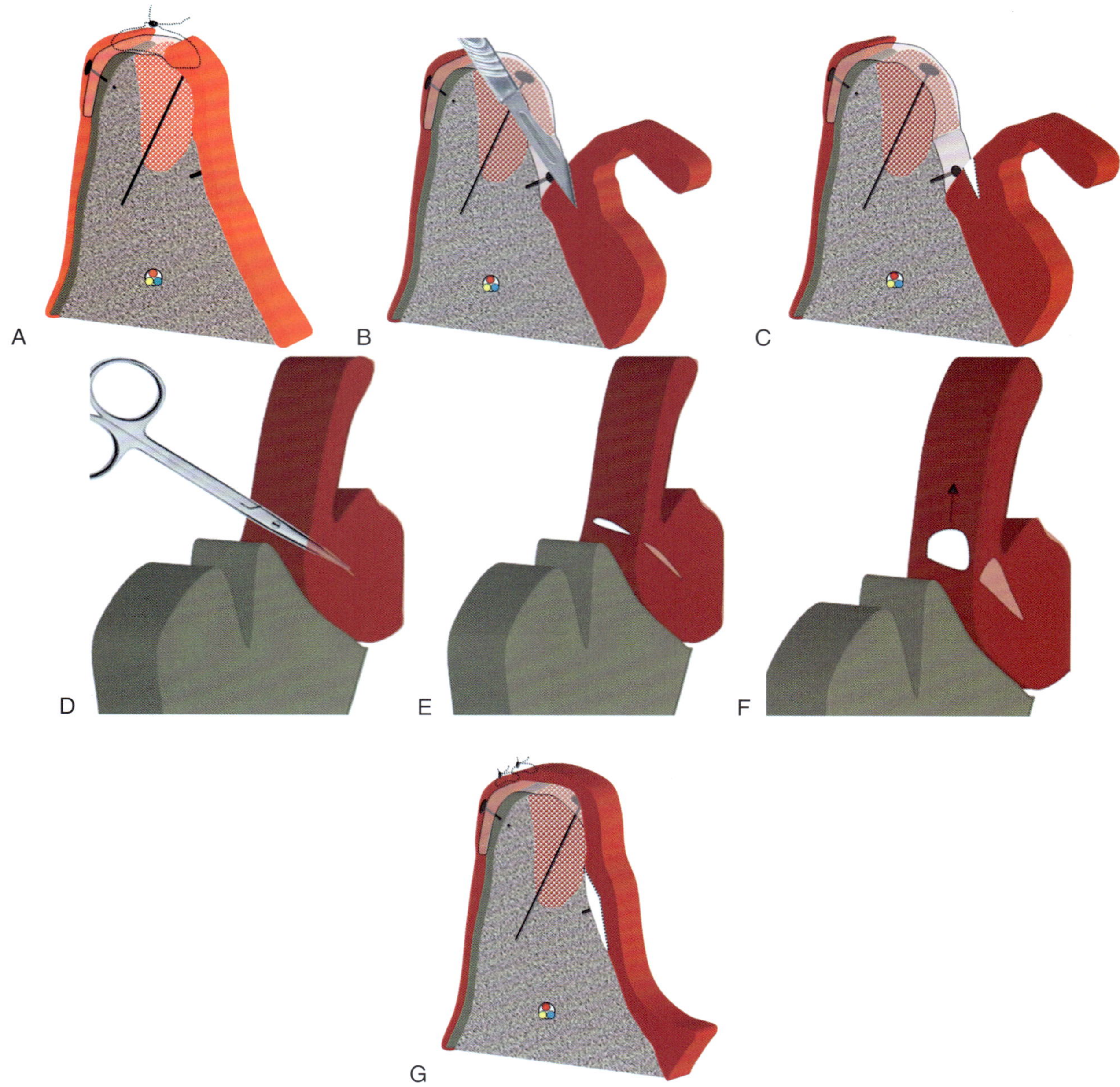

Fig 13.16 (A) Grafting of any bone defect increases the volume of the underlying hard tissue at the site, which may result in difficulty in achieving primary closure of the flap. The tension in sutures may result in suture line opening, which may cause the loss of graft and invasion of soft tissue into the defect area. A scalpel is inserted 1–2 mm deep through the periosteum underneath the facial flap and beyond the mucogingival junction. (B and C) Further, a horizontal incision is given parallel to the crestal incision. (D) Then, a soft tissue scissor is pushed into the facial flap for approximately 10 mm with the blades closed, parallel to the surface mucosa. The thickness of the facial flap is approximately 3–5 mm. The tissue scissors are opened, once at the proper depth. (E) This blunt dissection does not sever any blood vessels or nerves to the facial flap but does create a submucosal space or tunnel. (F and G) Once the submucosal space or tunnel has been created over and beyond the vertical release incisions, the facial flap can be advanced over the graft for tension free primary closure of the flap.

the periosteum of the flap so that it can be advanced to achieve the primary closure. There are two techniques for releasing the flap to achieve primary closure.

Submucosal space technique

This technique, developed by Misch in the early 1980s, is an effective method to expand tissue over larger grafts (greater than 15 × 10 mm in height and width) (Figs 13.16 and 13.17).

Advantage: A large degree of flap advancement can be achieved for a tension-free flap closure covering the large grafted sites.

Disadvantage: As the incision is given into the periosteum, the blood supply to the grafted region and overlying soft tissue is affected, which results in longer time taken for soft tissue healing.

Curvilinear-bevelled incision technique

This is another method of flap advancement. The cut back incisions are made at the vestibular ends of the vertical incisions and the flap is coronally advanced and sutured first at the crestal part, followed by suturing of the vertical incisions at the vestibular half by mobilizing mobile vestibular soft tissue together. Only a limited degree of

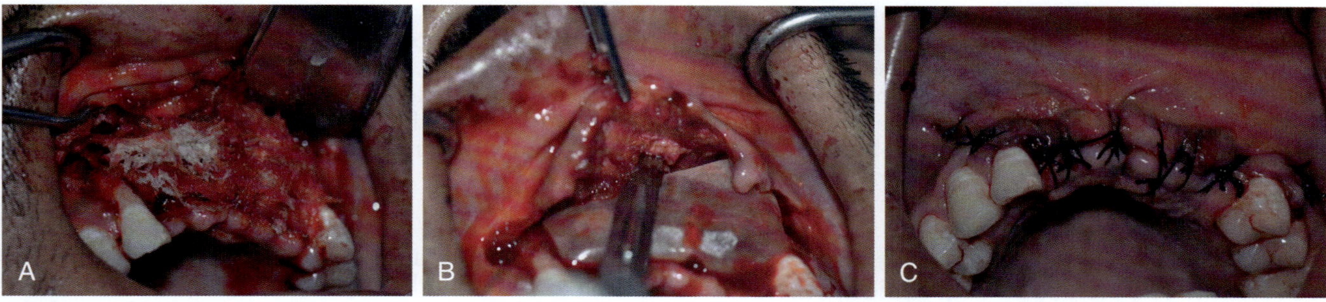

Fig 13.17 (A) Bone grafting has increased the volume of the hard tissue under the flap, which results in difficulty in achieving primary closure of the flap without tension in the sutures. (B) Thus a releasing incision is given through the periosteum of the facial flap for the easy coronal advancement of the flap and (C) to achieve primary closure without any tension in the flap.

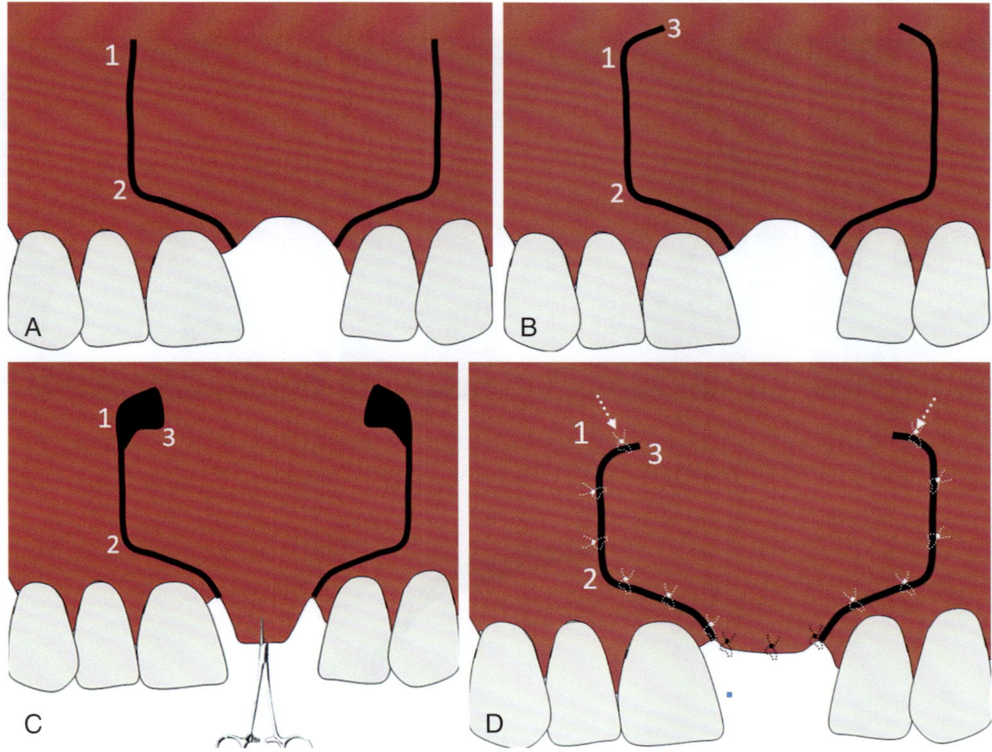

Fig 13.18 (A) Curvilinear-bevelled incision is given, and (B) extended with two cut back incisions at the vestibular ends. (C) The flap is advanced coronally and (D) sutured first at the crystal part with tension-free primary closure followed by suturing of nonkeratinized mobile vestibular tissue area. This technique can be followed for the smaller grafted regions as the coronal advancement of the flap with this technique is less than that obtained with the submucosal space technique but it has the advantage of not hindering the blood supply of the flap as the underlying periosteum remains intact to the flap.

flap advancement is possible with this technique when compared to the submucosal space technique. The advantage of this technique is that it does not hinder the blood supply to the grafted region and overlying soft tissue because no horizontal incisions are made through the periosteum (Fig 13.18A–D).

Graft immobilization/fixation

Graft stabilization is a must to achieve a predictable bone augmentation. If the particulate graft material or the bone block graft is not stable at the host site, it cannot develop the blood supply from the host bone for new bone regeneration. This can further result in the graft becoming encapsulated in fibrous tissue and often sequestrated. For barrier membrane or particulate graft to work effectively, no load should be placed on the soft tissue over the graft, because it may cause movement of the graft. If barrier membrane is used, it should be immobilized to the graft site by using bone tacks. The block bone graft should firmly be immobilized to the host bone using multiple fixation screws to avoid any micromovement during bone remodelling (Fig 13.19A–C).

Prevention of soft tissue ingression/barrier membranes

The epithelium and connecting tissue grows much faster than the new bone formation into a grafted area; hence, a barrier membrane is required to cover the bone graft to prevent the infiltration of the soft tissue into the graft site. A thick cortical plate of the block graft may act as a barrier membrane and often, the membrane is not required in the block grafting cases where a cortical block graft is used. If the periosteum of the flap over the grafted site is intact it can also act as natural barrier membrane and prevent epithelium and connective tissue infiltration into the graft.

Types of barrier membranes

There are various kinds of barrier membranes which are used in bone grafting and implant procedures. These membranes can either be the resorbable type (collagen membranes and pericardial membranes), which need to be completely covered by the soft tissue flap and are resorbed with time, or they are the nonresorbable type polytetrafluoroethylene (PTFE) membranes, which can be left exposed to the oral environment and need to be removed after the underlying graft has been consolidated (Fig 13.20A–C).

Resorbable collagen membrane

These membranes are used to cover the graft where the primary closure of the flap is possible. These membranes keep preventing soft tissue ingression into the graft during its resorption and new bone formation. These membranes slowly get resorbed in 6–10 months and do not have to be removed (Fig 13.21A–D).

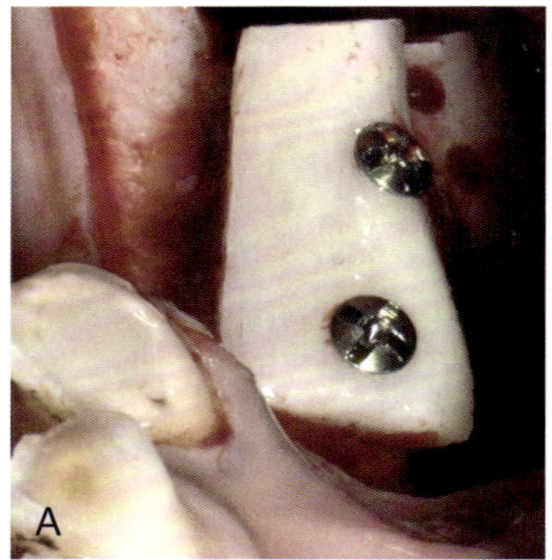

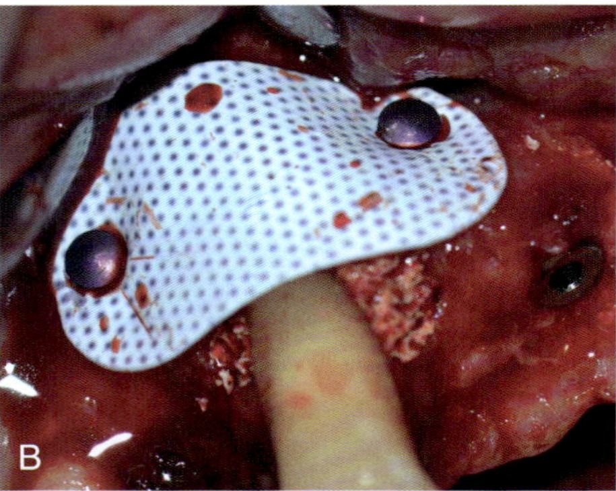

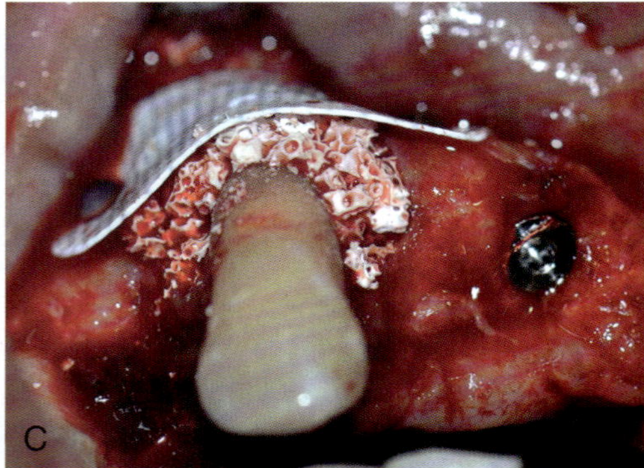

Fig 13.19 (A) Bone block graft firmly immobilized at the host site by using long fixation screws. (B and C) In another case, the membrane is stabilized using bone tacks to prevent its movement during the graft maturation.

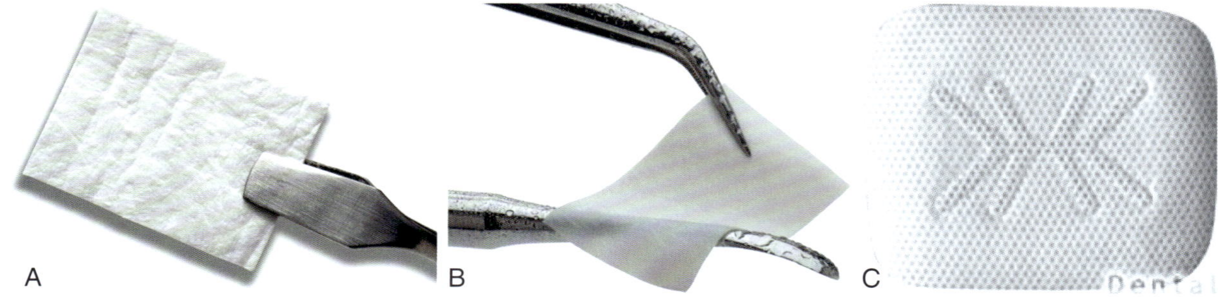

Fig 13.20 (A) Resorbable collagen membrane, (B) resorbable pericardium membrane from Zimmer Dental, and (C) nonresorbable PTFE Cytoplast TXT membrane.

Resorbable pericardium membrane

It is a biological three-layered membrane, which encases and protects the heart and can be used for guided tissue regeneration. The advantages of these membranes are flexible and adaptable, remodel/are resorbable, tough and resilient, suturable, and space creating.

Nonresorbable high-density PTFE barrier membrane

These are the nonresorbable type of membranes and so need to be removed after graft maturation. These membranes are very useful where soft tissue closure cannot be achieved because being nonresorbable these membranes can be left exposed to the oral environment (Fig 13.22A–F).

Bone graft vascularization

The nutrient blood vessels from the host bones are required to nourish the autogenous bone graft to keep its cells alive. The cortical bone should be perforated to grow the host blood vessels from the inner cancellous bone to the graft. These blood vessels from the host bone that enter the graft site also carry the bone forming cell (osteoblast) to populate the grafted site with osteoblast, which results in predictable new bone formation (Fig 13.23A and B).

Defect size

The size of the bone defect (width and height) is directly proportional to the period of bone maturation and the amount of autogenous bone needed in the graft.

Defect topography

Defect topography is a key factor affecting the bone augmentation procedure (Fig 13.24).

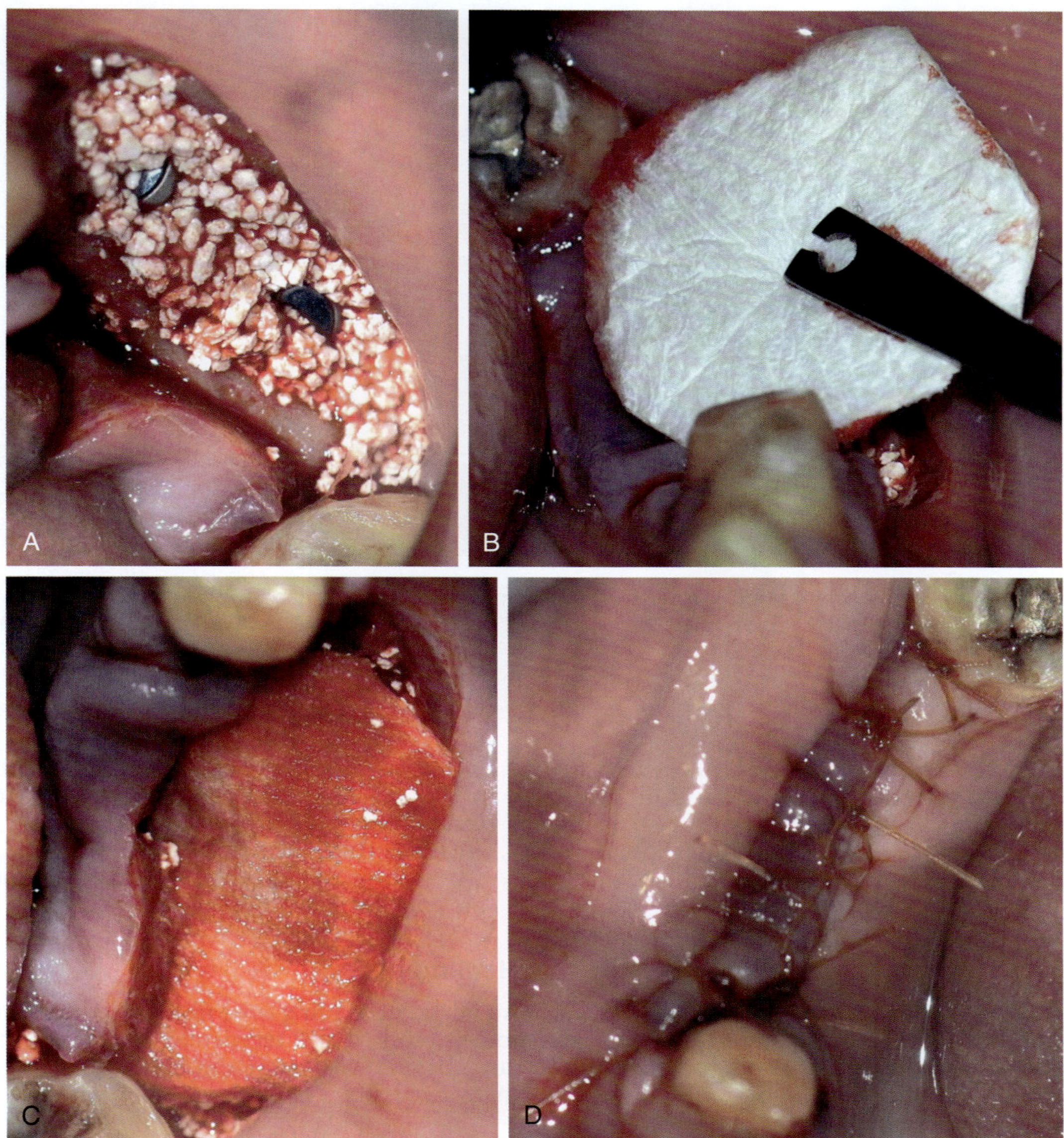

Fig 13.21 (A–D) The grafted site is covered with resorbable collagen barrier membrane and a primary closure of the soft tissue is achieved to completely cover the membrane.

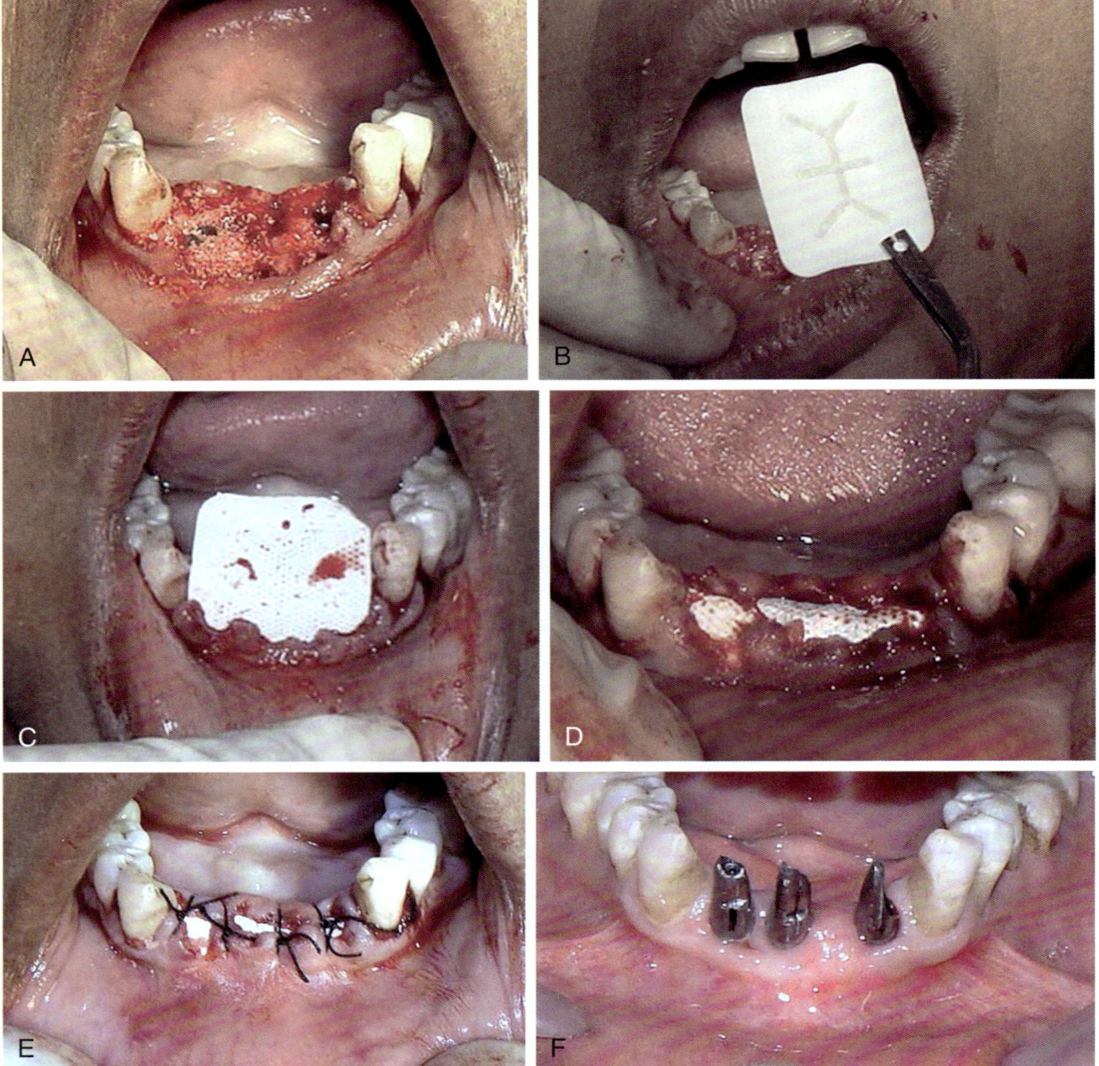

Fig 13.22 Graft to fill the peri-implant socket spaces is covered using titanium-reinforced nonresorbable TXT membrane and the flap is sutured with part of the membrane left exposed to the oral environment. The membrane is removed 6 weeks after the graft has consolidated. (A–F) The implants are uncovered after 4 months for prosthetic loading.

1. **Type of graft used.** The type of graft needed greatly depends on the number of walls present in the defect (Table 13.3).
2. **Space maintenance.** Tent screw and titanium-reinforced membrane can be used.
3. **Soft tissue closure.** Releasing incisions can be made to release the flap and achieve soft tissue closure.
4. **Graft immobilization.** Fixation screws should be used for graft immobilization.
5. **Graft vascularization.** Graft vascularization is directly proportional to the number of walls present in the defect. The decortications of host bone enhance vascularity to the graft.
6. **Growth factors.** Growth factors like PRGF, if mixed with graft, enhances bone formation in defects with compromise topography.
7. **BMPs.** Use of autogenous bone graft and decortication of the host bone site enhances the concentration of BMPs at the site.
8. **Healing time.** The more compromised the defect topography, the longer is the healing period required for bone formation.

Healing time

An adequate healing time must be provided for the graft to get resorbed and regenerate new bone at the site. The amount of healing time can be variable and depends on many factors like

1. Defect size
2. Topography of the defect
3. Amount of graft used

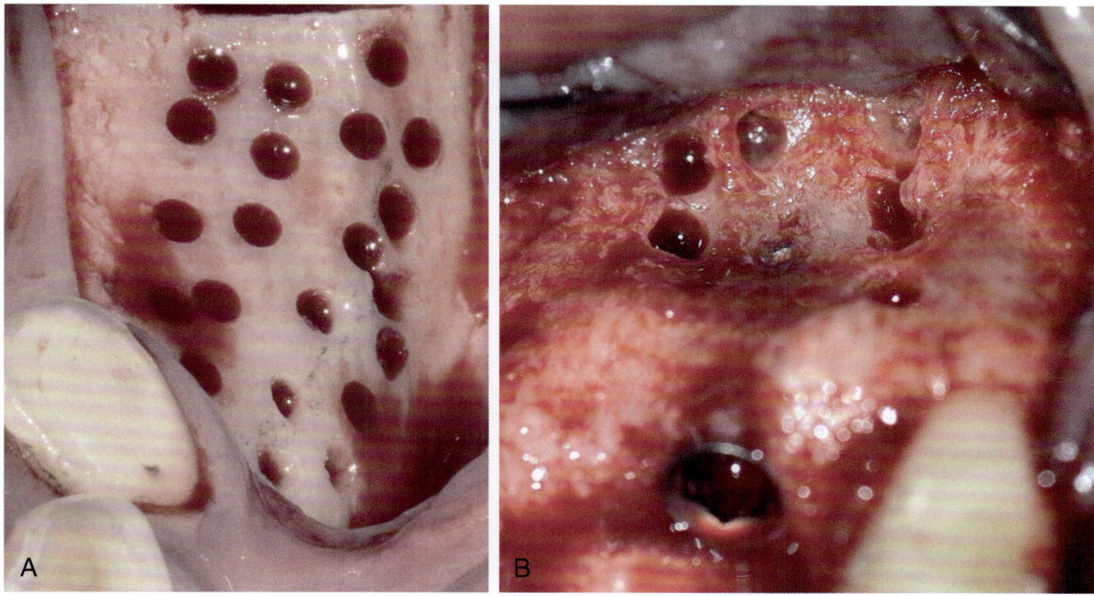

Fig 13.23 (A and B) The cortical bone at the host site is perforated using small round carbide bur before grafting, to achieve nutrient blood supply from the inner cancellous bone to the graft.

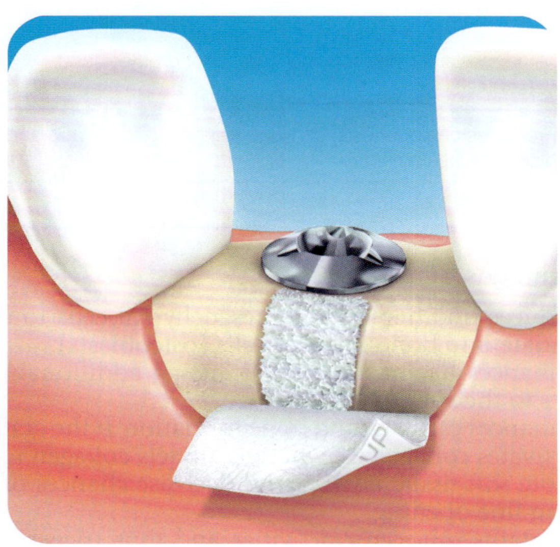

Fig 13.24 The type of the graft and barrier membrane which should be used largely depends on the topography of the bone defect. *(Courtesy: Geistlich Pharma AG, Switzerland).*

d. Type of graft material used.
e. Amount of autogenous bone used in the graft.
f. Host bone vascularity.
g. Number of bony walls surrounding the graft site.
h. Additional keys incorporated into the bone graft, such as growth factors.
i. Systemic diseases like diabetes, hyperparathyroidism, thyrotoxicosis, osteomalacia, osteoporosis, and Paget's disease affect the healing process. To avoid any error, as a general rule, 4–6 months healing is recommended for graft volumes less than 5 mm in dimension, and 6–10 months healing for graft volumes more than 5 mm in dimension.

Table 13.3 Types of bone graft used to augment different types of osseous defects

BONE DEFECT	GRAFT USED
Five bony wall defect	Any resorbable graft material (RGM)
Four bony wall defect	Autograft/RGM and membrane
Two/three bony wall defect	Autogenous bone + RGM and barrier membrane
One bony wall defect	Onlay block graft of autogenous bone

Bone graft material

Various types of bone graft materials have already been described in this chapter.

Growth factors

Wound healing involves a complex and incompletely understood array of cellular and molecular intracellular and extracellular events. However, it is known that platelets and the formation of a provisional matrix play a prominent and likely determinant role in the initiation and maintenance of wound healing. Platelets are naturally activated by exposure to damaged tissue. Primary haemostasis and initiation of the clotting cascade are just the beginning of the platelets' role in healing. Upon activation, platelets release their granular contents (α-granules) into the wound environment.

The contents of the platelet α-granule are of particular interest to wound healing as they contain a host of anabolic growth factors responsible for the initiation, propagation and maintenance of wound healing. These growth

Table 13.4 Synopsis of growth factors present in PRP

GROWTH FACTOR	SOURCE	FUNCTION
Transforming growth factor-beta (TGF-ß)	Platelets, extracellular bone matrix, T-lymphocytes, macrophages, monocytes and neutrophils	1. Stimulates undifferentiated mesenchymal cell proliferation 2. Regulates endothelial, fibroblastic and osteoblastic mitogenesis 3. Regulates collagen synthesis and collagenase secretion 4. Regulates mitogenic effects of other growth factors
Platelet-derived growth factor (PDGF)	Platelets, osteoblasts, monocytes, endothelial cells, macrophages and smooth muscle cells	1. Stimulates chemotaxis/mitogenesis of mesenchymal cells, osteoblasts, fibroblast, smooth muscle cells, macrophage and neutrophils 2. Regulates collagenase secretion and collagen synthesis
Platelet-derived epidermal growth factors (PDEGF)	Platelets, macrophages and monocytes	1. Stimulates endothelial chemotaxis/angiogenesis 2. Regulates collagenase secretion 3. Stimulates mitogenesis of epithelial/mesenchymal cells
Platelet-derived angiogenesis factor (PDAF)	Platelets and endothelial cells	1. Stimulates angiogenesis and vascular permeability 2. Stimulates mitogenesis of endothelial cells
Insulin-like growth factor (IGF)	Osteoblasts, macrophages, monocytes and chondrocytes	1. Stimulation of bone matrix synthesis 2. Replication of osteoblasts 3. Enhances the pace and quality of wound healing
Platelet factor-4 (PF-4)	Platelets	1. Enhances chemotaxis of neutrophils and fibroblasts 2. Acts as a potent antiheparin agent
Basic fibroblast growth factor (bFGF)	Platelets, macrophages, mesenchymal cells, chondrocytes and osteoblasts	1. Promotes growth and differentiation of chondrocytes and osteoblasts 2. Mitogenesis of mesenchymal cells, chondrocytes and osteoblasts
Connective tissue growth factor (CTGF)	Platelets	1. Promotes angiogenesis, cartilage regeneration, fibrosis and platelet adhesion

(*Source*: Peter AM, Everts, et al. Platelet-Rich Plasma and Platelet Gel: A review. J Extra Corpor Techn. 2006;38:174-187)

factors can be of various types like platelet-derived growth factor (PDGF), fibroblast growth factor (FGF), transforming growth factor (TGF), insulin-like growth factor (IGF), and many more. Individually and synergistically these growth factors stimulate progenitor cell localization to a wound, wound fibroblast expansion and subsequent wound matrix production. In concert with the provisional matrix or scaffolding, the growth factors initiate and propagate wound healing.

If explained in a very simplified manner, the human blood contains the platelets which remain suspended into the plasma. On activation, these platelets secrete the α-granules and these α-granules release the various growth factors which enhance the wound healing process. Thus, in bone augmentation procedures, if the plasma which is rich in the platelet count is applied over the graft site. On activation, it releases various growth factors which not only enhance the formation and mineralization of bone by inducing undifferentiated mesenchymal cells to differentiate into bone-forming cells but also enhance the pace of soft tissue healing at the surgical site (Table 13.4).

The human venous blood is made of four major components: red blood cells (RBCs), white blood cells (WBCs), platelets and plasma (Fig 13.25A and B) but the platelets are the greatest source of the growth factors. These factors have the characteristics of wound hormone, acting as a chemoattractant and recruiting the mesenchymal cells into the wound.

Advantages of using PRGF

1. Induces undifferentiated mesenchymal cells to differentiate into bone-forming cells (osteoblasts).
2. Enhances haemostasis by attracting additional platelets to the site.
3. Enhances cartilage and bone formation at the graft site.
4. Activates collagenase which remodels collagen to promote soft tissue healing and decrease chances of incision line opening.
5. Contains mitogenic activities and thus triggers capillary formation at the graft site, which generates a new blood supply to the graft from the host bone.
6. Enhances site debridement by inducing undifferentiated mesenchymal cells to differentiate into osteoclasts.
7. If mixed with autogenous bone graft it can accelerate mineralization by as much as 40% during the first year.
8. Provides a continued source of growth factors for bone regeneration and repairs.

Contraindications to the use of platelet-rich preparations

1. Platelet dysfunction syndrome
2. Critical thrombocytopaenia
3. Hypofibrinogenemia
4. Haemodynamic instability
5. Septicaemia

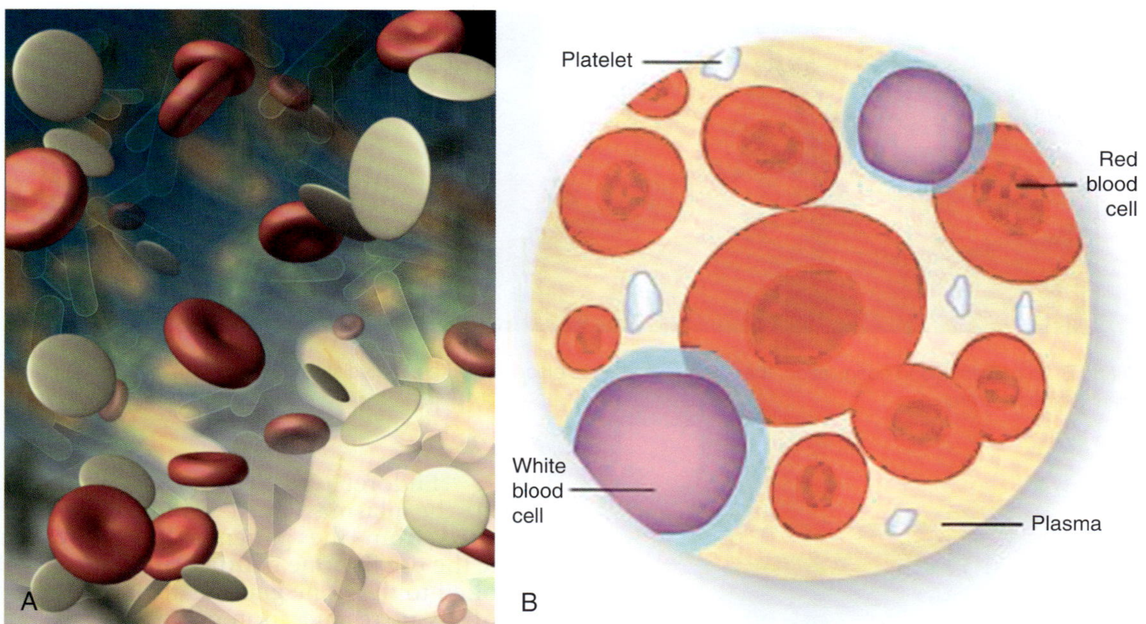

Fig 13.25 (A and B) Components of human blood.

6. Sensitivity to bovine thrombin (if using bovine thrombin with calcium to make platelet gel).

Types of growth factor preparations

Various types of platelet-rich preparations have been tried in the past but the most commonly used growth factor-rich preparations are:

1. Platelet-rich plasma (PRP)
2. Plasma rich in growth factors (PRGF)
3. Platelet-rich fibrin (PRF)

Platelet-rich plasma

It is defined as 'a sample of autologous blood with concentrations of platelets above baseline values'. Platelets play an instrumental role in the normal healing response via the local secretion of growth factors and recruitment of reparative cells.

The application of PRP has been documented in many fields. PRP was first promoted by M Ferrari in 1987 as an autologous transfusion component after an open heart operation to avoid homologous blood product transfusion. Since then, the PRP has been successfully used in various medical fields such as orthopaedics, sports medicine, dentistry, otolaryngology, neurosurgery, ophthalmology, urology, wound healing, cosmetic, cardiothoracic and maxillofacial surgery. In dentistry, PRP was first introduced by Marx et al. (1998) in combination with autologous bone grafts for the reconstruction of mandibular defects.

Preparation

Depending on the volume of PRP preparation desired, typically 20–50 ml of venous blood is withdrawn from the patient before the surgery into the tubes containing anticoagulant such as citrate dextrose-A. This blood is first centrifuged for 5 min at 1100 rpm which results in the separation of whole blood into two layers: the upper yellow plasma layer containing platelets, leukocytes and clotting factors and the lower red-coloured layer containing erythrocytes (RBCs). The yellow plasma layer is separated and the lower erythrocyte layer is discarded. The yellow plasma layer is again centrifuged at 2500 rpm for 10 min. This results in the separation of plasma into two layers: upper platelet poor plasma (PPP) and lower PRP. The upper PPP is discarded and the lower PRP is preserved for the use during bone augmentation procedure. Once the PRP is ready for use, it should be clotted by mixing it with an activator (thrombin and $CaCl_2$) just before using it. Once activated, it activates the platelets and the platelets start secreting growth factors immediately (90% within the first 10 min and rest in next 30 min). Within few minutes after activation, the PRP starts converting into a gel form and if immediately mixed into the graft it binds the graft particles together and improves its handling properties. This PRP gel cannot be used as the barrier membrane because it does not prevent the fibroblasts from invading a bone graft site over an extended period of time what the barrier membrane does. However, it may

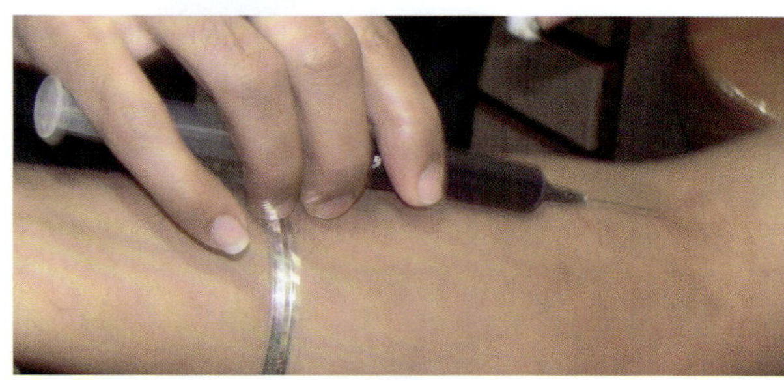

Fig 13.26 Venous blood is withdrawn from the patient from any superficial vein before the surgery using a 10 ml syringe.

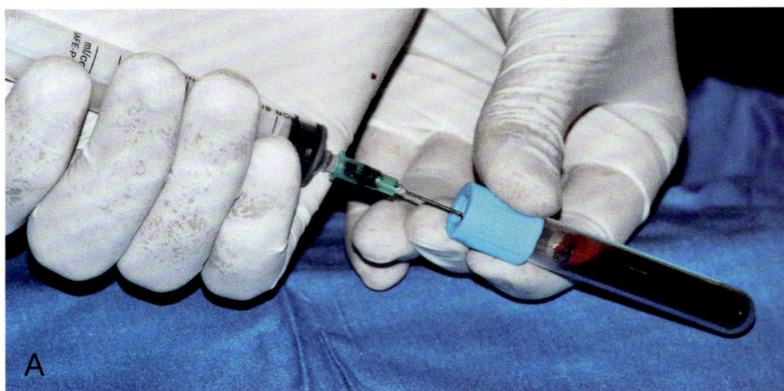

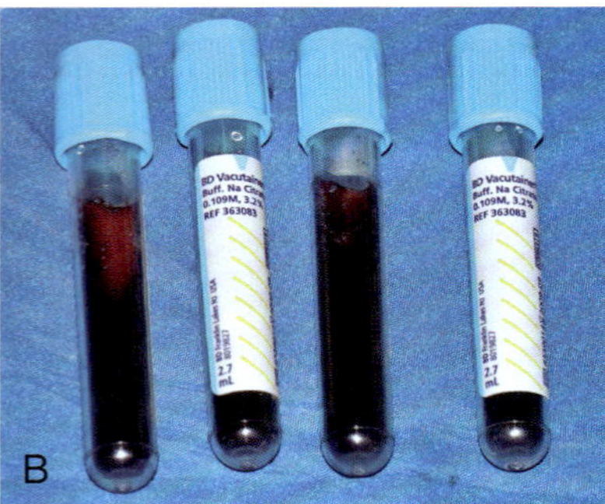

Fig 13.27 (A and B) To prevent blood coagulation, the withdrawn venous blood should be immediately poured into the vacuumed tubes containing an anticoagulant (sodium citrate).

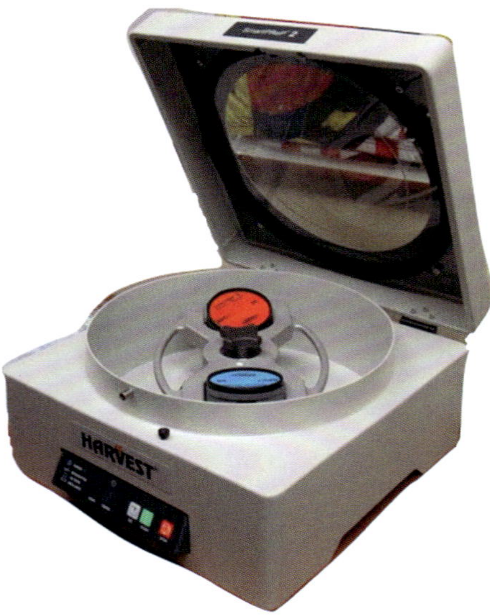

Fig 13.28 The tubes containing venous blood are placed in a centrifuge machine *(Courtesy: Harvest Technologies Corp.)* and the venous blood is centrifuged at 3500 rpm for approximately 20 min to separate the blood into three layers.

be applied over the barrier membrane. Because PRP gel also contains fibrinogen, it enhances the soft tissue healing by acting as a haemostatic agent and reducing the postoperative oedema and pain. Irrespective of the type of bone graft, when the PRP is added to the bone graft, it increases the rate, quality, and volume of bone formation at the grafted site.

Plasma rich in growth factors

In 1999, Eduardo Anitua proposed the use of PRGF. PRGF is based on obtaining a plasma preparation rich in platelets. These platelets contain the various growth factors such as TGF-β1, VEGF (vascular endothelial growth factor) and IGF which stimulate and speed up tissue regeneration.

When any tissue injury occurs, the human body releases proteins (cellular signals) to stimulate the process of repairing that injury. The PRP is the rich source of these proteins and growth factors. With PRGF®- Endoret® technology (BTI Biotechnology, Spain), the plasma which contains these proteins is separated from the patient's blood by centrifuging before the use in bone grafting surgery. Once this PRGF is applied to the bone grafting area, the bone as well as the soft tissue regeneration process at the graft site gets considerably accelerated. To carry out this process, a small amount of blood is withdrawn from the patient. This blood is centrifuged at a specific rotational speed and for a specific time to obtain the proteins essential for regeneration. These proteins are applied to the bone grafting area to enhance the pace of tissue regeneration. Thus in implantology, PRGF can be extracted out from the patient's own blood before the bone augmentation surgery and used with bone graft to enhance the bone regeneration potential of the graft. When the PRGF coagulum or membrane is placed under the flap or over the extraction socket, it also promotes the soft tissue healing. Clinically, PRGF can be differentiated from PRP in that it needs a smaller volume of blood and prepared by single spun only.

Preparation of PRGF

Step 1 – Venous blood withdrawal: Using a syringe, 10 ml of venous blood is withdrawn from the patient before surgery (Fig 13.26). The volume of blood withdrawal depends on the amount of PRGF required to be prepared. Usually for small to medium size grafting sites, 10 ml of blood is sufficient for PRGF preparation.

Step 2: Blood is poured into vacuum tubes containing anticoagulant (sodium citrate) (Fig 13.27A and B).

Step 3 – Centrifugation of blood: The tubes containing the venous blood are placed into a centrifuge machine and the blood is centrifuged at 3500 rpm for approximately 20 min to separate the blood into three layers (Fig 13.28). The upper layer contains the plasma, the middle layer contains WBCs, and lowermost layer contains the RBCs. The uppermost layer that contains plasma is of use and the other two layers (RBC and WBC) are of no use and hence should be discarded later. The plasma layer itself is further divided into three equal layers. The upper one-third plasma layer that contains no platelets, the middle one-third layer that contains platelets in poor concentration (PPP), and the lower one-third plasma layer that contains a high concentration of the platelets (Fig 13.29).

Lowest layer contains RBCs
Middle layer contains WBCs
Upper layer contains plasma

The lowest (RBCs) and middle (WBCs) layers are of no use in PRGF preparation and hence should be discarded.

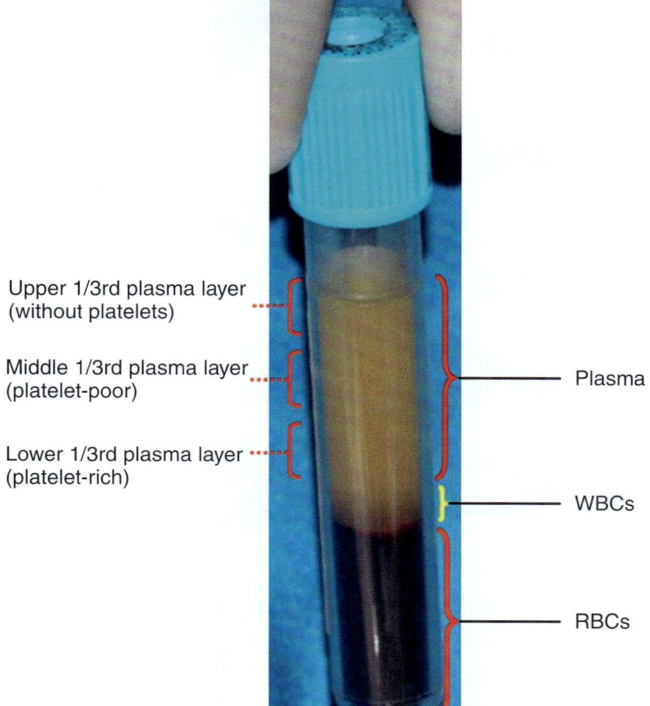

Fig 13.29 Centrifuged venous blood showing all the different layers of the blood.

Step 4 – Separation, activation and use of plasma layers: The uppermost plasma layer is further divided into three equal layers and separately withdrawn using the micropipette and stored in three different Borosil test tubes (Fig 13.30A–C).

1. The upper one-third plasma layer (plasma without platelets) – This layer contains no platelets, hence it is either discarded or can be used to irrigate the osteotomy site or to wash the implant surface before placing it into osteotomy site. This plasma can also be mixed in platelet-poor or platelet-rich plasma to raise their volume. Unlike the other two plasma layers this plasma layer is not activated by mixing the platelet activator ($CaCl_2$).
2. The middle one-third plasma layer (platelet-poor plasma) – This layer contains a very small concentration of platelets and hence is mixed with activator ($CaCl_2$) and placed in thermoblock for 20 min to make a coagulum (if placed in test tube) or a membrane (if placed in glass plate). The 15 µl activator is mixed in 1.0 ml plasma.

   This PRGF membrane is not a barrier membrane as it does not prevent the soft tissue growth into the bone graft for several weeks to months. However, it may be applied over the barrier membrane to reduce the postoperative pain and oedema and to enhance the pace of soft tissue healing (Fig 13.31A–E).
3. The lowermost one-third plasma layer (platelet-rich plasma) – This plasma layer is very rich in platelet concentration and of prime importance in guided bone regeneration.

   This layer is activated just before the graft application by the addition of calcium chloride ($CaCl_2$) to it and this activated plasma is mixed to the graft. Alternatively, this plasma is first mixed with the graft material and then the activator is added to it. It starts converting into a jelly form and the activated platelets start releasing various growth factors just within 15 min of its activation. The mixing of cancellous bone or particulated graft with PRGF also

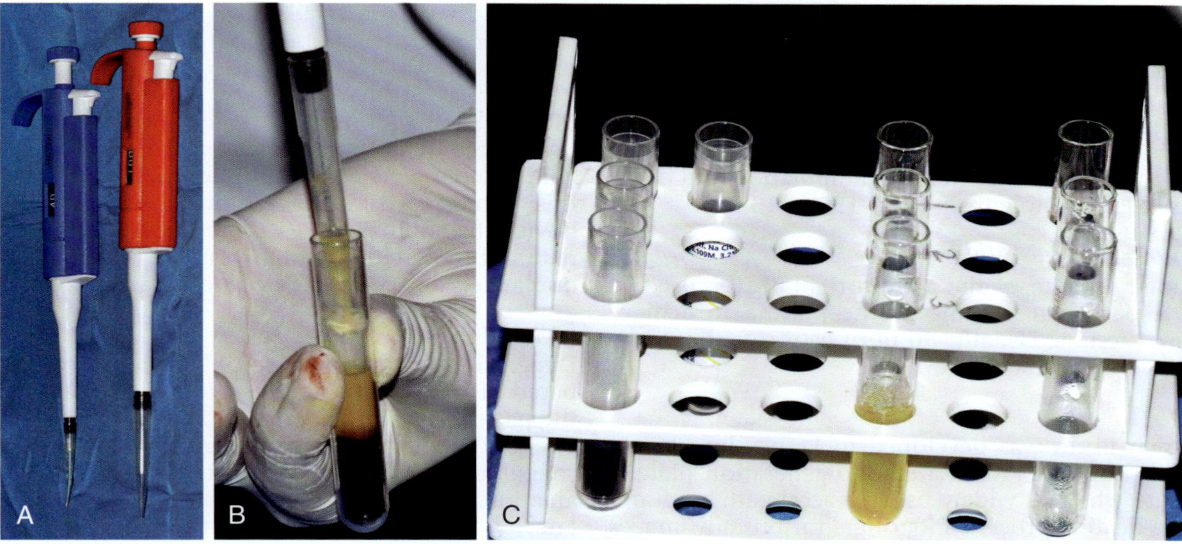

Fig 13.30 (A) Two small pipettes are used to transfer the plasma and to add the activator; (B) all three plasma layers are separately withdrawn and (C) stored into three individual Borosil tubes.

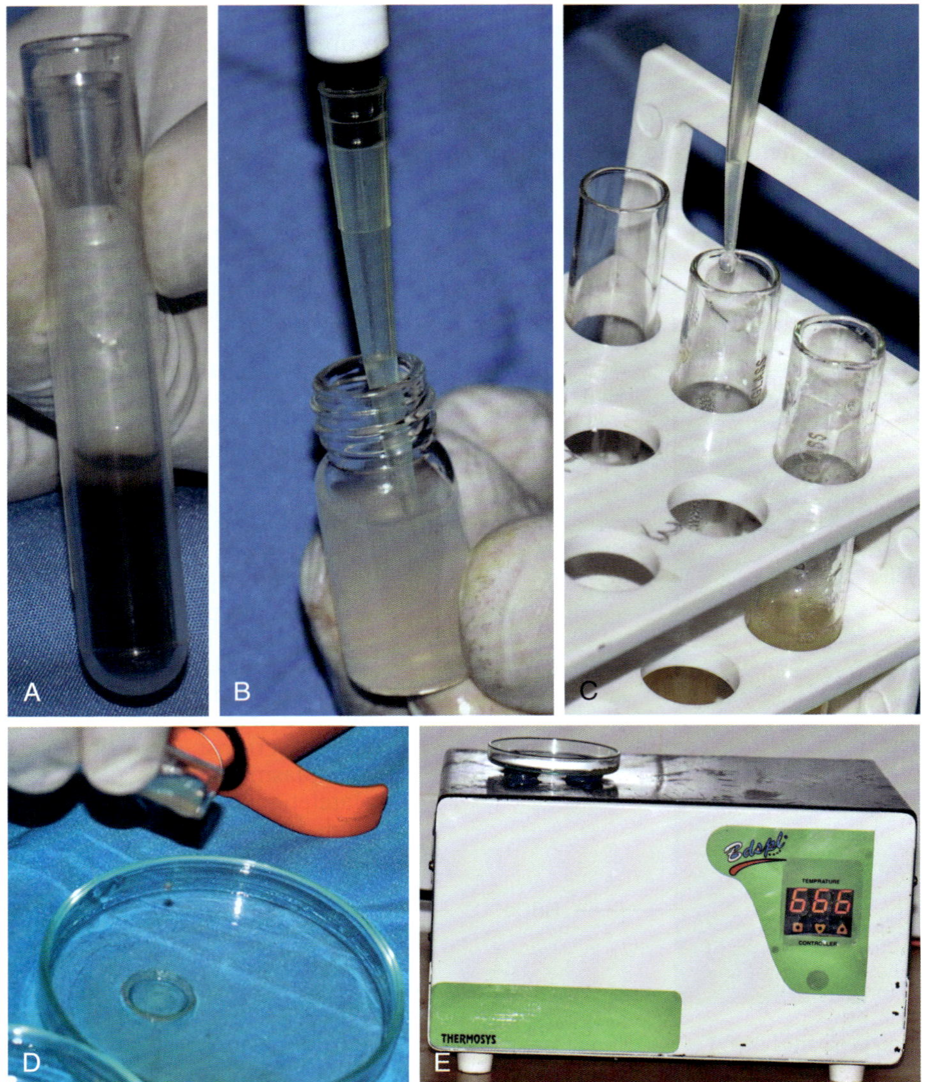

Fig 13.31 (A) The middle (WBC) and lower (RBC) layers are of no use, hence are discarded. (B and C) The activator (calcium chloride) added to the platelet-poor plasma. (D) The activated platelet-poor plasma can be poured into a Borosil glass plate and (E) placed over a thermoblock to make its membrane.

improves its healing properties as the PRGF acts as a 'biological' carrier and this mixture gives stability to the graft and facilitates manipulation and delivery to the recipient site (Figs 13.32–13.34).

Plasma and activator ratio

An accurate volume of the activator should be used to activate a particular volume of the plasma to achieve the desired results. Usually, 50 µl of activator should be mixed in 1 ml plasma (Table 13.5).

Platelet-rich fibrin

Platelet-rich fibrin was developed in France by Choukroun et al. in 2001. PRF is a second-generation platelet concentrate which is widely used to accelerate hard and soft tissue healing process. PRF offers various advantages over the better known PRP and PRGF and that include ease of preparation, ease of application, minimal expense and lack of biochemical modification as no bovine thrombin or anticoagulant is required to be mixed. Thus, PRF is a strictly (100%) autologous fibrin matrix containing a large quantity of platelet and leukocyte cytokines. Unlike other platelet concentrates such as PRP and PRGF, this technique does not require any anticoagulants or bovine thrombin. The PRF is prepared by centrifuging the natural blood without additives. The PRF is accumulated of platelets and releases cytokines in a fibrin clot.

Preparation

Depending on the amount of PRF required to be prepared, 10–20 ml of venous blood is withdrawn from the patient and immediately poured into the test tubes. The blood without any anticoagulant obviously starts to coagulate, thus the tubes are immediately transfused into an appropriate table centrifuge machine (PC-02, Process Ltd., Nice, France). When the tubes are removed from the centrifuge after 15 min spun, the blood is separated into three layers. The top layer contains the platelet poor plasma (PPP), middle layer contains fibrin clot (PRF), and lowest layer contains the RBCs.

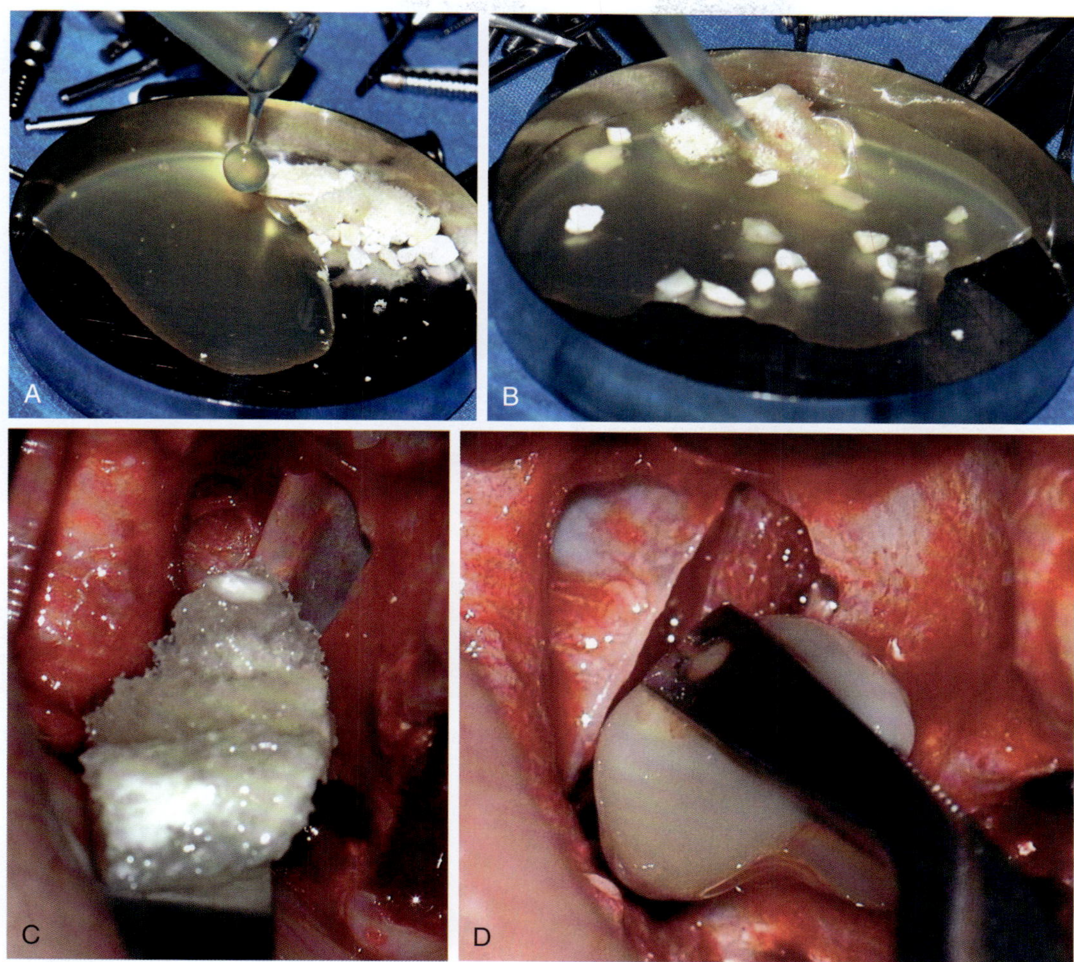

Fig 13.32 (A) The platelet-rich plasma is added to the bone graft material and (B) activated by adding the calcium chloride to it just before the graft is applied to the recipient site. (C) Besides releasing growth factors it also enhances the handling properties of the graft. (D) The membrane or coagulum formed from the platelet-poor plasma can be used to improve the soft tissue healing at the grafted site.

Unlike PRP, the PRF results from a natural and progressive polymerization which occurs during centrifugation. This fibrin clot (PRF) is grabbed and gently removed from the tube using tissue forcep. The fibrin clots are separated from the attached RBCs using scissor and stored in a sterile metal or Borosil bowl. Now this fibrin clot can be used in three ways:

1. The fibrin clot can be fragmented into several small pieces and mixed with the bone graft to enhance the bone regeneration potential of the bone graft.
2. It can be little compressed and placed into the bone defect/extraction socket or on top of the graft or collagen membrane to enhance the bone and soft tissue regeneration.
3. This fibrin clot can be compressed between two sterile Borosil plates for 1–2 min which results in the formation of an inexpensive autologous fibrin membrane with the constant thickness. This membrane remains hydrated for several hours for the use. The serum exudate which is produced on compressing the fibrin clot to form membrane can be used to hydrate the bone graft and to irrigate the osteotomy or the implant surface. When performing the bone grafting, this PRF membrane can be used to protect and stabilize the graft. This PRF membrane acts as fibrin bandage, protects the bone graft, accelerates the soft tissue healing and facilitates the rapid closure of the incision line.

The compressed fibrin plug or the PRF membrane can be used in the internal sinus elevation procedure. After fracturing up the sinus floor, if fibrin plug or the folded PRF membrane is inserted into the osteotomy it facilitates further the sinus membrane elevation using osteotomes without the membrane tear. In the lateral approach of sinus elevation, this PRF membrane can be placed under the elevated sinus membrane to facilitate its further elevation without tear and also to minimize the chances of membrane tear after the sinus has been successfully grafted due to the internal pressure on the sinus membrane. This membrane can be used to cover the small sinus membrane perforation and also to cover the lateral window after the sinus grafting.

Platelet-rich fibrin is an autologous fibrin matrix which contains a large quantity of platelet and leukocyte cytokines. The cytokines which remain incorporated within the fibrin mesh progressively release overtime (7–11 days), as the network of fibrin disintegrates. When applied, PRF

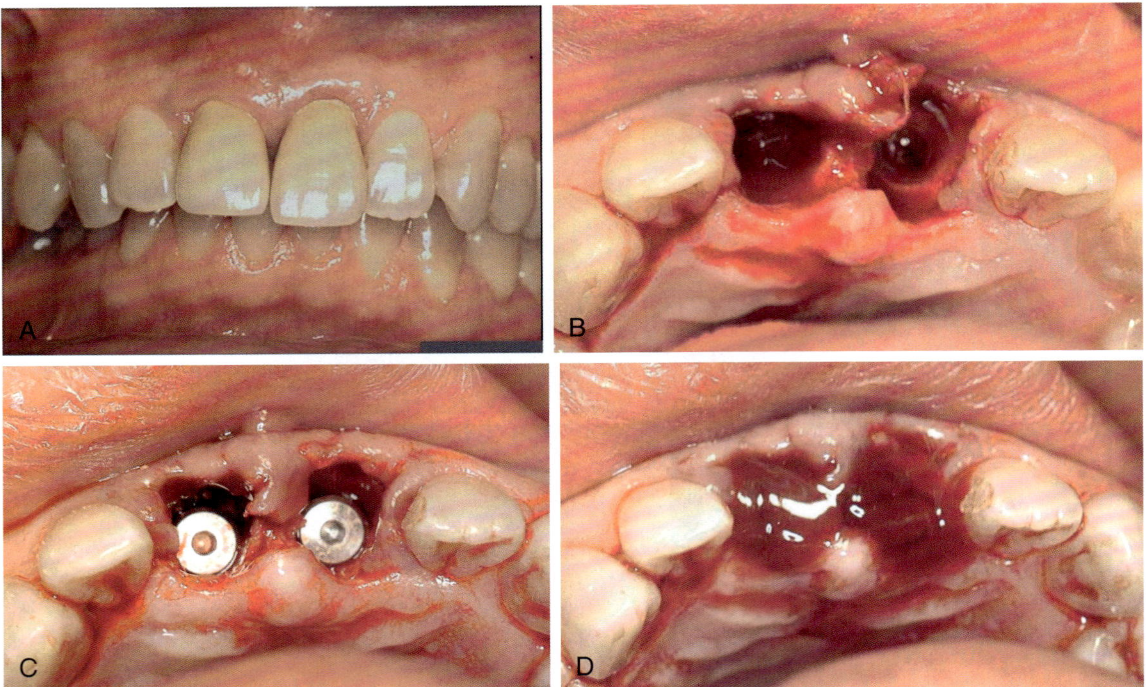

Fig 13.33 (A and B) Both the maxillary central incisors are extracted and the socket is irrigated with platelet-rich plasma (PRP). (C and D) Implants are inserted at the ideal position and the site is covered with PRP coagulum.

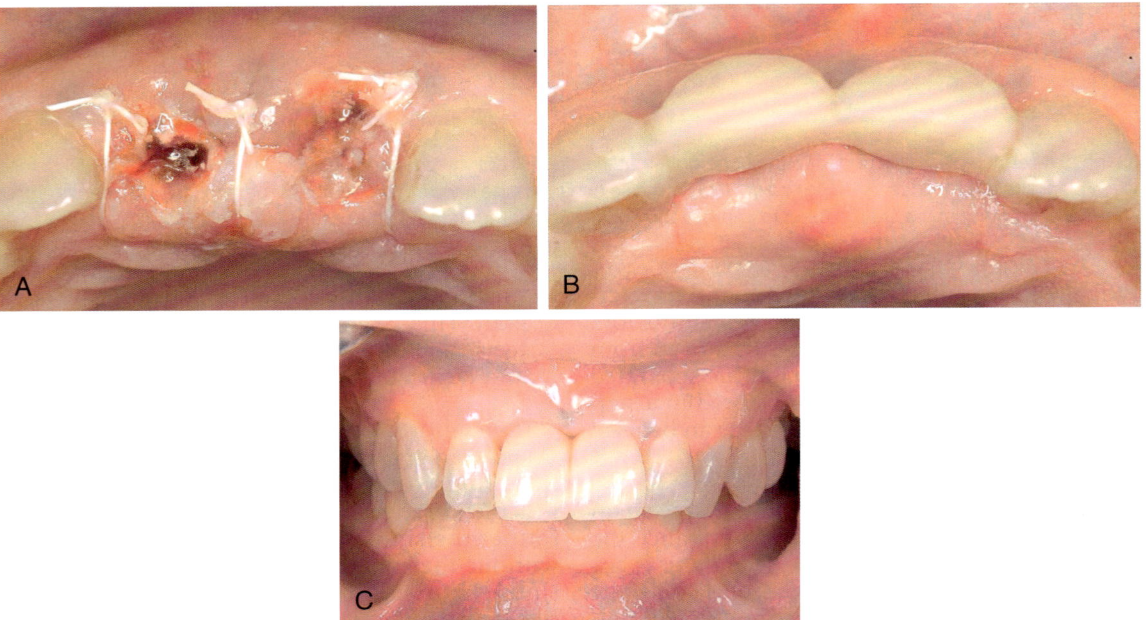

Fig 13.34 (A) Healing after 1 week shows a healthy regenerated soft tissue over the implant. (B) A provisional fixed prosthesis is given to guide the aesthetic soft tissue healing. (C) The final prosthesis on the implants shows predictable aesthetic soft tissue outcome *(Courtesy: Dr Jun Shimada, Japan).*

Table 13.5 Volume of activator required to activate different volumes of plasma

PLASMA VOLUME (μL)	ACTIVATOR ($CaCl_2$) VOLUME
300	1 drop
400–600	2 drops
600–900	3 drops

membrane acts much like a fibrin bandage, accelerates the wound healing, provides a significant postoperative protection to the surgical site and accelerates the integration and remodelling of the bone graft.

Advantages of PRF over PRP and PRGF

1. Ease of preparation
2. Ease of application
3. Less expense
4. Strictly autologous
5. No need of anticoagulant
6. No need of activator
7. No need of pippets
8. Preparation with single spin
9. Less chances of contamination
10. Can be stored for a longer period of time after preparation.

Step by step clinical presentation for production and use of PRF in bone augmentation (Figs 13.35–13.37)

Bone morphogenic proteins

These are different from platelet growth factors in that they can be found in the extracellular bone matrix itself and can induce mesenchymal cells to differentiate into osteoblasts. The autogenous cancellous bone is the richest source of BMPs but it can also be present in allografts. Thus, use of autogenous bone graft provides more BMPs at the grafted site.

Transitional prosthesis

No soft tissue-supported transitional prosthesis should be worn by the patient in the area of bone grafting during its healing time (4–6 months), as it can cause incision line opening, mobilization of the graft during healing, and distortion of the space of augmentation, which can further result in loss of graft, nonunion of block graft, and the formation of new bone with unfavourable contour and unsatisfactory quantity. Whenever possible a fixed transitional restoration can be given to the patient especially in an aesthetic region, which often also helps to contour the soft tissues and allow maturation before the final prosthesis fabrication.

Factors that impede bone regeneration

1. Failure of vascularity to the graft
2. Mechanical instability of the graft during bone regeneration
3. Oversized defect
4. Growth of soft tissue into the graft
5. Infection to the graft
6. Incorrect selection of the graft material.

Factors that promote bone regeneration

1. Use of autogenous (osteogenic) and/or allogenous (osteoinductive) bone in the graft
2. Use of growth factors (e.g. platelet-rich factor), which enhances osteogenesis and osteoinduction
3. BMPs.
4. Host bone quality
5. Space maintenance for the graft.

Armamentaria and materials required for bone grafting

Advances in instrumentation and grafting biomaterials have improved our ability to predictably reconstruct deficient hard tissue contours at multiple implant sites via minimally invasive intraoral approaches. Various types of armamentaria and materials are required to perform different kinds of bone grafting procedures (Fig 13.38A–O). Some bone grafting materials and membranes have already been described in this chapter. The additional armamentaria and materials specially required to perform any particular bone grafting procedure are described in the procedure-related chapters, but the basic armamentaria which the dentists more or less need to have to perform various bone grafting procedures are as follows:

1. Reduction handpieces (20:1 and 1:1)
2. Large and small round carbide burs
3. Straight carbide bur
4. Sharp chisels
5. Mallet
6. Bone rhonger
7. Bone mill
8. Bone collector
9. Trephines
10. Disc
11. Saws
12. Frios® Microsaw
13. Graft carrier
14. Graft bowl
15. Fixation screws
16. Screwdriver
17. Titanium mesh
18. Piezotome
19. Bone graft materials
20. Barrier membrane
21. Membrane stabilizing bone tack system
22. Retractors.

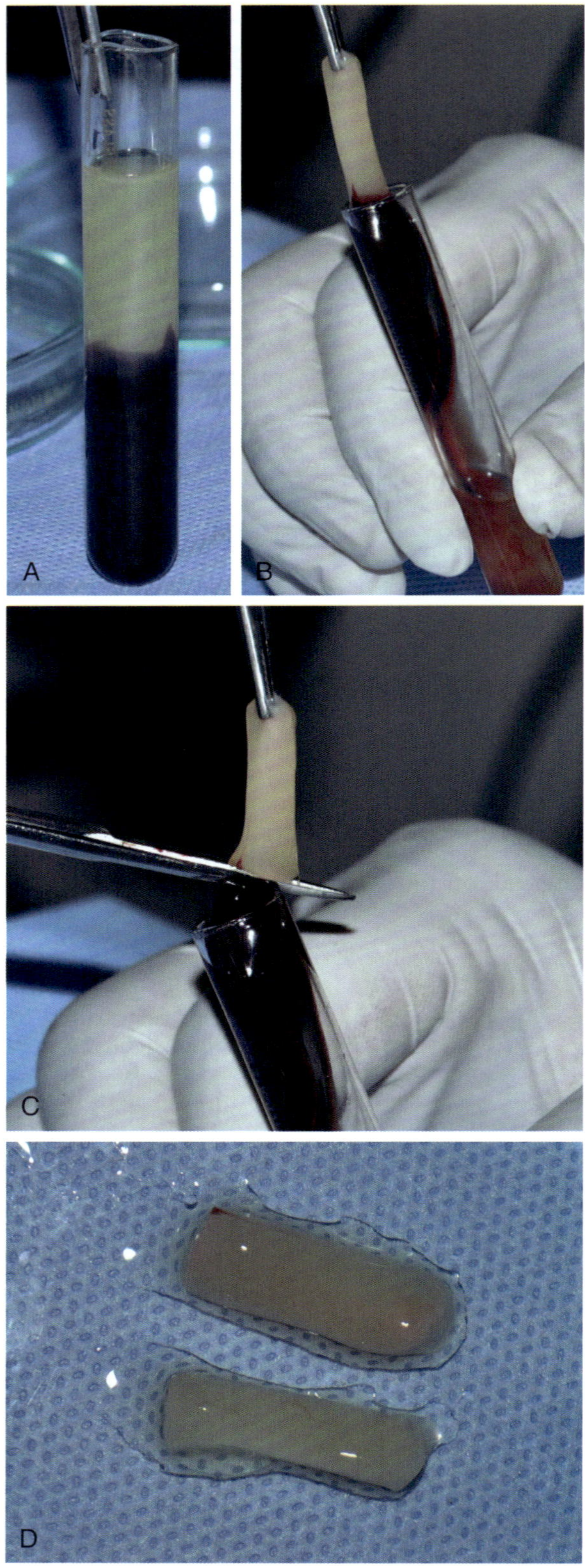

Fig 13.35 Depending on the volume of PRF need to be prepared, 10–20 ml of venous blood is withdrawn from patient and poured into the test tubes. Before the blood starts clotting, the test tubes are immediately transfused into an adequate table centrifuge machine. When the tubes are removed from the centrifuge after 15 min spun, the blood is separated into three layers. (A) The top layer contains the platelet poor plasma, middle layer contains fibrin clot (PRF), and lowest layer contains the red blood cells. (B) The fibrin clot (PRF) is grabbed and gently removed from the tube using tissue forceps. (C) The fibrin clot is separated from the attached red blood cells using scissor and (D) stored in a Borosil bowl.

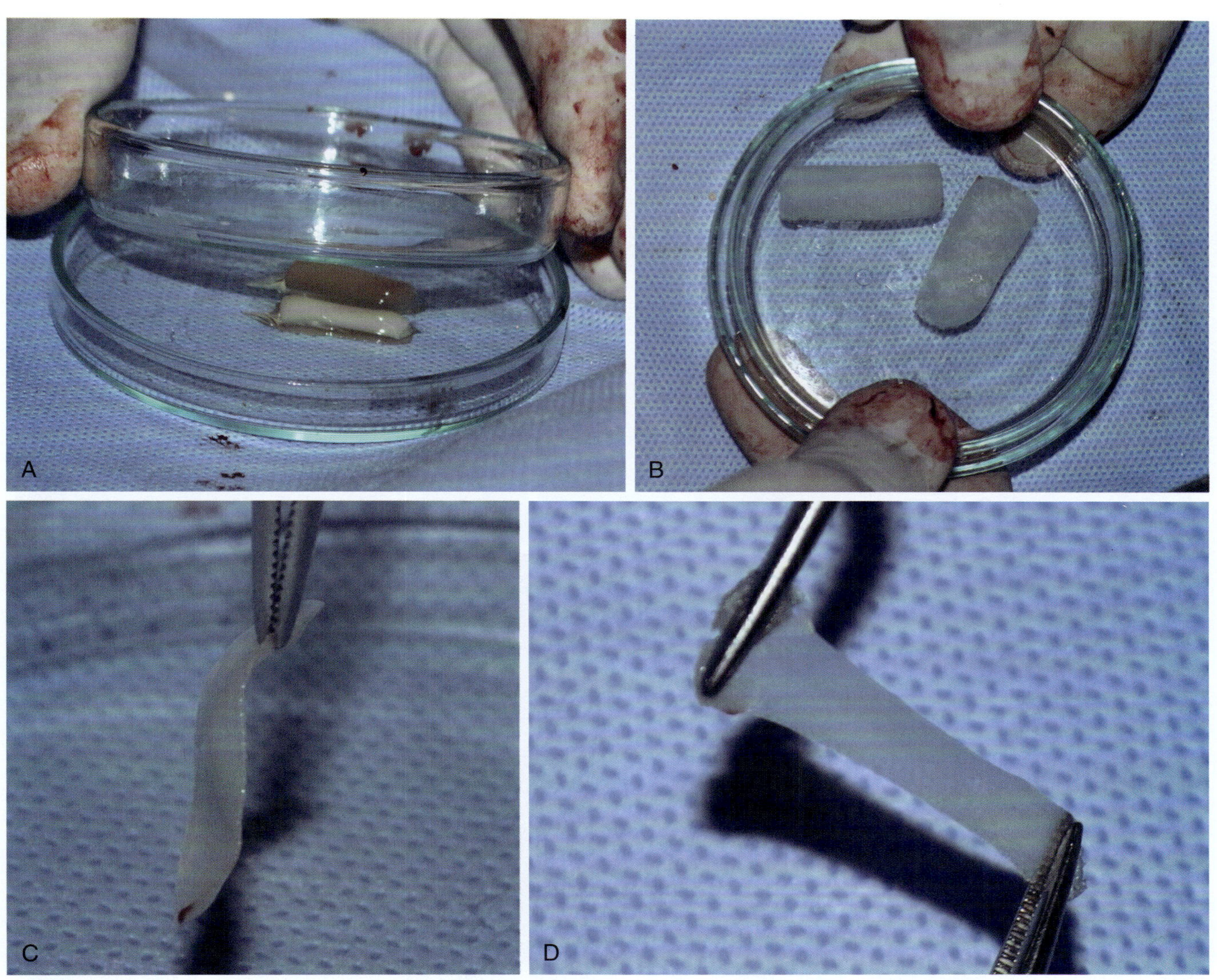

Fig 13.36 (A and B) To produce a fibrin membrane, the fibrin clots are compressed between two sterile Borosil plates for 1–2 min that results in the (C) formation of an inexpensive autologous fibrin membrane with the constant thickness. This membrane remains hydrated for several hours for the use. (D) The fibrin membrane is very elastic and resistant to tear.

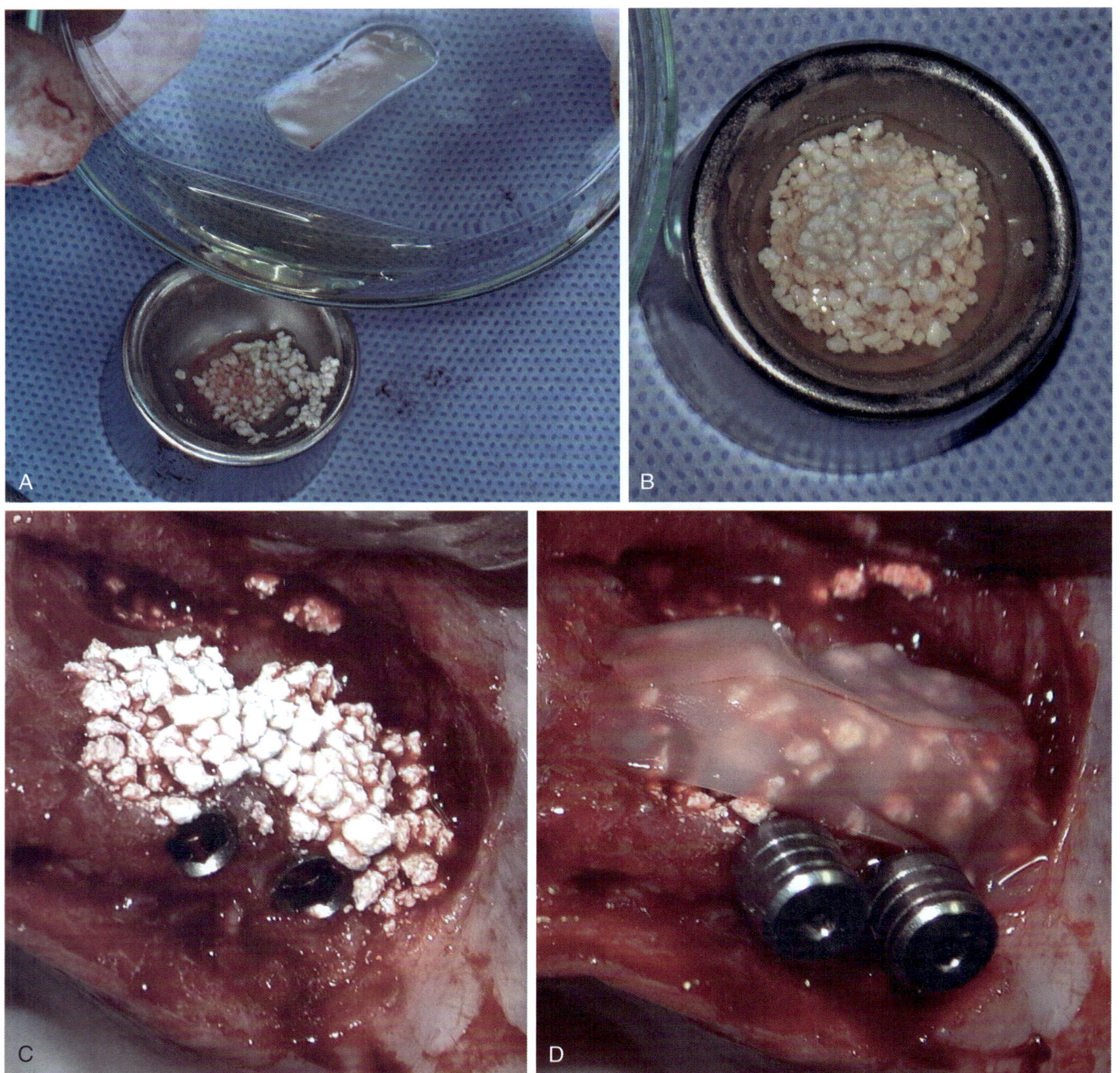

Fig 13.37 (A and B) The serum exudate which is produced on compressing the fibrin clot to form membrane can be used to hydrate the bone graft and to irrigate the osteotomy or the implant surface. Mixing the serum exudate with the bone graft enhances the bone regeneration pace and potential of the bone graft. (C and D) When performing the bone grafting, this PRF membrane can be used to protect and stabilize the graft. This PRF membrane acts as fibrin bandage, protects the bone graft, accelerates the soft tissues healing and facilitates the rapid closure of the incision line.

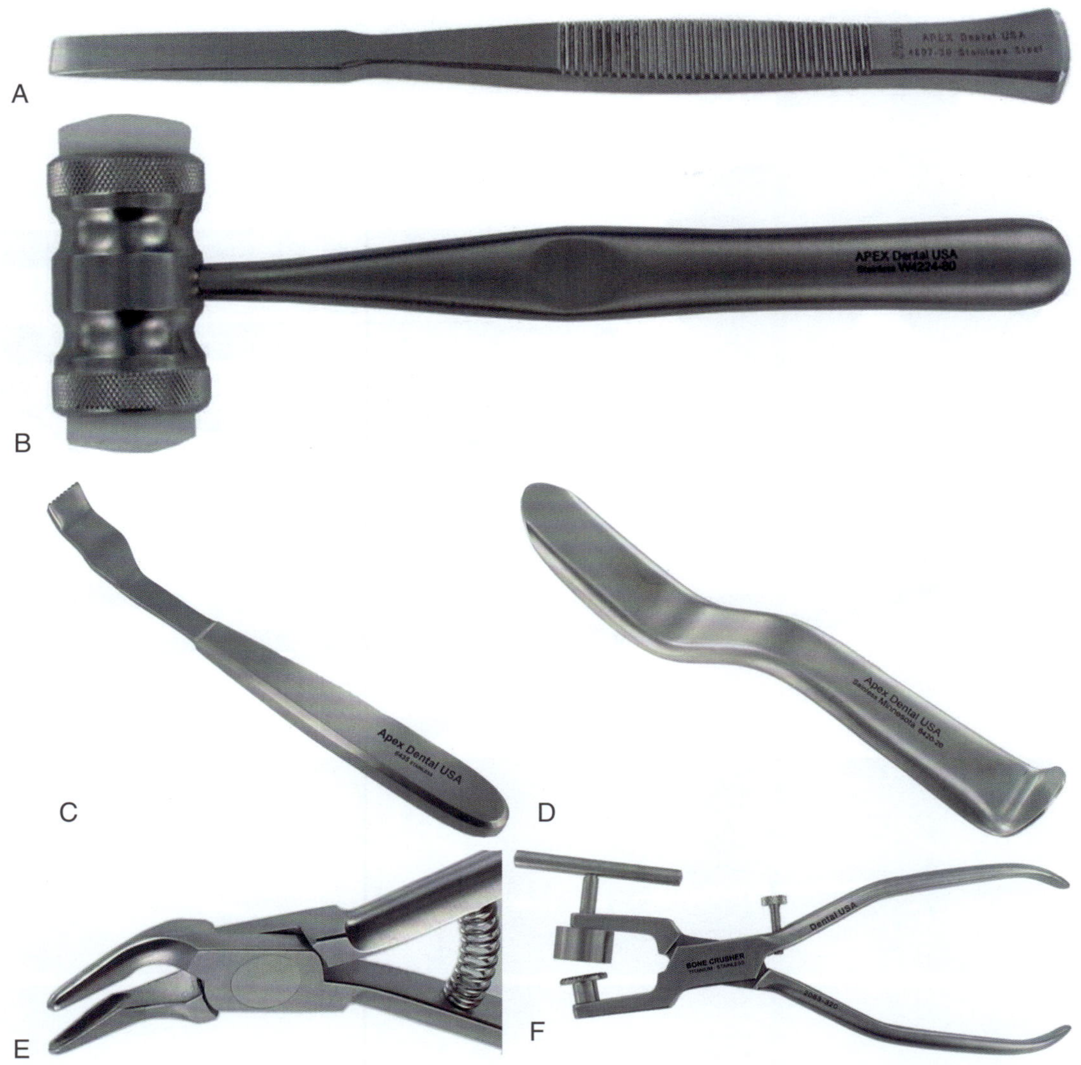

Fig 13.38 (A) Chisel used for bone splitting and to harvest autogenous bone. (B) Hammer. (C and D) Periosteum/flap retractors. (E) Bone rongeur used to nip the thin fibrosseous tissue from the ridge crest and to harvest the bone from the tuberosity. (F) Bone mill used to mill the large bone pieces to smaller pieces.

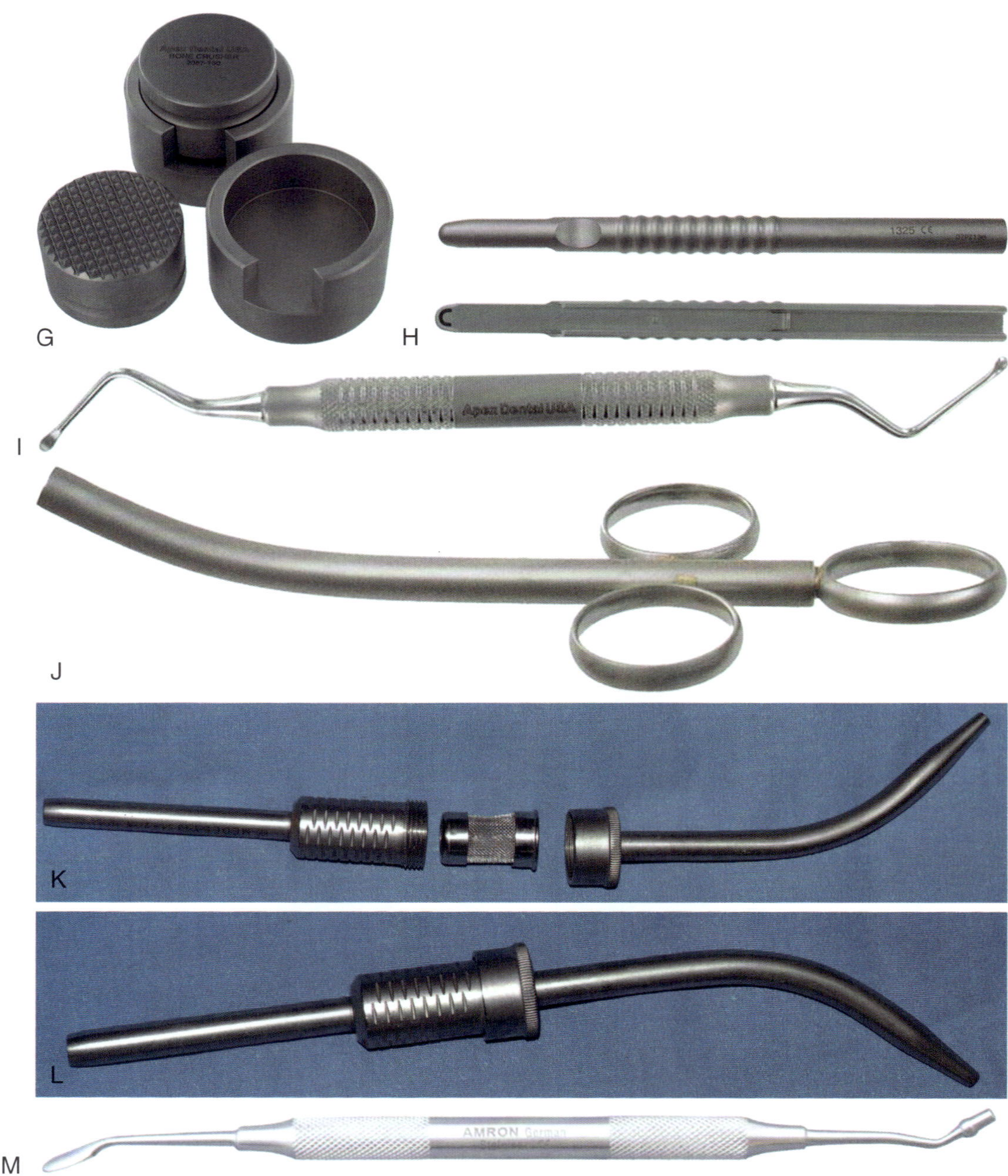

Fig 13.38, cont'd (G) Bone crusher used to crush the autogenous bone into the small particles. (H) Bone scrapper used to scrape out the small to medium amount of intraoral bone. (I) Bone curette used to curette out the granulation tissue from the extraction socket. (J) Bone carrier used to carry the bone graft to the host site. Bone collecting suction system (K and L) used to collect the bone which is usually washed out during the osteotomy preparation. (M) Bone carrier and packer.

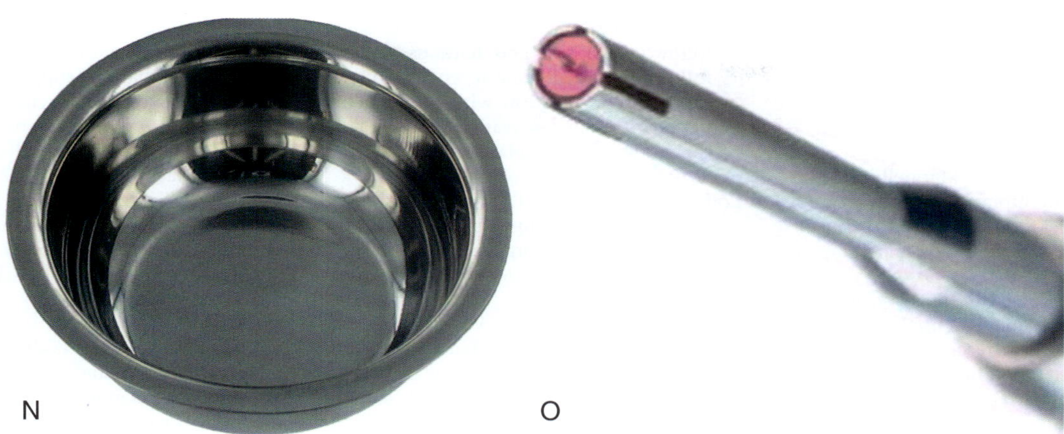

Fig 13.38, cont'd (N) Stainless steel bowl for mixing and storing bone graft material. (O) Bone tack used for barrier membrane stabilization. *(Courtesy: Apex Dental, USA, and Amron Dental)*.

Summary

Bone grafting has now become an integral part of implant practise. Depending on the type of bone graft used, there are three mechanisms of bone formation at the grafted site: osteoconduction, osteoinduction, and osteogenesis. Only autogenous bone has the ability to form bone by all three mechanisms and so it is considered to be the 'gold standard' in bone augmentation procedures. Most of the xenografts and synthetic graft materials only provide a bioactive and bioinert scaffold for bone formation by the process of osteoconduction. Thus the mixing of autogenous bone to bone substitutes enhances the bone growth potential of the bone substitutes. Bone grafting should never be attempted at infected sites as it does not only infect the graft but the low pH level at the infected site also resorbs the graft.The prevention of the soft tissue growth into the graft is paramount for bone formation of the desired quality and volume. It necessitates the use of barrier membrane to cover the graft for the prevention of soft tissue creeping into the graft. Adequate adaptation of the graft and its immobilization at the host site are the other points which an implant surgeon should keep in mind for the union of the graft to the host site and successful new bone regeneration. Space maintenance for the bone graft is also required to obtain a successful outcome and in some cases, it may require either the use of block graft or tent screws. The topography of the osseous defect should be closely evaluated and accordingly the type of graft should be selected. Achieving primary closure over the grafted sites is another problem which dentists face; the releasing incision should be given to the periosteum of the facial flap to coronally advance the flap to achieve a tension-free primary closure. When placing graft over the cortical plate, such as in the case of lateral bone augmentation using the block graft or particulate graft, the cortical bone of the host site should be perforated at multiple sites to obtain nourishment to the graft from the underlying spongiosa. The use of PRP or PRGF definitely enhances the bone formation potential of any graft. But the ease of preparation, completely autologous and cost-effective PRF definitely looks advantageous over the better known PRP or PRGF.

Further Reading

Araújo MG, Lindhe J. Ridge preservation with the use of Bio-Oss® Collagen: a 6-month study in the dog. Clin Oral Implants Res 2009;20:433–40.

Sartorii S, Silvestri M, Forni F, et al. Ten-year follow-up in a maxillary sinus augmentation using anorganic bovine bone (Bio-Oss). A case report with histomorphometric evaluation. Clin Oral Implants Res 2003;14(3):369–72.

von Arx T, Buser D. Horizontal ridge augmentation using autogenous block grafts and the guided bone regeneration technique with collagen membranes: a clinical study with 42 patients. Clin Oral Implants Res 2006;17(4):359–66.

Valentini P, Abensur DJ. Maxillary sinus grafting with anorganic bovine bone: a clinical report of long-term results. Int J Oral Maxillofac Implants 2003;18(4):556–60.

Urban IA, Lozada JL. A prospective study of implants placed in augmented sinuses with minimal and moderate residual crestal bone: results after 1 to 5 years. Int J Oral Maxillofac Implants 2010;25(6):1203–12.

Schwarz F, Bieling K, Latz T, et al. Healing of intrabony peri-implantitis defects following application of a nanocrystalline hydroxyapatite (Ostim) or a bovine-derived xenograft (Bio-Oss) in combination with a collagen membrane (Bio-Gide). A case series. J Clin Periodontol 2006;33(7):491–9.

Ruoff H, Terheyden H. Retrospective radiographic investigation of the long-term stability of xenografts (Geistlich Bio-Oss) in the sinus. Z Zahnärztl Impl 2009;25(2):160–9.

Becker ST, Terheyden H, et al. Prospective observation of 41 perforations of the Schneiderian membrane during sinus floor elevation. Clin Oral Implants Res 2008;19(12):1285–9.

Degidi M, Daprile G, Piattelli A. RFA values of implants placed in sinus grafted and non-grafted sites after 6 and 12 months. Clin Implant Dent Relat Res. 2009 Sep;11(3):178-82. Epub 2008 sep 9.

Pietursson BE, Tan WC, Zwahlen M, et al. A systematic review of the success of sinus floor elevation and survival of implants inserted in combination with sinus floor elevation. J Clin Periodontol 2008;35:216–40.

Schwarz F, Sculean A, et al. Two-year clinical results following treatment of peri-implantitis lesions using a nanocrystalline hydroxyapatite or a natural bone mineral in combination with a collagen membrane. J Clin Periodontol 2008;35(1):80–7.

Hämmerle CHF, Jung RE, Yaman D, et al. Ridge augmentation by applying bioresorbable membranes and deproteinized bovine bone mineral: a report of twelve consecutive cases. Clin Oral Implants Res 2008;19(1):19–25.
Zitzmann N, Schärer P, Marinello C. Long-term results of implants treated with guided bone regeneration: a 5-year prospective study. Int J of Oral Maxillofac Implants 2001;16(3).
Hämmerle CH, Lang NP. Single stage surgery combining transmucosal implant placement with guided bone regeneration and bioresorbable materials. Clin Impl Res 2001:21.
Hockers T, Abensur D, Valentini P, et al. The combined use of bioresorbable membranes and xenografts or autografts in the treatment of bone defects around implants – a study in beagle dogs. Clin Oral Impl Res 1999:10.
Benic GI, Jung RE, et al. Clinical and radiographic comparison of implants in regenerated or native bone: 5-year results. Clin Oral Implants Res 2009.
Simion M, Fontana F, Raspereini G, et al. Vertical ridge augmentation by expanded-polytetrafluoroethylene membrane and a combination of intraoral autogenous bone graft and deproteinized inorganic bovine bone (Bio-Oss). Clin Oral Implants Res 2007;18(5):620–9.
Canullo L, Trisi P, Simion M. Vertical ridge augmentation around implants using e-PTFE titanium-reinforced membrane and deproteinized bovine bone mineral (Bio-Oss): a case report. Int J Periodontics Restorative Dent 2006;26(4):355–61.
Artzi Z, Dayan D, Alpern Y, et al. Vertical ridge augmentation using xenogenic material supported by a configured titanium mesh: clinicohistopathologic and histochemical study. Int J Oral Maxillofac Implants 2003;18(3):440–6.
Thompson ID, Hench LL. Mechanical properties of bioactive glasses, glass-ceramics and composites. Proc Inst Mech Eng 1998;212:127–36.
Beitlitum I, Artzi Z, Nemcovsky CE. Clinical evaluation of particulate allogenic with and without autogenous bone grafts and resorbable collagen membranes for bone augmentation of atrophic alveolar ridges. Clin Oral Implants Res 2010;21(11):1242–50.
Maiorana C, Beretta M, Salina S, et al. Reduction of autogenous bone graft resorption by means of Bio-Oss coverage: a prospective study. Int J Periodontics Restorative Dent 2005;25:19–25.
Zitzmann N, Schärer P, Marinello C, et al. Alveolar ridge augmentation with Bio-Oss: a histological study in humans. Int J Periodontics Restorative Dent 2001;21:288–95.
Felice P, Marchetti C, et al. Vertical ridge augmentation of the atrophic posterior mandible with interposition bloc grafts: bone from the iliac crest vs. bovine inorganic bone. Clinical and histological results up to one year after loading from a randomized-controlled clinical trial. Clin Oral Implants Res 2009.
Dahlin C, Simion M, Hatano N. Long-term follow-up on soft and hard tissue levels following guided bone regeneration treatment in combination with a xenogeneic filling material: a 5-year prospective clinical study. Clin Implant Dent Relat Res 2010 Dec;12(4):263–70.
Rothamel D, Schwarz F, et al. Vertical ridge augmentation using xenogenous bone blocks: a histomorphometric study in dogs. Int J Oral Maxillofac Implants 2009;24(2):243–50.
Canullo L, Malagnino VA. Vertical ridge augmentation around implants by e-PTFE titanium-reinforced membrane and bovine bone matrix: a 24- to 54-month study of 10 consecutive cases. Int J Oral Maxillofac Implants 2008;23(5):858–66.
Testori T, Wallace SS, et al. Repair of large sinus membrane perforations using stabilized collagen barrier membranes: surgical techniques with histologic and radiographic evidence of success. Int J Periodontics Restorative Dent 2008;28(1):9–17.
Becker J, Al-Nawas B, et al. Use of a new cross-linked collagen membrane for the treatment of dehiscence-type defects at titanium implants: a prospective, randomized-controlled double-blinded clinical multicenter study. Clin Oral Implants Res 2009.
Hämmerle CHF, Chiantella GC, Karring T, et al. The effect of a deproteinized bovine bone mineral (Bio-Oss®) on bone regeneration around titanium dental implants. Clin Oral Implants Res 1998:9.
Hürzeler MB, Kohal RJ, Naghshbandi J, et al. Evaluation of a new bioresorbable barrier to facilitate guided bone regeneration around exposed implant threads. An experimental study in the monkey. Int J Oral Maxillofac Surg 1998:27.
Zitzmann N, Naef R, Schärer P. Resorbable versus nonresorbable membranes in combination with Bio-Oss for guided bone regeneration. Int J Oral Maxillofac Implants 1997;12.
Cao W, Hench LL. Bioactive materials. Ceramics Int 1996;22:493–507.
Billington RW, Willisams JA. Increase in compressive strength of glass ionomer restorative materials with respect to time. J Oral Rehabil 1991;18:163–8.
Nicholson JW. Glass ionomers in medicine and dentistry. Proc Inst Mech Eng 1998;212:121–6.
Brook IM, Hatton PV. Glass-ionomers: Bioactive implant materials. Biomaterials 1998;19:565–71.
Zitzmann N, Naef R, Schüpbach P, et al. Immediate or delayed immediate implantation versus late implantation when using the principles of guided bone regeneration. Acta Med Dent Helv 1996;1(10).
Galindo-Moreno P, Padial-Molina M, Fernandez-Barbero JE, et al. Optimal microvessel density from composite graft of autogenous maxillary cortical bone and anorganic bovine bone in sinus augmentation: influences of clinical variables. Clin Oral Implants Res 2010;21(2):221–7.
Merli M, Migani M, Esposito M. Vertical ridge augmentation with autogenous bone grafts: resorbable barriers supported by osteosynthesis plates versus titanium-reinforced barriers. A preliminary report of a blind, randomized, controlled clinical trial. J Oral Maxillofac Implants 2007;22(3):373–82.
Tadjoedin ES, de Lange GL, Bronckers ALJJ, et al. Deproteinized cancellous bovine bone (Bio-Oss) as bone substitute for sinus floor elevation. J Clin Periodontol 2003;30:261–70.
Hallmann M, Sennerby L, Lundgren S. A clinical and histologic evaluation of implant integration in the posterior maxilla after sinus floor augmentation with autogenous bone, bovine hydroxyapatite, or a 20:80 mixture. Int J Oral Maxillofac Implants 2002;17:635–43.
Galindo-Moreno P, Moreno-Riestra I, Avila G, et al. Effect of anorganic bovine bone to autogenous cortical bone ratio upon bone remodeling patterns following maxillary sinus augmentation. Clin Oral Implants Res 2011;22(8):857–64.
Chackartchi T, Iezzi G, Goldstein M, et al. Sinus floor augmentation using large (1–2 mm) or small (0.25–1 mm) bovine bone mineral particles: a prospective, intra-individual controlled clinical, micro-computerized tomography and histomorphometric study. Clin Oral Implants Res 2011;22(5):473–80.
De Souza Nunes LS, De Oliveira RV, Holgado LA, et al. Immunoexpression of Cbfa-1/Runx2 and VEGF in sinus lift procedures using bone substitutes in rabbits. Clin Oral Implants Res 2010;21(6):584–90; Epub 2010 Jan 23.
Mordenfeld A, Hallmann M, et al. Histological and histomorphometrical analyses of biopsies harvested 11 years after maxillary sinus floor augmentation with deproteinized bovine and autogenous bone. Clin Oral Implants Res 2010.
Marchetti C, Pieri F, et al. Impact of implant surfacei and grafting protocol on clinical outcomes of endosseous implants. Int J Oral Maxillofac Implants 2007;22(3):399–407.
Maiorana C, Sigurta D, Miranda A, et al. Sinus elevation with alloplasts or xenogenic materials and implants: an up-to-4-year clinical and radiologic follow-up. Int J Oral Maxillofac Implants 2006;21(3):426–32.
Wallace SS, Froum SJ, Cho SC, et al. Sinus augmentation utilizing anorganic bovine bone (Bio-Oss) with absorbable and nonabsorbable membranes placed over the lateral window: histomorphometric and clinical analyses. Int J Periodotics Restorative Dent 2005;25:551–9.
Del Fabbro M, Testori T, Francetti L, et al. Systematic review of survival rates for implants placed in the grafted maxillary sinus. Int J Periodontics Restorative Dent 2004;24:565–77.
John HD, Wenz B. Histomorphometric analysis of natural bone mineral for maxillary sinus augmentation. Int J Oral Maxillofac Implants 2004;19:199–207.

Hallmann M, Hedin M, Sennerby L, et al. A prospective 1-year clinical and radiographic study of implants placed after maxillary sinus floor augmentation with bovine hydroxyapatite and autogenous bone. J Oral Maxillofac Surg 2002;60:277–84.

Tawil G, Mawla M. Sinus floor elevation using a bovine bone mineral (Bio-Oss) with or without the concomitant use of a bilayered collagen barrier (Bio-Gide): a clinical report of immediate and delayed implant placement. Int J Oral Maxillofac Impl 2001;16:13–21.

Maiorana C, Redemagni M, Rabagliati M, et al. Treatment of maxillary ridge resorption by sinus augmentation with iliac cancellous bone, anorganic bovine bone, and endosseous implants: a clinical and histologic report. Int J Oral Maxillofac Implants 2000;15:873–8.

Valentini P, Abensur D, Wenz B, et al. Sinus grafting with porous bone mineral (Bio-Oss®) for implant placement: a study on 15 patients. Int J Periodontics Restorative Dent 2000;20:245–53.

McAllister B, Margolin M, Cogan A, et al. Eighteen-month radiographic and histologic evaluation of sinus grafting with anorganic bovine bone in the chimpanzee. Int J Oral Maxillofac Implants 1999:14.

Urist MR. Bone morphogenetic protein induced bone formation in experimental animals and patients with large bone defects. In: Evered D, Barnett S, editors. Cell and molecular biology of vertebrate hard tissue. London: CIBA Foundation; 1988.

Pelker RR, Friedlaender GE, Markham TC. Biomechanical properties of bone allografts. Clin Orthop Relat Res 1983;54.

Haas R, Mailath G, Dörtbudak O, et al. Bovine hydroxyapatite for maxillary sinus augmentation: analysis of interfacial bond strength of dental implants using pull-out tests. Clin Oral Implants Res 1998;9:117–22.

Hench LL, Wilson J. Surface active biomaterials. Science 1984;226:630–6.

Schrooten J, Helsen JA. Adhesion of bioactive glass coating to Ti6A14V oral implants. Biomaterials 2000;21:1461–9.

McAllister B, Margolin M, Cogan A, et al. Residual lateral wall defects following sinus grafting with recombinant human osteogenic protein-1 or Bio-Oss® in the chimpanzee. Int J Periodontics Restorative Dent 1998;18(3).

Hürzeler MB, Quiñones CR, Kirsch A, et al. Maxillary sinus augmentation using different grafting materials and dental implants in monkeys - part I. Evaluation of anorganic bovine-derived bone matrix. Clin Oral Implants Res 1997;8:476–86.

Valentini P, Abensur D. Maxillary sinus floor elevation for implant placement with demineralized freeze-dried bone and bovine bone (Bio-Oss®): a clinical study of 20 patients. Int J Periodontics Restorative Dent 1997:17.

Wetzel AC, Stich H, Caffesse RG. Bone apposition onto oral implants in the sinus area filled with different grafting materials. Clin Oral Implants Res 1995;6:155–63.

Mulliken JB, Glowacki J, Kaban LB, et al. Use of demineralized allogeneic bone implants for the correction of maxillocraniofacial deformities. Ann Surg 1981;194:366.

Köndell PA, Mattsson T, Astrand P. Immunological responses to maxillary on-lay allogeneic bone grafts. Clin Oral Implants Res 1996;7:373.

Urist MR. Bone: formation by autoinduction. Science 1965;150:893.

Osbon DB, Lilly GE, Thompson CW, et al. Bone grafts with surface decalcified allogeneic and particulate autologous bone: report of cases. J Oral Surg 1977;35:276.

Constantino PD, Freidman CD. Synthetic bone graft substitutes. Otolaryngol Clin North Am 1994;27:1037–73.

Perrott DH, Smith RA, Kaban LB. The use of fresh frozen allogeneic bone for maxillary and mandibular reconstruction. Int J Oral Maxillofac Surg 1992;21:260.

Marx RE, Carlson ER. Tissue banking safety: caveats and precautions for the oral and maxillofacial surgeon. J Oral Maxillofac Surg 1993;51:1372.

Goldberg VM, Stevenson S. Natural history of autografts and allografts. Clin Orthop Relat Res 1987;7.

Maletta JA, Gasser JA, Fonseca RJ, et al. Comparison of the healing and revascularization of onlayed autologous and lyophilized allogenic rib grafts to the edentulous maxilla. J Oral Maxillofac Surg 1983;41:487.

Cypher TJ, Grossman JP. Biological principles of bone graft healing. J Foot Ankle Surg 1996;35:413–7.

Triffitt JT. The stem cell of the osteoblast. In: Bilizekian J, Raisz L, Rodou G, editors. Principles of bone biology. San Diego, CA: Academic; 1996. pp. 39–50.

Toffler M, et al. Introducing choukroun's platelet rich fibrin (PRF) to the reconstructive surgery milieu. J Implant Adv Clin Dent September 2009;1(6):21–32.

Mazor H, Corso D, Prasad, et al. Sinus lift with platelet-rich fibrin as sole grafting material. J Periodontol December 2009;80(12):2056–64.

Crane D. Platelet rich plasma (PRP) matrix grafts practical. Pain Manag January/February 2008.

Ferrari M, Zia S, Valbonesi M, et al. A new technique for hemodilution, preparation of autologous platelet-rich plasma and intraoperative blood salvage in cardiac surgery. Int J Artif Org 1987;10:47–50.

Fuerst G, Gruber R, Tangl S, et al. Enhanced bone-toimplant contact by platelet released growth factors in mandibular cortical bone: a histomorphometric study in minipigs. Int J Oral Maxillofac Impants 2003;18(5):685–90.

Sánchez AR, Sheridan PJ, Kupp LI. Is PRP a perfect enhancement factor? A current review. Int J Oral Maxillofac Implants 2003;18(1):93–103.

Trisi P, Rebaudi A, Calvari F, et al. Sinus graft with biogran, autogenous bone, and PRP. A report of 3 cases with histology and micro CT. Int J Periodontics Restorative Dent 2006;26(2):113–25.

Marx RE. Platelet-rich plasma (PRP): what is PRP and what is not PRP? Implant Dent 2001;10:225–8.

Manimaran, Saisadan. Platelet rich plasma in implant dentistry - current trends. JIADS July–September, 2010;1(3):22–4.

Zechner W, Tangl S, Tepper G, et al. Influence of PRP on osseous healing of dental implants. Int J Oral Maxillofac Implants 2003;18(1):15–22.

Shanaman R, Filstein MR, Danesh-Meyer MJ. Localized ridge augmentation using GBR and platelet-rich plasma: case reports. Int J Periodontics Restorative Dent 2001;21(4):345–55.

You TM, Choi BH, Li J, et al. The effect of PRP on bone healing around implants placed in bone defects treated with Bio-Oss: a pilot study in the dog tibia. Oral Surg Oral Med Oral Pathol Oral Radiol Endod 2007;103(4):e8–12.

Froum SJ, Wallace SS, Tarnow DP, et al. Effect of platelet-rich plasma on bone growth and osseointegration in human maxillary sinus grafts: three bilateral case reports. Int J Periodontics Restorative Dent 2002;22(1):45–53.

Kim ES, Park EJ, Choung PH. Platelet concentration and its effect on bone formation in calvarial defects: an experimental study in rabbits. J Prosthet Dent 2001;86(4):428–33.

de Obarrio JJ, Araúz-Dutari JI, Chamberlain TM, et al. The use of autologous growth factors in periodontal surgical therapy: platelet gel biotechnology—case reports. Int J Periodontics Restorative Dent 2000;20(5):486–97.

Anitua E. Plasma rich in growth factors: preliminary results of use in the preparation of future sites for implants. Int J Oral Maxillofac Implants 1999;14(4):529–35.

Ito K, Yamada Y, Naiki T, et al. Simultaneous implant placement and bone regeneration around dental implants using tissue- engineered bone with fibrin. Clin Oral Implants Res 2006;17(5):579–86.

Buck BE, Resnick L, Shah SM, et al. Human immunodeficiency virus cultured from bone. Implications for transplantation. Clin Orthop Relat Res 1990;249.

Bone grafting simultaneous with implant placement

14

Ajay Vikram Singh   Peter Randelzhofer

CHAPTER CONTENTS HD

Introduction

Many patients seeking implant therapy show some osseous defects or deficient ridge dimensions, which need to be taken care of before implants can be placed with predictable success. With advancement in diagnostic and planning tools (e.g. the dental CT scan) and bone grafting materials, bone augmentation simultaneous with implant placement has become a routine procedure in implant practise. It is seen that more patients opt for the implant procedure if simultaneous grafting is offered, because it reduces the number of surgeries and the total treatment span of implant therapy, when compared to the two-stage procedure (first the grafting and then implant insertion after 4–6 months). The author suggests meticulous treatment planning using clinical pictures, model analysis, radiographs, and CT images to successfully perform bone augmentation simultaneous with implant placement. The implant surgeon should closely evaluate the type of osseous defect, the type of bone graft material required for predictable bone formation, space maintenance for the graft, prevention of soft tissue growth into the graft, nourishment for the graft, the amount and quality of host bone available for adequately stabilizing the implant, etc. to achieve predictable success in the procedure. For implant surgeons who are not very skilled at performing bone augmentation procedures, the author recommends reading of Chapter 13 Basics of bone grafting and graft materials and thoroughly understand the basic science of bone grafting, before attempting the bone augmentation procedure.

Advantages

1. Shortens the time span of the complete treatment
2. More acceptance by patients
3. Fewer visits are required
4. Reduces the treatment cost
5. Less volume of graft is required
6. Implant, if adequate primary stability is achieved, can be immediately restored in the aesthetics region
7. Autogenous bone can be collected from the implant osteotomy preparation and used to graft the bone defect.

Disadvantages

1. Increases the time span of the implant surgery
2. More chances of postoperative complications
3. Needs skilled approach to achieve a successful outcome.

Indications

1. Small to medium size bone defect
2. Peri-implant socket spaces in cases of immediate implant in fresh extraction socket
3. Ridge splitting with simultaneous implant placement
4. Sinus grafting with simultaneous implant placement
5. Adequate bone volume to engage the implant
6. Implant placement is possible within the osseous envelop of the defect
7. Adequate amount of thick, stable, and keratinized soft tissue is available to cover the graft site
8. Adequate blood supply for the graft from the host site.

Contraindications

1. Large size bone defect
2. Inadequate bone volume to engage the implant
3. Vertical bone augmentation is required
4. Inadequate blood supply for the graft from the host site
5. Space maintenance for new bone regeneration is difficult to achieve
6. Inadequate amount of thick, stable, and keratinized soft tissue available to cover the graft site.

CASE REPORT-1

Bone grafting of osseous defect of extraction socket simultaneous with implant placement *(Courtesy: Dr Peter Randelzhofer and Dr Gert de Lange)*

Aims of the therapy

1. Compensation of buccal bone wall resorption after tooth extraction by bone augmentation with Geistlich Bio-Oss® and Geistlich Bio-Gide®
2. Immediate implant placement to reduce overall treatment time in the aesthetic area
3. Preservation of the papillae (Figs 14.1–14.6).

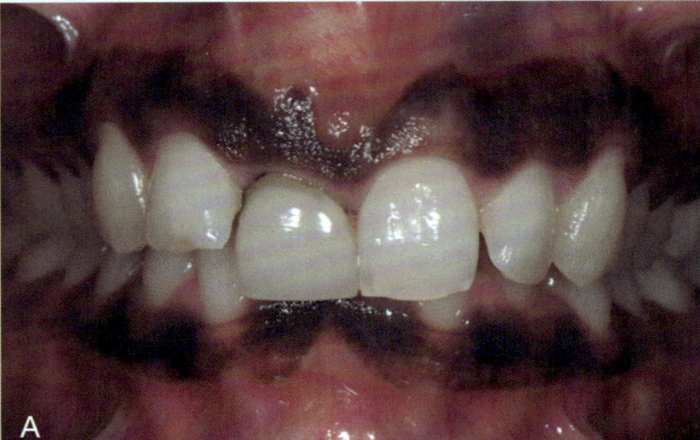

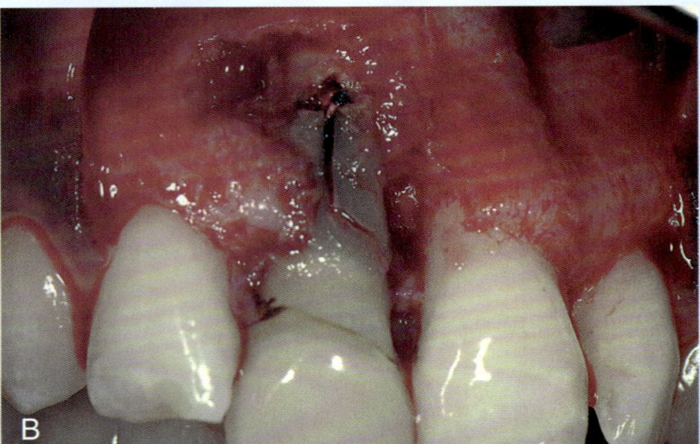

Fig 14.1 The patient presented with a thick, medium scalloped, gingival morphology. Tooth 11 presented with poor prognosis due to vertical root fracture. The tooth had slightly extruded resulting in a vertical gain of soft tissue. (A) The pigmented gingiva presented an extra challenge. (B) After careful flap elevation, a clear fracture of the root was visible. The vertical bone defect affected two-thirds of the buccal bone plate.

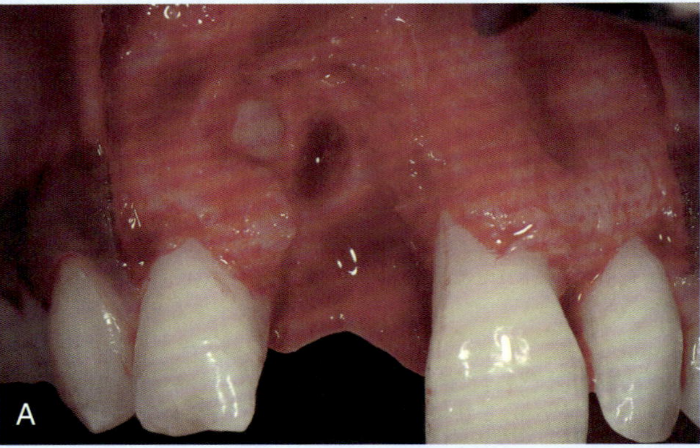

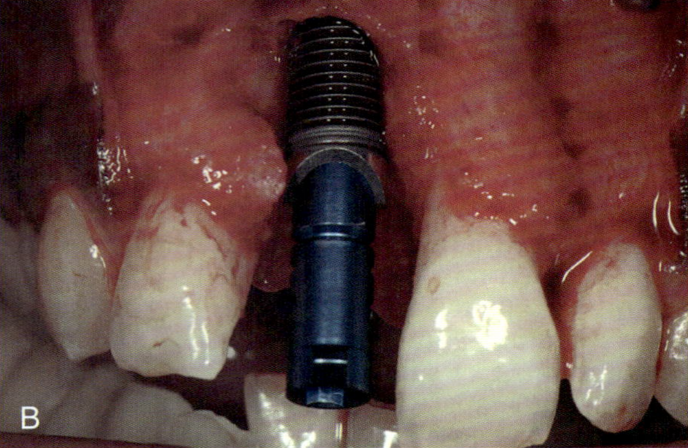

Fig 14.2 An extensive bone deficit became visible after tooth extraction. (A) It was accompanied by extensive attachment loss on tooth 21, which caused a high aesthetic risk due to possible loss of papillae after surgery. Inserted implant showed good primary stability. (B) Due to the pronounced bone defect, a closed healing approach was chosen.

CASE REPORT-1—cont'd

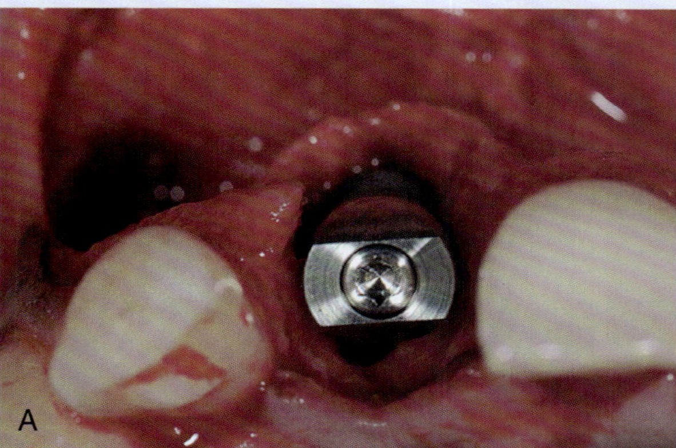

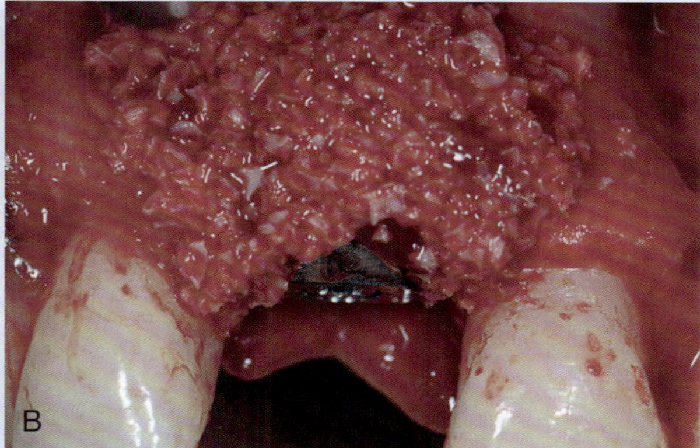

Fig 14.3 The implant was placed within the bordering sidewalls of the defect (within the osseous envelope) to maintain adequate space for the graft. (A) The gap distance from the implant surface to the buccal bone plate should be at least 2 mm. Autologous bone chips were harvested using a trephine drill from the retromolar area and were placed onto the implant surface. Geistlich Bio-Oss® was mixed with blood and applied onto the bone chips to prevent primary resorption of the autologous bone. (B) The regenerated hard tissue provided the basis for stable soft tissue architecture.

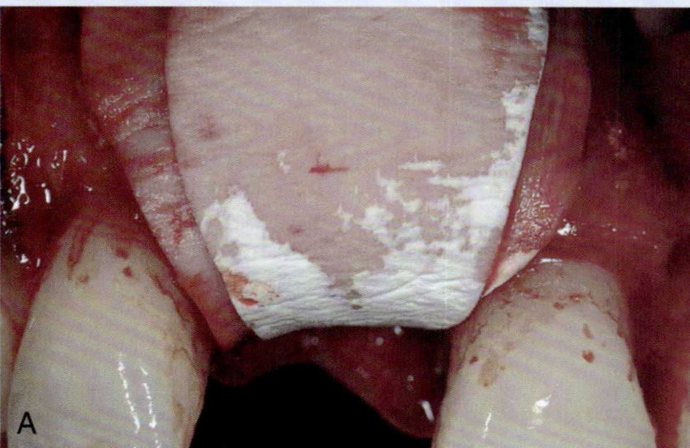

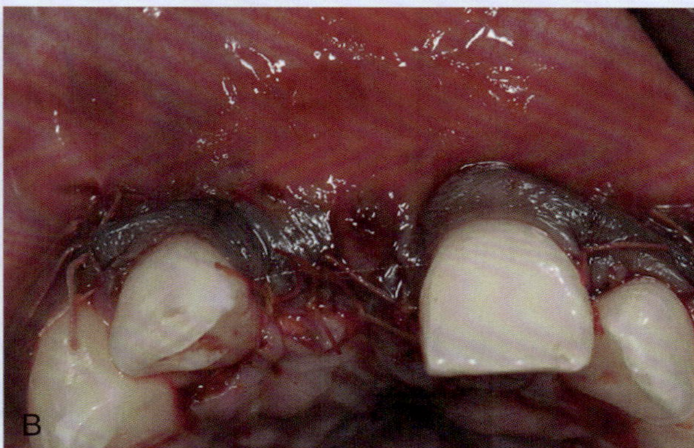

Fig 14.4 The augmented area was covered with the Geistlich Bio-Gide® membrane. (A) The membrane was placed in the double layer technique to provide stable protection for bone regeneration. For additional soft tissue augmentation, a connective tissue graft from the palate was sutured under the flap. In order to guarantee a tension-free closure the flap was mobilized by a split-flap technique. (B) Primary wound closure was achieved with resorbable vicryl sutures 6.0/5.0. During a second stage surgery, 4 months later, the pigmented gingiva was repositioned coronally by a split-flap technique to restore its natural shape (not shown).

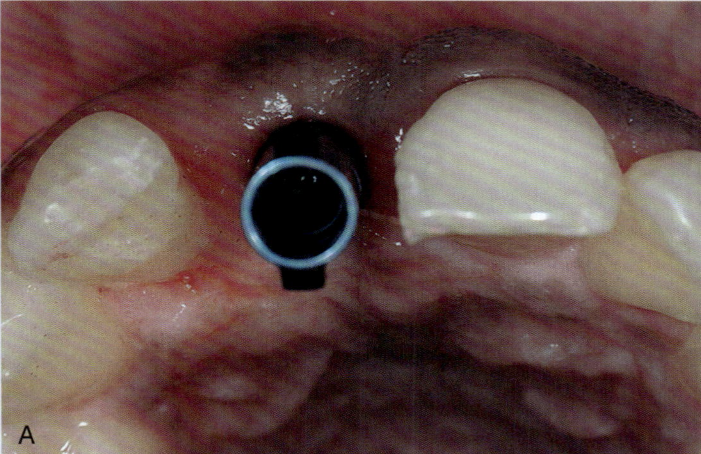

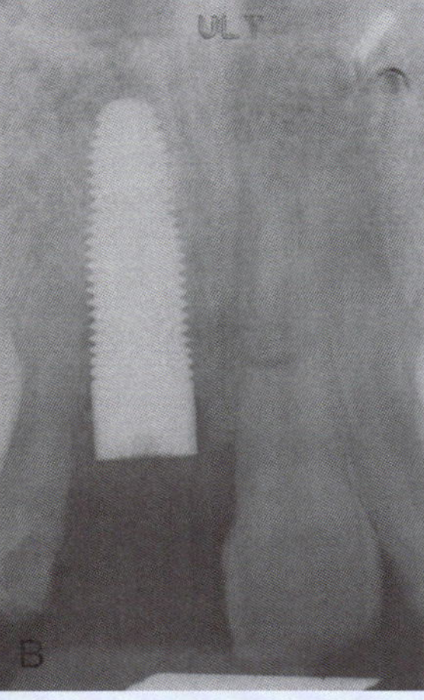

Fig 14.5 (A) Five months after implant placement: the distance from the implant to the buccal aspect of the alveolar ridge was still more than 2 mm, which was important for a stable long-term aesthetic result. (B) Control radiograph on reopening.

Continued

CASE REPORT-1—cont'd

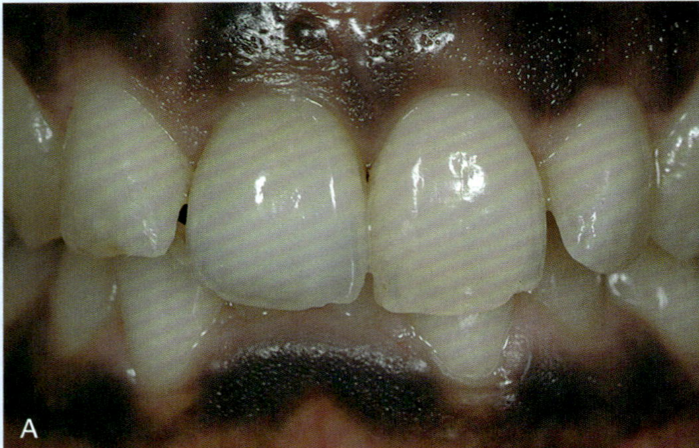

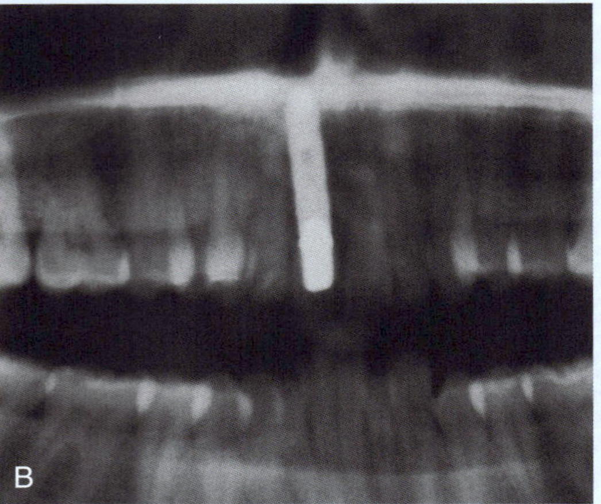

Fig 14.6 Clinical situation 1 month after crown placement: the gingiva showed a natural appearance, was nicely scalloped, and displayed no scar tissues. (A) The pigmented part could be maintained in shape and colour. (B) Control radiograph 1 year after implantation.

The technique presented in Case Report-1, has shown aesthetically pleasing results in more than 100 cases treated and documented in our clinic. It features immediate implant placement in cases with class 2 (medium size) buccal bone defects, with simultaneous ridge preservation technique followed by closed healing. A sound evaluation of the patient and the clinical situation is an important precondition for obtaining predictable results. The presented case displays an extra challenge in terms of soft tissue management due to the pigmentation of the gingiva. In such situations, scars are likely to become visible and the pigmentation line may be distorted.

CASE REPORT-2

Bone grafting simultaneous with immediate implant with open (transmucosal) healing *(Courtesy: Dr Peter Randelzhofer and Dr Gert de Lange)* (Figs 14.7–14.14).

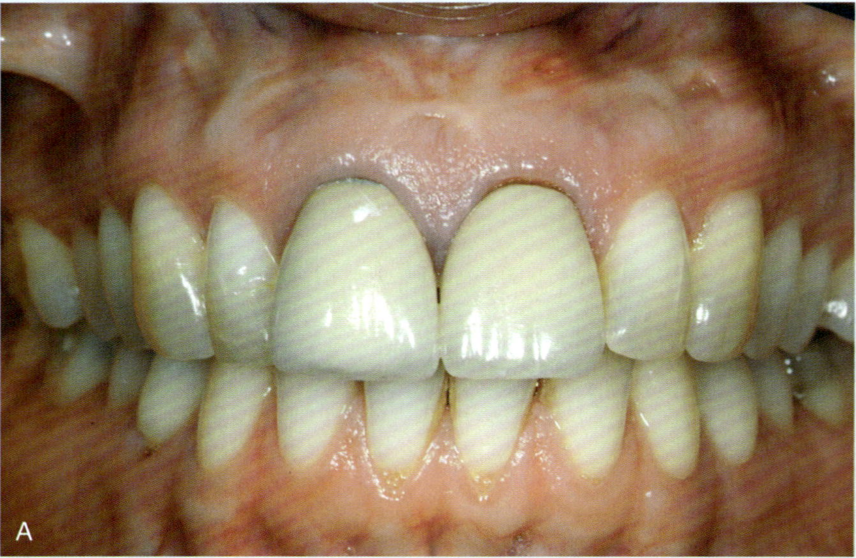

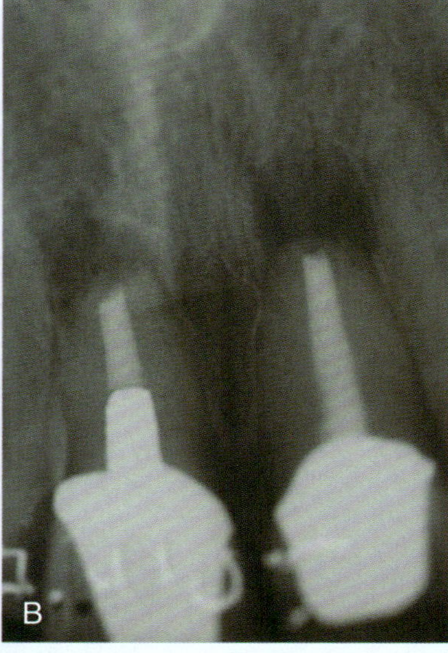

Fig 14.7 (A) Patient presented with a high smile line and thin biotype with two rather large central incisors with fistulae and poor prognosis. (B) Radiograph showed endodontic infections of both central incisors with expected osseous defect apical to the post-extraction socket.

CASE REPORT-2—cont'd

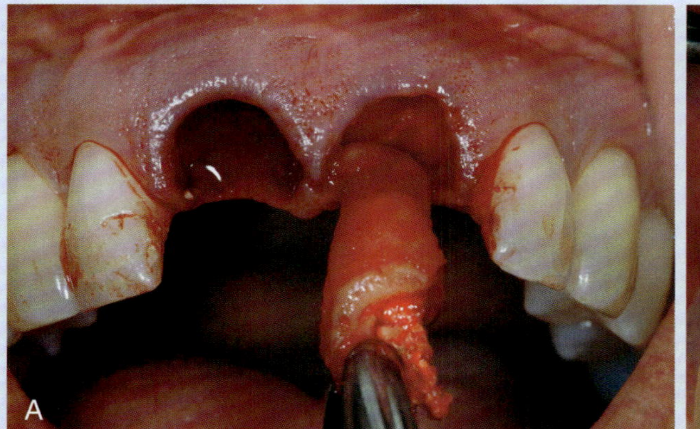

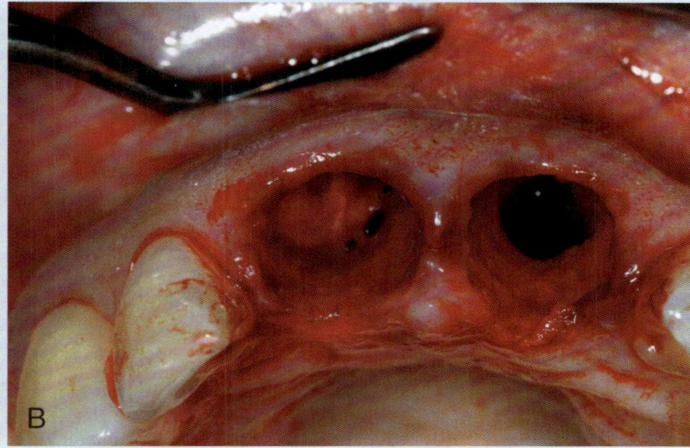

Fig 14.8 (A) Careful extraction of both central incisors was done, preserving marginal gingiva and papillae. (B) Palpation of the buccal wall showed bone defects connected with a granuloma in the socket.

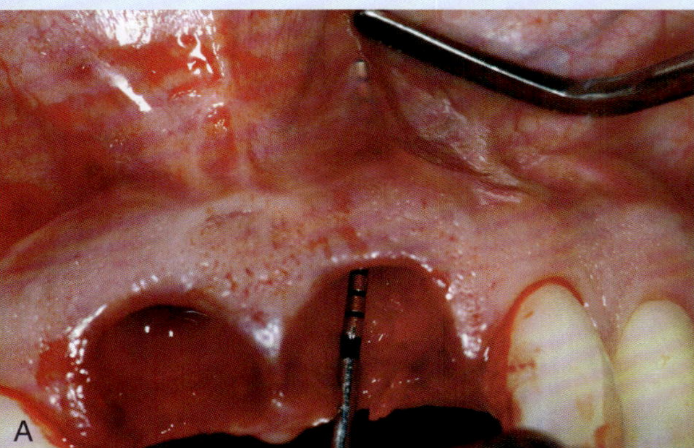

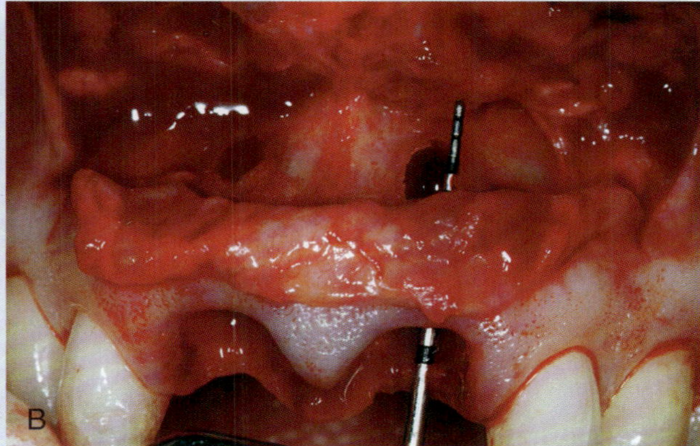

Fig 14.9 Inspection of the left socket showed apical soft tissue and hard tissue defects. (A) Note the thin central papilla. (B) After a vestibular half circle incision was made, the flap was deflected downwards and the buccal bone defects became visible for the right and left sockets.

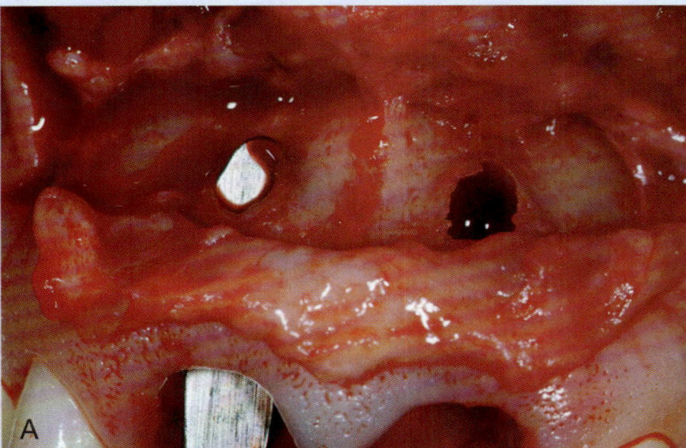

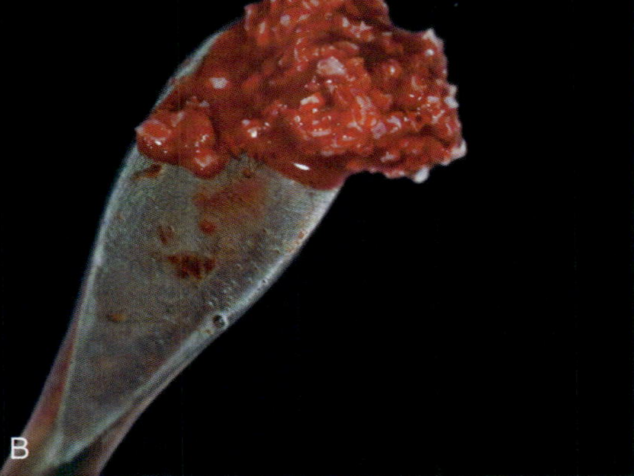

Fig 14.10 After removal of granuloma tissue and endodontic material, thorough cleaning of the bone was done using antibiotics. (A) There were large remaining bony defects of the buccal wall of both sockets. The buccal bone plate was restored using autologous bone particles collected from lower retromolar site and covered with Geistlich Bio-Oss®. (B) Geistlich Bio-Oss® particles were also used to fill the remaining buccal space between healing abutment and marginal gingiva for maximum soft tissue support.

Continued

CASE REPORT-2—cont'd

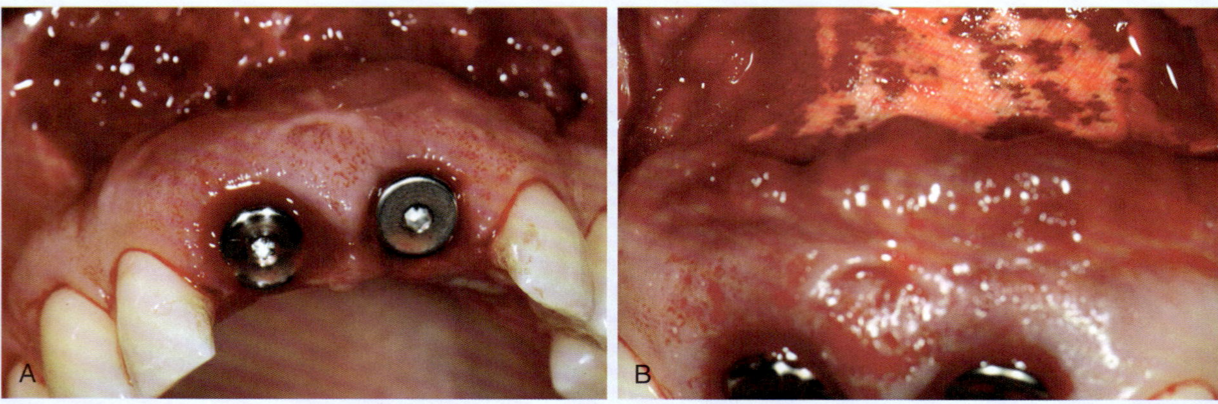

Fig 14.11 Two Camlog Screw Line implants were placed with primary stability of 35 Ncm. (A) Adequate supports of the marginal soft tissues was obtained by immediately placing a wide body healing abutment intended to prevent tissue collapse and to preserve the contour of the gingival margin. (B) For undisturbed bone regeneration, the augmented area was covered with Geistlich Bio-Gide® barrier membrane.

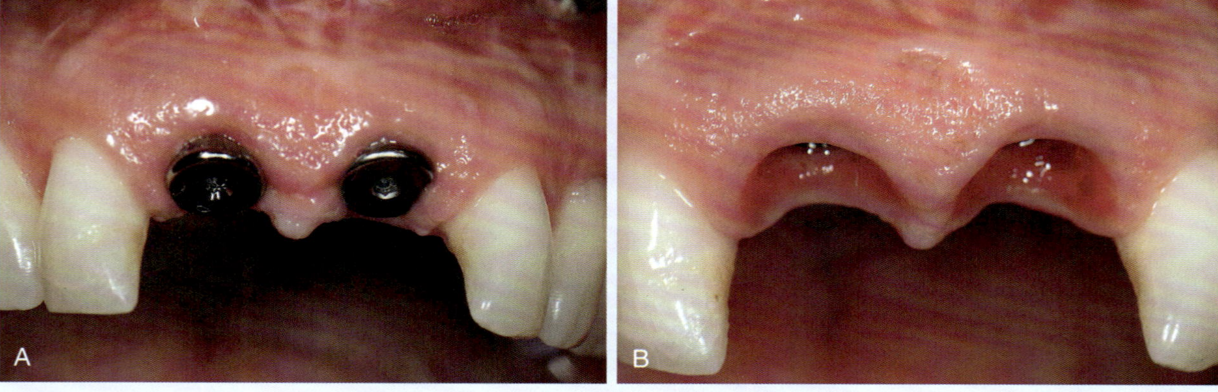

Fig 14.12 (A) One week after open healing, the soft tissues had adapted well. (B) Healing abutments which preserved the soft tissue well were removed 2 months after implant placement and replaced with provisional crowns of anatomical shape, which created nicely scalloped marginal gingiva and papillae.

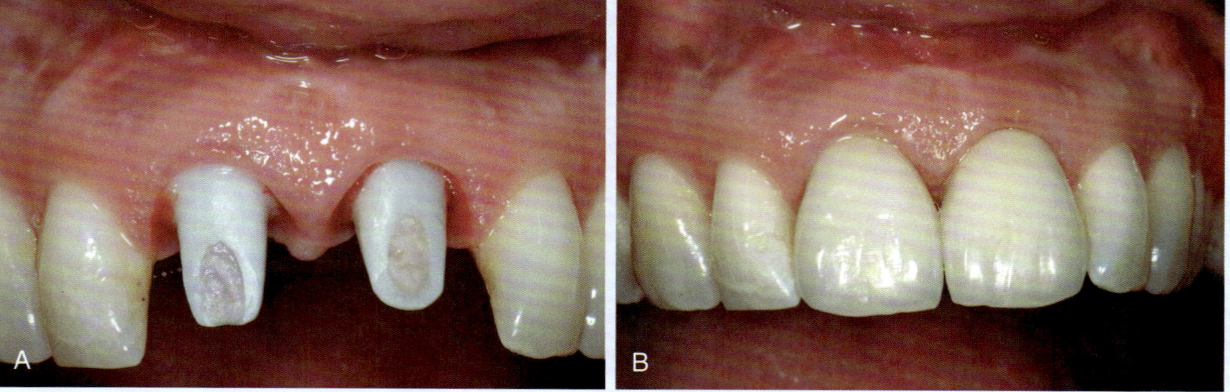

Fig 14.13 (A) Ceramic abutments were placed. Final zirconium crowns, which were smaller in the cervical region, were fixed on the abutments. (B) Note the total absence of tissue loss and gingival recession.

CASE REPORT-2—cont'd

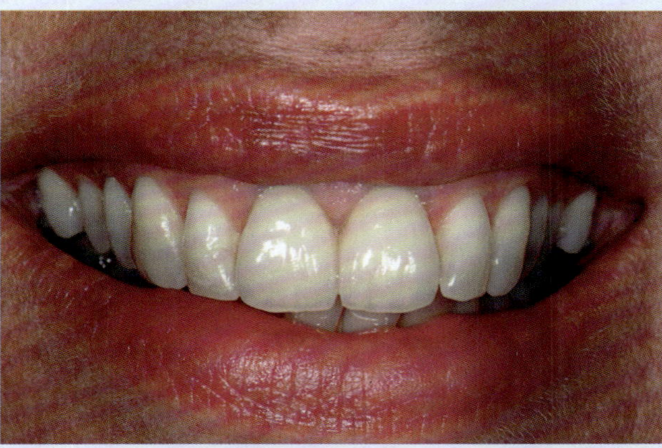

Fig 14.14 Patient presents with a nice smile, 12 months after implant placement.

The open healing procedure in Case Report-2 has also shown pleasing aesthetic results, despite the endodontic infections and the buccal bony defects present. Most clinicians remove the endodontically involved teeth first and wait for healing for several weeks or months. Then bone is augmented and after healing, the implant is placed. Finally, missing soft tissues are augmented to obtain a proper marginal contour. This approach involves repeated surgery and a treatment time of 9 months or more. Lifting fragile papillae especially, may result in attachment loss and soft tissue shrinkage, which will severely affect the aesthetic outcome in patients with a high smile line. These unwanted effects can be avoided by an apical approach via the vestibule. The frequently present apical infections and granuloma tissue can be removed with good visibility to clean the implant-receiving bony site. This more demanding technique gives sufficient access to the buccal bone defects for proper bone regeneration and/or soft tissue augmentation but does not affect gingival papillae. This method has been successfully used in more than 80 patients in the author's practise. A scientific evaluation study of efficacy and predictability is now in progress.

CASE REPORT-3

Bone defects are difficult to evaluate using only the radiograph, and often, surprisingly, are seen after the site is exposed to insert the implant (Fig 14.15A–J). The author strongly suggests meticulous treatment planning with bone mapping or dental CT scan to examine bone topography and the presence of any possible bone defect, before making the incision and elevating the flap. The implant surgeon should keep his grafting materials and armamentarium ready in each implant surgery case, to deal with such defects. *(Courtesy: Dentium Co. and Well Dental Clinic, Seoul, Korea.)*

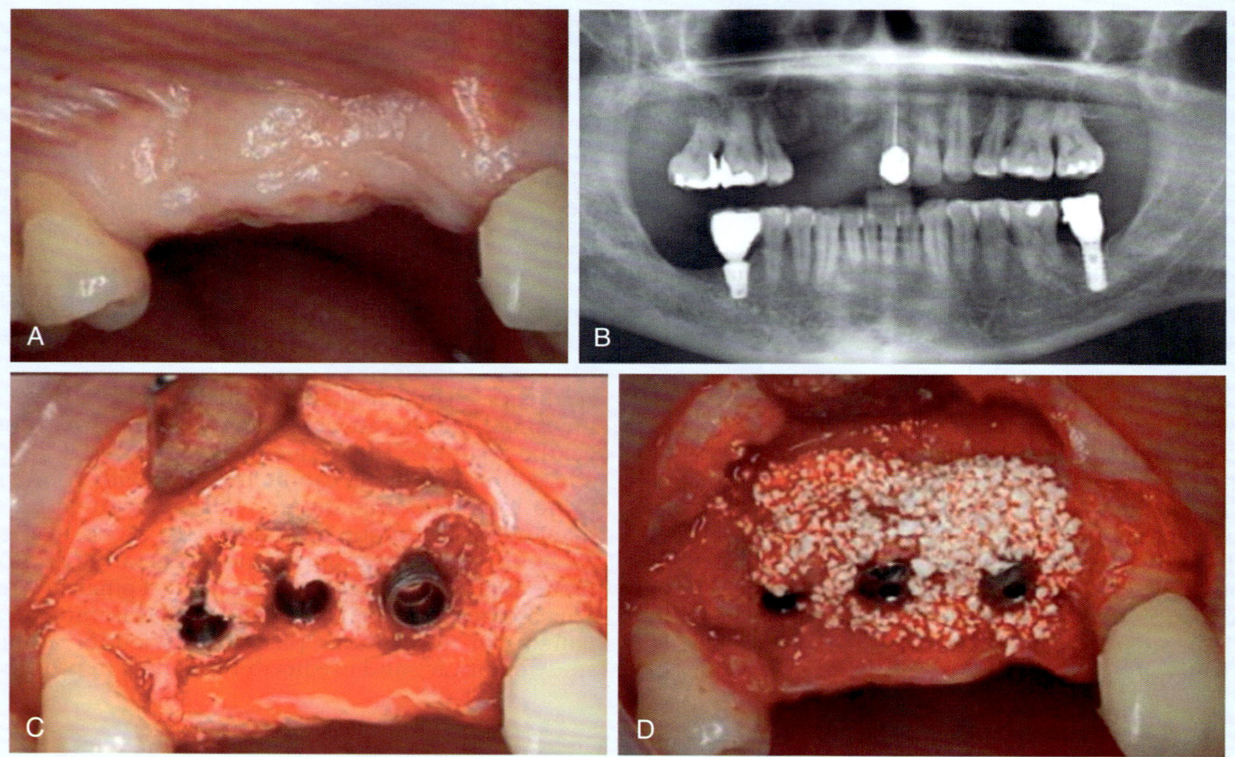

Fig 14.15 (A and B) Missing teeth numbers 11, 12, and 13. (C) The small bone defects are visible around the inserted implants, which need to be grafted. (D) The particulated (HA + β-TCP) bone graft (osteon) is used to graft the Peri-implant defects and (E) a collagen barrier membrane is used to cover the grafted site. Flaps are sutured back. (F) Post implantation radiograph. (G) Implants are uncovered and temporized after 4 months (H and I) the implants are finally restored using metal-free zirconium prosthesis. (J) Post loading radiograph.

CASE REPORT-3—cont'd

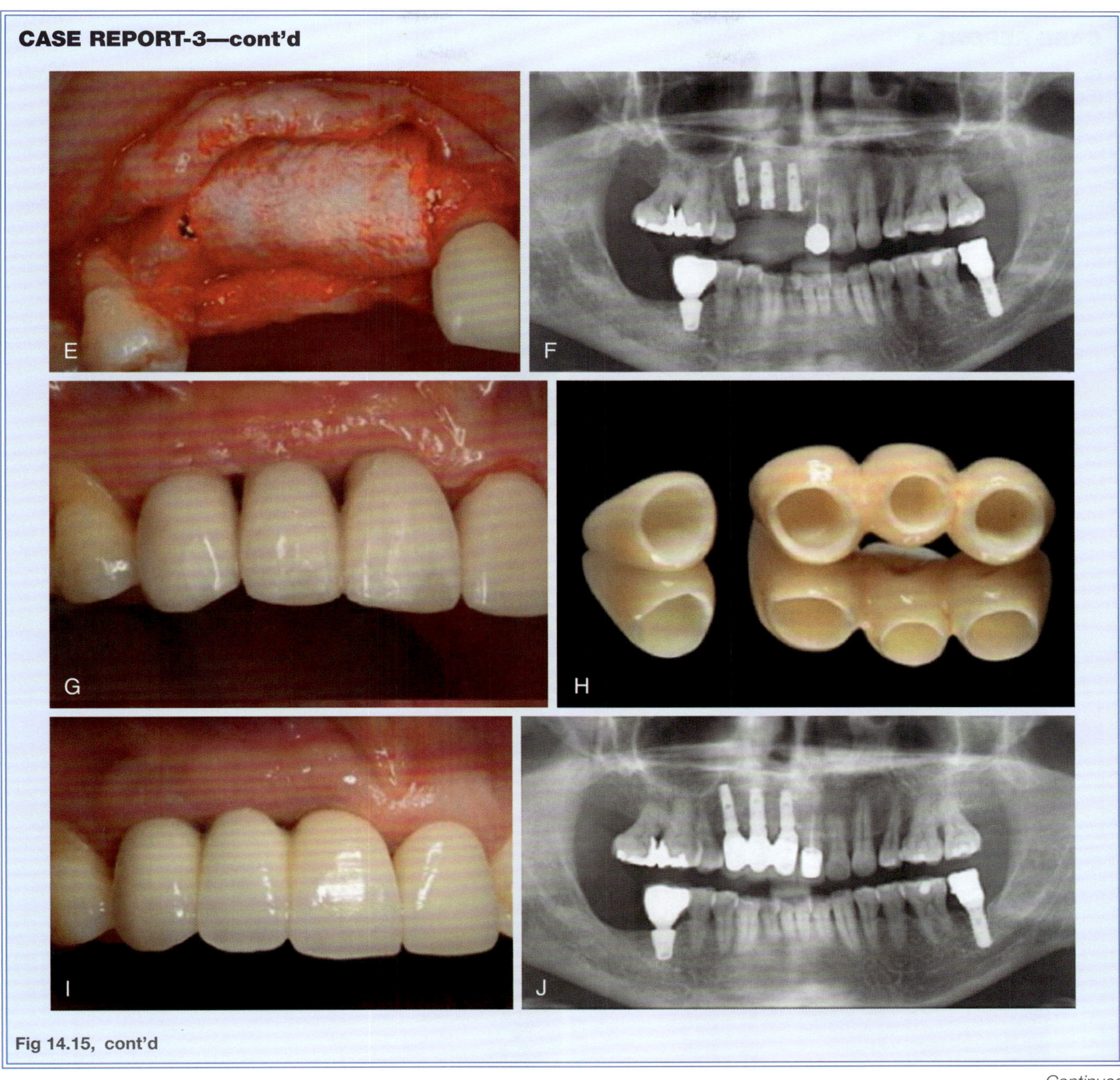

Fig 14.15, cont'd

Continued

CASE REPORT-4

Grafting of small osseous defects simultaneous with implants placement *(Courtesy: Dentium Co. and Well Dental Clinic, Soul, Korea)* (Figs 14.16 and 14.17)

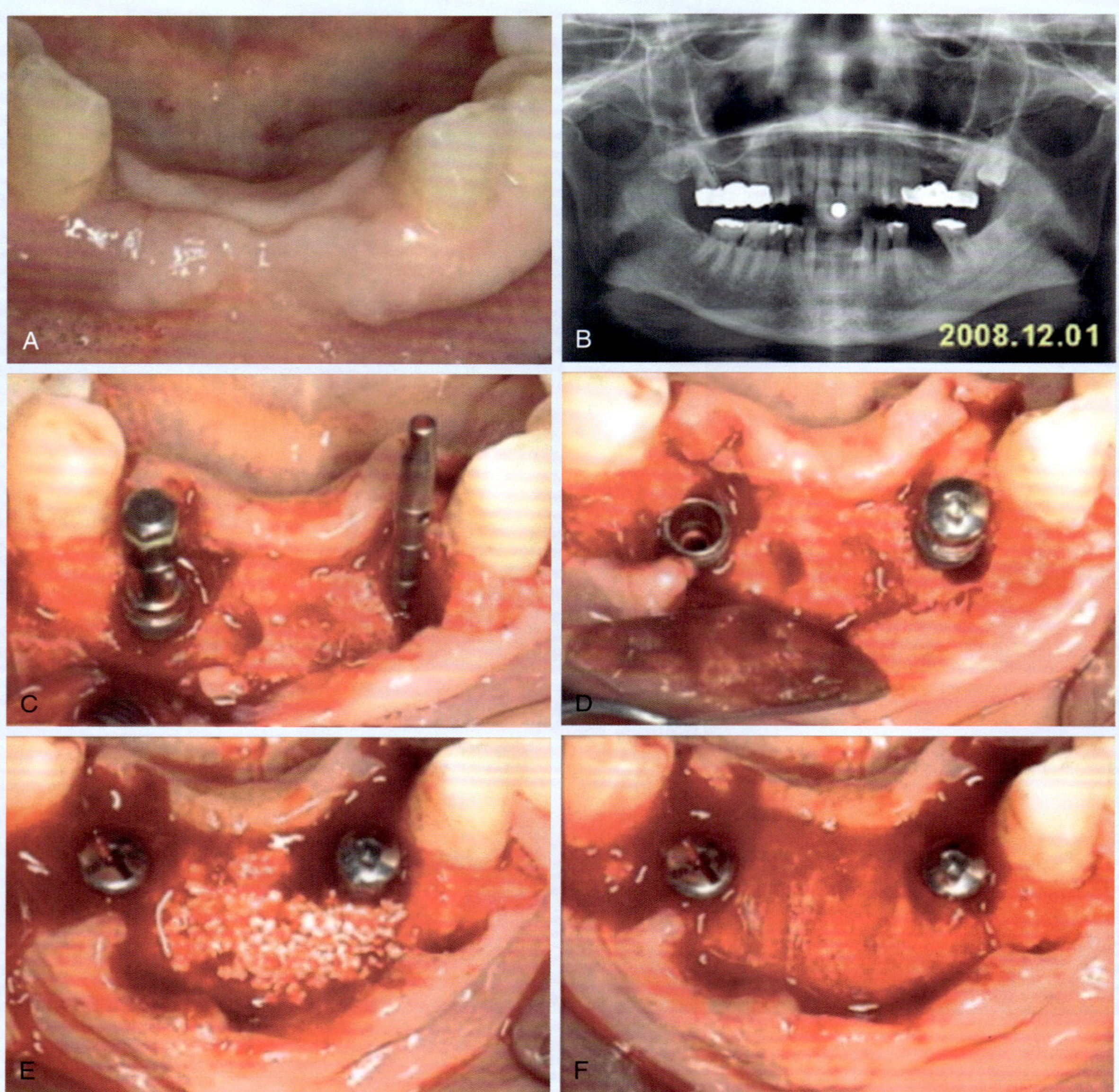

Fig 14.16 (A and B) Missing mandibular incisors. (C and D) Small osseous defects are visible after insertion of the implants, which were grafted using (E and F) osteon bone substitute and covered with collagen barrier membrane.

CASE REPORT-4—cont'd

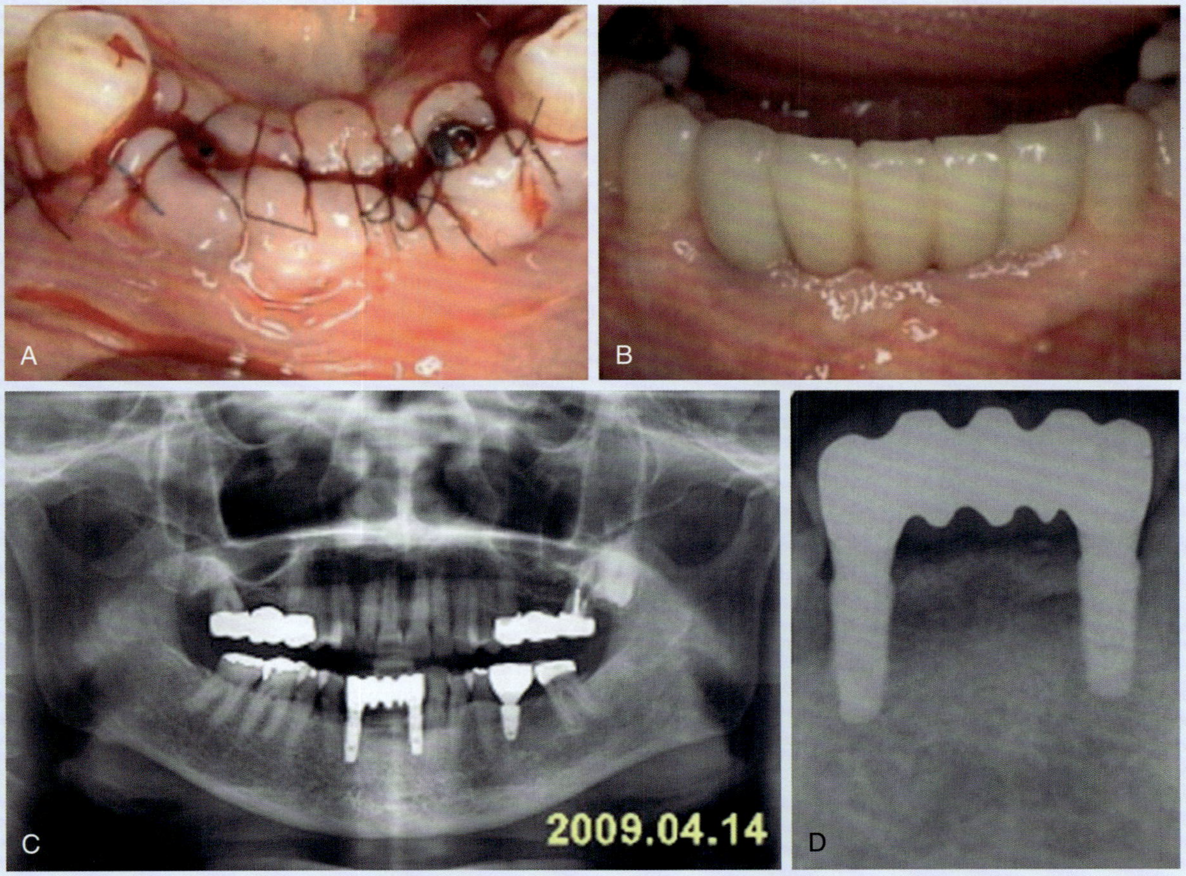

Fig 14.17 (A) Flap is sutured back. (B and C) Implants are uncovered and restored after 4 months. (D) Radiograph 1 year after implant restoration shows stable crestal bone level.

CASE REPORT-5

A 57-year-old healthy female with history of trauma to the face 8 years earlier, presented to the Oral Surgery and Implantology Center of Dr Len Tolstunov, San Francisco, CA, USA. The patient was referred by the general dentist for evaluation of a failing upper left canine. On presentation, the patient complained of cuspid mobility and periodic discharge from a wound high in the vestibule.

The patient's history of the present condition was significant for the trauma that happened 8 years ago, when she was hit with a fist to the left anterior maxilla. The upper left canine was affected by the blow, the patient felt it was loose but she did not go to a dentist and let it heal on its own. The patient felt a bump deep in the vestibule next to the tooth for many years and there was occasional discharge. The patient finally decided to see a dentist and an oral surgeon, due to recent increased swelling and pain in the area of the traumatized tooth.

The patient's aesthetic profile consisted of a low smile line, oval teeth and a thick, flat gingival biotype. There was an open gingival flap exposing the necrotic apical two-thirds of the root of the canine, which was probed deep in the vestibule with no discharge from the wound (Fig 14.18A). The cuspid had mobility 2 plus.

Radiographic examination consisted of the periapical, panoramic, and cone beam computed tomography (CBCT) scans that demonstrated (old) mid root fracture, previous root canal treatment, and severe apical bone loss around the tooth with just a small amount of structural bone support left on the palatal and buccal crestal area (Fig 14.18B). The tooth was literally 'hung in the air.' There was also a significant amount of alveolar bone width deficiency. The patient was

Continued

CASE REPORT-5—cont'd

diagnosed with a previously traumatized and fractured non-restorable upper left cuspid with severe three-dimensional bone loss.

The recommendations for the patient's condition included a staged approach with an extraction of the cuspid, a bone graft followed by the placement of an endosseous implant 4–6 months later, followed by a restorative phase with a ceramic restoration. The patient also needed a provisional appliance.

The patient rejected a staged treatment due to her busy schedule and asked that the practitioner should attempt to do both surgical stages in one. The patient's consent was taken and she was scheduled for surgery.

The surgery consisted of extraction of the affected tooth, bone grafting and implant placement at the same time under intravenous (IV) sedation. After the IV sedation was started and local anaesthesia was given, the crestal full-thickness flap with a distal releasing incision was reflected. Severe buccal bone loss and exposure of the unsupported and fractured canine tooth were visualized (Fig 14.18C). Using a periotome and with careful, slow dissection, the tooth was removed leaving a single buccal crestal bone bridge with a large and deep fenestration extending to the apical region of the elevated tooth (Fig 14.18D and E). The palatal bone was intact. The internal connection parallel-walled implant (Biomet 3i, Osseotite, Certain, 4 × 13 mm) was guided carefully with a surgical stent into the palatal and apical bone at about 25°, making sure it has an adequate primary implant stability (30 Ncm), platform 2 mm below the cementoenamel junction (CEJ) of the adjacent teeth, and an ideal restorative draw or projection (Fig 14.18F and G). Entire bone defect was grafted using composite bone grafting material (Bio-Oss [Osteohealth Co.], 0.5 g and Puros [Zimmer], 0.5 ml) (Fig 14.18H). The bone graft was covered using a barrier collagen membrane (Fig 14.19A) and the reflected buccal flap was repositioned back and closed primarily with 4-0 chromic gut suture. The patient recovered well after the surgery and was followed up in both surgical and restorative offices where a temporary fixed provisional bridge from the lateral incisor to the first premolar was made (in addition, the patient required several maxillary temporary crowns including both incisors, two premolars and a molar. The postoperative radiograph demonstrated an ideal implant position (Fig 14.19B).

Surgical stage 2 was done 6 months after the first stage, under local anaesthesia. Temporary 3i healing abutment of 2 mm height was placed (Fig 14.19C and D). The implant was well-osseointegrated. A large amount of bone was regenerated in the previous bone defect, in the buccal and apical regions. The soft tissue healed nicely not only in the crestal region but also deep in the vestibule where the original open post-traumatic chronic wound was present. The provisional prosthesis was modified in the cervical region to guide the soft tissue to heal with a scalloped aesthetic profile (Fig 14.19E and F).

A permanent porcelain fused to metal (PFM) crown was placed 2 months later and demonstrated excellent aesthetics, function, phonetics, and comfort (Fig 14.19G and H). The implant continued to function well 2 years after completion of the case.

Unique features of the case

Advanced (severe) localized bone loss (of traumatic and infectious origin) was reconstructed fully with the help of a (composite) cancellous graft. A ledge of a preserved natural bone on the buccal side served as anchor in the rebuilding of the missing bone with a help of guided tissue regeneration (GTR) on the buccal side and above (apically). Although this was mainly two-dimensional reconstruction (correction of the width deficiency), the amazing possibilities of cancellous bone graft and membrane (GBR and GTR) can be truly appreciated. Function and aesthetics were completely rehabilitated in this complex post-traumatic implant treatment case. *(Courtesy: Dr Len Tolstunov, DDS, California.)*

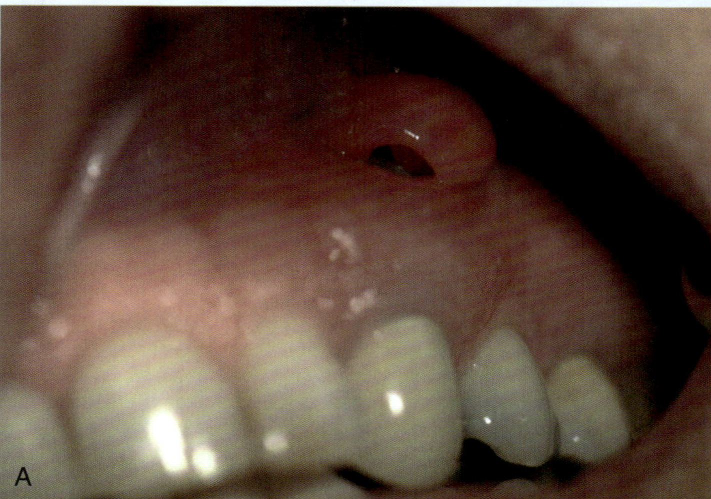

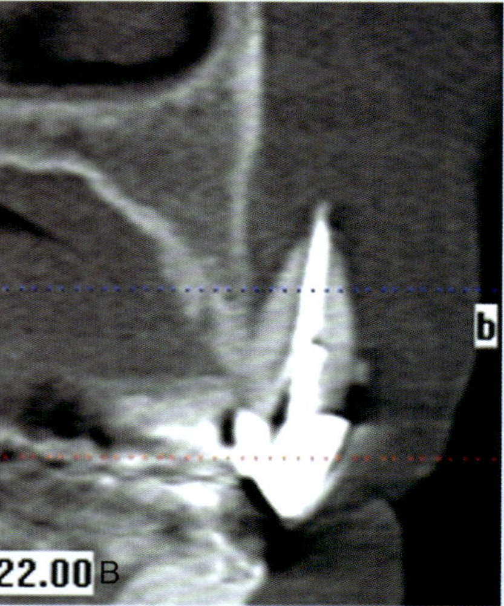

Fig 14.18 (A and B) Maxillary left canine with the large hard and soft tissue defect.

CASE REPORT-5—cont'd

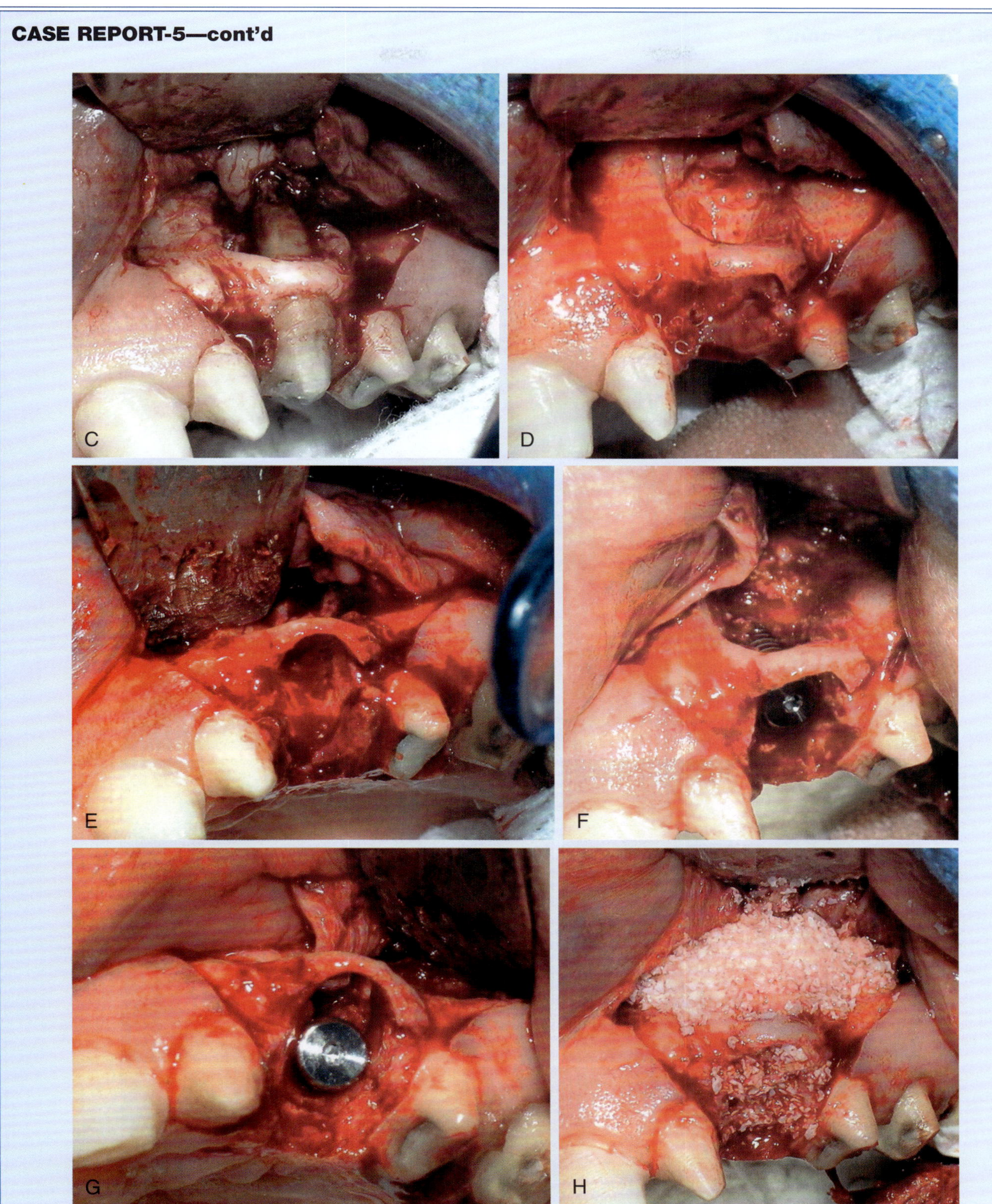

Fig 14.18, cont'd (C–E) A large osseous defect is visible after careful flap elevation and tooth extraction. All the granulation tissue was curetted out and site was disinfected using tetracycline powder. (F and G) The osteotomy was prepared and the implant was placed within the bony envelope and at the correct prosthetic position. (H) The facial wall defect as well as the Peri-implant socket spaces were grafted using Bio-Oss (Osteohealth Co.), 0.5 g and Puros (Zimmer), 0.5 ml.

Continued

CASE REPORT-5—cont'd

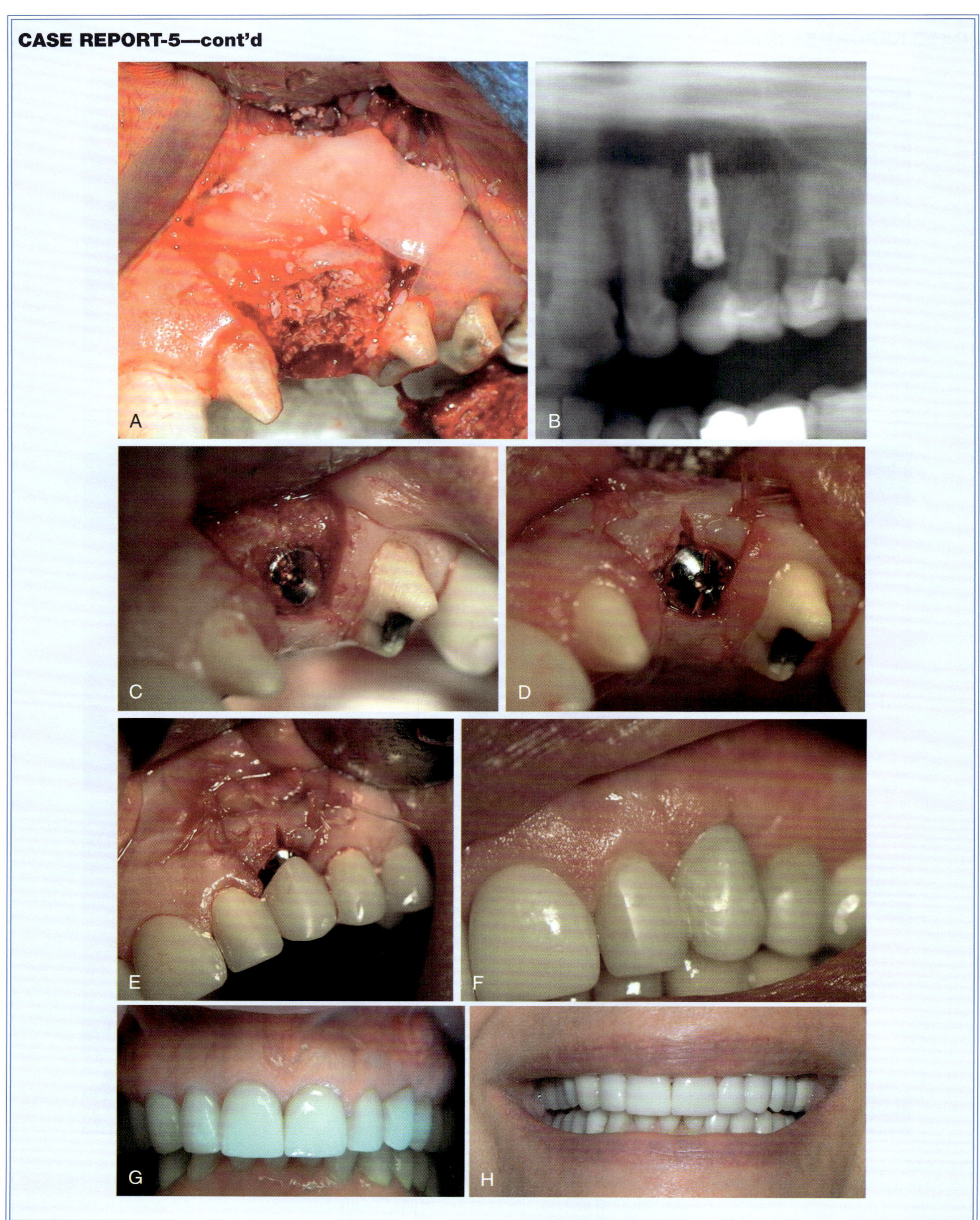

CASE REPORT-5—cont'd

Fig 14.19 The graft is covered by barrier membrane (A) and the flap is sutured back for submerged healing of the implant. Post implantation radiograph (B). Surgical stage 2 was done 6 months after the first stage under local anaesthesia. Temporary 3i healing abutment of 2 mm height was placed (C and D). The implant was well osseointegrated. The large amount of bone regenerated the previous bone defects in the buccal and apical regions. The soft tissue healed nicely not only in the crestal region but also deep in the vestibule where the original open post-traumatic chronic wound was present. The provisional prosthesis was modified in the cervical region to guide the soft tissue to heal with a scalloped aesthetic profile (E and F). A permanent PFM crown was placed 2 months later and demonstrated excellent aesthetics, function, phonetics, and comfort (G and H). (Restorative dentist: Dr Sam Itani, Blende Dental Group, San Francisco, CA, USA.)

CASE REPORT-6

Grafting of facial perforation and periodontal defect with adjacent tooth

A 45-year-old female patient presented with missing maxillary incisors. Careful intraoral examination revealed swelling and purulent discharge from the soft tissue pocket around the right canine, which otherwise was neither mobile nor caused pain to the patient (Fig 14.20A). The dental CT scan confirmed the presence of a large osseous defect with the canine and also facial concavity along the ridge morphology, which could result in perforation through the facial concavity if implants were placed at the correct prosthetic axis (Fig 14.20B and C). The placement of implants at teeth numbers 22 and 11 (away from the periodontal defect with the canine) was planned, with simultaneous grafting of the perio-osseous defect with canine. The perio pocket was drained and irrigated using citric acid and parenteral form of clindamycin to kill the residual pathogens in the pocket. After the pocket healed and no purulent discharge was seen after several dressings, the mucoperiosteal flaps were elevated to expose the bony ridge and perio-defect with canine (Fig 14.20D). All the granulation tissue was carefully curetted out from the periodontal defect and defect was disinfected using clindamycin (Fig 14.20E and F). Osteotomies for both the implants were prepared using a prosthetic guide, and implants were placed at the correct position and angulation (Fig 14.20G and H). It resulted in a small perforation through the facial concavity with the left implant (Fig 14.20I). The bone around the perforation was decorticated using small round carbide bur to receive the nourishment for the graft from the underlying spongiosa (Fig 14.20J).

A small amount of autologous bone was harvested from the adjacent site using a sharp chisel and used to cover the exposed implant threads (Fig 14.21A–C). Further, a bone substitute (HA + β-TCP) was used to fill the concavity as well as the periodontal defect (Fig 14.21D and E). The grafted periodontal defect was covered with a cytoplast TXT membrane, which was immobilized using membrane tacks (Fig 14.21E–G).

More graft was added under the membrane to keep it tented for the time adequate for new bone formation (Fig 14.22A). The flap was released and sutured back with primary closer (Fig 14.22B). Implants were uncovered after 4 months, and showed new bone regeneration at the dehiscence area (Fig 14.22C and D). Final abutments were inserted (Fig 14.22E) and a PFM prosthesis was fixed over the implants (Fig 14.22F and G).

Continued

CASE REPORT-6—cont'd

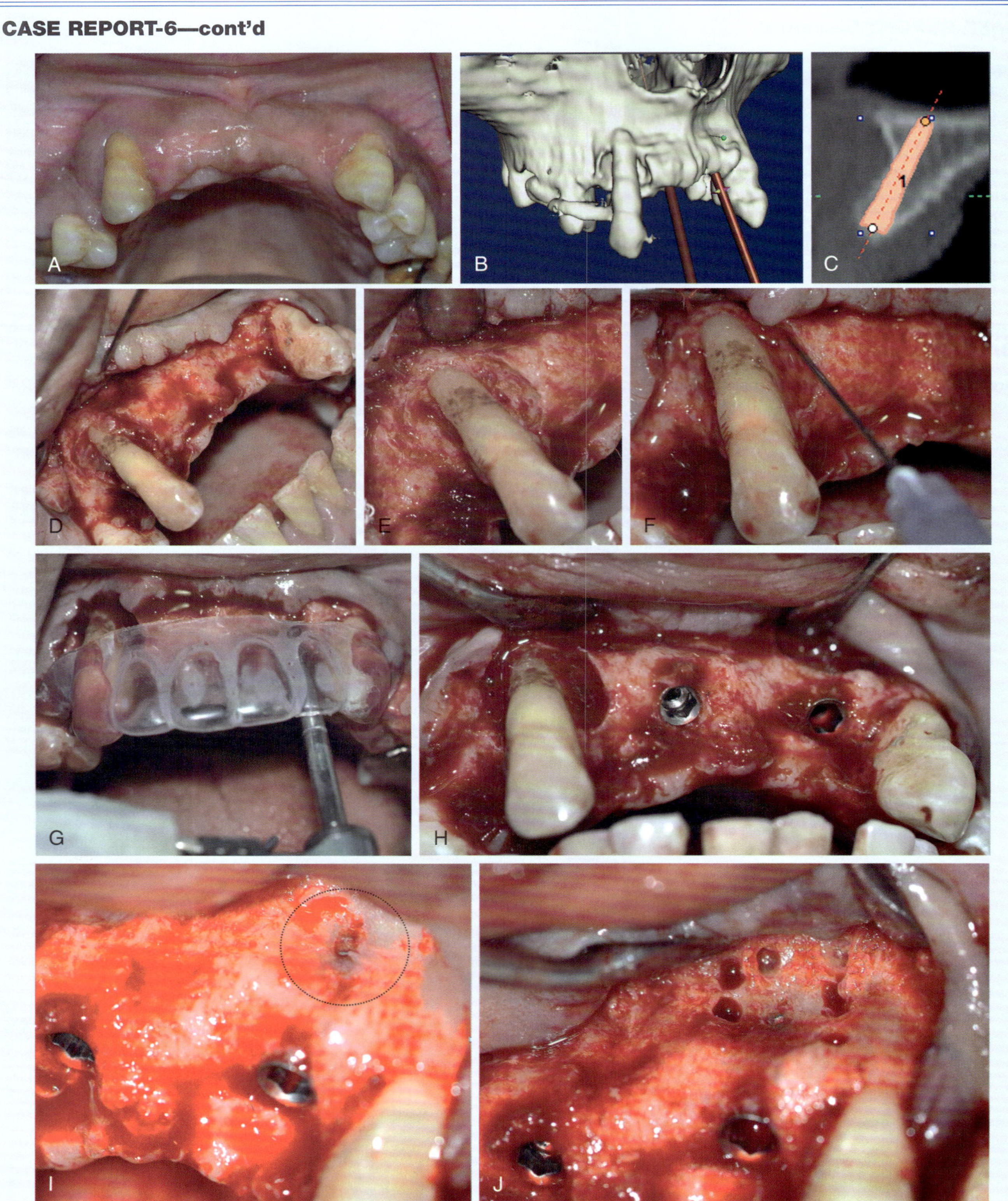

Fig 14.20 (A) Missing maxillary incisors. (B and C) CT images show large facial concavities and a large periodontal osseous defect around the right canine. (D–F) The flap was elevated, granulation tissue was curetted out from the periodontal defect, and the defect was disinfected using clindamycin. (G and H) Osteotomies for the implants were prepared using a prosthetic guide and implants were placed at the correct position and angulation. (I) It resulted in a small perforation through the facial concavity with the left implant. (J) The bone around the perforation was decorticated using a small round carbide bur, to receive the nourishment for the graft from the underlying spongiosa.

CASE REPORT-6—cont'd

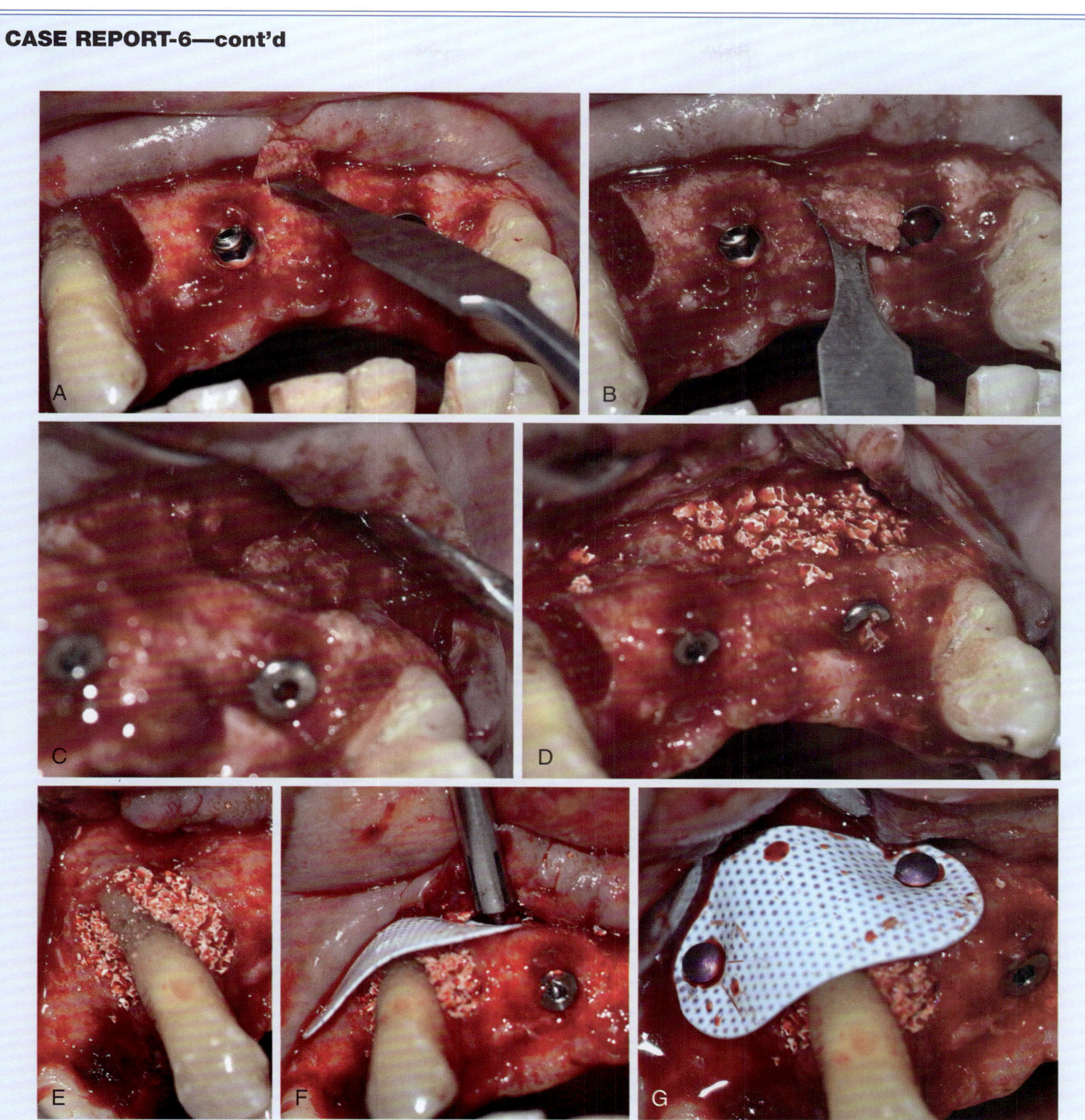

Fig 14.21 (A–C) A small amount of autologous bone was harvested from the adjacent site using a sharp chisel and used to cover the exposed implant threads. (D and E) Further, a bone substitute (HA + β-TCP) was used to fill the concavity as well as the periodontal defect. (E–G) The grafted periodontal defect was covered with a Cytoplast TXT membrane, which was immobilized by using membrane tacks.

Continued

CASE REPORT-6—cont'd

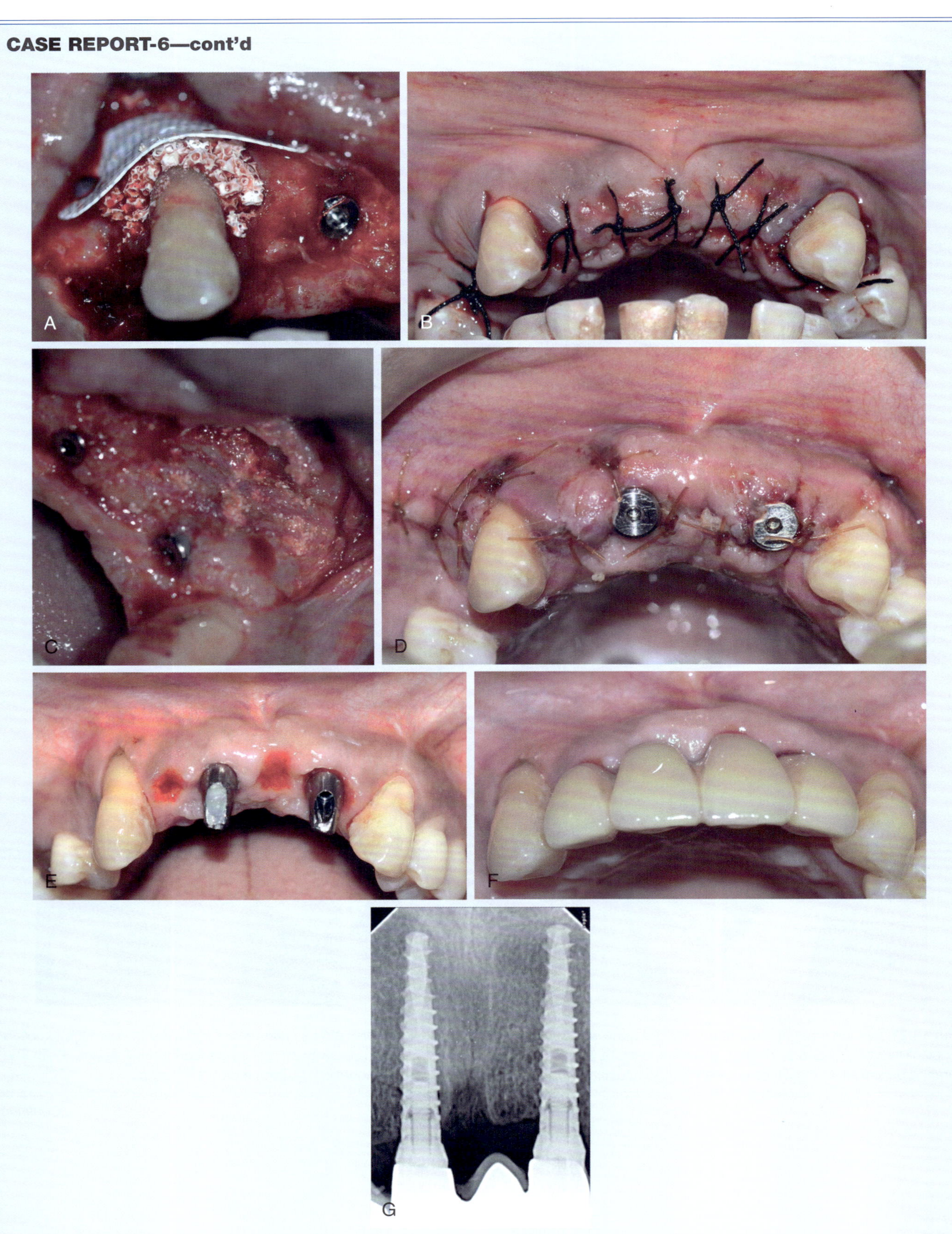

Fig 14.22 (A) More graft was added under the membrane to keep it tented for adequate amount of new bone formation. (B) The flap was released and sutured back with primary closer. (C and D) Implants were uncovered after 4 months, showing new bone regeneration at the dehiscence area. (E) Final abutments in place. (F) Final prosthesis in place. (G) Post loading radiograph.

CASE REPORT-7

Restoration of trauma case with bone augmentation simultaneous with implant placement

A 25-year-old male patient presented with a history of having lost upper front teeth in a road accident 3 months ago (Fig 14.23A). Intraoral examination revealed that the left maxillary canine was intact but had intruded and shifted outward (Fig 14.23B). The radiographs could not provide any relevant information about possible bone defect on the exposure of the site (Fig 14.23C and D), but the author had been treating many trauma cases with implants and most of the cases had shown some degree of bone defect, so all preparations were made to graft defects, if found after flap elevation. The orthodontic correction of the shifted canine and replacement of the lost teeth with implants was offered to the patient as the first treatment option, but because of long time span required to complete the

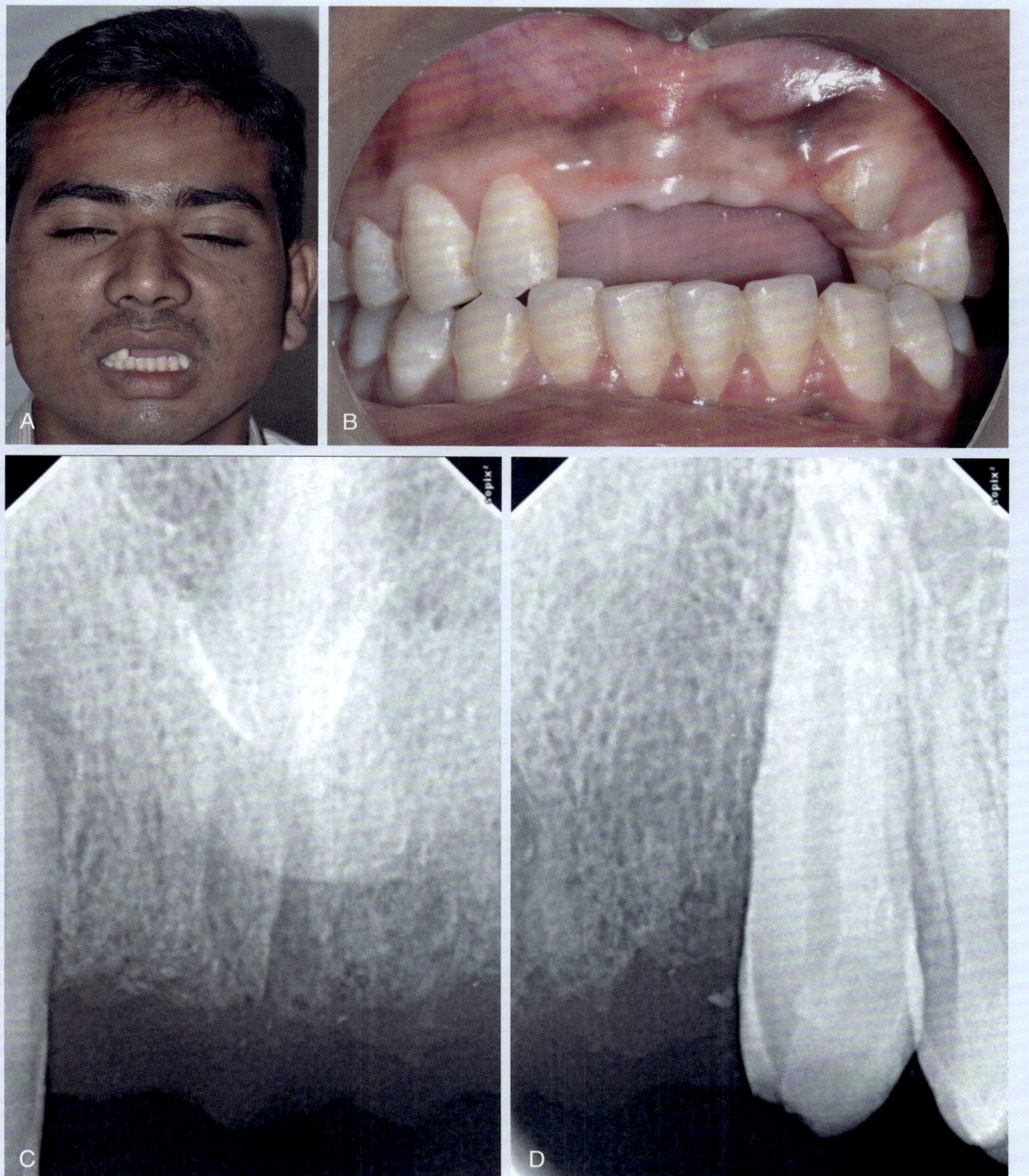

Fig 14.23 (A) A 25-year-old male patient presented with the history of having lost the upper front teeth in a road accident 3 months previously. (B) The intraoral examination revealed the intact left maxillary canine but it had intruded and shifted outward. (C and D) The radiographs could not provide any relevant information about possible bone defects.

Continued

CASE REPORT-7—cont'd

treatment, the patient opted to extract and replace the shifted canine by implant therapy.

All preparations were done for atraumatic extraction of the canine and prosthetically guided implant placement as well as simultaneous grafting of any bone defect. When the mucoperiosteal flap was elevated, the site showed a large osseous defect with canine and multiple defects along the facial wall of the ridge. The soft tissue growth into the traumatized hard tissue, which leads to disruption of the periosteum of the facial flap was seen, because blunt dissections were needed when elevating the flap to adequately expose the site (Fig 14.24A). The canine was carefully extracted, to preserve the available osseous architecture around it, to place the implant within the osseous envelope and provide space for the bone graft (Fig 14.24B).

During thorough removal of the fibrosseous tissue, the fibro sseous tissue was removed from the ridge, and a small autogenous bone block was harvested from the subnasal region using a bone saw (Fig 14.25A–C). The prefabricated prosthetic guide supported over the adjacent teeth was used to guide the osteotomy preparation for three implants (Fig 14.25D). Three implants at the correct prosthetic position were placed with adequate primary stability (more than 35 Ncm) (Fig 14.26A and B).

The implant at the canine position was placed within the bony envelope of the osseous defect of the socket. A small amount of bone was collected during the osteotomy preparation using a bone collector in suction line. This autogenous bone was grafted into the canine defect, which was further grafted using the previously harvested bone block. The site was further grafted using demineralized freeze dried allograft (Grafton) to reinforce the thin facial wall with multiple small bone defects (Fig 14.27A–D). The grafted site was covered using a collagen barrier membrane, and a releasing incision was given through the periosteum to achieve primary closure (Fig 14.28A and B). The implants were uncovered after 4 months and restored using PFM prosthesis. The desired aesthetic and functional results were achieved and implants were in function after 1 year with stable crestal bone around the implants (Fig 14.29A–E).

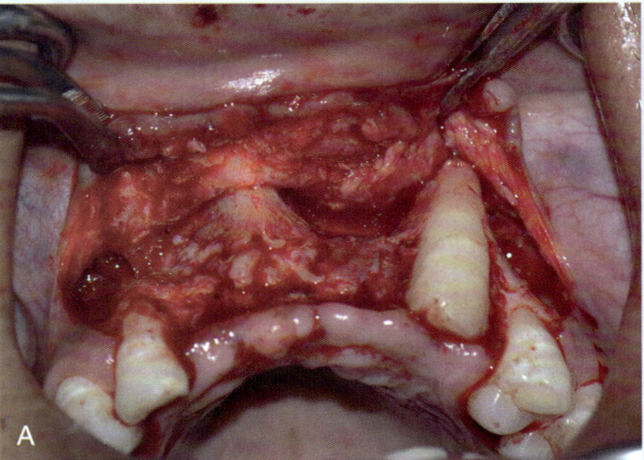

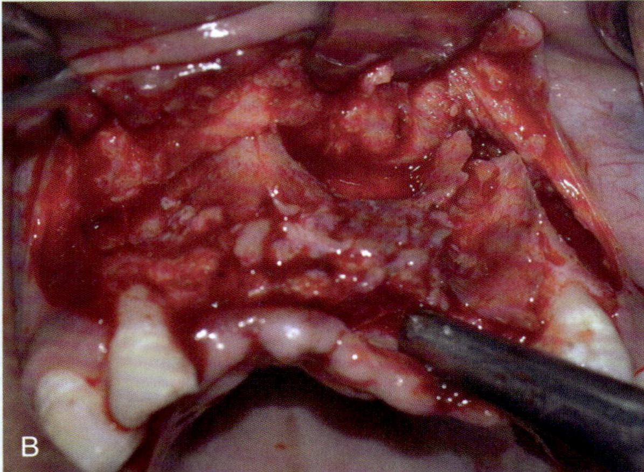

Fig 14.24 (A) Mid-crestal as well as vertical incisions were given and the site was exposed with mucoperiosteal flap elevation by giving blunt dissections through the soft tissue attachments into the osseous defects. (B) The canine was carefully extracted to preserve the thin socket walls which could be used to provide space maintenance and blood supply to the graft.

CASE REPORT-7—cont'd

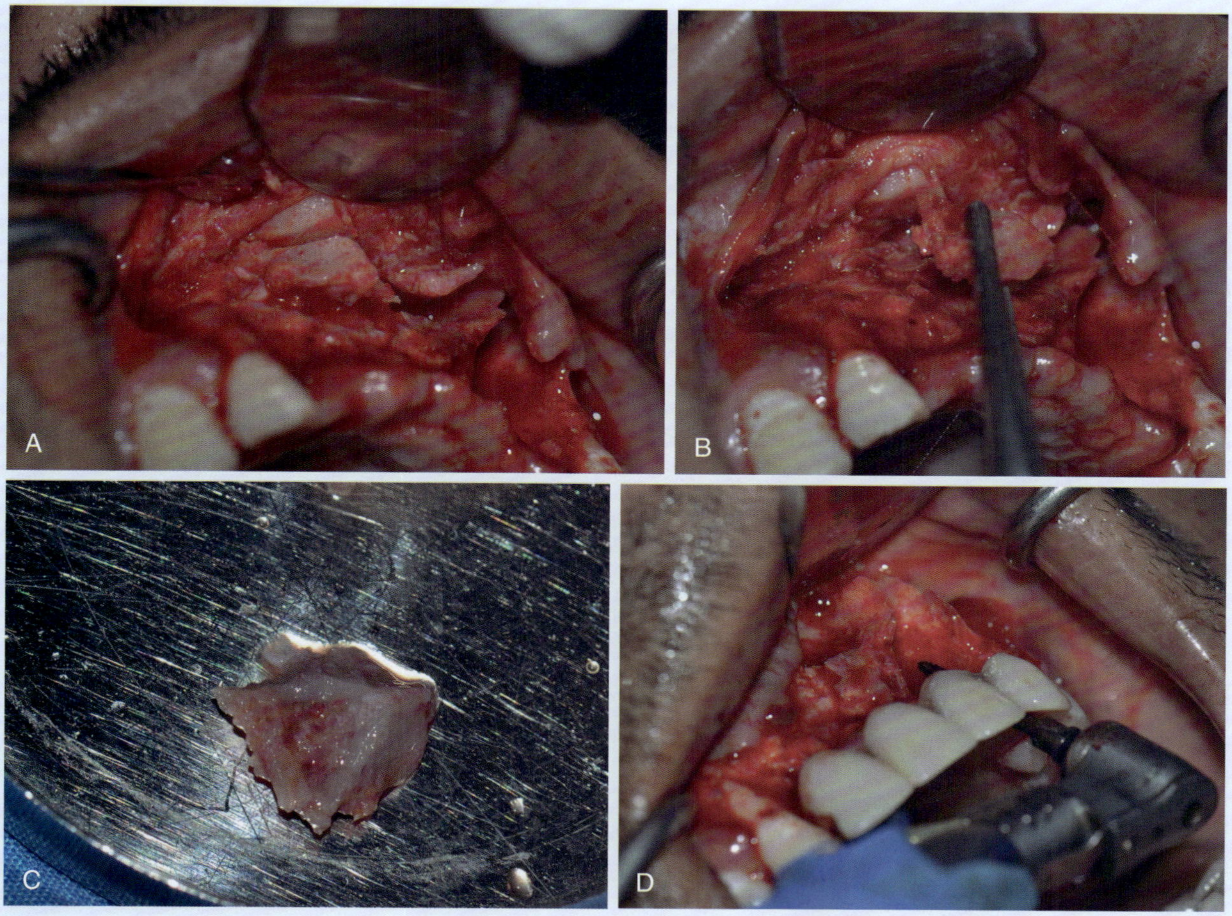

Fig 14.25 (A–C) The fibrosseous tissue was removed from the ridge and a small autogenous bone block was harvested from the subnasal region using the bone saw. (D) The prosthetic guide was seated over the adjacent teeth and the osteotomies for the implants were prepared through the guide.

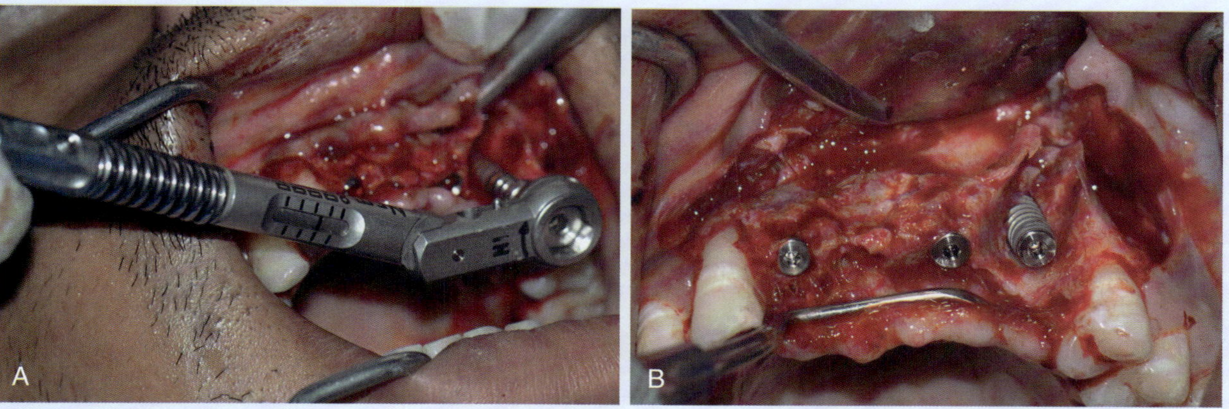

Fig 14.26 (A and B) Three implants were inserted at the correct prosthetic positions and with adequate primary stability.

Continued

CASE REPORT-7—cont'd

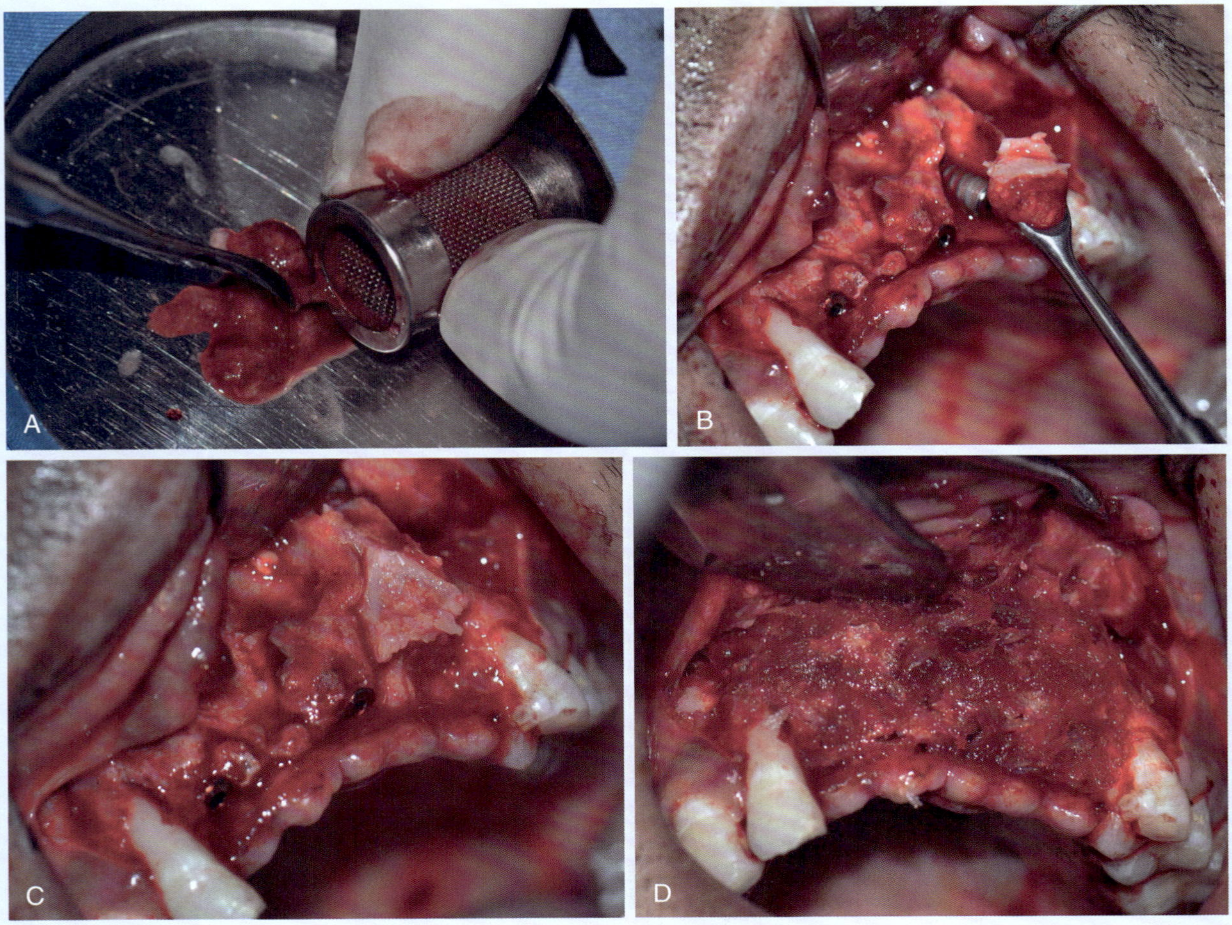

Fig 14.27 (A and B) The small amount of autogenous bone which was collected during osteotomy preparation using bone collecting suction, was used to graft the large osseous defect at the canine position (C) covered by the bone block which was shaped to fit in the defect. (D) Further, the demineralized freeze dried allograft (Grafton) was used to graft the whole site to fill all the osseous deficiencies and to regain the natural appearance of ridge topography.

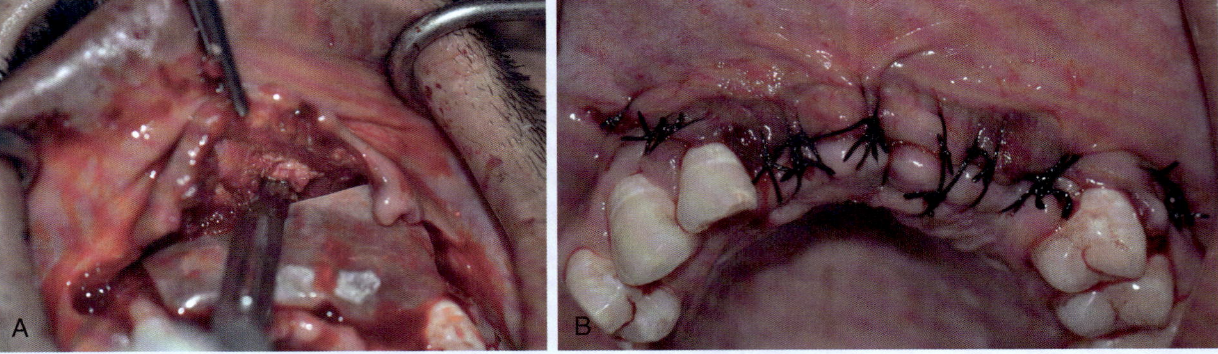

Fig 14.28 A collagen barrier membrane was used to cover the grafted site. Because the grafting increased the hard tissue volume thus to achieve primary closure of the flap, (A) releasing incision was given through the periosteum of the flap from underneath and apical to the muco-epithelial junction. (B) The primary closure of the flap was achieved. No soft tissue-supported provisional prosthesis was given to the patient, to avoid pressure on the grafted site which may have resulted in the displacement of the graft from its position.

CASE REPORT-7—cont'd

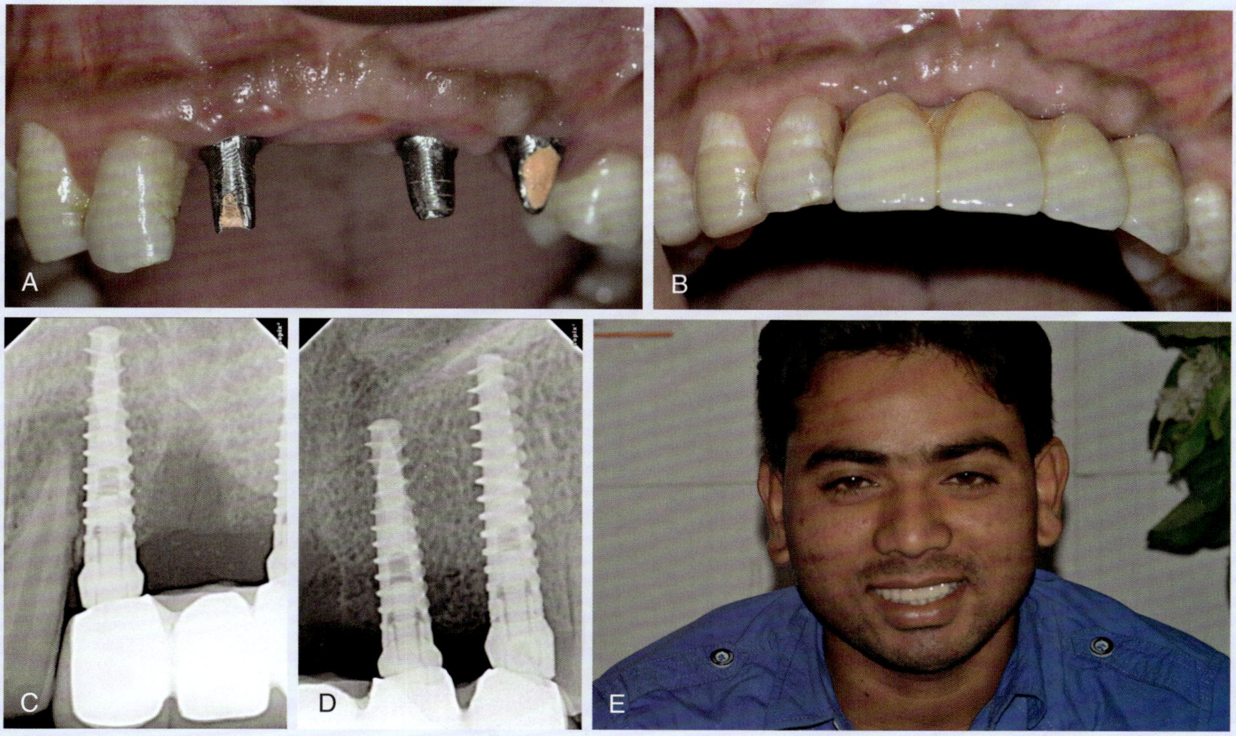

Fig 14.29 (A and B) The implants were uncovered 4 months after placement and restored with porcelain fused to metal (PFM) prosthesis. (C and D) Radiographs 1 year after implant loading, showing stable crestal bone level around the implants. (E) Patient with a pleasant smile. (The patient consented to the publication of his picture in literature.)

Subperiosteal tunnelling technique

The conventional techniques of lateral or vertical augmentation of ridge defects or perforations that occur during osteotomy preparation, need extensive mucoperiosteal flap elevation to completely visualize the host site for graft placement. These conventional techniques are well documented for success rate in bone augmentation for new bone regeneration, but there are also various problems that the dentist faces with these techniques, such as difficulty in stabilizing the graft at site, extensive flap elevation leading to reduced blood supply to the region, need of a barrier membrane to cover the graft, problem in achieving primary closure of the flap, suture line opening, and more postoperative discomfort to the patient. To overcome these problems, the subperiosteal tunnelling approach for lateral and vertical bone augmentation is found to be more comfortable and successful in many cases. In this approach, a small vertical incision is given at the distant location and a subperiosteal tunnel is created to reach over the defect. Further, through this tunnel, controlled periosteal elevation is done to create a desired subperiosteal pouch over the defect. The bone graft material is carried through the tunnel and deposited over the defect within the created subperiosteal pouch and the vertical incision line is sutured (Fig 14.30A–E). In this technique, mixing platelet-rich plasma into the graft enhances the handling properties of the graft, keeps the graft at the desired localized position, prevents graft dispersion from the site, and enhances the bone regeneration potential of the bone graft.

Advantages

1. Minimally invasive technique.
2. Less technique sensitive.
3. Cost effective as no barrier membrane is used.
4. Fewer complications (e.g. suture line opening, loss of graft, infection, etc.) compared to open augmentation techniques.

Disadvantages

1. Graft takes longer time to get resorbed and to regenerate new bone in the area, as decortication of the host site is difficult to perform in most cases.
2. It is a blind procedure that needs proper radiographic and CT imaging planning to evaluate the size and location of the defect.
3. Needs a very controlled surgical hand for successfully performing the procedure.
4. Tearing of the periosteum during its elevation from the defect area, may cause soft tissue growth in the graft.

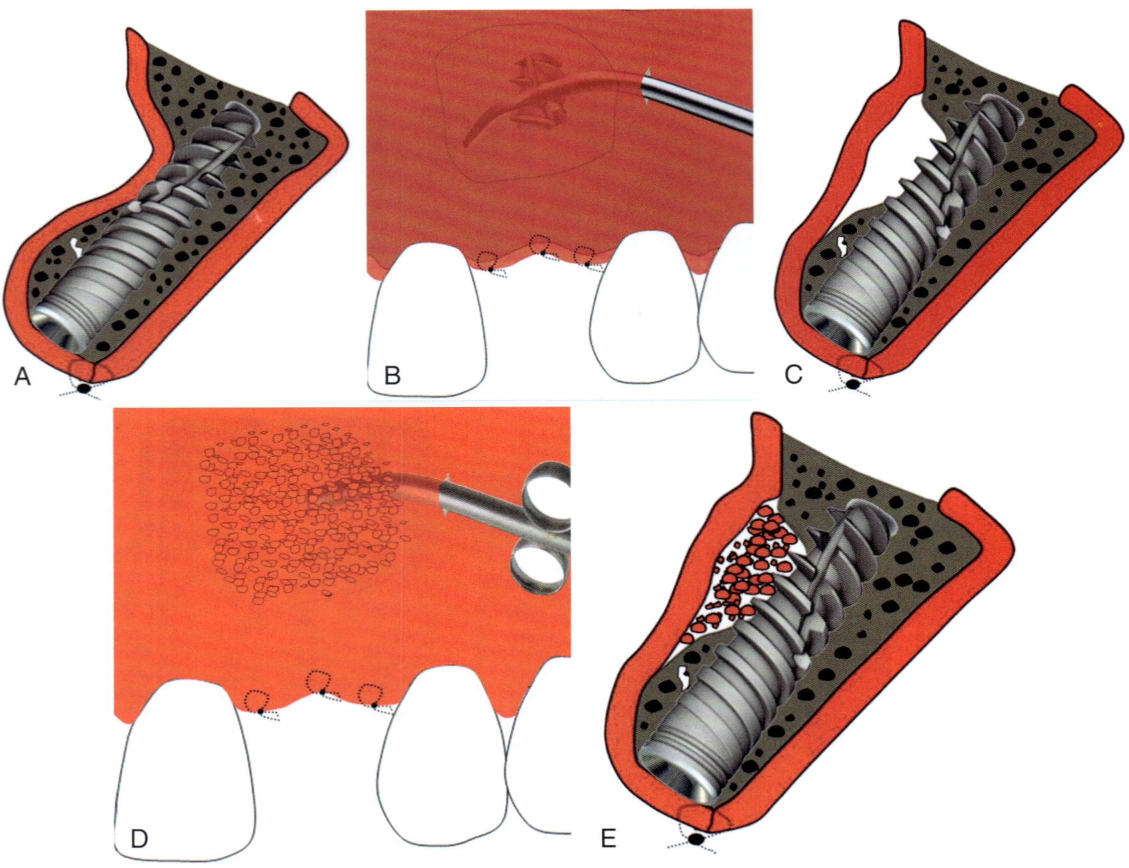

Fig 14.30 Diagrammatic presentation of subperiosteal tunnelling approach. (A) Cross-sectional view of the ridge showing the immediately placed implant, which has resulted in perforation through the facial concavity. (B) A small vertical incision is given through the facial mucosa at a distant location (minimum 8–10 mm away from the defect) and a subperiosteal tunnel is created, using an appropriate curette, to reach over the defect. (C) The periosteum is elevated from the defect as well as from the small area of the peripheral bone, to create a subperiosteal pouch over the defect. (D and E) The graft is carried to the created subperiosteal pouch through the tunnel and deposited over the defect. The incision line is sutured.

Indications

1. Lateral bone augmentation of facial concavities along with ridge morphology.
2. Grafting of perforation that occurs through the facial cortical plate, well above the crest.
3. Augmentation of the apical bone defects with immediate implant in extraction cases.
4. Lateral bone augmentation of thin maxillary or mandibular ridge in the crestal half with a favourable bed for graft placement (favourable defect).
5. Vertical bone augmentation of the ridge with adequate buccolingual base to place the graft and to receive the nourishment.

Contraindications

1. Bone dehiscence during implant placement in the crestal half of the ridge.
2. Bone defects where adequate base for graft placement is not available. For example, need of vertical bone augmentation in a pencil-thin mandibular ridge.
3. Trauma cases where the periosteum is not intact and the soft tissue has badly grown into the bone defects.

CASE REPORT-8

Lateral bone augmentation by tunnelling approach (Fig 14.31A–P).

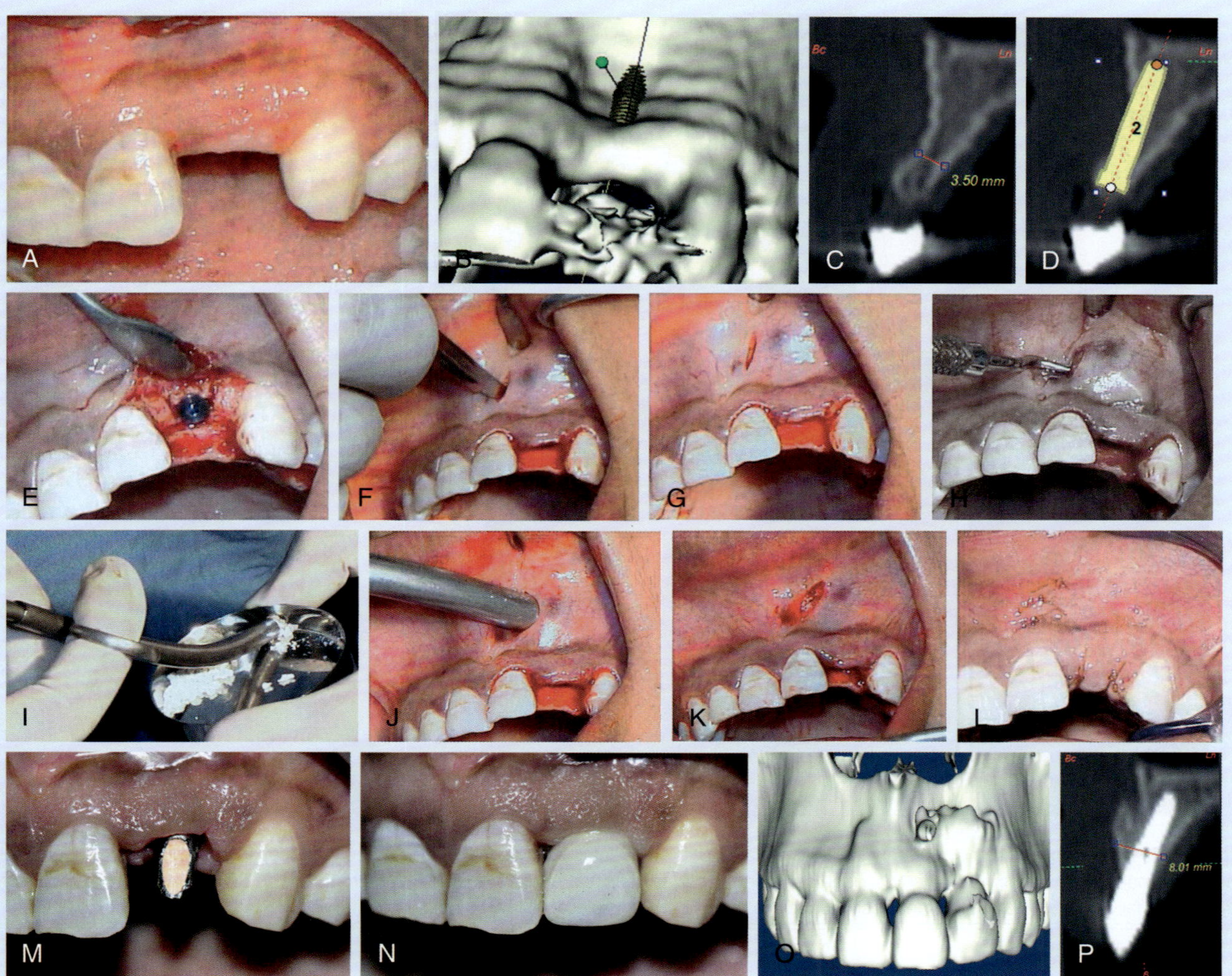

Fig 14.31 (A) Site of the missing maxillary lateral incisor, which clinically presented as the presence of adequate ridge dimensions for implant placement. (B and C) But, CT images showed the inadequate faciopalatal bone dimension with deep facial concavity, (D) which was inadequate even for the placement of a narrow diameter implant. A mid-crestal incision was made and the flap was minimally elevated (limited to the attached and stable facial mucoperiosteum) to expose the ridge crest. (E) The implant was inserted at the ideal prosthetic position. The inserted implant achieved adequate primary stability but the dehiscence which occurred through the facial concavity needed to be grafted. (F and G) A small vertical incision was given through the facial mucosa, a little away from the dehiscence. (H) A subperiosteal tunnel was created to elevate the periosteum at the facial concavity. (I–K) The bone substitute (HA + β-TCP) mixed with plasma rich in growth factors (PRGF) was carried through the tunnel and deposited at the facial concavity. (L) Both the incision lines were sutured with primary closer. (M and N) Implant was uncovered and restored after 4 months. (O and P) Post loading CT images show the island of new bone formation at the concavity area.

CASE REPORT-9

Vertical bone augmentation by the tunnelling approach (Figs 14.32 and 14.33).

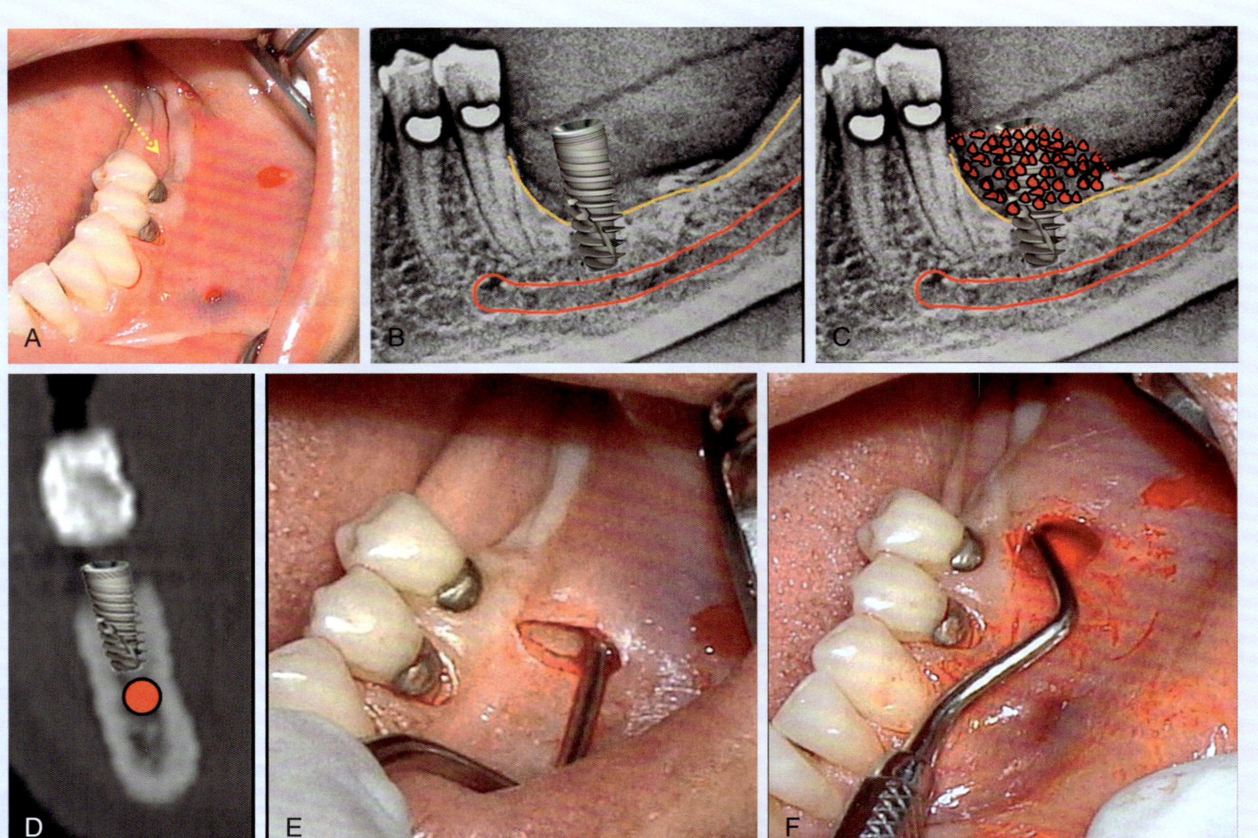

Fig 14.32 (A) The implant for the missing first molar is planned. (B–D) Dental radiograph and CT scan cross-section show inadequate bone height above the mandibular canal; hence vertical bone augmentation was necessary before implant insertion. (E and F) Small vertical incision was given through the facial mucosa at the distant position and the periosteum was elevated from the ridge crest through the subperiosteal tunnel.

CASE REPORT-9—cont'd

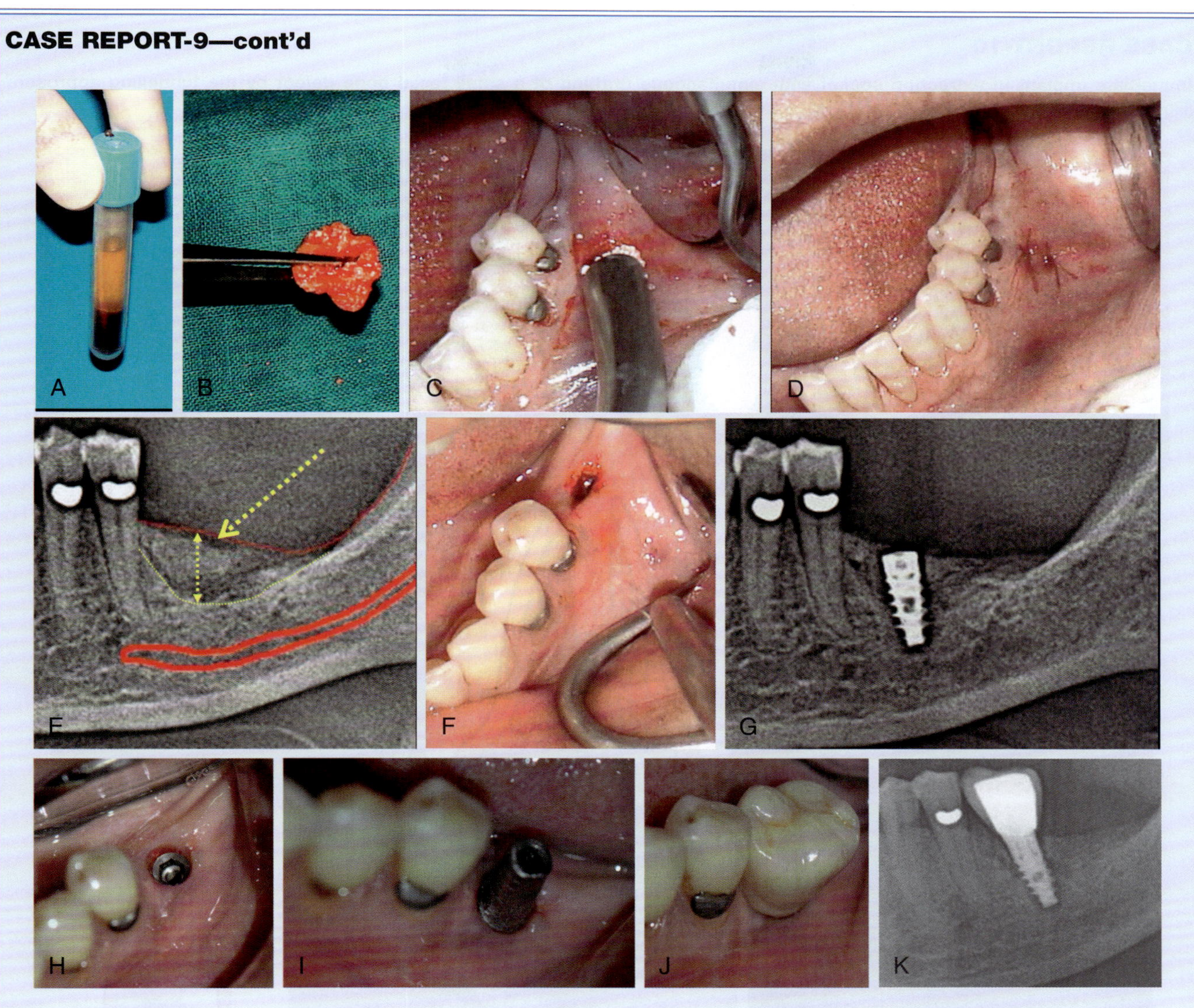

Fig 14.33 (A and B) PRGF is prepared from the patient's venous blood and was mixed with bone substitute. (C and D) The bone graft was deposited into the created subperiosteal pouch on the ridge crest and the incision line was sutured. (E) Post-grafting radiograph shows approximately 10 mm of vertical bone augmentation. (F and G) The implant was inserted after 6 months with mini incision technique. (H–J) Implant was uncovered and restored after 4 months. (K) The follow-up radiograph after 1 year shows the homogenous consolidation of newly regenerated bone with no crestal bone resorption with the implant in function.

CASE REPORT-10

Immediate implant in extraction socket with simultaneous grafting of a small facial bone defect by the tunnelling approach (Figs 14.34–14.36).

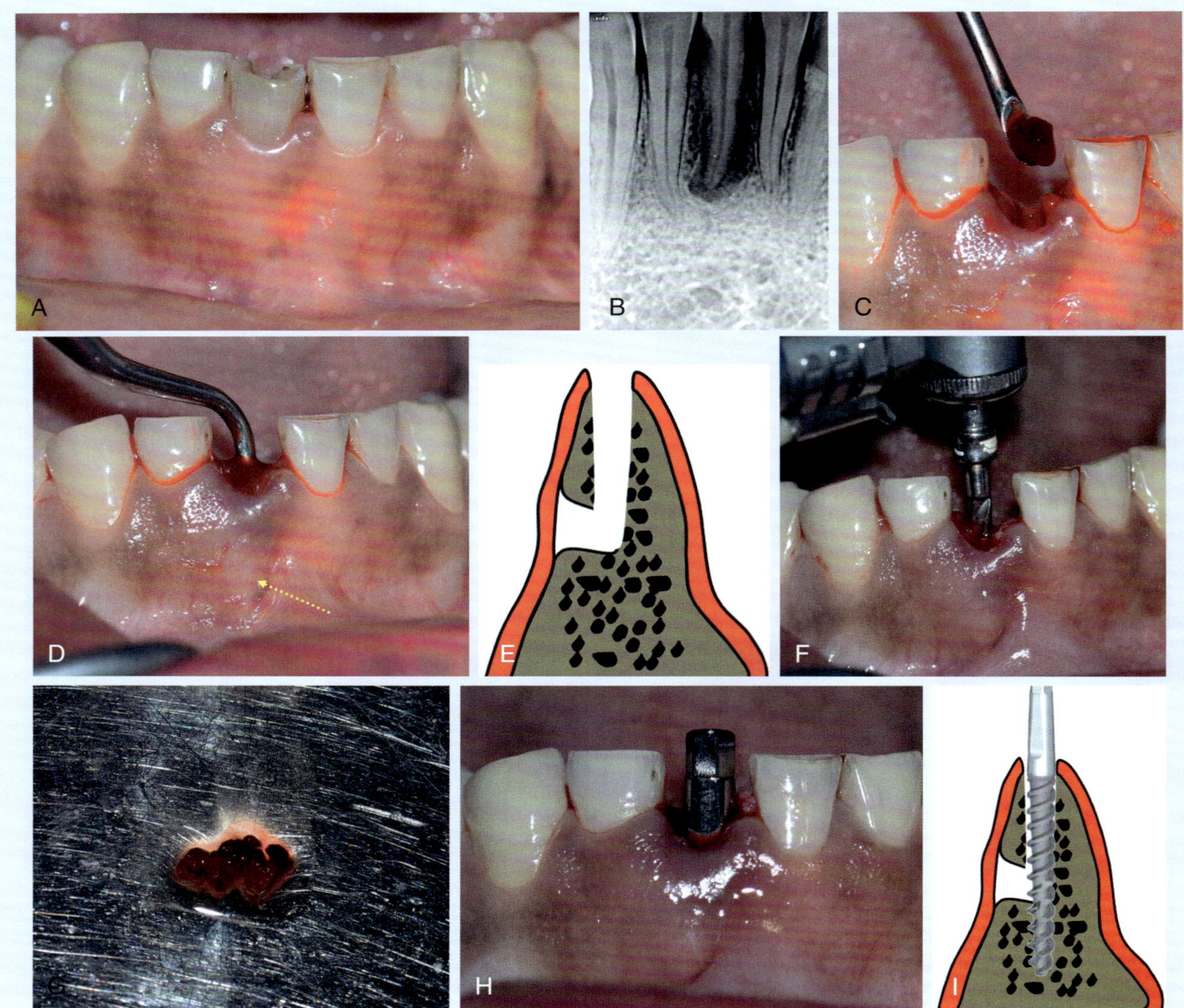

Fig 14.34 (A) Mandibular central incisor with history of chronic periapical infection and recurrent drainage through intraoral sinus. (B) Dental radiograph shows large periapical radiolucent lesion affecting half the root length. (C) The tooth was atraumatically extracted and all the granulation tissue was curetted from the socket. (D and E) A small osseous defect was felt through the facial ball of the socket in the apical region. (F) The socket was disinfected using the parenteral form of clindamycin for 5 min to kill the residual pathogens, and then implant osteotomy was prepared in the usual fashion. (G) A small amount of autogenous bone was collected from the drills. (H and I) A single body narrow diameter implant (3 × 15 mm One™ implant from Adin) was inserted at the ideal position. The implant achieved adequate primary stability (more than 35 Ncm).

CASE REPORT-10—cont'd

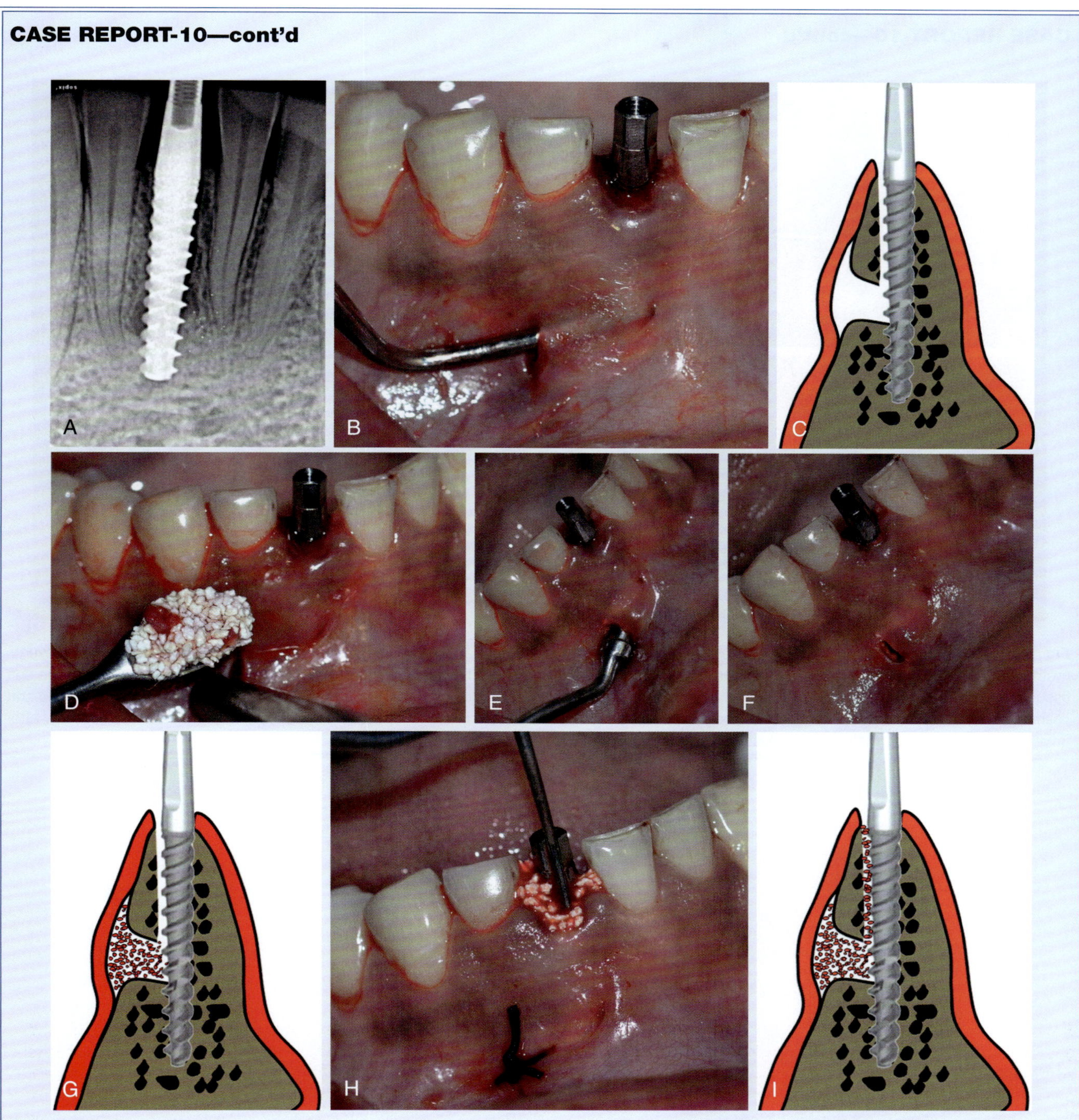

Fig 14.35 (A) The post-implantation radiograph showed that the implant apex had been stabilized into 3 mm healthy bone apical to the radiolucency. (B and C) A small vertical incision was given through the facial mucoperiosteum at the distant position and a subperiosteal tunnelling approach was taken to elevate the periosteum from the defect and to create a small subperiosteal pouch at the defect area. (D–G) Bone substitute mixed with autogenous bone, was deposited in and over the facial defect through the subperiosteal tunnel. (H and I) The incision line was closed with a single suture and the Peri-implant socket spaces were also loosely filled with graft.

Continued

CASE REPORT-10—cont'd

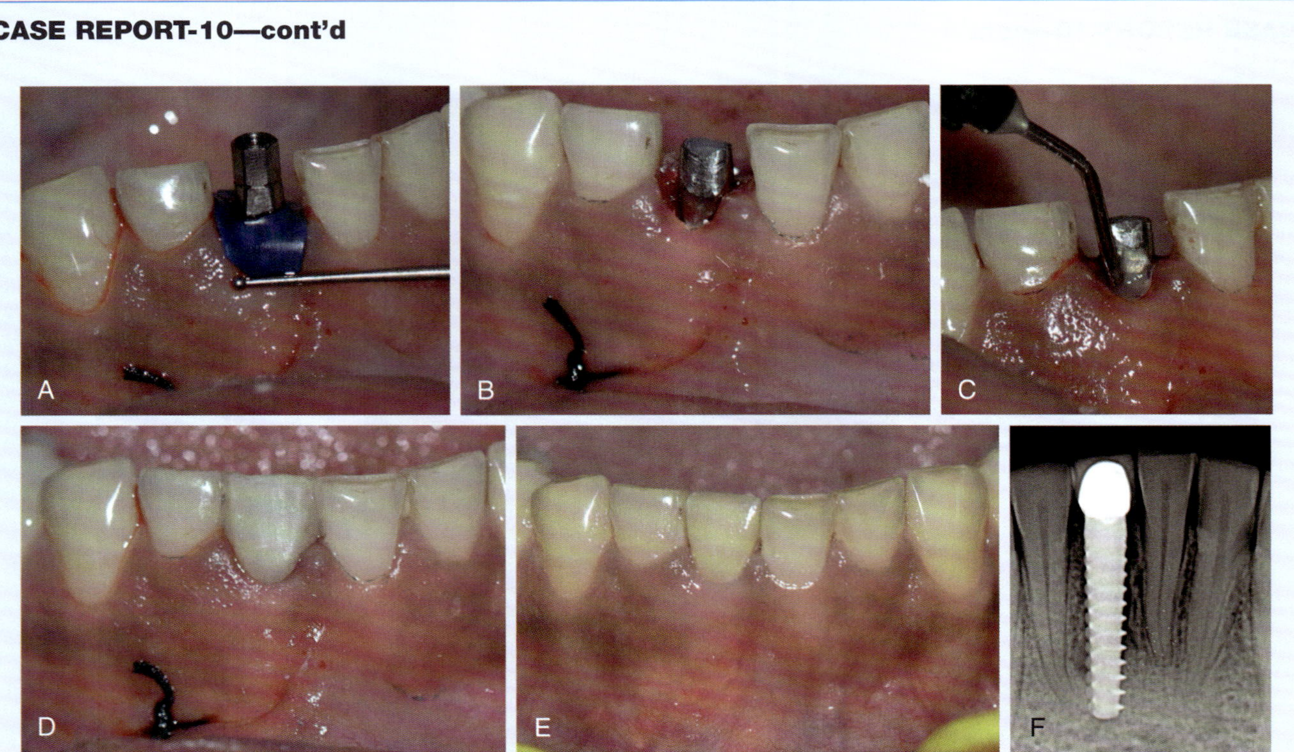

Fig 14.36 A small piece of rubber dam was used to cover the socket and the abutment was prepared in the mouth. (A and B) This prevents metal dust from entering the grafted Peri-implant socket spaces. (C) Further, the flow composite was used around the abutment to seal the soft tissue area of the socket. A provisional crown was fixed over the implant. (D) This prevents the loss of graft from the socket, supports the soft tissue papillae, and also creates an aesthetic soft tissue emergence profile around the implant prosthesis. (E) Implant was loaded early, after 3 weeks, using ceramic prosthesis. (F) Post loading radiograph.

CASE REPORT-11

Immediate implant with simultaneous grafting of Peri-implant socket spaces (Fig 4.37A–M).

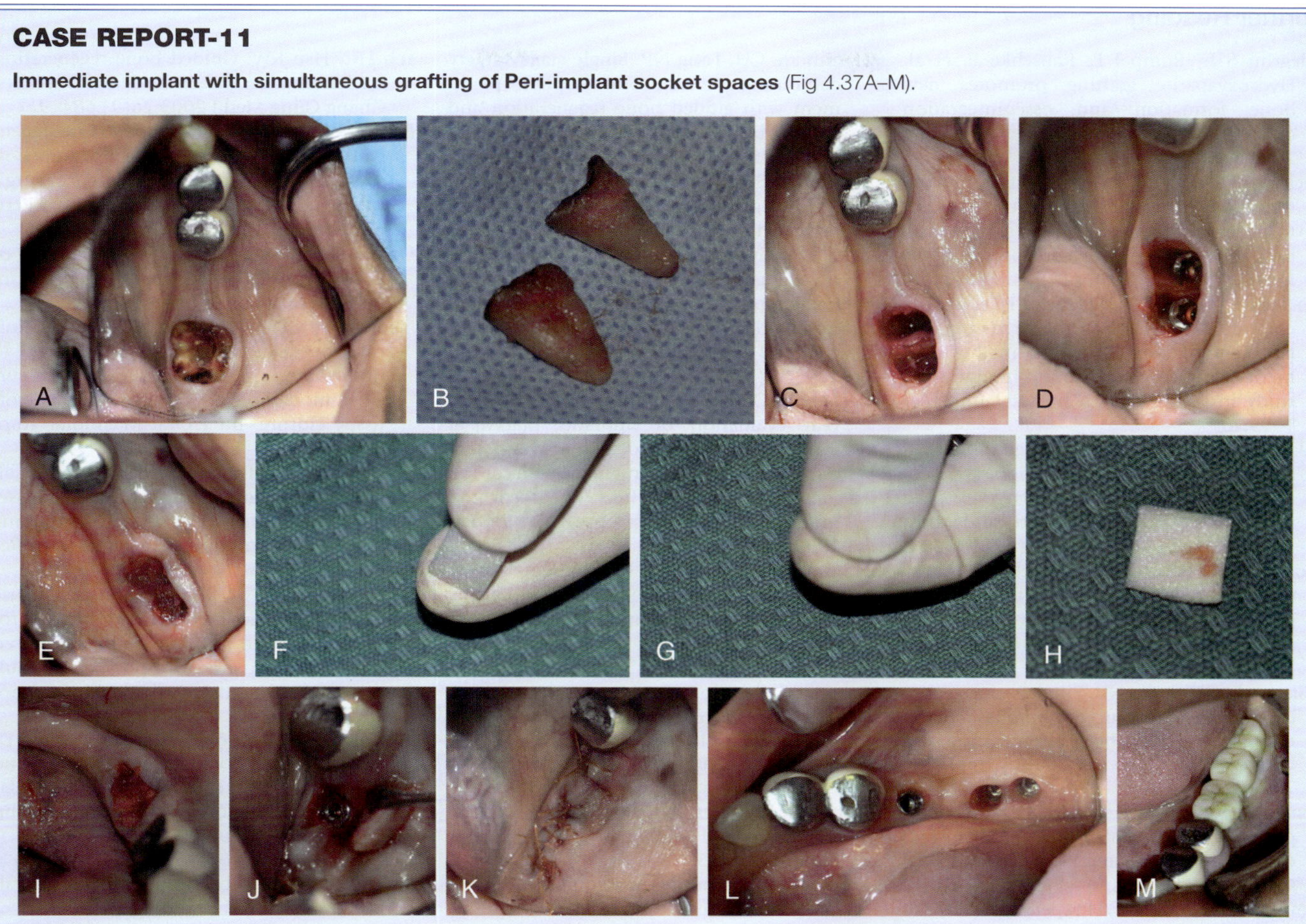

Fig 14.37 (A) Grossly decayed, non-restorable mandibular molar with missing tooth, anterior to it. (B and C) The tooth was extracted with minimum trauma to preserve the osseous architecture of the socket. Implants were placed in both the root sockets with adequate primary stability. (D) The elliptical shape of the sockets resulted in large Peri-implant socket spaces which needed to be grafted. (E) The Peri-implant socket spaces were grafted using demineralized allograft putty (Grafton). (F–H) A piece of gelatine sponge was compressed between two fingers to make it denser. This gelatine sponge was placed over the graft and marginal soft tissue, released and mobilized to achieve primary closure. (I–K) Another implant was placed at the anterior site. (L and M) Implants were uncovered after 4 months and restored using full zirconia (monolithic) prosthesis.

Summary

Bone grafting simultaneous with implant placement has now become a routine procedure in implantology. The implant surgeon should develop the skills to graft peri-implant osseous defects with minimally invasive techniques to achieve a successful outcome. It is seen that bone grafting simultaneous with implant placement is a more technique-sensitive procedure and requires varied approaches for different types of bone defects. The basics of the bone grafting that are described in the previous chapter, should be followed to obtain the desired outcome. The selection of the appropriate bone graft and approach for bone grafting are key for a successful outcome. Meticulous treatment planning should be done in cases with possible osseous defects, to evaluate the type of defect, volume of graft required, bone available for implant placement, surgical approach, etc. Whenever possible, autogenous bone should be mixed with bone substitutes. Effort should be made to avoid tears in the periosteum during the flap elevation, and if it has occurred or if the size of the defect is larger than envisaged, barrier membrane should be used to prevent soft tissue creeping into the graft. The implant should be placed simultaneous with grafting only if it can be placed well within the bony envelope and can achieve adequate primary stability. The subperiosteal tunnelling technique is found to be the minimally invasive technique for grafting and can be performed in cases of facial perforations, facial defects, favourable vertical defects, and where lateral bone augmentation is required. Each case differs from the other, so meticulous treatment planning using radiographs and CT images and the skilled approach of the surgeon are paramount for success in such cases.

Further Reading

Allegrini S Jr, Rumpel E, Kauschke E, et al. Hydroxyapatite grafting promotes new bone formation and osseointegration of smooth titanium implants. Ann Anat 2006;188(2):143–51.

Becker W, Becker BE, Polizzi G, et al. Autogenous bone grafting of bone defects adjacent to implants placed into immediate extraction sockets in patients: a prospective study. Int J Oral Maxillofac Impl 1994a;9:389–96.

Hockers T, Abensur D, Valentini P, et al. The combined use of bioresorbable membranes and xenografts or autografts in the treatment of bone defects around implants – a study in beagle dogs. Clin Oral Impl Res 1999:10.

Lekholm U, Sennerby L, Roos J, et al. Soft tissue and marginal bone conditions at osseointegrated implants that have exposed threads – a 5-year retrospective study. Int J Oral Maxillofac Impl 1996;11(5):599–604.

Zitzmann N, Schärer P, Marinello C. Long-term results of implants treated with guided bone regeneration: a 5-year prospective study. Int J Oral Maxillofac Impl 2001;16(3).

Hämmerle CH, Lang NP. Single stage surgery combining transmucosal implant placement with guided bone regeneration and bioresorbable materials. Clin Impl Res 2001:21.

Benic GI, Jung RE, et al. Clinical and radiographic comparison of implants in regenerated or native bone: 5-year results. Clin Oral Impl Res 2009.

Simion M, Fontana F, Raspereini G, et al. Vertical ridge augmentation by expanded-polytetrafluoroethylene membrane and a combination of intraoral autogenous bone graft and deproteinized inorganic bovine bone (Bio Oss). Clin Oral Impl Res 2007;18(5):620–9.

Gher ME, Quintero G, Assad D, et al. Bone grafting and guided bone regeneration for immediate dental implants in humans. J Periodontol 1994;65:881–991.

Hämmerle CH, Lang NP. Single stage surgery combining transmucosal implant placement with guided bone regeneration and bioresorbable materials. Clin Oral Impl Res 2001;12:9–18.

Nyman S. Bone regeneration using the principle of guided tissue regeneration. J Clin Periodontol 1991;18:494–8.

Artzi Z, Dayan D, Alpern Y, et al. Vertical ridge augmentation using xenogenic material supported by a configured titanium mesh: clinicohistopathologic and histochemical study. Int J Oral Maxillofac Impl 2003;18(3):440–6.

Becker W, Dahlin C, Lekholm U, et al. Five-year evaluation of implants placed at extraction and with dehiscence and fenestration defects augmented with ePTFE membranes: results from a prospective multicenter study. Clin Impl Dent Rel Res 1999;1:27–32.

Hammerle CH, Jung RE. Ridge augmentation procedures. In: Lindhe J, Lang NP, Karring T, editors. 5th ed. Clinical periodontology and implant dentistry, vol. 2. Munksgaard: Blackwell Publication; 2008. pp. 1090–2.

Boronat A, Carrillo C, Penarrocha M, et al. Dental implants placed simultaneously with bone grafts in horizontal defects: a clinical retrospective study with 37 patients. Int J Oral Maxillofac Impl 2010;25(1):189–96.

Hermann JS, Buser D. Guided bone regeneration for dental implants. Curr Opin Periodontol 1996;3:168–77.

Kahnberg K-E. Grafting procedures. In: Kahnberg K-E, Rasmusson L, Zellin G, editors. Bone grafting techniques for maxillary implants. Munksgaard: Blackwell Publishing Co.; 2005. pp. 14–23.

Nemcovsky CE, Artzi Z, Moses O, et al. Healing of dehiscence defects at delayed-immediate implant sites primarily closed by a rotated palatal flap following extraction. Int J Oral Maxillofac Impl 2000a;15:550–8.

Yeh HC, Hsu KW. Guided bone regeneration for fenestration defects in dental implants. Chang Gung Med J 2003;26(9):684–9.

Becker W, Becker BE. Guided tissue regeneration for implants placed into extraction sockets and for implant dehiscence: surgical techniques and case reports. Int J Periodont Restor Dent 1990;10:376–91.

Dahlin C, Linde A, Gottlow J, et al. Healing of bone defects by guided tissue regeneration. Plast Reconst Surg 1988;81:672–6.

Nemcovsky CE, Moses O, Artzi Z, et al. Clinical coverage of dehiscence defects in immediate implant procedures: three surgical modalities to achieve primary soft tissue closure. Int J Oral Maxillofac Impl 2000b;15:843–52.

Schliephake H, Dard M, Planck H, et al. Guided bone regeneration around endosseous implants using a resorbable membrane vs a PTFE membrane. Clin Oral Impl Res 2000;11:230–41.

Becker W, Dahlin C, Becker BE, et al. The use of e-PTFE barrier membranes for bone promotion around titanium implants placed into extraction sockets: a prospective multicenter study. Int J Oral Maxillofac Impl 1994b;9:31–40.

Hürzeler MB, Quinõnes CR, Hutmacher D, et al. Guided bone regeneration around dental implants in the atrophic alveolar ridge using a bioresorbable barrier. Clin Oral Impl Res 1997;8:323–31.

Landsberg C, Grosskopf A, Weinreb M. Clinical and biological observations of demineralized freeze-dried bone allograft in augmentation procedures around dental implants. Int J Oral Maxillofac Impl 1994;9:586–92.

Canullo L, Trisi P, Simion M. Vertical ridge augmentation around implants using e-PTFE titanium-reinforced membrane and deproteinized bovine bone mineral (Bio-Oss): a case report. Int J Periodont Restor Dent 2006;26(4):355–61.

Block grafting for dental implants

15

Ajay Vikram Singh Jun Shimada

CHAPTER CONTENTS HD

Introduction

'Block grafting is a procedure where a block of autogenous or allogenous bone is secured at the bone defect area to regenerate new bone at the host site'.

Reconstruction of alveolar ridge defects or deficiencies requires bone grafting before or at the time of implant placement. Various types of osseous defects occur due to various reasons such as prolonged edentulism, trauma, congenital anomalies, periodontal disease, and infection, and they often require to be corrected by various types of hard and soft tissue reconstruction procedures. If a defect is small and contains favourable topography (defect with four or five bony walls), it can be possible to graft it using particulate graft before or at the time of implant insertion, but the presence of a defect with three or fewer bony walls, mandates grafting using bone block to regenerate the desired bone dimensions before implant placement.

The use of autogenous bone grafts for ridge augmentation is well documented and has shown a high success rate over many years. The autogenous bone block is still considered to be a gold standard for jaw reconstruction. Allogenic bone blocks of various sizes are also commercially available to be used for the patients who either do not have adequate bone to harvest or are not willing to undergo the bone harvesting procedure.

The use of iliac crest autogenous bone block with the osseointegrated implants was originally presented by Branemark and associates et al, and has been extensively used for maxillofacial reconstruction procedures. The iliac crest graft is usually used for the reconstruction of large maxillofacial defects and often used for the full arch ridge reconstruction in implantology. To harvest iliac graft, the patient needs to be hospitalized, as this procedure is performed under general anaesthesia. Besides, it gives discomfort to the patient for months and costs are high compared to the mandibular block.

Misch and associates et al. first described the use of intraoral sites such as mandibular symphysis and ramus to harvest bone blocks, which can be used to reconstruct small to medium size ridge defects for implant placement. The intraoral donor sites offer several advantages over the extraoral sites, including less discomfort, close proximity of donor and recipient sites, less cost, no hospitalization, capability to be performed under local anaesthesia, ease of surgical access, and decreased donor site morbidity.

Indications

1. Bone defects with less than five bony walls.
2. Vertical bone augmentation is required using onlay graft.
3. Defect outside the alveolar housing preventing ideal implant placement.
4. Defects involving the buccal crest in aesthetic area.
5. A long-lasting scaffold for soft tissue support in the aesthetic region is required.

Contraindications

1. Inability to fix the block graft.
2. Compromised surrounding bone.

3. Inadequate donor site availability.
4. Inadequate soft tissue envelopes.
5. Patient is not fit for the procedure.

Advantages

1. Small to large defects can be grafted with quite predictable results.
2. More predictable qualitative and quantitative new bone regeneration outcomes than with the particulated graft alone.
3. Cost effective, as the autogenous block can be harvested from the patient's own body and also the use of membrane can be avoided when using cortical or corticocancellous block, because the cortical bone serves the purpose of barrier membrane and prevents soft tissue invasion into the graft area.
4. Horizontal as well as vertical bone augmentation can be done using block graft.

Disadvantages

1. Time consuming and more invasive procedure.
2. Technique-sensitive procedure.
3. Requires another surgical site to harvest bone blocks.
4. Donor site morbidity.
5. Multiple surgical steps.
6. Simultaneous implant insertion is not possible – takes a long time to complete the treatment.

Types of block grafts

1. Based on structural form

a. Cortical
b. Cancellous
c. Corticocancellous

2. Based on source

a. Autogenous block graft (autograft)
b. Allogenic block graft (allograft).

Autogenous block grafts

Autogenous block grafts are harvested from the patient's own body and immediately transported to the host site.

Donor sites

Extraoral sites

Branemark et al. originally presented the use of the iliac crest autologous bone blocks to regenerate new bone for dental implant placement. A few other extraoral sites like the iliac crest, tibia, ribs, and calvarium have also been used to harvest the large amounts of autogenous bone required for grafting intraoral bone defects and deficiencies. However, most of these procedures need to be performed under general anaesthesia and are not very comfortable for the patient; thus the use of bone blocks has been avoided to graft the small intraoral defects.

Intraoral sites

To make the block grafting procedure easy and comfortable for the patient, Misch et al. presented the use of mandibular symphysis and ramus block bone grafts for use in dental implants in 1992. As this intraoral bone harvesting can easily be performed under local anaesthesia and needs no hospitalization of the patient, it is being performed by many implant surgeons to graft small intraoral bone defects.

Block allografts

The block allografts are harvested from cadavers, processed in the bone banks and made available to be used for intraoral bone grafting. These blocks are available in different sizes and forms like cortical, corticocancellous, and cancellous blocks and are very useful in the cases where there is no availability of intraoral bone at any site that can be harvested, or where the surgeon is not skilled in harvesting autogenous bone blocks.

Advantages of using block allografts

1. Saves operating time by eliminating the need for a secondary surgical procedure to obtain an autogenous graft.
2. Functions as a natural biological scaffold, allowing for complete incorporation over time.
3. Remodels with the patient's own bone.
4. Processed and terminally sterilized by Tutoplast process.
5. Three to five years of shelf life/room temperature storage.

Armamentarium required for block grafting

Various types of armamentaria are used to perform the block grafting procedure. Depending on various factors like ease of use, cost and availability of the armamentarium, and the specific approach required in a particular case, etc. surgeons have multiple choices of armamentaria such as bone saws, carbide burs, Piezotome, and bone discs to harvest autogenous bone blocks. Various types of carbide burs and bone saws have been conventionally used to harvest autogenous blocks (Fig 15.1A–C), and still continue to be the first choice of many surgeons. Use of bone saws and carbide burs need a skilled approach to avoid any inadvertent soft tissue injury. The use of new generation armamentaria, such as Frios microsaw (Fig 15.2) and piezosurgery unit (Fig 15.3A and B), offer several advantages over the burs and oscillating saws, like more controlled and precise bone cutting and the least possibility of soft tissue injuries. The only disadvantage with these new generation block harvesting systems is the increased cost to the patient. The other armamentaria like block holding forceps (Fig 15.4) and block fixing kit (Fig 15.5) are required to modify and immobilize the block at the host site. The bone block fixation system contains various drills, mini screws and screwdrivers. Usually 1.5 or 2.0 mm diameter screws are used, which can be 6–18 mm long (Figs 15.1–15.5).

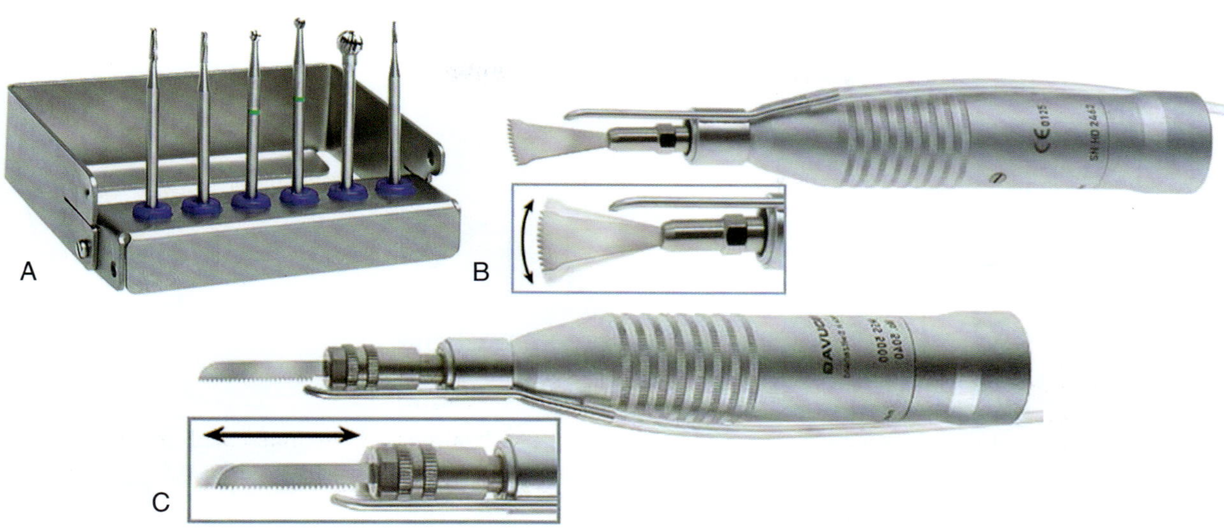

Fig 15.1 (A) Pikos block grafting bur kit. (B) Oscillating saw for bone harvesting. (C) Reciprocating saw for bone harvesting. *(Courtesy: Salvin Dental Specialties, USA).*

Step by step surgical technique

Step 1: A mucoperiosteal flap is elevated to expose the host site.

Step 2: A small round or straight fissure carbide bur is used to create inlay preparation and to make the small perforations through the cortex at the host site. This enhances the blood supply to the bone block from the underlying spongiosa of the host site.

Step 3: The mucoperiosteal flap is elevated to expose the donor site and a bone block of the desired shape, but 1–1.5 mm smaller in size than the prepared recipient site, is harvested.

Step 4: Block graft should be stored in blood, saline, or nonactivated platelet-rich plasma.

Step 5: A small amount of additional autogenous bone can also be scraped out from the donor site and stored in blood, saline, or nonactivated platelet-rich plasma.

Step 6: The block graft is tried over the prepared recipient site for its intimate adaptation. The further preparation of the recipient site, if required, is preferred over the shaping of the block graft.

Step 7: Two to three holes are prepared through the block graft for the fixation screws, using a straight carbide bur.

Step 8: The block graft is transported to the recipient site, adapted at the desired three-dimensional positions (preferably the cancellous face of the block towards the host bone), and the holes in the block are extended into the host site to the desired depth, using the same straight fissure bur. At the time of extending the holes through the block, the block is held at the position using the block-holding forceps. Further, the block is immobilized at the recipient site using two to three fixation screws.

Step 9: The particulated autogenous bone that has been harvested from the donor site, is mixed with synthetic or xenograft (Bio-Oss) and delivered at the host site to fill the deficiencies around the bone block.

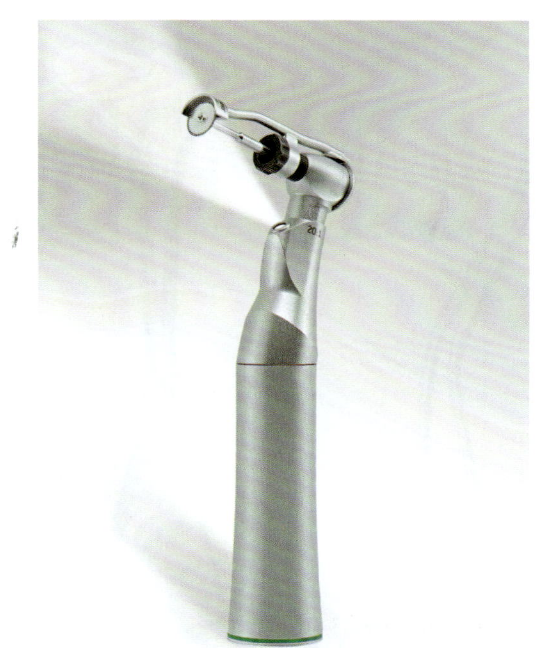

Fig 15.2 Frios Microsaw (Dentsply Friadent) is a very useful tool for intraoral corticocancellous block harvesting. Its 0.25 mm diamond disc allows precise preparation of donor sites. Its tissue guard controls depth of osteotomy and protects the soft tissue from injury. Its conservative axis minimizes surgical trauma. The horizontal cuts made using contra-angle and vertical curves are made using a straight handpiece.

Step 10: A barrier membrane can be used to cover the whole grafted site. The surgeon can avoid the barrier membrane in selective cases, because the cortical part of

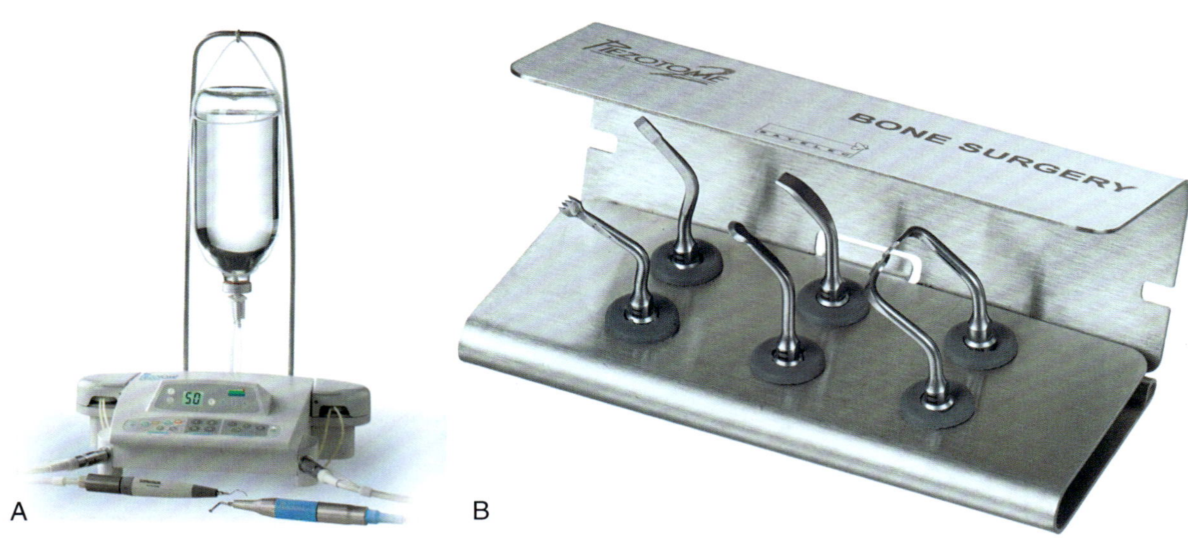

Fig 15.3 (A and B) Piezotome with bone surgery kit. Bone surgery kit comprising six ultrasonic tips (three saws and three scalpels) adapted to the different cases that arise in the intraoral environment, used for clinical treatments such as bone harvesting, osteoplasty, crest expansion, preparation of the implant site, accessing the lower alveolar nerve, etc. The use of the piezosurgery unit offers many advantages such as fast, fine, and selective cut (cuts only bone without any injury to the soft tissue), and fast healing. *(Courtesy: Setlec, France).*

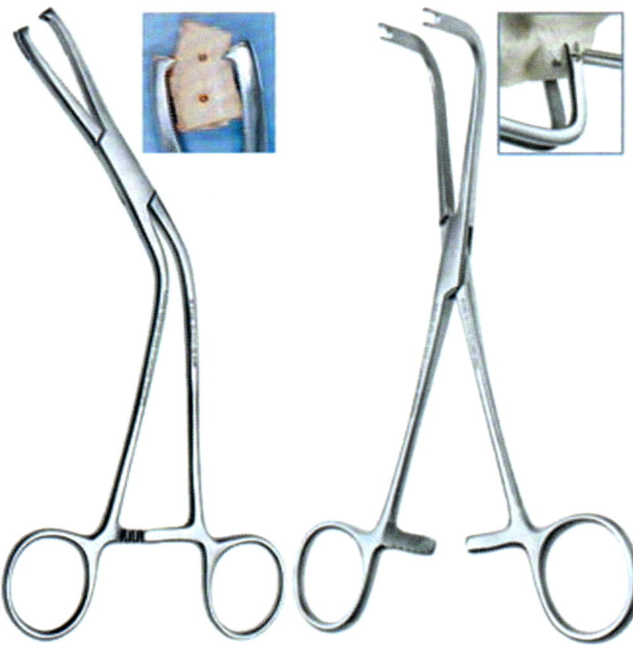

Fig 15.4 Anterior and posterior cortical block clamps with slotted tips. *(Courtesy: Salvin Dental Specialties, USA).*

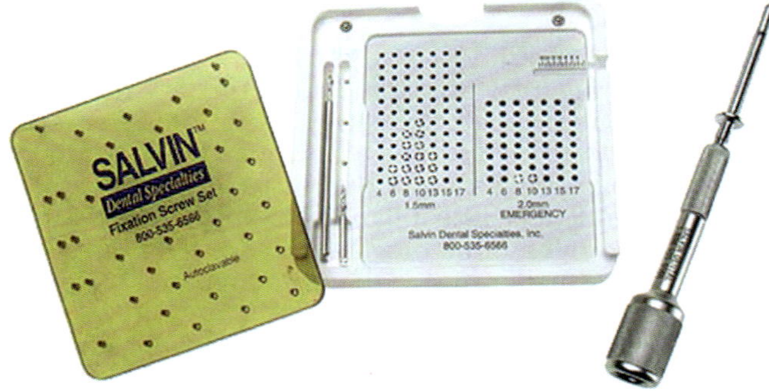

Fig 15.5 Bone blocks fixation system containing drills, mini screws and screwdriver. Usually 1.5 or 2.0 mm diameter screws are used, which can be 6–18 mm long. *(Courtesy: Salvin Dental Specialties, USA).*

the block graft itself prevents the soft tissue creeping into the grafted region. The barrier membrane should be used, if a large region around the block is grafted using particulate graft.

Step 11: Verify the passive flap closer over the grafted site and if required, the flap is released and coronally advanced to cover the grafted site for a watertight primary closure.

Step 12: The site is left to heal for 4–6 months without any functional loading over the grafted site (no softtissue-supported prosthesis should be used). The site is uncovered after the graft has united with the host bone, with the phases of resorption and apposition at the graft and host bone interfaces. This process may however take 4–6 months. The fixation screws are removed and implants are inserted in the consolidated new bone.

CASE REPORT-1

Step by step clinical presentation of block grafting using autogenous block from the mandibular ramus buccal shelf (Figs 15.6–15.22).

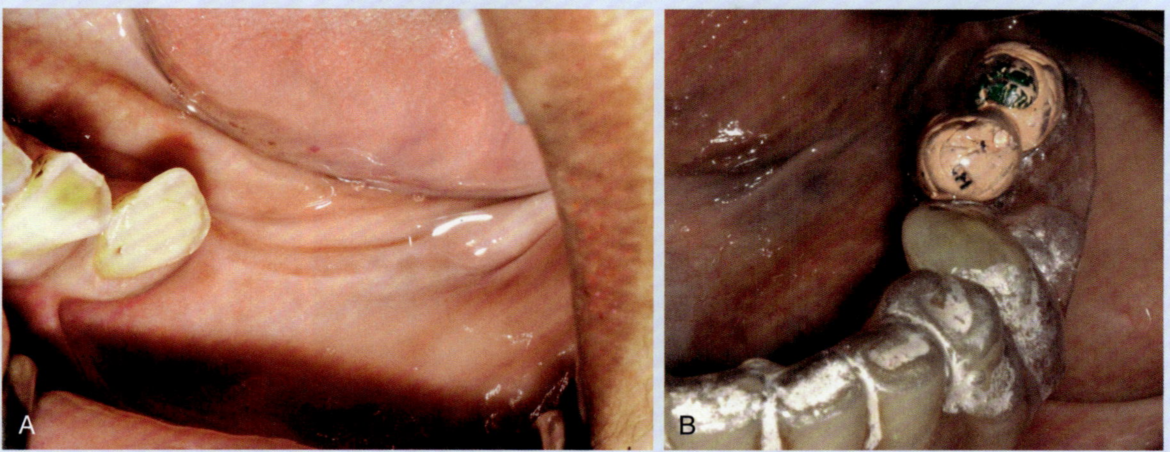

Fig 15.6 Clinical view of the edentulous ridge of missing molars. (A) Patient was seeking implant-supported fixed prosthesis. (B) A radiographic template is fabricated to plan the appropriate positions for implant placement at molar sites.

Continued

CASE REPORT-1—cont'd

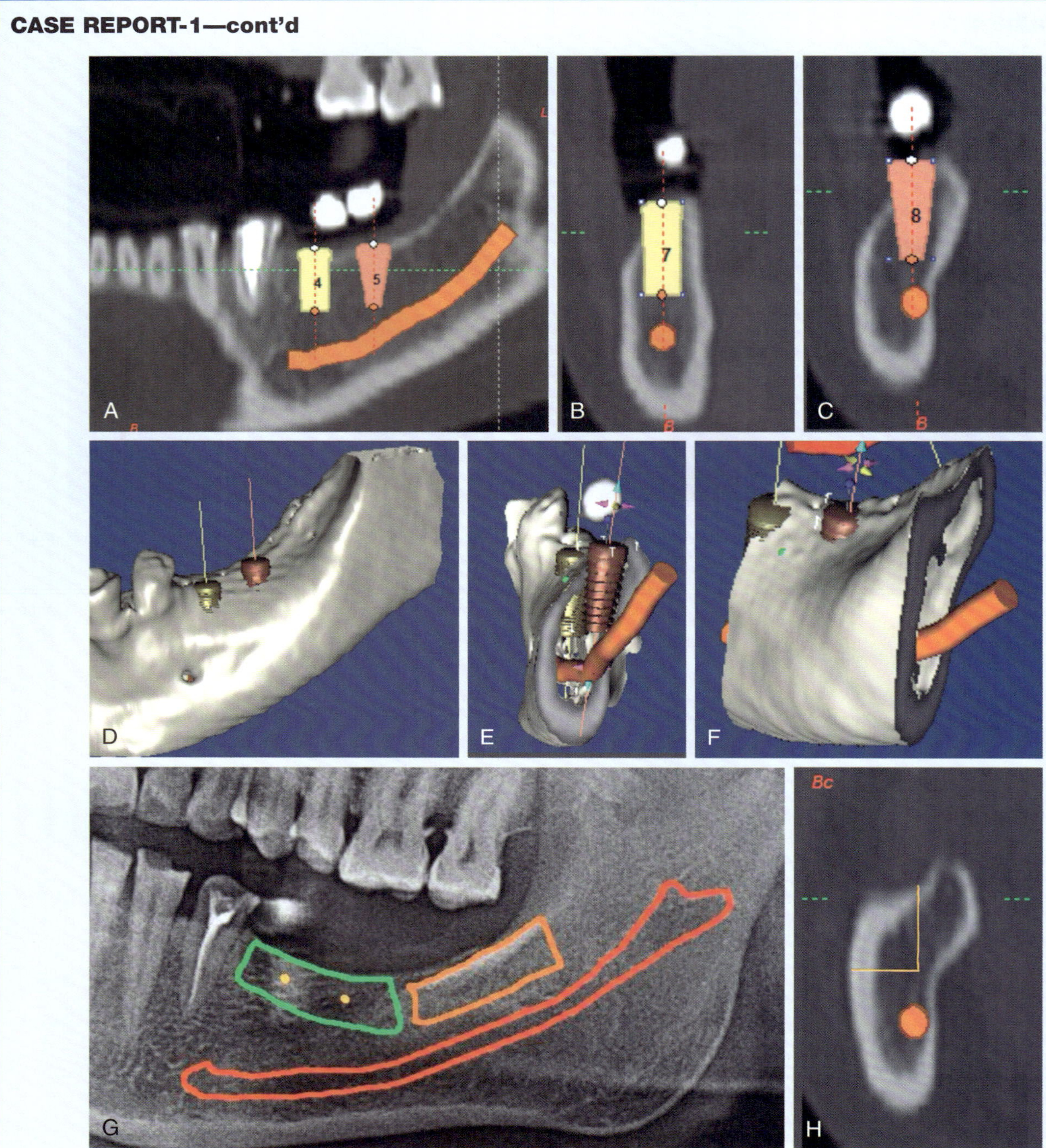

Fig 15.7 (A–F) When two regular diameter implants were planned to replace the teeth no. 46 and 47 using CT planning software, the various CT views showed the deficient buccolingual bone dimensions at the crestal part of the ridge. The block grafting was planned to reconstruct the lost bone dimensions. (G and H) The ramus buccal shelf area was chosen as the donor site.

CASE REPORT-1—cont'd

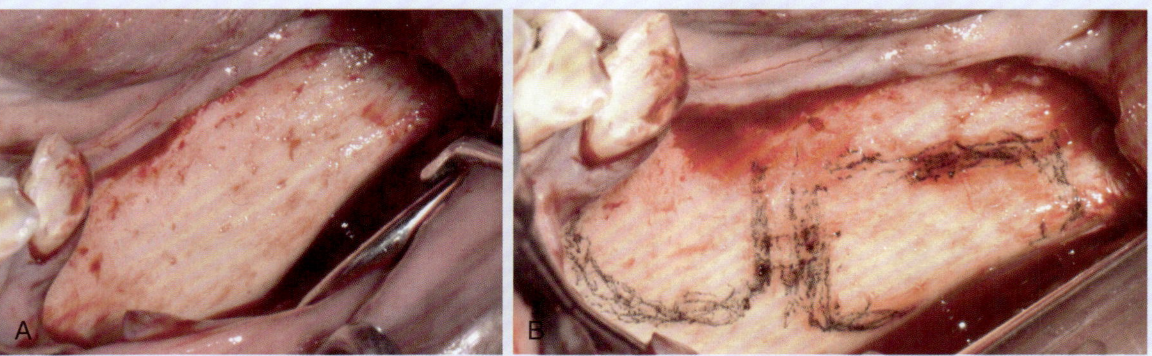

Fig 15.8 (A) A mid-crestal incision was given and the mucoperiosteal flap was elevated to expose the recipient as well as the donor sites. (B) The host and donor sites were separately marked using a sterile HB pencil.

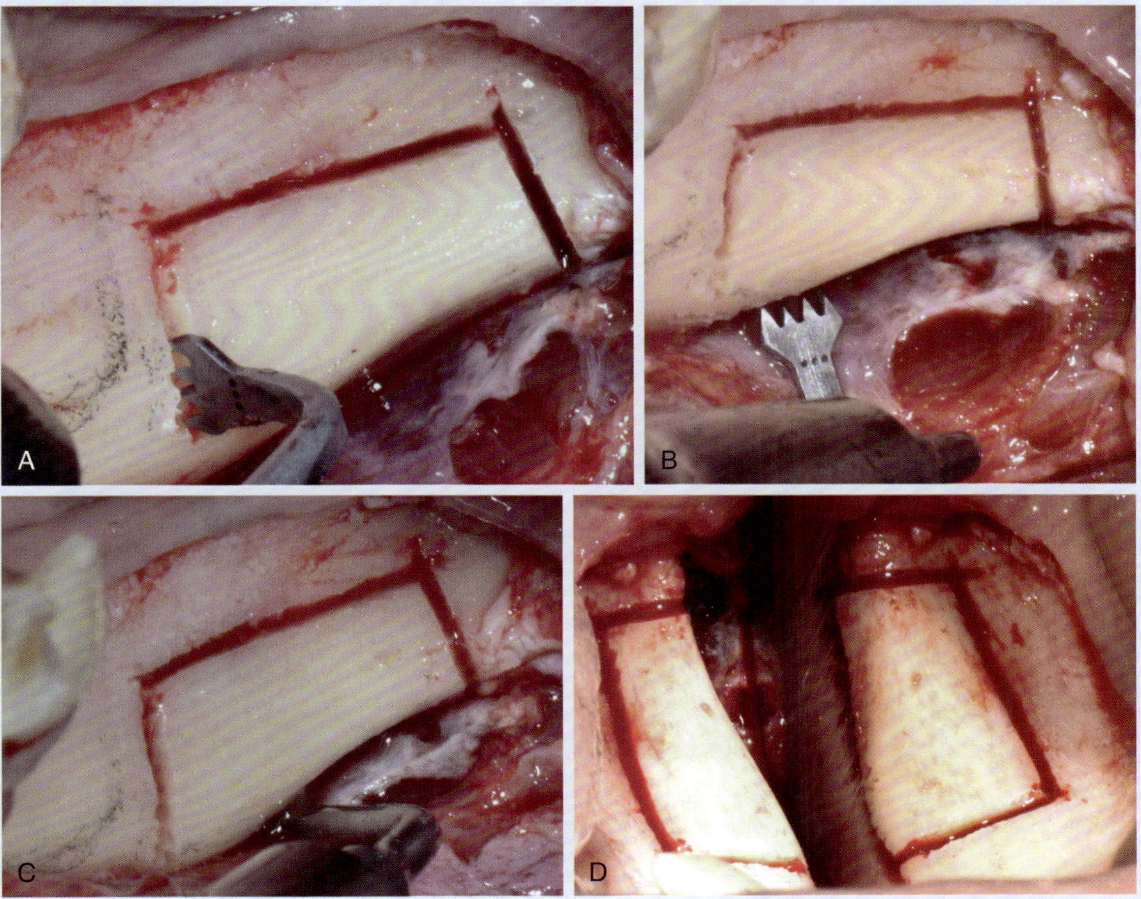

Fig 15.9 (A–D) The different types of Piezotome bone surgery saws were used to prepare a rectangular osteotomy at the ramus buccal shelf area under copious chilled saline irrigation. Care should be taken to avoid any injury to the inferior alveolar nerve. The osteotomy preparation should be done minimally to reach the underlying spongiosa. By completely bypassing the high density cortex all around, it is easy to separate the block from the site.

Continued

CASE REPORT-1—cont'd

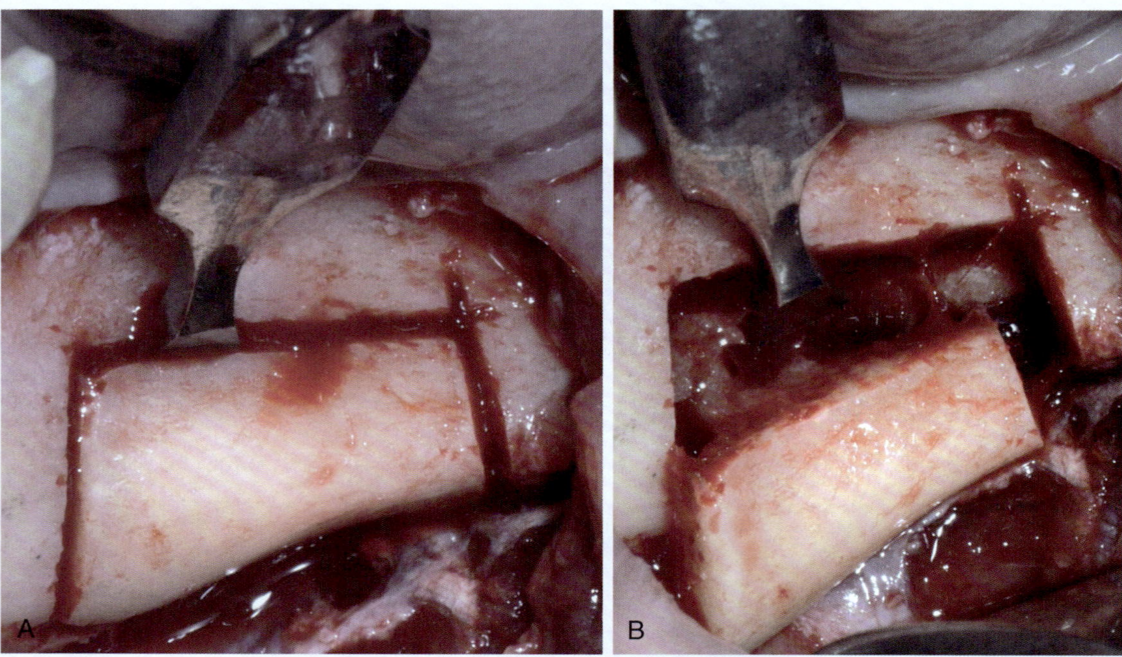

Fig 15.10 (A and B) Once the rectangular osteotomy is completed deep enough to reach the underlying cancellous bone, bone chisels or osseous splitters are used to laterally separate the bone block.

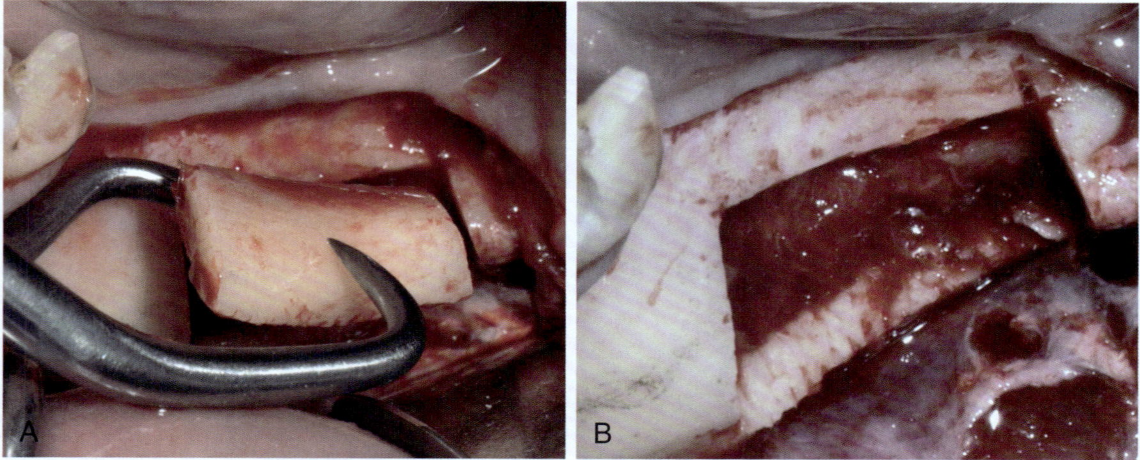

Fig 15.11 (A) Block-holding forceps can be used to hold the block. (B) Donor site as seen after the block removal. If the mandibular nerve comes out attached to the inner surface of the block, it should be carefully detached using any blunt instrument before removing the block from the site.

CASE REPORT-1—cont'd

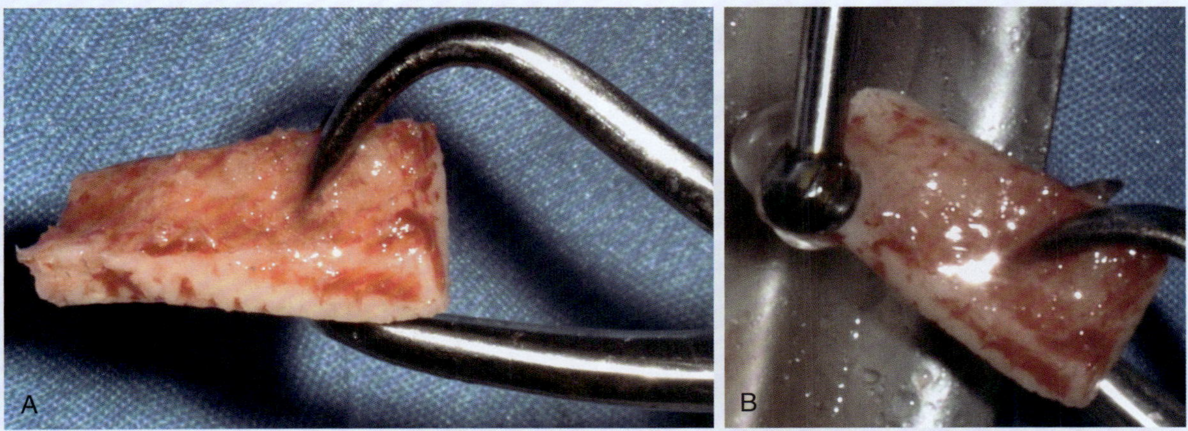

Fig 15.12 (A) The block harvested from the mandibular ramus buccal shelf mostly contains the cortical bone with very little or no cancellous bone. (B) As and if required, the block is shaped using a large round carbide bur to fit the host site. All the sharp edges of the block should be smoothened for easy and effective adaptation of the overlying soft tissue without any perforation or tearing.

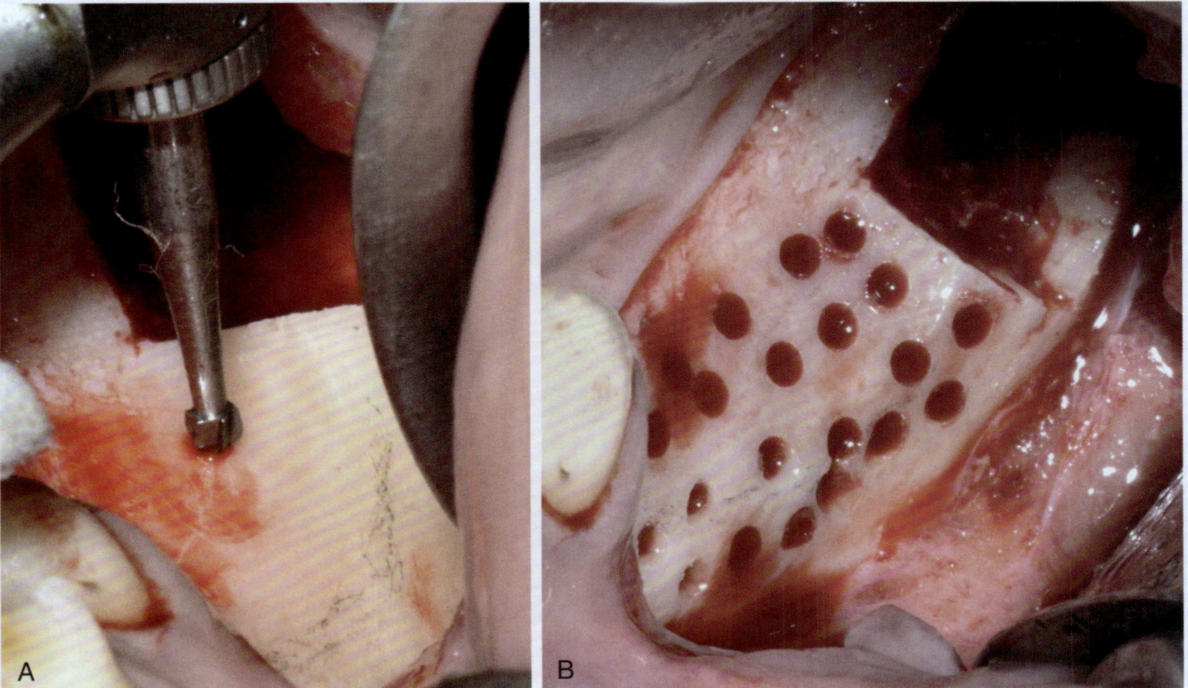

Fig 15.13 (A and B) A small round carbide bur is used to prepare multiple holes through the cortex at the host site to receive the nutrient blood supply from the host bone to nourish and keep alive the transplanted autogenous block graft cells.

Continued

CASE REPORT-1—cont'd

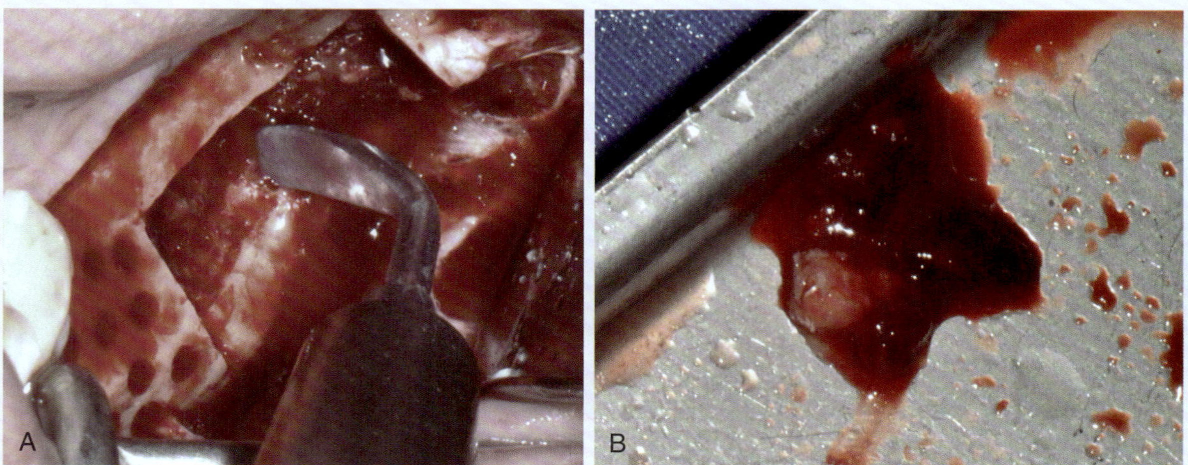

Fig 15.14 (A and B) A small amount of cancellous bone can be scraped out from the donor site using a piezotome bone scraper.

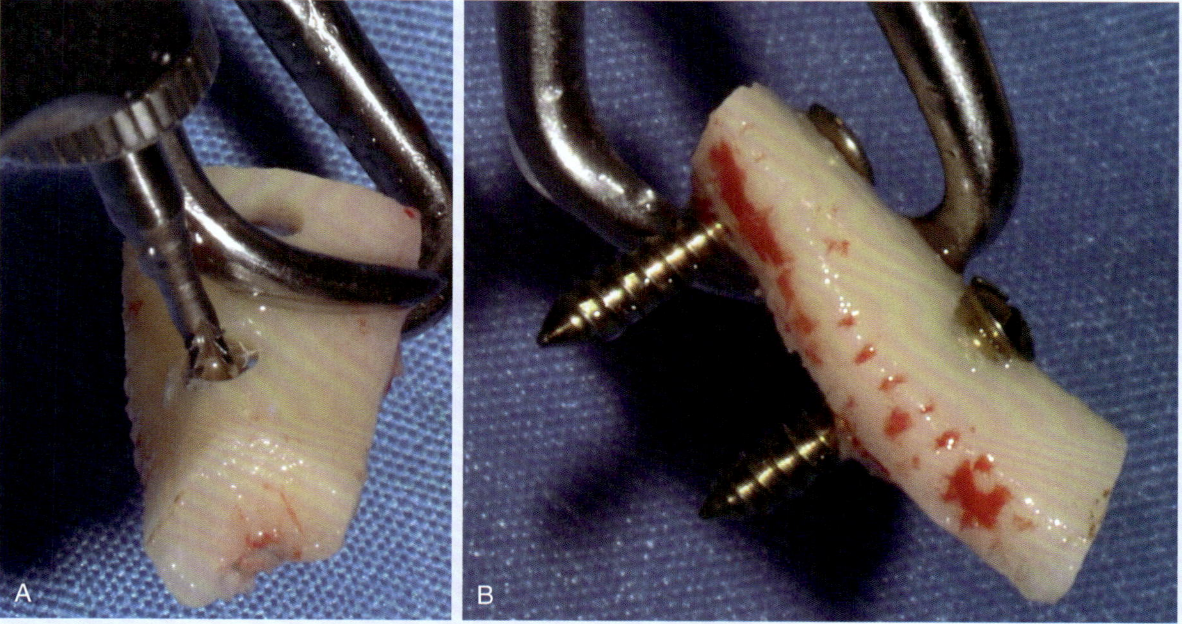

Fig 15.15 (A and B) Two holes are prepared through the block using a long carbide bur and two block fixation screws are inserted.

CASE REPORT-1—cont'd

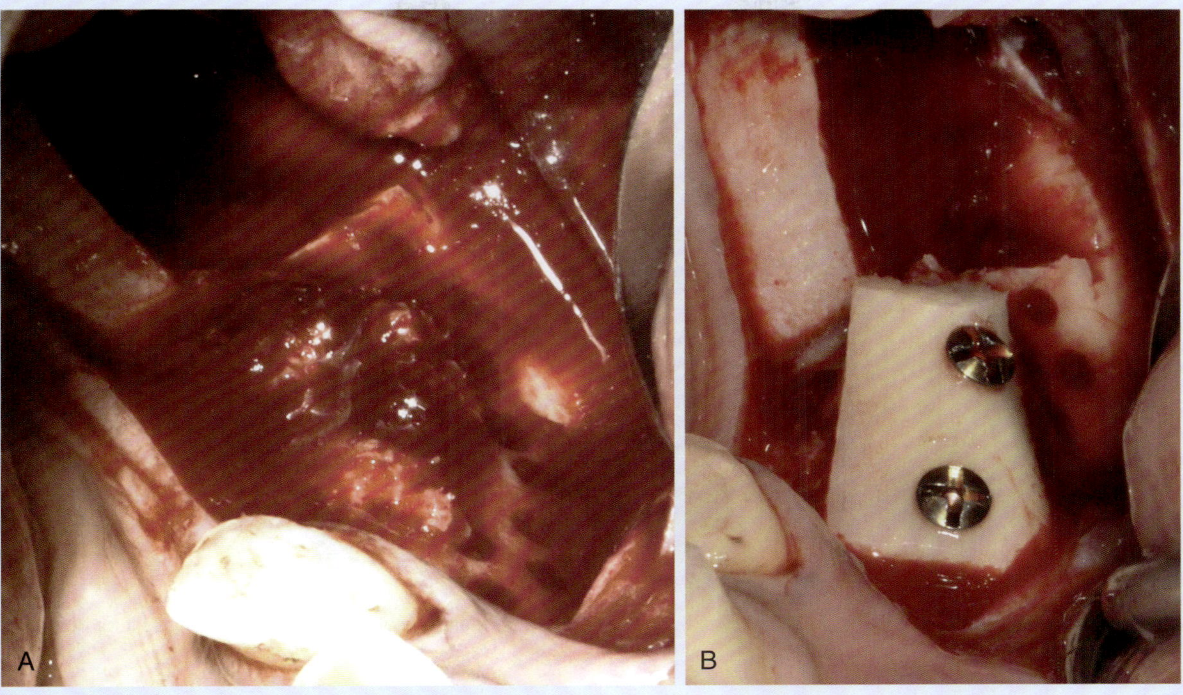

Fig 15.16 (A) The cancellous bone is delivered at the host site to fill the gaps between the inner surface of the block and the host bone. (B) Now the block is placed over the host site and firmly immobilized using fixation screws.

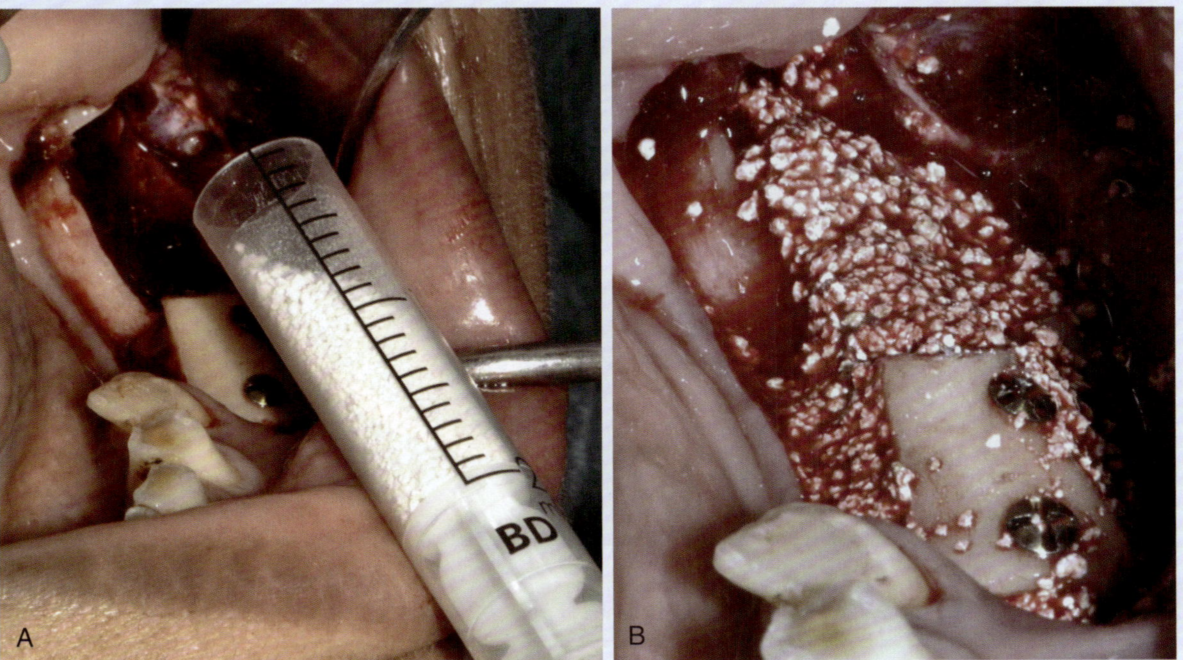

Fig 15.17 (A and B) The particulate graft (HA + β-TCP) is used to fill the spaces and deficiencies around the bone block as well as to fill the donor site.

Continued

CASE REPORT-1—cont'd

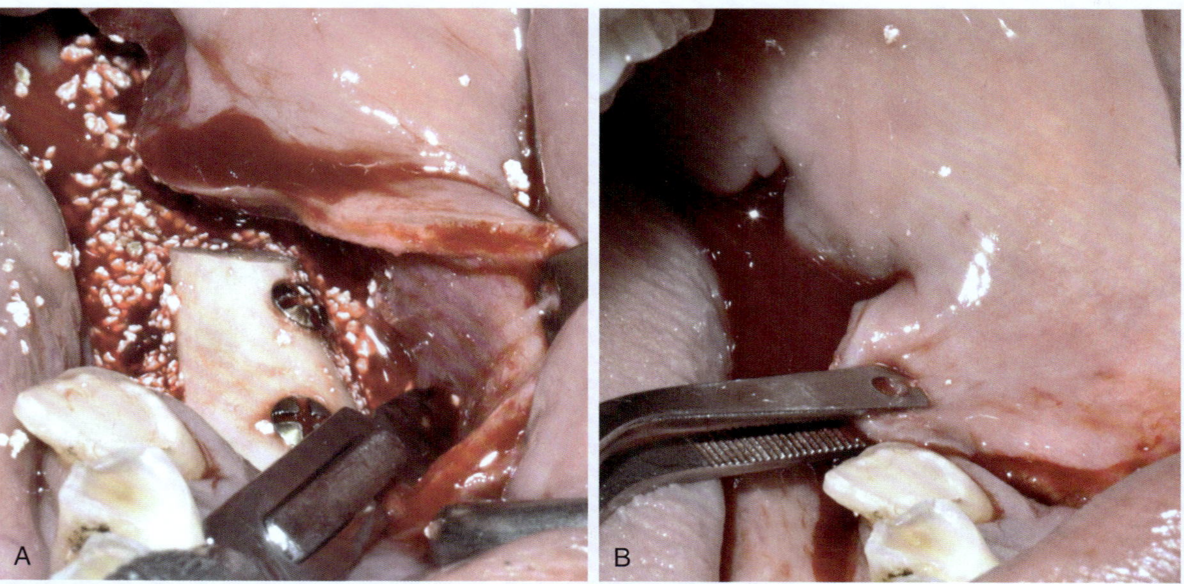

Fig 15.18 (A and B) Horizontal releasing incisions are given through the periosteum underneath the facial flap to release it for coronal advancement and to achieve tension-free primary closure.

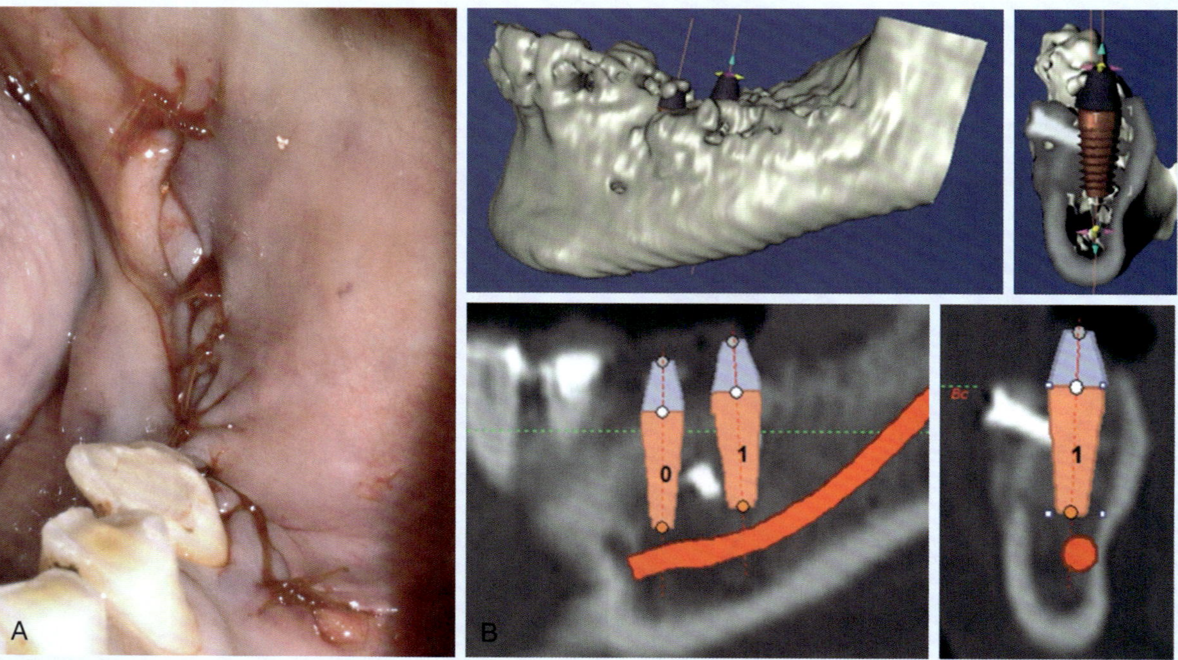

Fig 15.19 (A) The flap is sutured to achieve a watertight closure. (B) The dental CT 4 months after block grafting, showing newly regenerated bone dimensions, which are now adequate for regular to wider diameter implant placement.

CASE REPORT-1—cont'd

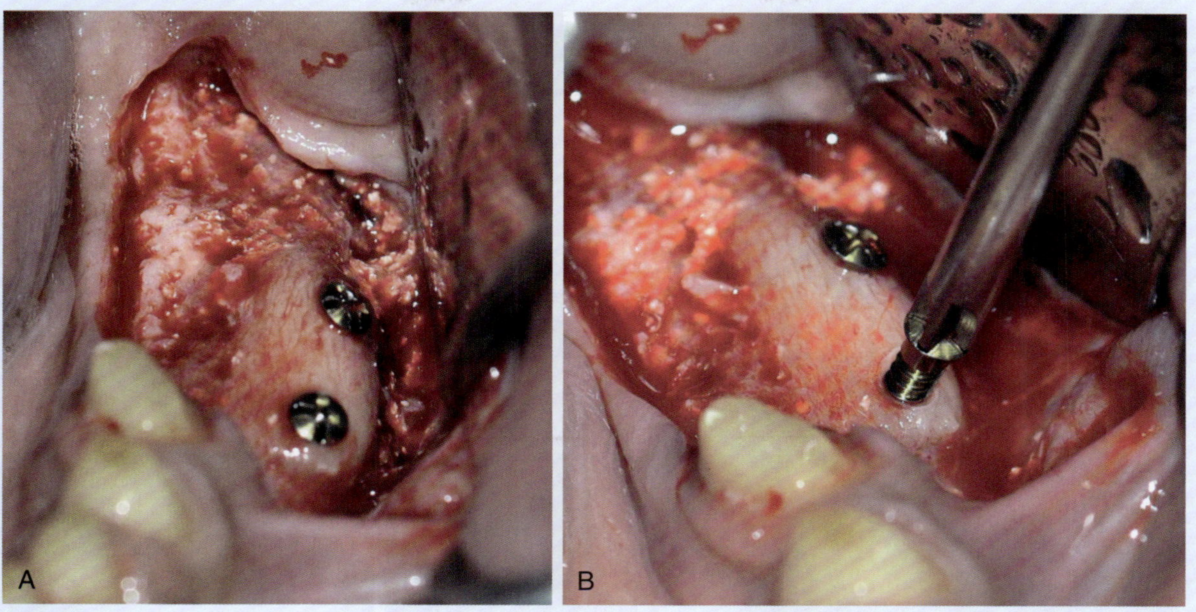

Fig 15.20 (A and B) The mucoperiosteal flap is elevated to expose the grafted site and the fixation screws are removed using screwdriver. The block as well as the particulate graft has been consolidated and the site is ready to receive the implants.

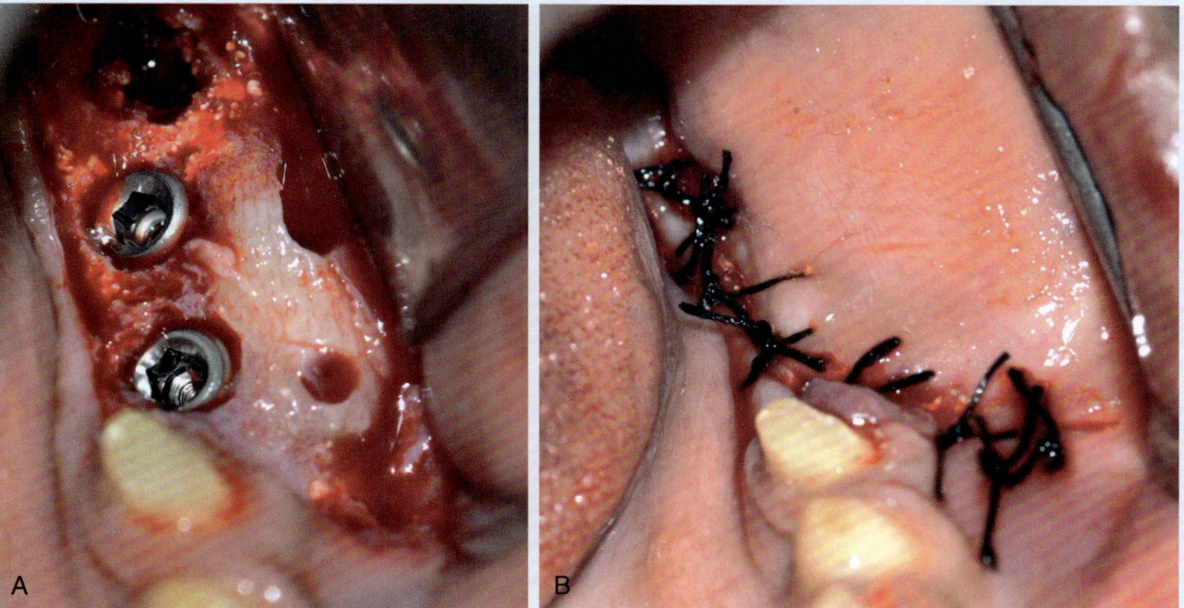

Fig 15.21 (A and B) Two wider diameter implants (5 x 10 and 6 x 10 mm) are inserted at the ideal prosthetic positions and flap is sutured back for submerged healing of the implants.

Continued

CASE REPORT-1—cont'd

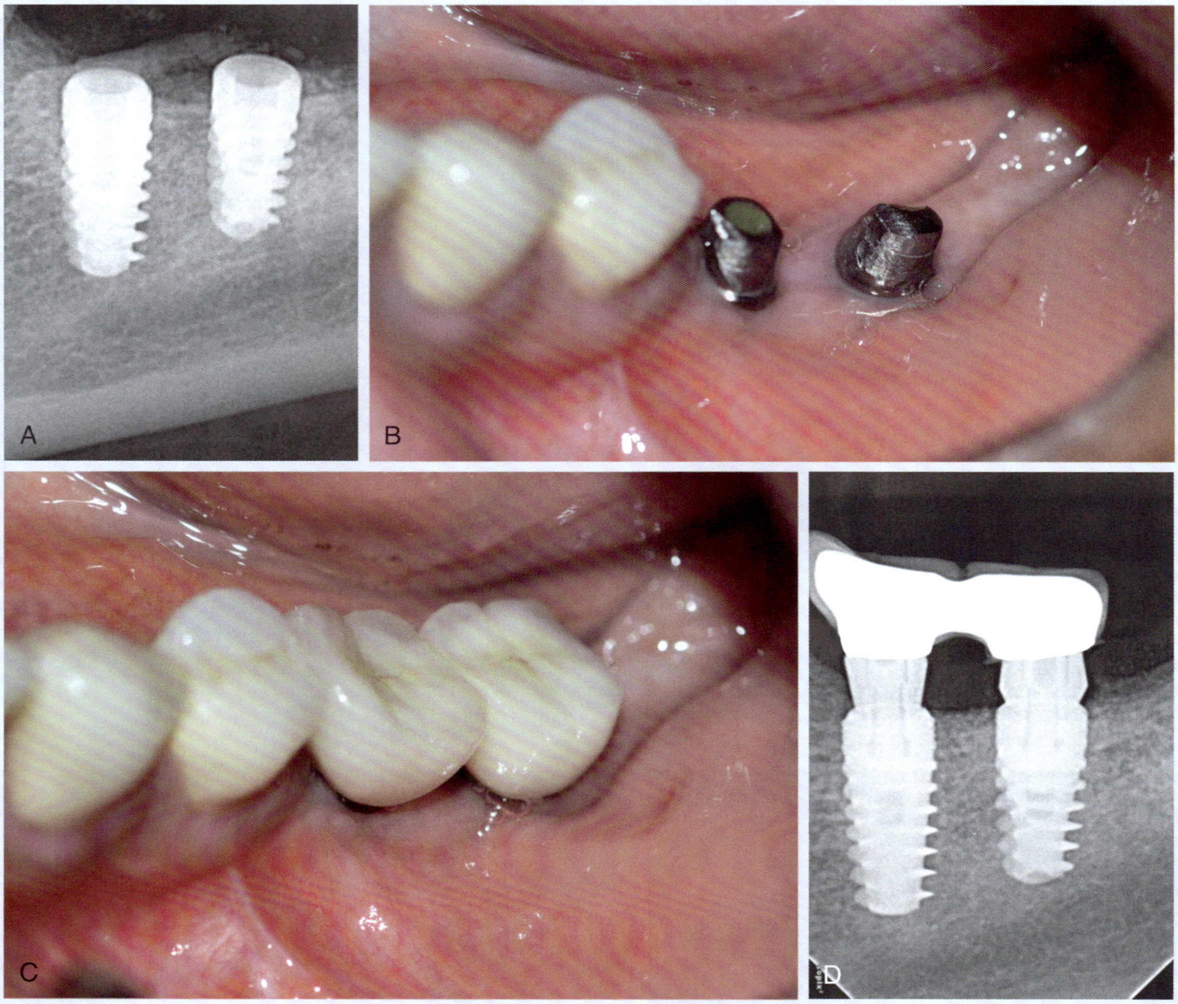

Fig 15.22 (A) Post-implantation radiograph. (B and C) Implants are uncovered after 3 months and restored using metal-free zirconium crowns along with the crowns over the worn out adjacent teeth. (D) The radiograph 1 year after loading shows stable bone around the implant.

'J' block grafting: For ridge defects with a thin ridge crest that widens apically especially in the aesthetic region, the 'J' shaped block graft can be the right choice, as it adapts well over such defects and regenerates the bone in the desired shape. The 'J' block can either be harvested from the mandibular symphysis of the patient, or an allogenic bone block of 'J' shape can be used for this purpose (Fig 15.23A and B).

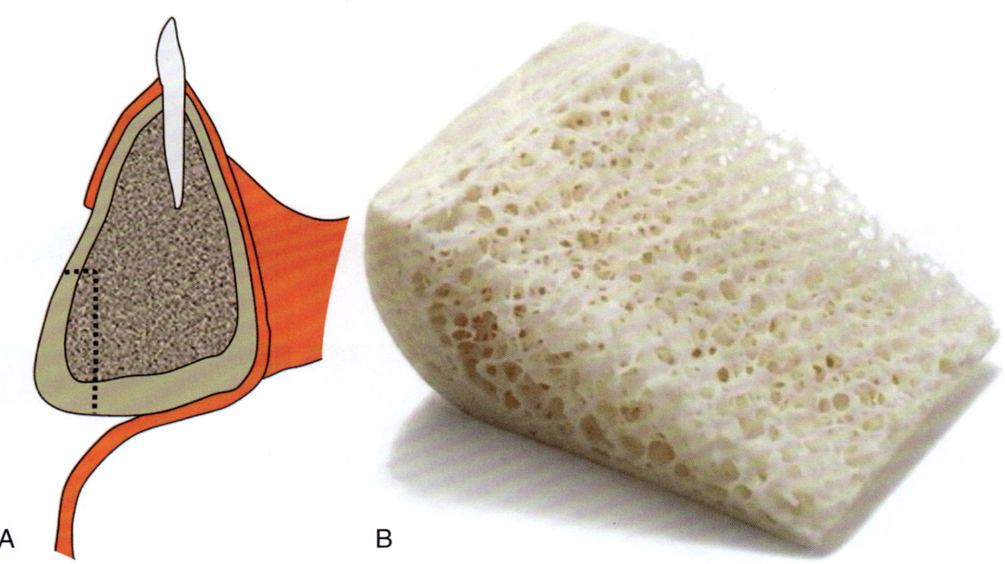

Fig 15.23 (A) A corticocancellous 'J' block can either be harvested from the mandibular symphysis of the patient or (B) a 'J' block allograft can be used to reconstruct the ridge with thin ridge crest that widens as it proceeds apically *(Courtesy: Zimmer Dental Inc.)*.

CASE REPORT-2

Reconstruction of premaxilla with large osseous defect using autogenous 'J' blocks harvested from the mandibular symphysis

A 28-year old male patient presented with a four-unit dental bridge, which had been placed 1 year previously to replace two maxillary central incisors. The patient complained of continued ridge loss under the bridge which had caused an unaesthetic appearance, phonetic problem, and also discomfort to the patient (Fig 15.24A). On giving the detailed history, the patient attributed the tooth loss to large endo-perio lesions developed after a trauma, which resulted in recurrent pain, swelling, draining abscess, periodontal bone loss, and teeth mobility. The dentist extracted two central incisors and replaced them with the dental bridge.

The dental CT images of the region showed the loss of almost all the bone structure with large amount of soft tissue growth into the ridge (Fig 15.24B–E). The situation was almost contradictory to any possibility of hard and soft tissue reconstruction for implant insertion. The patient's consent for the procedure was obtained, after his current situation and the possible outcomes of the reconstruction process were explained to him.

The case was planned for reconstruction using 'J' blocks harvested from the mandibular symphysis. The bridge was removed and a mid-crestal incision, which extended to two vertical incisions, was given. The facial mucoperiosteal flap was elevated by giving blunt dissections through the soft tissue, which had grown deep into the ridge. The mucoperiosteum on the palatal aspect of the defect was left intact to provide stability to the defects (Fig 15.25A). The fibrosseous tissue from the defects was removed using sharp tissue curettes.

The mucoperiosteal flap was elevated to expose the mandibular symphysis and two 'J' shaped corticocancellous bone blocks were harvested using a rotary carbide bur (Fig 15.25B and C). The blocks were stored in normal saline (Fig 15.25D) and the donor site was sutured after placing absorbable collagen sponge into the donor sites (Fig 15.25E and F). Now the prevention of soft tissue growth into the graft was one of the challenges, so the pieces of collagen barrier membrane were placed into the defects and pushed to the palatal side to prevent any soft tissue creeping into the graft from the palatal side (Fig 15.26A–C). The bone blocks were shaped and placed to exactly fit into the defects (Fig 15.26D and E). A titanium mesh was placed over the blocks and stabilized using small bone screws in the subnasal bone (Fig 15.26F). The freeze dried demineralized allograft (Grafton) was mixed with platelet-rich plasma (Fig 15.27A) and added over the blocks (Fig 15.27B). The entire grafted site was covered with the titanium mesh (Fig 15.27C) and flap was sutured back (Fig 15.27D). The CT images after 6 months showed the desired volume of new bone regeneration at the grafted site (Fig 15.27E–G). The site was exposed again after 8 months healing (Fig 15.27H), the titanium mesh was removed, implants were inserted (Fig 15.27I) and the flap was sutured back with primary closure (Fig 15.27J). The implants were uncovered after 4 months (Fig 15.27K) and restored using zirconium prosthesis (Fig 5.27L–N).

Continued

CASE REPORT-2—cont'd

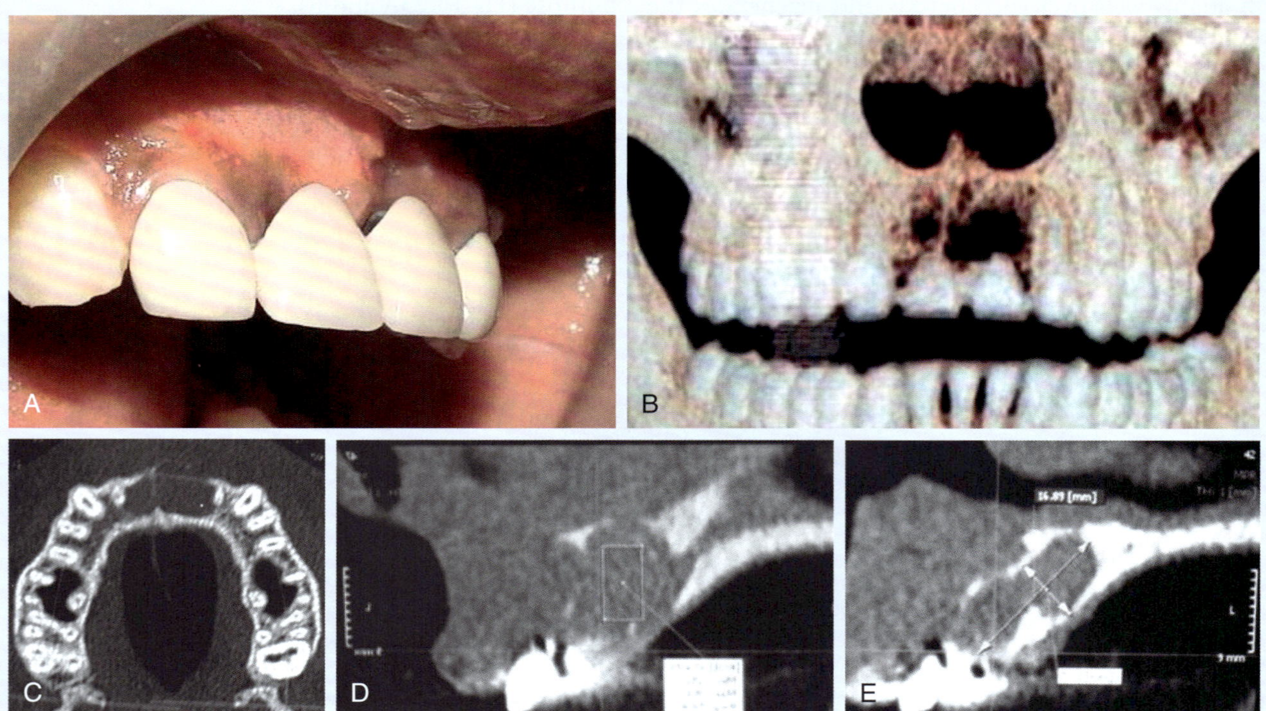

Fig 15.24 (A) Clinical view of the case with complaints of continuous ridge loss under the bridge, placed to replace teeth numbers 11 and 21. Patient gave a history of tooth loss because of large endo-perio lesions which resulted in recurrent pain, swelling, draining abscess, periodontal bone loss, and teeth mobility. (B–E) Dental CT images revealed severe bone loss in the region, which absolutely contradicted any possibility of implant placement.

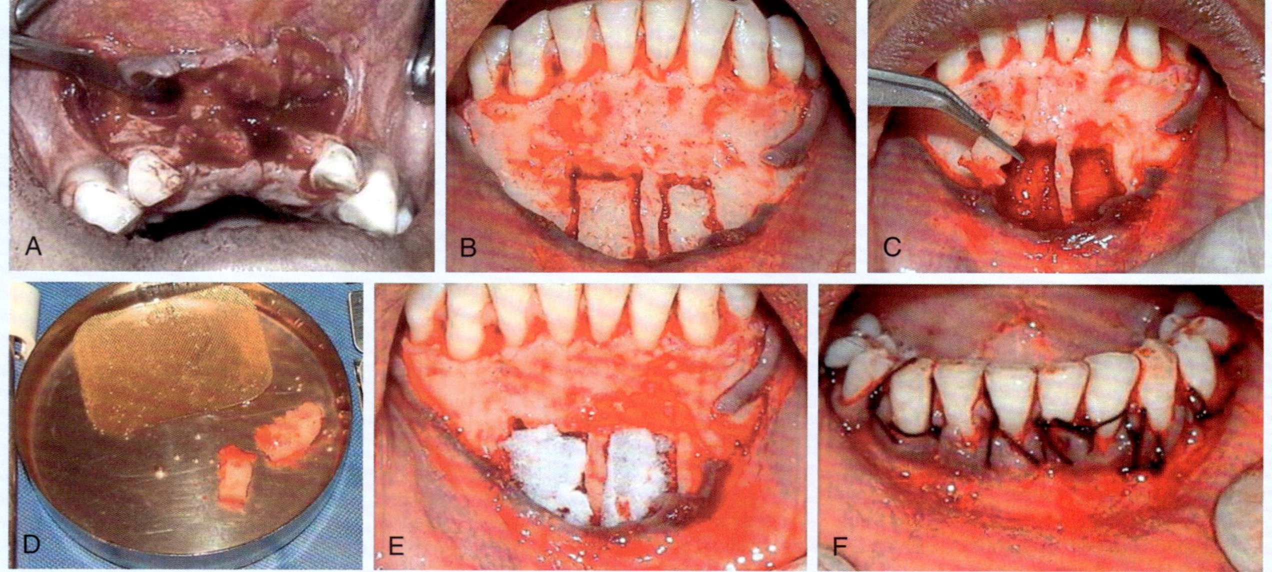

Fig 15.25 (A) The flap was elevated to expose the host site and all the soft tissue, which had grown into the defects, was curetted out. (B–D) Two bone blocks of the same sizes as the defect were harvested from the mandibular symphysis region and stored in normal saline. (E) Small pieces of absorbable collagen sponge were placed at the donor site and (F) the flap was sutured back.

CASE REPORT-2—cont'd

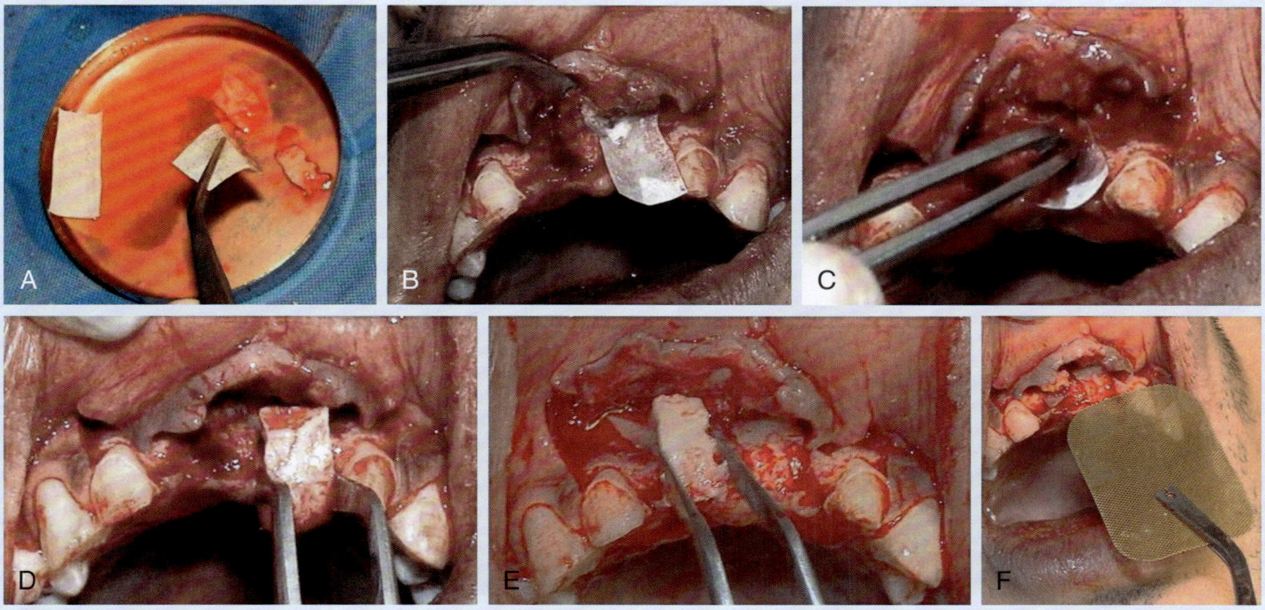

Fig 15.26 (A–C) Pieces of collagen barrier membrane were placed into the defects and pushed to the palatal side to prevent any soft tissue creeping into the graft from the palatal side. (D and E) The bone blocks were placed into the defects. (F) A titanium mesh was placed over the blocks and stabilized using small bone screws in the subnasal bone.

Continued

CASE REPORT-2—cont'd

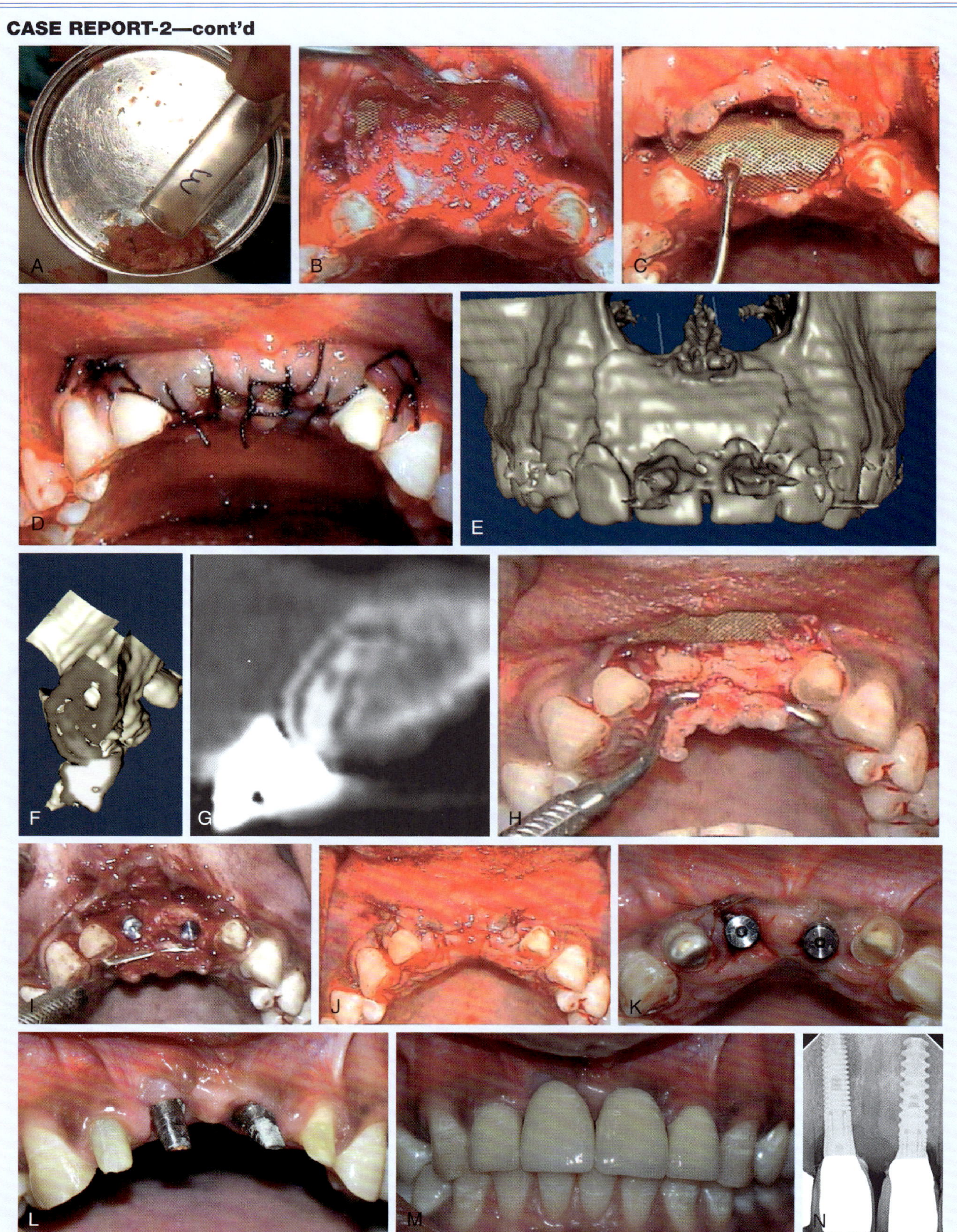

Fig 15.27 (A) The freeze-dried demineralized allograft (Grafton) was mixed with platelet-rich plasma and (B) added over the blocks. (C) The entire grafted site was covered with titanium mesh and (D) the flap sutured back. (E–G) The CT images after 6 months showed new bone regeneration at the grafted site. (H) The site was exposed again, titanium mesh was removed, and (I) implants were inserted. (J) The flap was sutured back with primary closure. (K) The implants were uncovered after 4 months and (L and M) restored. (N) The radiograph 1 year after loading showed stable bone around the implants.

CASE REPORT-3

Reconstruction of premaxilla with vertical bone augmentation using onlay block grafts, lateral bone augmentation using particulate graft, and grafting of the anterior third of the maxillary sinus (Figs 15.28–15.30).

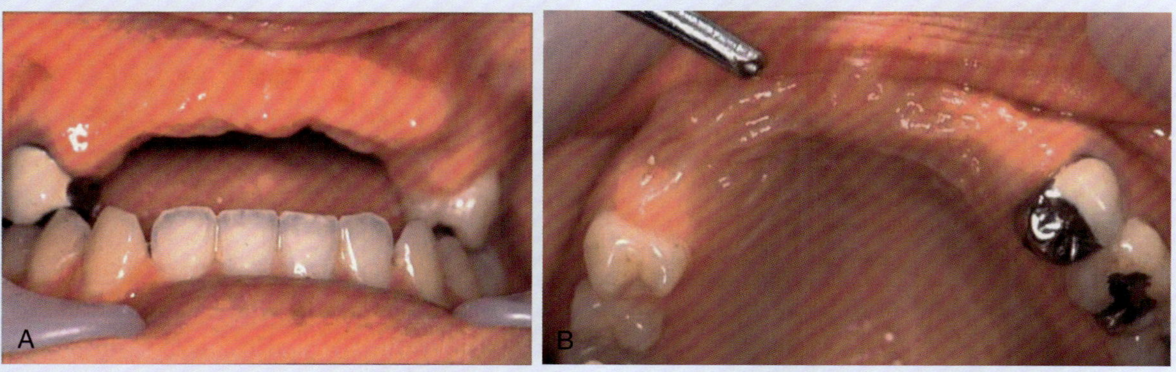

Fig 15.28 (A and B) Clinical view of maxillary anterior edentulous ridge showing vertical as well as horizontal ridge defect.

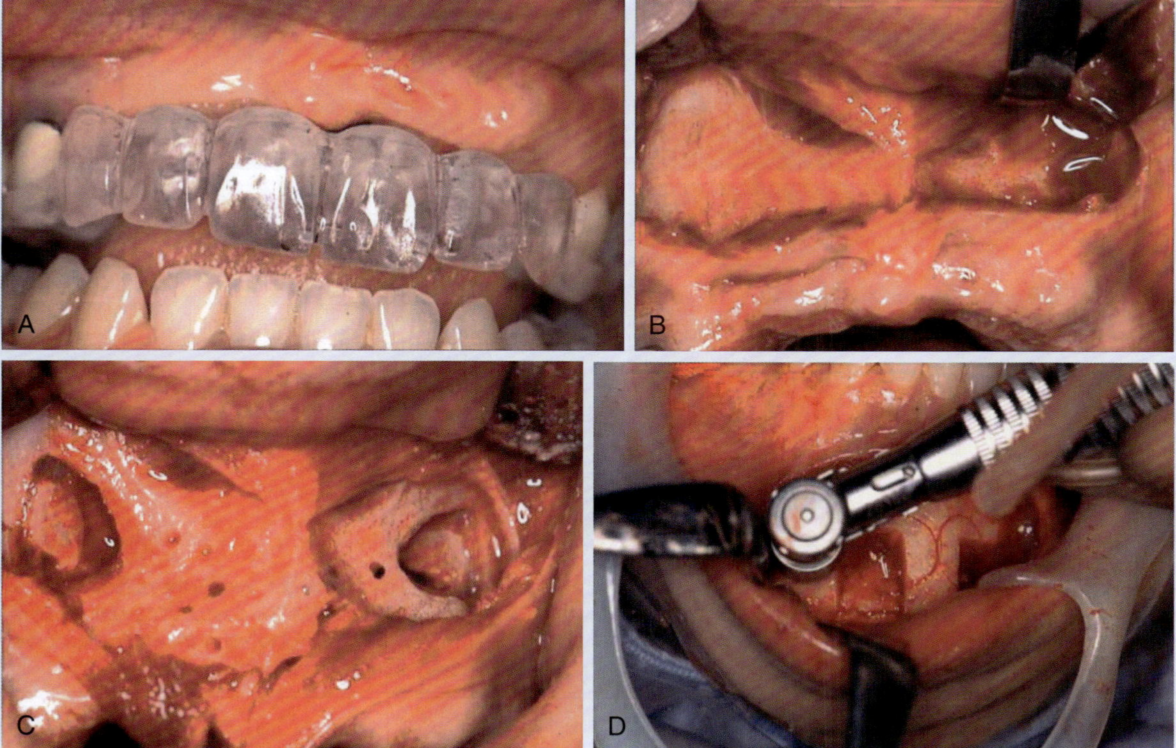

Fig 15.29 (A) A surgical guide was fabricated showing ideal teeth positions of the future prosthesis. (B) A vestibular incision was given to expose the labial cortex and ridge crest. The labial cortical plate was micro-perforated using small round carbide bur. (C) The lateral windows were prepared and sinus membrane elevated to graft the anterior one-third of the maxillary sinus cavity. (D) Two rectangular bone blocks were harvested from the mandibular symphysis.

Continued

CASE REPORT-3—cont'd

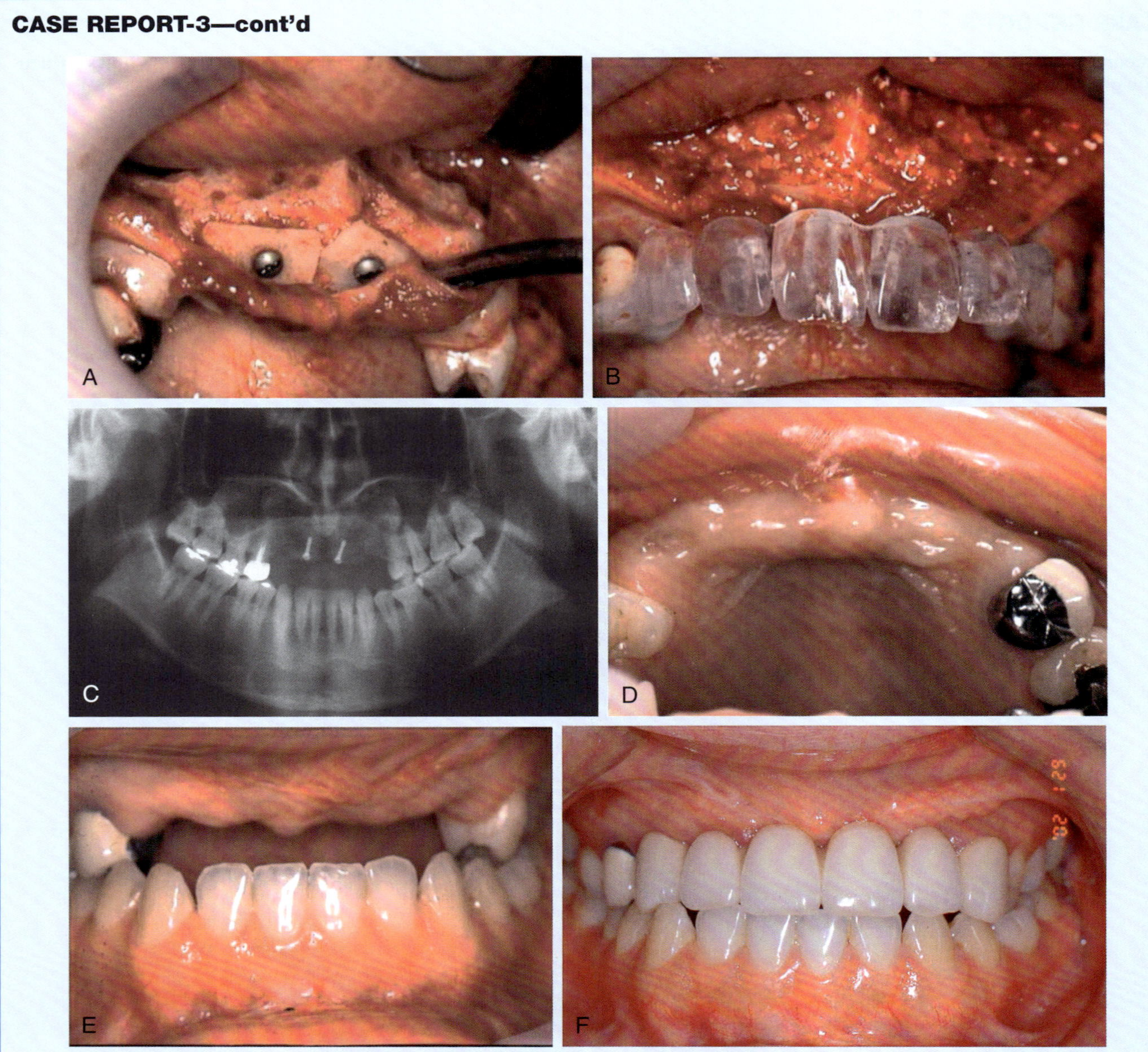

Fig 15.30 (A) The blocks were fixed onto the ridge crest to obtain vertical augmentation to the desired height, and (B) the particulated bone substitute was used to fill the elevated sinus cavities as well as to laterally augment the labial part of the ridge. (C) The post grafting panoramic radiograph showed the bone blocks, grafted anterior part of the sinuses, and donor site. (D and E) The healing after 4 months showed noticeable amount of vertical and horizontal new ridge dimensions. (F) The implant-supported prosthesis showed an acceptable aesthetic profile.

CASE REPORT-4

Reconstruction of maxillary defect using the autogenous cortical block harvested from the ascending ramus of mandible (Figs 15.31–15.39).

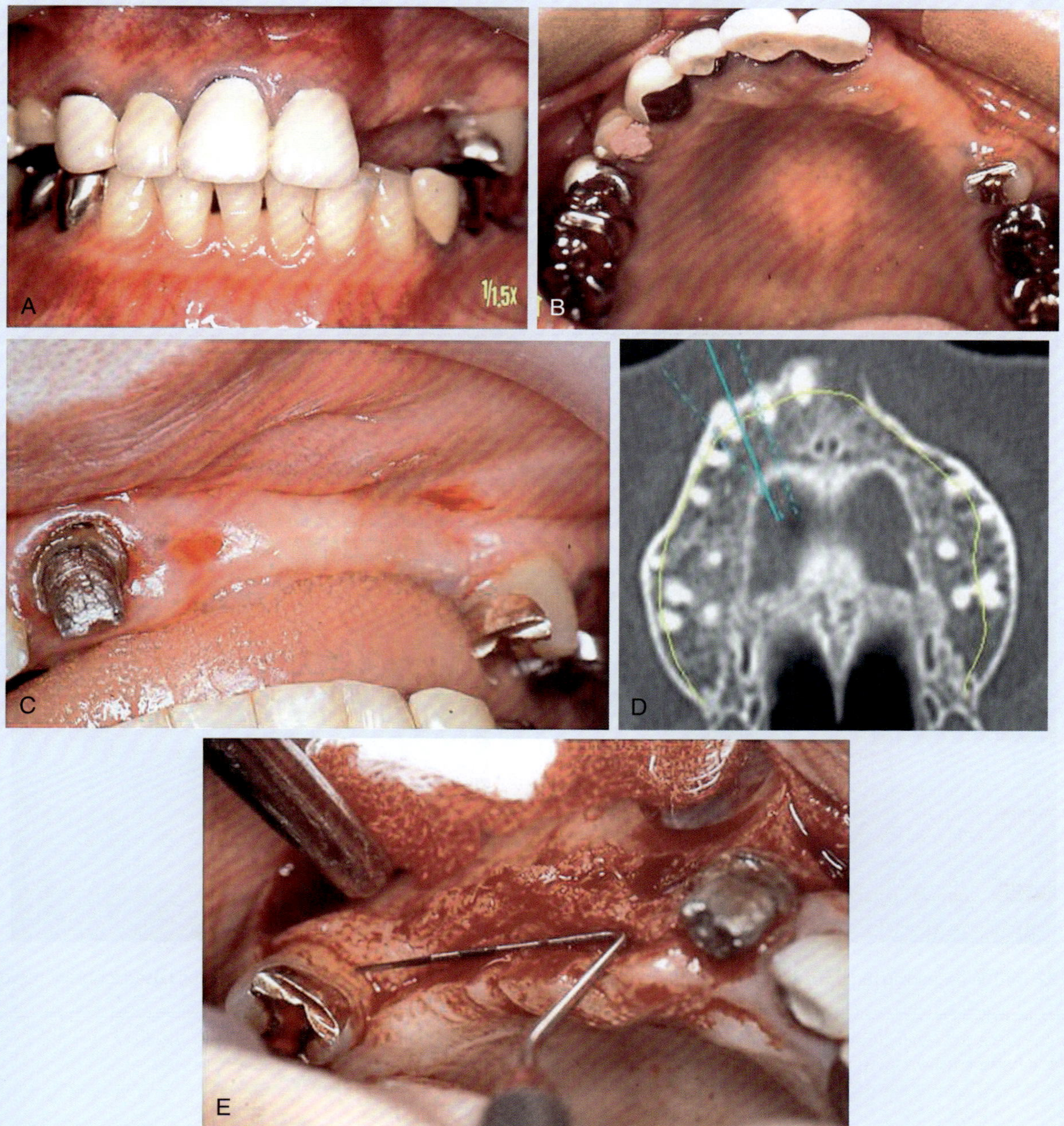

Fig 15.31 (A–C) Clinical view of edentulous region of maxilla showing the horizontal ridge defect. (D) The axial view of the dental CT showing a large ridge defect. (E) The mucoperiosteal flap was elevated to expose the ridge crest and buccal cortex.

Continued

CASE REPORT-4—cont'd

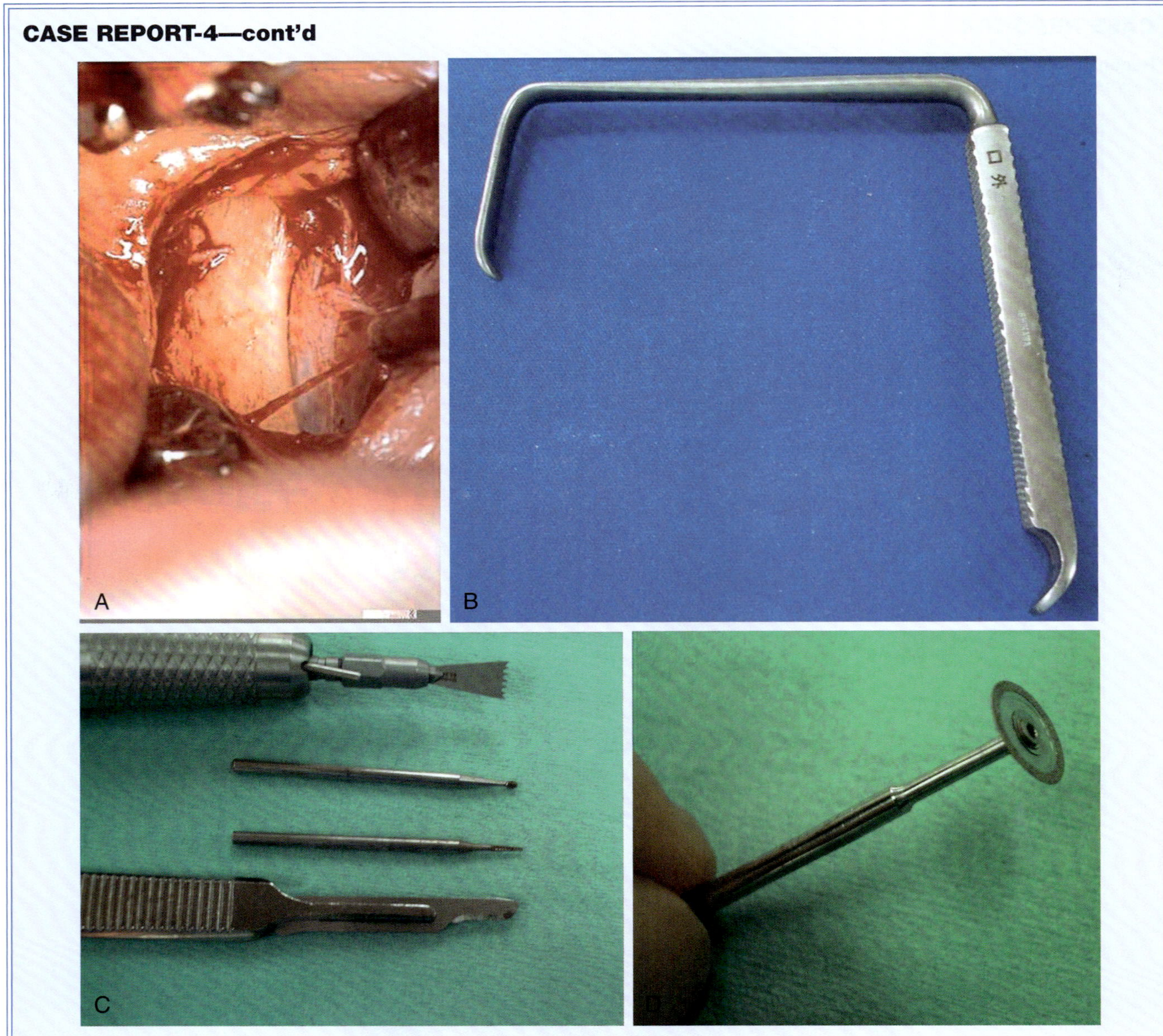

Fig 15.32 (A) The ascending ramus of the mandible was exposed to harvest the bone block. (B–D) The armamentaria used for block harvesting.

CASE REPORT-4—cont'd

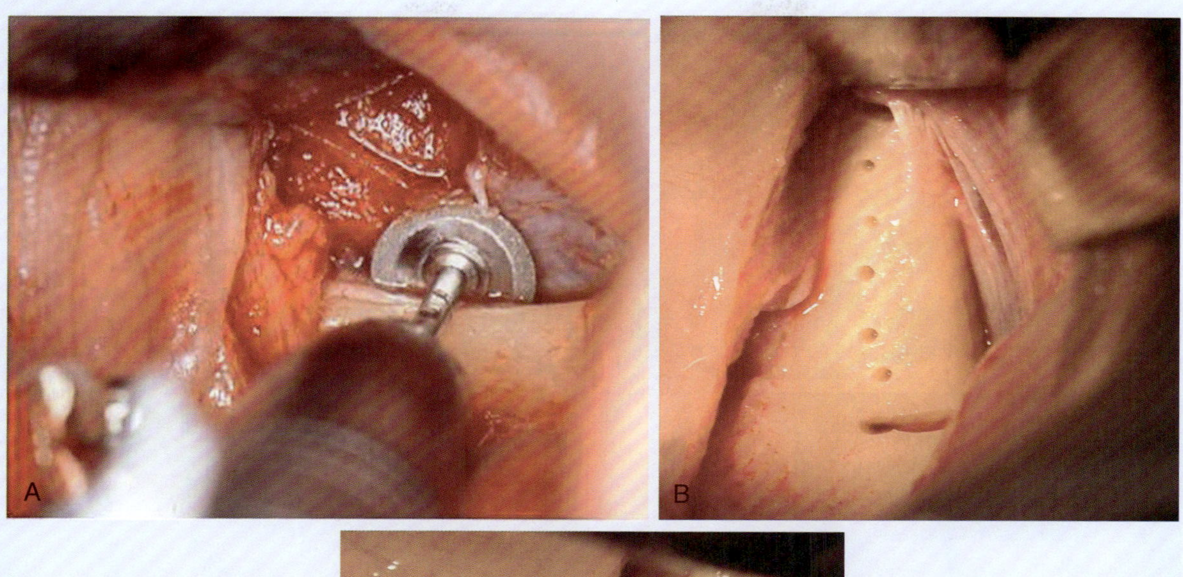

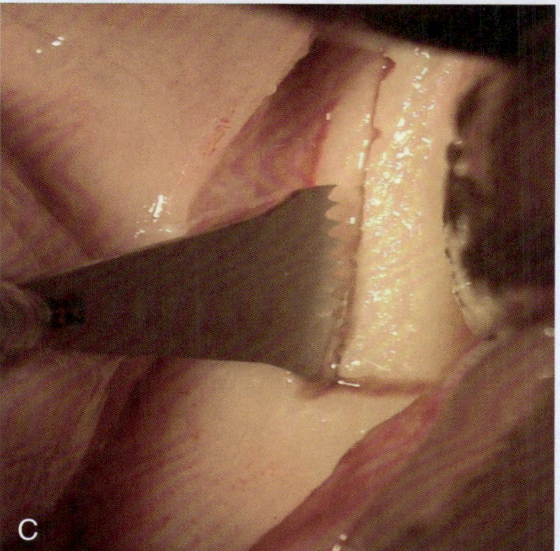

Fig 15.33 (A and B) A disc was used to prepare inferior horizontal osteotomy and two vertical cuts (C) while the oscillating saw was used to prepare superior horizontal osteotomy.

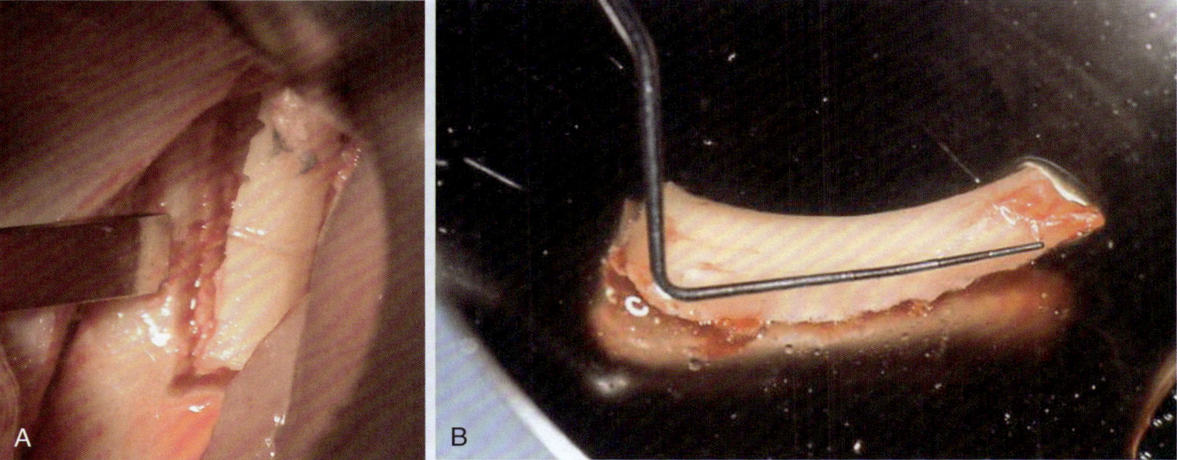

Fig 15.34 (A) The block was separated from the donor site using a sharp chisel, and (B) measured to fit the host site.

Continued

CASE REPORT-4—cont'd

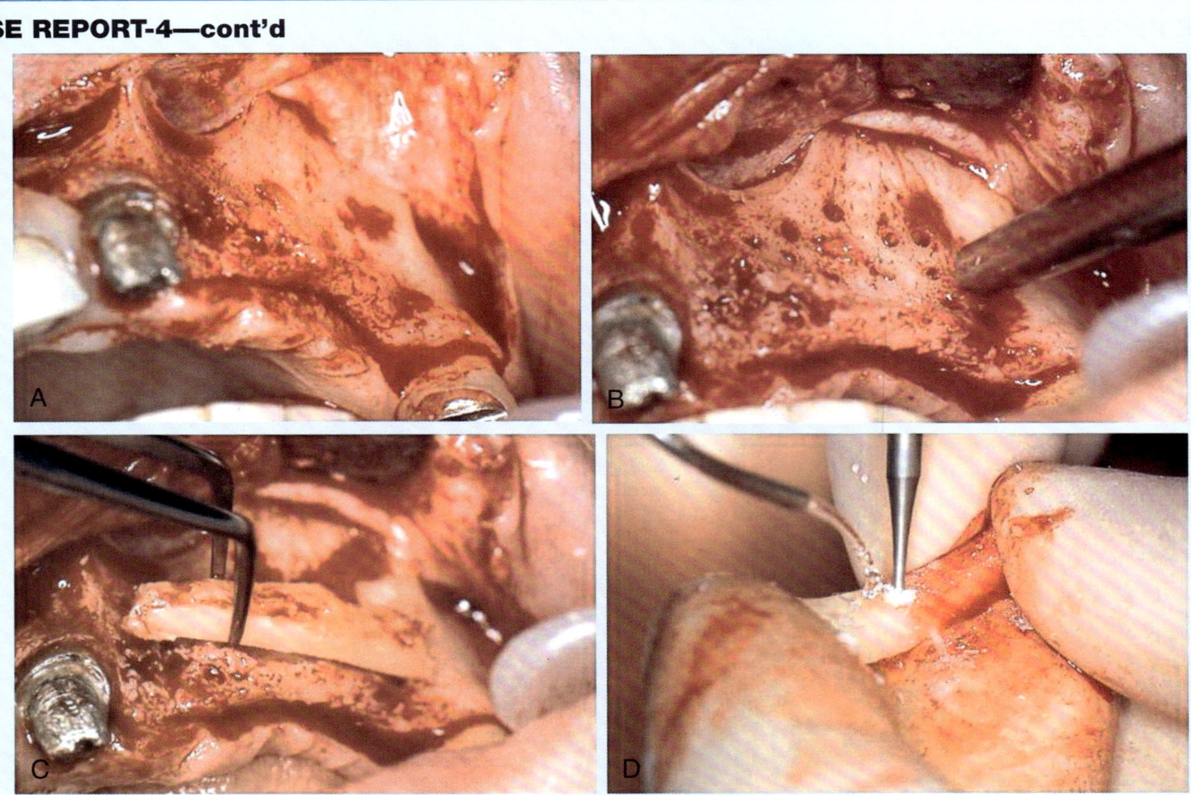

Fig 15.35 (A and B) The host site was microperforated to access the rich blood supply from the underlying spongiosa as well as for the desired union of the block with the host site. (C) The block was tried on the host site to assure its desired adaptability. (D) Two screw holes are prepared through the block using a straight carbide bur.

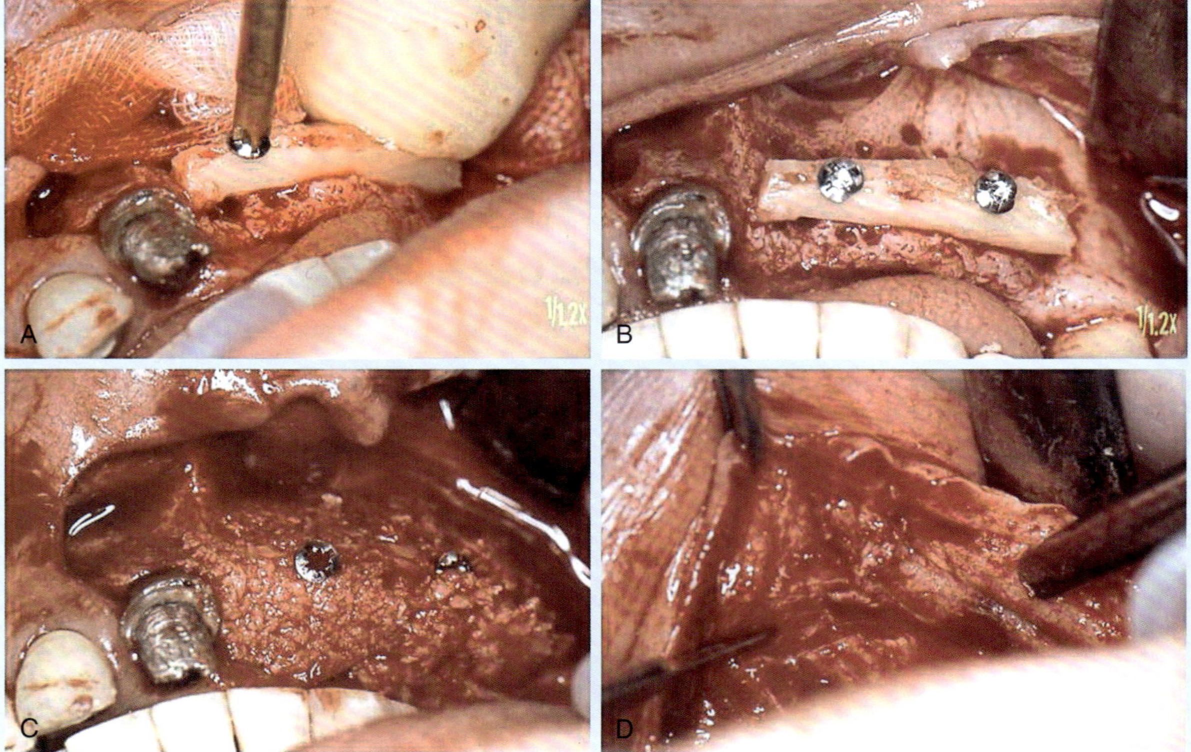

Fig 15.36 (A and B) The block was immobilized on the host site using long fixation screws. (C) Further, the particulated graft was used to fill the deficient areas. (D) The releasing incisions were given into the periosteum of the buccal flap.

CASE REPORT-4—cont'd

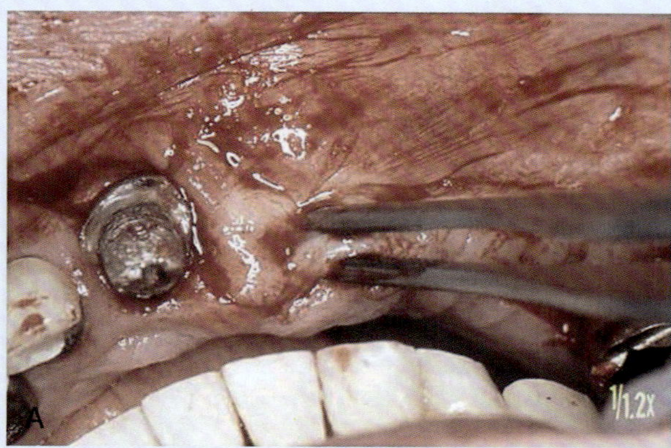
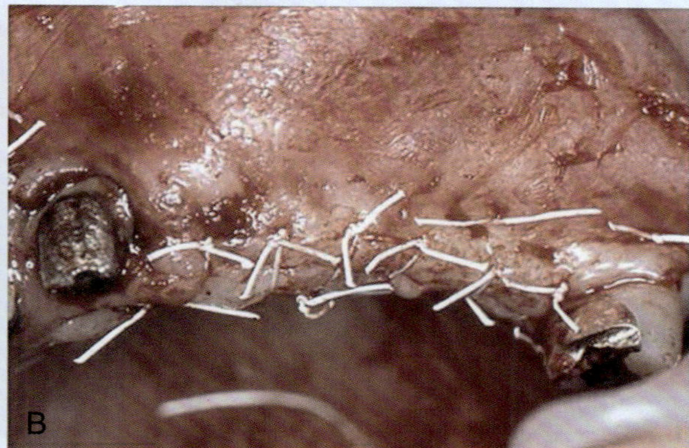

Fig 15.37 (A and B) The mucoperiosteal flap was coronally advanced and sutured to achieve a watertight closure.

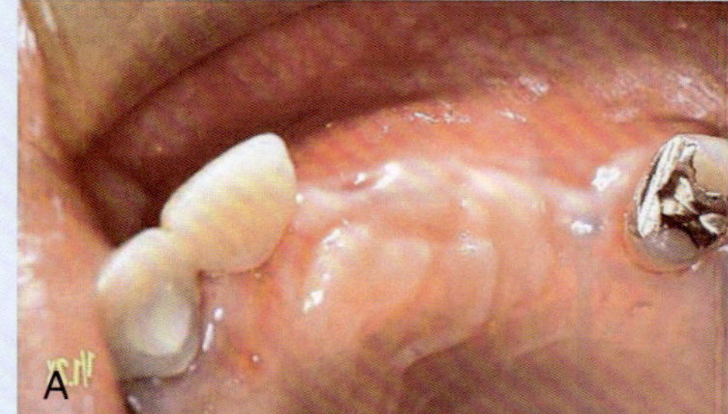
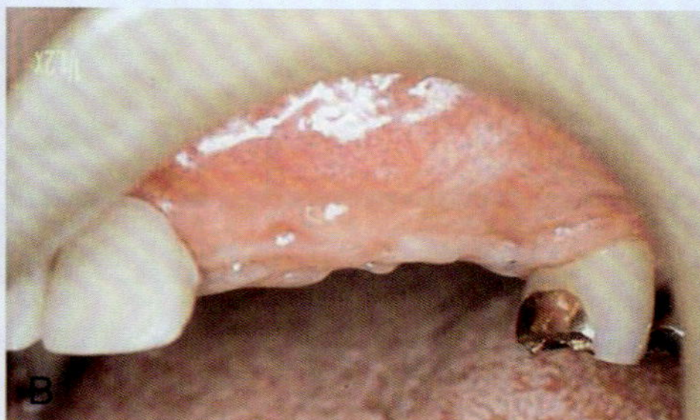
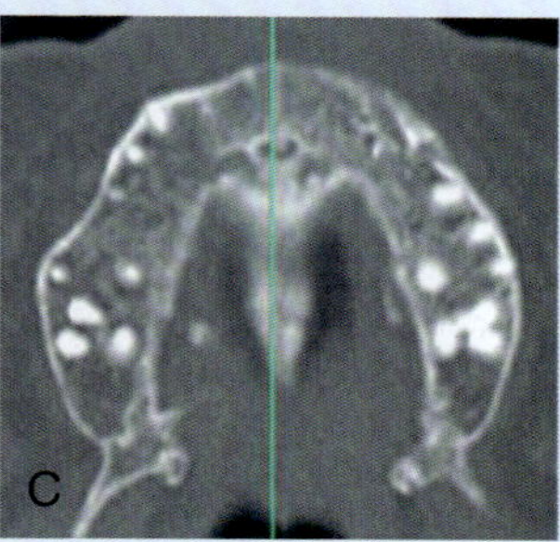

Fig 15.38 (A and B) Healing after 4 months shows remarkable improvement in three-dimensional ridge morphology. (C) The axial view of the dental CT scan shows reconstructed ridge defect.

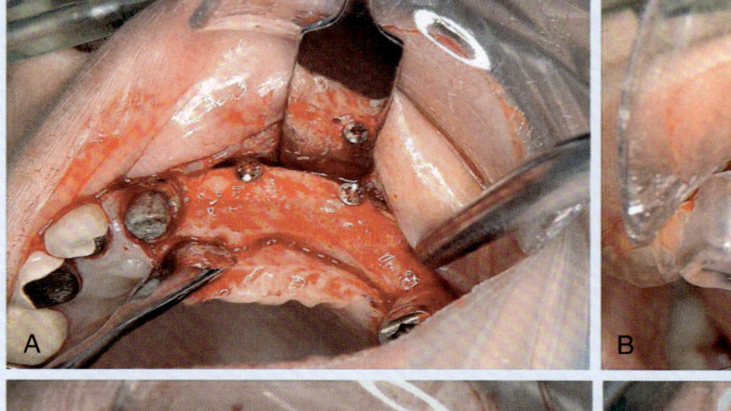
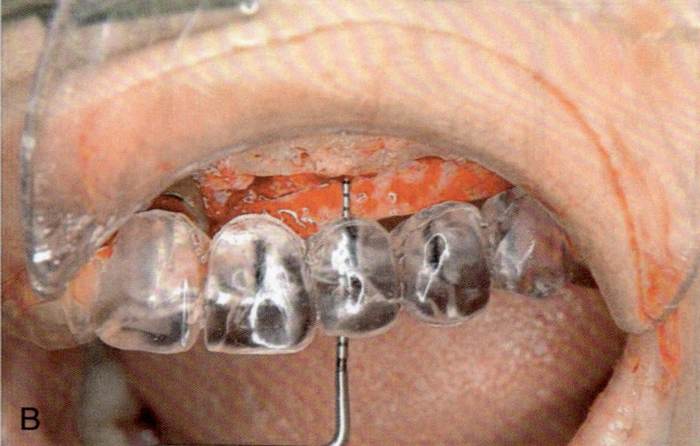
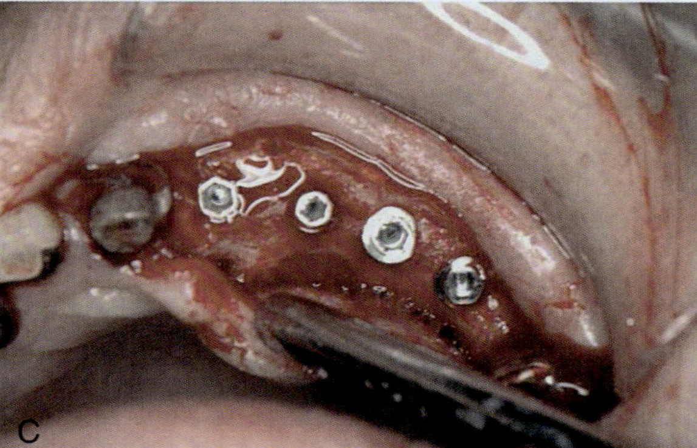
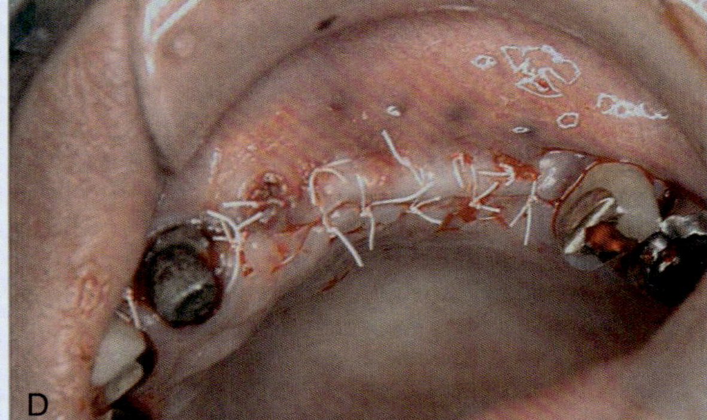

Fig 15.39 (A) Site was exposed after 4 months and fixation screws are removed. (B–D) Implants were inserted using a prosthetic guide and the flap was sutured back.

CASE REPORT-5

Reconstruction of vertical bone defect of the mandibular molar region using onlay block graft (Figs 15.40–15.43).

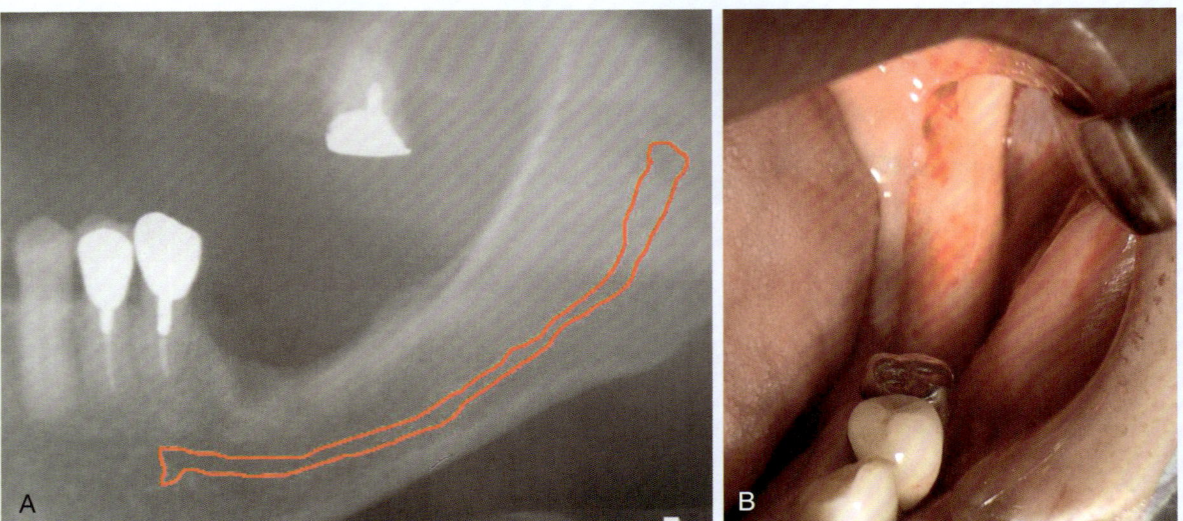

Fig 15.40 (A) Radiograph shows a large vertical bone defect in the posterior mandibular region, which had resulted in insufficient vertical bone dimensions above the mandibular canal to insert adequately long implants. (B) The host site as well as the ascending ramus of the mandible was uncovered.

CASE REPORT-5—cont'd

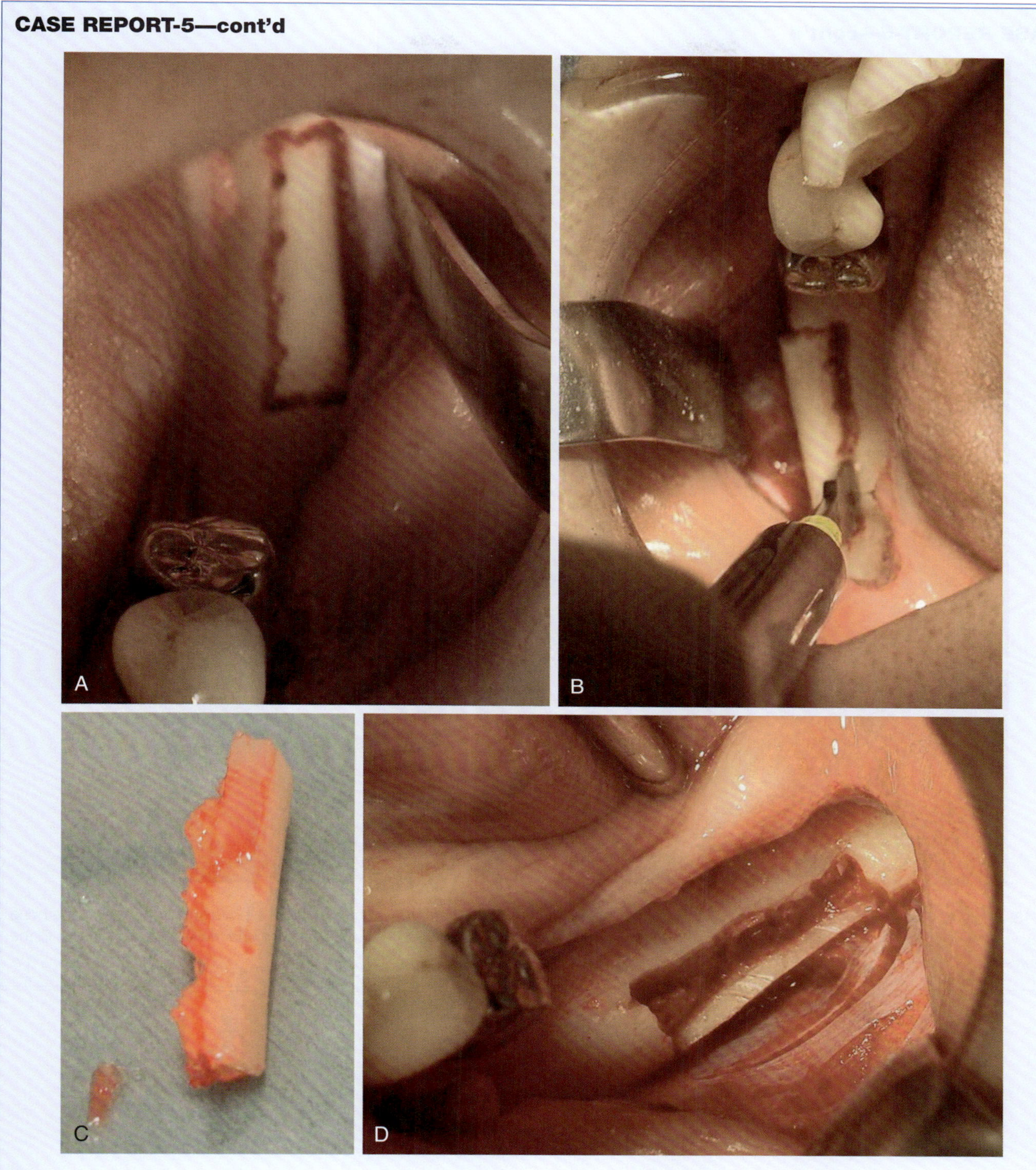

Fig 15.41 (A–D) A large corticocancellous bone block was harvested from the ascending ramus of the mandible.

Continued

CASE REPORT-5—cont'd

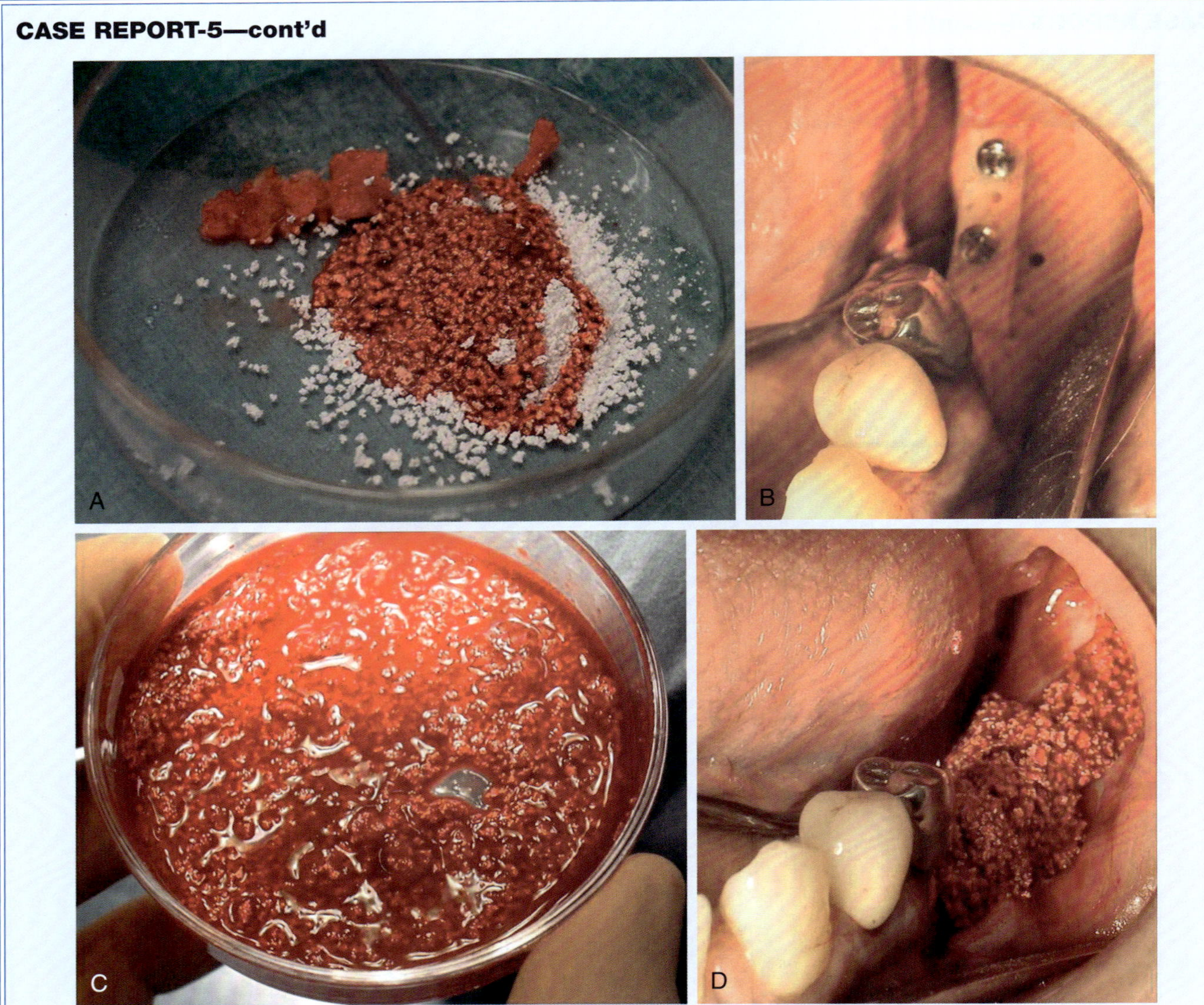

Fig 15.42 (A) A small amount of cancellous bone was also harvested from the donor site and mixed with the bone substitute. (B–D) The bone block was fixed on top of the ridge crest and the particulated graft, mixed with blood, was added over and around the block as well as, to fill the donor site.

CASE REPORT-5—cont'd

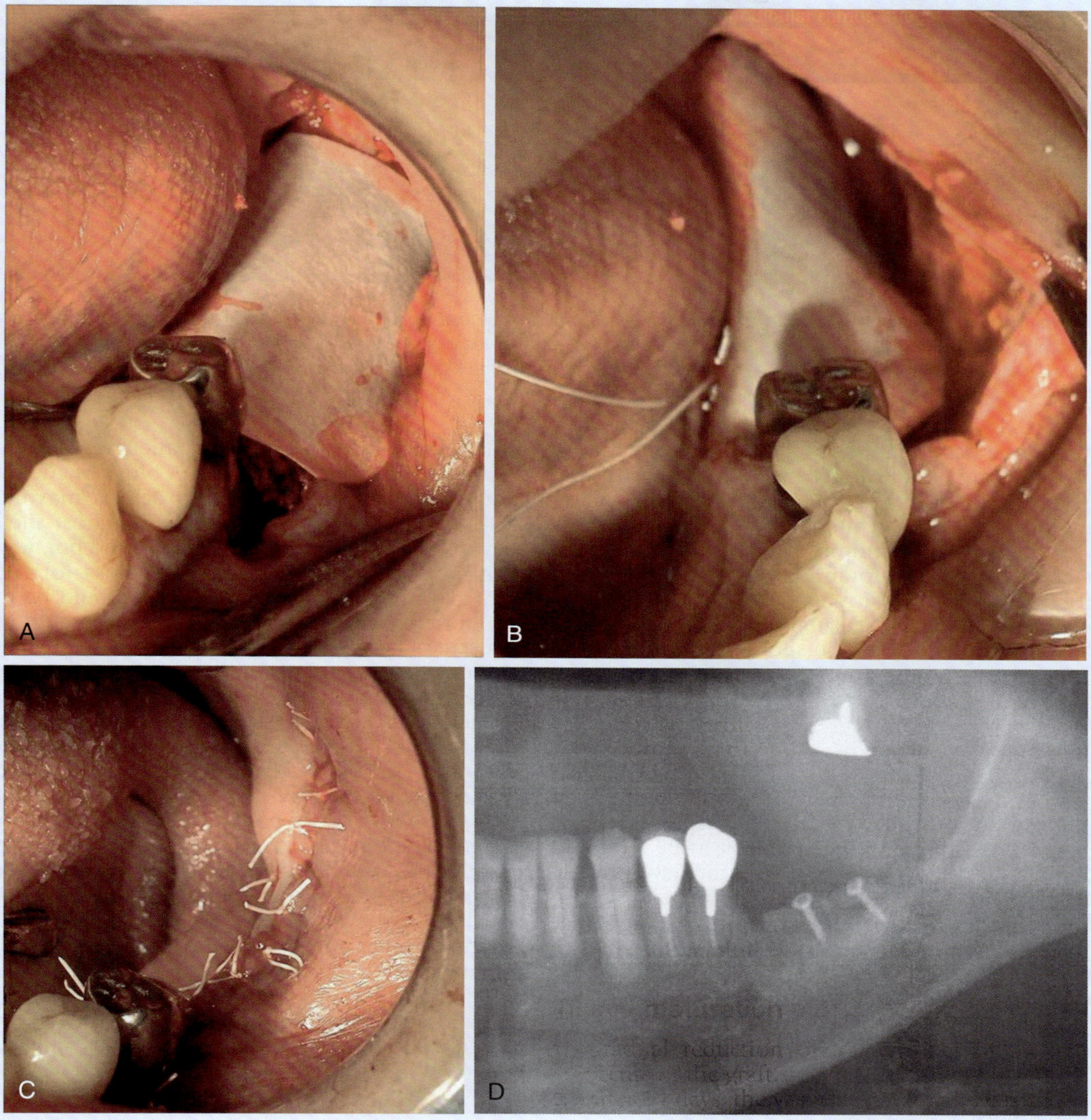

A B C D

Fig 15.43 (A) The grafted site was covered using a collagen barrier membrane. (B and C) The flap was released and sutured to achieve watertight closure. (D) Post-grafting radiograph shows the vertical bone augmentation using bone block.

Continued

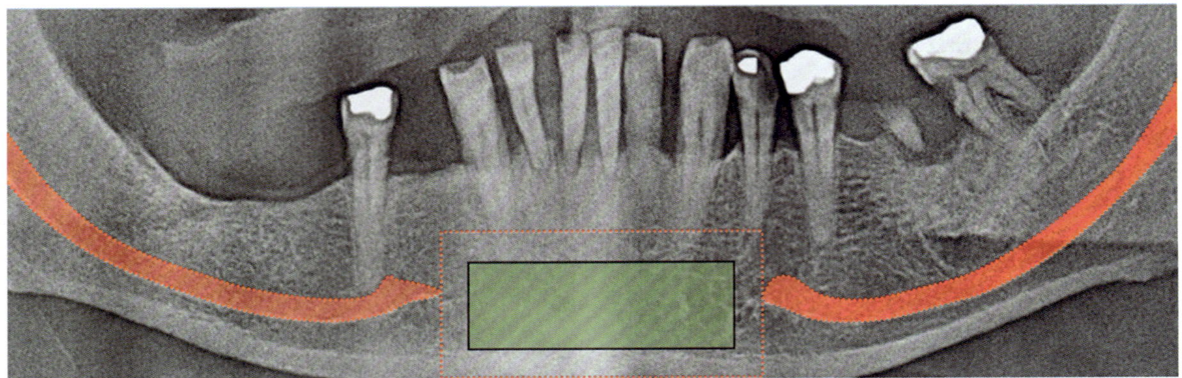

Fig 15.44 When harvesting the block graft from the mandibular symphysis region, care should be taken to avoid any injury to the vital structures like mental nerve and root apices. The outer margins of the block osteotomy (presented in green) should remain a minimum of 5 mm away from the root apices, mental nerve, and basal margin of the mandible (presented with red dotted block) (Rule of 5).

Rule of 5: When harvesting the block from the mandibular symphysis, care should be taken to avoid any injury to the vital structures, such as mental nerve and roots of the mandibular anteriors. The margins of the osteotomy should be prepared a minimum of 5 mm away from all the structures like mental foramina, root apices of mandibular anteriors, and basal margin of the mandible. In cases where the mandibular canal is showing the anterior loop, osteotomy preparation should end 5 mm anterior to the anterior-most margin of the anterior loop (Fig 15.44).

Summary

Block grafting can be a preferred option in ridge defects where the particulate graft does not look to be a definitive option. The desired results can be achieved using block graft in cases of large defects with vertical or lateral bone deficiency. The autogenous bone block is known to be the gold standard and can be harvested from the various intraoral sites, such as mandibular symphysis, mandibular ramus, and buccal shelf, to be used to augment small to medium-sized defects. Meticulous planning should be done to perform the procedure with minimum postoperative discomfort to the patient and to obtain the desired results from the grafting. A block of adequate size should be harvested and shaped to achieve maximum and closest adaptation at the host site. The host site should be microperforated using the small round bur, to provide nutrition from the underlying spongiosa for the transplanted graft cells to survive. Efforts should be made to immobilize the block graft using a minimum of two fixation screws because the use of only one screw may cause rotational movement of the block and result in nonunion of the graft to the host site. The particulate graft, either autogenous bone harvested from the host site or bone substitute, should be used to fill the spaces and deficiencies around the block. The barrier membrane can be used in selective cases where the periosteum is not intact, or in cases where a lot of particulate graft has been used to augment the defect. The fixation screws should passively pass through the block, as the lateral pressure from the screws may result in block fracture from the screw hole. The sharp edges of the graft should be smoothened out to avoid any tear of the overlying soft tissue and the consequent exposure of the block to the oral environment. However, if it has occurred, the exposed part of the block graft should be reduced using a carbide trimmer, and the site left to heal by the process of secondary intension.

Further Reading

Pikos MA. Block autografts for localized ridge augmentation: part II. The posterior mandible. Implant Dent 2000;9(1):67–75.

Bahat O, Fontanessi RV. Efficacy of implant placement after bone grafting for three-dimensional reconstruction of the posterior jaw. Int J Periodontics Restorative Dent 2001;21:220–31.

Misch CM, Misch CE. The repair of localized severe ridge defects for implant placement using mandibular bone grafts. Implant Dent 1995;4:261–7.

Triaca A, Minoretti R, Merli M, et al. Periosteoplasty for soft tissue closure and augmentation in preprosthetic surgery: a surgical report. Int J Oral Maxillofac Implants 2001;16:851–6.

Hernández-Alfaro F, Pages CM, García E, et al. Palatal core graft for alveolar reconstruction: a new donor site. Int J Oral Maxillofac Implants 2005;20:777–83.

McCarthy C, Patel RR, Wragg PF, et al. Dental implants and on lay bone grafts in the anterior maxilla: analysis of clinical outcome. Int J Oral Maxillofac Implants 2003;18:238–41.

Pikos MA. Alveolar ridge augmentation with ramus buccal shelf autografts and impacted third molar removal. Dent Implantol Update 1999;4(10):27–31.

Hernández-Alfaro F, Martí C, Biosca MJ, et al. Minimally invasive tibial bone harvesting under intravenous sedation. J Oral Maxillofac Surg 2005;63:464–70.

Proussaefs P, Lozada J, Kleinman A, et al. The use of ramus autogenous block grafts for vertical alveolar ridge augmentation and implant placement: a pilot study. Int J Oral Maxillofac Implants 2002;17:238–48.

Bahat O, Fontanesi FV. Complications of grafting in the atrophic edentulous or partially edentulous jaw. Int J Periodontics Restorative Dent 2001;21:487–95.

Pikos MA. Block autografts for localized ridge augmentation: part I. The posterior maxilla. Implant Dent 1999;8(3):279–84.

Tecimer D, Behr MM. Use of autogenous bone grafting to reconstruct a mandibular knife edge ridge before implant surgery: a case report. J Oral Implantol 2001;27:98–102.

Misch CE. Contemporary implant dentistry. 2nd ed. St. Louis (MO): Mosby; 1999. p. 443–4.

Pikos MA. Alveolar ridge augmentation using mandibular block grafts: clinical update. Alpha Omegan 2000;93(3):14–21.

Pikos MA. Facilitating implant placement with chin grafts as donor sites for maxillary bone augmentation: part I. Dent Implantol Update 1995;6(12):89–92.

Pikos MA. Posterior maxillary bone reconstruction: importance of staging. Implant News and Views 1999;1(3)(1):6–8.

Kleinheinz J, Büchter A, Kruse-Lösler B, et al. Incision design in implant dentistry based on vascularization of the mucosa. Clin Oral Implants Res 2005;16:518–23.

Pikos MA. Buccolingual expansion of the maxillary ridge. Dent Implantol Update 1992;3(11):85–7.

Wheeler SL. Implant complications in the esthetic zone. J Oral Maxillofac Surg 2007;65(7 Suppl. 1):93–102. Review. Erratum in: J Oral Maxillofac Surg. 2008;66:2195–6.

Frost H. The biology of fracture healing: an overview for clinicians. Part I. Clin Orthop Relat Res 1989;248:283–92.

Li J, Wang HL. Common implant-related advanced bone grafting complications: classification, etiology, and management. Implant Dent 2008;17:389–401.

Collins TA. Onlay bone grafting in combination with Branemark implants. Oral Maxillofac Surg Clin North Am 1991;3:893–902.

Collins TA, Nunn W. Autogenous veneer grafting for improved esthetics with dental implants. Compend Contin Educ Dent 1994;15:370–6.

Bedrossian E, Tawfilis A, Alijanian A. Veneer grafting: a technique for augmentation of the resorbed alveolus prior to implant placement. A clinical report. Int J Oral Maxillofac Implants 2000;15:853–8.

Pikos MA. Facilitating implant placement with chin grafts as donor sites for maxillary bone augmentation: part II. Dent Implantol Update 1996;7(1):1–4.

Perry T. Ascending ramus offered as alternate harvest site for onlay bone grafting. Dent Implantol Update 1997;3:21–4.

Sethi A, Kaus T. Ridge augmentation using mandibular block bone grafts: preliminary results of an ongoing prospective study. Int J Oral Maxillofac Implants 2001;16:378–88.

Capelli M. Autogenous bone graft from the mandibular ramus: a technique for bone augmentation. Int J Periodontics Restorative Dent 2003;23:277–85.

Kainulainen VT, Sàndor GK, Carmichael RP, et al. Safety of zygomatic bone harvesting: a prospective study of 32 consecutive patients with simultaneous zygomatic bone grafting and 1-stage implant placement. Int J Oral Maxillofac Implants 2005;20:245–52.

Proussaefs P, Lozada J. The use of intraorally harvested autogenous block grafts for vertical alveolar ridge augmentation: a human study. Int J Periodontics Restorative Dent 2005;25:351–63.

Gapski R, Wang HL, Misch CE. Management of incision design in symphysis graft procedures: a review of the literature. J Oral Implantol 2001;27:134–42.

Schuler R, Verardi S. A new incision design for mandibular symphysis bone-grafting procedures. J Periodontol 2005;76:845–9.

Schwartz-Arad D, Levin L. Intraoral autogenous block onlay bone grafting for extensive reconstruction of atrophic maxillary alveolar ridges. J Periodontol 2005;76:636–41.

Koymen R, Karacayli U, Gocmen-Mas N, et al. Flap and incision design in implant surgery: clinical and anatomical study. Surg Radiol Anat 2009;31:301–6.

Frost H. The regional acceleratory phenomenon: a review. Henry Ford Hosp Med J 1983;31:3–9.

Jensen OT, Pikos MA, Simion M, et al. Bone grafting strategies for vertical alveolar augmentation. Peterson's principles of oral and maxillofacial surgery. 2nd ed. Ontario: BC Decker; 2004. pp. 223–32.

Jensen J, Sindet-Pedersen S. Autogenous mandibular bone grafts and osseointegrated implants for reconstruction of the severely atrophied maxilla: a preliminary report. J Oral Maxillofac Surg 1991;49:1277–87.

Marx RE. Biology of bone grafts. In: Kelly JPW, editor. OMS knowledge update. Rosemont (IL): American Association of Oral and Maxillofacial Surgeons; 1994. RCN3–17.

Ridge splitting for implant placement

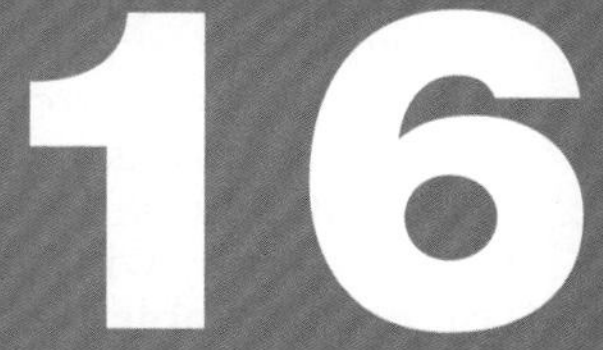

Ajay Vikram Singh Angelo Troedhan

CHAPTER CONTENTS HD

Introduction

Deficiencies in the width or height of the alveolar ridge in the maxilla and the mandible, can severely limit the use of dental implants in both edentulous and partially edentulous patients. Ridge-width problems can be solved through a variety of methods, including the use of alveolar distraction, osteogenesis, onlay bone grafts, titanium reinforced membranes, ridge splitting and ridge expansion. Whether implants are placed immediately or at a later stage after healing, ridge splitting through the use of bone-splitting osteotomes or other cutting/chiseling apparatus expand the ridge, often in conjunction with bone grafting. Careful displacement of the buccal plate is essential when ridge splitting is used, because abnormal bone healing may result from undue trauma to the plate.

According to Dr Ady Palti, several specifically designed instruments (e.g. bone chisels for bone splitting and osteotomes for bone spreading) enable techniques for placing implants in the lateral region of the maxilla, where the alveolar ridge is not wide enough. Palti explains that 'these techniques make it possible to condense the bone laterally, resulting in a higher bone density and an improved primary stability of the implant, and to augment the alveolar ridge locally, thus creating a stable vestibular and palatine lamella of 1.5–2 mm'. He adds that these criteria are important to ensure long-term successes in implantology and, moreover to shorten the period of osseointegration.

The ridge splitting technique was originally proposed by Dr Simion et al and later on modified by Dr Scipioni et al, and Dr Nivins and Dr Stein. This technique is performed to widen a narrow ridge to place adequate diameter implants. As the name indicates, the implant dentist splits the two collapsed cortical plates apart to achieve adequate buccolingual ridge dimensions for ideal diameter implant placement between two cortical plates. The bone graft is packed to fill the spaces between the cortical plates after implant insertion. The site is covered with resorbable collagen membrane and the flap sutured back with a primary closure. With advancements in implant science and armamentarium, several modifications have been made to conventional ridge splitting techniques and can selectively be performed in any particular case.

Causes of bone loss

1. Traumatic avulsion of anterior teeth often causes severe injury to the thin facial cortical plate, which in turn gets resorbed and results in inadequate ridge width for adequate diameter implant insertion (class 2 ridge).
2. A large chronic periapical/periradicular abscess often causes the resorption of the labial cortical plate, and the extraction of such teeth results in a narrow ridge with a severe undercut along the facial aspect of the ridge (class 3 ridge).
3. Periodontal bone defects.
4. Disuse atrophy with long-term edentulism.
5. Use of removable partial prosthesis/flipper for a long time.

Author's classification for the edentulous ridge morphology of the anterior maxilla

Edentulous ridge morphology of the premaxilla can be classified based on its cross-sectional topography.

Class 1 – Ideal ridge

The ideal diameter implant can be inserted without any ridge modification and grafting procedure (Fig 16.1A).

Class 2 – Deficient ridge crest

Deficient ridge width at the crest needs ridge expansion or lateral bone grafting at the crestal region for ideal diameter implant placement (Fig 16.1B).

Management for ideal implant insertion

1. Lateral bone augmentation and delayed implant insertion
2. Ridge splitting and simultaneous implant insertion.

Class 3 – Adequate ridge at crest but with severe facial concavity

This condition does not require any ridge modification or grafting at the crestal region but the facial concavity needs to be grafted before implant placement (Fig 16.1C).

Management for ideal implant insertion

1. Lateral bone augmentation in the facial concavity and delayed implant insertion
2. Implant insertion with simultaneous bone augmentation of the facial concavity.

Class 4 – Deficient ridge crest with severe facial concavity

Deficient ridge crest with severe undercuts along the facial aspect, needs to be grafted along with ridge splitting and expansion (Fig 16.1D).

Management for ideal implant insertion

1. Lateral bone augmentation and delayed implant insertion
2. Ridge splitting with mid-crestal horizontal and two vertical cuts on facial plate and simultaneous implant insertion with bone augmentation to fill the large spaces between expanded cortical plates
3. Ridge splitting to expand the crestal one-third followed by implant insertion and lateral bone augmentation over the undercut, preferably by tunnelling technique.

Indications

Compromised bone width for ideal implant placement

Ridge splitting and expansion are performed to widen the thin ridge and the implant is immediately inserted between two expanded cortical plates (Fig 16.2A and B).

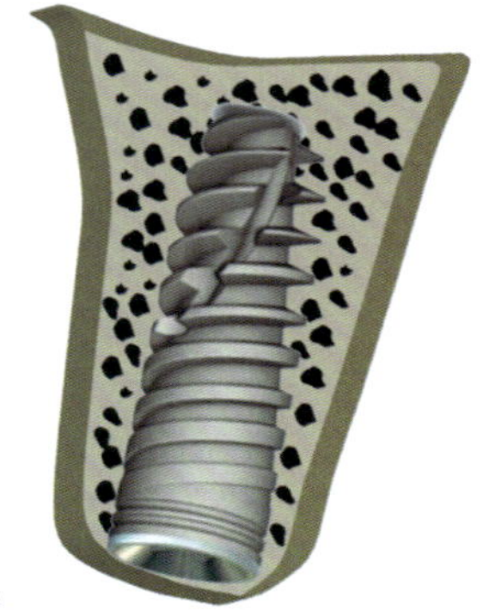

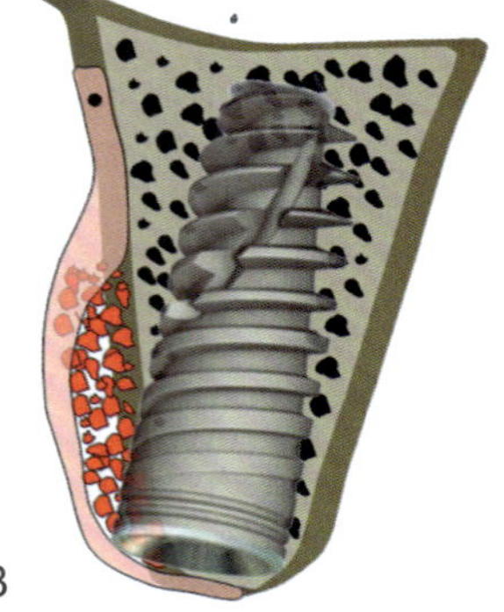

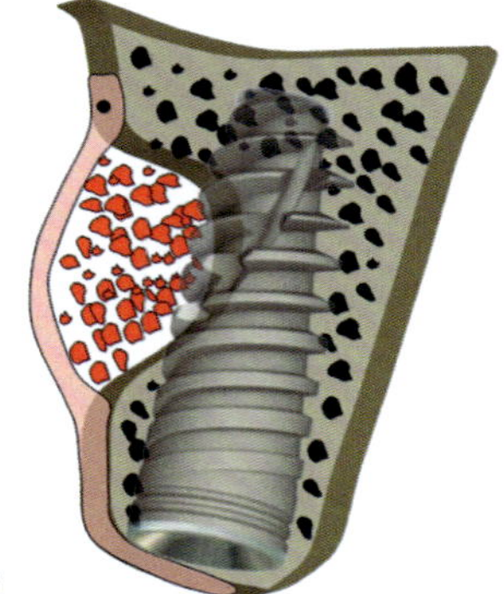

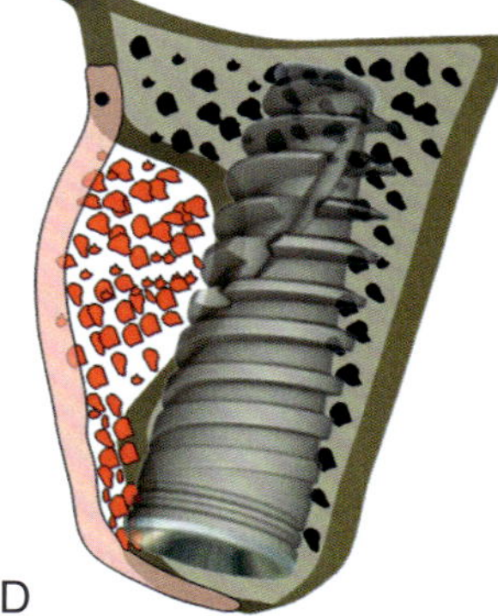

Fig 16.1 Author's classification for the edentulous ridge morphology of the anterior maxilla. (A) Abundant bony ridge for ideal implant insertion without any bone augmentation (class 1). (B) Bony ridge deficient at the crest, needs bone augmentation with or prior to implant placement (class 2). (C) Bony ridge with facial concavity at the middle one-third, needs bone augmentation with or prior to implant insertion (class 3). (D) Bony ridge with the combination of crestal bone deficiency and facial concavity, needs bone augmentation with or prior to implant insertion (class 4).

Porous cortical and coarse/fine trabecular bone (D3/D4 bone)

Bone splitting can be performed with a greater rate of success in the bone with medium density (e.g. maxillary bone). Ridge splitting in the hard bone (e.g. mandible) often leads to sudden and complete splitting/fracture of the cortical plate during its expansion. But with the newer protocols described later in this chapter, one can manage to perform ridge splitting in the high density bone as well.

Presence of both cortical plates with observable interposed cancellous bone

Ridge splitting should not be performed in cases where any of the cortical plate is missing or if there are large osseous defects in the bone.

Absence of severe undercuts

Severe undercut along the ridge morphology may result in sudden fracture of the cortical plate at the undercut area during its expansion (Fig 16.3A–C). Newer protocol is described later in the chapter to manage such ridge situations.

Improvement of facial profile is a necessity to improve the aesthetics

Often the available bone width is adequate to insert adequate diameter implant but the concavity in the ridge morphology, especially in the aesthetic region, needs to be improved with lateral bone augmentation or ridge expansion to improve the facial aesthetics along with the implant restoration (Fig 16.4).

Contraindications

1. Presence of dense cortical bone (D1 bone)
2. Compromised buccal cortical plate
3. Absence of cancellous bone between two cortical plates
4. Presence of severe undercuts
5. Inadequate ridge width (<3 mm) to perform ridge splitting
6. Insufficient mesiodistal space of edentulous area (<7 mm) – if mesiodistal dimension of the edentulous ridge area is less than 7 mm, ridge splitting with two vertical cuts should not be performed as either of these cuts can harm the roots of adjacent teeth, or because there is inadequate bone between two cuts, which is often very difficult to expand.

Comparative features of block grafting versus ridge splitting procedures

If performed with the proper case selection, treatment planning, and skilled approach, ridge splitting offers several advantages over the conventional block grafting procedure (Table 16.1).

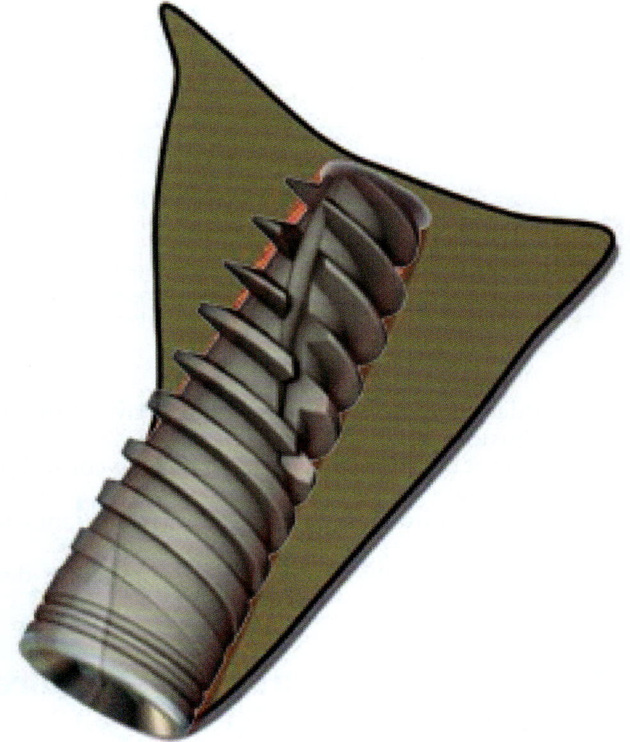

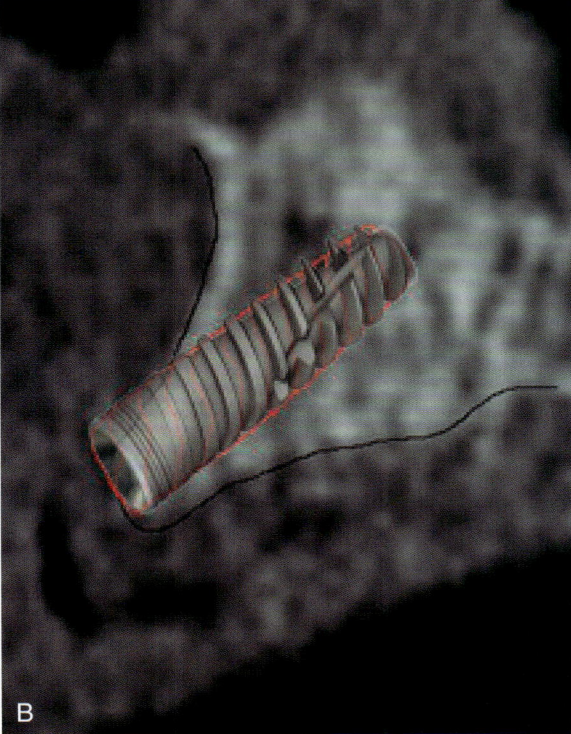

Fig 16.2 (A and B) Placement of an implant with adequate size in the ridge with compromised buccolingual ridge dimensions may result in bone dehiscence. The ridge splitting and expansion should be performed to obtain adequate bone width before implant placement.

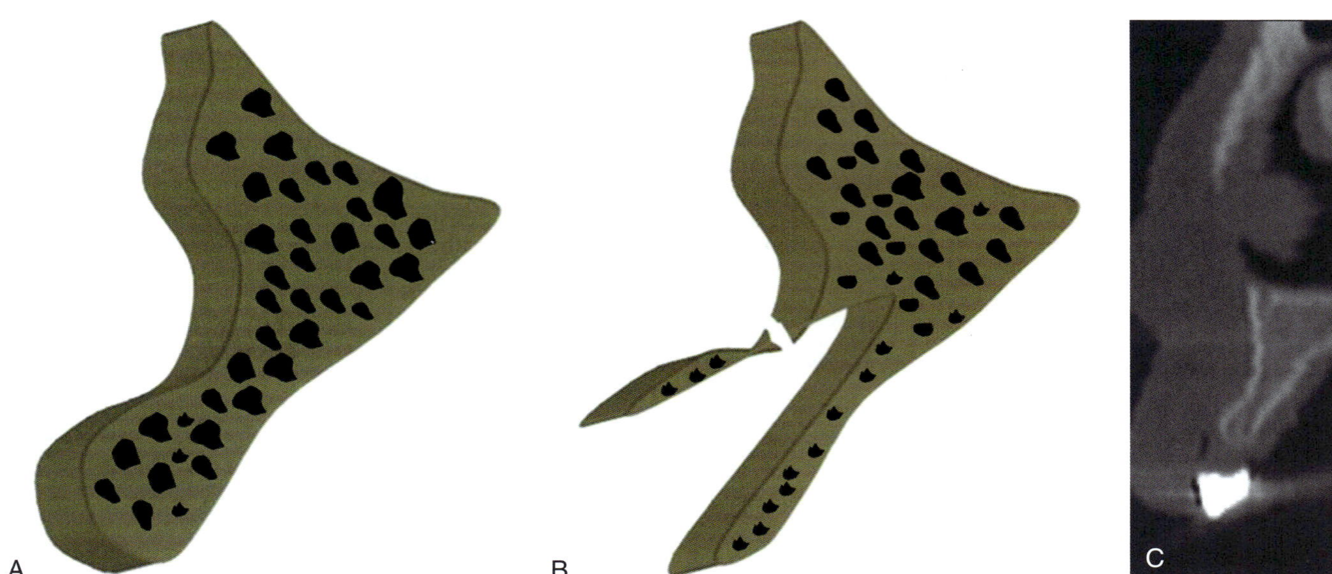

Fig 16.3 (A–C) Severe undercut along the ridge morphology may result in sudden fracture of the cortical plate at the undercut area during its expansion.

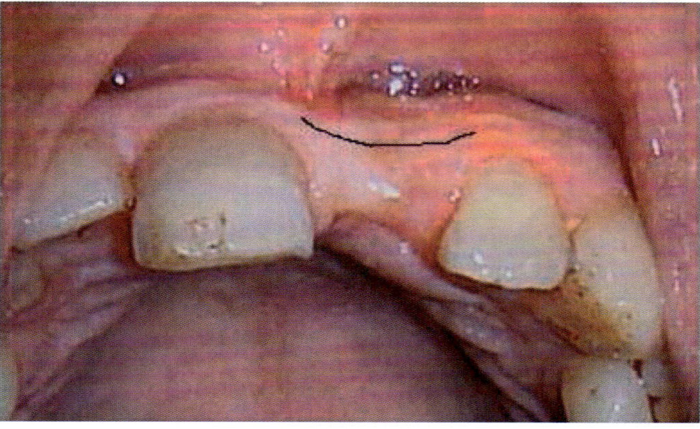

Fig 16.4 Concavity in ridge morphology in the aesthetic region often needs to be improved with lateral bone augmentation or ridge expansion to improve facial aesthetics.

Table 16.1 Comparison between block grafting and ridge splitting

BLOCK GRAFTING	RIDGE SPLITTING
Takes more time	Takes less time
More invasive	Less invasive
More technique-sensitive	Less technique-sensitive
Needs another site to harvest autogenous bone block	Not required
More surgical steps	Fewer surgical steps
Simultaneous implant insertion is not possible	Simultaneous implant insertion is possible
Takes a long span of time to complete the treatment	Takes shorter time span to complete the treatment

Advantages

1. It can be performed as an alternative to the block grafting in selected cases.
2. Simultaneous implant placement is done.
3. It does not usually require expensive armamentarium; can be performed using ridge splitters.
4. Implant with adequate diameter can be placed.
5. It enhances hard and soft tissue profile.
6. Bone density around implants is increased.
7. Interposed graft receives rich blood supply for maturation.

Disadvantages

1. Crestal bone resorption: The 'bounce back' pressure of the expanded resilient cortical plate against the implant platform may lead to its resorption.
2. Sudden fracture of cortical plate may occur during expansion.
3. It cannot be performed if one of the two cortical plates is missing.
4. It may require graft materials and membranes to fill the voids/spaces.
5. Skilled approach is required to obtain the desired results.

Materials and instruments required for ridge splitting (Fig 16.5A–C)

1. Razor sharp osseous splitters
2. Bone spreading osteotomes (D-shaped)
3. Good bone expanders

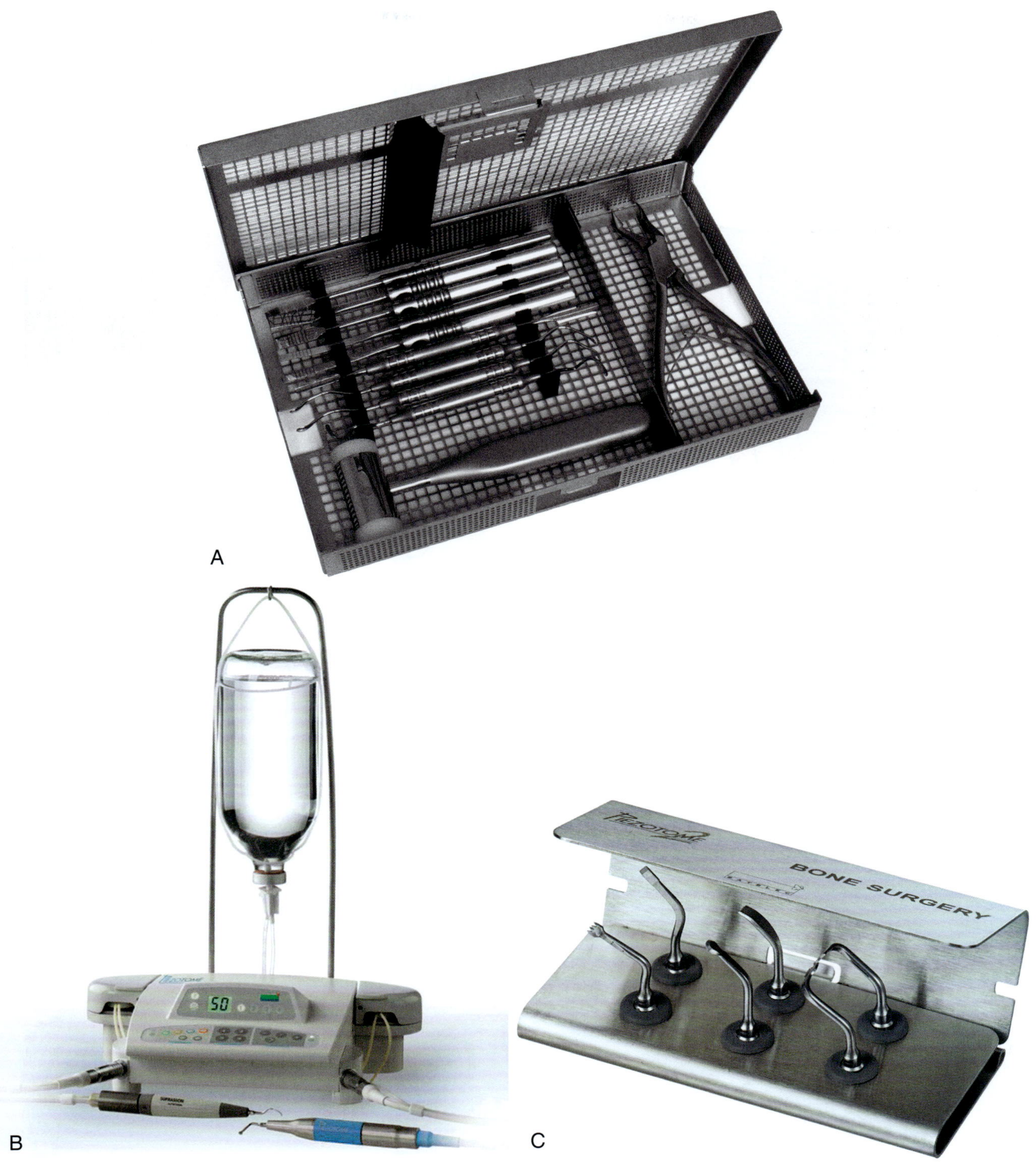

Fig 16.5 (A) Palti's ridge splitting kit containing various types of ridge splitters and accessories required to perform ridge splitting procedures, (B) piezotome saw along with (C) bone surgery kit (from Satelec, France) can be used to prepare horizontal and vertical osteotomies more precisely than rotary burs, before ridge splitting and expansion using splitters.

4. A balanced mallet
5. Thin straight fissure bur
6. Piezo surgery unit
7. Graft placement instruments
8. Good regenerative materials (bone graft and membrane)

Conventional technique of ridge splitting

Step by step diagrammatic presentation of ridge-splitting technique is shown in Figs 16.6–16.9.

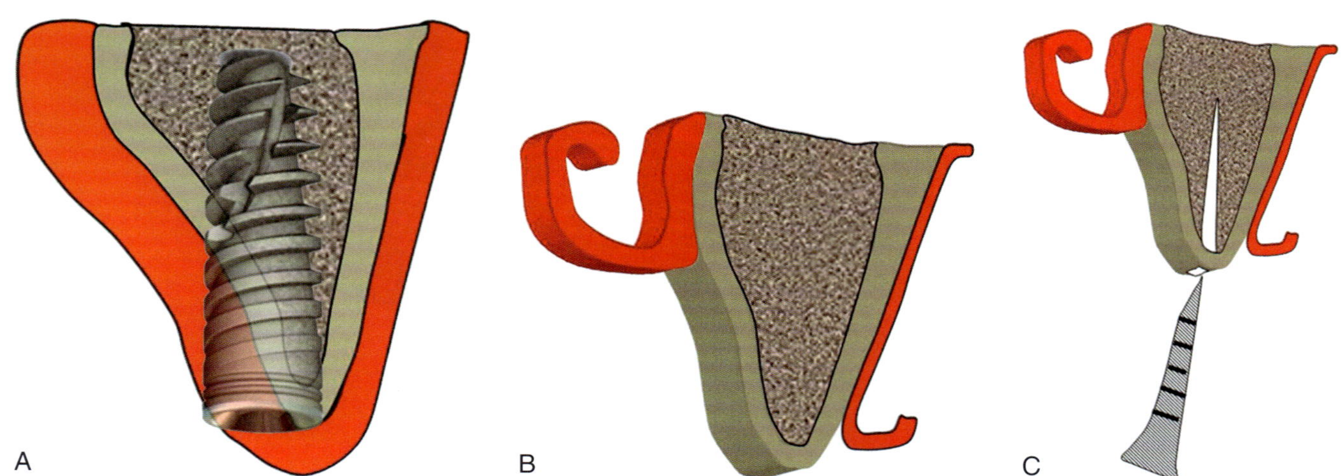

Fig 16.6 Cross-sectional 3D view of the maxillary anterior edentulous ridge showing narrow ridge crest. (A) Any attempt to place the implant may result in dehiscence at the crestal region. (B) The mid-crestal incision is made and mucoperiosteal flaps are elevated to expose the ridge crest as well as the facial cortical bone. (C) A mid-crestal horizontal cut is made and deepened several millimetres, using sharp chisel/piezo saw/straight fissure bur.

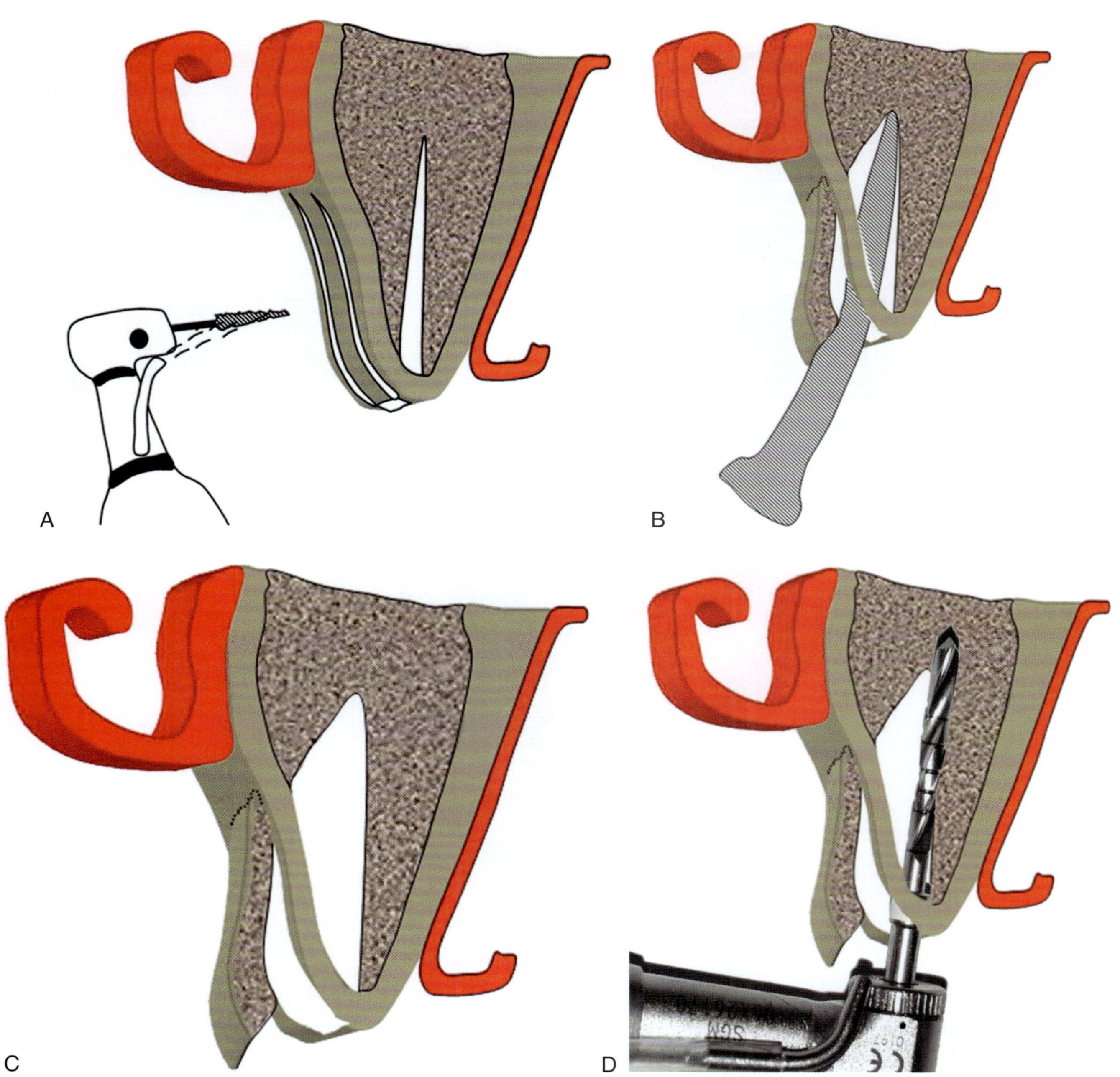

Fig 16.7 (A) A thin long straight fissure bur/piezo saw/osseous splitters are used to make two vertical cuts deep enough to reach the underlying cancellous bone and apically to reach beyond the narrow bone or facial undercut, if present. (B) Different sized osseous splitters are then sequentially used to widen the seam and pry apart the two cortical plates. The facial plate should be supported with the finger or any appropriate instrument during its expansion to counteract the expansion forces and to prevent its sudden fracture. (C) Fully spread cortical plates with a large degree of separation can be seen. The implant osteotomy is prepared in usual fashion. Drills should be used in contact with hard and stable palatal plate far away from the spread facial plate and deeper to reach at least 3–4 mm. (D) Apical to the split ridge, to achieve adequate implant stability at its apex.

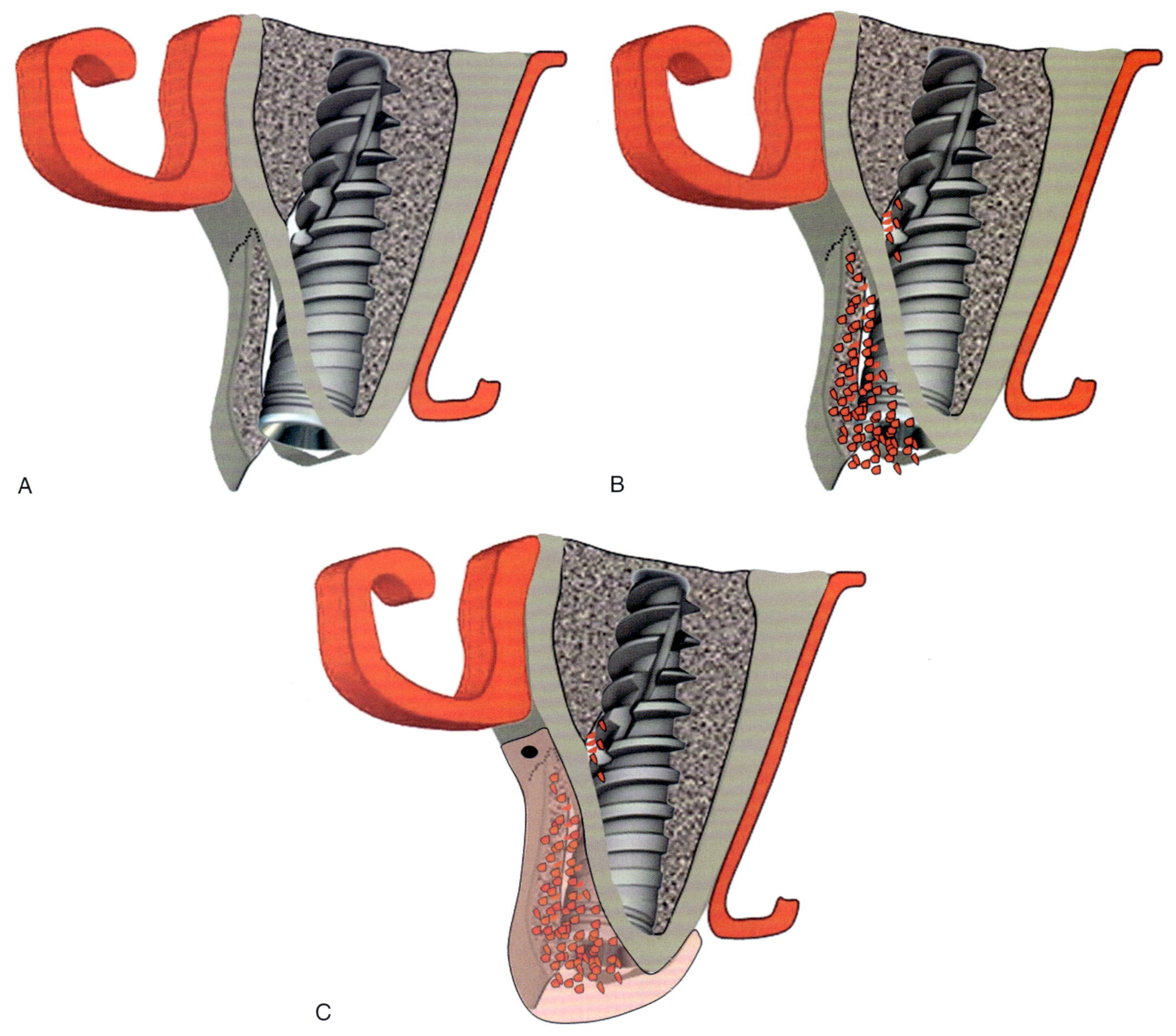

Fig 16.8 (A) Implant is inserted at the correct position; implant should preferably be submerged 1.0 mm apical to the ridge crest. (B) All the spaces between the implant and expanded cortical plates should be grafted using bone graft. (C) The grafted site should be covered using barrier collagen membrane, which can be immobilized using bone tacks.

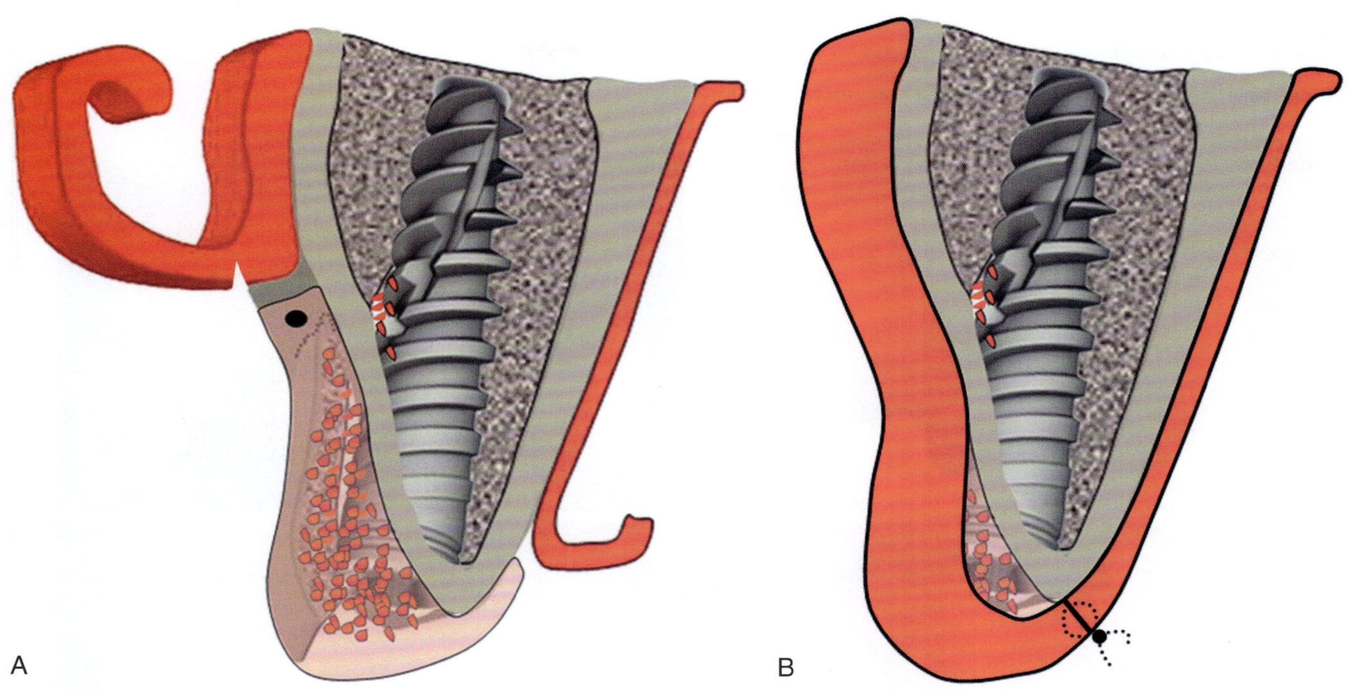

Fig 16.9 (A) Releasing incisions are made into the periosteum underneath the facial flap and (B) the flap is sutured back with primary closure. Implant should be uncovered only after a minimum of 4 months.

CASE REPORT-1

Ridge splitting with simultaneous implant placement to restore maxillary central incisors (Figs 16.10–16.12).

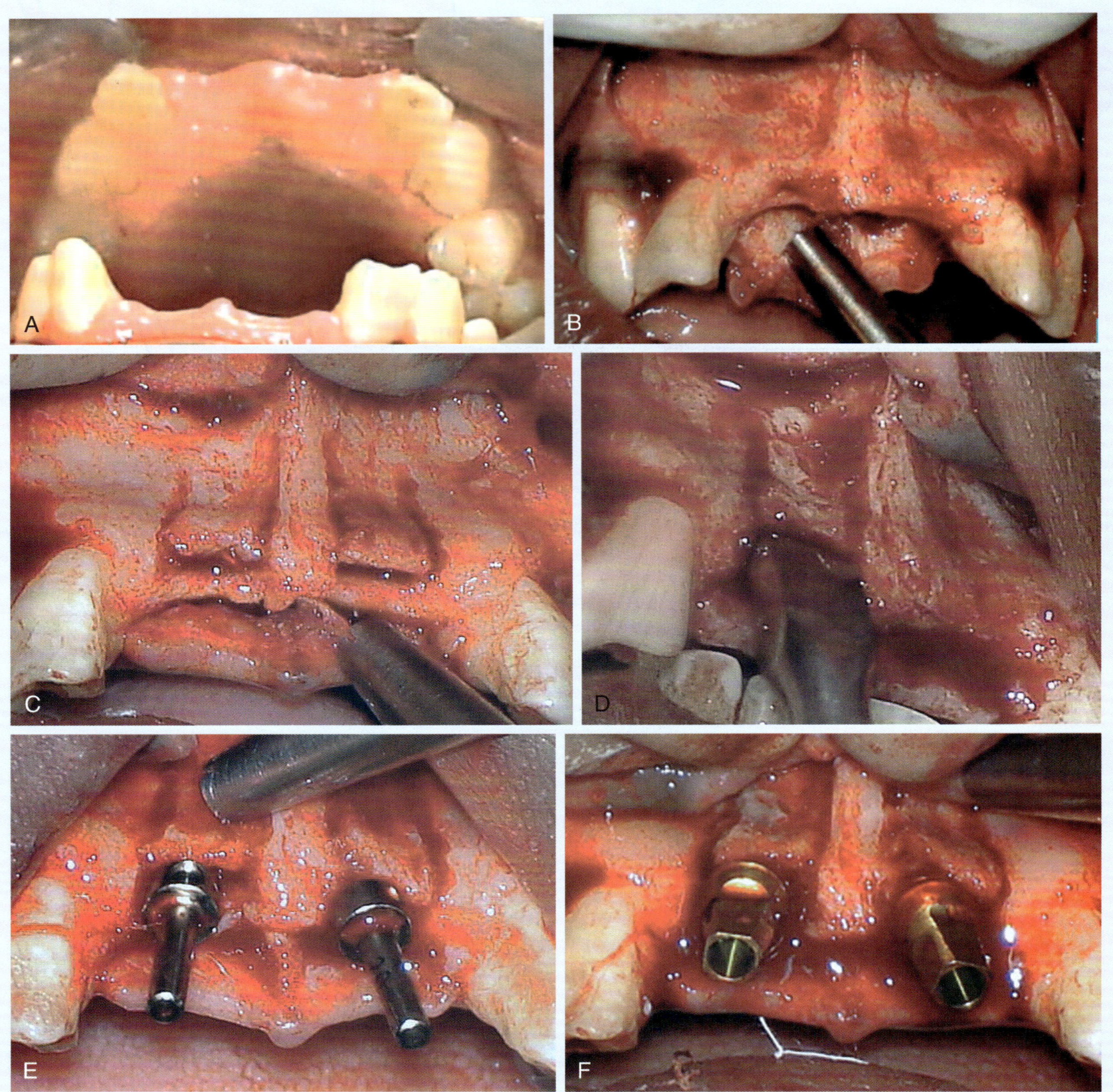

Fig 16.10 (A) Edentulous site of the missing maxillary central incisors show a labial concavity in ridge morphology, which is indicative of the possibility of inadequate bone width. (B) As can be seen after flap elevation, any attempt to place implant would result in dehiscence at the osteotomy opening or the fenestration at the facial concavity. A thin long straight fissure bur is used to make a mid-crestal horizontal cut to resect the bony trabeculae and deepen the seam. Seam should come within 2 mm of adjacent teeth, but no closer. Further, two vertical cuts are made on the labial cortical plate using sharp osseous splitters or the same bur. All cuts should be deep enough to reach the underlying cancellous bone. (C) The vertical cuts should be extended apical to the concavity at the facial bone to achieve maximum expansion without sudden fracture of the labial plate from the concavity. (D) The bone expenders used to widen the seam and pry the plates apart. (E) The osteotomy is prepared using pilot drill and parallel guide pins inserted to check the parallelism. (F) The further expansion and osteotomy preparation is done using bone spreaders and implants (3.5 x 12 mm) are inserted with adequate initial stability.

CASE REPORT-1—cont'd

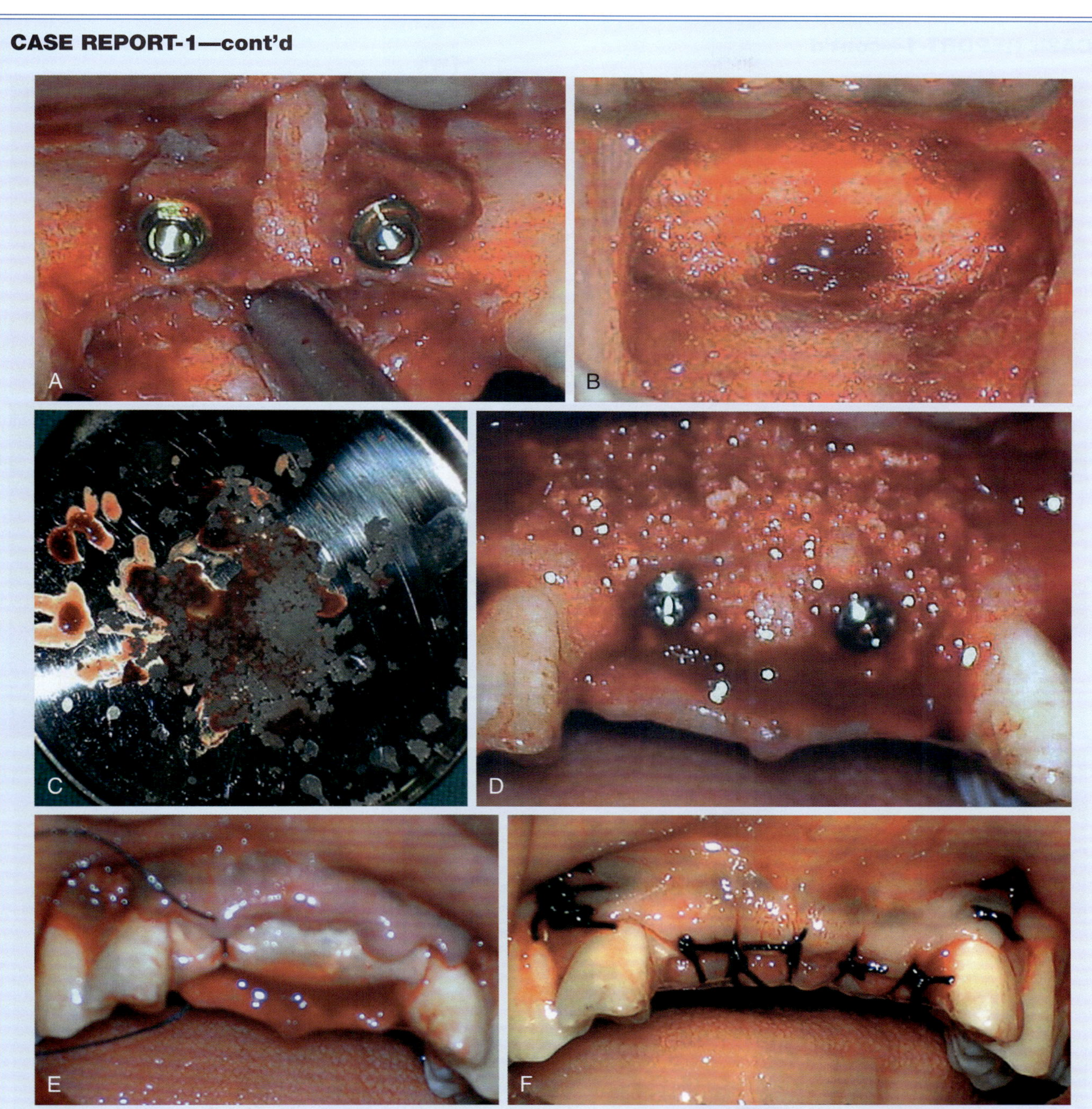

Fig 16.11 (A) The peri-implant spaces can be seen between two fully spread cortical plates which need to be grafted. (B and C) Autogenous bone is harvested from the mandibular symphysis, crushed and mixed with bovine bone material (Bio-Oss). (D) The site is grafted to fill the spaces and to reinforce the thin facial cortical plate. (E) A collagen barrier membrane is used to cover the graft. (F) Periosteum is released and the flap is sutured with primary closure.

Continued

CASE REPORT-1—cont'd

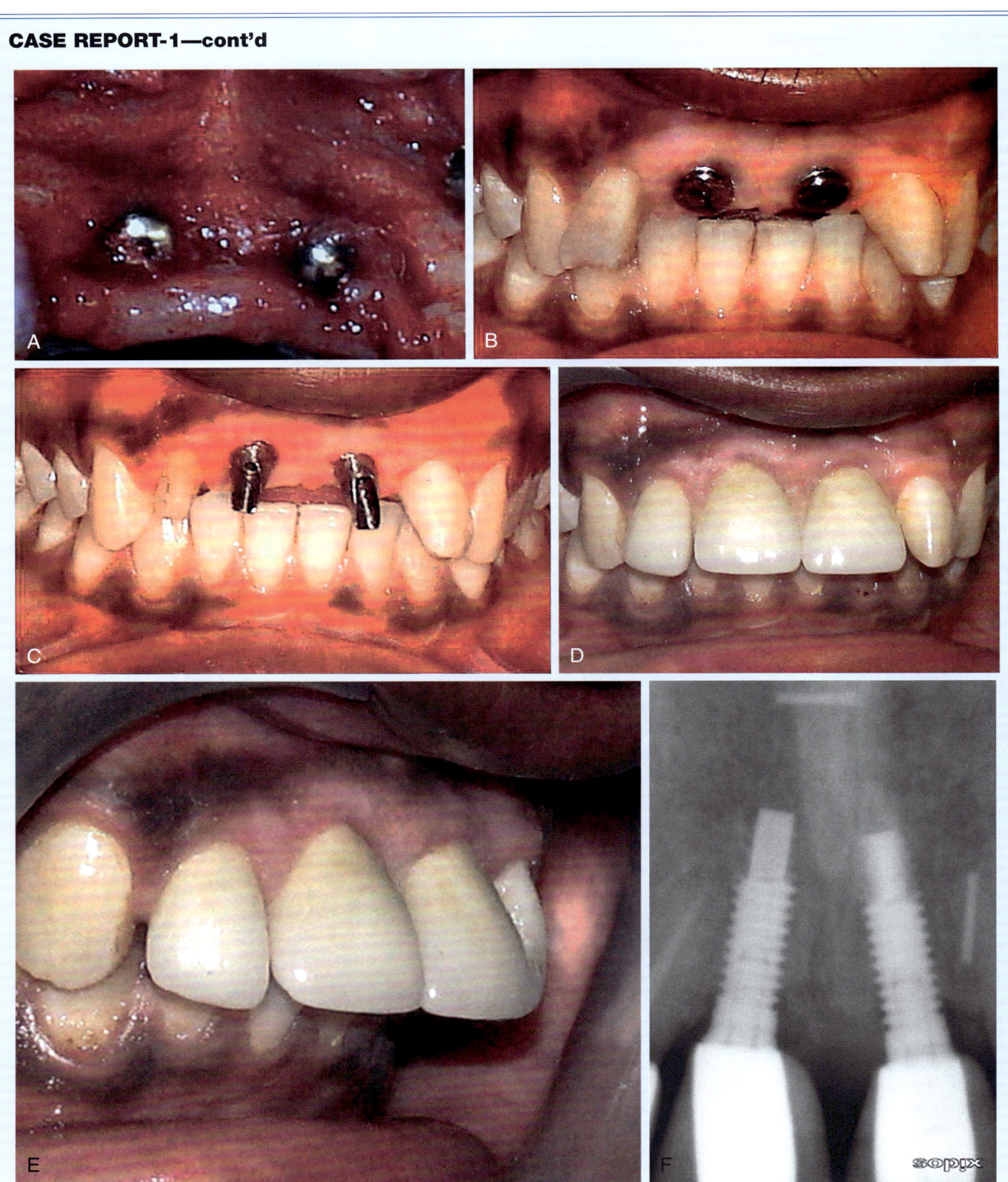

Fig 16.12 (A) Site uncovered after 4 months shows complete bone regeneration. (B) The gingival formers are in place. (C) The final abutments are in place. (D and E) Final prosthesis fixed over the implants shows adequate soft tissue aesthetics around the prosthesis. (F) The follow-up radiograph after 3 years shows stable crestal bone around the implants.

Minimal incision techniques for ridge splitting and expansion

Minimal incision techniques for ridge splitting and expansion can be performed in selective cases using appropriate armamentarium and skills.

Ridge splitting in the ridge with class 2 ridge morphology (thin ridge crest without any facial concavity)

The ridge with the class 2 ridge morphology is the most appropriate ridge for the ridge splitting procedure because

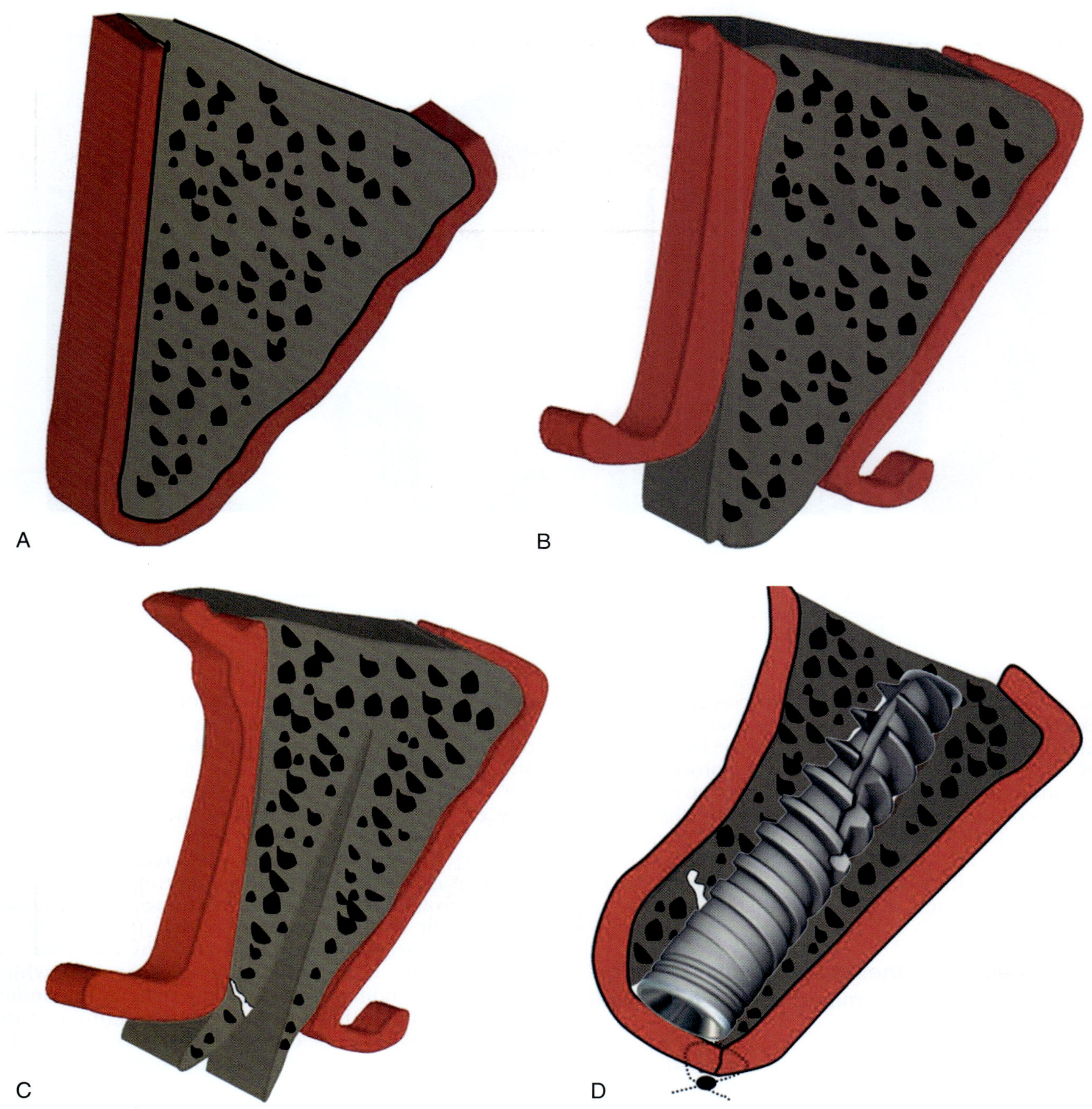

Fig 16.13 (A) Cross-sectional 3D view of the anterior maxillary ridge with inadequate crestal bone width but without any severe undercut in ridge morphology (class 2 ridge morphology). (B) A mid-crestal incision is made and flaps are minimally elevated only to expose the ridge crest. A mid-crestal cut is made and deepened to several millimetres using the piezo saw or sharp thin and long straight fissure bur. (C) Ridge splitters are then used to split and expand the narrow ridge crest. (D) Once the narrow ridge crest has been adequately expanded, the osteotomy is prepared in usual fashion using drills, and the implant is inserted.

CASE REPORT-2

Ridge splitting and expansion of class 2 ridge using piezotome and ridge splitters (Figs 16.14–16.16).

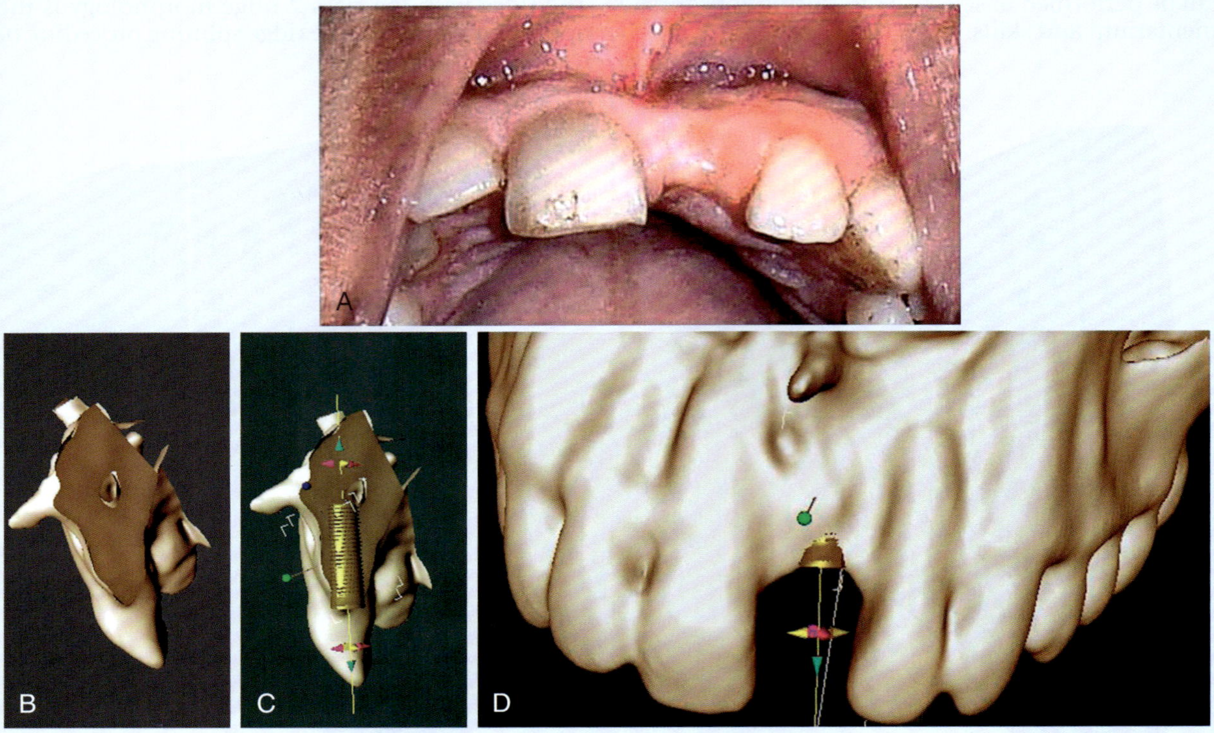

Fig 16.14 (A) Preoperative clinical view of missing tooth number 21 shows the narrow ridge crest. (B) Cross-sectional 3D view of dental CT scan showing inadequate bone width at the ridge crest. (C and D) Implant insertion without ridge splitting or lateral bone augmentation procedure may result in dehiscence at the crestal region and subsequent implant thread exposure.

the ridge widens faciopalatally as it proceeds apically. This results in minimum chances of ridge perforation during implant drilling or sudden fracture of the facial plate during the ridge splitting and expansion procedure. Thus, minimum flap elevation is required if ridge expansion is being performed without vertical cuts along the facial cortical plate. Only the crestal part of the ridge is expanded in such cases to accommodate the implant platform within the ridge crest dimensions and in most of such cases bone grafting is not required (Fig 16.13A–D).

Ridge splitting in the ridge with class 4 ridge morphology (compromised crestal bone width with facial concavity)

Such type of ridges are known to be a little difficult for the performance of the ridge splitting procedure because a severe undercut can be found along the facial aspect of the ridge, which may cause the sudden fracture of the facial cortical plate during ridge splitting and expansion. The dehiscence of the ridge through the facial cortical plate and subsequent implant surface exposure may also result in the undercut region. Thus the best way of dealing with such cases is ridge splitting and expansion of the ridge crest with the minimal flap elevation, followed by grafting of the undercut region with the subperiosteal tunnelling technique. The benefit of this approach is that the periosteum remains intact with the facial plate in the undercut region during ridge splitting and expansion, which prevents the sudden fracture of the plate at the undercut region. Other benefits are that the grafting of the undercut region can be done with a minimally invasive approach and there is no need to use barrier membrane (Figs 16.17–16.19).

CASE REPORT-2—cont'd

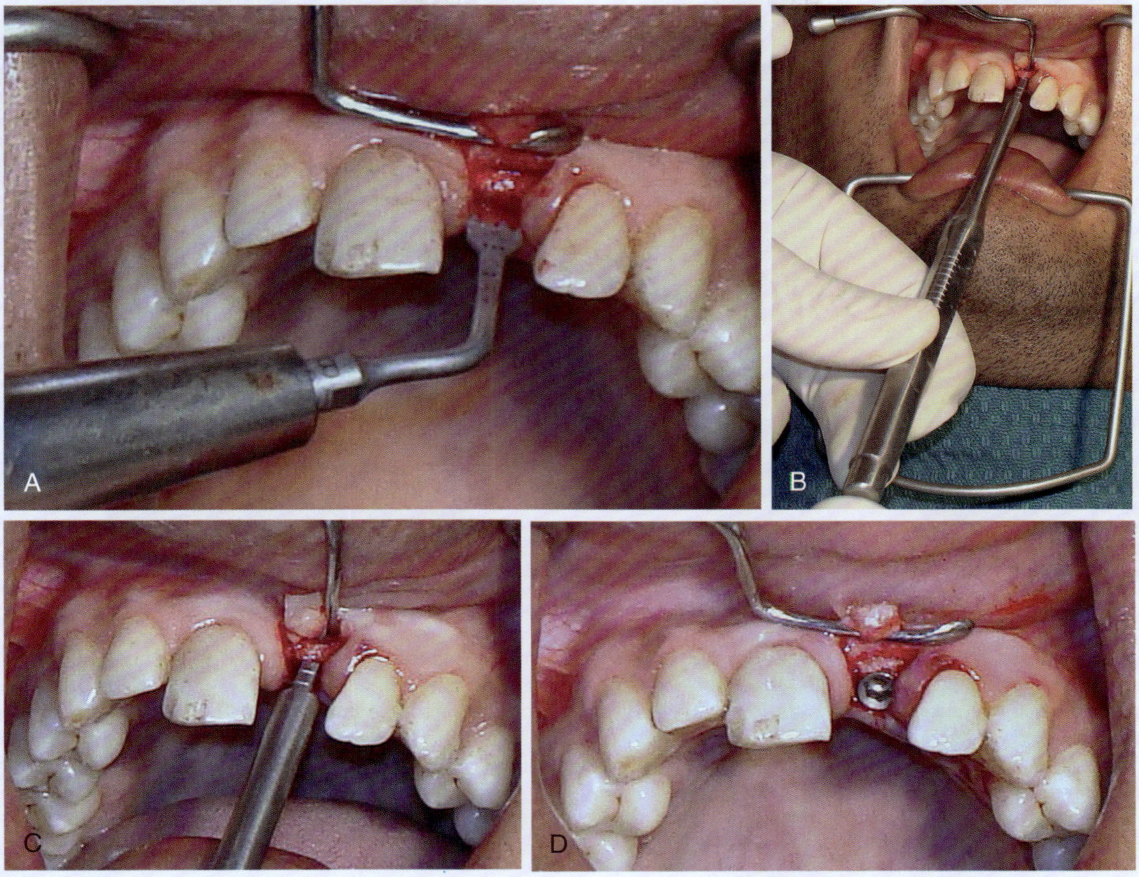

Fig 16.15 The papilla preservation incision is made and a small flap is elevated only to expose the ridge crest. (A) A mid-crestal cut is made and deepened to several millimetres using the piezo saw. (B and C) The ridge splitters are then used to split and expand the narrow ridge crest. (D) Once the narrow ridge crest has been expanded, the osteotomy is prepared using drills and the implant is inserted.

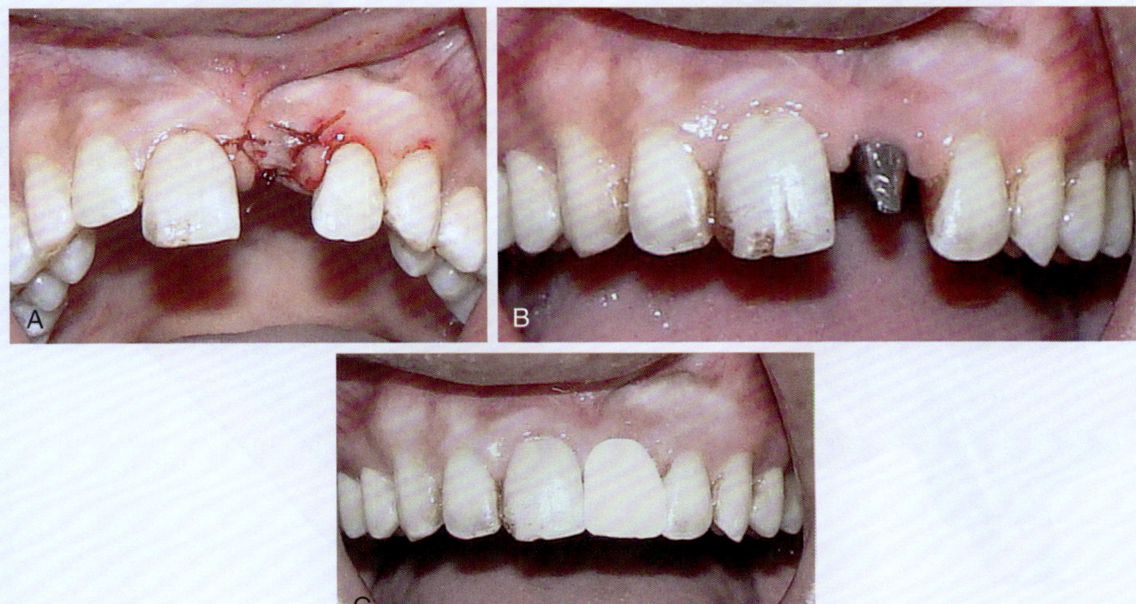

Fig 16.16 (A) As there were no peri-implant spaces to graft, the flap is sutured back without using any graft and membrane. (B and C) Implant is uncovered and restored after 3 months.

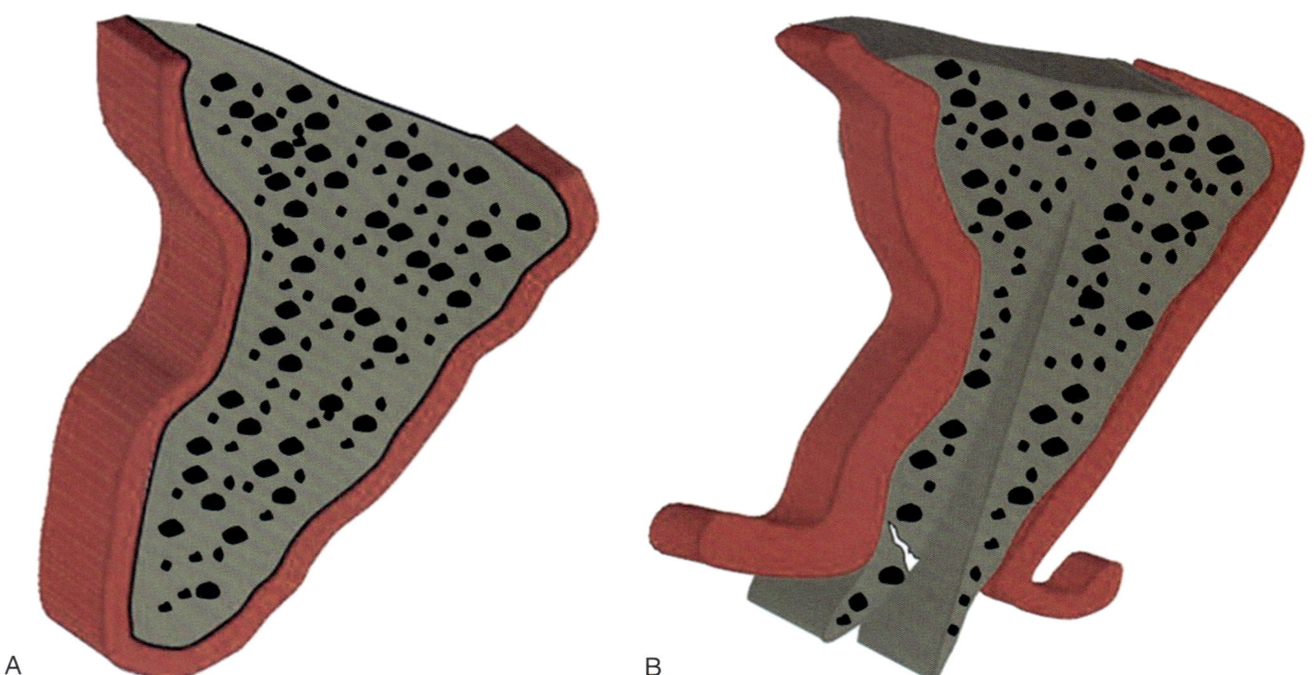

Fig 16.17 (A) Cross-sectional 3D view of the anterior maxillary bone shows compromised crestal bone width and severe facial undercut. Any attempt to place implant may lead to dehiscence of the facial bone at the crestal as well as at the undercut region. Ridge splitting using conventional flap technique can result in sudden and complete fracture of the facial cortical plate from the undercut area during its expansion. A mid-crestal incision is made and flaps are minimally elevated to expose only the ridge crest. A mid-crestal cut is made and deepened to several millimetres to reach beyond the facial undercut using the piezo saw or sharp thin and long straight fissure bur. (B) The ridge splitters are used to split and expand the narrow ridge crest only.

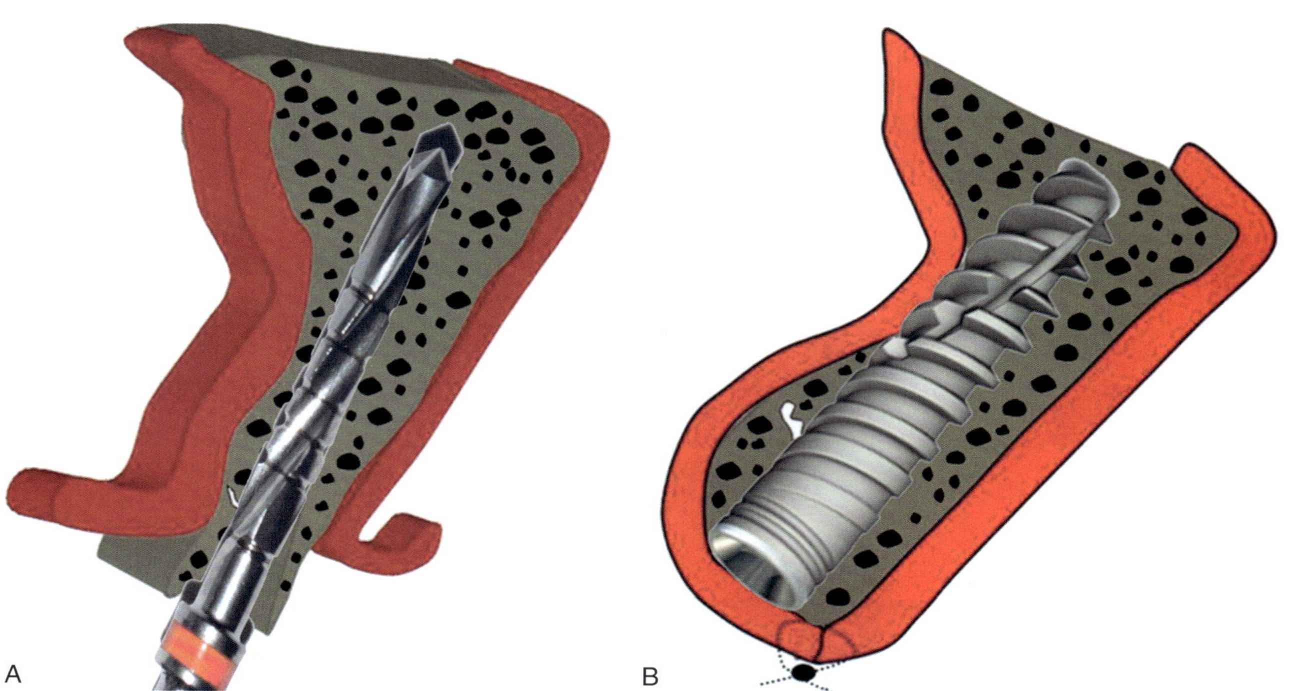

Fig 16.18 (A) Once the narrow ridge crest is expanded, implant osteotomy is prepared in the usual fashion using drills. (B) Implant is inserted and flaps are sutured back. Implant insertion may either cause the dehiscence or thinning of the facial bone which may resorb later at the facial concavity. Hence, it needs to be grafted.

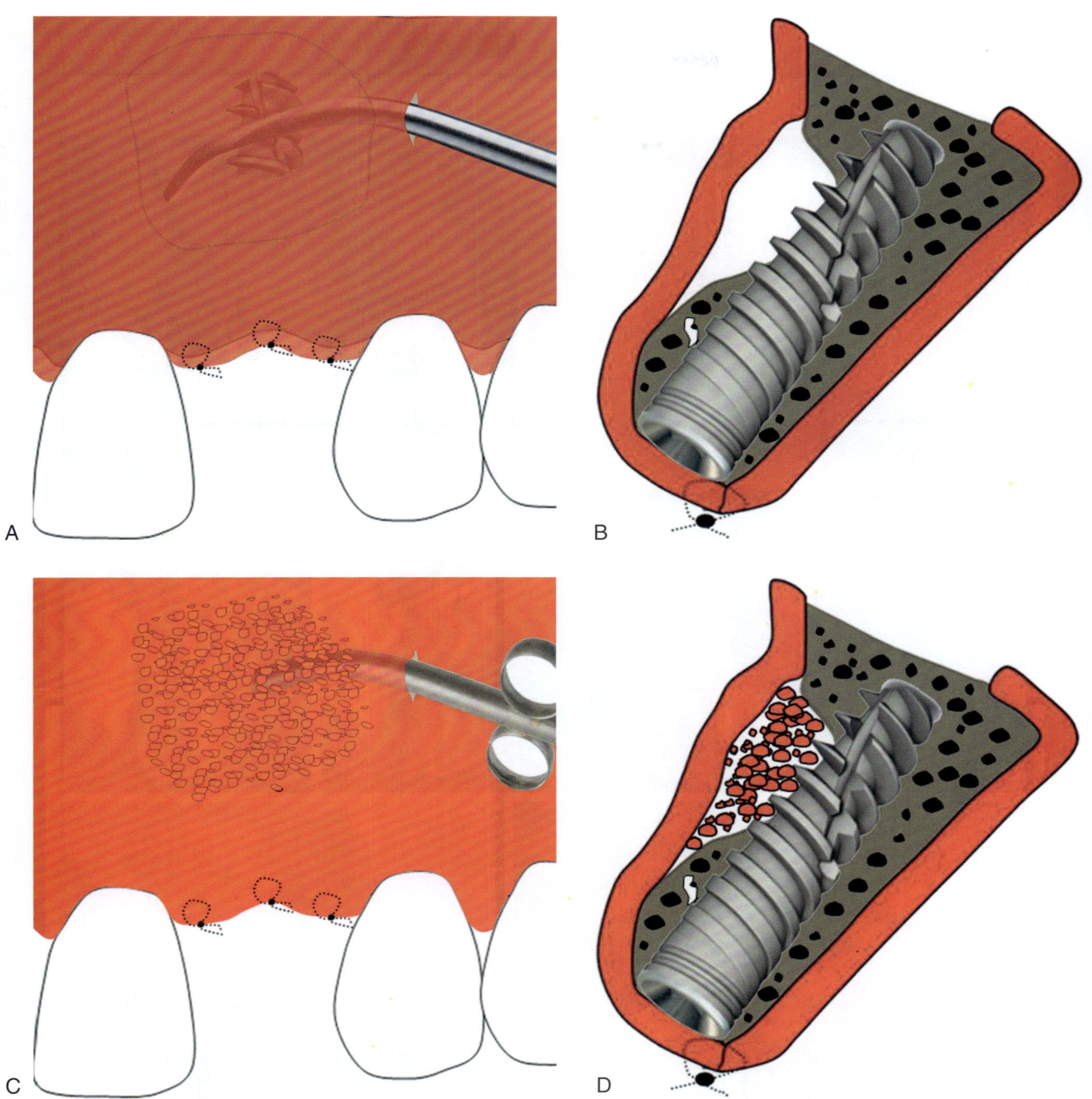

Fig 16.19 (A and B) A small vertical incision is made at a distant position and the periosteum is elevated at the undercut area with subperiosteal tunnelling technique. (C and D) The site is grafted through the tunnel and the incision line is sutured.

CASE REPORT-3

Ridge splitting, implant placement, and simultaneous lateral bone grafting in the class 4 ridge (Figs 16.20–16.25).

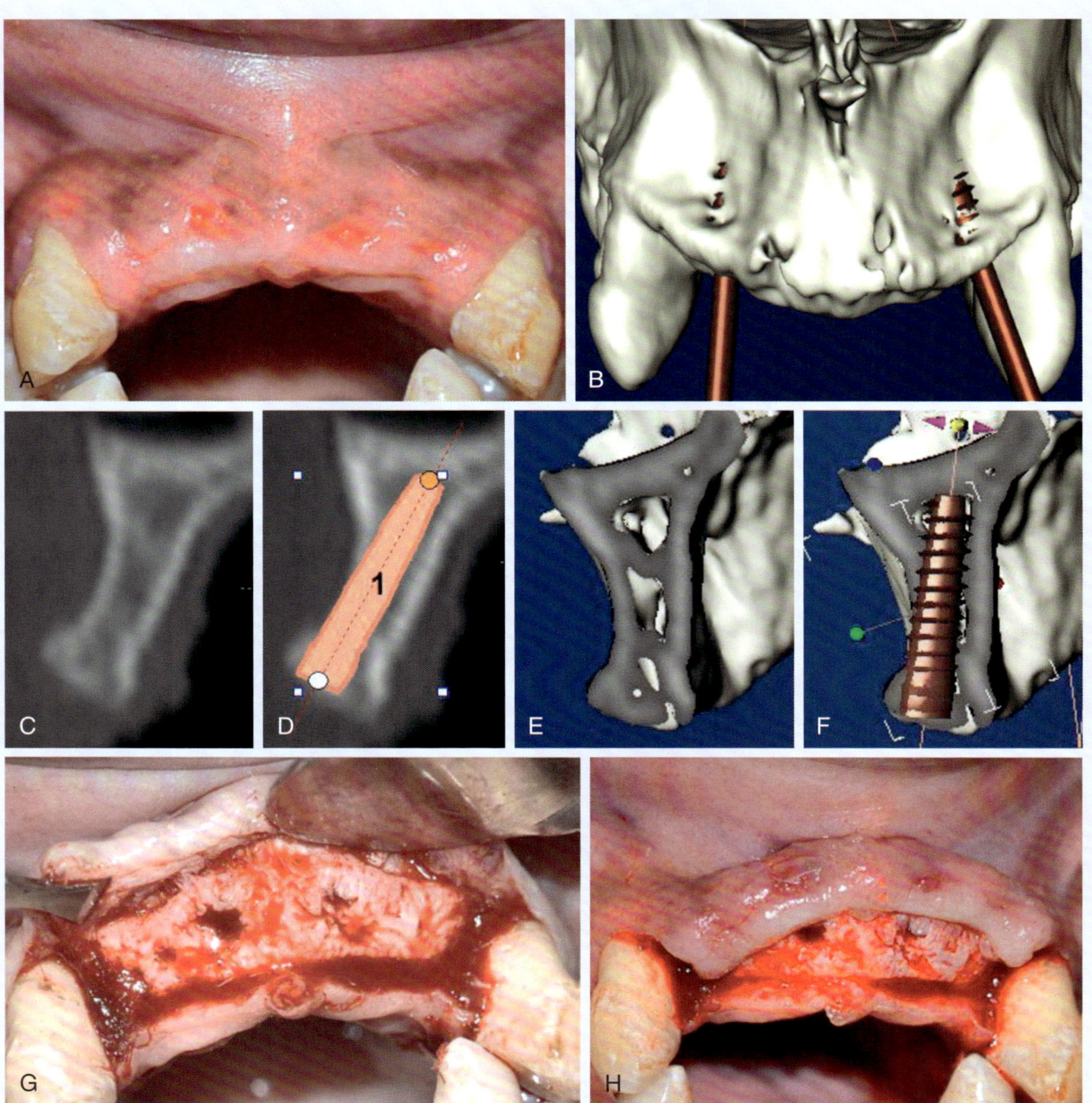

Fig 16.20 (A) Clinical view of edentulous maxillary anterior region, a 4-unit bridge supported by two implants is planned. (B–F) The 3D and cross-sectional views of the dental CT scan are showing facial undercuts (concavities) in the ridge morphology; thus any attempt to place implant at the correct prosthetic axis may result in dehiscence of the facial bone at the undercut region. (G) An incision, slightly palatal, is made and the facial flap is minimally elevated to expose the ridge crest. (H) The facial periosteum should not be elevated beyond the muscle attachment to the ridge.

CASE REPORT-3—cont'd

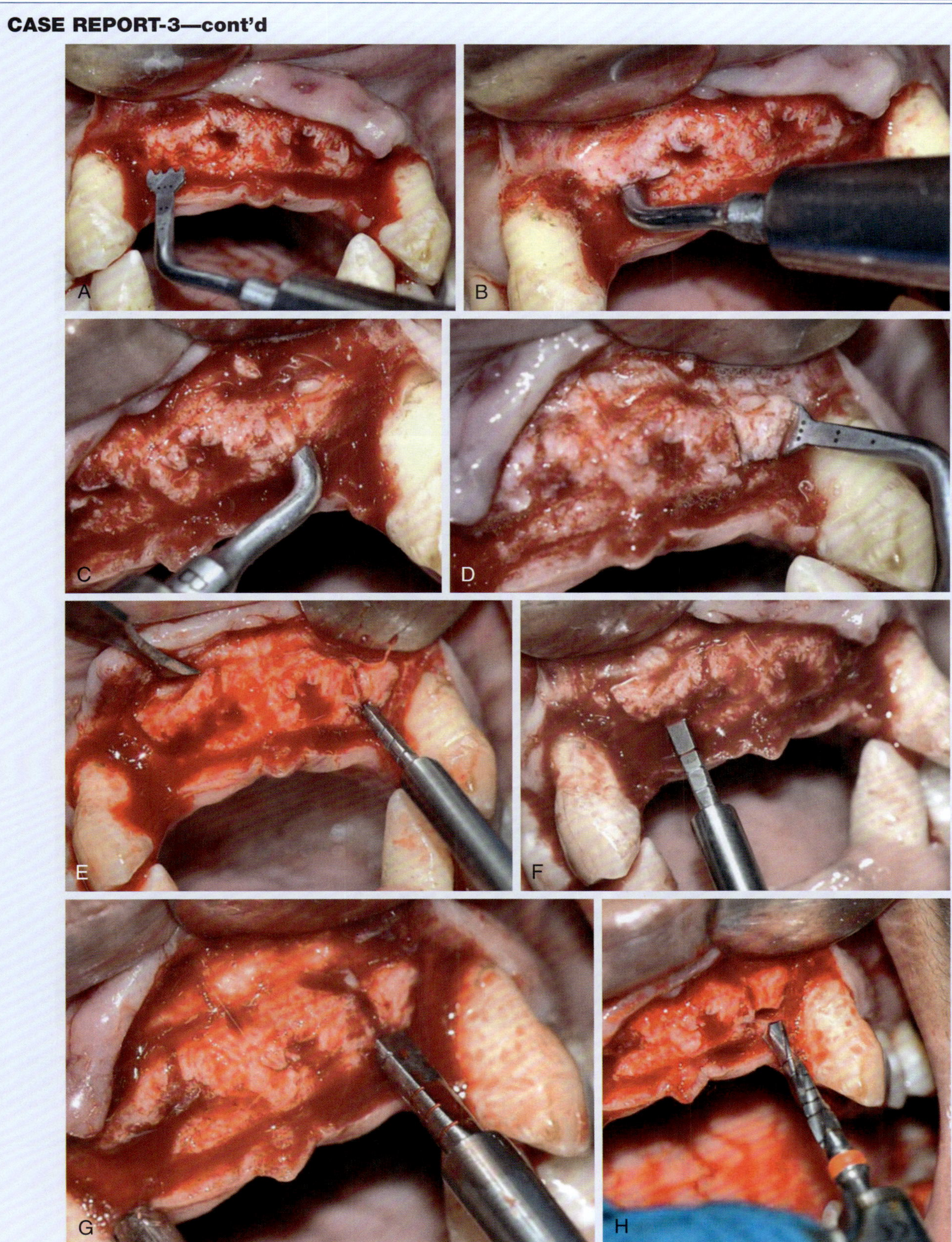

Fig 16.21 (A–C) Two separate crestal cuts are made at the planned implant sites and deepened several millimetres to reach beyond the facial undercut, using the piezo saw. (D) Two small vertical cuts are also made on the labial side of the ridge crest using the same saw. (E–G) The ridge splitters are then used to split and expand the narrow ridge crest. (H) After the ridge crest has been adequately expanded, the osteotomy is prepared using drills to the planned depth.

Continued

CASE REPORT-3—cont'd

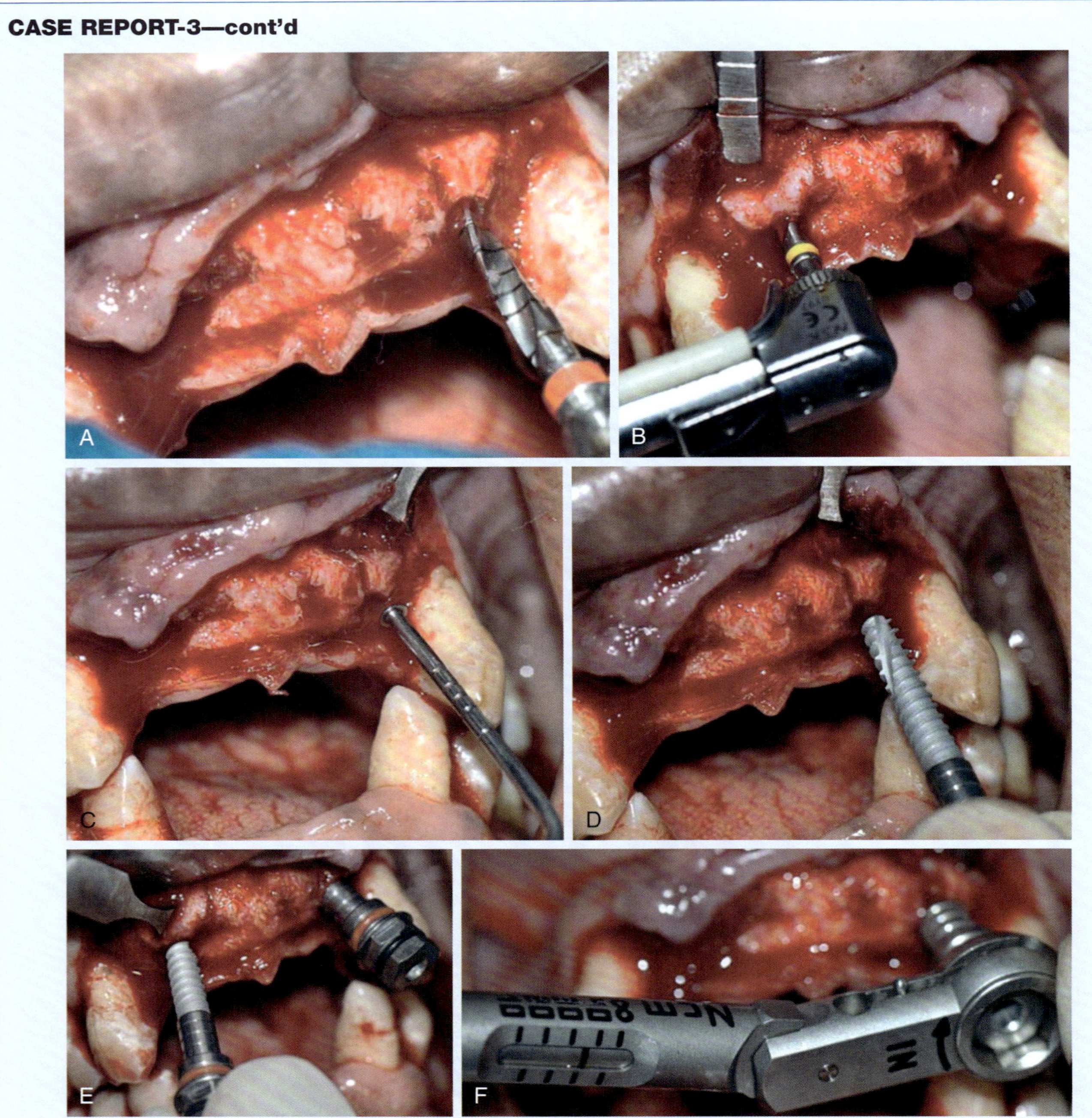

Fig 16.22 (A and B) The expanded labial cortical plate should be supported with the finger or any instrument even during implant osteotomy preparation to prevent its sudden fracture. (C) Once the implant osteotomy is completed, a special probe (DGI probe) can be used to evaluate any labial dehiscence. (D and E) Again, the expanded labial cortical plate should be supported with any instrument during implant insertion to avoid sudden fracture. (F) Implant stability can be checked using the torque ratchet, which reached up to 35 Ncm in this case.

CASE REPORT-3—cont'd

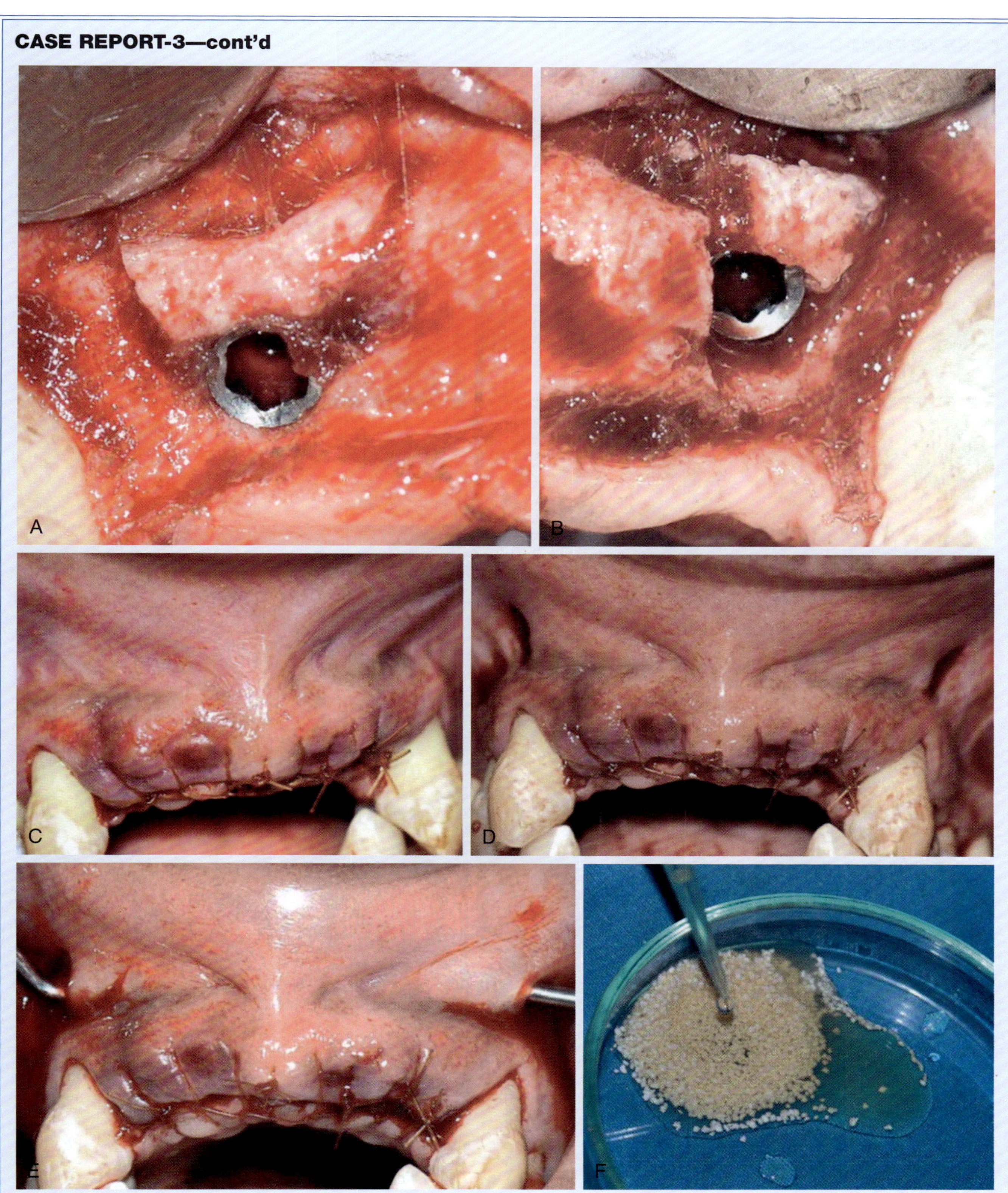

Fig 16.23 (A and B) Inserted implants at their final positions. (C) Flap is sutured back with watertight primary closure, (D) two small vertical incisions are made at distant locations on the labial mucosa and (E) the periosteum is elevated from the facial concavities with the subperiosteal tunnelling technique. (F) The small particle sized synthetic hydroxyapatite graft is mixed with PRGF (plasma rich in growth factors) prepared from the patient's venous blood. The PRGF not only enhances the new bone regeneration potential of the graft material but also enhances the handling properties of the graft, as it acts like a glue to bond the graft particles together and prevent their dispersion from the grafted site.

Continued

CASE REPORT-3—cont'd

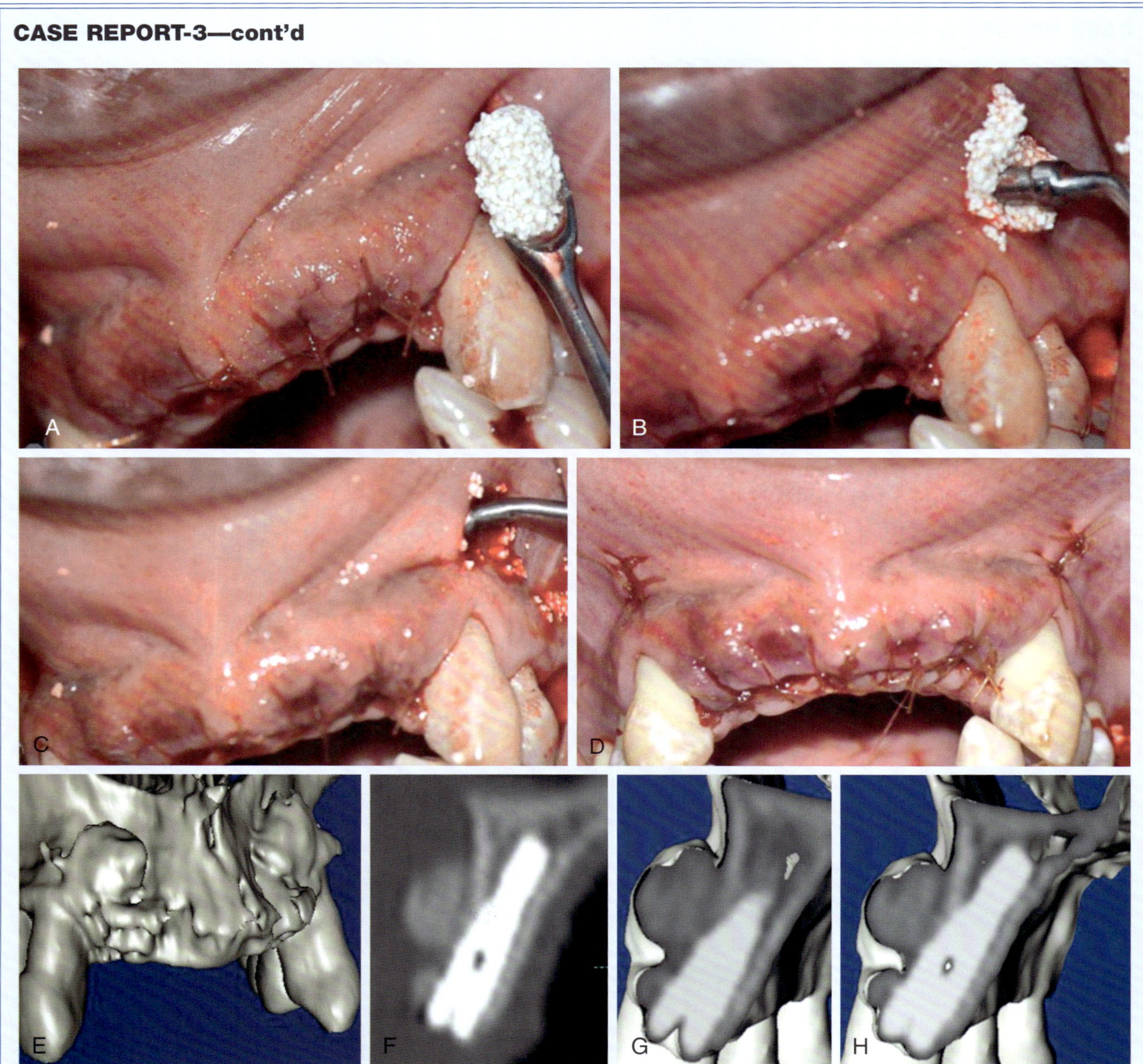

Fig 16.24 (A–D) Both the facial concavities are grafted by carrying the bone graft through the subperiosteal tunnels, and incision sites are sutured. (E–H) The islands of the new bone formation on the facial aspect of the inserted implants can be seen in the dental CT scan 4 months after implant insertion.

CASE REPORT-3—cont'd

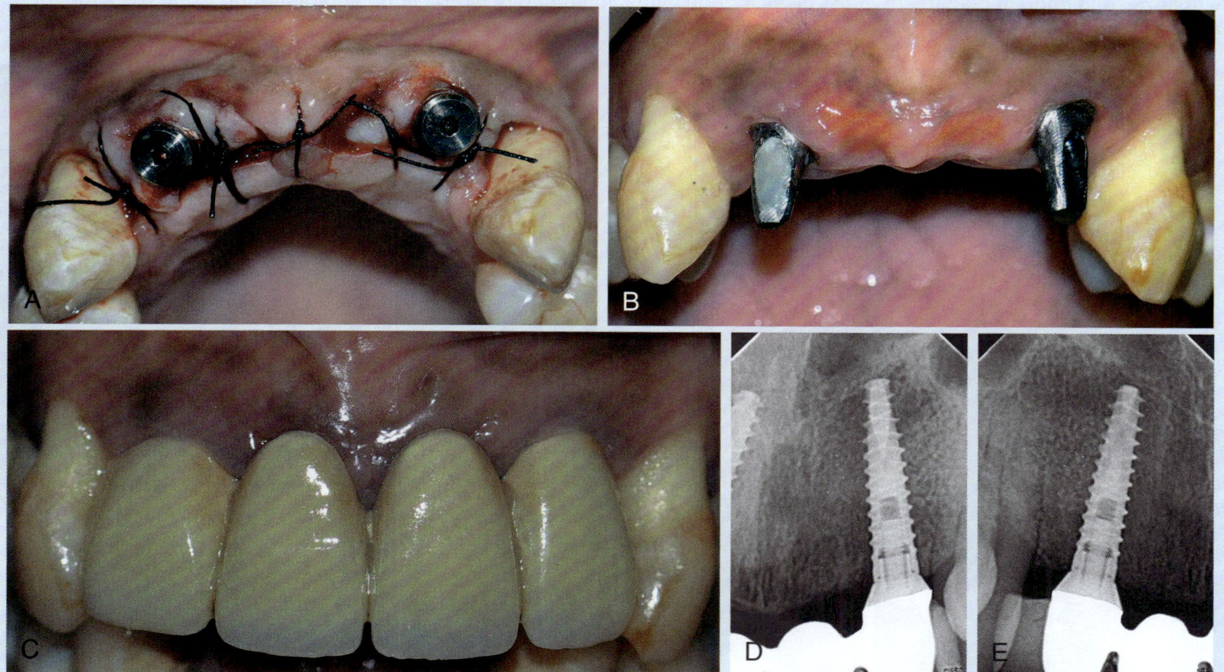

Fig 16.25 (A) Implants are uncovered after 4 months and (B and C) restored using a 4-unit ceramic bridge. The desired aesthetic and functional results have been achieved. The graft has been consolidated and has taken an aesthetic shape so that the facial concavities are not visible now. This has enhanced the soft tissue aesthetics apical to the restoration. (D and E) The radiographs taken 11 months after final restoration show stable bone at the crest.

CASE REPORT-4

Ridge splitting and implant placement in the class 4 ridge with simultaneous lateral bone augmentation using the subperiosteal tunnelling technique (Figs 16.26–16.28).

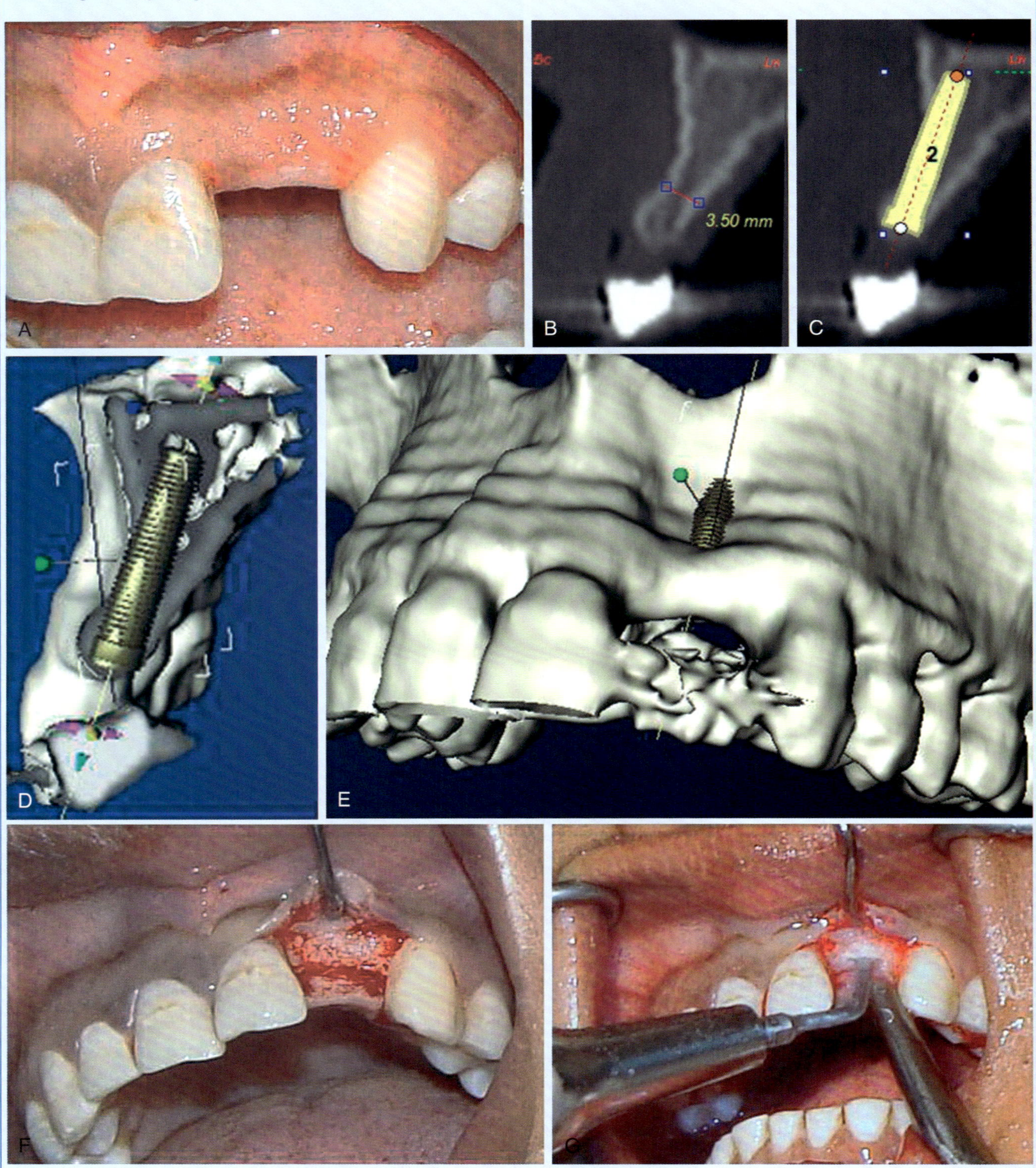

Fig 16.26 (A) Missing tooth number 22. Three-dimensional and cross-sectional views of the dental CT scan show severe facial concavity in the ridge morphology, and (B–E) any attempt to place implant may lead to dehiscence of the facial bone at the undercut region. (F) An incision, slightly palatal, is made and the facial flap is minimally elevated to expose only the ridge crest. (G) A piezo saw is used to make a small mid-crestal horizontal cut deep enough to reach apical to the facial concavity.

CASE REPORT-4—cont'd

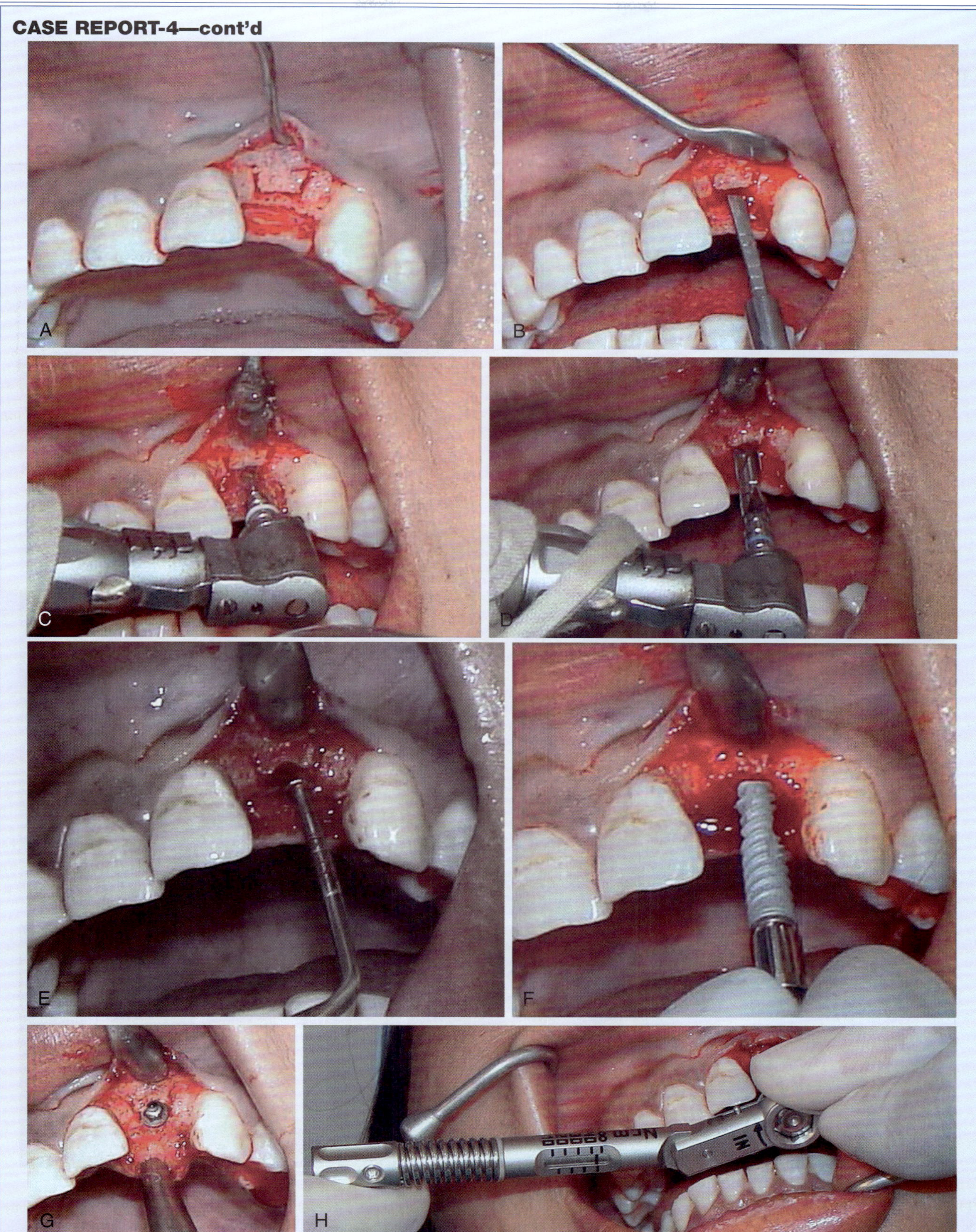

Fig 16.27 (A) Two small vertical cuts are made at the facial ridge contour and (B) ridge splitters are then used to split and expand the facial plate at the crestal region. (C and D) After achieving adequate ridge expansion, the osteotomy is prepared, using drills. (E) A dehiscence at the facial concavity is clearly evaluated using a depth probe and (F and G) the implant is inserted. (H) The initial stability of the implant is checked using the torque ratchet, which has reached to more than 35 Ncm.

Continued

CASE REPORT-4—cont'd

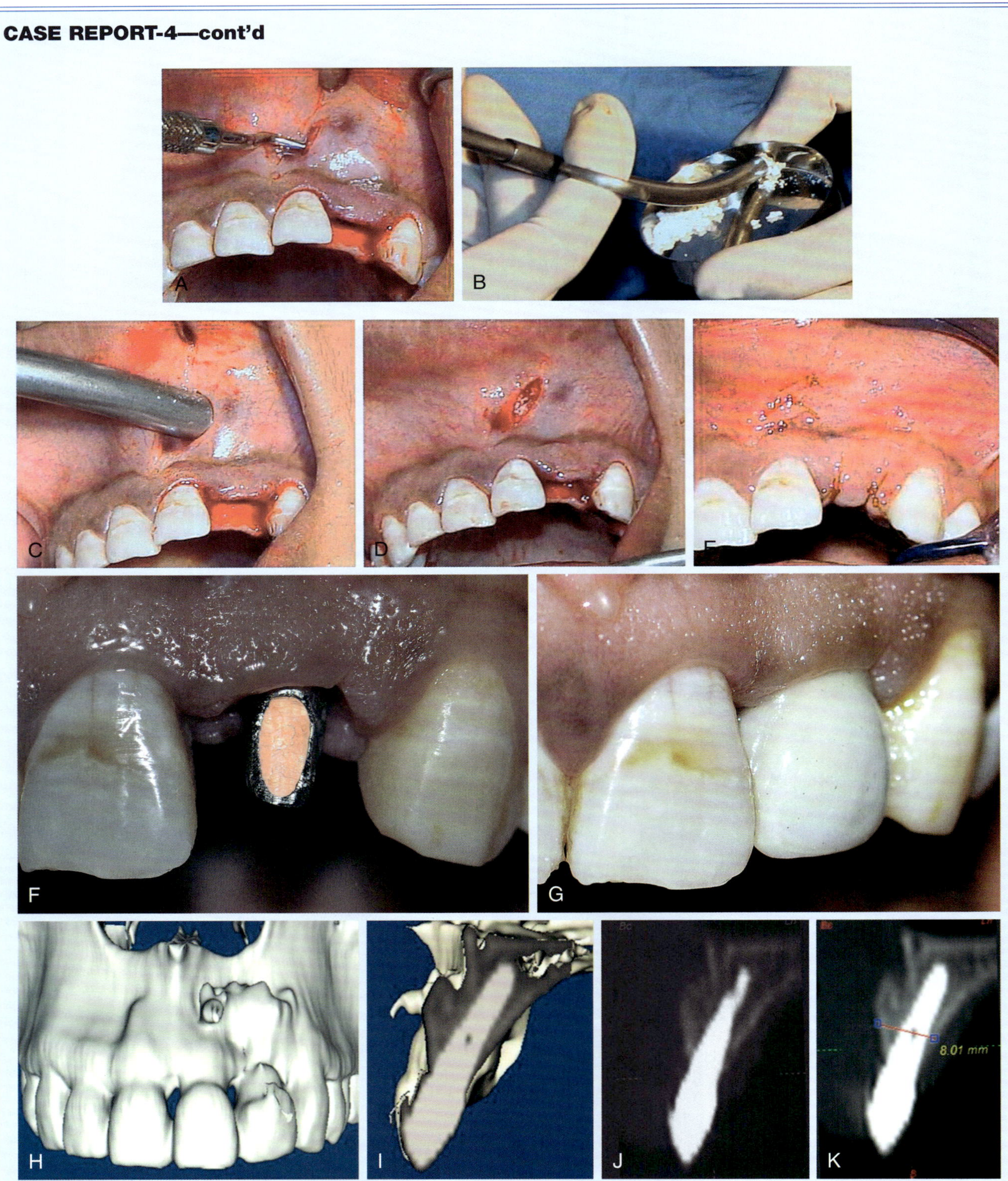

Fig 16.28 (A–E) A small vertical incision is made through the facial mucosa at a distant location and the periosteum from the facial concavity is elevated through subperiosteal tunnelling to create a subperiosteal pouch. Bone substitute (HA + β-TCP) mixed with platelet-rich plasma is deposited at the concavity and incision lines are sutured. (F and G) The implant is uncovered and restored after 4 months. (H–K) Postloading CT images are showing an island of new bone formation over the dehiscence site.

Ridge splitting and expansion in the posterior maxilla

Reduced subantral bone height due to vertical resorption of the long-time edentulous posterior maxilla and the pneumatization of the maxillary sinus are very common complaints and have successfully been treated with the sinus grafting procedures. As the maxilla resorbs towards the hard palate, the resorbed maxillary posterior ridge is often found inadequate in width to insert the regular diameter implant. The osteoplasty of the vertically resorbed narrow ridge further increases the height of the implant prosthesis and hence often needs ridge splitting and expansion to insert a regular diameter implant at the correct faciopalatal position (Fig 16.29A–D).

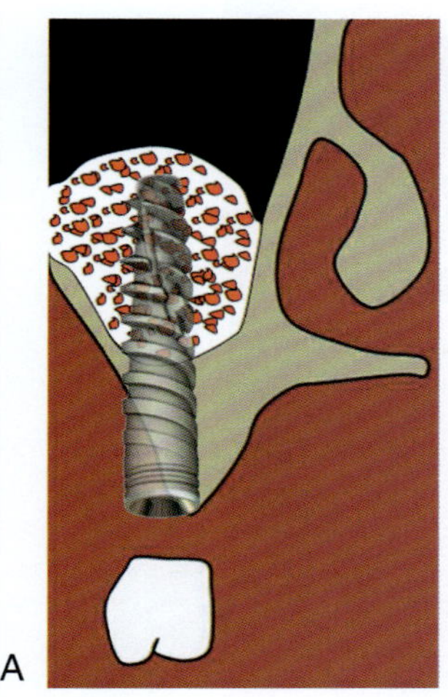

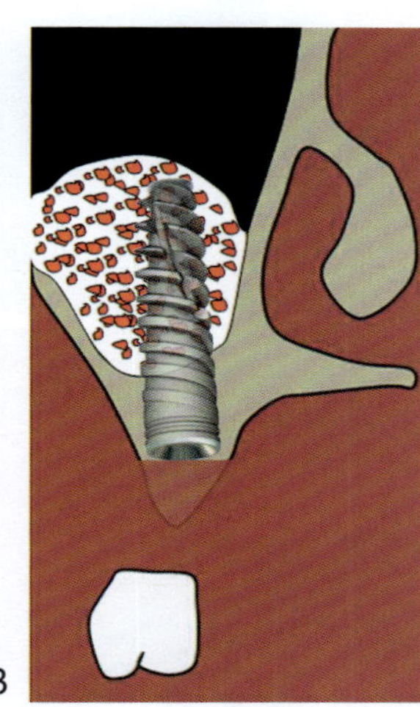

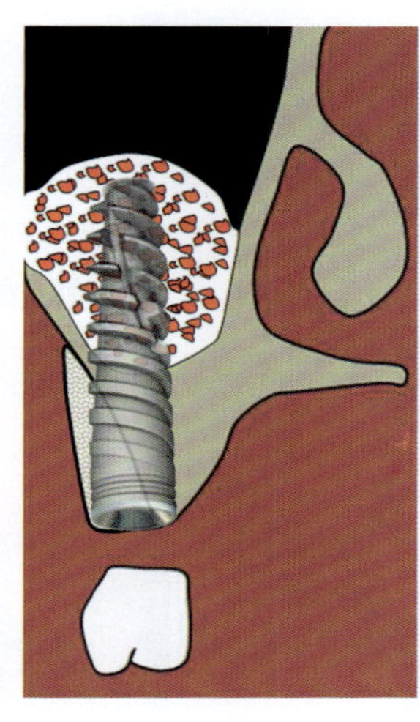

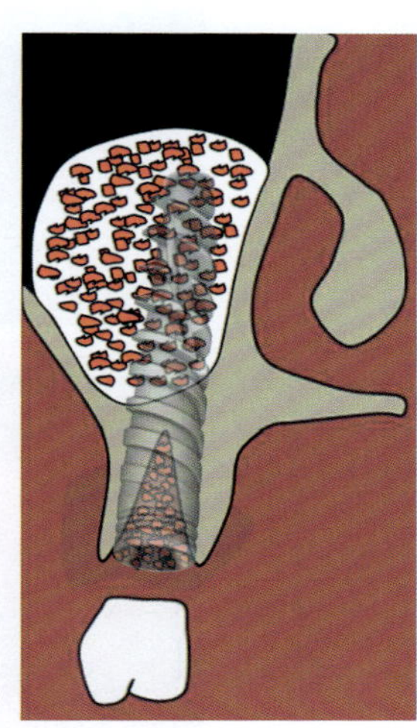

Fig 16.29 (A) Maxilla resorbed towards the hard palate, thus, placing an implant in the narrow ridge crest of posterior maxilla with sinus grafting can result in dehiscence at the facial cortical plate. (B) Vertical ridge reduction can be done at the time of implant placement surgery to obtain the desired bone width for implant placement but it can result in various problems, such as further reduction in the subantral bone height available to stabilize the implant, increase in the crown–implant ratio, and facial cantilevering of the future prosthesis. (C) Such ridge should be managed either with lateral bone augmentation using block graft during or before sinus grafting and implant insertion or (D) by ridge splitting and expansion and simultaneous implant placement.

CASE REPORT-5

Ridge splitting in the posterior maxilla along with sinus grafting and implant placement (Fig 16.30A–M).

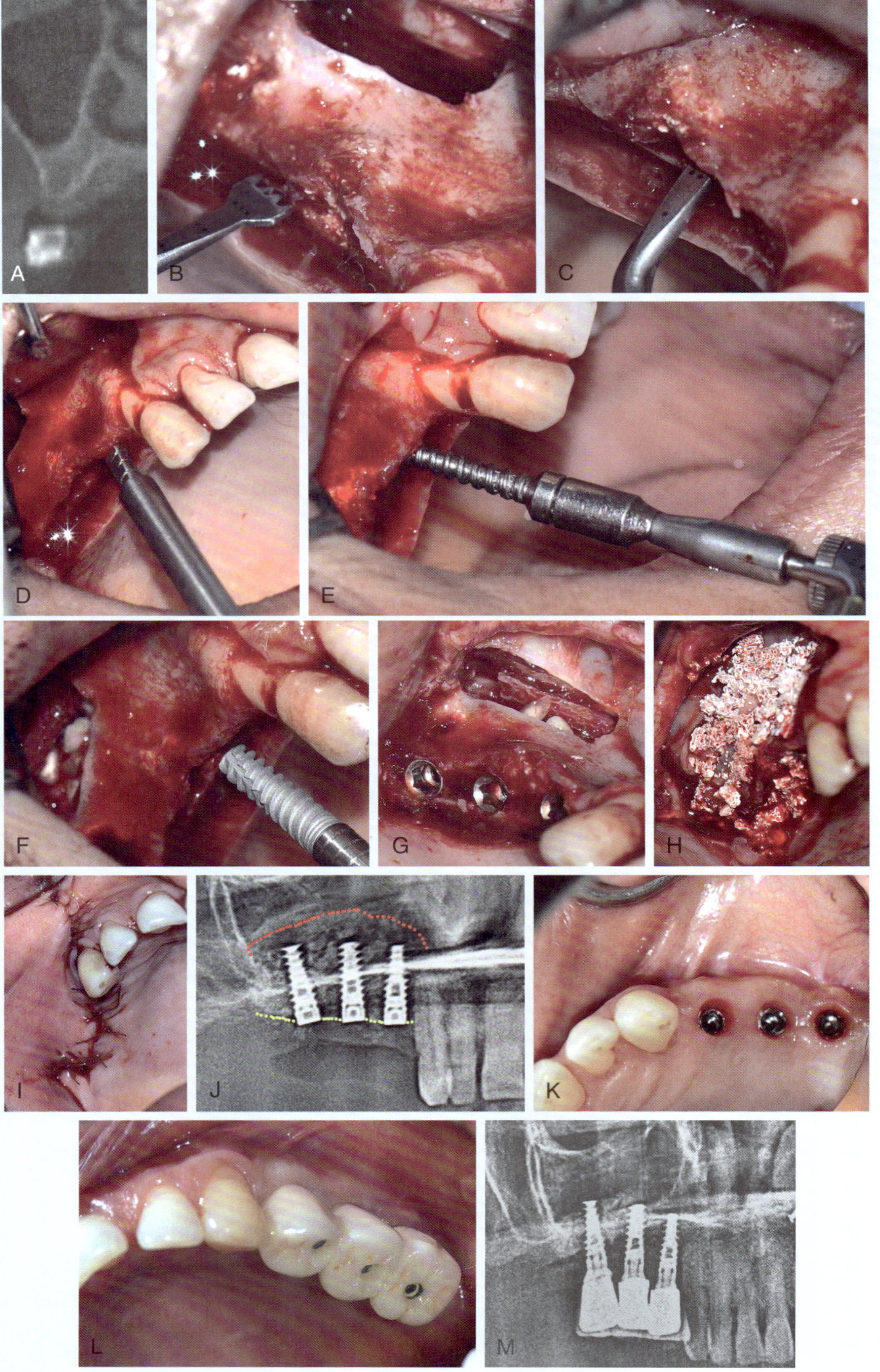

CASE REPORT-5—cont'd

Fig 16.30 (A) Cross-sectional CT view of the posterior maxilla shows narrow ridge crest and reduced subantral bone height. (B and C) Sinus elevation is performed with the lateral window approach and a piezo saw is used to make a deep mid-crestal cut. (D) The ridge splitters are sequentially used to split and pry the cortical plates apart. (E) A rotary ridge expander is used for further expansion of the plates. (F) The elevated sinus floor is grafted using allografts mixed with autogenous bone and three regular diameter self-tapping implants are inserted. (G) All the implants at their final positions. (H) The peri-implant spaces between two expanded cortical plates are grafted and the some amount of graft is also deposited on the facial aspect to reinforce the thin facial plate. (I) The flap is sutured back to achieve a watertight primary closure. (J) Postimplantation radiograph shows ideal implant insertions and grafted sinus. (K and L) Implants are uncovered 6 months after the implant placement surgery and soft tissue grafting is performed to further enhance the soft tissue emergence for implant restoration. (M) Postloading radiograph. The implants have been in function for more than one-and-half years without any noticeable crestal bone resorption.

CASE REPORT-6

Ridge split of the complete maxillary arch for full-arch implant-supported restoration (Fig 16.31A–F).

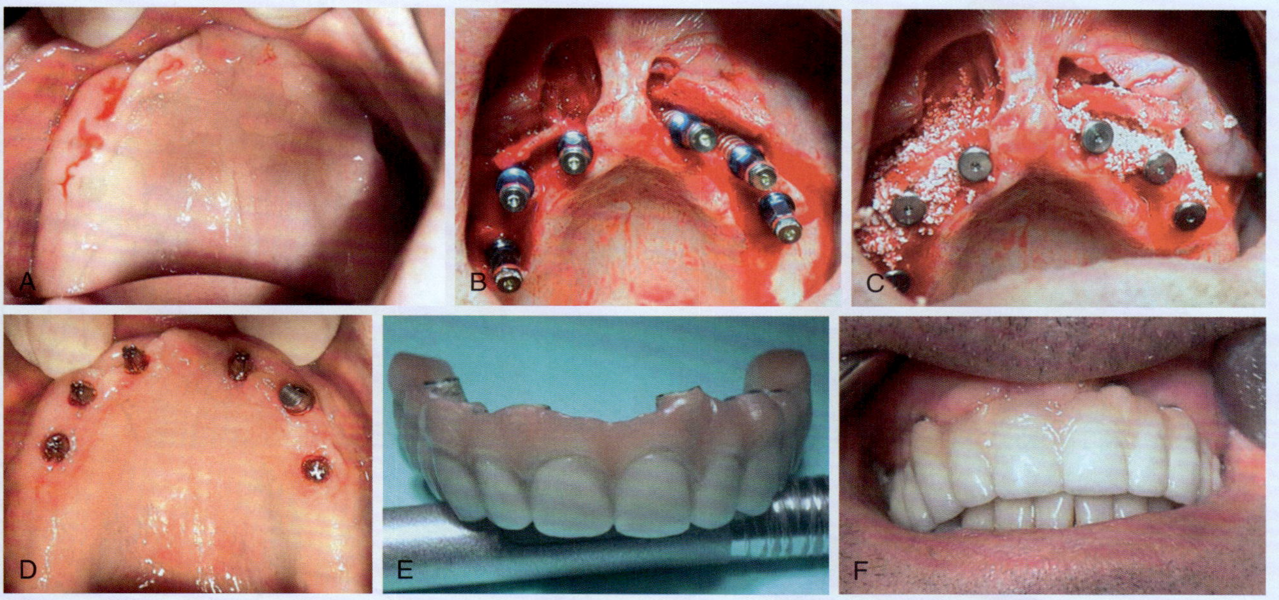

Fig 16.31 (A) The edentulous maxillary ridge, which shows the narrow ridge morphology. (B) Multiple ridge splits are performed and six implants are inserted. (C) All the peri-implant spaces are filled using bone graft. (D–F) Implants are uncovered after 6 months using the tissue punch and restored using fixed ceramic prosthesis.

Ridge-splitting procedure in the mandibular ridge

Due to higher bone density and the presence of thick cortical plates, ridge splitting has never been easy to perform in the mandibular ridge, but with recent advances in armamentarium and clinical skills, ridge splitting can successfully be performed, following many protocols, in the mandibular ridge. Ridge splitting in the mandibular ridge should be performed very carefully and special techniques are followed to avoid the complete split of the cortical plate. Depending on the particular case and the surgeon's skills, ridge splitting in the high density mandibular ridge can be performed with a two-stage procedure or with a single-stage procedure.

1. Two-stage technique
2. Single-stage technique

Two-stage ridge-splitting technique

In the two-stage ridge-splitting procedure, the mucoperiosteal flap is elevated to expose the ridge crest as well as the facial cortical plate and a rectangular osteotomy of planned dimensions is prepared through the ridge crest and facial cortex, similar to osteotomy preparation at the time of bone block harvesting. The osteotomy all around should be prepared deep enough to reach the underlying spongiosa. The flap is sutured back and site is left to heal for 3–4 weeks. In the healing period of 4 weeks, the woven bone formation occurs along the prepared osteotomy seam, which is soft and makes ridge expansion easy to perform, without sudden fracture of the facial cortex. After 4 weeks, a horizontal crestal incision, slightly facial to the mid-crest or facial to the previously prepared mid-crestal osteotomy seam is made, and the flap is elevated lingually. The facial mucoperiosteum should not be elevated as its attachment with the rectangular osteotomy prevents the sudden fracture of the facial plate during its expansion. Moreover, its continued attachment provides the necessary nourishment to the expended facial plate. After exposing the previously prepared, mid-crestal, horizontal osteotomy, ridge splitters are sequentially used to carefully split and expend the facial cortical plate. After achieving desired amount of expansion, the osteotomy of the implant is prepared and the implant of the desired dimensions is inserted. The peri-implant spaces between two cortical plates are grafted using bone substitutes and covered with the barrier membrane. The lingual flap is coronally advanced and sutured. The implants are uncovered after 4–6 months and restored.

Step by step diagrammatic presentation of the two-stage ridge-splitting procedure is shown in Figs 16.32 and 16.33.

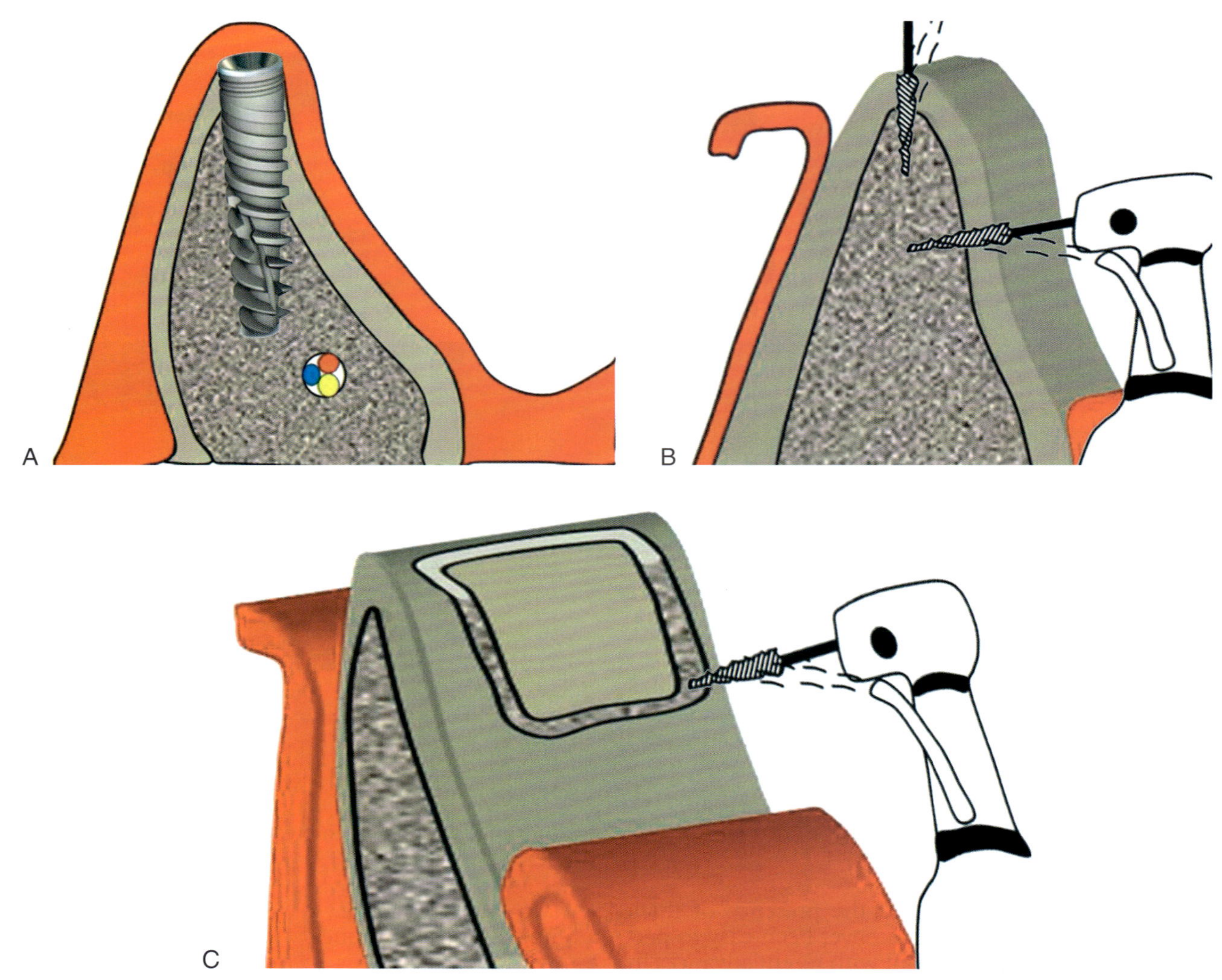

Fig 16.32 (A) Cross sectional 3D view of the posterior mandibular ridge shows inadequate bone width for ideal diameter implant placement. Buccal and lingual flaps are elevated to expose the ridge crest and facial cortical plate. (B and C) A rectangular window osteotomy is prepared using a rotary bur or the piezo saw through the ridge crest and high-density buccal cortical plate, deep enough to reach the underlying cancellous bone. The superior horizontal cut should be made mid-crestal and the inferior one at least 5–6 mm above the mandibular canal or 3–4 mm short of the apex of the future implant, so that the implant can be engaged apically in 3–4 mm of unsplit bone and chances of any nerve injuries are avoided. Two thin vertical osteotomies are prepared at the planned position depending on the planned future implant position.

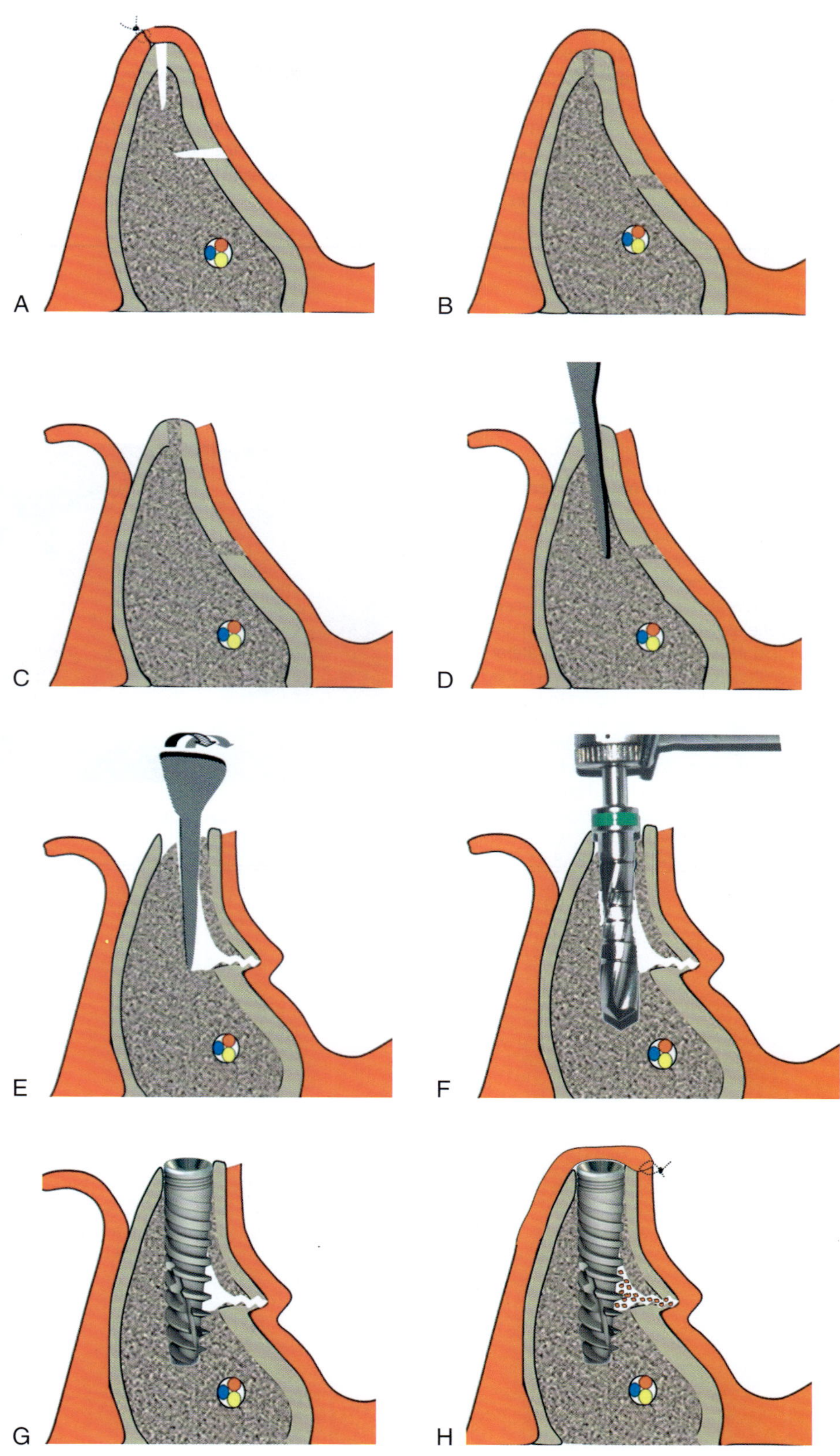

Fig 16.33, cont'd

Fig 16.33 (A and B) The flaps are sutured back and site is left to heal for 3–4 weeks to re-establish blood supply to the cortical bone and for the formation of low-density woven bone at the osteotomy seam. (C) The site is re-exposed after 3–4 weeks by making a crestal incision 2–3 mm buccal to the previously prepared mid-crestal horizontal osteotomy and only the lingual flap is elevated. (D) The previously prepared mid-crestal seam is deepened using either straight fissure bur or piezo saw. (E) The buccal plate is carefully splitted and expanded facially using sharp osseous splitters. The buccal cortex is outfractured as wider ridge splitters or implant drills are used, but its attachment to the buccal periosteum maintains its nourishment and long-term viability. (F) Further, the implant osteotomy is prepared, 3–4 mm apical to the ridge split. (G) The implant is inserted. (H) The peri-implant spaces between the cortical plates are filled using bone graft; the lingual flap is released and sutured back. The site is allowed to heal for a minimum of 4 months before implant uncovery and restoration.

CASE REPORT-7

Two-stage ridge-splitting procedure and implant placement in the posterior mandible. A 42-year-old male, referred for the replacement of missing teeth numbers 46 and 47 using implants, showed limited bone height above the mandibular canal in the diagnostic radiograph. The CT planning of the edentulous region showed only 8–10 mm of bone height above the canal, the CT cross-sections of the bone showed narrow bone at the crestal region, which could lead to dehiscence if implants were inserted without lateral bone augmentation or ridge-splitting procedure. The lateral bone augmentation using autogenous bone block was going to be a more time-consuming and invasive procedure as it needed another site to harvest the block, so the decision was taken to perform ridge splitting. It was decided to adopt the two-stage protocol, because the facial cortical plate was very dense and thick and presented the probability of complete separation, if the one-stage ridge splitting and expansion technique was used (Figs 16.34–16.41).

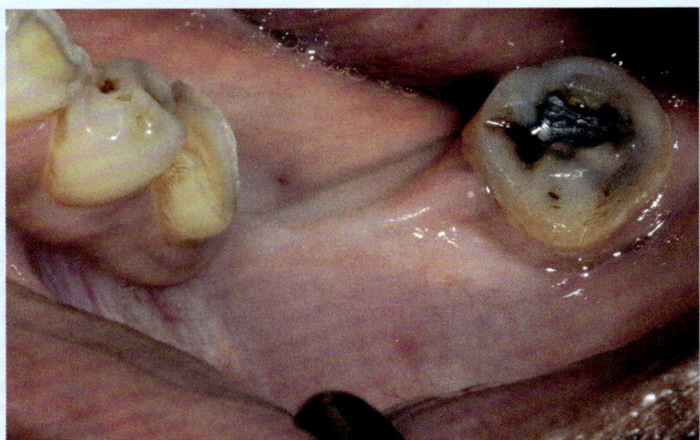

Fig 16.34 Clinical view of edentulous ridge.

CASE REPORT-7—cont'd

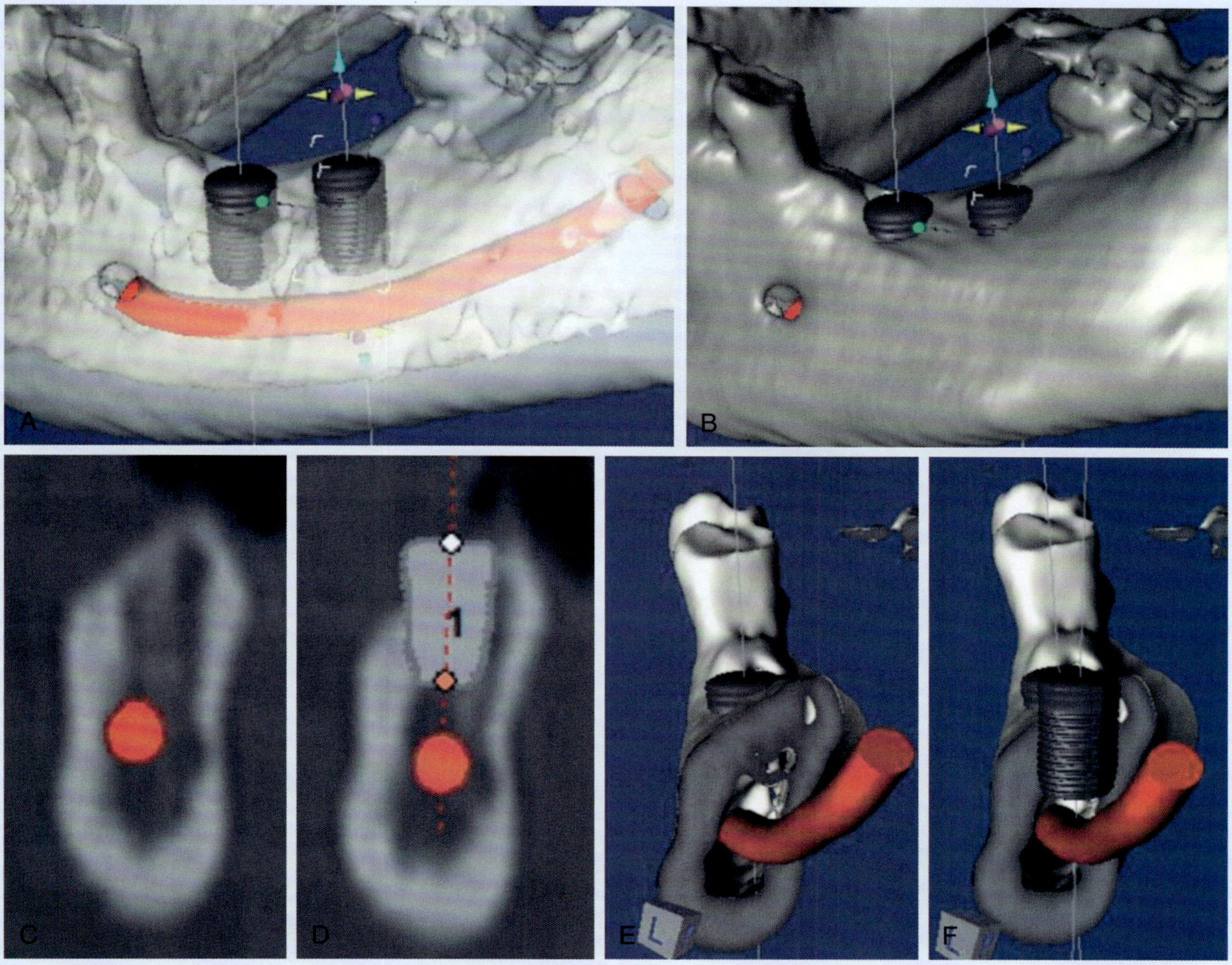

Fig 16.35 (A–F) Different views of CT planning of the site with implant simulation show inadequate bone width at the crestal region for the insertion of the implants.

Continued

CASE REPORT-7—cont'd

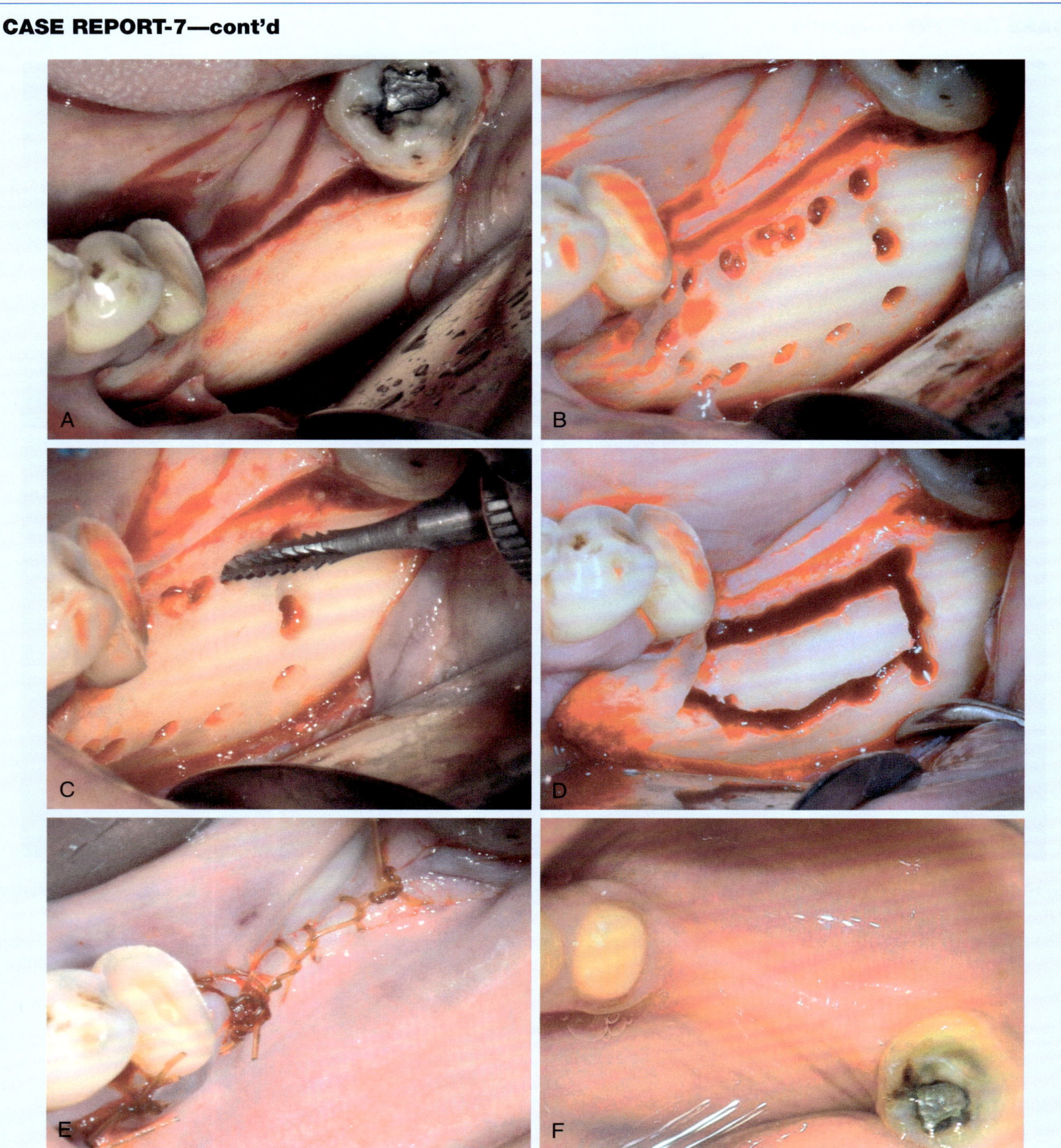

Fig 16.36 (A) Mid-crestal incision is made and a mucoperiosteal flap is elevated to expose the ridge crest and buccal cortical plate. (B) Small round carbide bur is used to make a series of holes through the cortex, deep enough to reach the underlying cancellous bone. (C and D) A straight carbide bur is used to prepare an osteotomy window through the buccal cortex. (E) Flap is sutured back. (F) Clinical view after 3 weeks shows complete soft tissue healing. Re-establishment of blood supply to the buccal cortical plate from the periosteum and woven bone formation along the seam of osteotomy preparation occurs in 3–4 weeks.

CASE REPORT-7—cont'd

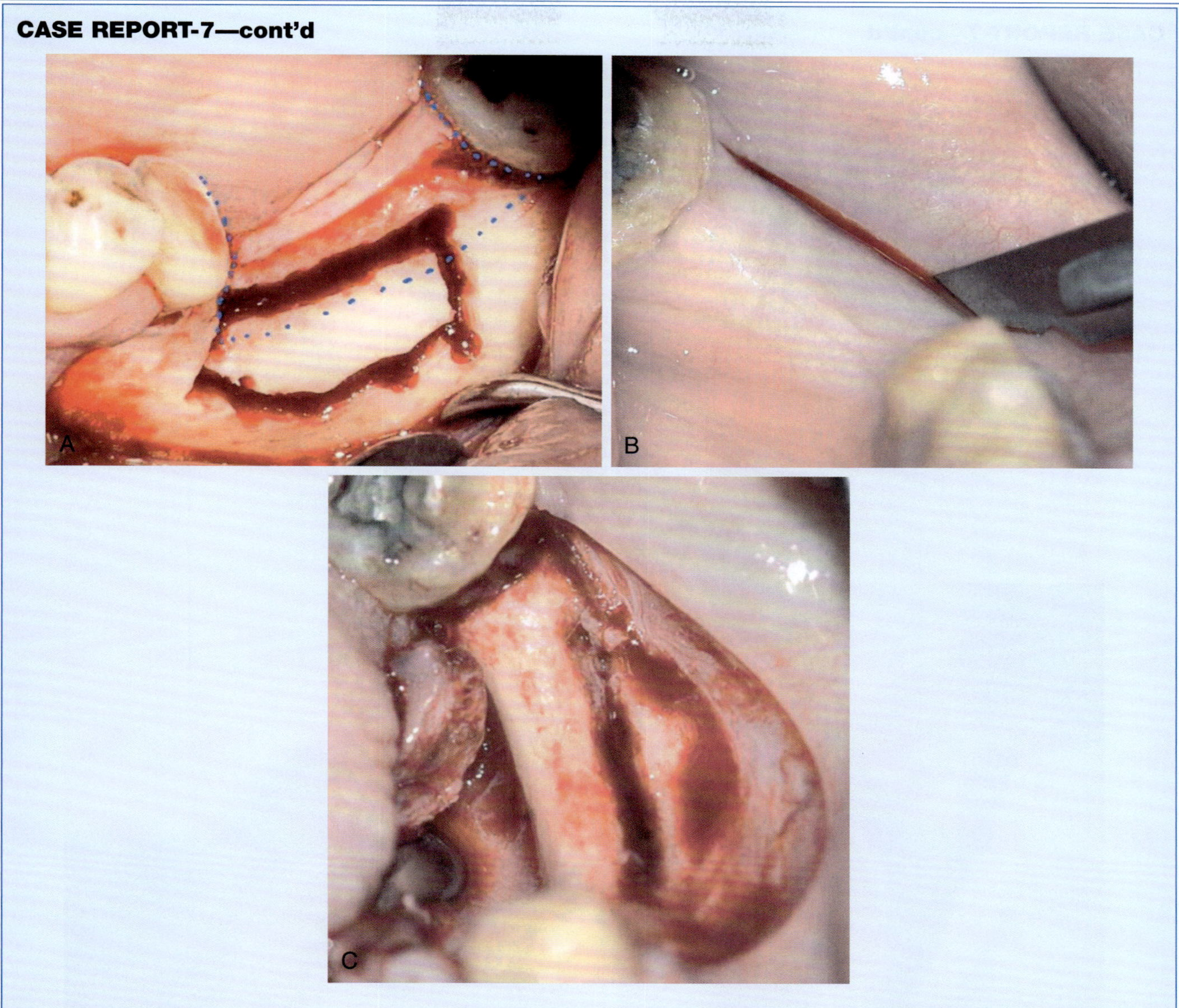

Fig 16.37 (A) Incision line for the second stage surgery is planned by taking reference from the previous picture of the first stage surgery. (B) Incision is made 3–4 mm buccal to the mid-crestal osteotomy. (C) Lingual flap is elevated to expose the ridge crest and horizontal osteotomy.

Continued

CASE REPORT-7—cont'd

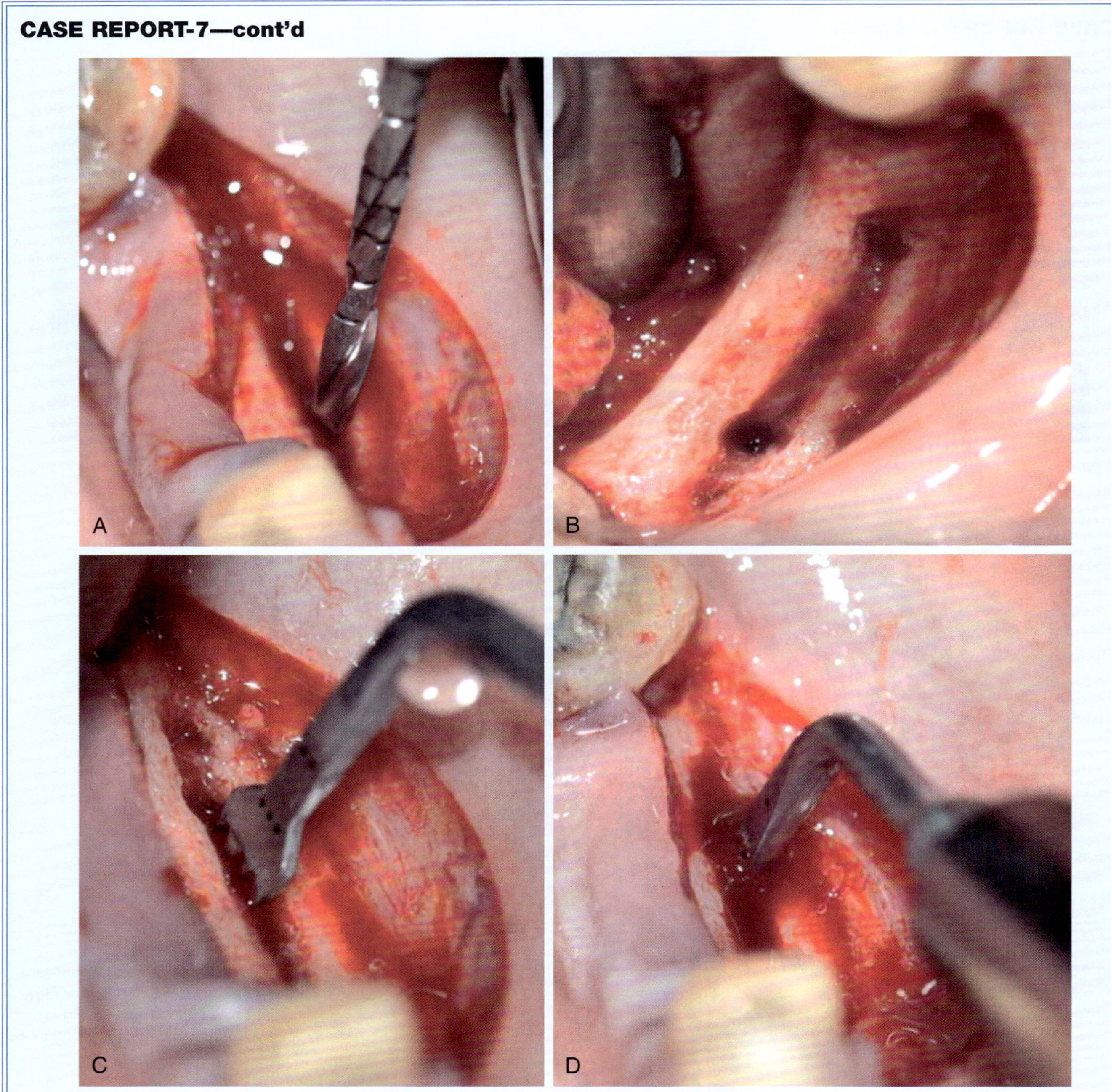

Fig 16.38 (A and B) Pilot drill is used for initial implant osteotomy preparation to partial depth. (C and D) The piezo saw is used to re-prepare the horizontal osteotomy channel to a similar depth as in the previous surgery.

CASE REPORT-7—cont'd

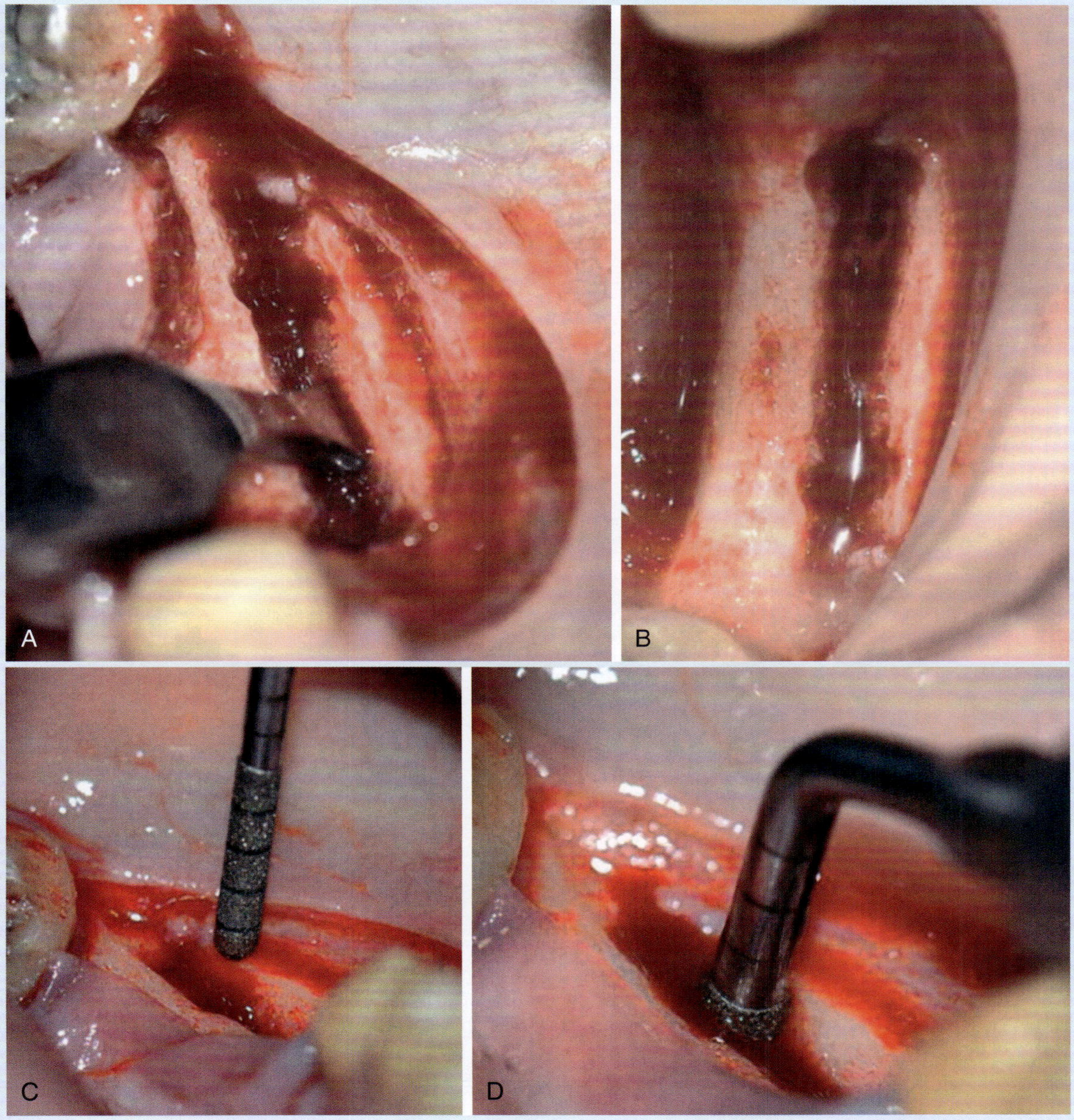

A B C D

Fig 16.39 (A and B) Sharp osseous splitters are used to split the buccal cortical plate and to expand it facially. (C and D) Since the mandibular canal is close to the planned implant apex, different diameter diamond tips of the piezotome are sequentially used to prepare the implant osteotomies to the complete depth, to prevent any nerve injury and to insert implants close to the mandibular canal.

Continued

CASE REPORT-7—cont'd

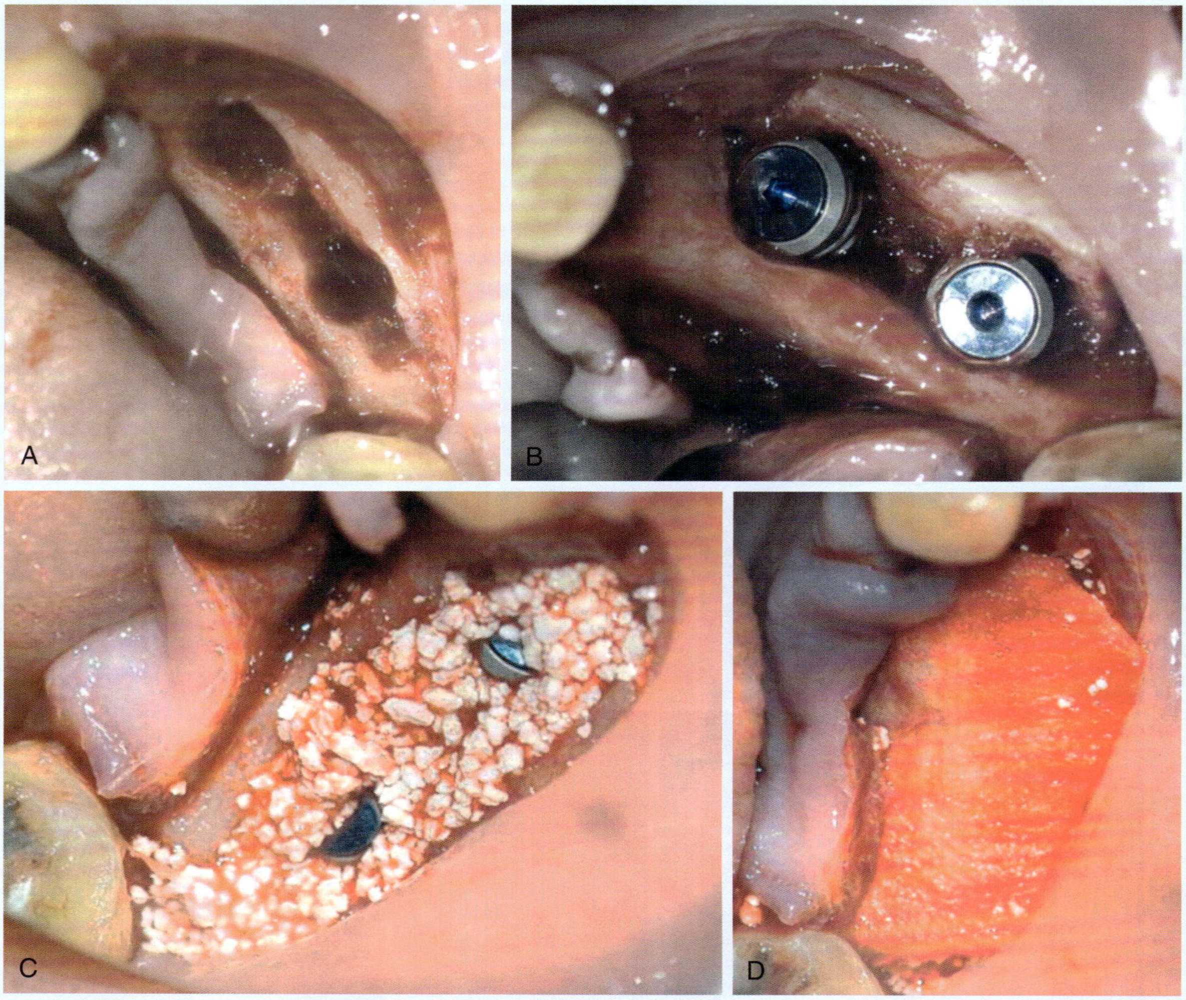

Fig 16.40 (A) Finally prepared implant osteotomies. Efforts were made to prepare the osteotomies with the maximum pressure towards the more stable lingual cortical plate. (B) Two large diameter and short length (5 × 10 mm) implants were inserted with adequate initial stability (more than 30 Ncm). (C) HA + β-TCP graft was used to fill the peri-implant spaces between the two expanded cortical plates. (D) A collagen barrier membrane was used to cover the graft site.

CASE REPORT-7—cont'd

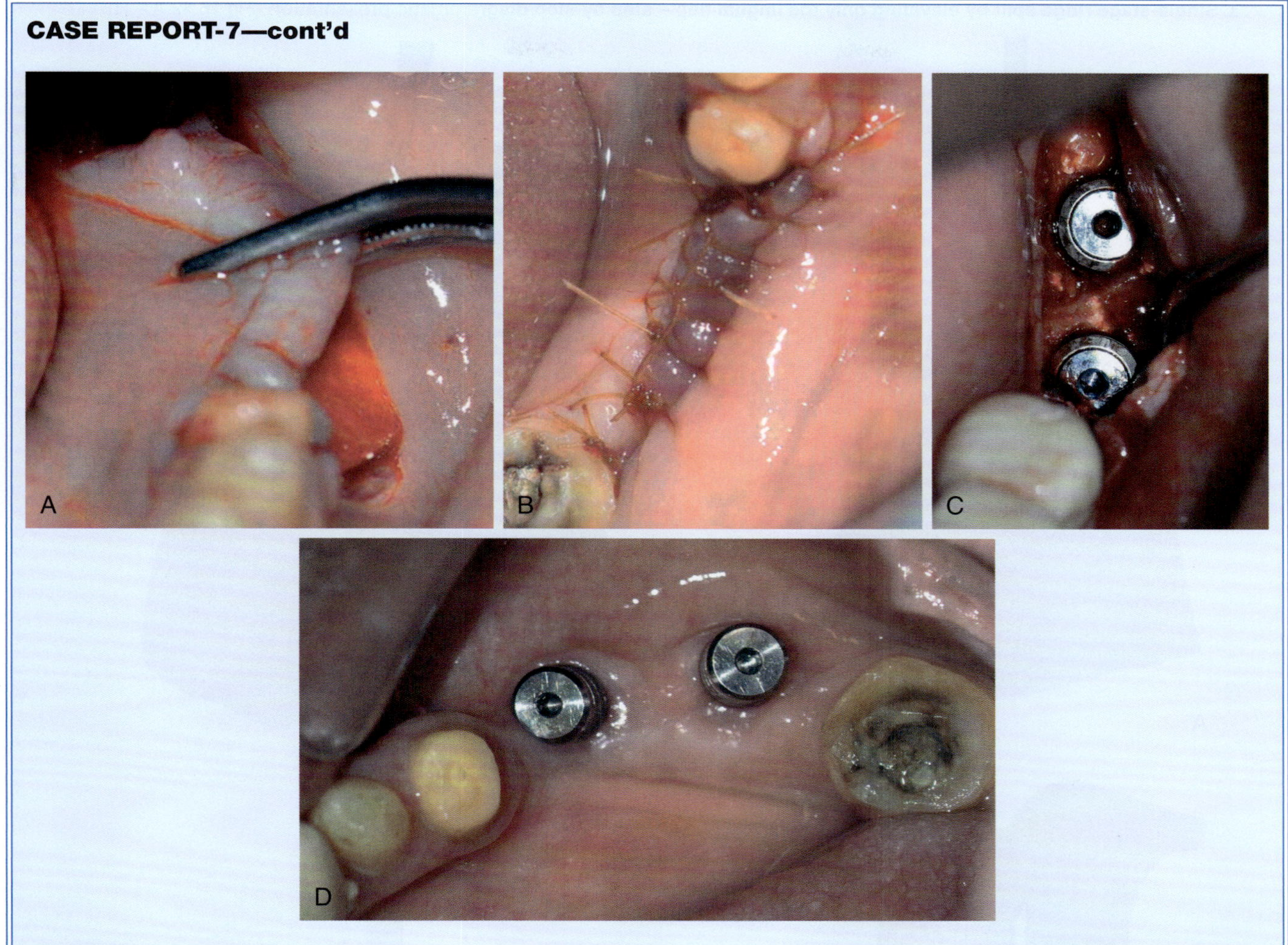

Fig 16.41 (A and B) The lingual flap is coronally advanced and the flap sutured back with a watertight primary closure. (C) The implants uncovered after 4 months, show complete bone regeneration around the implants. (D) Implants are ready for the prosthetic loading.

Single-stage ridge-splitting technique

With advancement in the oral surgery armamentarium such as the piezotome unit, the single-stage ridge split is possible in the high density mandible, but should be performed using the appropriate tools and with a well-planned skilled approach, to achieve the desired results. There can be two protocols for performing the single-stage ridge split in the mandibular ridge.

a. Single-stage ridge split by elevating only lingual flap
b. Single-stage ridge split by elevating the buccal flap

a. Single-stage ridge split by elevating only the lingual flap – step by step diagrammatic presentation (Fig 16.42 A – H).

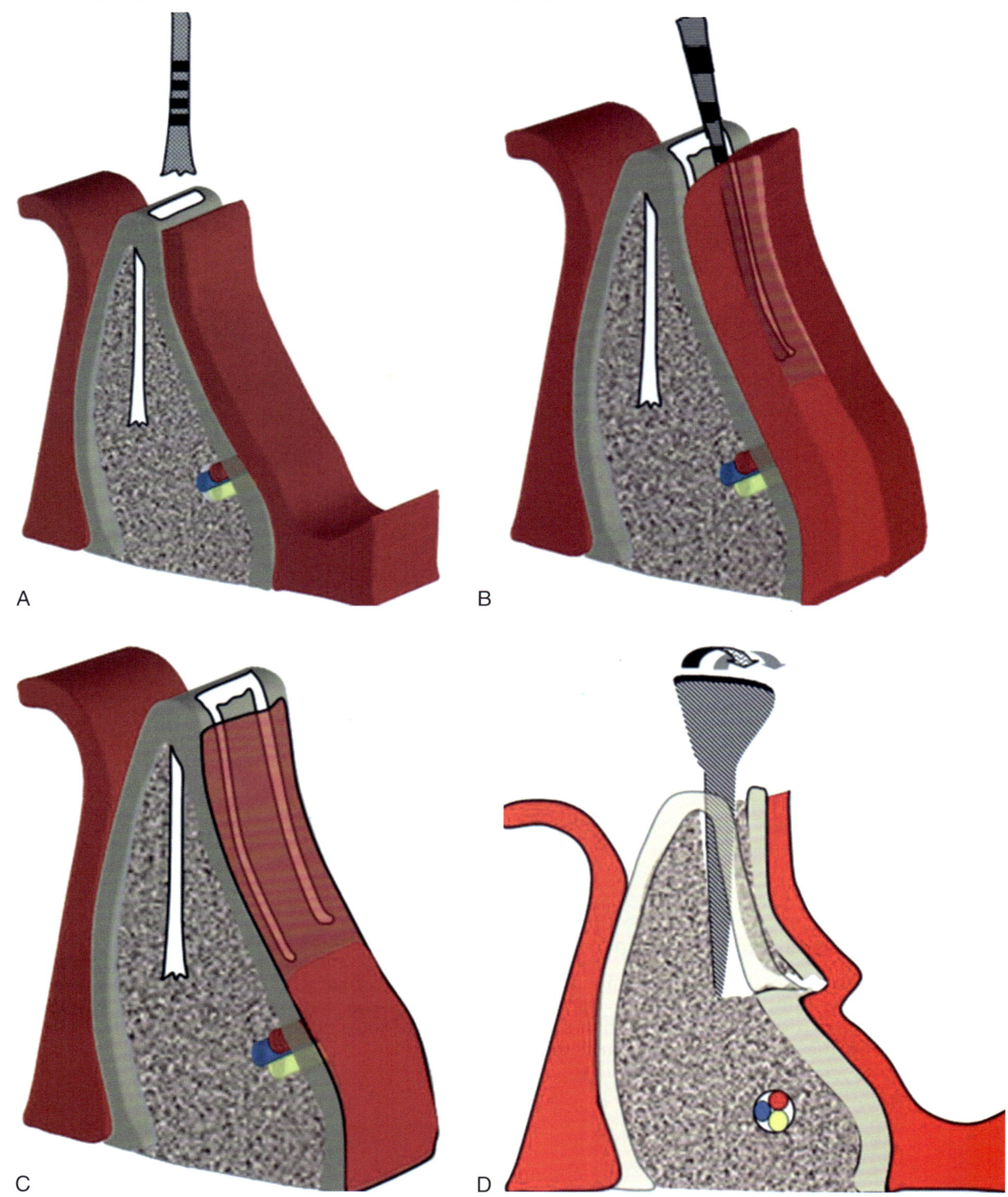

Fig 16.42 An incision is made slightly buccal to the mid-crest and the lingual flap is elevated to uncover the ridge crest. Two small vertical incisions can also be made, which are extended buccally only 2–3 mm. (A) This assists in easy expansion of the buccal cortical plate. A mid-crestal horizontal and deep osteotomy channel is prepared using the piezo saw. (B and C) Now two vertical cuts are made lateral to the buccal cortical plate with the side-cutting LC1 tip of the piezo saw (which does not cut the soft tissue), so that these two vertical cuts can be made in the buccal bone without damaging the overlying periosteum. (D) The ridge splitters are then used to split and expand the buccal cortical plate, which remains attached to the overlying periosteum.

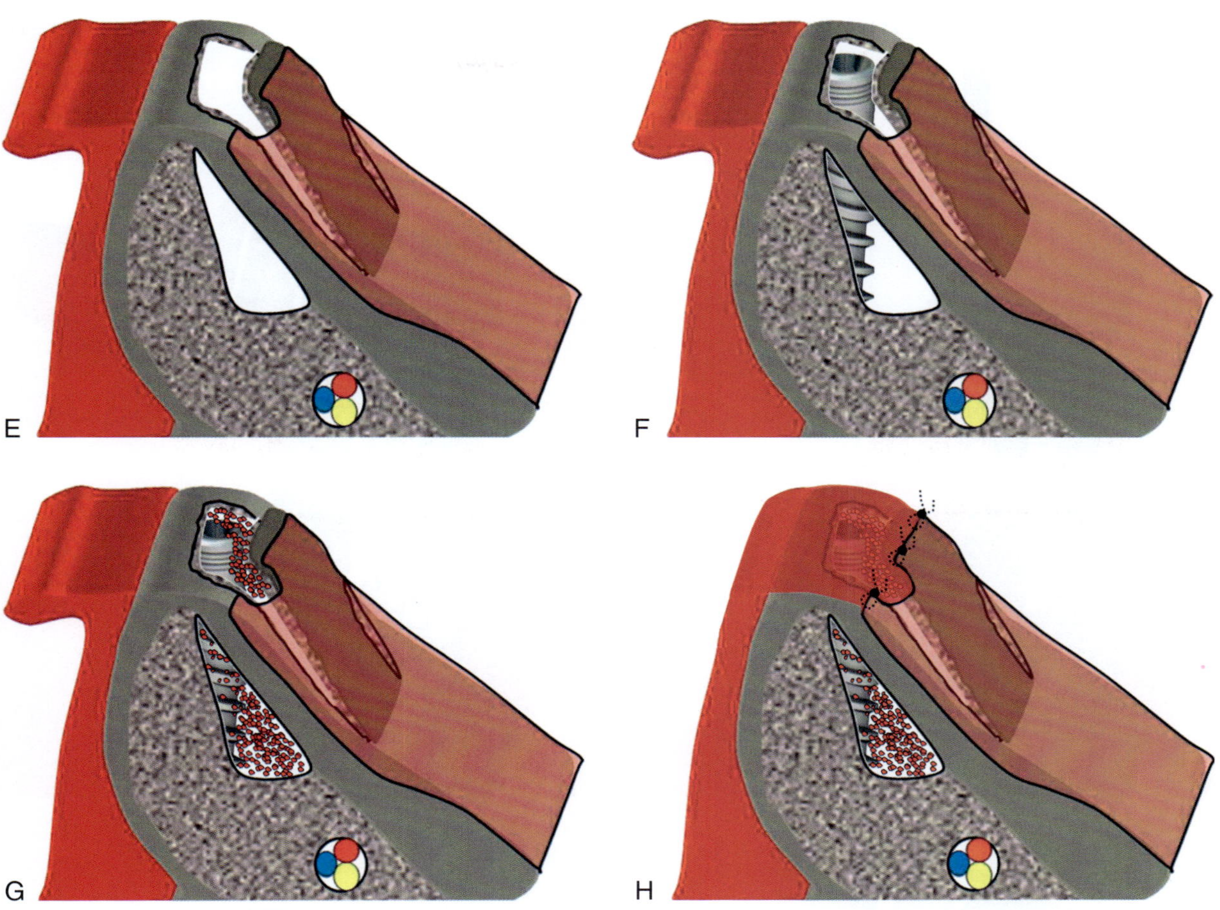

Fig 16.42, cont'd (E) After achieving the desired expansion, (F) the implant osteotomy is prepared using implant drills and the implant is inserted. (G) The peri-implant spaces between the two cortical plates can be grafted using bone substitute. (H) The lingual flap is coronally advanced and sutured to achieve primary closure.

b. Single-stage ridge split by elevating the buccal flap – step by step diagrammatic presentation (Fig 16.43 A – H).

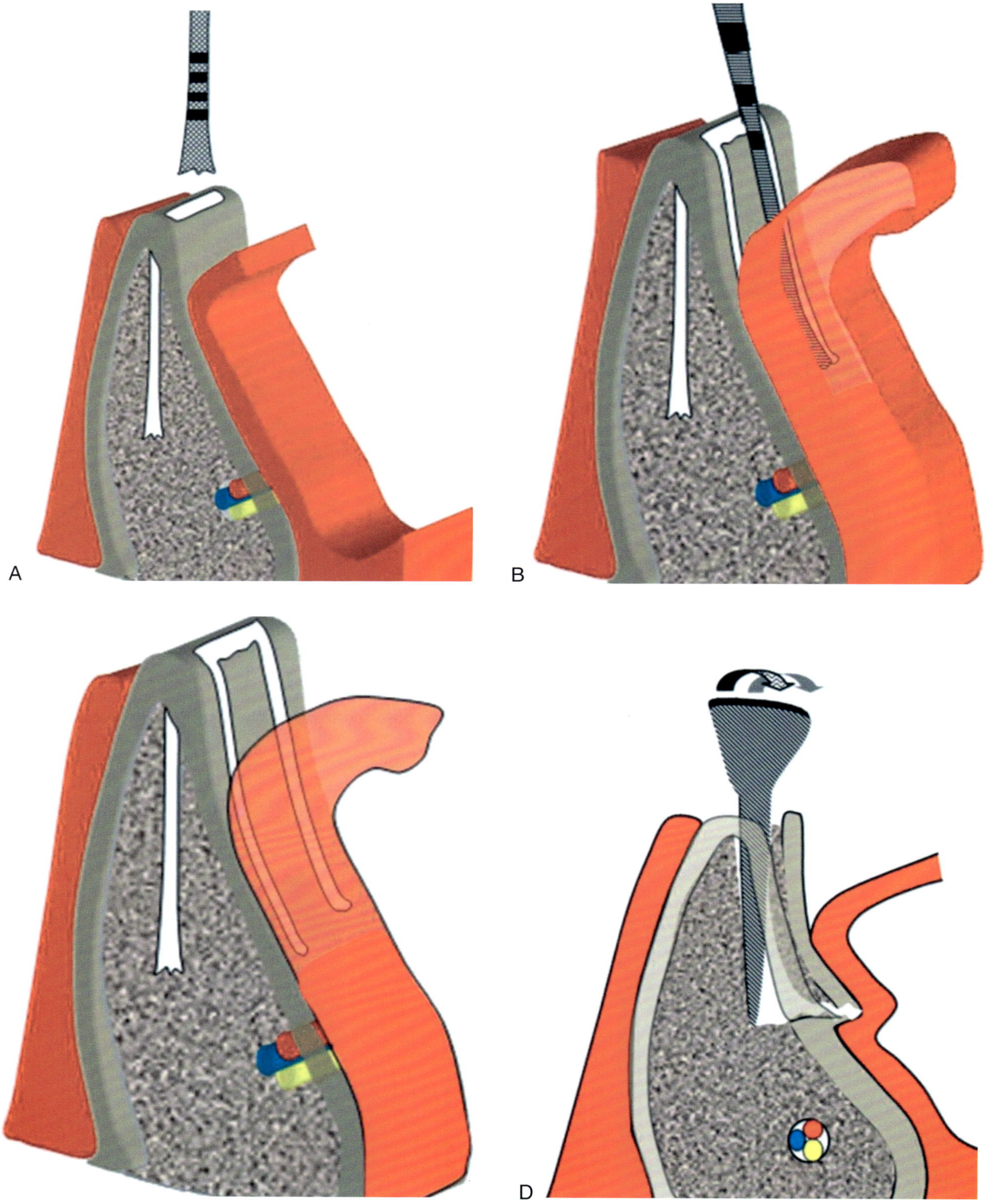

A

B

C

D

Fig 16.43 An incision slightly lingual to the mid-crest is made and the buccal flap is elevated to expose the ridge crest. Two small vertical incisions are made buccally to minimally elevate the facial flap to partially expose the buccal cortical plate. (A) A mid-crestal horizontal deep osteotomy channel is prepared using a piezo saw. (B and C) Two vertical cuts are made lateral to the buccal cortical plate using the side-cutting LC1 tip of the piezo saw. (D) The ridge splitters are used to split and expand the buccal cortical plate attached to the overlying periosteum.

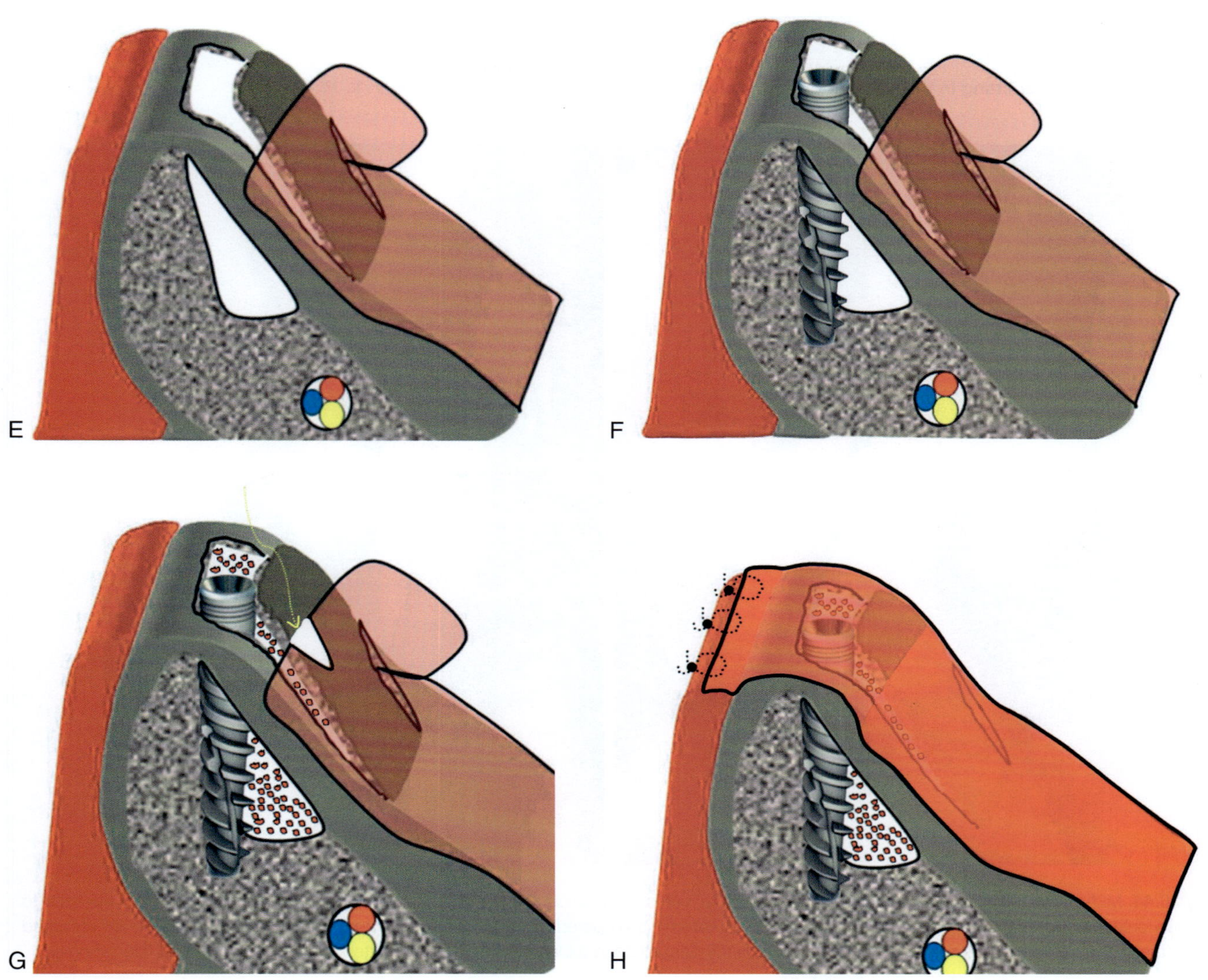

Fig 16.43, cont'd (E) After achieving the desired amount of ridge expansion, (F) the implant osteotomy is prepared using implant drills and the implant is inserted. (G) The peri-implant spaces between two cortical plates are grafted using bone graft material. (H) A releasing incision is made in the periosteum of the buccal flap and flap is sutured back with primary closure.

CASE REPORT-8

Single-stage ridge splitting in the posterior mandible with simultaneous implant insertion (Figs 16.44–16.46).

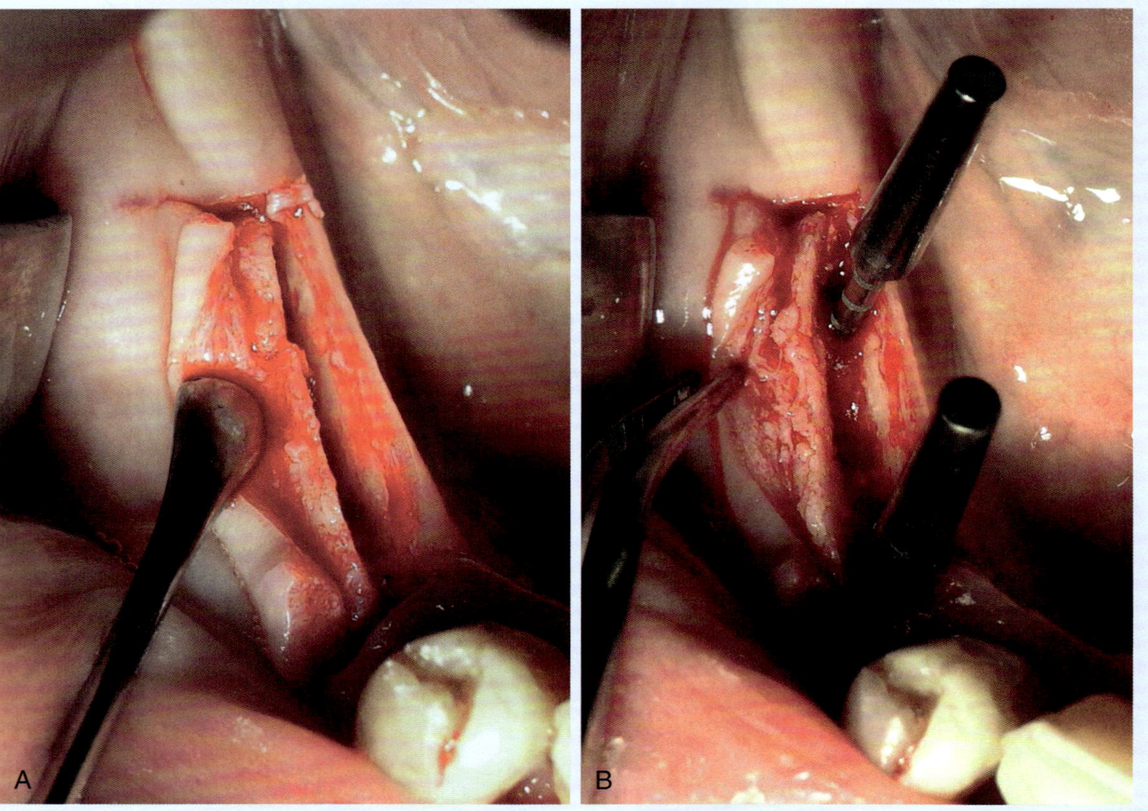

Fig 16.44 Mid-crestal incision is made along with two minimal vertical extensions on the buccal aspect. The buccal flap is minimally elevated to expose only the ridge crest. (A) A mid-crestal horizontal osteotomy is prepared using the piezo saw and two vertical osteotomies are prepared using the LC1 tip of the piezotome unit. (B) After obtaining the desired ridge expansion using ridge splitters, implant sites are carefully prepared.

CASE REPORT-8—cont'd

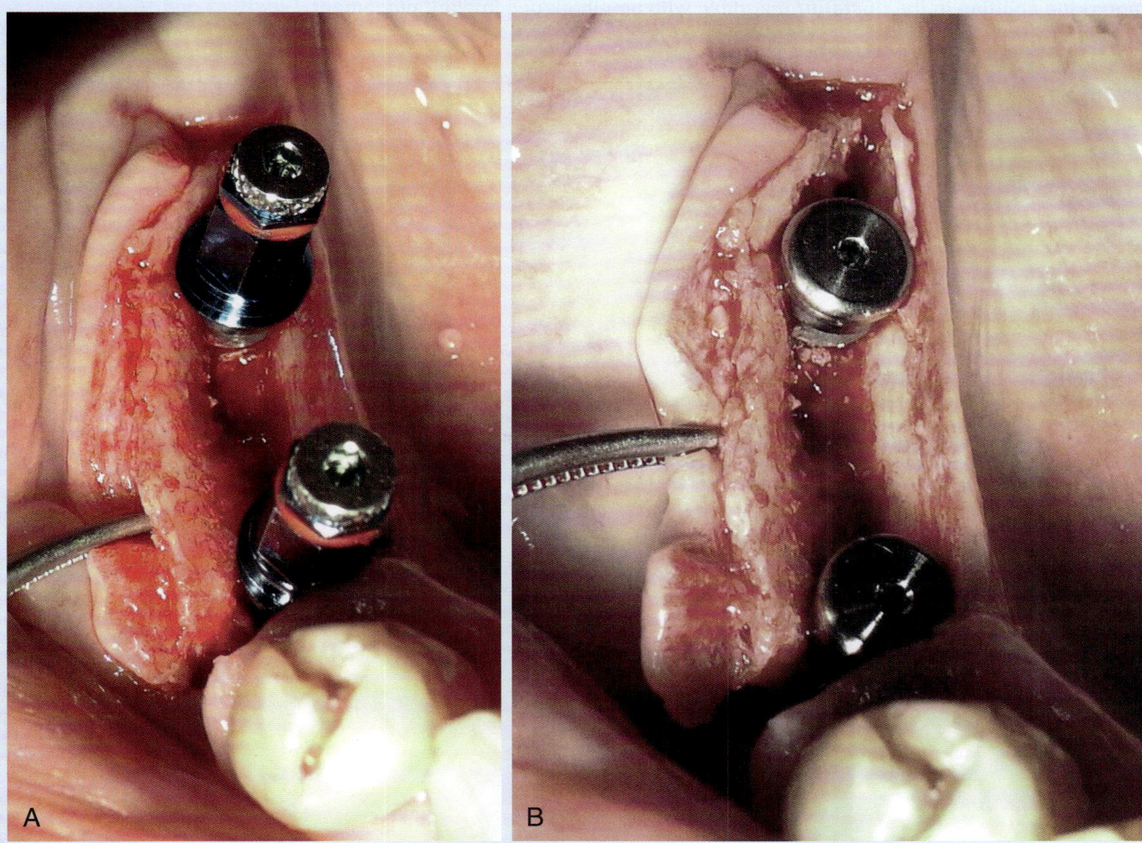

Fig 16.45 (A and B) Two implants are inserted after achieving adequate amount of ridge expansion and osteotomy preparation.

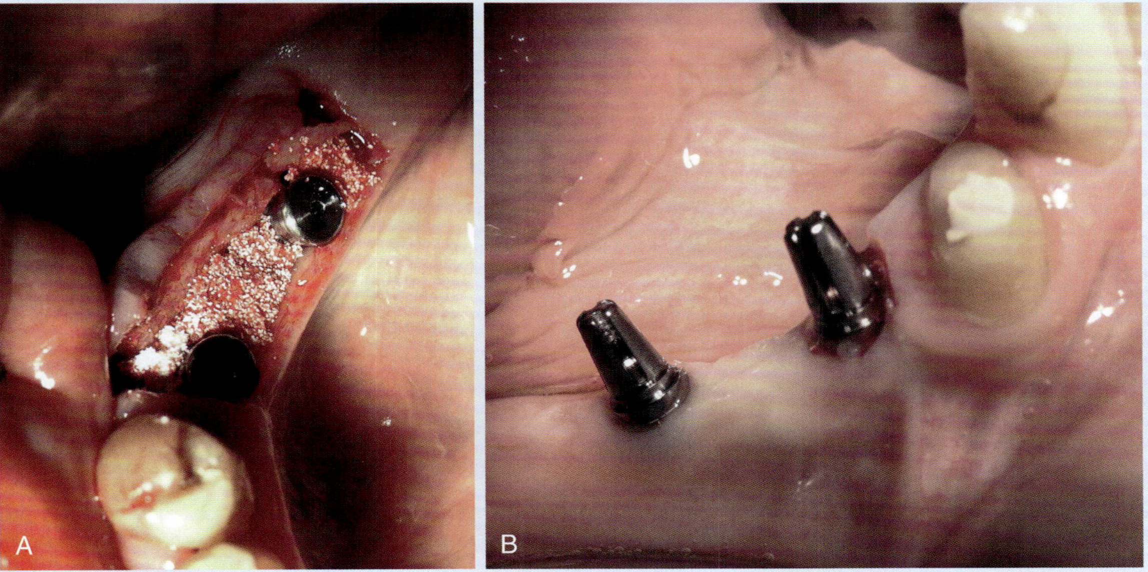

Fig 16.46 (A) The peri-implant spaces between two cortical plates are grafted using bone substitute and the flap is sutured with primary closure. (B) Implants are uncovered using tissue punch after 4 months and final abutments are inserted for restoration.

CASE REPORT-9

Single-stage ridge splitting in the posterior mandible with simultaneous implant placement (Figs 16.47 and 16.48).

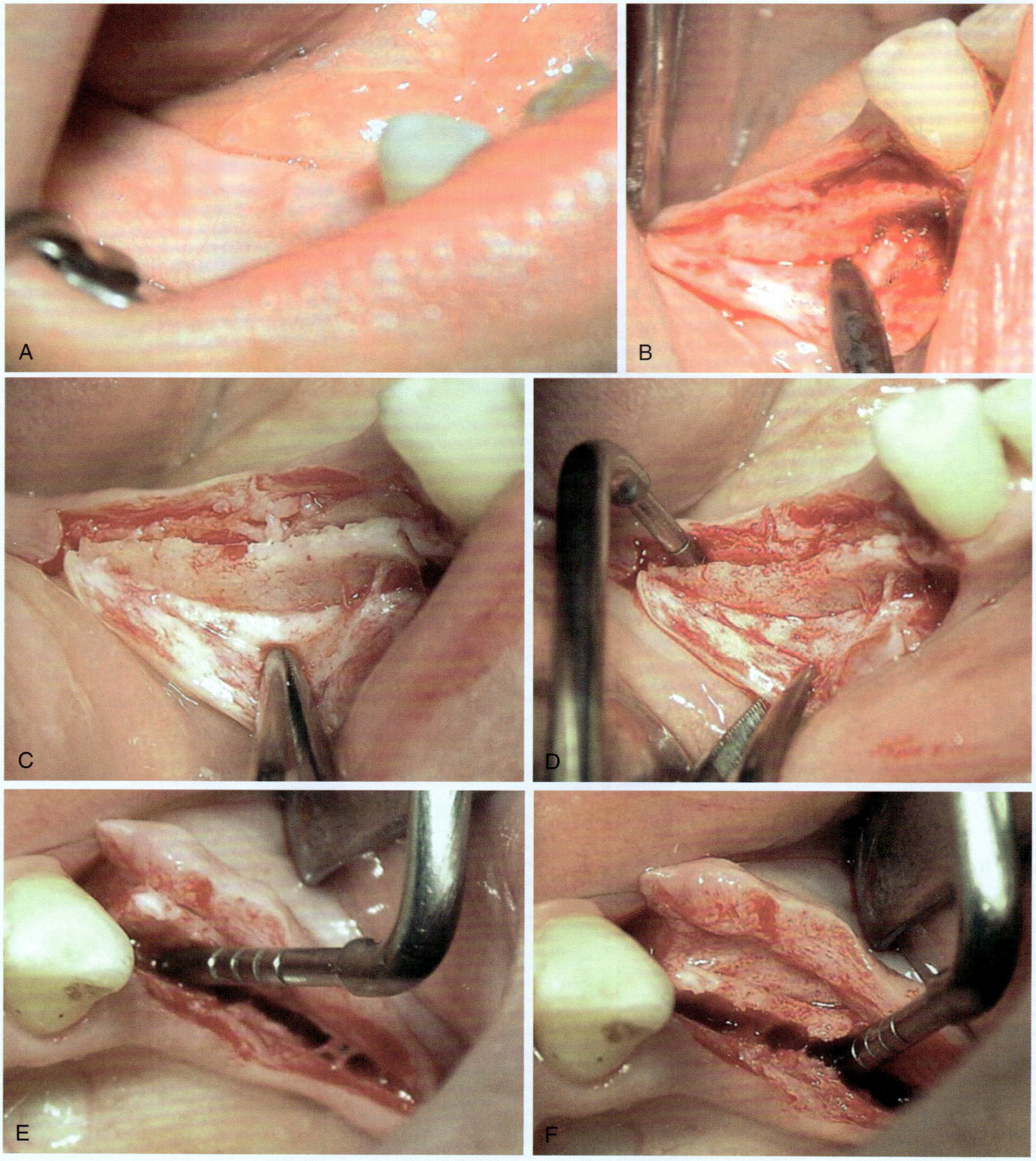

A B C D E F

Fig 16.47 (A) Clinical view of the mandibular edentulous ridge shows narrow ridge morphology. A horizontal incision slightly lingual to the mid-crest along with two small facial vertical incisions are made. (B) The facial flap is elevated to expose the ridge crest and part of the buccal cortical plate. (C) A piezo saw is used to prepare a deep mid-crestal horizontal osteotomy with two vertical cuts through the buccal cortical plate. (D–F) A set of ridge splitters and expanders is used to split and expand the buccal cortical plate, which is still attached to the periosteum at its apical half.

CASE REPORT-9—cont'd

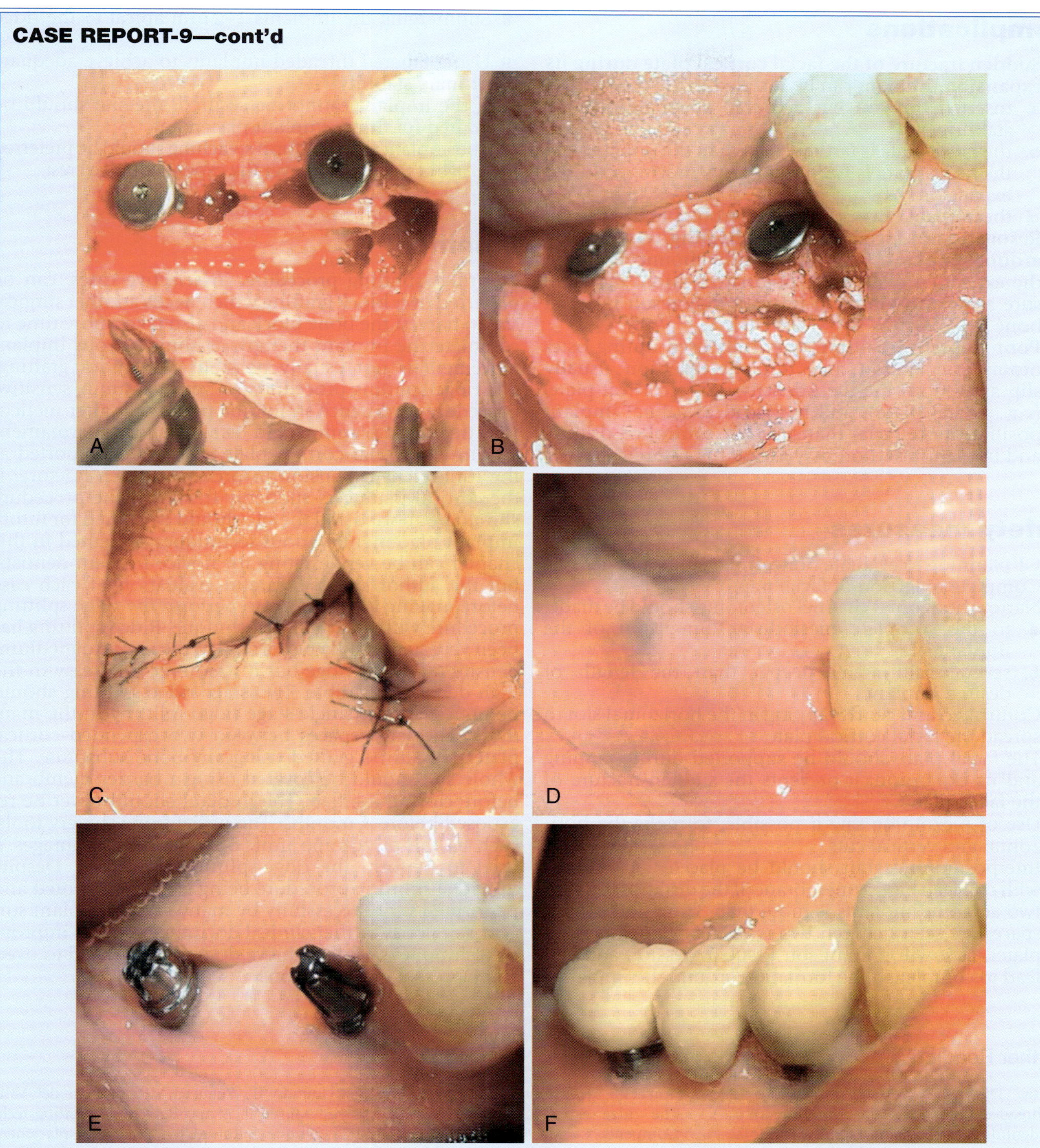

Fig 16.48 (A) After achieving a large degree of expansion, the implant osteotomies are prepared and two regular diameter implants are inserted. (B) The spaces between the two cortical plates are filled with graft and more amount of graft is deposited on the buccal cortical plate. (C) The periosteum is released and the flap is sutured back to achieve primary closure. (D) Healing as seen after 3 weeks. (E and F) Implants are uncovered and restored after 4 months.

Complications

1. **Sudden fracture of the facial cortical plate during its expansion.** Implant can be inserted if:
   a. inserted implant has achieved adequate primary stability
   b. the facial plate is farther facial than the implant, e.g. the facial plate is fractured after achieving required expansion
   c. the implant can be inserted at favourable angulation.
2. **Resorption of facial plate after healing/remodelling around implant.** Because of elastic 'bounce back' of the expanded plate to its original position, the pressure against the inserted implant may result in facial bone resorption.
3. **Poor implant position.** The drills used during osteotomy preparation and implant insertion usually slip away from the high density stable cortical plate, (e.g. palatal plate), and may lead to a final implant position more facial than ideal. A controlled drilling and implant insertion may avoid this complication.

Safety measures

1. CT planning to evaluate bone dimensions and density.
2. Complete reflection of facial flap.
3. Narrow horizontal channel osteotomy should be made:
   a. to the complete mesiodistal dimension of the implant site
   b. several millimetres deeper than the length of desired implant.
4. Controlled and gentle tapping in the horizontal slot to spread the facial cortical plate.
5. The facial plate should be supported during tapping and its expansion; it prevents the sudden fracture of the facial plate.
6. Use of piezotome saw if possible, to make the horizontal and vertical cuts.
7. Interpositioning graft should be placed and covered with collagen barrier membrane, if the distance between two adjacent implants is more than 3 mm and if wide spaces are seen between two widely expanded cortical plates, as it will prevent soft tissue ingression and will lead to complete bone formation around the implants.
8. Submerging the implants 1–2 mm apical to the ridge crest.
9. Using tapered threaded implants to achieve adequate primary stability.
10. If the implant cannot be secured, the site should be grafted for future implant placement.
11. The implant with platform switching should be preferred to avoid the pressure over the expended ridge crest.

Summary

The ridge-splitting procedure, in selective cases, can be preferred over block grafting which needs another surgical site to harvest the bone block and also takes more time to complete the implant therapy, as simultaneous implant placement is not usually possible with block grafting. The ridge-splitting procedure is a very technique-sensitive procedure, and hence should be performed after meticulous treatment planning and using the correct armamentarium. The facial cortical plate should be supported at the time of its expansion to prevent sudden fracture. If the cortical plate gets suddenly fractured, the procedure should be aborted and the site should be grafted for future implant placement. Various techniques presented in this chapter can be very exciting for novice implant dentists, but the author suggests careful evaluation of each case before making the decision to perform the ridge-splitting procedure with a particular technique. Ridge splitting has been very successfully performed in the poor- to medium-density maxillary ridge but it has never been easy in the high-density mandible. Two-stage ridge splitting should be preferred over single-stage ridge splitting in the mandible. The large spaces between two expended cortical plates should be grafted using any bone substitute. The whole site should be covered using a barrier membrane before closing the flap. The implant should never be re-exposed before 4 months. The newer bone surgery tools, such as the piezotome unit, offer several advantages if used to perform the ridge-splitting procedure. Despite the ridge-splitting procedure being well documented and performed very successfully by many skilled implant surgeons, it needs further clinical documentation to improve its techniques to fully achieve desired results and to overcome present complications.

Further Reading

Tarnow DP, et al. Immediate loading of threaded implants at stage one surgery in edentulous arches. Int J Oral Maxillofac Implants 1997;12:319–24.

Scipioni A, Bruschi GB, Calesini G. The edentulous ridge expansion technique: a five-year study. Int J Periodontics Restorative Dent 1994;14(5):451–9.

Simoni M, Baldoni M, Zaffe D. Jaw bone enlargement using immediate implant placement associated with a split-crest technique and guided tissue regeneration. Int J Periodontics Restorative Dent 1992;12:462–73.

Summers RB. The osteotome technique. Part 2. The ridge expansion osteotomy (REO). Compend Contin Educ Dent 1994;15:422–36.

Sethi A, Kaus T. Maxillary ridge expansion with simultaneous implant placement in. Int J Oral Maxillofac Implants 2000;15:491–9.

Bernhart T, Weber R, Mailath G, et al. Use of crestal bone for augmentation of extremely knife-edged alveolar ridges prior to implant placement: report of 3 cases. Int J Oral Maxillofac Implants 1999;14:424–7.

Guirado JL, Yuguero MR, Carrión del Valle MJ, et al. A maxillary ridge-splitting technique followed by immediate placement of implants: a case report. Implant Dent 2005;14(1):14–20.

Palti A, Hoch T. A concept for treatment of various dental bone defects. Implant Dent 2002;11(1):73–8.

Reilly DT, Burstein AH. The elastic and ultimate properties of compact bone tissue. J Biomech 1975;80:393–405.

Ferrigno N, Laureti M. Surgical advantages with ITI TE implants placement in conjunction with split crest technique. 18-month results of an ongoing prospective study. Clin Oral Implants Res 2005;16(2):147–55.

Basa S, Varol A, Turker N. Alternative bone expansion technique for immediate placement of implants in the edentulous posterior mandibular ridge: a clinical report. Int J Oral Maxillofac Implants 2004;19(4): 554–8.

Chiapasco M, Ferrini F, Casentini P, et al. Dental implants placed in expanded narrow edentulous ridges with the Extension Crest device. A 1–3-year multicenter follow-up study. Clin Oral Implants Res 2006;17(3):265–72.

Tinti C, Parma-Benfenati S. Clinical classification of bone defects concerning the placement of dental implants. Int J Periodontics Restorative Dent 2003;23:147–55.

Chiapasco M, Zaniboni M, Boisco M. Augmentation procedures for the rehabilitation of deficient edentulous ridges with oral implants. Clin Oral Implants Res 2006;17(Suppl. 2):136–59.

Collins TA. Onlay bone grafting in combination with Branemark implants. Oral Maxillofac Surg Clin North Am 1991;3:893–902.

Jensen J, Sindet-Pedersen S. Autogenous mandibular bone grafts and osseointegrated implants for reconstruction of the severely atrophied maxilla: a preliminary report. J Oral Maxillofac Surg 1991;49:1277–87.

Misch CM, Misch CE. The repair of localized severe ridge defects for implant placement using mandibular bone grafts. Implant Dent 1995;4:261–7.

Shulman LB. Surgical considerations in implant dentistry. J Dent Educ 1988;52:712–20.

Summers RB. Maxillary implant surgery. The osteotome technique. Part 1. Compend Contin Educ Dent 1994;15:152–62.

Summers RB. The osteotome technique. Part 3. Less invasive methods of elevating the sinus floor. Compend Contin Educ Dent 1994;15:698–708.

Summers RB. The osteotome technique. Part 4. The future site development. Compend Contin Educ Dent 1995;11; 1090–1025.

Davarpanah M, Martinez H, Tecucianu JF, et al. The modified osteotome technique. Int J Periodontics Restorative Dent 2001;21:559–607.

Garg AK, Morales MJ, Navarro I, et al. Autogenous mandibular bone grafts in the treatment of the resorbed maxillary anterior alveolar ridge: rationale and approach. Implant Dent 1998;7(3):169–76.

Triplett RG, Schow S. Autologous bone grafts endosseous implants: complementary techniques. J Oral Maxillofac Surg 1996;54:486–94.

Montazem A, Valauri DV, St-Hilaire H, et al. The mandibular symphysis as a donor site in maxillofacial bone grafting: a quantitative anatomic study. Int J Oral Maxillofac Implants 2000;58:1368–71.

Scipioni A, Brushi GB, Calesini G. The edentulous ridge expansion technique: a 5-year study. Int J Periodontics Restorative Dent 1994;14:451–9.

Misch CM. Comparison of intraoral donor sites for onlay grafting prior to implant placement. Int J Oral Maxillofac Implants 1997;12:767–76.

Distraction osteogenesis in implantology

17

Tetsu Takahashi

CHAPTER CONTENTS HD

Introduction

Following tooth loss, alveolar ridge bone height and width deficiencies limit the application of dental implants. Alveolar deficiency can be classified both by anatomic findings and the desired clinical approach (Fig 17.1).

Class I – horizontal deficiency
Class II – vertical deficiency
Class III – both horizontal and vertical deficiency.

To augment these alveolar deficiencies, traditionally autogenous onlay bone grafts have been performed. Ridge augmentation is required not only for functional but also for aesthetic reasons in implant-supported restoration for an atrophic, narrow alveolar process. Bone grafting with autogenous bone or bone materials, guided bone regeneration (GBR), and ridge expansion techniques have been used for this purpose. However, these procedures have disadvantages, such as the need for surgical intervention and harvesting bone, unpredictable bone resorption, and difficulty in achieving soft tissue coverage.

Ilizarov established the concept of distraction osteogenesis (DO) for orthopaedic surgery in the early 1950s. Subsequently, the idea was introduced to the field of oral and maxillofacial surgery by McCarthy and associates in 1992. In 1996, DO was introduced as an effective new technique for vertical alveolar ridge augmentation, and since then the vertical alveolar DO technique is applied widely to correct alveolar ridge defects or atrophy. Unlike GBR or bone grafts, the DO technique does not need a donor site or the simultaneous lengthening of surrounding soft tissues.

Vertical alveolar distraction

In 1996, Chin et al developed a vertical alveolar distraction device, LEAD system (Stryker Leibinger, Kalamazoo, MI), consisting of a threaded rod, a threaded transport plate, and a stabilizing unthreaded base plate (Fig 17.2).

In 1998, Hidding et al developed the TRACK system (Tissue Regeneration by Alveolar Callus distraction –Köln) distraction device (KLS Martin, GmbH, Tutlingen, Germany), consisting of titanium microplates welded onto the sliding mechanism of the distraction screw (Fig 17.3).

Basic concepts of vertical alveolar distraction are the same as those of Ilizarov (Fig 17.4A–C).

Alveolar reconstruction is achieved by a bone transport technique whereby the transport segment is moved using a special distractor such as the LEAD system or the TRACK system.

Surgical technique

Alveolar distraction surgery is typically performed as an in-office procedure utilizing local anaesthesia and intravenous sedation. A horizontal vestibular incision is used to expose the bone at the level of the planned horizontal osteotomy. The periosteum is only minimally exposed because of its role in blood supply to the segmented bone (Fig 17.5).

The bone plates of the distraction device (Track 1.0) are contoured to the surface of the bone. The plates are also bent to give the proper distraction vector, which is chosen based on the desired direction of the distraction, the final bone segment position, and avoidance of occlusal

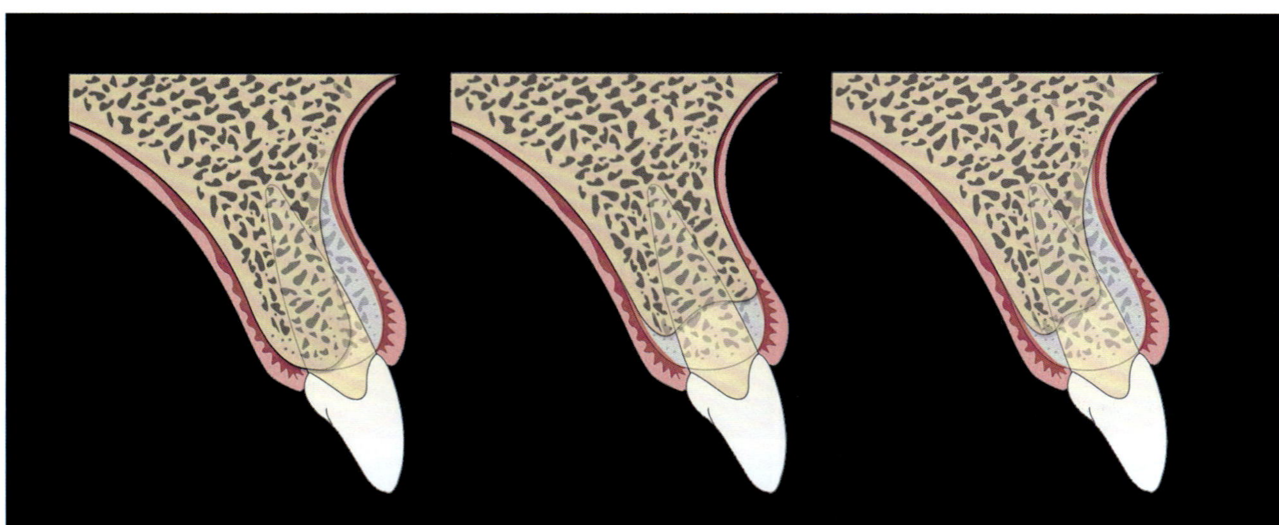

Fig 17.1 Seibert's alveolar defect classification (Class I, Class II and Class III).

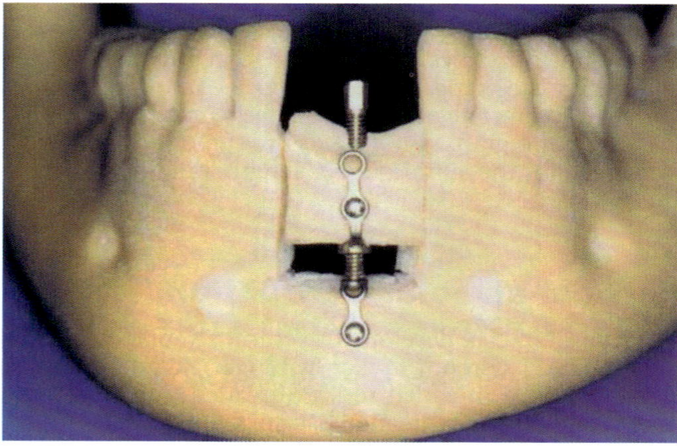

Fig 17.2 LEAD distraction device (Stryker Leibinger, Kalamazoo, MI).

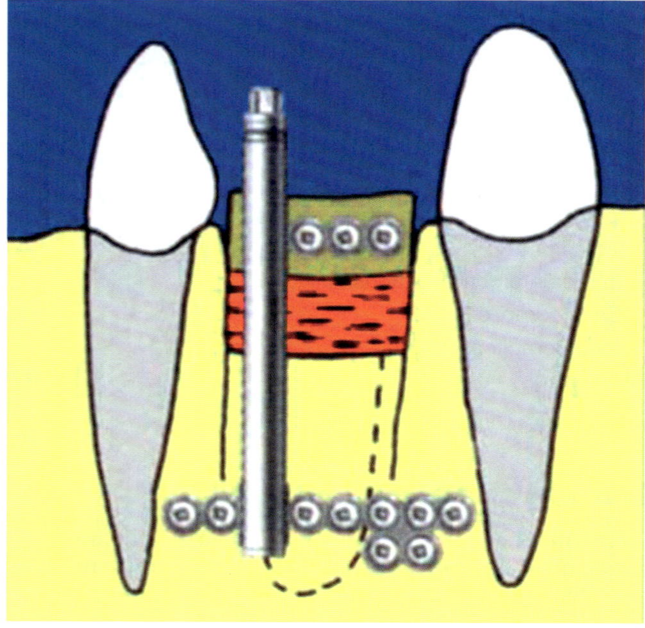

Fig 17.3 TRACK system (KLS Martin, GmbH, Tutlingen, Germany).

interference (Fig 17.6). Once the device is contoured, it is attached using one screw for each plate, so that the intended osteotomy line can be marked, followed by device removal. Using a reciprocating bone saw, osteotomy is then performed horizontally and vertically (Fig 17.7), and the distractor is re-attached (Fig 17.8). At this point, the device should be functionally tested through its range of activation in order to detect any intraoperative tilting/lodging in the underlying areas, to ensure even transport of the osteomized segment (Fig 17.9).

The distractor is then deactivated to its initial position, and the flap is closed in a meticulous manner (Fig 17.10). After 7–10 days of latency period allowing the healing of the wound, the distractor is activated by rotating the threaded rod at a rate of 0.4–0.8 mm (one to two turns, respectively) per day until obtaining the planned length (Fig 17.11).

After a 2–3 month consolidation period, the distraction device is removed, and the placement of the implants is performed (Fig 17.12). Subsequently, the final implant-supported prosthesis is then fabricated (Fig 17.13).

Horizontal alveolar distraction

A horizontal DO for correcting a narrow alveolar ridge has also been published. Nosaka et al reported horizontal alveolar ridge distraction in a dog model and observed woven bone in the distraction gap at 12 weeks and new mature lamellar bone at 24 weeks. Funaki et al also mentioned the method of horizontal DO using a titanium mesh plate that gradually expands the buccal plate horizontally, which is very similar to ridge expansion osteotomy or the bone-splitting technique without interposition grafting. Horizontal alveolar distraction using a titanium mesh plate is an excellent augmentation technique for the placement of implants

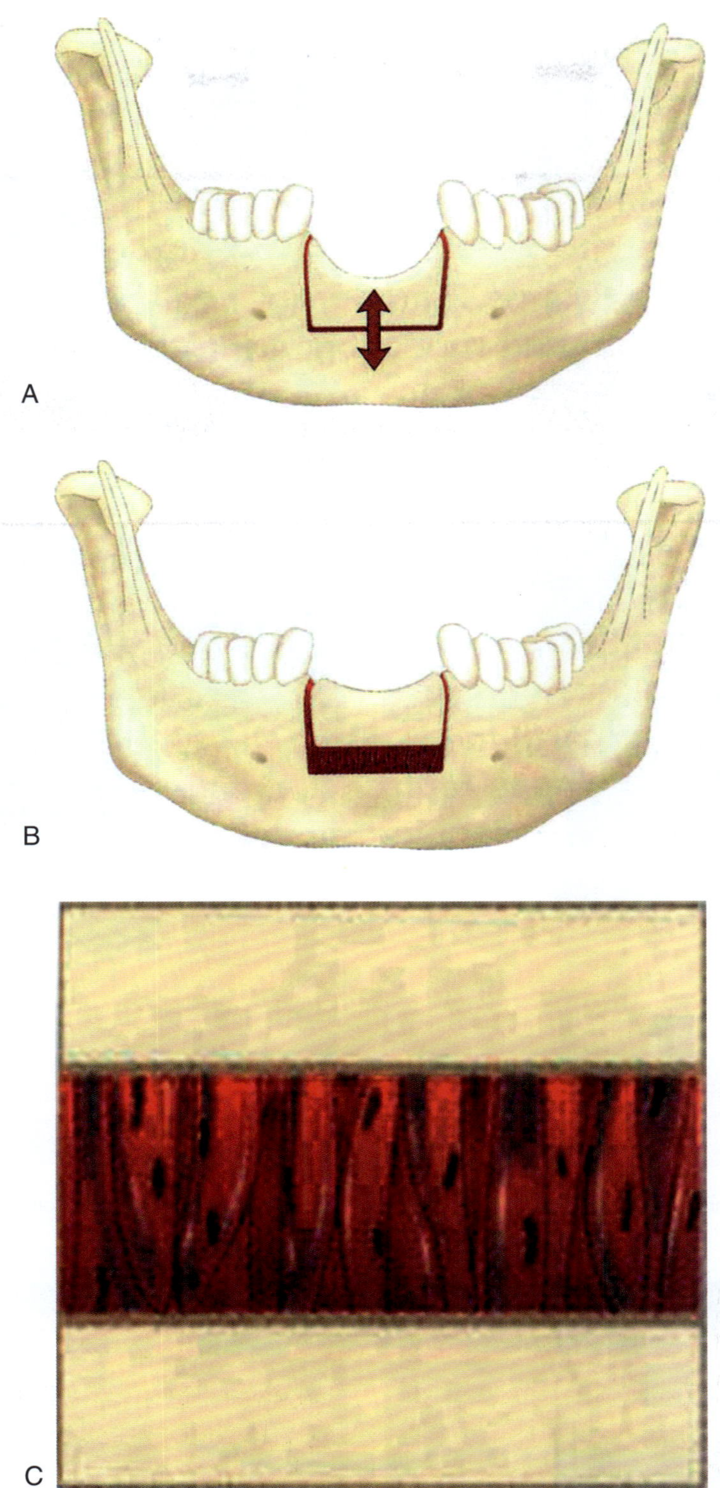

Fig 17.4 (A–C) Mechanisms of alveolar DO.

in a narrow alveolar ridge. However, previous in vivo studies were reported the transport segment underwent resorption and it requires appropriate bone volume to make a transport segment by performing an osteotomy, which placed a heavy burden on the patient. Recently the idea of osteogenesis by periosteal distraction or elevation without corticotomy for bone augmentation has been suggested. These methods indicate a new technical aspect of DO or tissue expansion, with controlled guided formation of new bone.

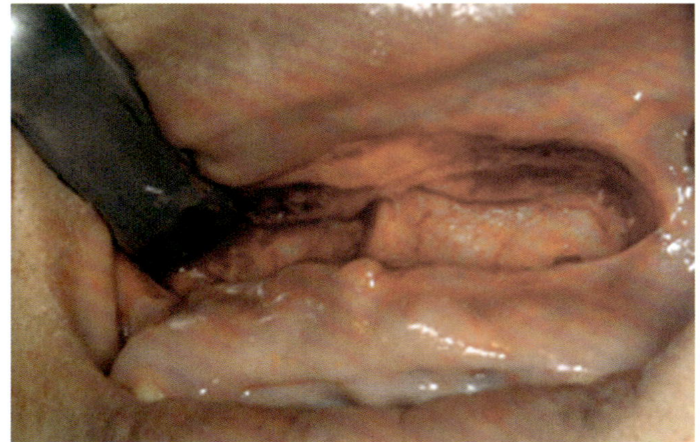

Fig 17.5 A horizontal vestibular incision.

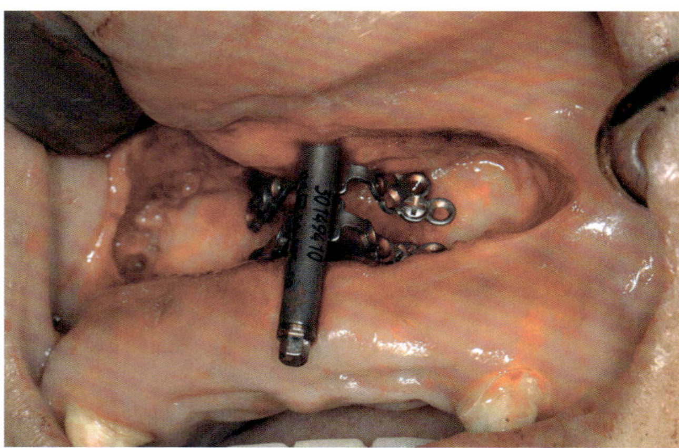

Fig 17.6 Pre-setting of Track 1.0 distraction device.

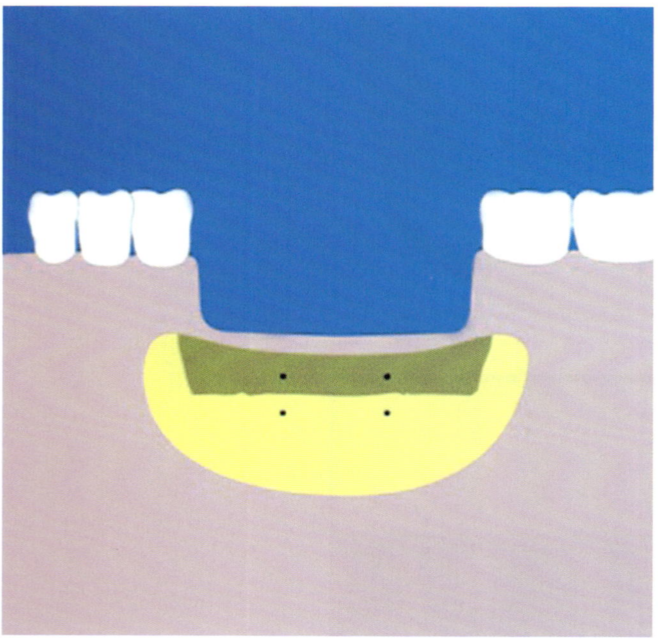

Fig 17.7 Preparation of transport segment – osteotomy.

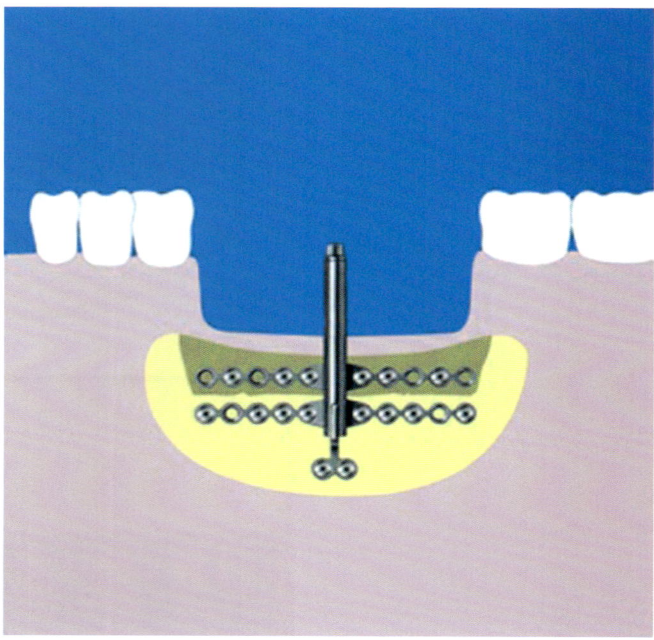

Fig 17.8 Fixation of the distraction device.

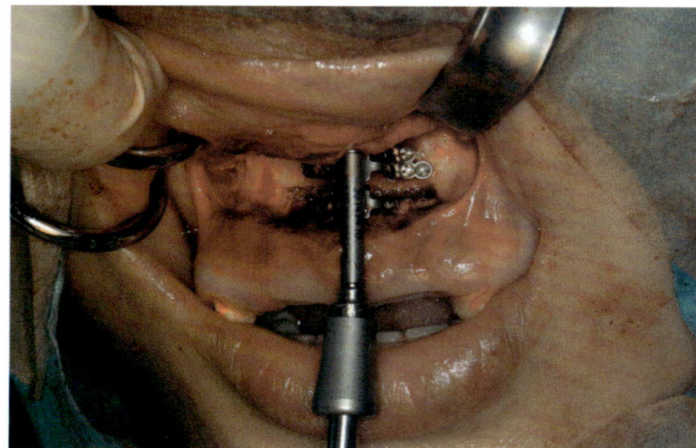

Fig 17.9 Distraction test.

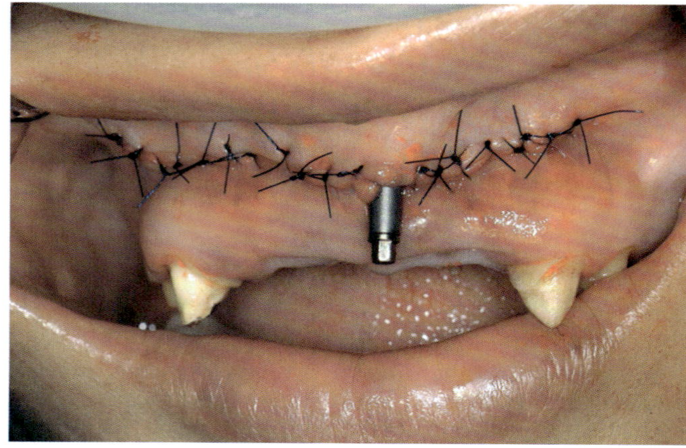

Fig 17.10 Flap closure.

Devices

Horizontal alveolar distraction devices have been previously reported. 'Calluspreader' was developed by Gaggle et al. (Fig 17.14A and B).

The concept of horizontal distraction is quite similar to the vertical alveolar distractor. The author and associates developed a horizontal distraction device consisting of a 0.3-mm-wide commercially pure (CP) titanium mesh plate and a pure titanium distraction screw, 2 mm in diameter and 12 mm in length (Alveo-Wider®, Okada Medical Instrument Supply Co. Ltd., Tokyo, Japan) (Fig 17.15A–E).

Most of the transport segment of horizontal distraction is thin, and the segment was difficult to be fixed with a distraction device. The mesh type device used a titanium microscrew (1.2 mm in diameter) placed in the transport segment and stabilized it to the remaining mandible. The mesh structure has many holes to insert microscrews and it is an advantage to have many choices to insert the screws, especially when an inadvertent fracture occurs to the transport segment. This device is worked at a rate of 0.4 mm (0.45 mm for the prototype) from one turn, using an original driver distraction speed of 0.4–0.8 mm/day.

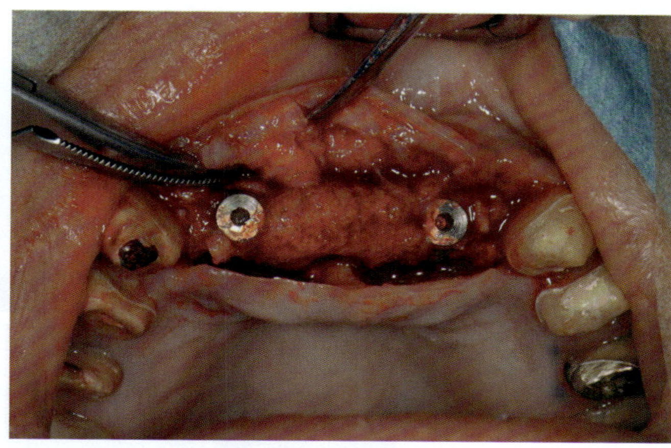

Fig 17.12 Implant placement after distractor removal.

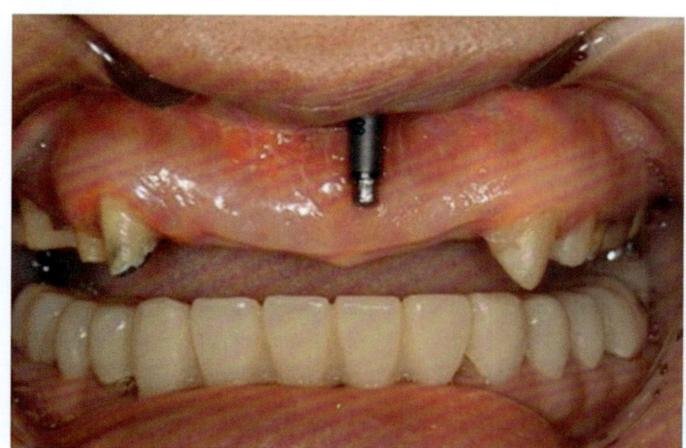

Fig 17.11 Distractor activation.

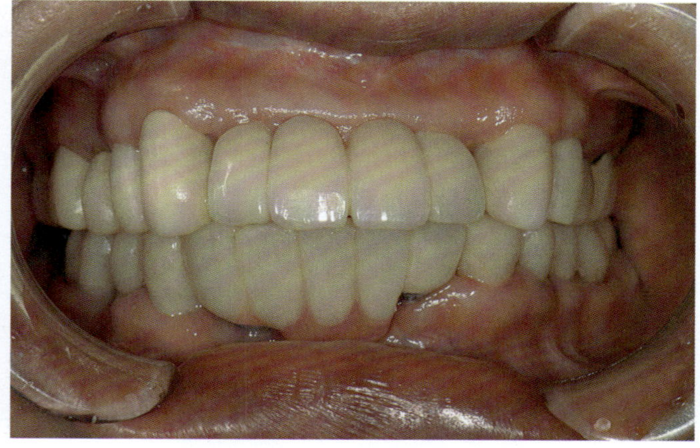

Fig 17.13 Final superstructure.

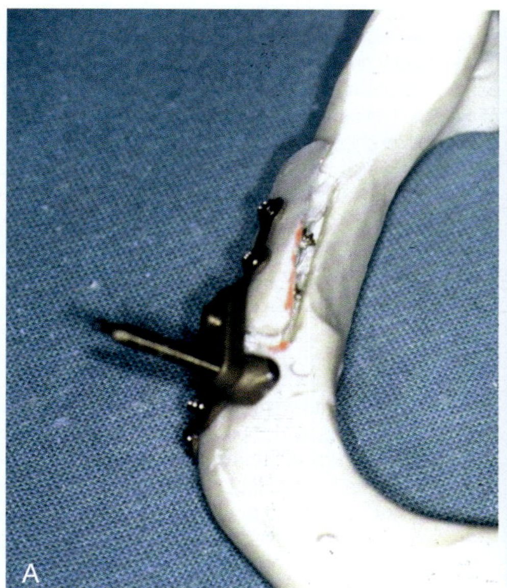

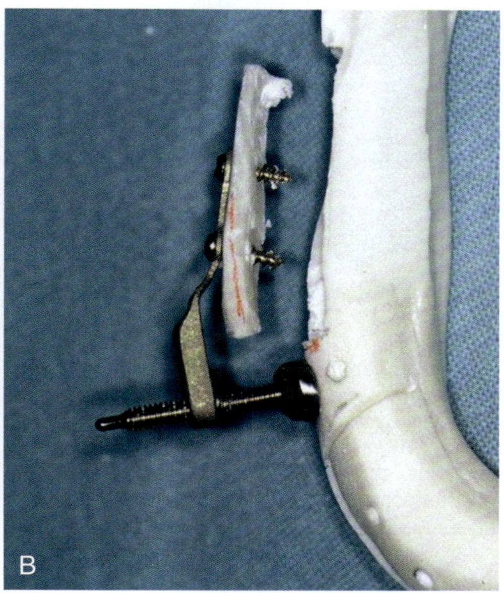

Fig 17.14 (A) Horizontal alveolar DO device 'Calluspreader', (B) transport segment was moved laterally followed by activation of Calluspreader.

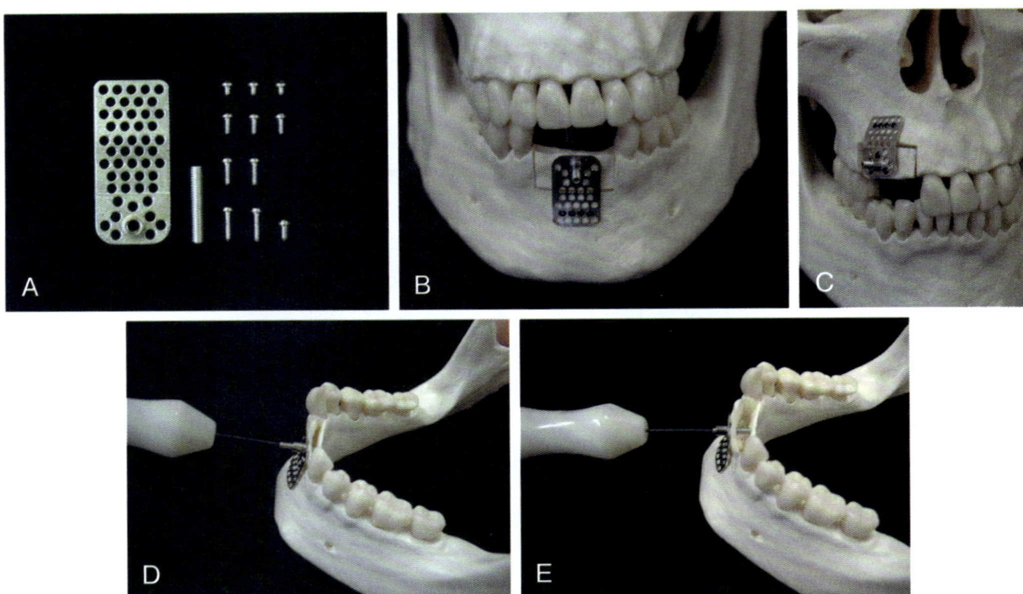

Fig 17.15 (A) Custom horizontal alveolar distraction device Alveo-Wider® of 2 mm titanium miniplate (Okada Medical Instrument Supply Co. Ltd., Tokyo, Japan). (B) Front view of Alveo-Wider® appliance for the anterior mandible. (C) Alveo-Wider® appliance for maxillary premolar region. (D) Distraction activation is done by turning distraction screw using driver. (E) Transport segment was moved laterally followed by activation.

CASE REPORT-1

A healthy 51-year-old female presented with the chief complaint of masticatory dysfunction. She had been using removable partial dentures for the maxilla and mandible, and had been suffering from instability of the mandibular denture because of advanced periodontitis involving the abutment teeth (right mandibular lateral incisor and canine). After these teeth were extracted, she insisted on having an implant-supported prosthesis instead of a removable denture. However, her mandibular alveolar ridge showed extremely thin (Fig 17.16A), and a CT scan (Aquilion, Toshiba Medical Co., Japan) revealed that her anterior alveolar ridge was extremely thin, being 2 mm wide at a level 3 mm from the apex of the alveolar crest (Fig 17.16B).

The initial plan was to perform buccal onlay bone grafting from the ilium for implant placement. However, the patient refused to undergo bone grafting. Therefore, horizontal DO of the anterior mandibular ridge was chosen to augment the alveolar ridge after conventional implant placement in the posterior molar region bilaterally.

Surgical procedure

The patient was anaesthetized with local anaesthetic and intravenous sedation. A crestal incision was made, and extended vertically mesial to the first molar region. The mucoperiosteum was reflected, exposing the labial surface of the mandible. First, a vertical osteotomy was performed using a reciprocating bone saw (Fig 17.17A). This was followed by a horizontal osteotomy to the depth of the buccal plate using an oscillating saw (Fig 17.17B). Finally, a splitting osteotomy was completed using a reciprocating bone saw and a thin-bladed osteotome, and the transport bone was then displaced labially by a horizontal green stick fracture apically (Fig 17.18A). In this manner, a transport bone segment was made from the central to the canine region bilaterally (Fig 17.18B). A horizontal distraction device, consisting of a 0.3-mm-wide CP titanium mesh plate, and a pure titanium distraction screw 2 mm in diameter and 12 mm in length (Alveo-Wider®), was attached bilaterally using a titanium microscrew (1.2 mm in diameter) placed in each transport segment and stabilized to the remaining mandible (Fig 17.19A). The wounds were closed with 4-0 Gore-Tex® suture (Johnson & Johnson, Somerville, NJ) with the distraction screws penetrating from the flaps (Fig 17.19B).

Postoperative protocol

After 7 days to allow for soft tissue healing and early revascularization, the distraction devices were activated by turning the distraction screws 0.225 mm twice a day, for 14 consecutive days on the left side and for 12 days on the right side. In all, the alveolar process of the anterior mandibular region was widened to 6 mm, at a level 3 mm from the apex of the alveolar crest on both sides. During distraction, there were no apparent problems except a small dehiscence observed in the middle of the flap. The patient was instructed to rinse her mouth daily with chlorhexidine chloride solution. After consolidation period of 3 months, the devices were removed, and it was confirmed that the distracted areas were completely filled with newly formed bone. Post distraction, a CT scan (Newtom, Italy) confirmed that the alveolar process had widened to 5.8–6 mm at 3 mm from the apex of the alveolar crest (Fig 17.20A–C).

Two months after distraction device removal, four 13-mm-long standard Astra Tech Implants (Astra Tech AB, Göteborg, Sweden), all 3.5 mm in diameter, were placed in the distracted areas with good initial stability (Figs 17.21 and 17.22).

Four months after implant placement, the implants were uncovered, and abutments were connected. A bone-anchored fixed definitive prosthesis was then fabricated and put in place (Fig 17.23). No significant marginal bone resorption was seen around the implant almost 7 years after implant placement. The patient has been using this prosthesis with good function and great satisfaction.

CASE REPORT-1—cont'd

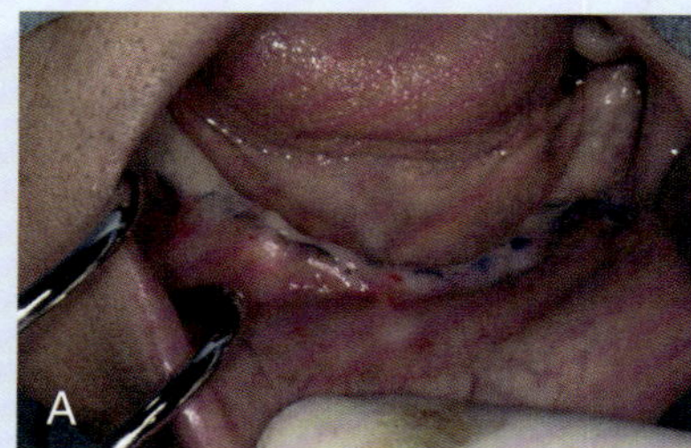

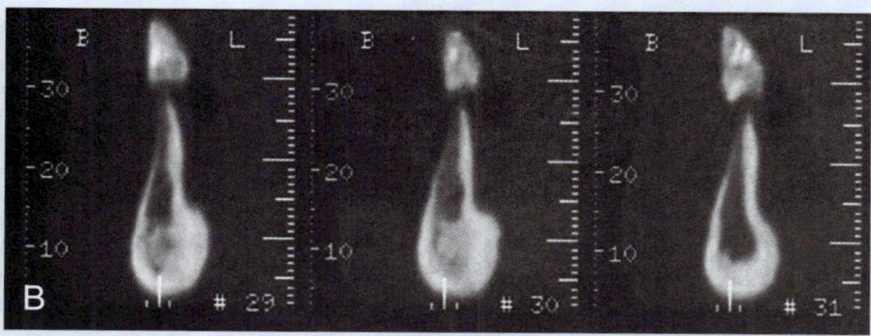

Fig 17.16 (A) Preoperative intraoral view of the extremely atrophic mandible. (B) Preoperative cross-sectional CT scan views showing extremely thin bony ridge in the mandibular symphyseal region.

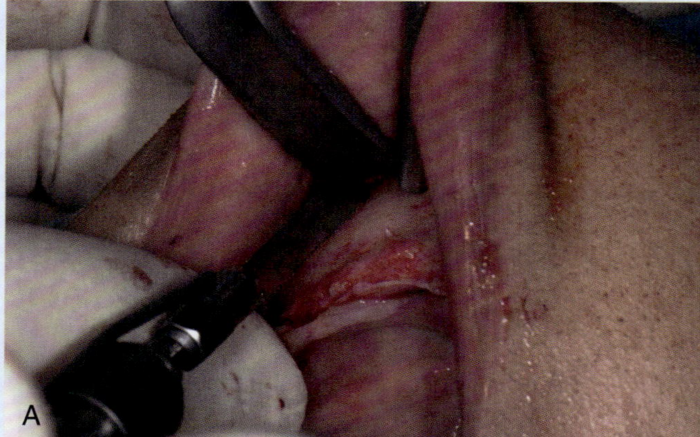

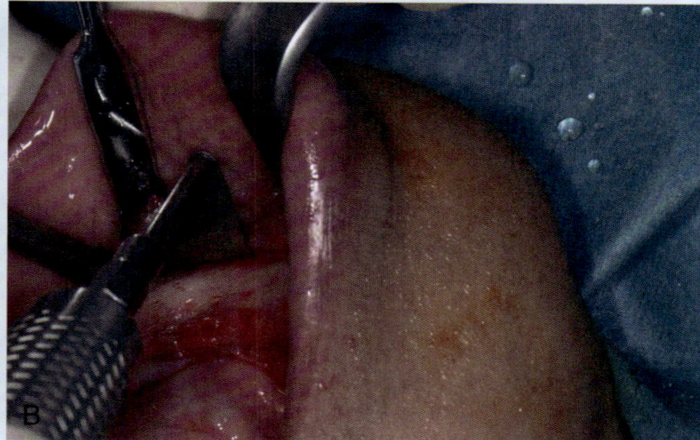

Fig 17.17 (A) Vertical corticotomy using microreciprocating saw. (B) Horizontal corticotomy using microoscillating saw. Horizontal cut was only performed to labial cortex.

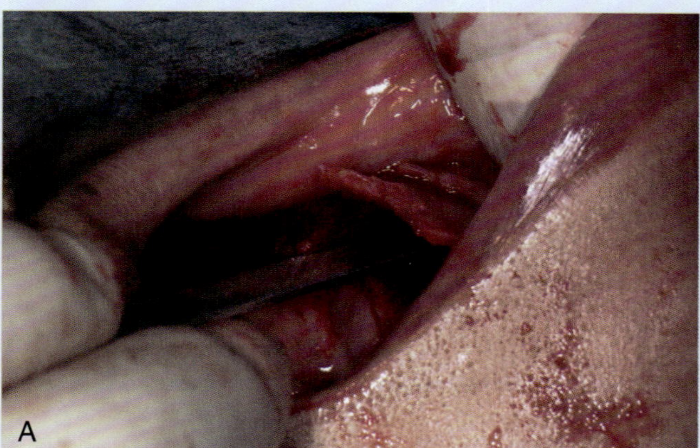

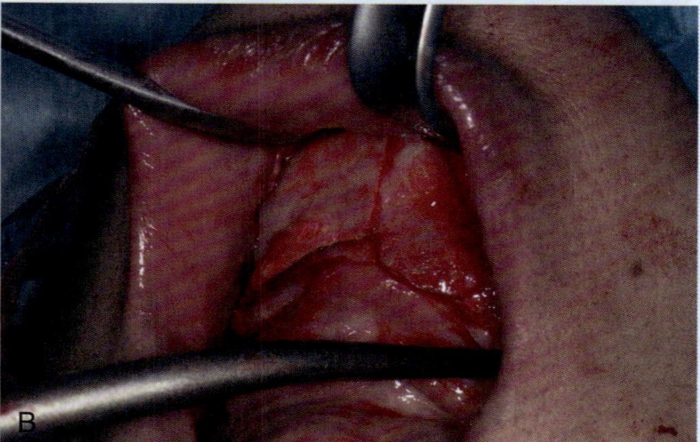

Fig 17.18 (A) Splitting osteotomy using microreciprocating saw and thin osteotome. (B) Bilateral transport segments were created by separation at the midline.

Continued

CASE REPORT-1—cont'd

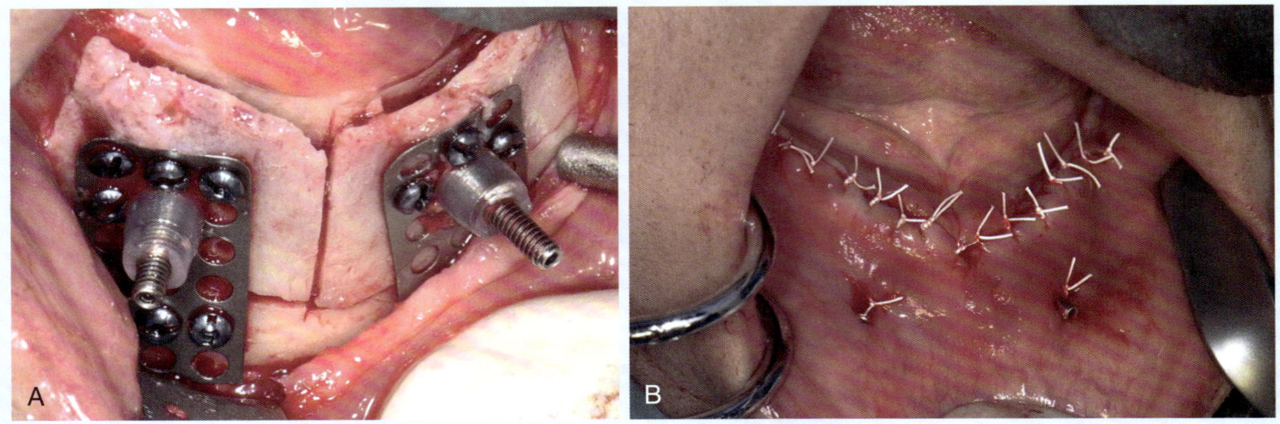

Fig 17.19 (A) Two distraction devices (Alveo-Wider®) were set and thin transport segment was fixed with three microscrews in each side. (B) The wounds were closed with 4-0 Gore-Tex® suture with the distraction screws penetrating from the flaps.

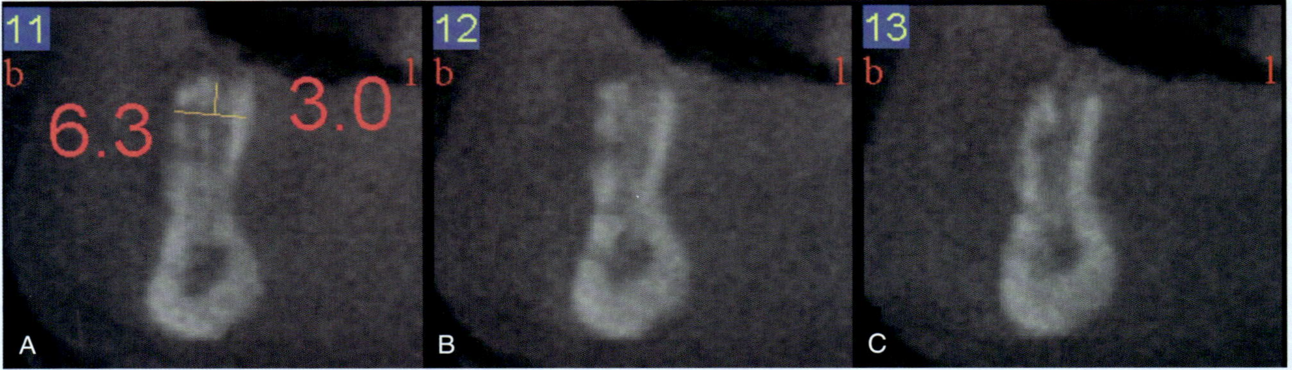

Fig 17.20 (A–C) CT findings of distracted area at postoperative 3 months.

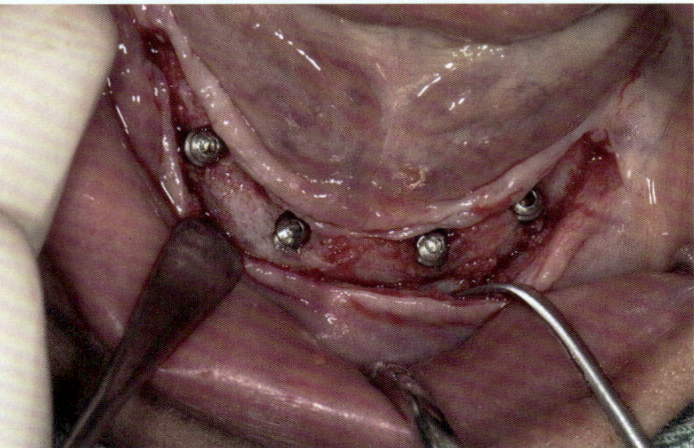

Fig 17.21 Implant placement in the distracted area.

CASE REPORT-1—cont'd

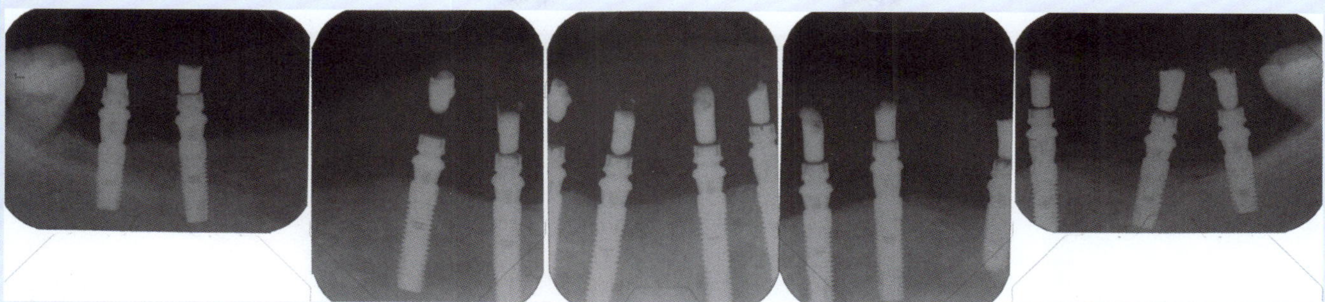

Fig 17.22 Intraoral radiographic findings after implant placement.

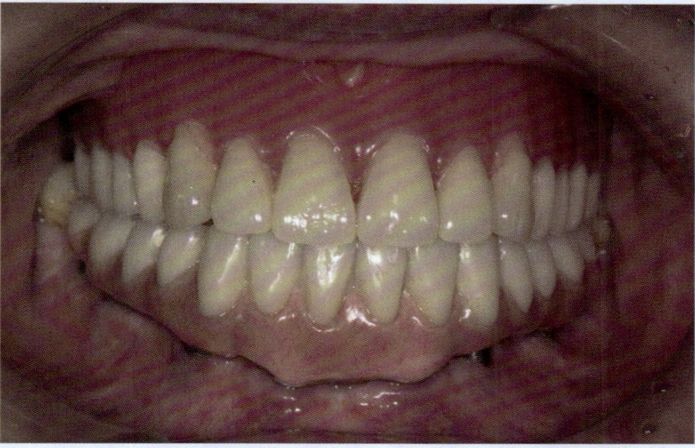

Fig 17.23 Definitive prosthesis was set at postoperative 9 months.

CASE REPORT-2

A healthy 21-year-old female presented with the chief complaint of masticatory dysfunction. She lost her teeth (12–15) in a traffic accident and insisted on having an implant-supported prosthesis instead of a removable denture. CT scan revealed that her alveolar ridge was knife-edged in shape, being 3 mm wide at a level of 3 mm from the apex of the alveolar crest (Fig 17.24).

Surgery was planned with alveolar widening using Alveo-wider® and simultaneous septoplasty under general anaesthesia.

Surgical procedure

A crestal incision was made and extended vertically mesial to the central incisor. The mucoperiosteum was reflected, exposing the labial surface of the maxilla. First, a vertical osteotomy was performed using a reciprocating bone saw. In the same manner as case 1, a transport bone segment was made from the central to the second premolar region. A horizontal distraction device was attached using titanium microscrews placed in the transport segment and stabilized to the remaining maxilla (Fig 17.25).

After checking the movement of the device from trial activation, the wounds were closed with 5-0 nylon suture with the distraction screws penetrating from the flaps.

Postoperative protocol

After 7 days latency period, the distraction devices were activated by turning the distraction screws 0.2 mm twice a day for 24 consecutive days. During distraction, there were no apparent problems on the device and surrounding tissues. The patient was instructed to rinse her mouth daily with chlorhexidine chloride solution. After consolidation for 3 months, the devices were removed, and it was confirmed that the distracted areas were completely filled with newly formed bone. A CT scan revealed that bone regeneration was approximately 500–800 HU showing excellent bone quality (Fig 17.26).

Two months after distraction device removal, two 13-mm-long (diameter 3.5 mm) and two 15-mm-long (diameter 4.5 mm) standard Astra Tech implants (Astra Tech AB, Goteborg, Sweden) were placed in the distracted areas with sufficient initial stability (Fig 17.27A). Three months after implant placement, the implants were uncovered, and abutments were connected. A bone-anchored fixed definitive prosthesis was then fabricated and put in place (Fig 17.27B). Six years after implant placement, marginal bone loss around the implants is minimal, showing excellent clinical outcome.

CASE REPORT-2—cont'd

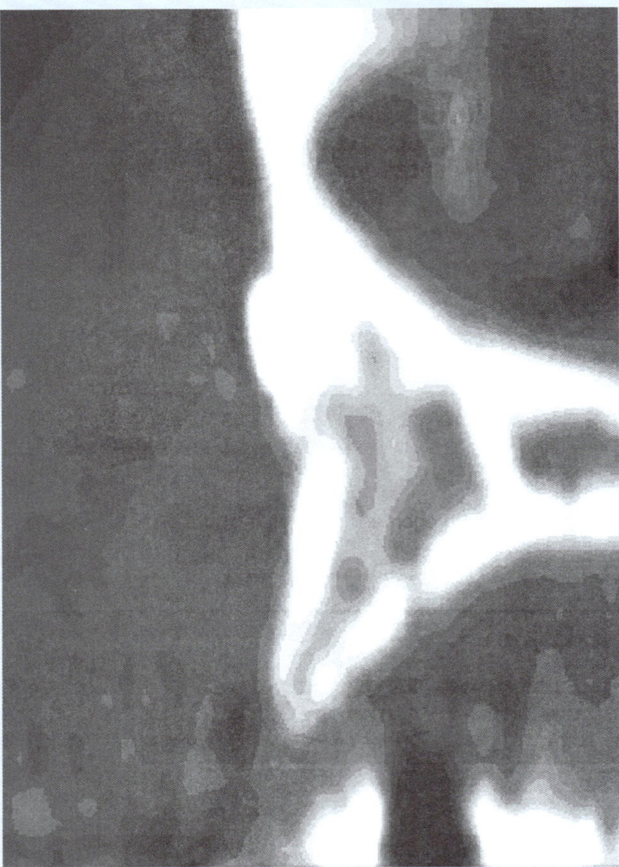

Fig 17.24 Preoperative CT finding. Horizontal defect was seen at right maxillary incisor to premolar region.

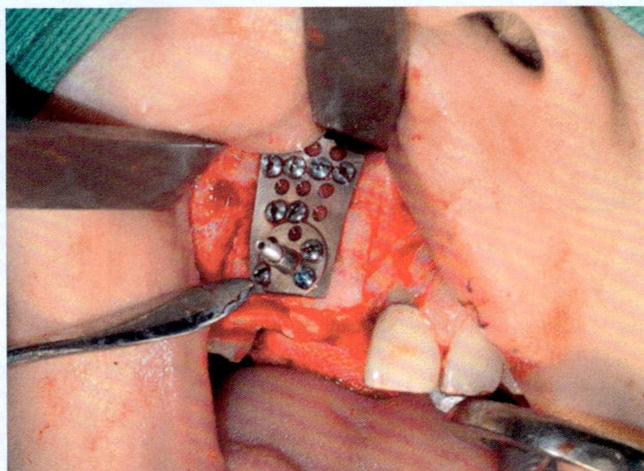

Fig 17.25 Distraction device was fixed using microscrews.

CASE REPORT-2—cont'd

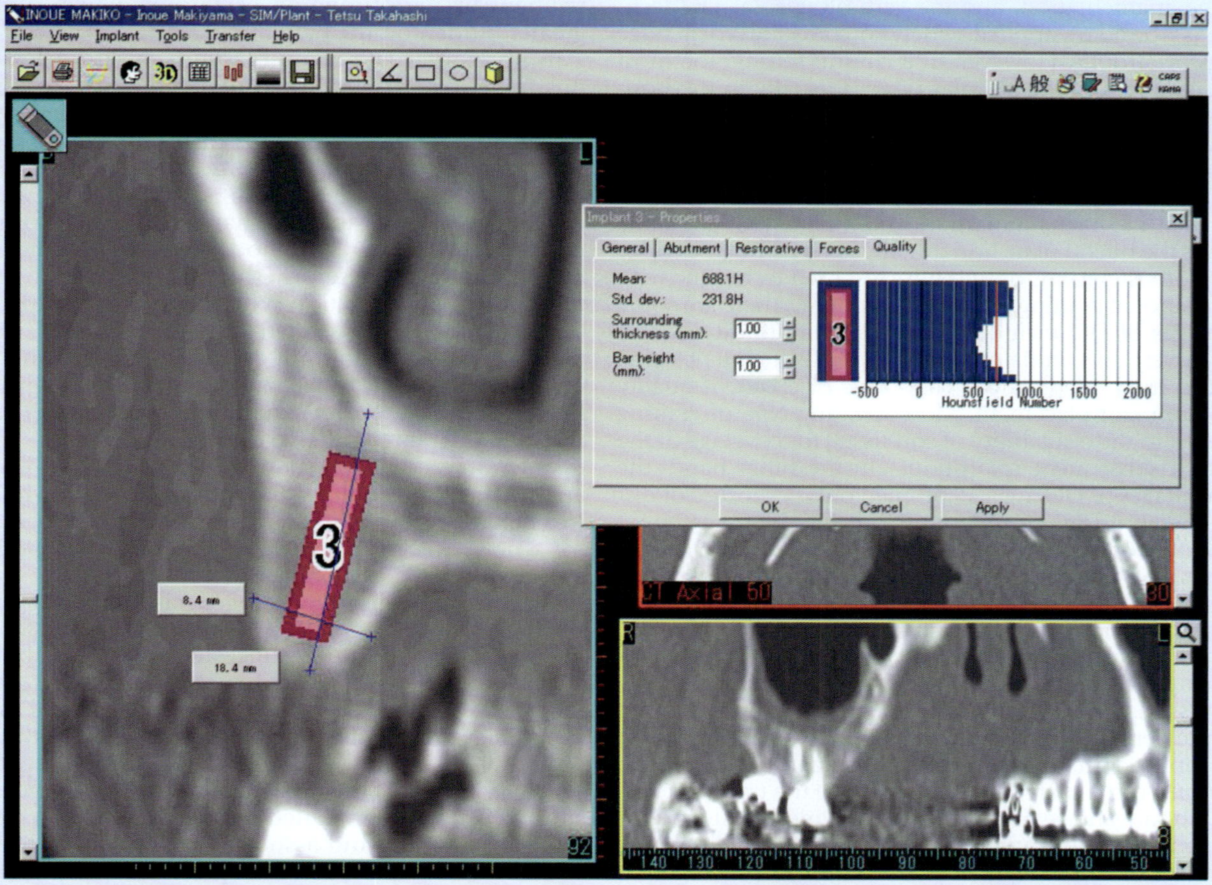

Fig 17.26 CT finding (SimPlant) 3 months after distraction before implant insertion.

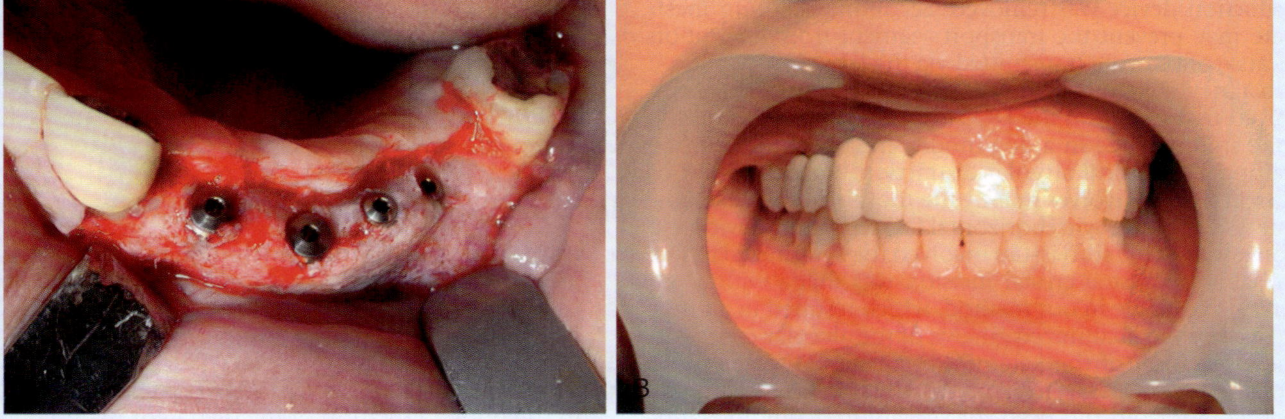

Fig 17.27 (A) Implant insertion at distracted area. Please note the augmented area after distraction. (B) Definitive prosthesis was set at postoperative 11 months.

Discussion

In 1996, DO was introduced as an effective new technique of ridge augmentation, and the vertical alveolar DO technique is nowadays applied widely to correct alveolar ridge defects or atrophy. However, in a clinical setting, the most substantial loss of the alveolar ridge is usually in the horizontal dimension. Although case reports and case series of horizontal DO for correcting a narrow alveolar ridge have been published, the method of horizontal DO for a narrow alveolar ridge has not been established. The method of horizontal DO using a titanium mesh plate that gradually expands the buccal plate horizontally is very similar to ridge expansion osteotomy, or the split-crest (SC) technique with interpositional grafting. Compared with SC, there are some advantages of DO including the lack of morbidity from a graft harvest site, initial stability of bone fragment using titanium mesh plate, and a vital bone of excellent quality for the implant placement. Moreover, any type of grafting is limited to the availability of soft tissue for coverage of the graft and subsequent resorption. On the other hand, the disadvantages of DO are also pointed out – exposure of distraction device, long treatment period, and the necessity for a secondary operation for the removal of distraction device.

Compared with vertical DO, there are some technical difficulties with the horizontal DO. First, a splitting osteotomy is necessary and a splitting osteotomy for a thin alveolar ridge can be technique-sensitive with the risk of cracking or fracturing the transport segment, even when the osteotomy is successful. Second, the transport segment must be freed from the periosteum, because the splitting osteotomy must be completed in addition to the horizontal osteotomy. A titanium mesh plate is used to stabilize the transport segment. The advantage of using a titanium mesh plate for this purpose is that the titanium mesh is strong enough for stabilizing the transport segment, even if the transport segment cracks or fractures after the splitting osteotomy. While there was a crack in the right transport segment in Case Report 2, the crack had completely disappeared by the time the distraction device was removed. Second, a titanium mesh plate may prevent the transport segment from resorption because of pressure transmitted via the labial soft tissue.

In a previous study by the author and associates, the keratinized tissue gain on the DO side was greater than on the bone splitting side in a dog model. In conventional bone grafting and vertical alveolar distraction, the elongation of the soft tissues involves mainly the movable mucous membrane. In contrast, with horizontal DO using this device, the elongation of the soft tissues involved the keratinized tissue, probably because a crestal incision was made within the keratinized tissue in our method, which resulted in a direct increase in the keratinized gingiva of the alveolar crest area. The elongation of the keratinized soft tissue seems to be a major advantage of horizontal DO using this technique, that would avoid the need for surgery to acquire keratinized tissue for cosmetic purposes. In addition, the physical stress, costs, and treatment period could be reduced.

Horizontal periosteal expansion osteogenesis

Distraction osteogenesis is a biological process that leads to new bone formation between segments that are gradually separated, and it continues as long as the strained tissue is activated incrementally. However, it requires appropriate bone volume to make a transport segment by performing an osteotomy, which induces a greater burden on the patient.

In horizontal DO using titanium mesh device, previous in vivo studies reported that the transport segment had undergone resorption at 12 weeks and 24 weeks in a dog model. This resorption of the transport segment probably occurred because the periosteum was completely reflected from the transport segment and was not pedicle. A possible mechanism of bone formation of this horizontal DO method, seems to mainly depend on periosteum. Therefore, this method is not conventional 'bone distraction', but 'periosteal expansion'. Garcia-Garcia also asserted that this method was not true bone distraction, but 'dynamic guided bone regeneration'. The role of the transport segment appeared to be as a continuously expanding space-maker. Nonetheless, the author believes that horizontal alveolar distraction using a titanium mesh plate is an excellent augmentation technique for the placement of implants in a narrow alveolar ridge. This method may open a door to 'a new concept of bone augmentation by periosteal expansion'.

Recently the idea of osteogenesis by periosteal distraction or elevation without a corticotomy for bone augmentation has been suggested. These methods are based on the concept that tensile strain on the periosteum, which causes tenting of the subperiosteal capsule, is sufficient to produce bone formation, without corticotomy or local harvesting of the bone. These studies indicate a new technical aspect of DO or tissue expansion, with the controlled guided formation of new bone. The author and associates investigated the utility of periosteal expansion osteogenesis (PEO), the same concept as periosteal DO or elevation, using a highly purified β-TCP block, instead of titanium devices, in a dog model.

Complications

Complications of DO can be classified into immediate, early and late complications.

Immediate complications

1. Damage to the dentition including pulp necrosis and loosening
2. Inability to find the screw-holes after performing the osteotomy for the device
3. Damage to the orthodontic appliance
4. Severe undercuts along the ridge topography, resulting in the poor adaptation of the distractor plate
5. Fracture of the distractor plate or fixation screw.

Early complications

1. Postoperative infection
2. Distractor loosening
3. Pressure necrosis of bone around the fixation screws
4. Paraesthesia, if nerve injury has occurred during distractor fixation.

Late complications

1. Occlusal disharmony
2. Relapse
3. Incorrect vector
4. Tooth elongation by elastic traction
5. Premature bony consolidation
6. Facial nerve damage
7. Condylar resorption
8. Alterations in the articulation
9. Atypical facial pain
10. Injury through the distractor
11. Fibrous union
12. Quadriparesis
13. Maxillary sinus perforation
14. Parotid fistula
15. Alterations in speech.

Summary

Alveolar distraction osteogenesis is a viable clinical alternative for alveolar ridge augmentation. This technique, when applied for alveolar ridge augmentation, is characterized by the absence of donor site morbidity and ample bone volume augmentation, with simultaneous expansion of the surrounding soft tissues. Specifically, horizontal alveolar distraction osteogenesis using a titanium mesh plate is an excellent augmentation technique for the placement of implants in a narrow alveolar ridge. This method may shed a light on 'a new concept of bone augmentation by periosteal expansion'. Further basic and clinical studies are necessary concerning the indications, limitations, and probable complications of using horizontal distraction to expand a narrow alveolar ridge.

Further Reading

Collins TA, Brown GK, Johnson N, et al. Team management of atrophic edentulism with autogenous inlay, veer, and split grafts and endosseous implants: case reports. Quintessence Int 1995;26:76–93.

Artzi Z, Nemcovsky CE. The application of deproteinized bovine bone mineral for ridge preservation prior to implantation: clinical and histological observations in a case report. J Periodontol 1998;69:1062–7.

Jovanovic SA, Nevins M. Bone formation utilizing reinforced barrier membranes. Int J Periodont Restor Dent 1995;15:56–69.

Ilizarov GA. The tension-stress effect on the genesis and growth of tissue: part 1. The influence of stability of fixation and soft tissue preservation. Clin Orthop 1989;238:249–81.

Ilizarov GA. The tension-stress effect on the genesis and growth of tissue: part 2. The influence of the rate and frequency of distraction. Clin Orthop 1989;239:263–85.

McCarthy JG, Schreiber J, Karp N, et al. Lengthening the human mandible by gradual distraction. Plast Reconstr Surg 1992;89:1–8.

Chin M, Toth B. Distraction osteogenesis in maxillofacial surgery using internal devices: review of five cases. J Oral Maxillofac Surg 1996;54:45–53.

Hidding J, Lazar F, Zölller JE. The vertical distraction of the alveolar bone. J Craniomaxillofac Surg 1998;26(Suppl. 1):72.

Nosaka Y, Kitano S, Wada K, et al. Endosseous implants in horizontal alveolar ridge distraction osteogenesis. Int J Oral Maxillofac Implants 2002;17:846–53.

Funaki K, Takahashi T, Yamauchi K. Horizontal alveolar ridge augmentation using distraction osteogenesis: comparison with a bone-splitting method in a dog model. Oral Surg Oral Med Oral Pathol Oral Radiol Endod 2009;107:350–8.

Kessler P, Bumiller L, Schlegel A, et al. Dynamic periosteal elevation. Br J Oral Maxillofac Surg 2007;45:284–7.

Schmidt BL, Kung L, Jones C, et al. Induced osteogenesis by periosteal distraction. J Oral Maxillofac Surg 2002;60(10):1170–5.

Sencimen M, Aydintug YS, Ortakoglu K, et al. Histomorphometrical analysis of new bone obtained by distraction osteogenesis and osteogenesis by periosteal distraction in rabbits. Int J Oral Maxillofac Surg 2007;36:235–42.

Yamauchi K, Takahashi T, Funaki K, et al. Periosteal expansion osteogenesis using highly purified beta-tricalcium phosphate blocks: a pilot study in dogs. J Periodontol 2008;79:999–1005.

Gaggl A, Rainer H, Chiari FM. Horizontal distraction of the anterior maxilla in combination with bilateral sinus lift operation—preliminary report. Int J Oral Maxillofac Surg 2005;34:37–44.

Laster A, Rachmiel A, Jensen O. Alveolar width distraction osteogenesis for early implant placement. J Oral Maxillofac Surg 2005;63:1724–30.

Takahashi T, Funaki K, Shintani H, et al. Use of horizontal alveolar distraction osteogenesis for implant placement in a narrow alveolar ridge: a case report. Int J Oral Maxillofac Implants 2004;19:291–4.

Jensen OT, Cockrell R, Kuhlke L, et al. Anterior maxillary alveolar distraction osteogenesis: a prospective 5-year clinical study. Int J Oral Maxillofac Implants 2002;17:52–68.

Gaggl A, Schultes G, Karcher H. Vertical alveolar ridge distraction with prosthetic treatable distractors: a clinical investigation. Int J Oral Maxillfac Surg 2000;15:701–10.

Holbein O, Neidlinger-Wilke C, Suger G, et al. Ilizarov callus distraction produces systemic bone cell mitogens. J Orthop Res 1995;13(4):629–38.

Garcia-Garcia A, Somoza-Martin M. Bone distraction versus dynamic guided bone regeneration. J Oral Maxillofac Surg 2005;63:724.

Suhr MAA, Kreusch Th. Technical considerations in distraction osteogenesis. Int J Oral Maxillofac Surg 2004;33:89–94.

18 Sinus grafting for dental implants

Ajay Vikram Singh   Angelo Troedhan

CHAPTER CONTENTS HD

Introduction

Treatment of the posterior edentulous maxilla has been and continues to remain a challenge for the implant surgeon, because of reasons like pneumatization of the maxillary sinus, poor bone density and volume, and difficult access. Further, the bone which forms around the osseointegrated implants in this region does not show very high density; thus in several cases the implant which has successfully osseointegrated may lead to failure after loading in this region.

Much research has been done on the management of implant therapy in the posterior maxilla and researchers have advocated many techniques of sinus grafting, several types of bone grafts to generate new bone in the elevated sinus floor, and various treatment protocols in the posterior maxilla to obtain successful and long-term implant therapy in this region. Sinus grafting is the procedure commonly practised by most implant dentists to deliver a stable and long-term, implant-supported prosthesis in the posterior maxilla. Various approaches for the safe and easy sinus elevation have been advocated and several types of armamentariums and graft materials have been tried in this field to obtain maximum success in the procedure.

Limitations with the posterior maxilla

1. Poor bone density (type 4/D4) – challenging to achieve adequate initial stability of the implant.
2. Reduced bone height because of sinus pneumatization and vertical bone resorption of ridge crest.
3. Reduced bone width because of lateral resorption of posterior maxilla towards the hard palate, which also results in final prostheses with facial cantilevering.
4. Area of less visibility and access.
5. Proximity with sinus floor, posterior superior artery, etc.

Guidelines for successful implant therapy in the posterior maxilla

1. Longest and widest possible implant insertion.
2. Bicortical implant stabilization – implant platform is stabilized in hard crestal bone and its apex in the high-density sinus floor to achieve adequate initial implant stability.
3. Using more implants for the multiple unit prosthesis.
4. Implants with the sharp, self-engaging, deeper threads should be preferred to achieve high primary stability in low-density trabecular bone.
5. Implants with faster osseointegrating surfaces, like the hydroxyapatite-coated surface implants or the sand blasted and acid etched (SLA) surface implants, should be preferred.
6. Implant can be submerged 1 mm apical to the ridge crest to prevent its premature loading and micromovement during its healing phase.
7. Lateral bone condensation using a special set of osteotomes to achieve high-density bone around the inserted implant.
8. Longer submerged healing period for the implant.
9. Progressive bone loading.

These guidelines can be valuable if the patient has minimum average bone dimensions under the sinus floor to insert the wider and longer implant; but after the loss of the maxillary molars and premolars, the maxillary sinus expands and lowers down ('pneumatization'), resulting in reduced subantral bone height, which is often found inadequate to insert adequately long implants. Further, long-time edentulism of the posterior maxilla also leads to vertical ridge resorption, which further deteriorates the situation for the insertion of long implants and also increases the crown–implant height ratio. Postextraction buccal resorption of the posterior maxilla also reduces the bone available to place wider diameter implants (Fig 18.1A and B).

History

To manage these problems and to offer an optimal implant therapy in the posterior maxilla, a sinus-lift procedure was first performed by Dr Hilt Tatum Jr in 1974 during his period of preparation to begin sinus grafting. The first sinus graft was performed by Tatum in February 1975 in Lee County Hospital in Opelika, Alabama. This was followed by the placement and successful restoration of two endosteal implants. After this, suitable instruments were developed to manage the lining elevation from the different anatomical surfaces encountered in sinuses. Tatum first presented the concept at the Alabama Implant Congress in Birmingham, Alabama in 1976 and presented the evolution of the technique during multiple podium presentations each year until 1986, when he published an article describing the procedure. Dr Philip Boyne was introduced to the procedure when he was invited, by Tatum, to be 'The Discusser' of a presentation on sinus grafting given by Tatum at the American Academy of Implant Dentistry. Boyne and James authored the first publication on the technique in 1980, when they published case reports of autogenous grafts placed into the sinus and healed for 6 months prior to the placement of blade implants.

The sinus floor elevation procedure is one of the most common surgeries performed in implant dentistry. Since its first description, numerous articles have been published to describe different grafting materials used to graft the elevated sinus floor, modifications to the classic technique, and comparisons between different techniques.

Sinus floor elevation and bone grafting into the sinus has produced predictable results enabling clinicians to

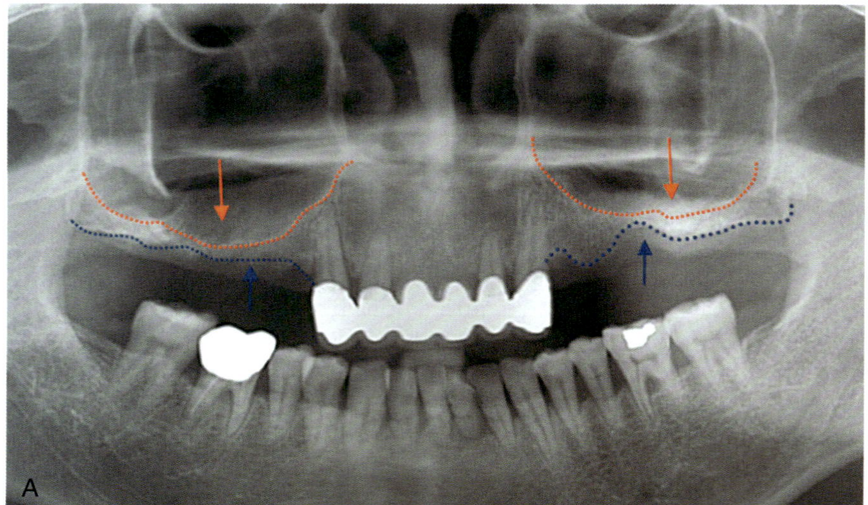

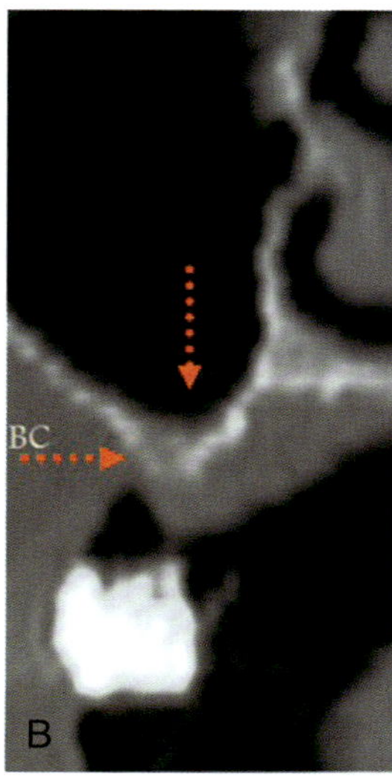

Fig 18.1 (A) Panoramic radiograph shows reduced subantral bone height because of pneumatization of maxillary sinuses and vertical bone resorption, (B) cross-sectional view of the maxillary sinus showing sinus pneumatization and buccal bone resorption, which leads to reduced bone height and width.

place longer implants for more stable prostheses and better long-term outcomes.

Maxillary sinus anatomy

The maxillary sinus is a pyramid-shaped cavity with its base adjacent to the nasal wall and apex pointing to the zygoma. The size of the sinus is insignificant until the eruption of permanent dentition. The average dimensions of the adult sinus are 2.5–3.5 cm wide, 3.6–4.5 cm tall, and 3.8–4.5 cm deep. It has an estimated volume of approximately 12–15 cm. Anteriorly, it extends to the canine and premolar area. The sinus floor usually has its most inferior point near the first molar region. The size of the sinus increases with age if the area is edentulous. The extent of pneumatization varies from person to person and from side to side. Nonetheless, this process often leaves the bony lateral and occlusal alveolus paper-thin in the posterior maxilla. The maxillary sinus bony cavity lined with the sinus membrane, is also known as the 'schneiderian membrane.' This membrane consists of ciliated epithelium like the rest of the respiratory tract. It is continuous with, and connects to, the nasal epithelium through the ostium in the middle meatus. The membrane has a thickness of approximately 0.8 mm. Antral mucosa is thinner and less vascular than nasal mucosa (Fig 18.2A–C).

The blood supply to the maxillary sinus is primarily derived from the posterior superior alveolar artery and the infraorbital artery, both being branches of the maxillary artery. There are significant anastomoses between these two arteries in the lateral antral wall. The greater palatine artery also supplies the inferior portion of the sinus. However, because the blood supplies to the maxillary sinus area are from terminal branches of peripheral vessels, significant haemorrhage during the sinus-lift procedure is rare. Nerve supply to the sinus is derived from the superior alveolar branch of the maxillary (V2) division of the trigeminal nerve.

Indications for sinus grafting

1. Residual subantral bone is less than 10 mm in height.
2. Residual subantral bone is less than 5 mm in width – sinus lifting and grafting can be performed to insert a narrow diameter but longest possible implant, to gain more implant bone contact area for optimal results in implant therapy.
3. Maxillary sinus is free of any acute or chronic infection (sinusitis) or pathology (cyst).

Contraindications for sinus grafting

1. Heavy smoking – smoking is a relative contraindication for sinus grafting as many studies have shown more failures of sinus grafting and implants in smokers. However, smokers can successfully be treated with sinus grafting and implant therapy but the patient should refrain from smoking at least 15 days before sinus graft surgery and for 4–6 weeks after surgery.
2. Acute sinus infection.
3. Significant recurrent history of chronic sinusitis.
4. Uncontrolled diabetes.
5. Maxillary sinus hypoplasia (MSH) – in these patients, the sinus drainage system is chronically compromised and is associated with malformed uncinate process.
6. Cystic fibrosis (CF) – cystic fibrosis is a genetic disease which represents 92–100% chronic sinusitis rate. Patients with cystic fibrosis exhibit significant rates of sinus polyp formation and fungal sinusitis.
7. Maxillary sinus malignant tumours.
8. Big nose variant – patients having inferior turbinate and/or meatus pneumatization.

Pre- and post-medication for the sinus graft procedure

Antibiotics

1. Amoxicillin–clavulanic acid combination is the drug of choice for sinus procedures (e.g. tab. Augmentin, 1 g) – One tablet twice a day starting 1 day before surgery and continued 5 days after surgery.
2. If the patient is allergic to penicillin, then either cefuroxime axetil (1 tab. Ceftin, 500 mg b.i.d.) or clindamycin (1 tab. Dalacin C, 300 mg t.i.d.) can be prescribed for the patient.
3. Antibiotics like clindamycin (inj. Dalacin-C, 300 mg) can also be added with the graft material used for filling the elevated sinus cavity. It significantly reduces the chances of postoperative infection complications.

Analgesics

Any analgesic combination which contains codeine (tab. Tylenol 3) can be prescribed, one tablet 1 h before surgery and one 1 t.i.d. continued for 5 days after surgery. Codeine is a potent antitussive and so it reduces coughing, which may exert additional pressure on the elevated sinus membrane and can cause its tear and the introduction of bacteria into the graft.

Anti anxiety/sedatives

Sinus grafting is a technique-sensitive and time-consuming procedure; thus a sedative like alprazolam (tab. Alprax, or Valium, 2 mg) should be given to the patient:

1. One tablet in the night before surgery to reduce anxiety, so that patient can sleep comfortably at night before the surgery.
2. One tablet in the morning before the surgery, which reduces the patient's anxiety so that the patient remains calm and comfortable during the surgery. It also enhances the effect of the analgesia.
3. One tablet at night after the surgery; it reduces excessive movement of the patient, which may cause the complications.

Corticosteroids

A short-term dose of a steroid like dexamethasone (tab. Decadron, 4 mg) can be prescribed for sinus graft patients.

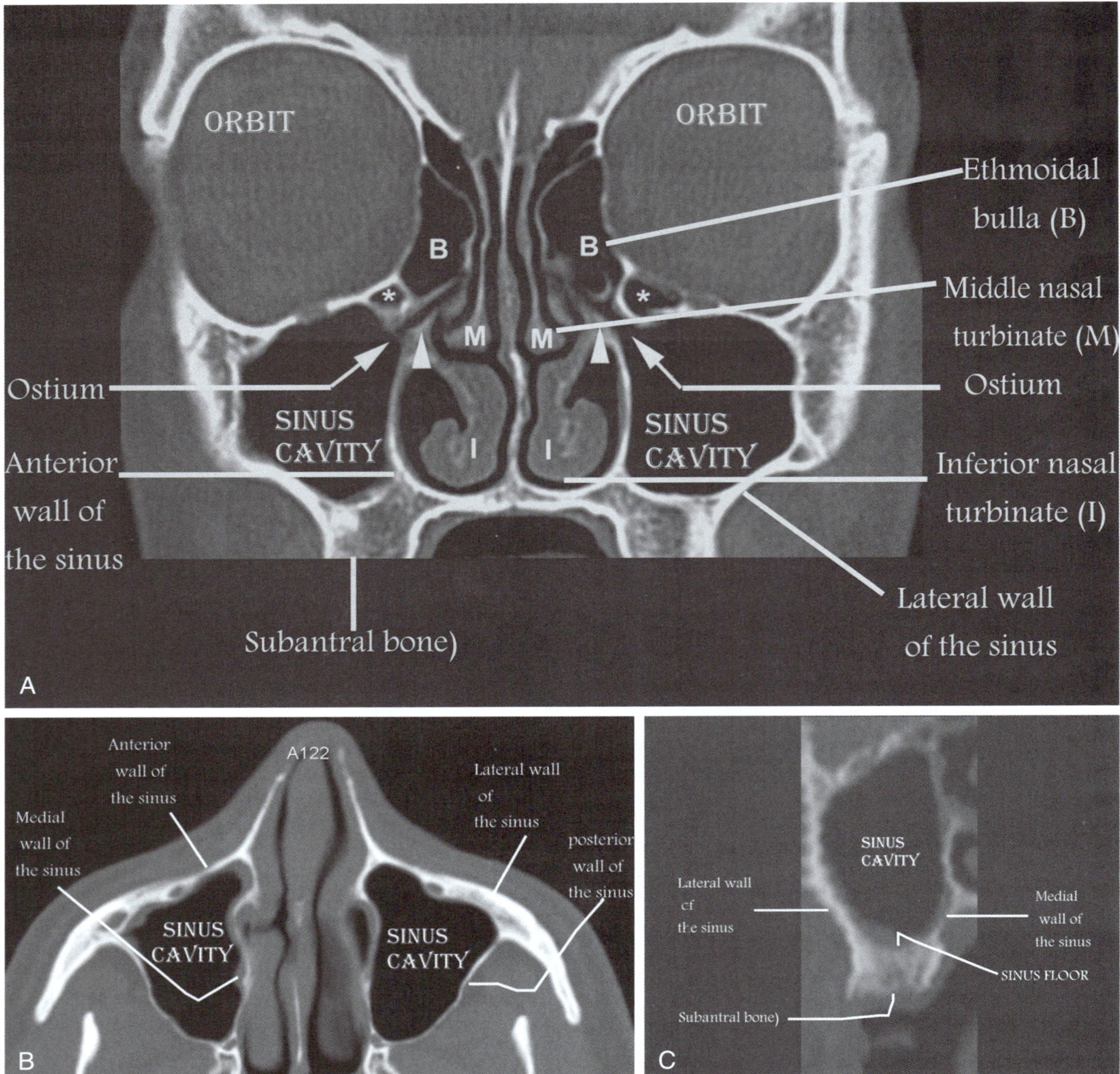

Fig 18.2 (A) Facial, (B) axial, and (C) cross-sectional views of the maxillary sinus region show three-dimensional anatomies of the maxillary sinus and surrounding structures.

1. Steroids reduce the inflammation of soft tissue and so the chances of postoperative swelling, pain, and incision line opening are reduced.
2. Ensures the patency of the ostium and minimizes any inflammation in the sinus before surgery.

   Two tablets (8 mg) (tab. Decadron, 4 mg) in the morning, the day before surgery.

   Two tablets (8 mg) (tab. Decadron, 4 mg) in the morning, before the surgery.

   One tablet (4 mg) on the next day, i.e. on the morning after the surgery.

   One tablet (4 mg) on the third day morning, (48 h) after the surgery.

Multivitamins

Vitamin B complex + zinc + Lactobacillus combination (Cap. BC-Z-LB, once a day) for 5 days after the surgery. It enhances postoperative healing process and maintains gastric flora during the intake of antibiotics.

Antibacterial oral rinse

Chlorhexidine gluconate 0.12% (Periogard mouth rinse) should be used just before the surgery and twice a day for 2 weeks after the surgery. It significantly reduces the microbial flora in the oral cavity and the chances of post-surgery complications.

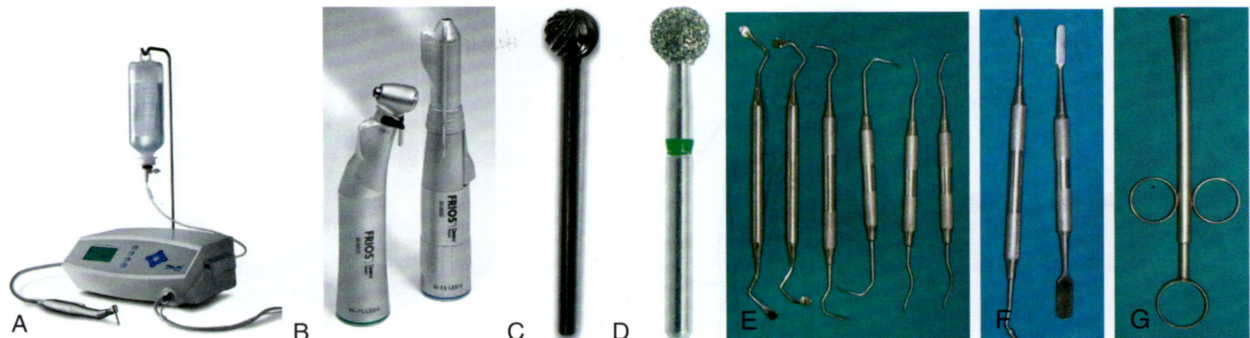

Fig 18.3 (A) Implant motor (physiodispensor) is also used for lateral sinus window preparation. (B) Either contra-angle or straight handpieces (1:1) (C and D) can be used with large round carbide or diamond bur to prepare the osteotomy in the lateral wall of the sinus. (E) A special set of sinus curettes/elevators is then used to carefully elevate the sinus membrane. (F and G) Special instruments can be required to carry the graft into the elevated sinus floor and to fill it adequately and effectively.

Cryotherapy

Ice or cold dressings on the face and cold oral liquids should be used for 24–48 h after sinus graft surgery. It minimizes the postoperative inflammatory swelling.

Hot fomentations

Heat may be applied to the region 48 h after surgery, to increase blood and lymph flow; it clears the area of inflammatory consequences and also reduces any ecchymosis present.

Conventional surgical techniques

There are two main conventional approaches to the maxillary sinus floor elevation procedure, which have been modified to a large extent with the invention of new armamentariums for safe and effective elevation of the schneiderian membrane.

Lateral approach for sinus grafting

This procedure was first performed by Tatum in February 1975. A crestal incision is given along with two vertical extensions and a trapezoidal mucoperiosteal flap is elevated to expose the lateral aspect of the posterior maxilla. Then the osteotomy is completed by preparing a rectangular/oval window in the lateral bony wall of the maxillary sinus to expose the sinus membrane. The osteotomy can be prepared with the rotary handpiece using a large round carbide or diamond bur. The diamond bur should be preferred over the carbide bur because the carbide bur has more tendency to tear the delicate sinus membrane. The newer piezosurgery unit can also be used for the safe preparation of the window osteotomy and the elevation of the sinus membrane, as it does not cut the soft tissue and thus chances of the sinus membrane tearing are minimized. Once the osteotomy is completed to expose the sinus membrane, the bony window can gently be tapped with the back of the mouth mirror handle, to visualize the complete preparation and to break the small and thin bony bridges still left between the window bone and the surrounding lateral wall of sinus. The sinus membrane is then gently lifted up from the bony floor by using a special set of sinus curettes. Marx and Garg suggested that a cottonoid soaked with a carpule of 2% lidocaine with 1:100,000 epinephrine should be left in the space created for 5 min, to limit bleeding and allow better visualization for further dissection. It is important to free up the sinus membrane in all directions (anteriorly, posteriorly, and medially) before attempting to intrude the sinus elevators medially to elevate the sinus membrane from the sinus floor to the desired height. At the time of sinus membrane elevation, the sharp margins of the curette/sinus elevator should always be maintained on the bony floor to avoid inadvertent membrane tear. The curette should never be placed blindly into the access window. A space is created after the sinus membrane has been elevated by the intruded sinus elevators. This space is then grafted using various bone substitutes alone or mixed with autogenous bone. Care should be taken not to overfill the elevated sinus floor, because it may cause membrane necrosis.

The medial part of the sinus is grafted first. The graft material used can be either an autograft, an allograft, a xenograft, an alloplast, a growth-factor infused collagen matrix, or combinations thereof. After the implants have been placed, the remaining lateral part of the sinus defect is grafted and the window can be covered with a collagen barrier membrane to prevent any soft tissue growth in the grafted sinus.

Armamentaria required for lateral approach are shown in Fig 18.3A–G.

Step by step diagrammatic and clinical presentation of the conventional lateral window approach is given in Figs 18.4–18.11.

Simultaneous or delayed implant placement

Depending on the residual subantral bone height to stabilize the implant, the implant surgeon may decide either on simultaneous or delayed implant insertion in sinus grafting cases. Implants are placed either simultaneously with the graft (one-stage lateral antrostomy) or after a delayed period of up to 6–12 months, to allow

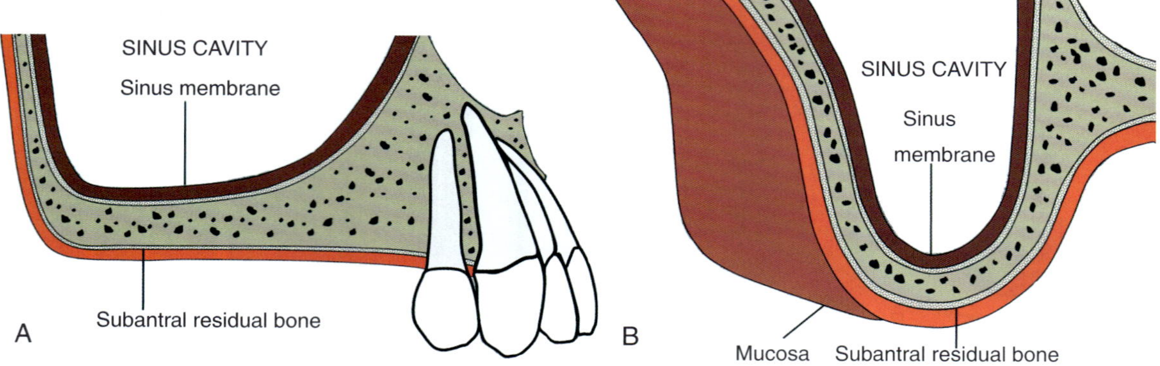

Fig 18.4 (A) Lateral and (B) cross-sectional views of posterior maxilla showing sinus cavity (sinus antrum) and subantral residual bone, which is inadequate in height to insert adequately long implants.

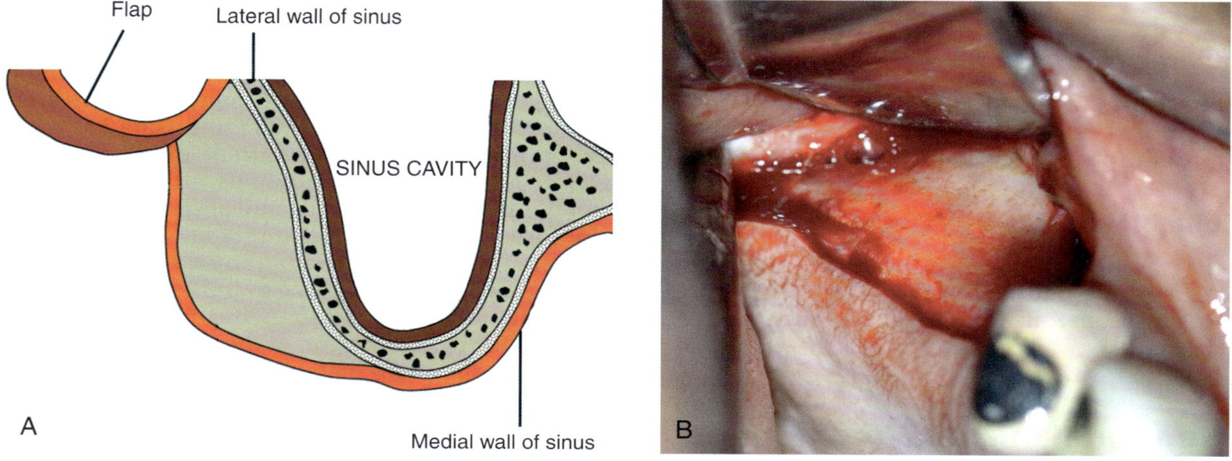

Fig 18.5 (A and B) A mid-crestal incision along with two facial vertical extensions are made and a trapezoidal mucoperiosteal flap is elevated to expose the lateral wall of the maxillary sinus.

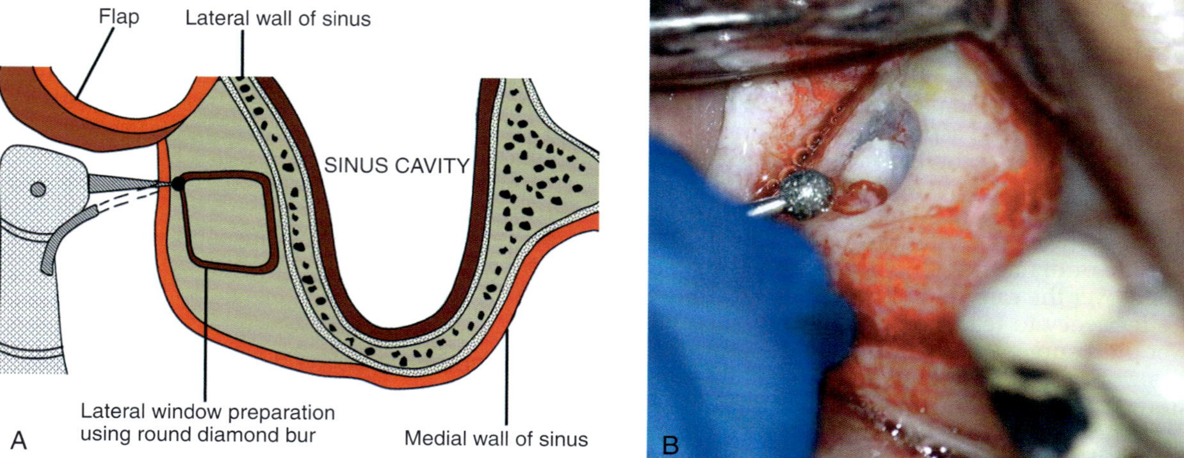

Fig 18.6 (A and B) A rectangular or oval osseous window is carefully prepared on the lateral wall of the sinus using a large round diamond bur to expose the sinus membrane without perforating it.

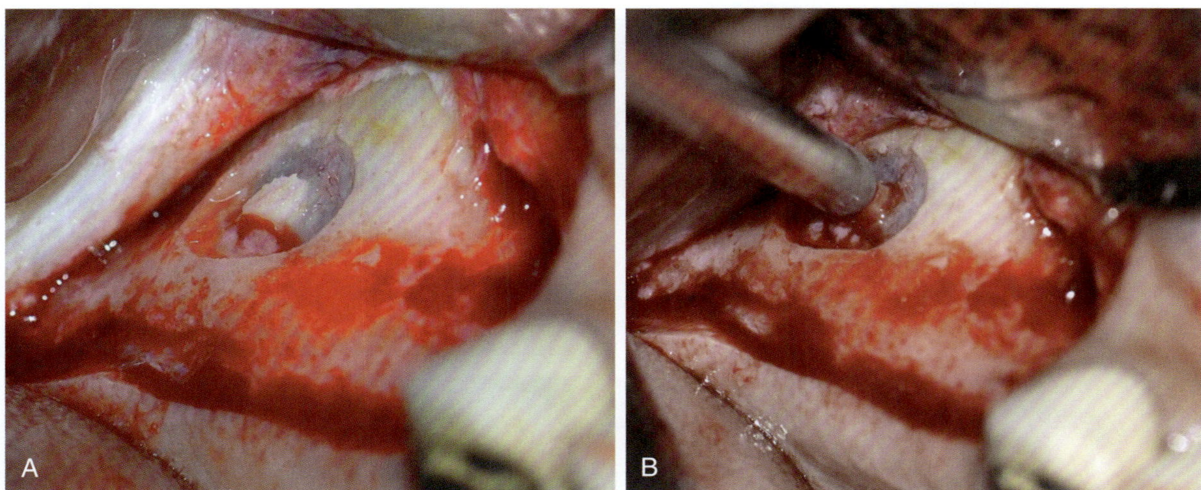

Fig 18.7 (A and B) Once the osteotomy is completed to expose the sinus membrane, the bony window can gently be tapped with the back of the mouth mirror handle to visualize the complete preparation and to break the small and thin bony bridges still left between window bone and surrounding bone.

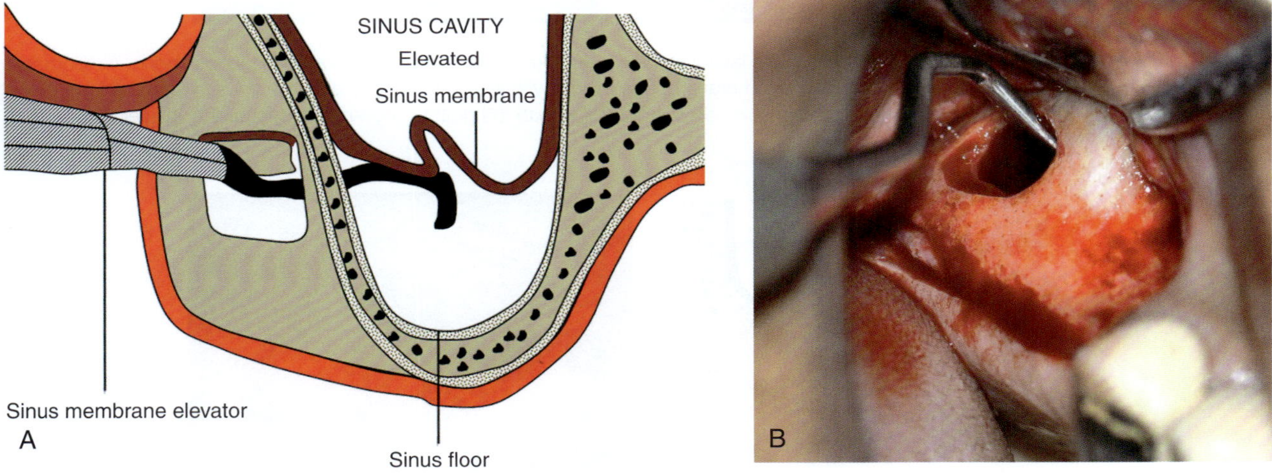

Fig 18.8 (A and B) The schneiderian membrane is carefully elevated to the desired height using a special set of sinus curettes.

for graft maturation (two-stage lateral antrostomy). The initial bone thickness at the alveolar ridge seems to be a reliable indicator in deciding between these two methods. If the subantral bone height is 4 mm or less, initial implant stability could be jeopardized. Therefore, a two-stage lateral antrostomy should be carried out. If the residual bone present below the sinus floor is sufficient in dimension and quality to adequately stabilize the implant, the implant can be inserted at the time of sinus grafting.

Graft materials for the sinus grafting

Numerous research papers have been published to evaluate the prognosis of implants under various grafting materials. Autogenous bone remains the gold standard in bone grafting. Iliac crest, chin, anterior ramus, and tuberosity have all been mentioned as common autogenous donor sites in maxillary sinus lift. Hydroxyapatite (HA), mixed with autogenous bone or used alone, has also been shown to be a viable alternative. Based on past research and clinical trials, the demineralized bone matrix (FDBM, Grafton), which is osteogenic in nature, can be a viable alternative for autogenous bone if used with Bio-Oss or tricalcium phosphate (TCP). Bio-Oss or HA + β-TCP has shown remarkable results in sinus grafting even if used alone (Fig 18.12A–H). Mixing platelet-rich growth factors like platelet rich plasma (PRP)/platelet-derived growth factor (PDGF)/plasma rich growth factor (PRGF)/platelet rich fibrin (PRF) to the sinus graft material increases the amount, quality, and pace of new bone formation in the grafted sinus.

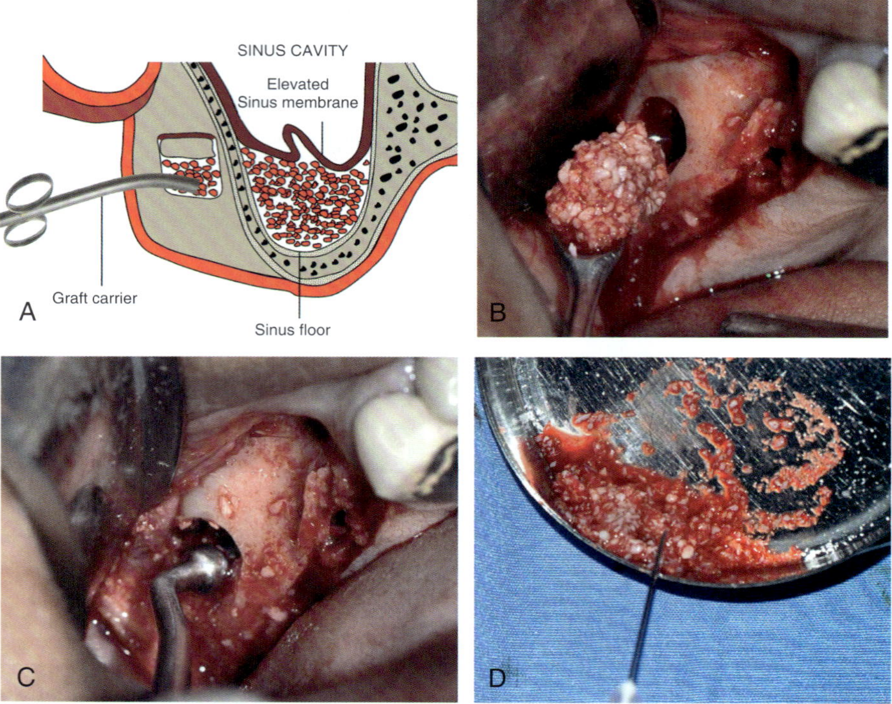

Fig 18.9 (A–C) The elevated sinus floor is grafted through the lateral window using bone substitutes mixed with autogenous bone. A resorbable collagen membrane can be placed under the elevated sinus membrane before filling it with the graft as it protects the sinus membrane from being torn by the graft particles. (D) A parenteral antibiotic like clindamycin can also be mixed with the graft to prevent any postoperative infection.

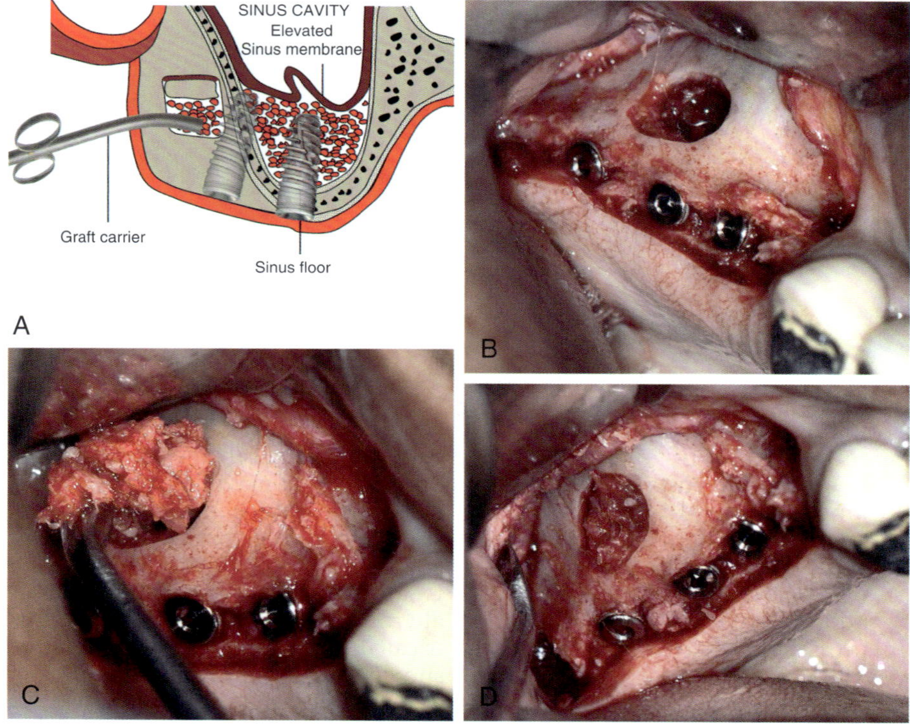

Fig 18.10 Once the elevated sinus floor has been loosely filled with the graft, the implant osteotomies are prepared in the usual fashion and implants are inserted. (A–D) The rest of the sinus is further grafted until it is all loosely packed with the graft. If subantral bone height is inadequate to stabilize the immediately inserted implants, the surgeon can only graft the sinus and choose to go for delayed implant placement when the new bone has regenerated in the grafted sinus floor after 6–8 months.

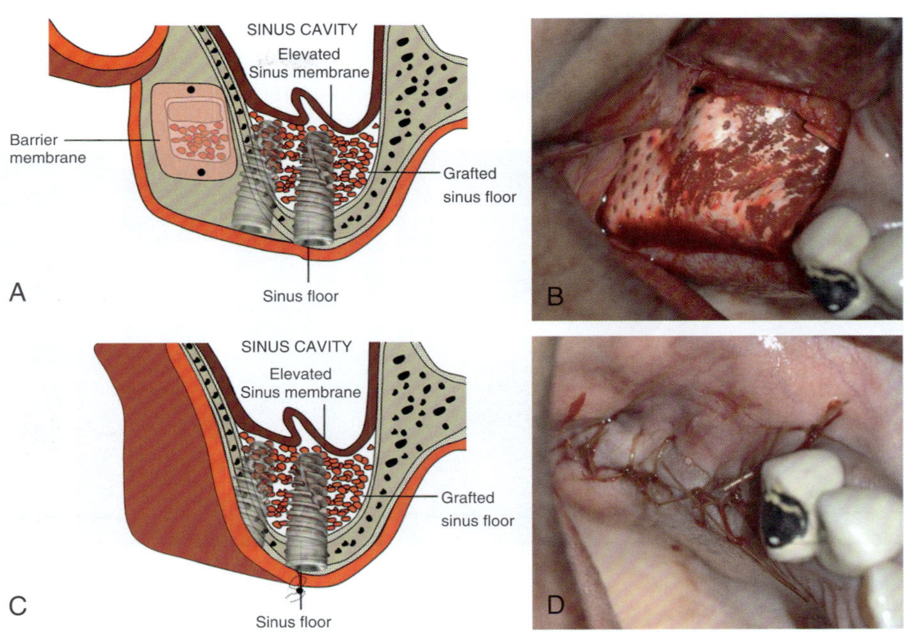

Fig 18.11 (A and B) A resorbable collagen barrier membrane can be placed to cover the lateral window to prevent soft tissue ingression into the grafted sinus. (C and D) Flap is sutured back with a primary closure. Implants are uncovered and restored after new bone formation has occurred in the entire grafted sinus in 6–8 months.

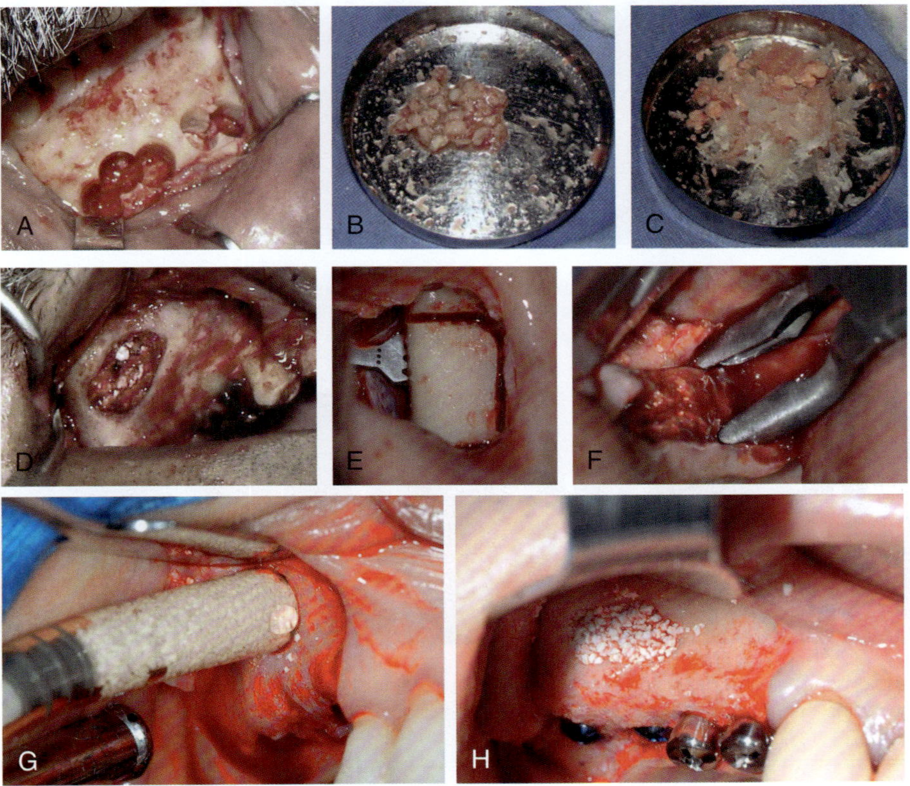

Fig 18.12 (A and B) Autogenous bone can be harvested from the mandibular symphysis using trephines, crushed and mixed with demineralized bone matrix or (C and D) any synthetic graft like HA or HA + β-TCP mixture and used to graft the sinus. (E) The other intraoral sources of autograft can be mandibular buccal shelf or (F) maxillary tuberosity. (G and H) The mixture of the HA (70%) and β-TCP (30%) has also been used to successfully graft the sinus cavity, with predictable success rate.

CASE REPORT-1

Sinus grafting with lateral approach and delayed implant insertion (Figs 18.13–18.18).

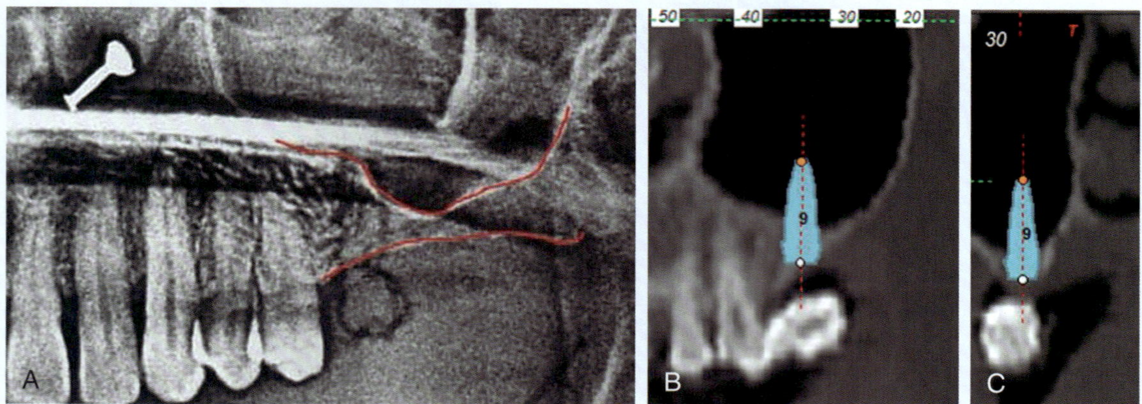

Fig 18.13 (A) Preoperative dental radiograph shows inadequate subantral bone height to insert implant; thus sinus grafting and delayed implant placement are planned to replace missing first molar. (B and C) The lateral and cross-sectional CT images with simulated implant placement show absolute need of sinus grafting procedure for adequately long implant placement.

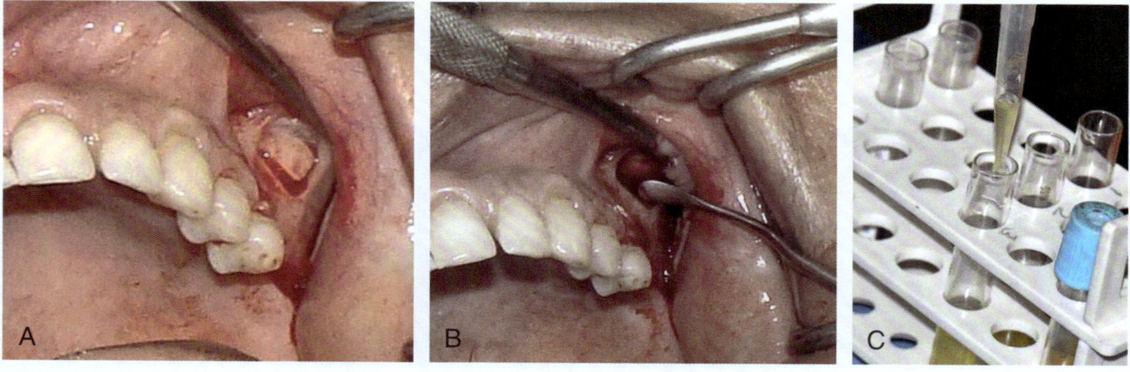

Fig 18.14 (A) A trapezoidal flap is elevated to expose the anterolateral wall of the sinus and an oval window is prepared using a large round diamond bur to expose the sinus membrane. (B) Further, the Schneiderian membrane is carefully elevated using a set of sinus elevators. (C) The PRGF (plasma rich in growth factors) is prepared from the patient's venous blood.

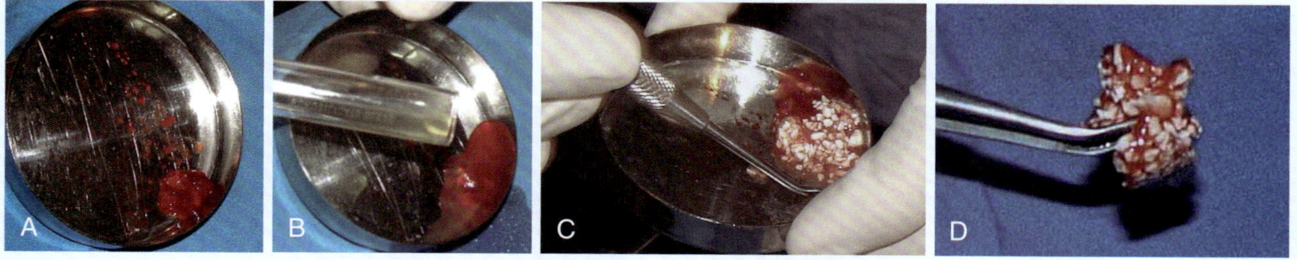

Fig 18.15 (A–D) Autogenous bone, which is harvested from the maxillary tuberosity of the same side, is mixed with PRGF and bone substitute (HA + β-TCP). Besides enhancing the bone regeneration potential of the bone graft, PRGF also binds the graft particles together and improves its handling properties.

CASE REPORT-1—cont'd

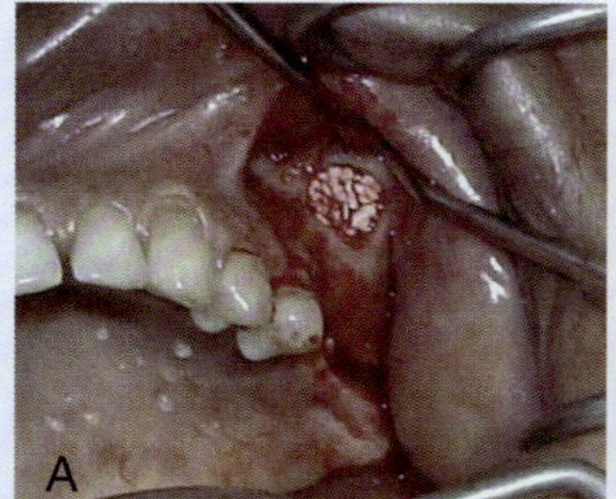
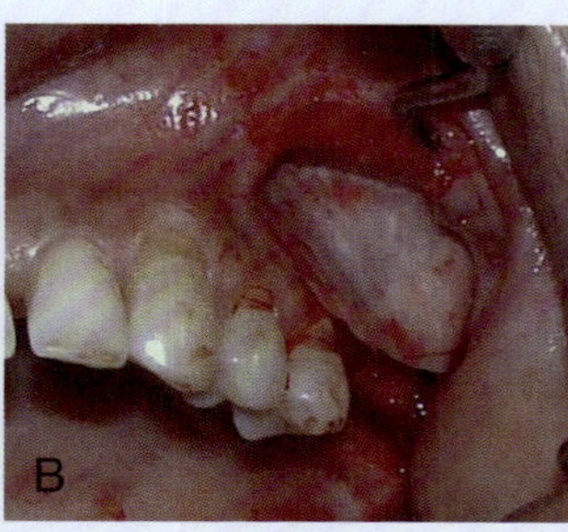
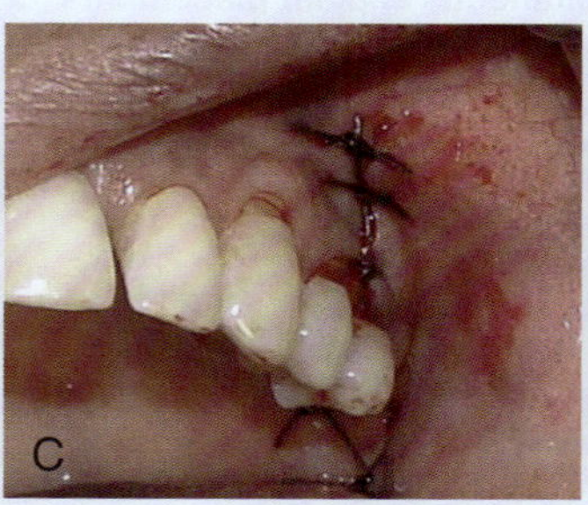
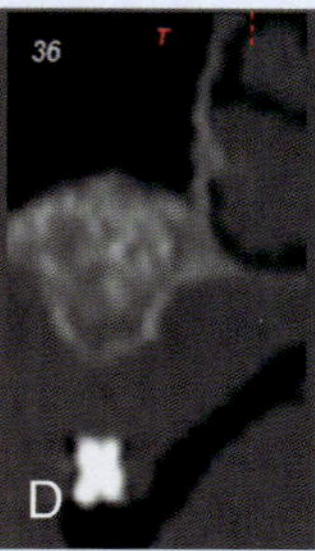
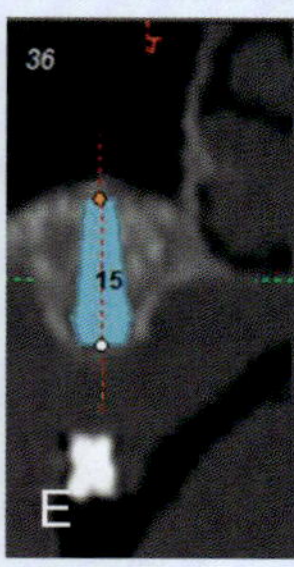

Fig 18.16 (A) Elevated maxillary sinus is grafted and (B) covered with a barrier collagen membrane. (C) Flap is sutured with primary closure. (D and E) CT cross-sectional images show new bone formation in the grafted sinus after 6 months, which seems sufficient for the insertion of an adequately long implant.

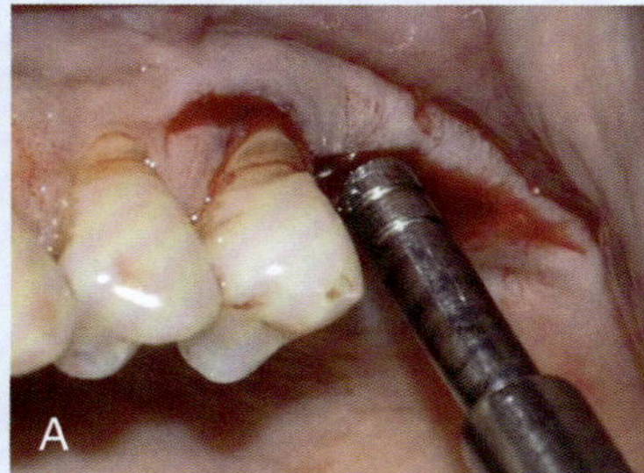
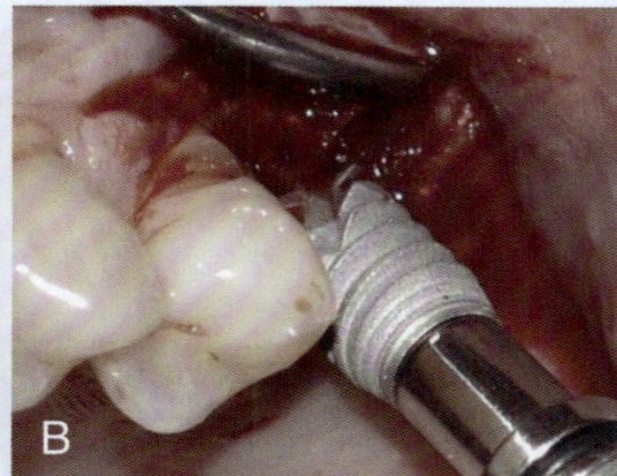
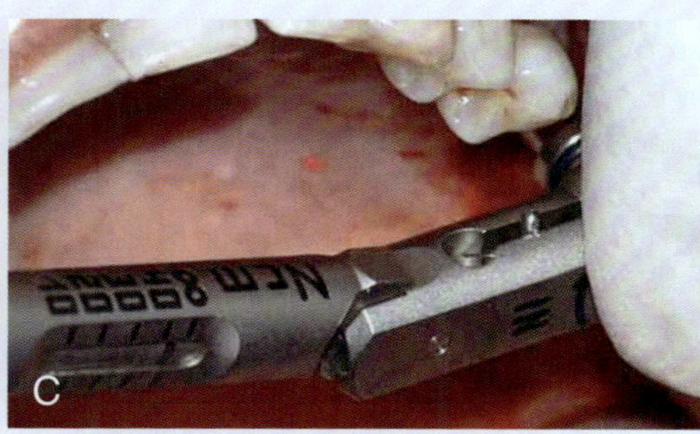

Fig 18.17 (A) The implant osteotomy is prepared after 6 months using only osteotomes to laterally condense the bone and (B) implant (5 × 13 mm) is inserted. (C) Inserted implant shows adequate primary stability evaluated with the torque ratchet (more than 35 Ncm).

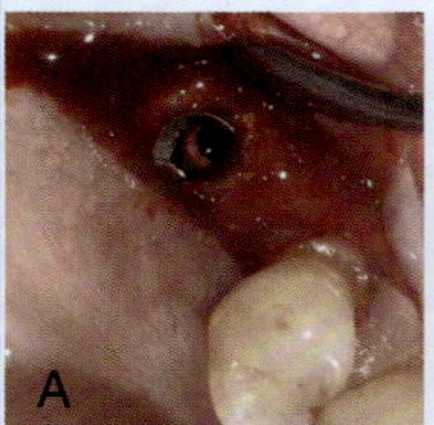
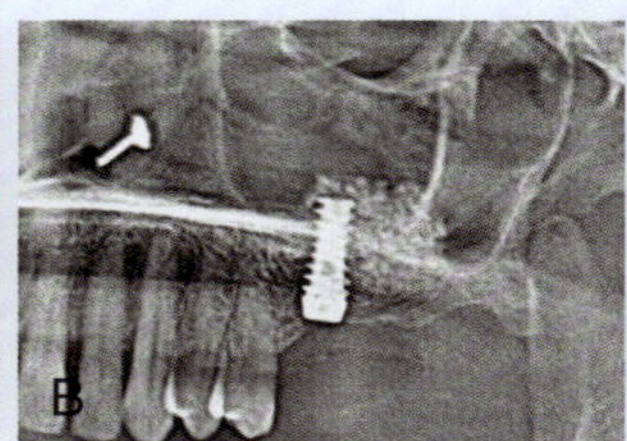
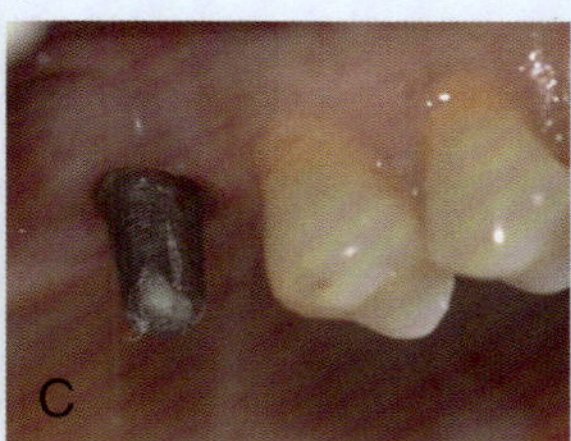
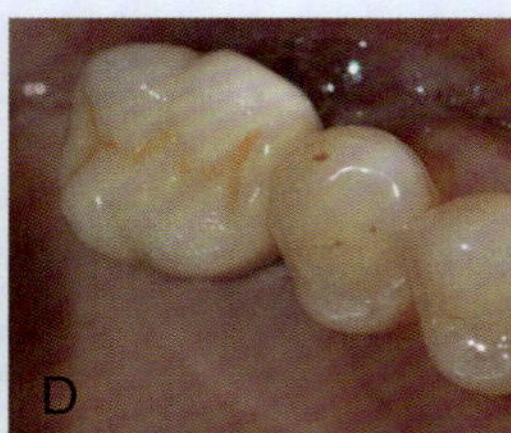
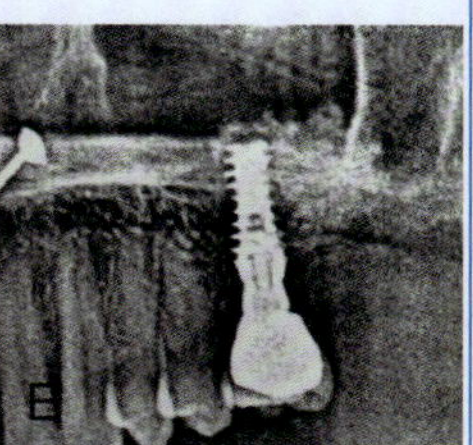

Fig 18.18 (A) Clinical view of inserted implant and (B) postimplantation radiograph. (C and D) Implant uncovered and restored after 6 months. (E) Radiograph 1 year after loading shows stable bone around the implant.

CASE REPORT-2

Bilateral sinus grafting with simultaneous implant placements *(Courtesy: Dr Ata Garajei, DMD and Dr Amin Yamani, DDS, Tehran, Iran)* (Figs 18.19–18.25).

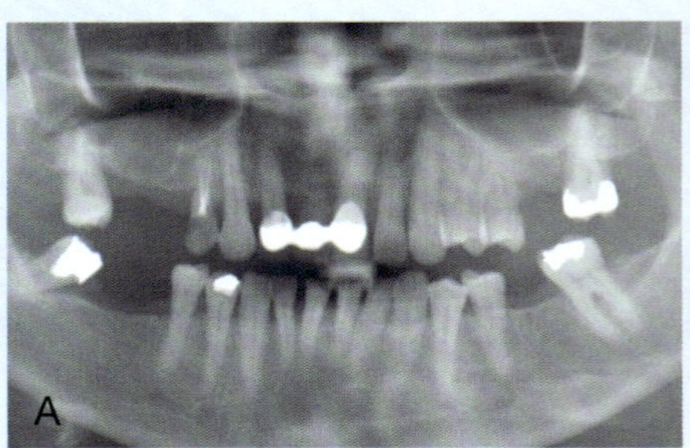
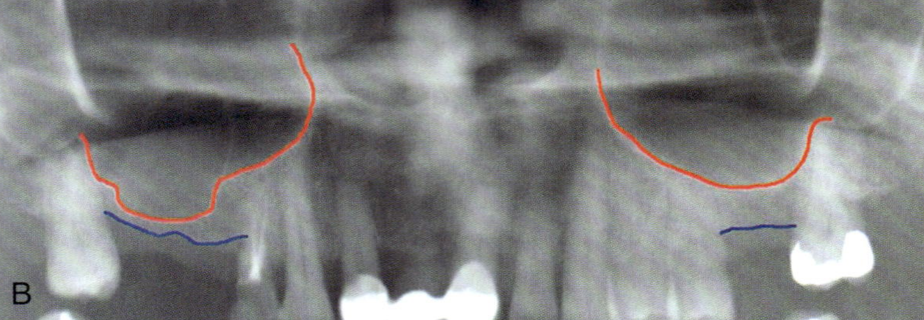

Fig 18.19 (A and B) Long-time missing teeth numbers 15, 16 and 26 have resulted in lowering down of the sinus floor, which in turn leads to reduced subantral bone height insufficient to insert implants; thus, sinus grafting procedure and simultaneous implant insertion is planned.

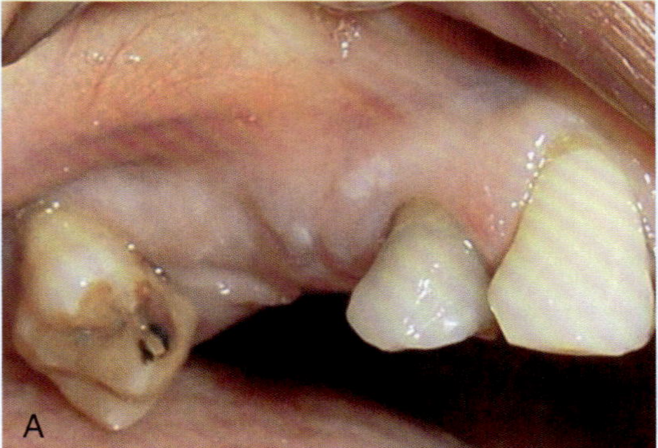
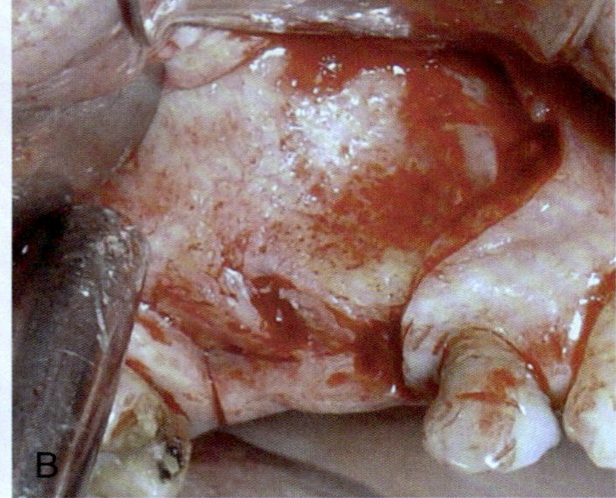

Fig 18.20 (A and B) A trapezoidal flap is elevated to expose the lateral wall of the sinus on the right side of maxilla.

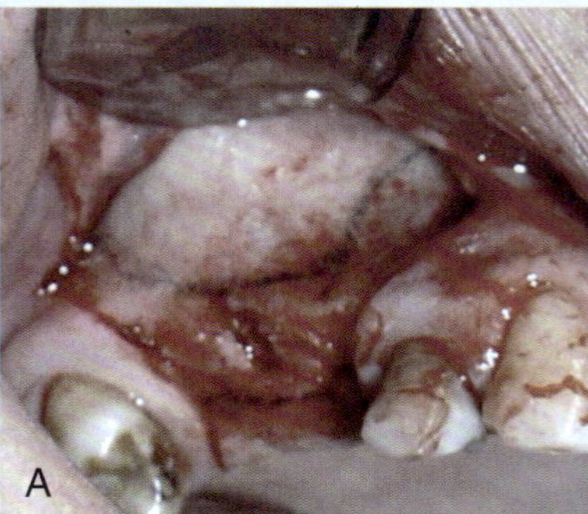
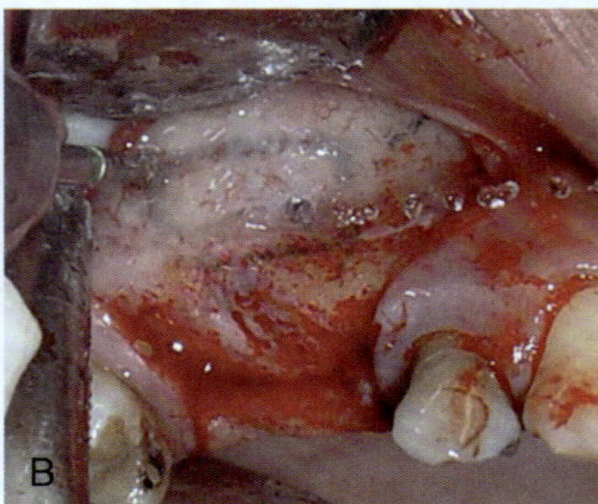
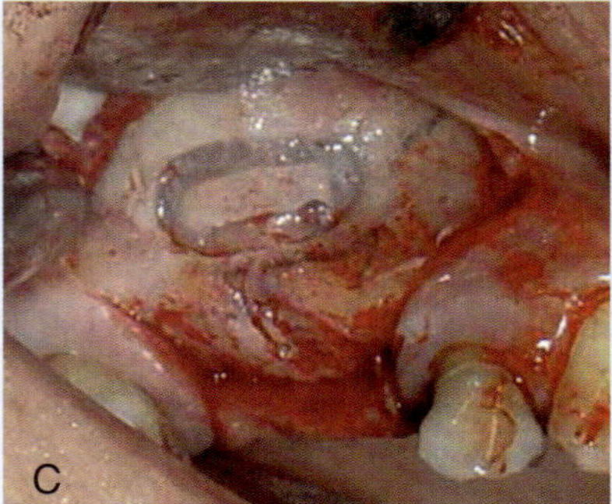

Fig 18.21 (A) The sinus lining path is approximately marked using sterile HB pencil using the radiograph as reference. This avoids the problem of window preparation at an incorrect position. (B) An oval window is prepared on the lateral wall of the sinus using a large round diamond bur to expose the membrane. A (C) greyish colour sinus membrane can be seen through the scored window.

CASE REPORT-2—cont'd

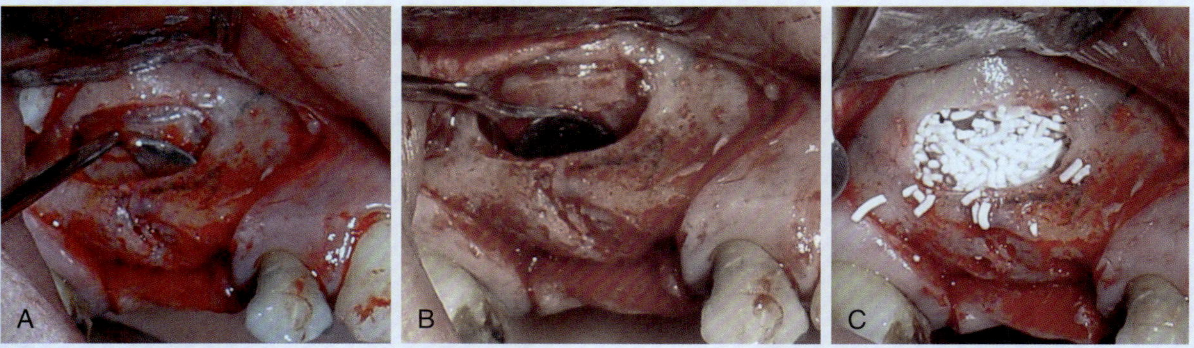

Fig 18.22 (A and B) The sinus membrane is carefully elevated using a set of sinus curettes and (C) the elevated sinus floor is grafted using a mixture of HA and β-TCP.

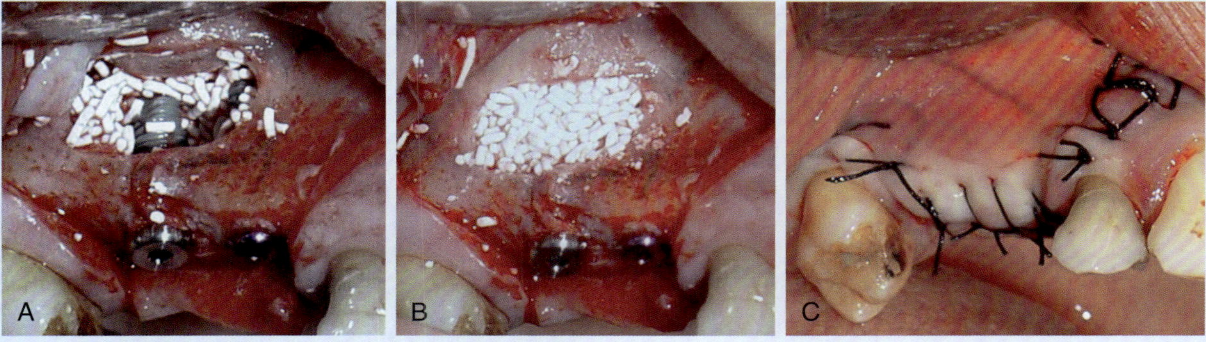

Fig 18.23 (A) The implant osteotomies are prepared and implants are inserted in usual fashion. (B) Graft is further filled into the sinus over the implants and (C) the flap is sutured back.

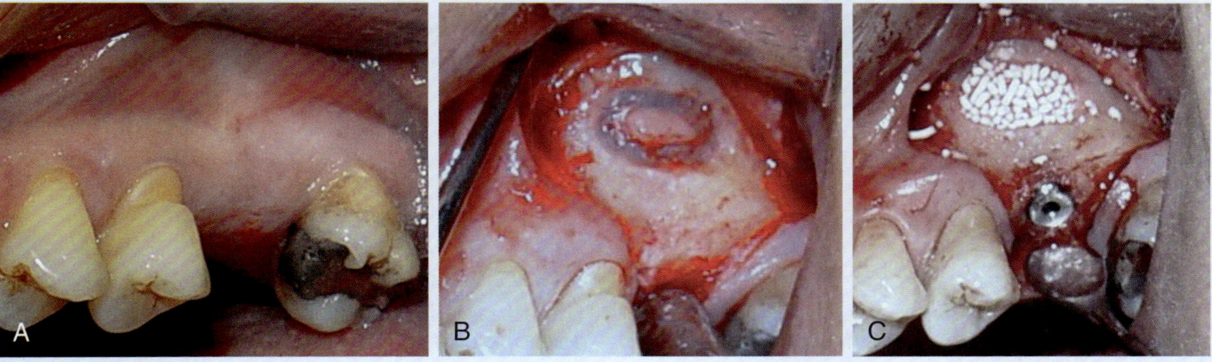

Fig 18.24 (A–C) Sinus grafting and implant insertion are performed in a similar fashion on the left side.

Continued

CASE REPORT-2—cont'd

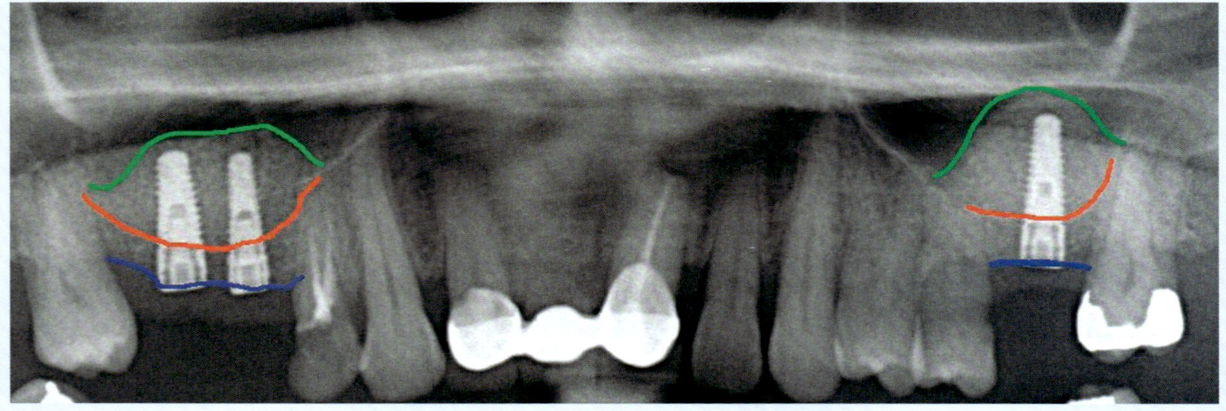

Fig 18.25 Postoperative radiograph shows elevated and grafted sinuses with inserted implants.

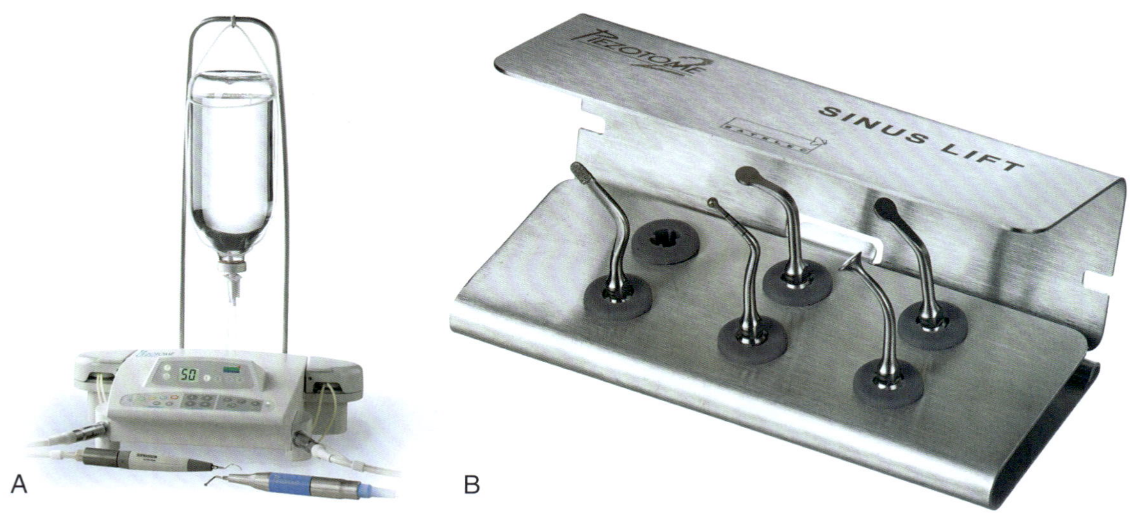

Fig 18.26 (A) Piezosurgery unit (piezotome from Satelec, France), sinus lift kit containing special tips for lateral window preparation and (B) sinus membrane elevation.

Advances and modifications in the lateral approach of sinus lifting

With advancements in technology and armamentariums, several modifications have been proposed in the conventional lateral sinus window technique, which was originally proposed by Tatum. A few of these advancements, which facilitate easy and safe sinus lifting through the lateral approach are described here.

Lateral approach of sinus lifting using piezosurgery unit

The ultrasonic piezosurgery unit has specifically been developed for cutting bony tissue with minimal damage to the soft tissue. High-frequency oscillations between 24 and 29.500 Hz, modulated with a low frequency between 10 and 60 Hz, enable efficient and controlled use and improve healing of the tissue (Figs 18.26 and 18.27).

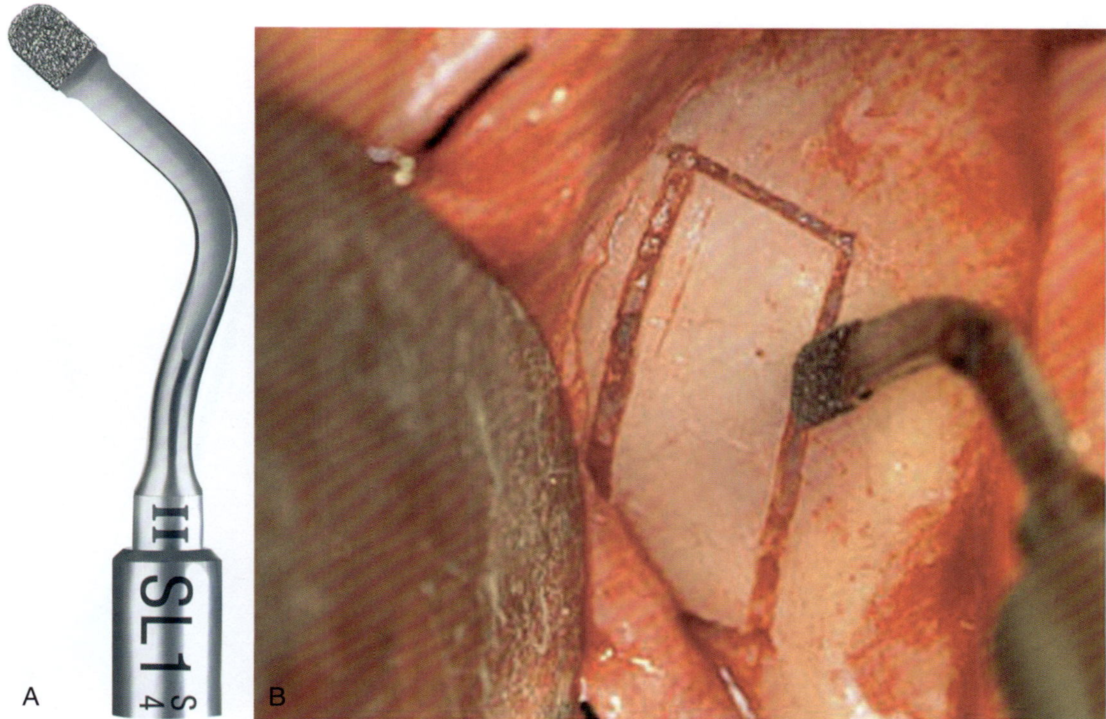

Fig 18.27 Application of the various piezo tips: SL1 Tip is a diamond-coated tip for vestibular bone window cut and for attenuation of sharp angles. (A and B) A rectangular window can easily be scored using this tip, without tearing the sinus membrane.

Continued

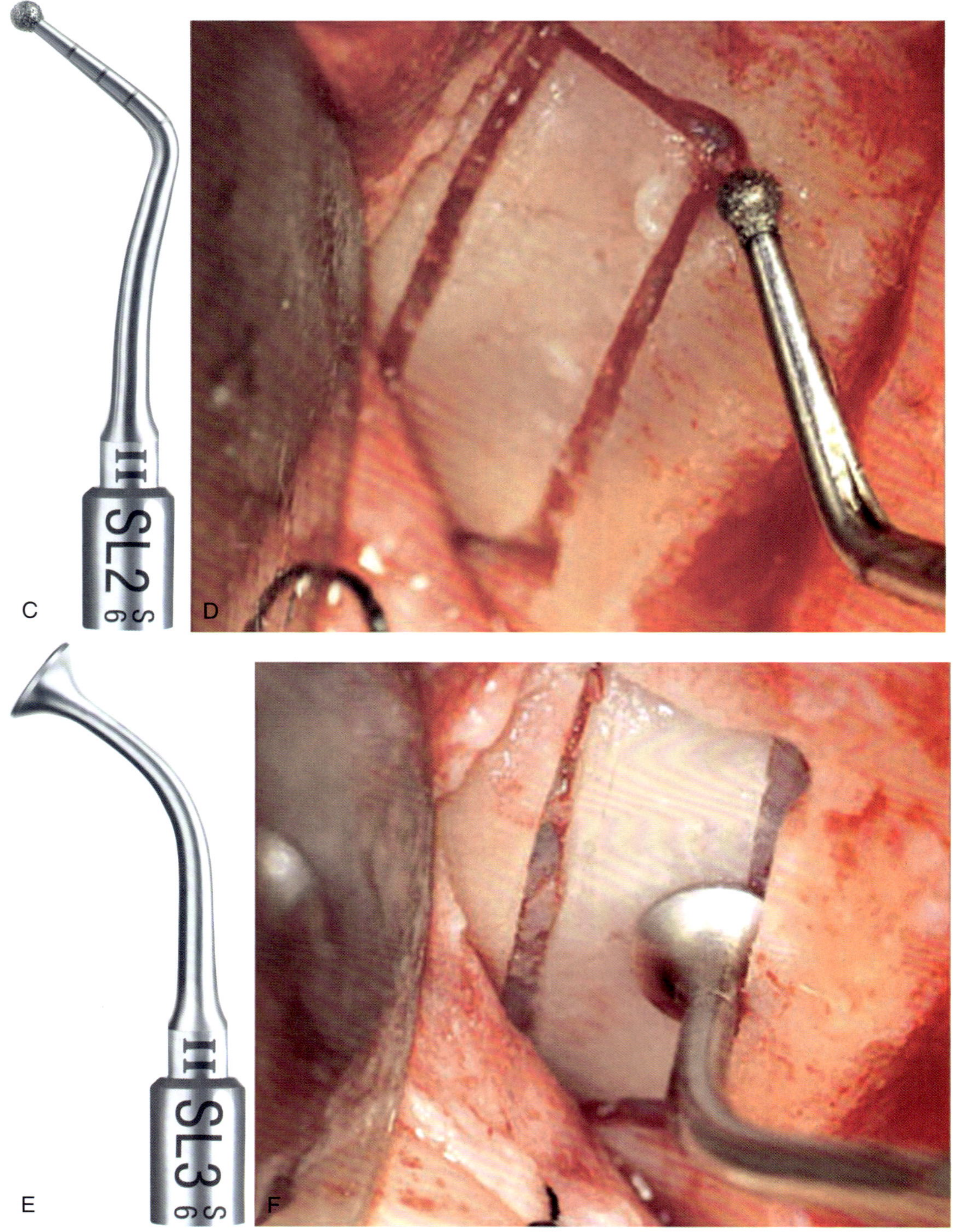

Fig 18.27, cont'd SL2 Tip is a diamond-coated ball tip for smoothing the vestibular bone window; precise osteoplasty using this tip at the prepared osteotomy corners to remove the sharp bony edges, reduces the chances of membrane tear during elevation. (C and D) Ball diameter: 1.5 mm, laser marked every 2 mm. (E and F) SL3 Tip is a flat-ended noncutting tip used for detaching the Schneiderian membrane from the window edge. (G and H) SL4 Tip is a noncutting spatula, oriented at 90°, used for detaching the Schneiderian membrane inside the sinus.

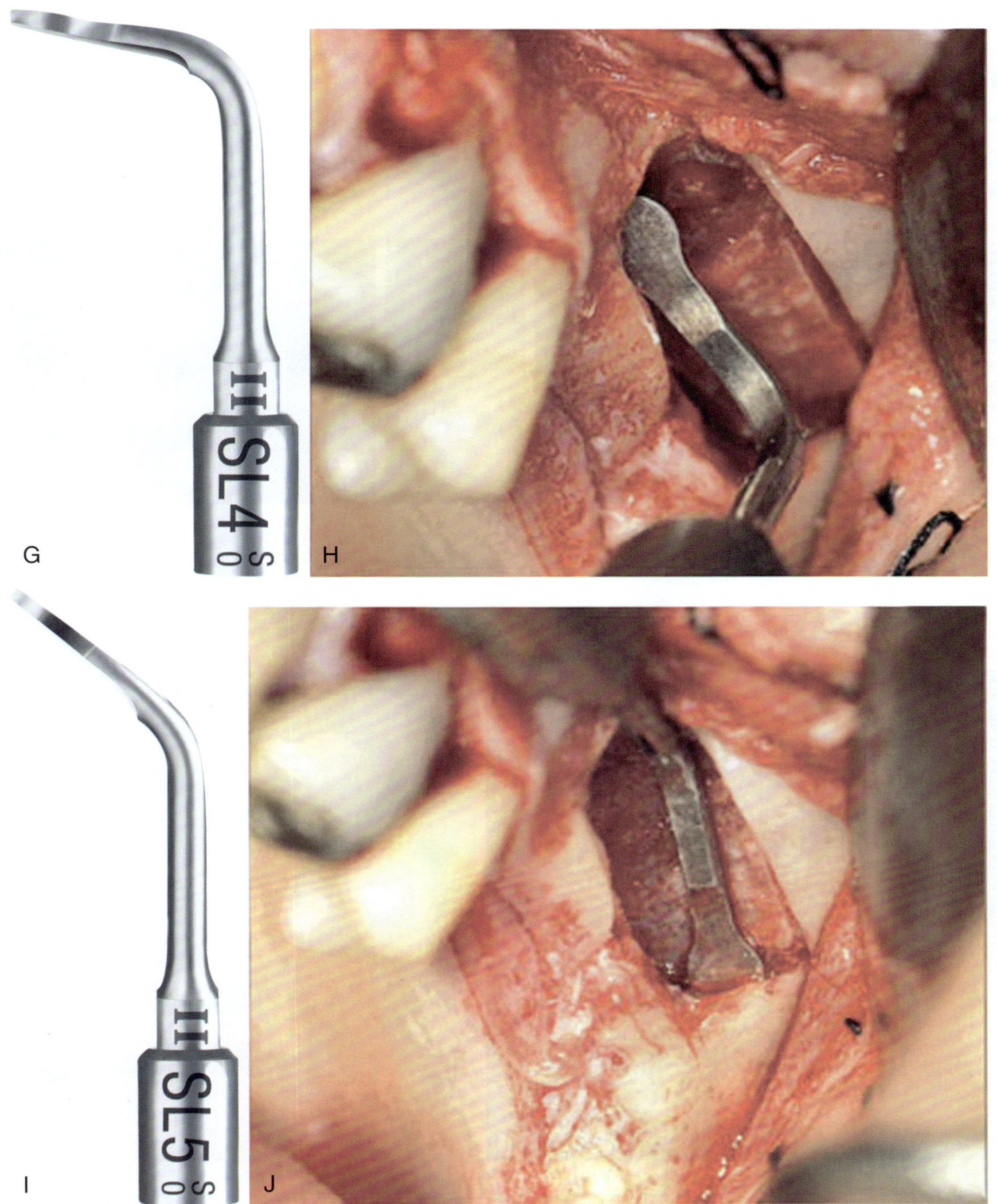

Fig 18.27, cont'd (I and J) SL5 Tip is a noncutting spatula, oriented at ±135°, used for detaching the Schneiderian membrane inside the sinus and for removing anatomical structures. *(Courtesy: Dr Pierre Marin, Implantologist–private practice, Bordeaux, France)*

CASE REPORT-3

Sinus elevation using piezotome with simultaneous implants insertion

A 62-year-old female patient presented with teeth numbers 14, 16, 17 missing and tooth number 15 misaligned and mobile. The patient was medically fit for the sinus grafting surgery. Tooth number 15 was extracted and socket grafting was performed 3 months before the sinus graft surgery (Figs 18.28–18.39).

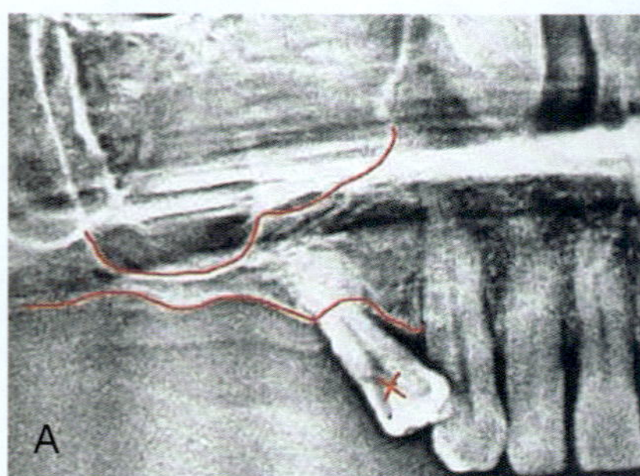

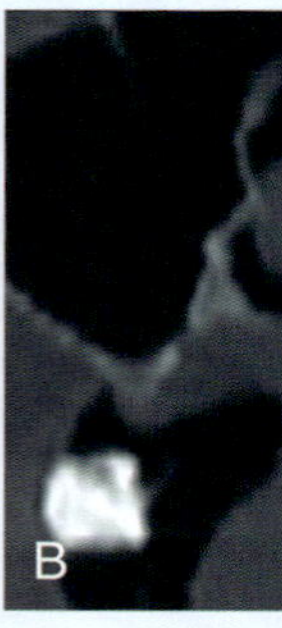

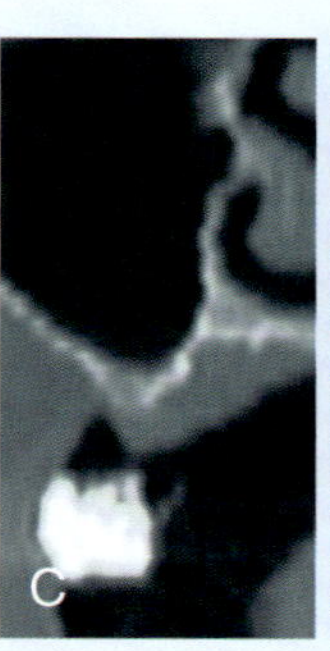

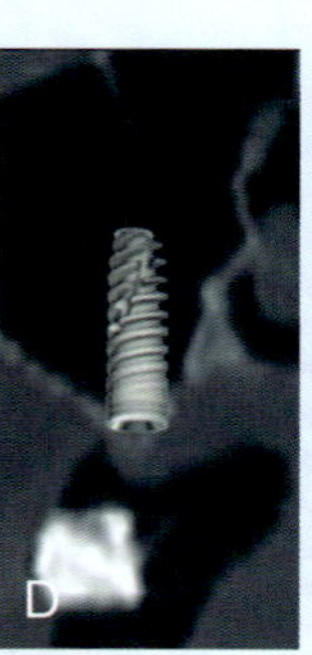

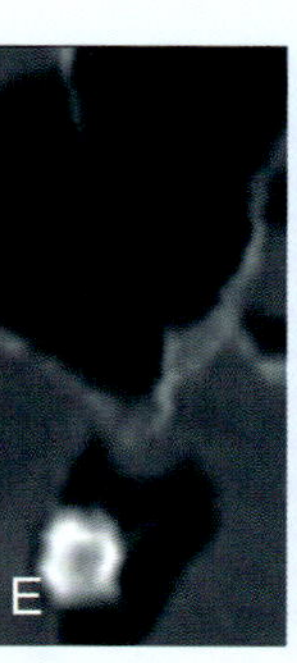

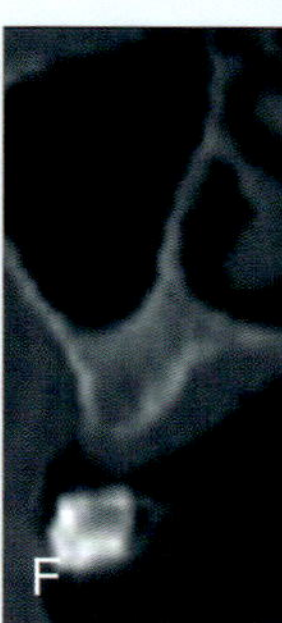

Fig 18.28 (A) Patient's radiograph shows very limited subantral bone height. (B–F) Cross-sectional CT images of the edentulous area show very limited bone height and ridge width. It indicates need for sinus grafting and simultaneous ridge splitting to insert implants with adequate diameter and length.

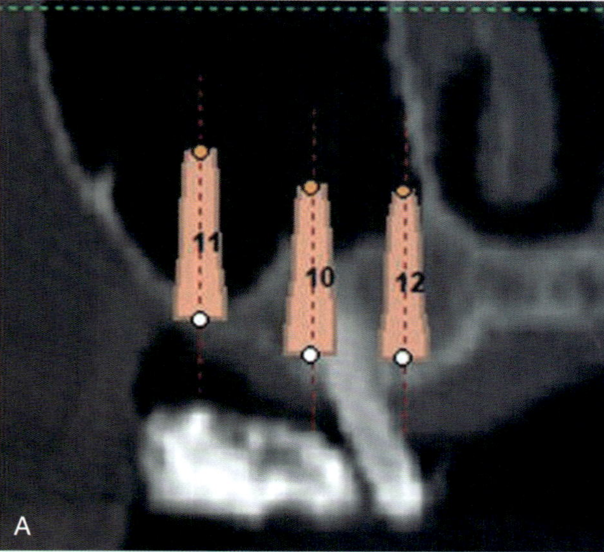

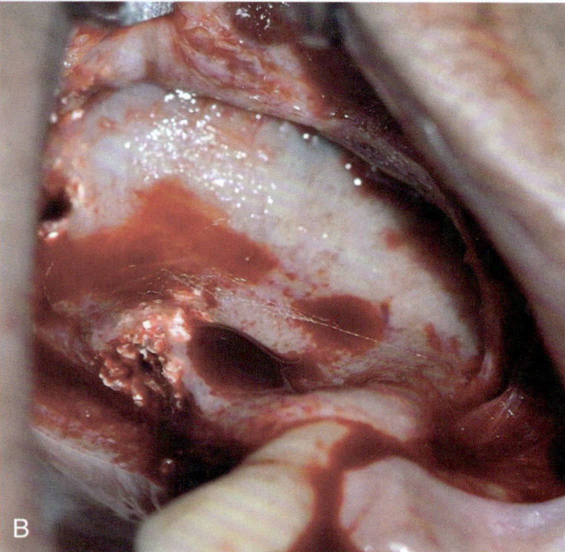

Fig 18.29 (A) Three simulated implants (3.75 × 13 mm) were planned using implant planning software. (B) Trapezoidal flap is elevated to expose the lateral wall of the sinus. The previously grafted socket of the tooth number 15 can be seen.

CASE REPORT-3—cont'd

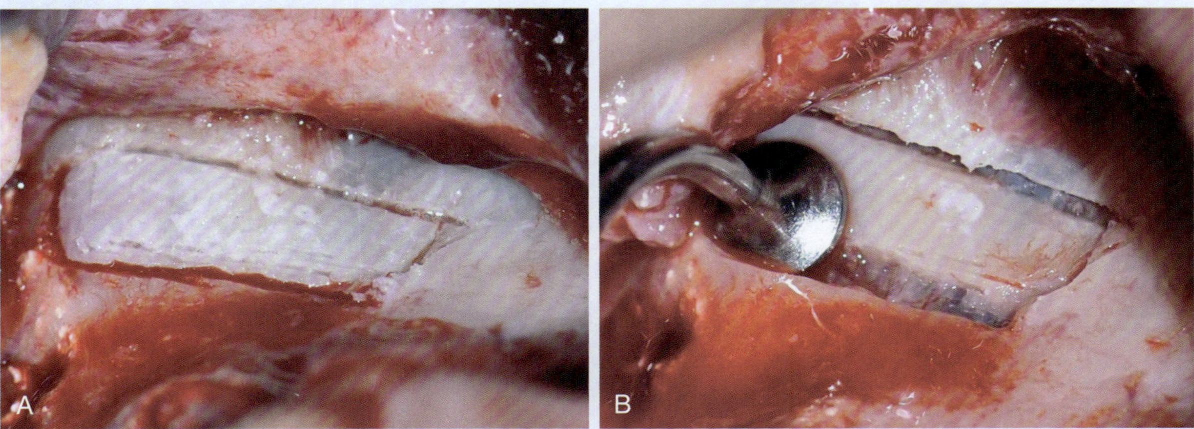

Fig 18.30 (A) A rectangular osseous window is prepared on the lateral wall of the sinus using SL1 and SL2 tips of the piezotome. (B) The SL3 tip is then used to detach the Schneiderian membrane from the window edges.

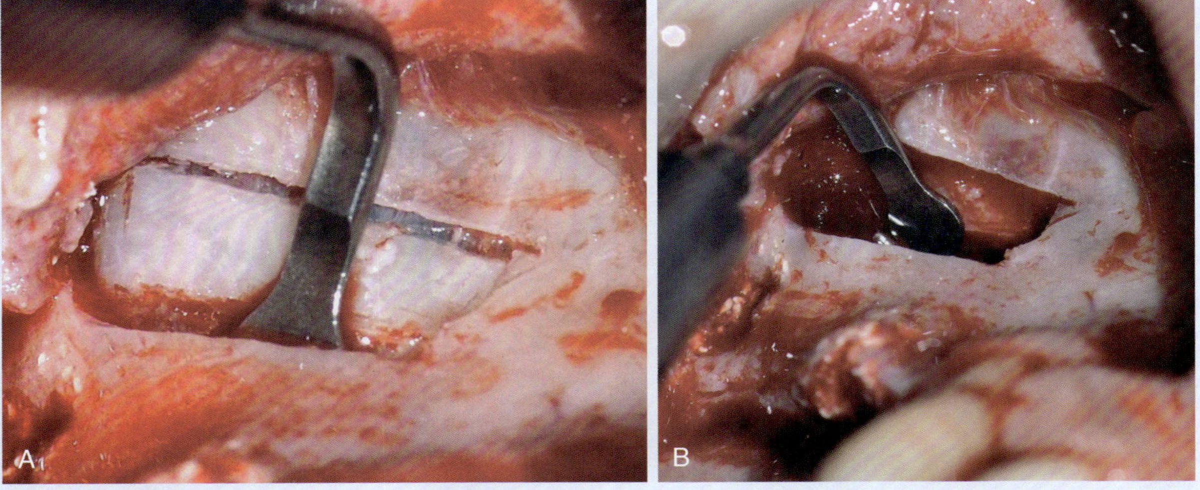

Fig 18.31 (A and B) The SL4 tip is then used to carefully free the membrane from the inferior, posterior, and anterior wall of the sinus, and to elevate it to the desired height.

Continued

CASE REPORT-3—cont'd

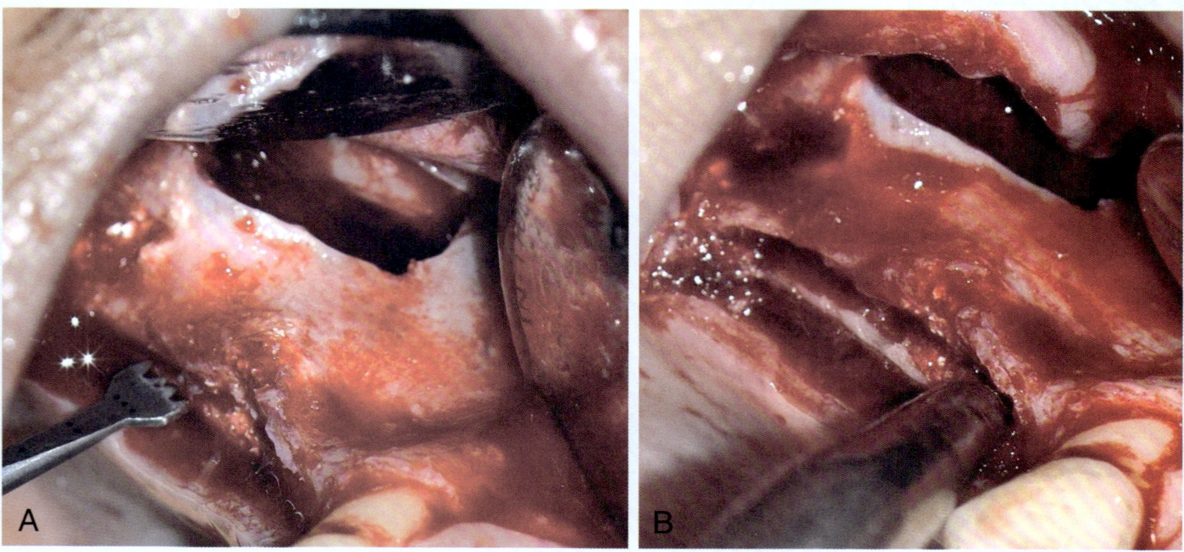

Fig 18.32 (A and B) A mid-crest osteotomy channel is created using the piezo saw and the ridge is splitted to pry the buccal and palatal plates apart, using the razor sharp osseous splitters.

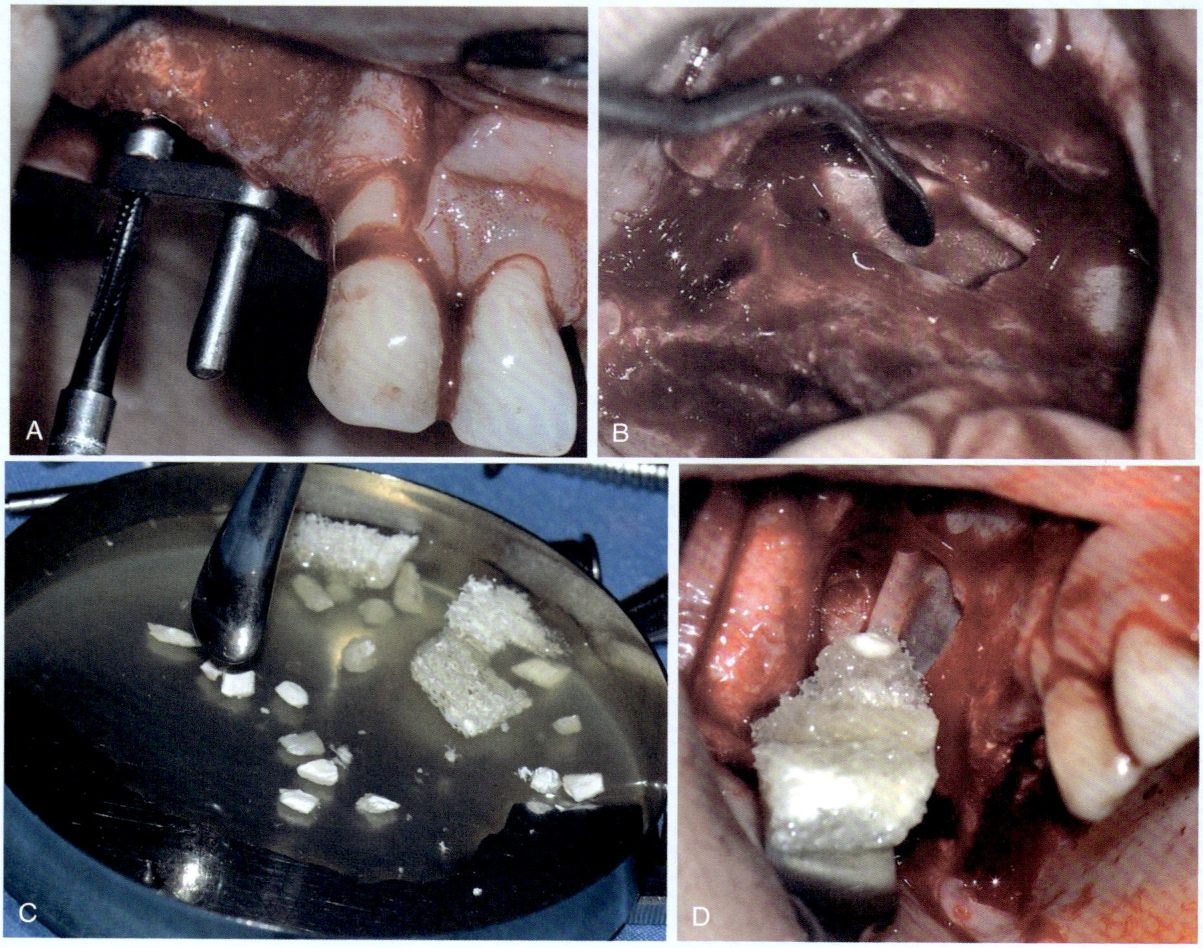

Fig 18.33 (A) Implant osteotomies are prepared using a ParaGuide. (B) A collagen barrier membrane is placed underneath the elevated sinus membrane to prevent its inadvertent tearing during grafting. (C) The corticocancellous allograft is mixed with PRGF. (D) First, the collagenous spongy soft bone is placed under the membrane. It gives a cushion effect against the expansion of the sinus membrane when the patient respires through the nose and prevents membrane tear.

CASE REPORT-3—cont'd

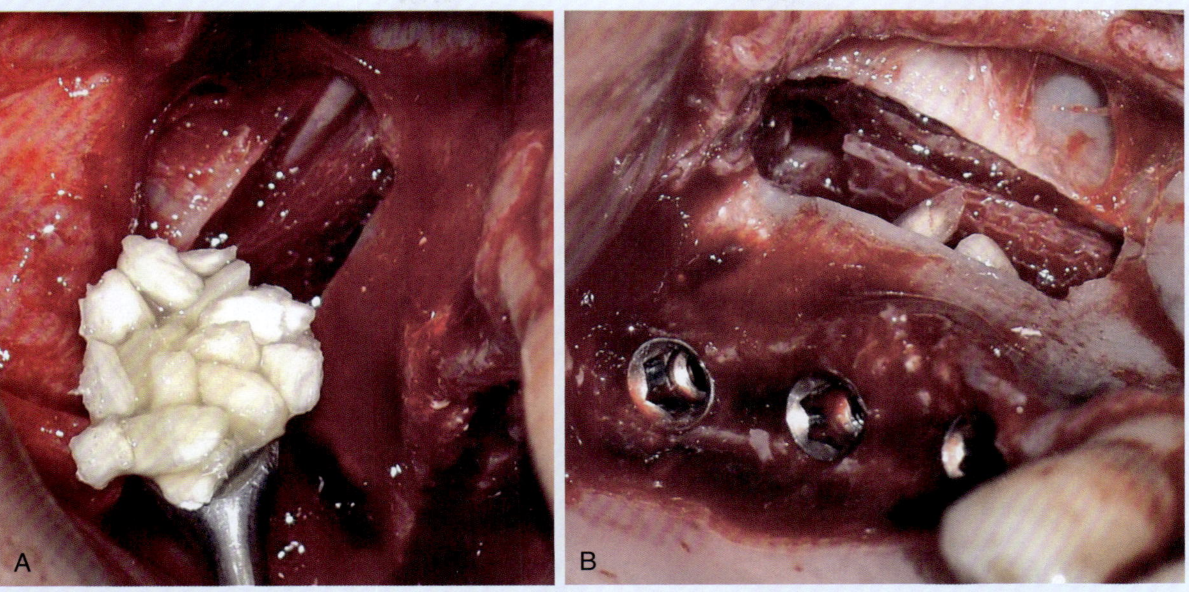

Fig 18.34 (A) The sinus is further grafted using cortical chips and (B) once the medial half of the sinus has been grafted, three implants are (3.75 × 15 mm) inserted.

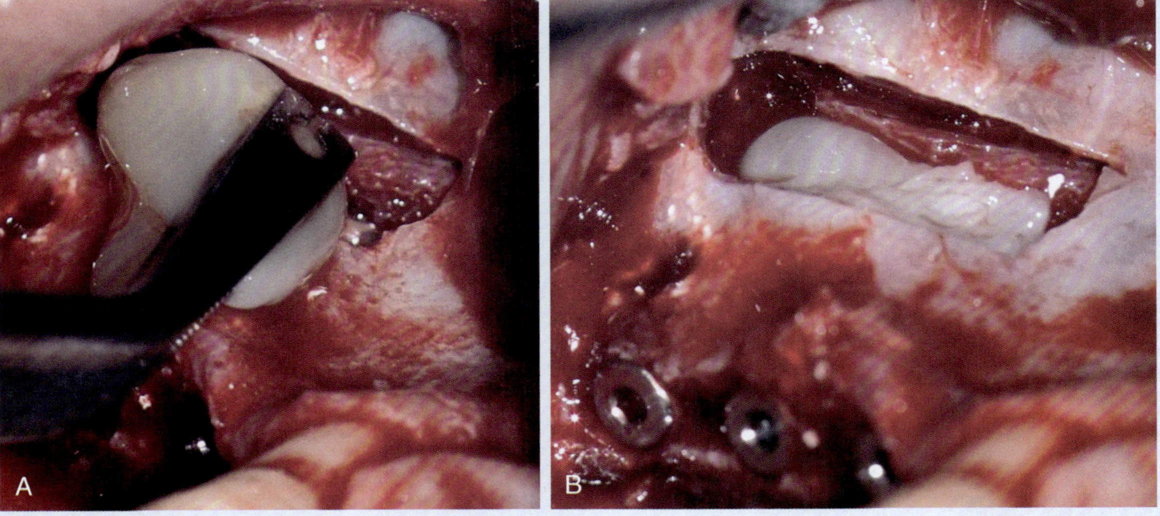

Fig 18.35 (A and B) Sinus cavity is further filled with the PRGF coagulum.

Continued

CASE REPORT-3—cont'd

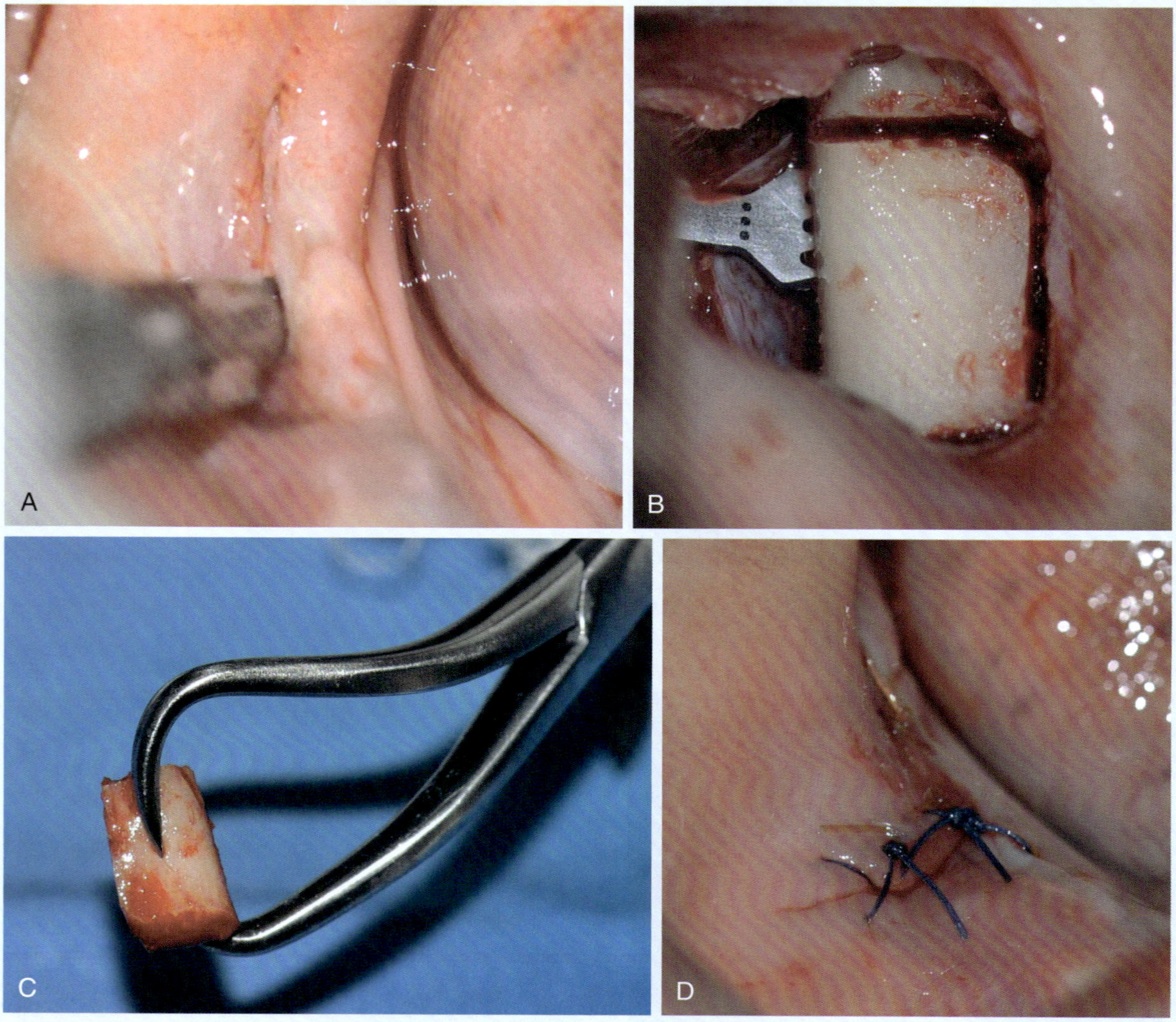

Fig 18.36 (A–D) A vertical incision is given to expose the mandibular buccal shelf region and a corticocancellous block is harvested using piezo saw, and the flap is sutured back.

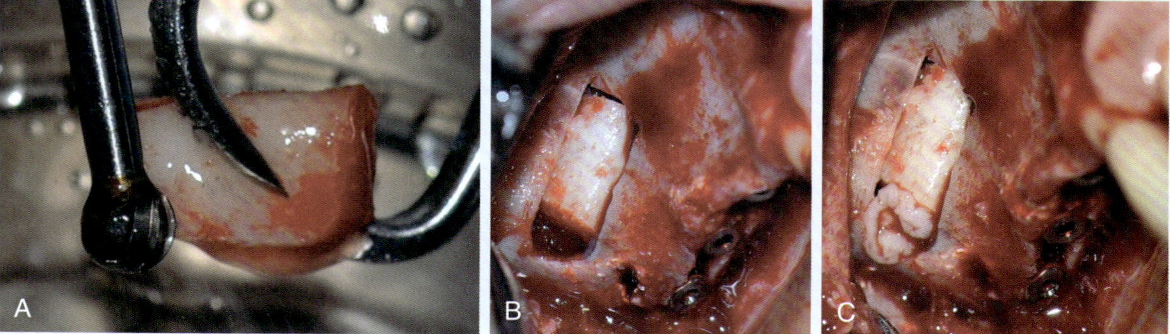

Fig 18.37 (A) The block is shaped to fit the sinus window using a large carbide trimmer. (B) The block is inserted to graft the lateral half of the sinus cavity as well as to close the window. (C) The rest of the window opening is closed using PRGF membrane.

CASE REPORT-3—cont'd

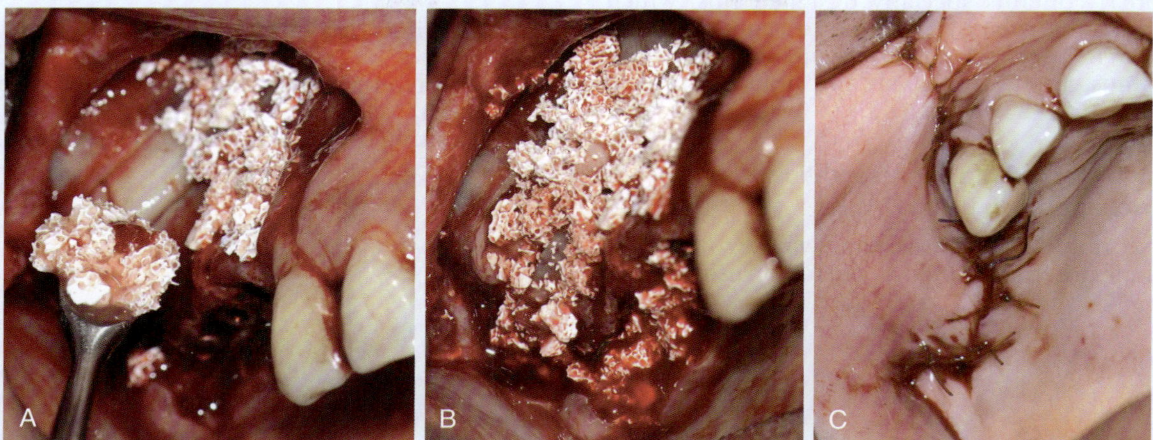

Fig 18.38 (A and B) The synthetic particulate graft (HA + β TCP) mixed with PRGF is used to graft the peri-implant spaces and for lateral bone augmentation. (C) Flap is sutured back with watertight sutures.

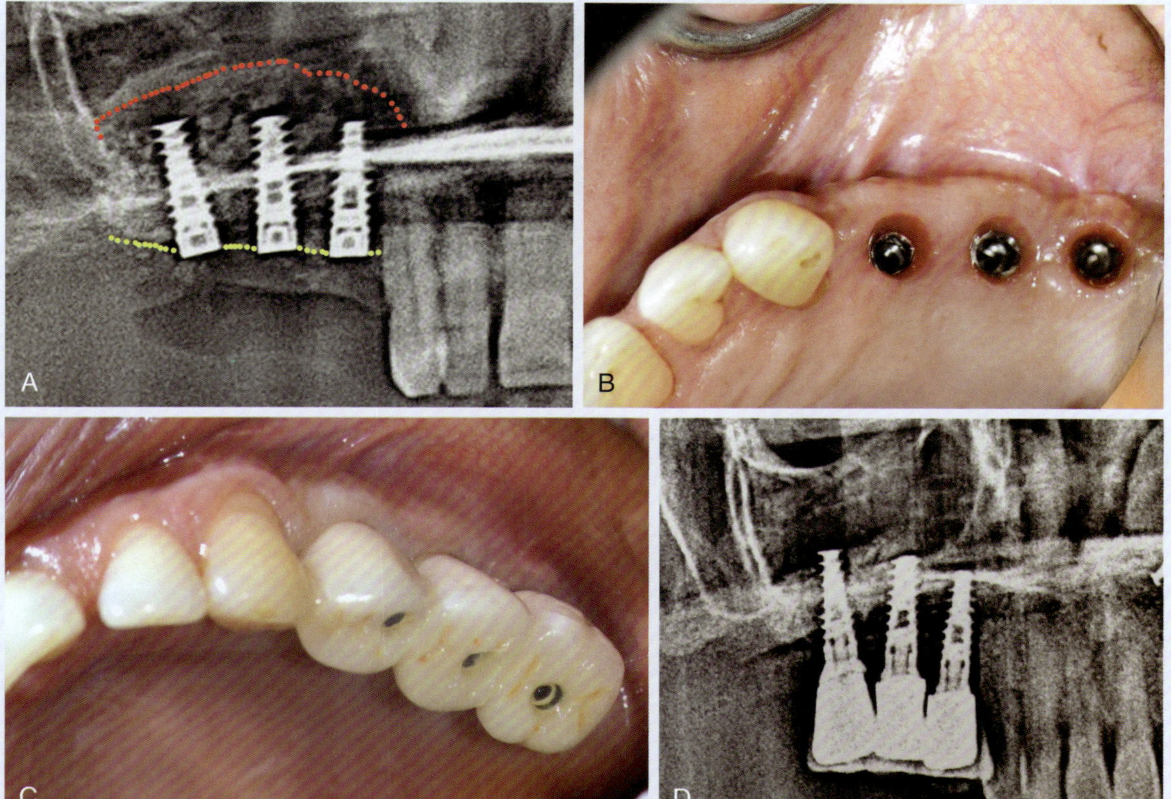

Fig 18.39 (A) Postoperative radiograph shows grafted sinus floor and inserted implants. (B and C) Implants are uncovered and restored after 8 months. (D) Radiograph 1 year after loading shows consolidated sinus graft.

Lateral approach of sinus lifting using DASK

The DASK sinus elevation kit (from Dentium Co. Ltd., Seoul, Korea) contains specially designed tips, which are used with the rotary handpiece to score the osseous window to approach the sinus membrane. It also contains sinus curettes to elevate the sinus membrane (Fig 18.40).

Step by step diagrammatic presentations of the lateral approach using DASK

Step 1 – scoring the lateral osseous window. There are two techniques for lateral window preparation using DASK:

1. Wall-off technique (Fig 18.41A–C)
2. Grind-out technique (Fig 18.42A and B).

Step 2 – sinus membrane elevation (Fig 18.43A and B).
Step 3 – osteotomy preparation for the implant (Fig 18.44A and B).
Step 4 – grafting of the elevated sinus floor and implant placement (Fig 18.45A–D).

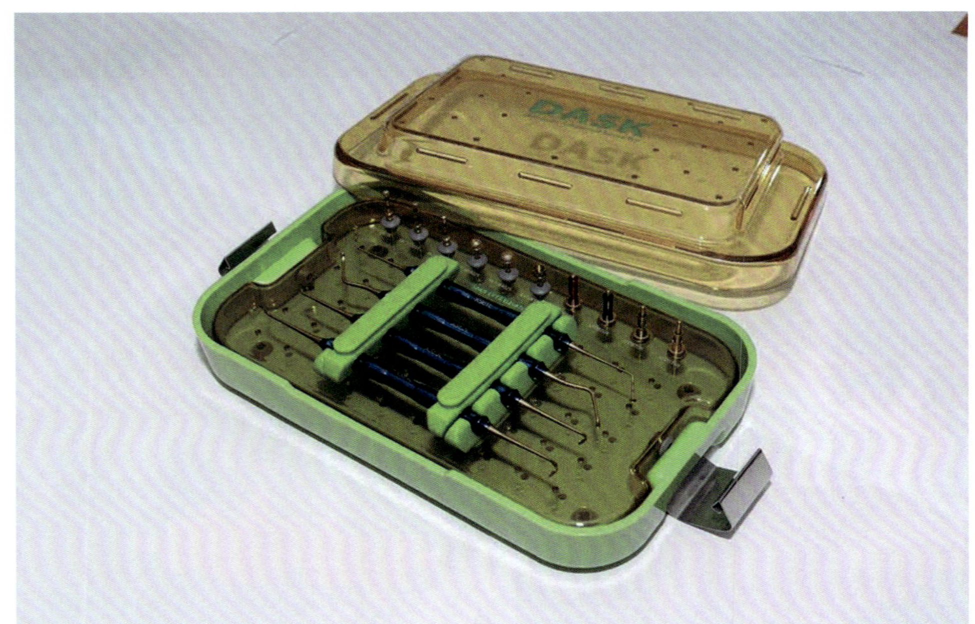

Fig 18.40 The DASK kit (Dentium Co. Ltd. Korea) is very useful, has gained high popularity, and is being widely used for the lateral window as well as crestal approach of sinus elevation procedure.

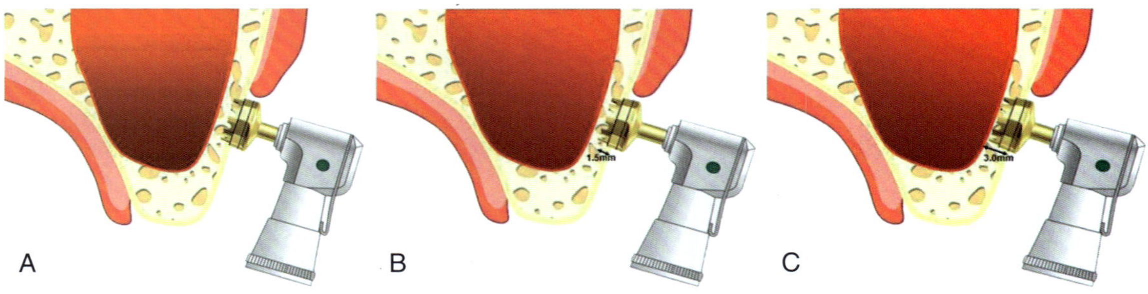

Fig 18.41 (A–C) **Wall-off technique-** After elevating the mucoperiosteal flap to expose the ridge and lateral wall of the sinus, a special DASK drill attached to a rotary handpiece is used to carefully score a circular osseous window at the lateral osseous wall of the sinus, without any tear to the underlying Schneiderian membrane. Once the drill has reached the membrane, the scored round bony wall is carefully removed (wall-off) from the underlying sinus membrane and the membrane is elevated using a special set of sinus curettes.

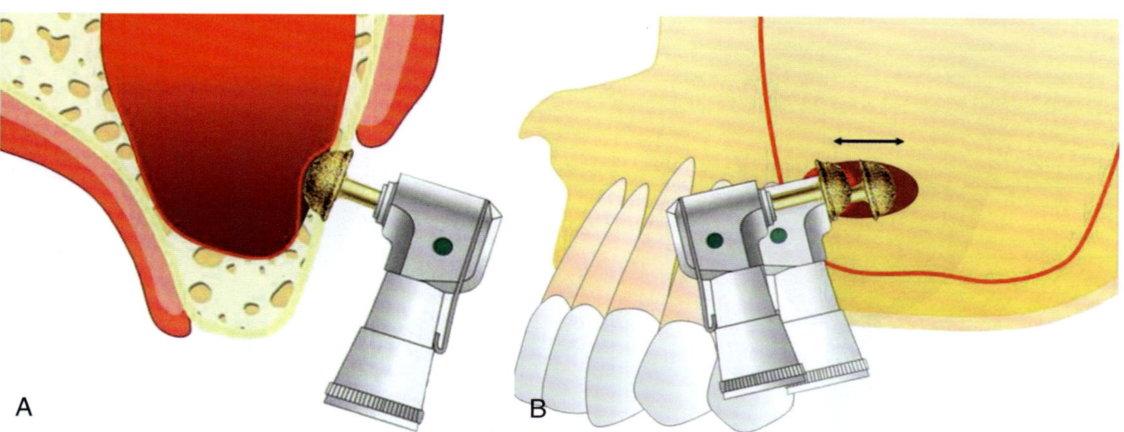

Fig 18.42 (A and B) **Grind-out technique-** A special large coarse diamond DASK drill is used to grind the lateral wall of the sinus with a sweeping action to reach the underlying sinus membrane. Once the sinus membrane is exposed, it is elevated using a special set of sinus curettes.

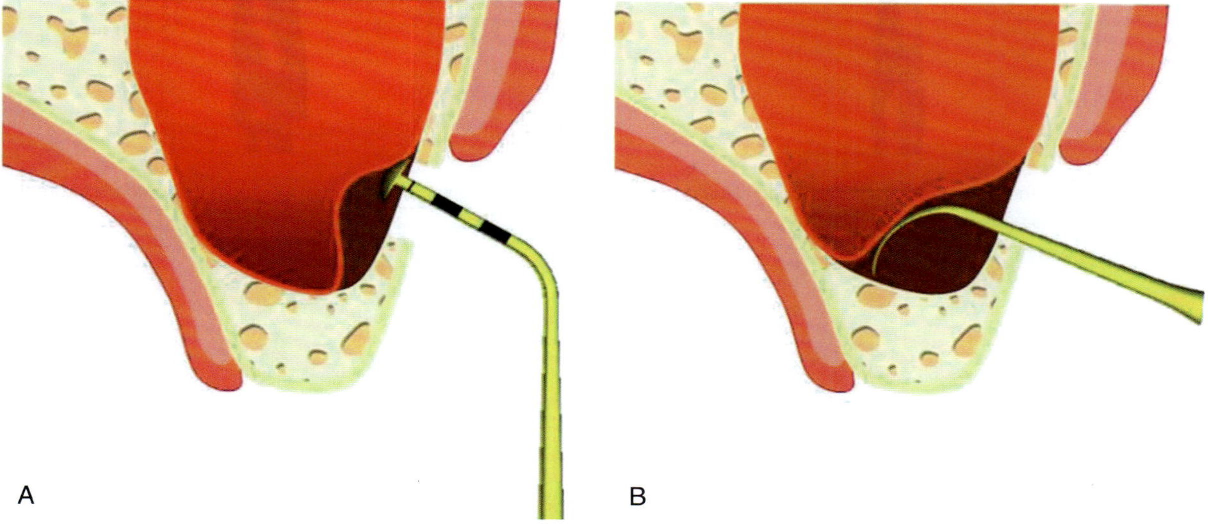

Fig 18.43 (A) After exposing the sinus membrane either with wall-off or grind-out technique, a special DASK tip is used to detach the membrane from the prepared window margins. (B) Once the membrane has successfully been detached all around from the prepared osseous window, a special set of curettes (sinus elevators) is used to elevate the Schneiderian membrane to the desired height.

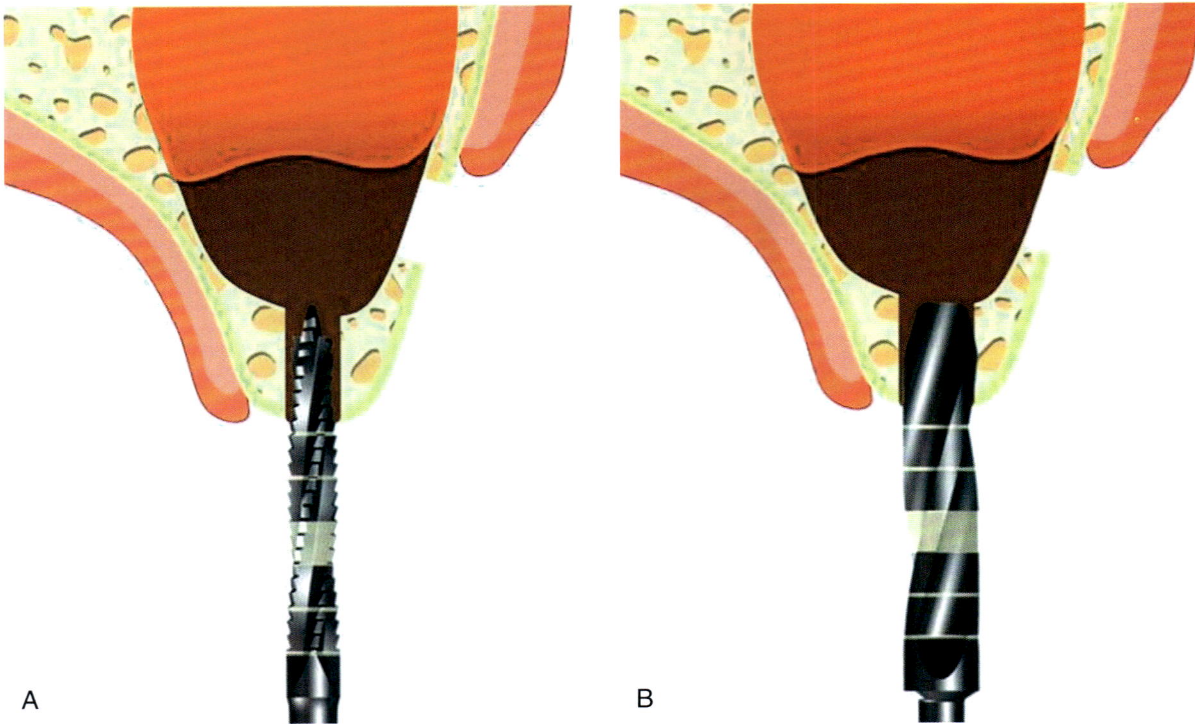

Fig 18.44 (A and B) After the sinus membrane has been elevated to the desired height, the osteotomy for the implant is prepared from the crestal approach using drills of the particular implant system.

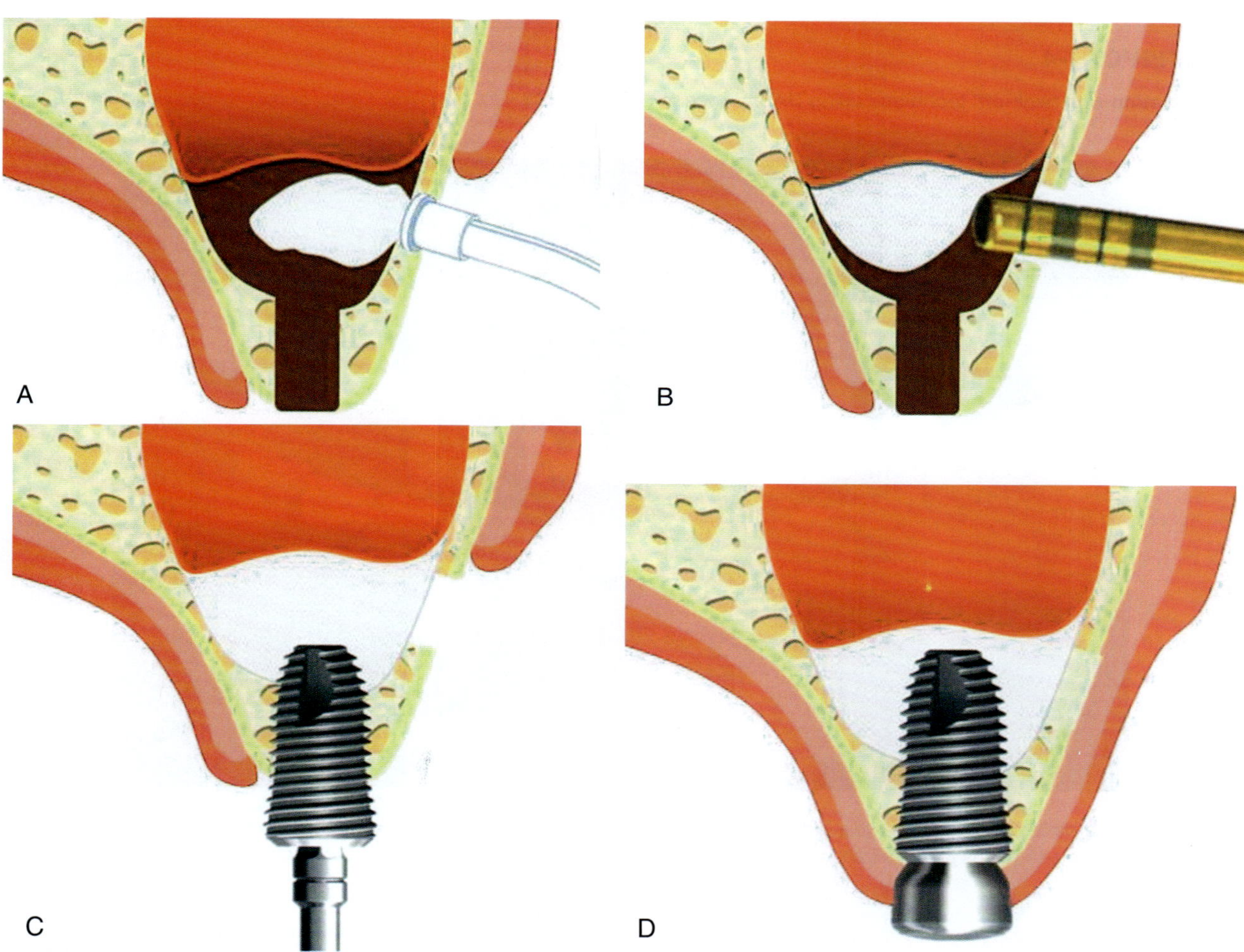

Fig 18.45 (A–D) Once the implant osteotomy has been prepared, the elevated sinus floor is grafted through the lateral window using bone graft and the implant is inserted. Usually the implant is placed and left for submerged healing but in selective cases where the inserted implant has achieved adequate initial stability (more than 30 Ncm) and the force factors are minimum, the implant can be left for open healing by placing the long healing abutment on top of the implant.

CASE REPORT-4

Sinus elevation with 'wall-off' technique using DASK *(Courtesy: Dentium Co. Ltd. and Well Clinic, Seoul, Korea)* (Figs 18.46–18.55).

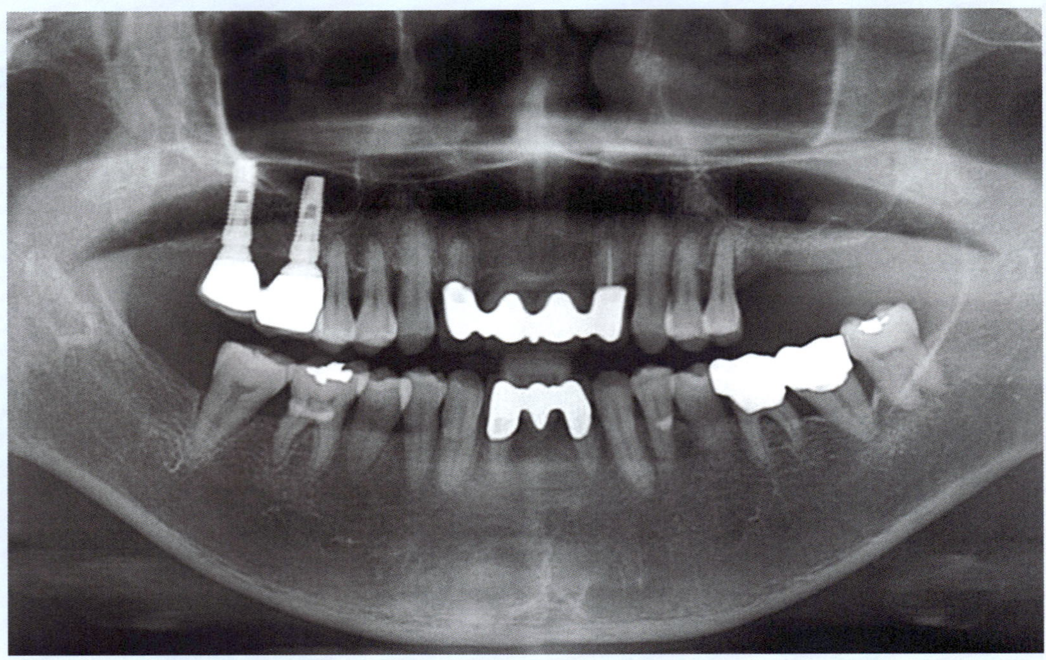

Fig 18.46 Preoperative radiograph of a 59-year-old female patient shows missing upper left molar with limited subantral bone height because of vertical bone resorption and sinus pneumatization. Sinus grafting and simultaneous implant placement were planned.

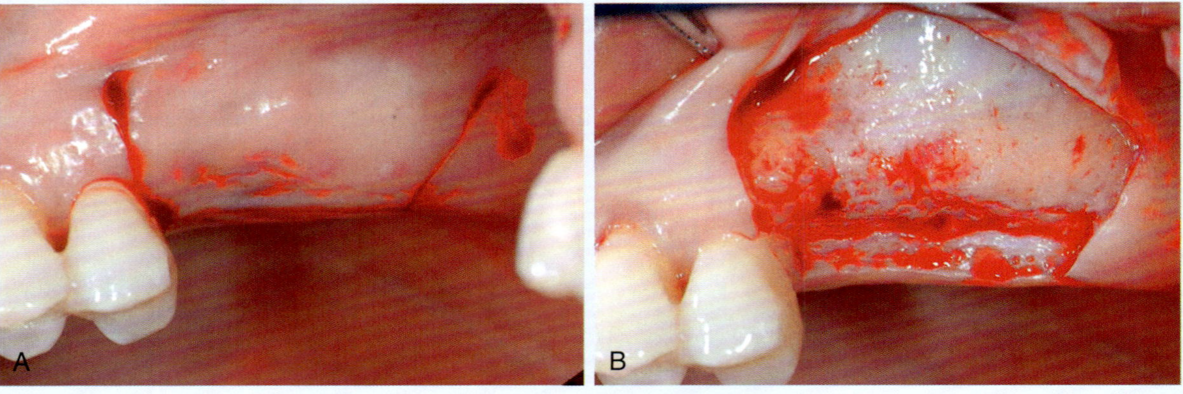

Fig 18.47 (A and B) A trapezoidal flap is elevated to expose the ridge crest and lateral wall of the sinus.

CASE REPORT-4—cont'd

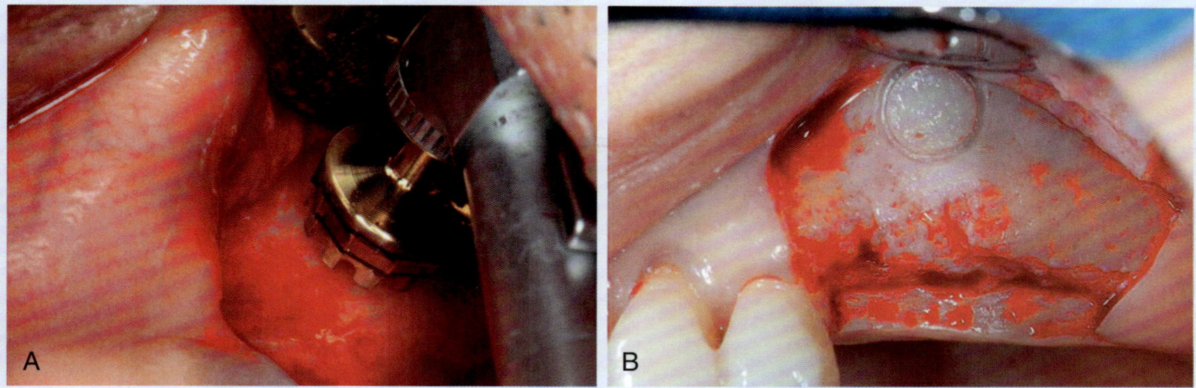

Fig 18.48 (A and B) A lateral window is carefully prepared using DASK drill.

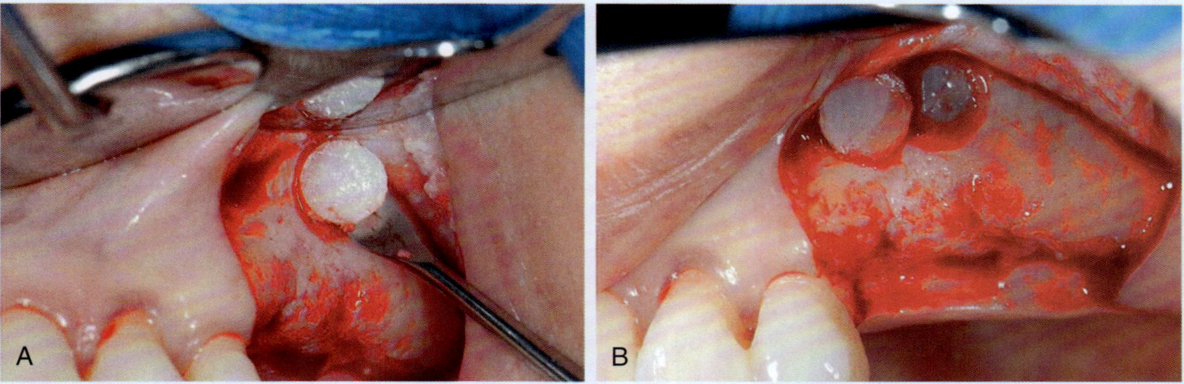

Fig 18.49 (A) The prepared lateral window wall is carefully taken off (wall-off) using an elevator. (B) The bluish-hued underlying Schneiderian membrane can be seen without any tear.

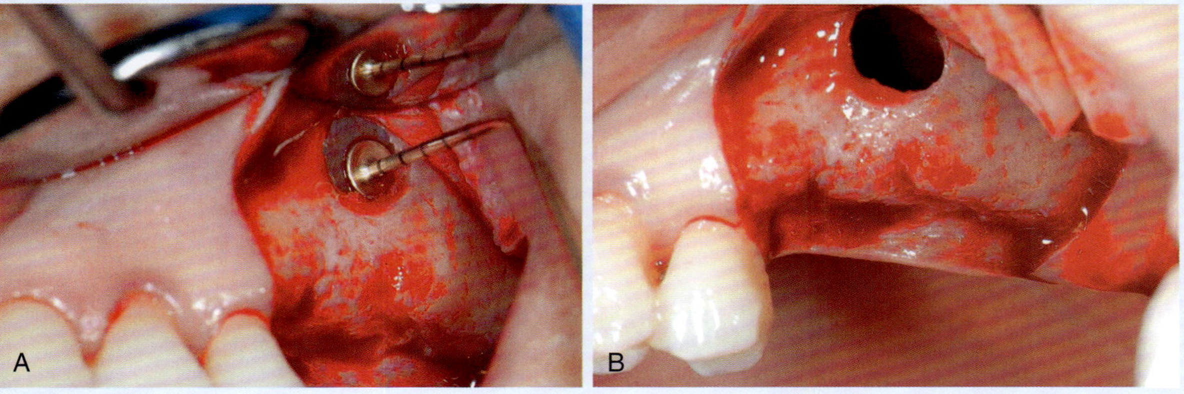

Fig 18.50 (A) A special instrument from the DASK kit is used to detach the sinus membrane from the prepared window margins. After the membrane has been successfully detached from window margins, it is elevated to the planned height using the sinus elevators. (B) Finally the elevated sinus membrane can be seen through lateral window.

Continued

CASE REPORT-4—cont'd

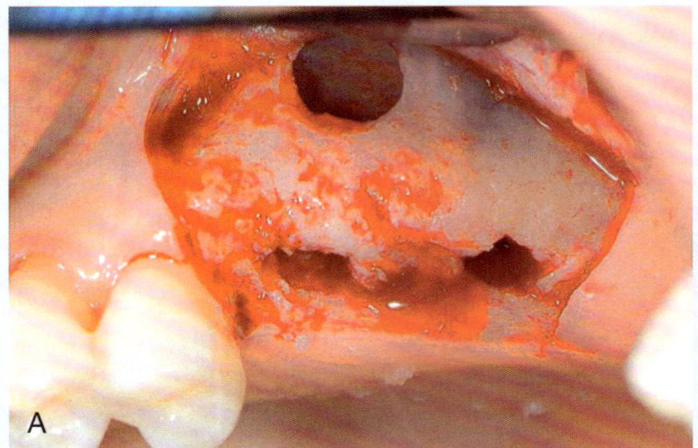

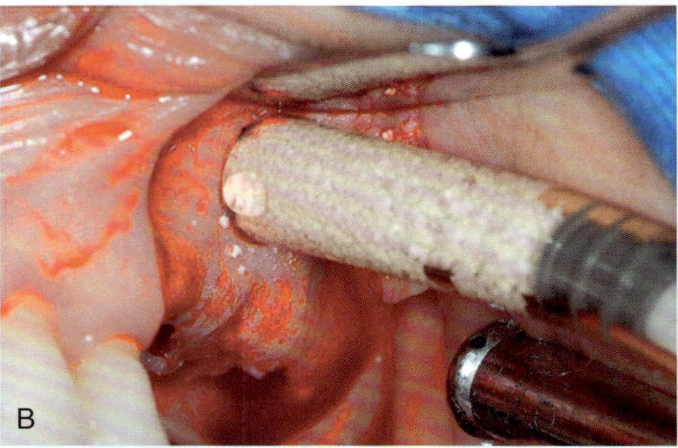

Fig 18.51 Implant osteotomies are prepared from the crestal approach in the usual fashion. (A) The elevated Schneiderian membrane can be seen through the prepared window. (B) The medial half of the elevated sinus floor is grafted through the lateral window using the Osteon sinus graft (HA + β-TCP).

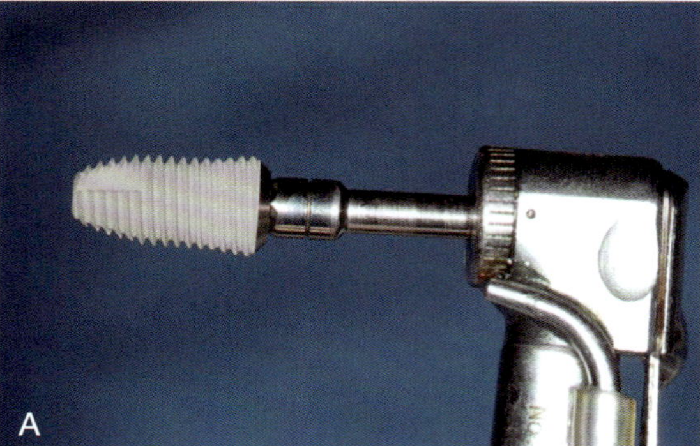

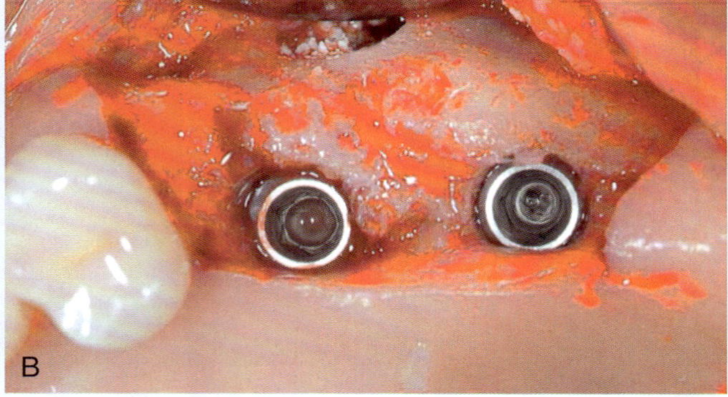

Fig 18.52 (A and B) Two SuperLine (4.5 × 10 mm.) implants (from Dentium Co. Ltd.) are inserted with adequate primary stability.

CASE REPORT-4—cont'd

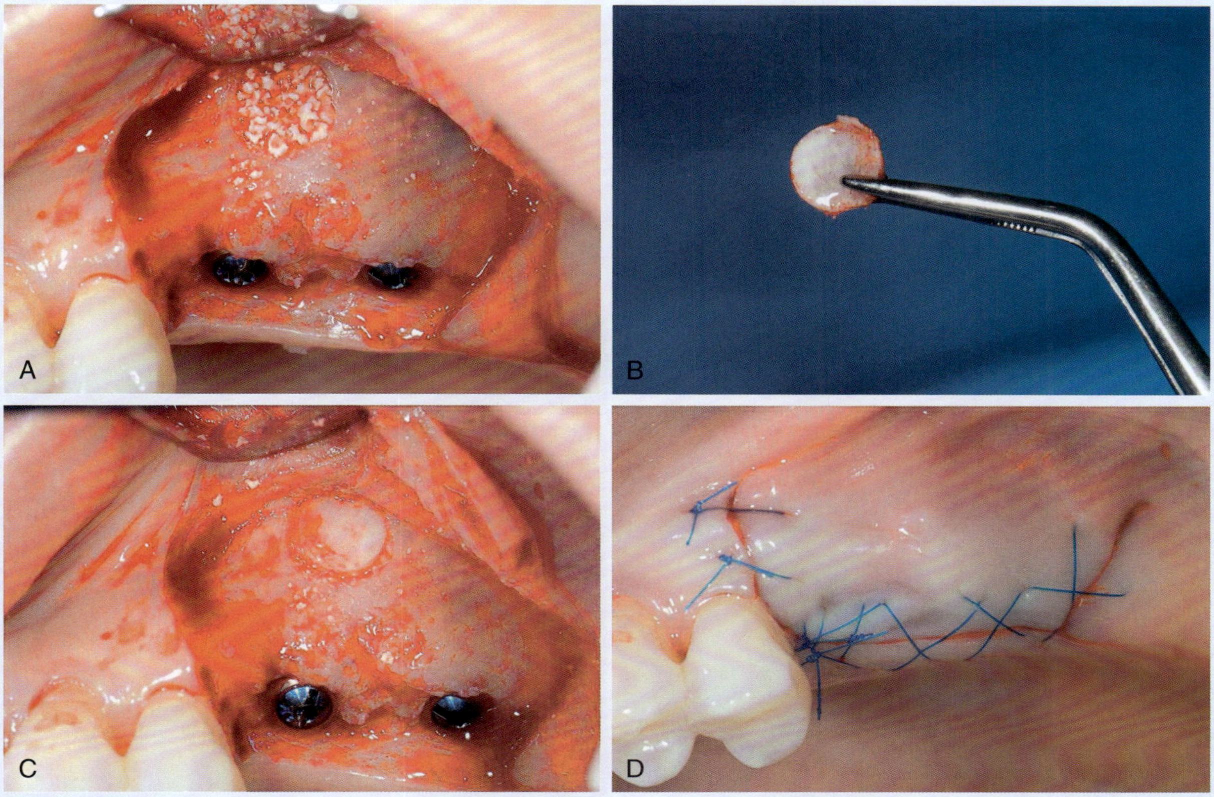

Fig 18.53 (A) More Osteon graft is deposited to loosely fill the sinus cavity. (B and C) The bony island is repositioned to close the grafted sinus window. (D) The flap is sutured back for the submerged healing of the implant and sinus graft maturation.

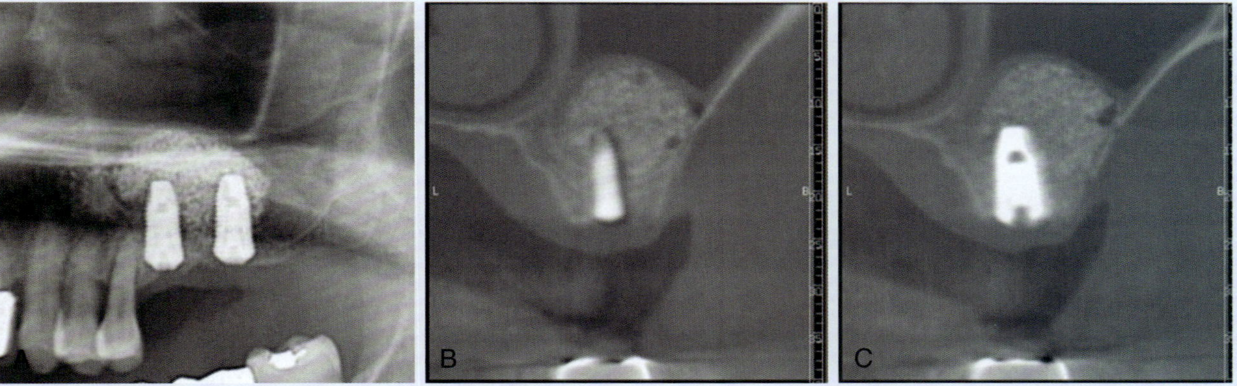

Fig 18.54 (A) Post-sinus-grafting radiograph. (B and C) Dental CT images show 3D view of the grafted sinus floor and immediately inserted implant.

Continued

CASE REPORT-4—cont'd

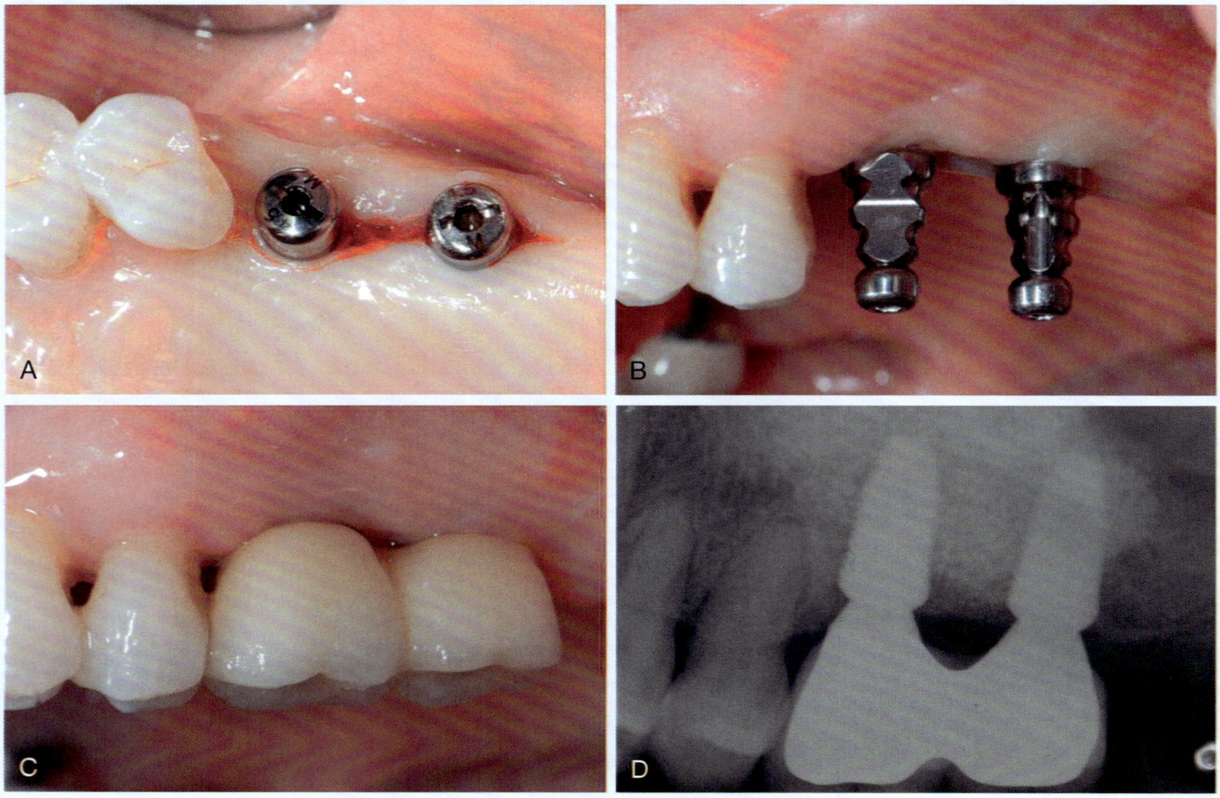

Fig 18.55 (A) Implants are uncovered after 6 months and (B and C) restored using screw-retained, metal-free zirconium prosthesis. (D) Post-implant loading radiograph.

CASE REPORT-5

Sinus elevation with 'grind out' technique using DASK *(Courtesy: Dentium Co. Ltd. and Well Clinic, Seoul, Korea)* (Figs 18.56–18.61).

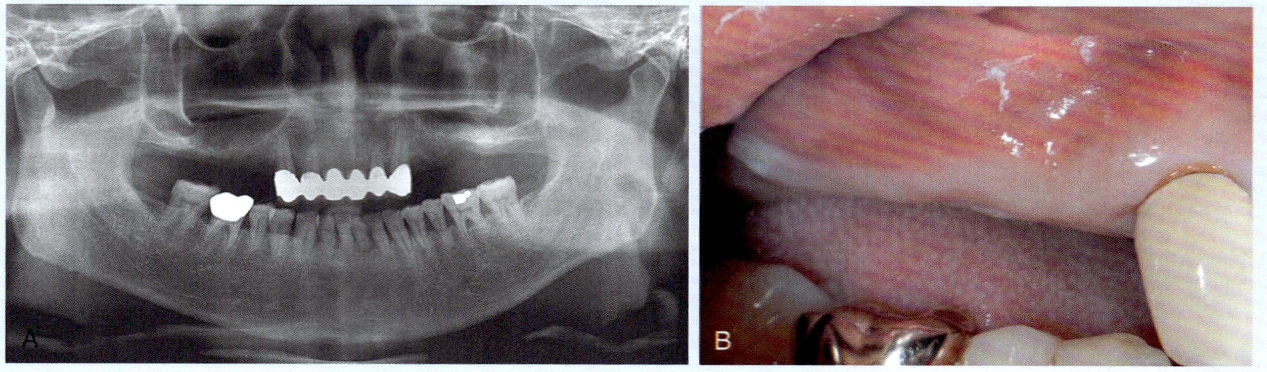

Fig 18.56 (A) Preoperative panoramic radiograph of a 59-year-old male shows bilaterally missing premolar and molars. (B) Preoperative clinical view of the right posterior edentulous maxilla.

CASE REPORT-5—cont'd

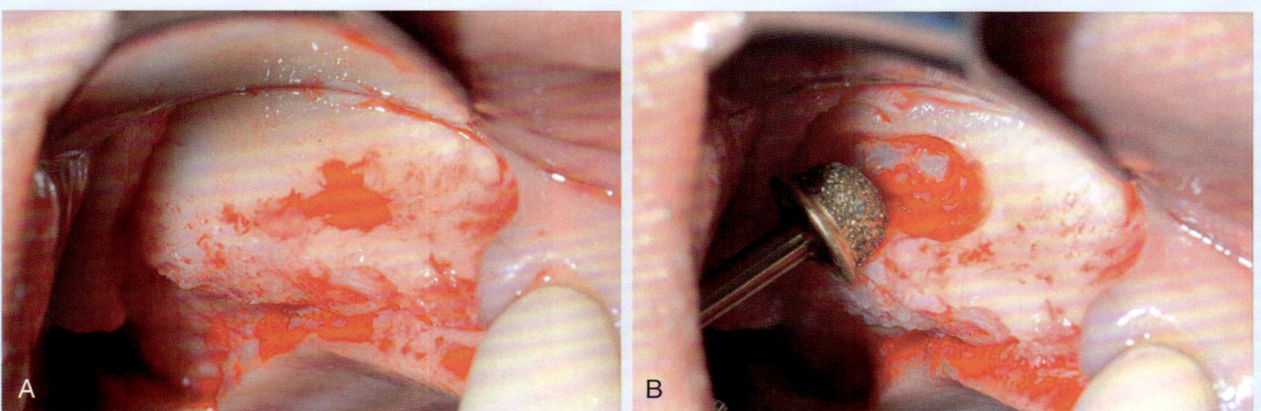

Fig 18.57 (A) The trapezoidal flap is elevated to expose the lateral wall of the sinus. (B) Large diameter coarse diamond DASK attached to the rotary handpiece is carefully used to grind the lateral wall of the sinus with a sweeping motion.

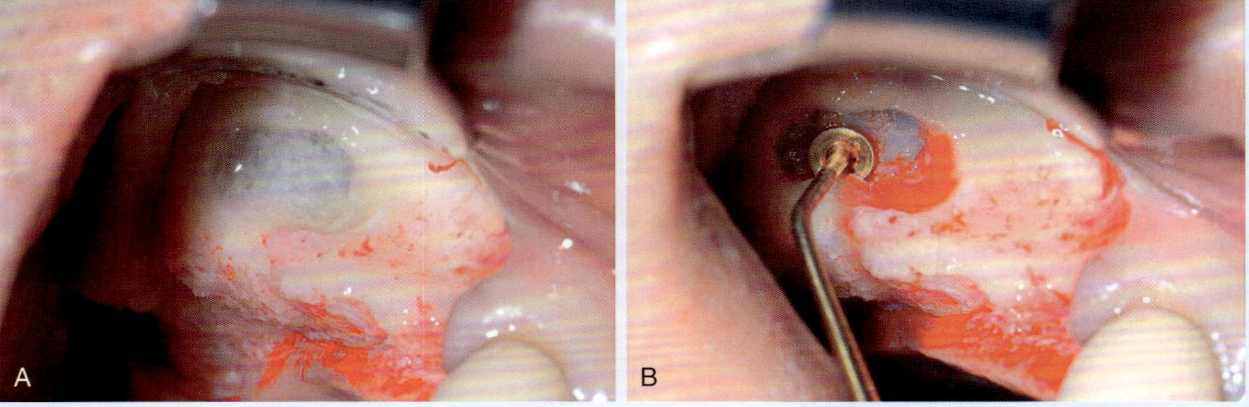

Fig 18.58 (A) Exposed bluish-hued Schneiderian membrane can be seen through the ground lateral window. (B) Sinus membrane is carefully detached from the window margins and elevated using sinus elevators.

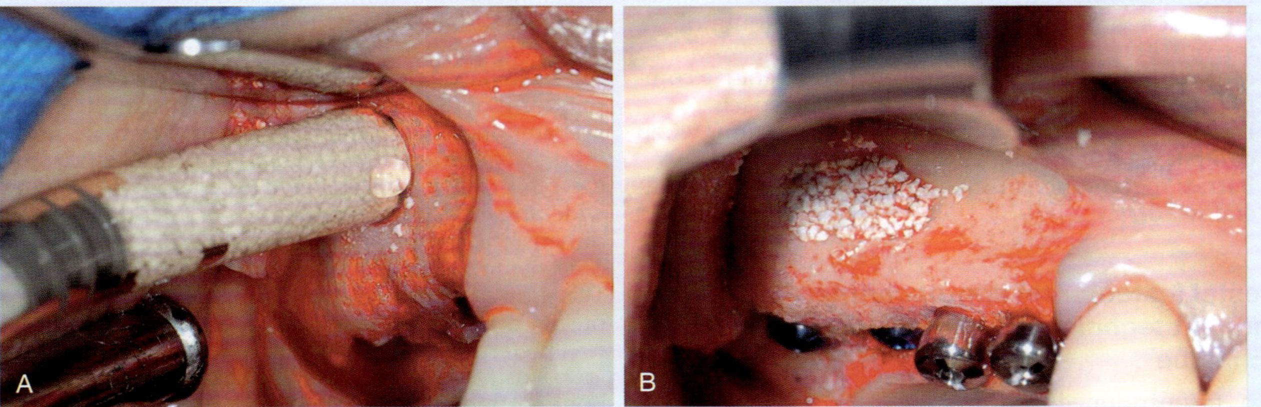

Fig 18.59 (A) Osteon sinus graft (HA + β-TCP) is introduced into the elevated sinus through the lateral window to graft the medial half of the sinus. (B) Implants are inserted and more Osteon graft is added to the remaining lateral half of the sinus. The graft should loosely fill the sinus cavity.

Continued

CASE REPORT-5—cont'd

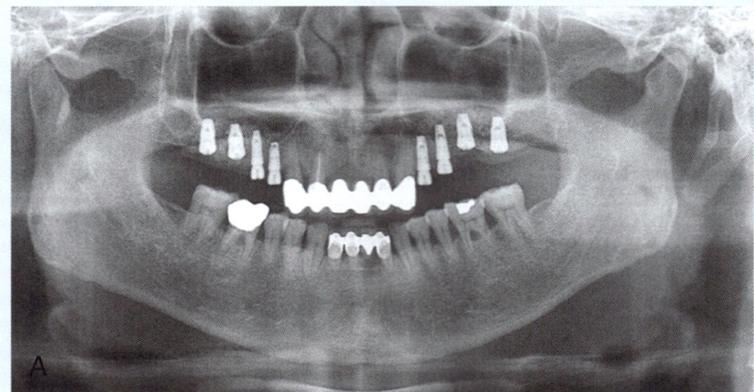

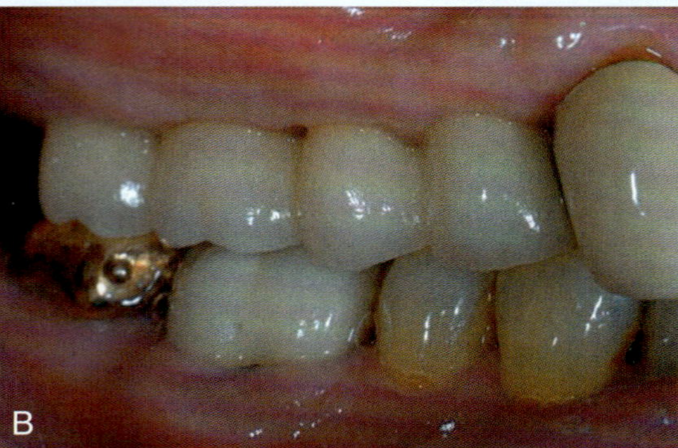

Fig 18.60 (A) Post-sinus-graft and postimplantation radiograph shows bilateral sinus grafting and implantation using DASK technique. (B) Implants are restored after a 6-month healing period.

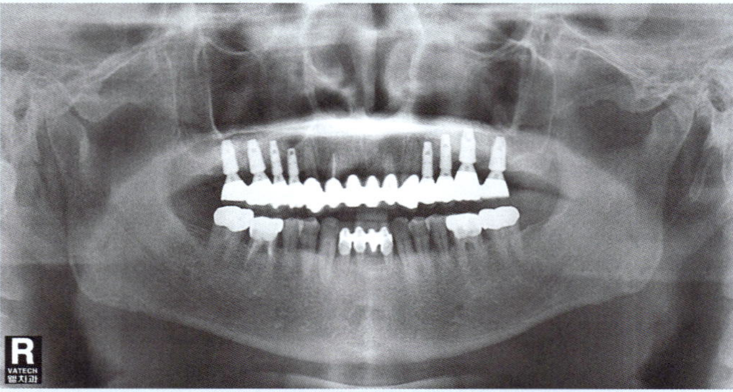

Fig 18.61 Postloading radiograph.

Disadvantages of the lateral approach

1. It requires a large flap elevation for surgical access, which reduces the blood supply to the lateral wall of the sinus.
2. Difficult access in patients with reduced mouth opening or stiff perioral musculature.
3. More chances of sinus rupture and postoperative complication, compared to the subcrestal approach.
4. Large amount of graft is required to fill the sinus when compared with the subcrestal approach.
5. Barrier membrane is usually needed to cover the lateral window.

Crestal (osteotome) approach/internal sinus-lift technique/Summer's osteotome technique

It was first performed by Hilt Tatum in 1974 and published in 1994. To perform this technique, first the residual bone height under the sinus floor is measured with the help of radiographs and dental CT scans. A minimum 8–10 mm of bone height should be present under the sinus floor to perform this procedure following the conventional osteotome technique. The newer intralift and other advanced techniques are possible even if the subantral residual bone is less than 4 mm in height. This technique begins with a crestal incision. Summer suggested that the crestal incision should be extended distally, in selective cases, to the tuberosity area where autogenous bone can be harvested. A full-thickness flap is elevated to expose the alveolar ridge crest. A pilot drill of 2 mm diameter is used to start the osteotomy preparation, which should be ended 2 mm short of sinus floor. A confirmatory radiograph can be taken by inserting the pilot drill in the prepared osteotomy. Now either the widening drills or a set of Summer's osteotomes of varying dimensions can be sequentially used to widen the osteotomy site to the same level (2 mm short of the sinus floor). The choice of using osteotomes or widening drills depends on the density of the residual bone; in poor-density bone it is preferred to use osteotomes to laterally condense the low-density bone and enhance the density of the trabecular bone around the inserted implant. An osteotome of diameter a little less than the planned implant body, is inserted in the prepared osteotomy site and gently tapped to reach the same level. Now the osteotome is tapped gently to fracture up the sinus floor. Once the largest osteotome has expanded the implant site, the particulated bone substitutes, alone or mixed with autogenous bone, are added to the osteotomy as the grafting material. Summer suggested a 25% autogenous bone with 75% hydroxyapatite mix; however, a variety of other graft materials have also been successfully used. The final stage of sinus floor elevation is completed by reinserting the largest osteotome in the implant site with the graft material in place. This causes the added bone graft to exert pressure onto the sinus membrane and to further elevate it. Additional grafting material can subsequently be added and tapped in to achieve the desired amount of sinus membrane elevation. Once the desired height of sinus elevation is gained and grafted, the implant fixture is inserted. The implant fixture should be slightly larger in diameter than the osteotomy created by the final osteotome. The inserted implant becomes the final osteotome, which keeps tenting up the elevated maxillary sinus membrane.

Step by step diagrammatic and clinical presentation of the conventional crestal approach of sinus lifting (Summer's osteotome technique) is shown in Figs 18.62–18.69.

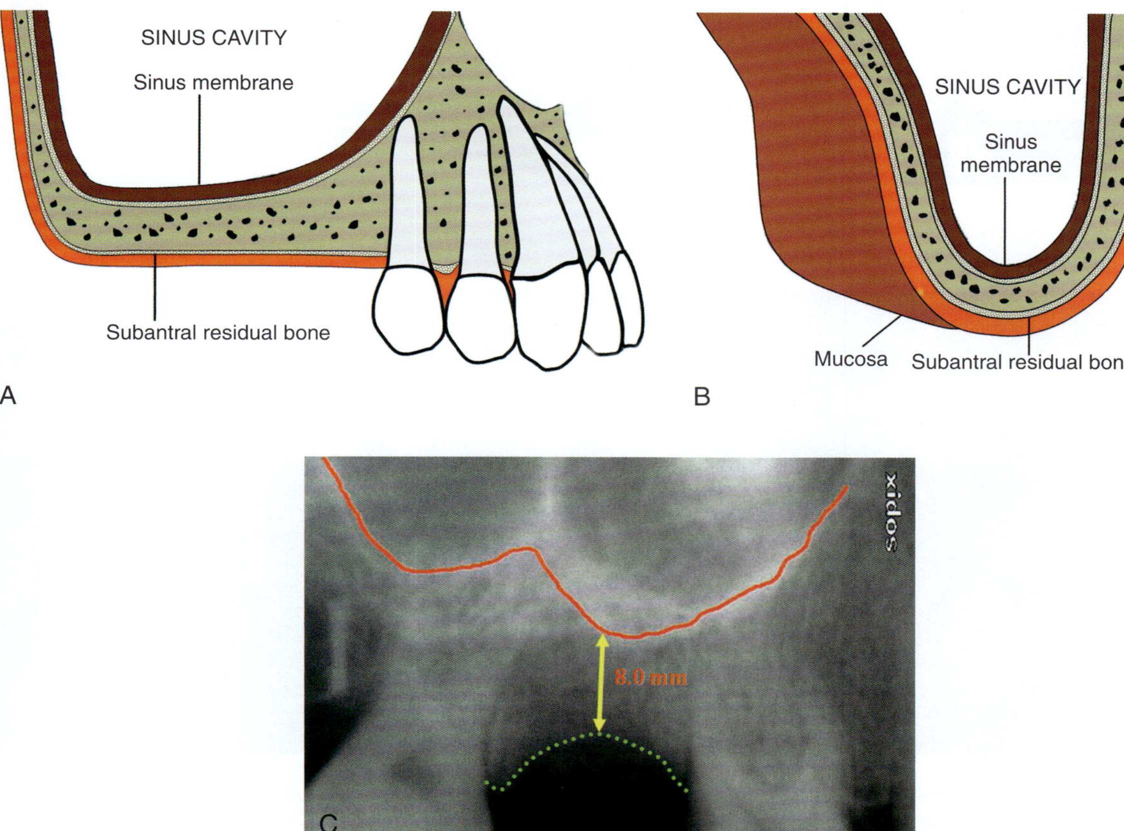

Fig 18.62 (A and B) Facial and cross-sectional views of posterior edentulous maxilla showing limited subantral bone height, which is not sufficient for adequately long implant placement. (C) Preoperative radiograph shows 8 mm subantral bone height.

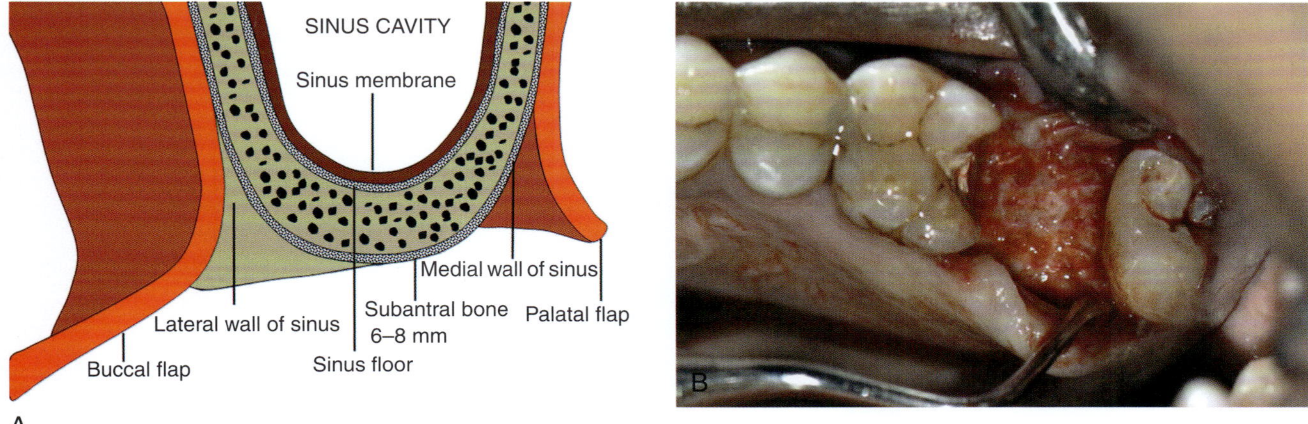

Fig 18.63 (A and B) Mid-crestal incision is made and flaps are elevated to expose the ridge crest.

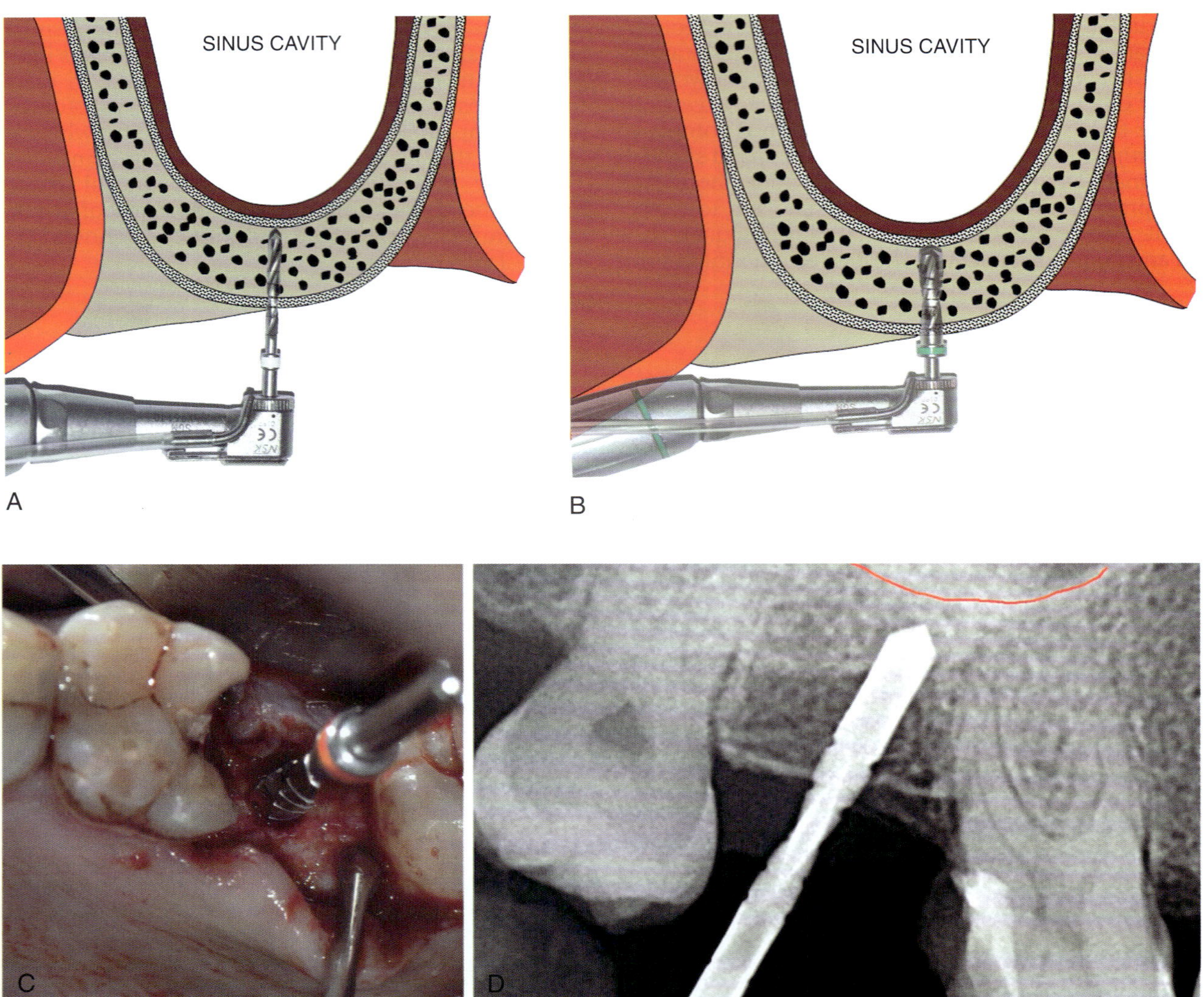

Fig 18.64 (A–D) Osteotomy for the implant is prepared in the usual fashion using all the drills 2.0 mm short of sinus floor, which can be verified with the dental radiographs with the drill in place.

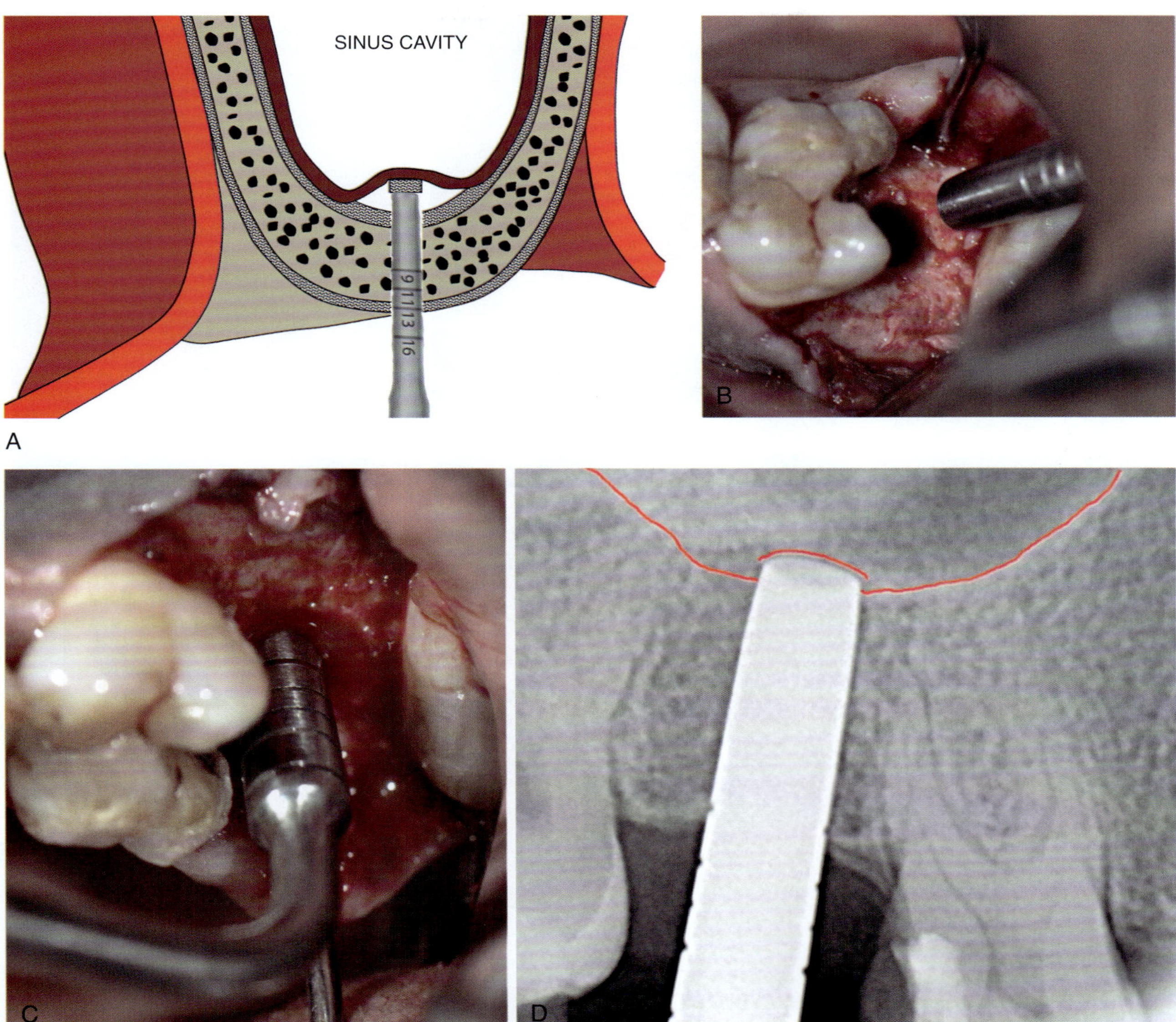

Fig 18.65 (A–D) Once the implant osteotomy is completely prepared 2 mm short of the sinus floor, an appropriate sized sinus-lifting osteotome is inserted and carefully tapped to fracture up the sinus floor, and also lift up the Schneiderian membrane. After fracturing the bony floor of the sinus, a collagen membrane or collagen plug (Collaplug, Zimmer Dental) can be inserted into the osteotomy before further lifting the sinus membrane. It prevents the inadvertent rupture of the delicate Schneiderian membrane. After achieving the required height of sinus elevation, a blunt implant probe can be inserted to evaluate the height of the sinus elevation that has been achieved and also to check if any rupture have occurred in the membrane.

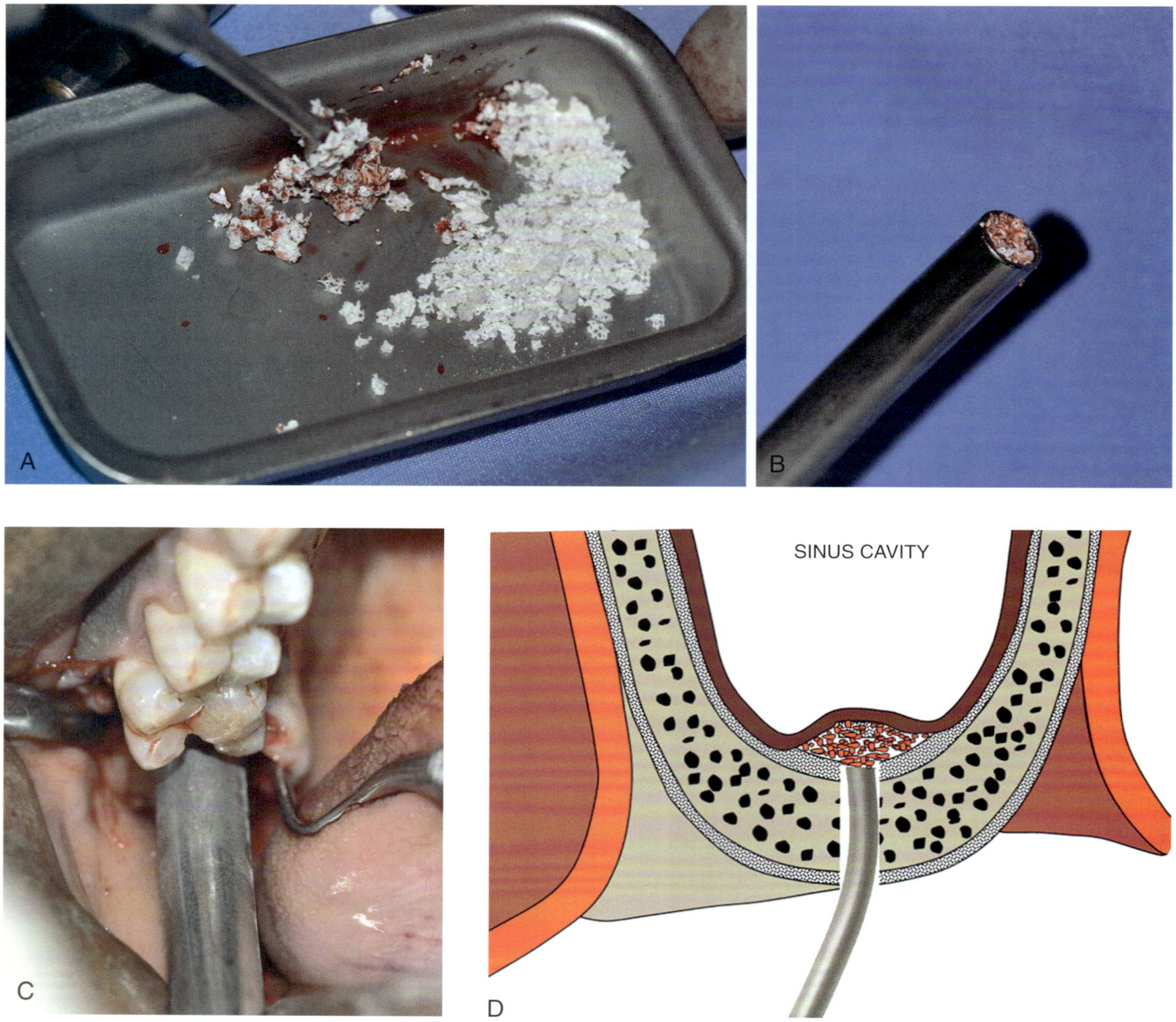

Fig 18.66 (A–D) The bone substitute alone or mixed with autogenous bone is carried into the osteotomy using the bone carrier, and deposited under the lifted sinus floor.

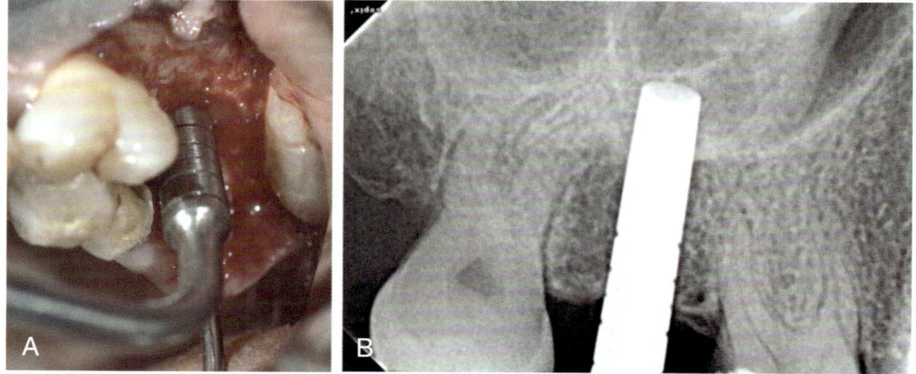

Fig 18.67 (A and B) The same osteotome can be used to push the graft up and further lift the grafted sinus floor to prepare space for the implant.

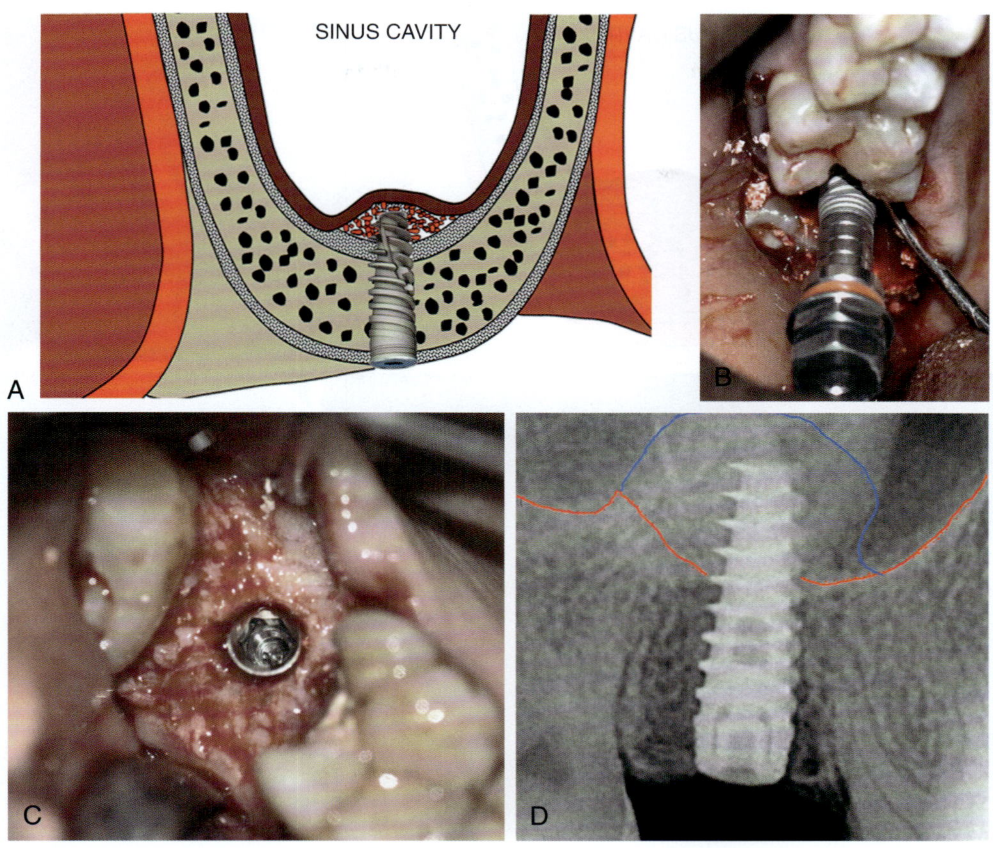

Fig 18.68 (A–D) Once the sinus floor is successfully lifted and grafted, an adequately long implant is inserted.

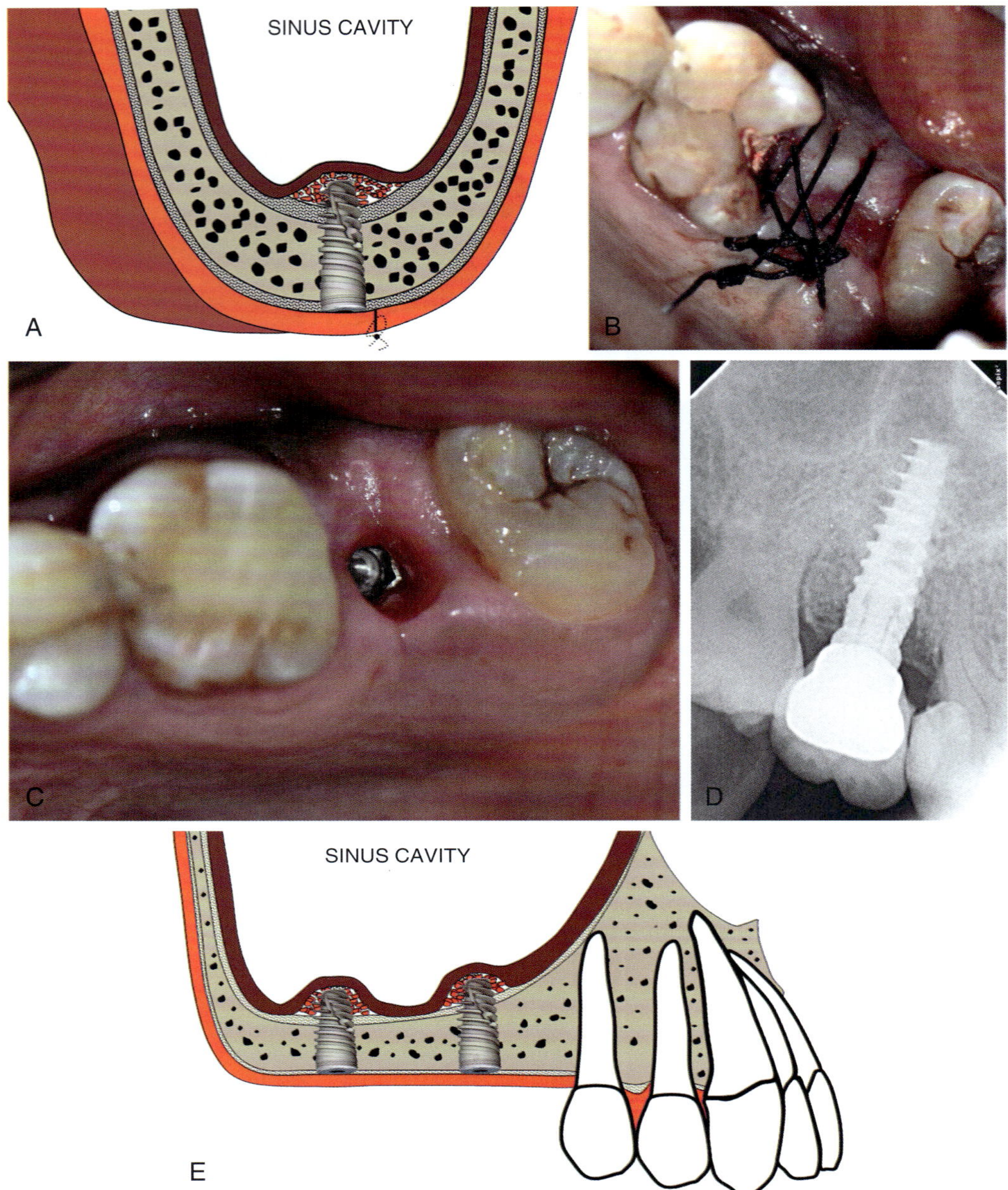

Fig 18.69 (A and B) The flap is sutured back with primary closure. (C and D) The implant is exposed and restored after new bone regeneration has occurred in the grafted sinus in 4–6 months. (E) Multiple implants can also be inserted with internal sinus-lifting performed individually for each implant.

Advantages of the crestal approach/Summer's osteotome technique

1. Less invasive procedure.
2. Improves maxillary bone density, which allows greater initial stability of implants.
3. Less amount of grafting material is required to fill the lifted sinus membrane.
4. No barrier membrane is required.
5. Limited flap elevation is required which maintain blood supply to the lateral wall of the sinus.

Disadvantages of the crestal approach/Summer's osteotome technique

1. Initial implant stability is unproven, if the residual bone height is less than 6 mm.
2. Limited height of sinus elevation is possible when compared to the lateral approach.
3. With this approach there could also be a higher chance of misaligning the long axis of the osteotome during sequential osteotomy.
4. Tapping can cause mental trauma to the patient.

Recent advancements and modifications in the crestal approach of the sinus lifting

Bicortical engagement without sinus grafting

If the subantral residual bone is more than 6–8 mm in height and more than 10 mm in width, a large diameter (6–7 mm) and short length (7–9 mm) implant can be inserted with bicortical engagement (in the crest bone as well as into the antral floor). The engagement of the implant in the high-density sinus floor results in higher initial stability of the implant. Moreover, a slightly longer implant can be placed by this procedure. After the osteotomy has been prepared 1–2 mm short of the sinus floor, the implant is inserted so that its apex itself fractures up the thin sinus floor and lifts up the membrane; thus the apical part of the implant gets firmly engaged in the sinus floor. No graft is used in this technique. In cases of high-density sinus floor, the author suggests the use of an adequate size osteotome to fracture up the sinus floor before implant insertion. However, if the implant surgeon is not willing to use the osteotome, the diamond-coated DASK drill can be used as an alternative to grind up the remaining part of the sinus floor, followed by implant placement (Figs 18.70–18.72).

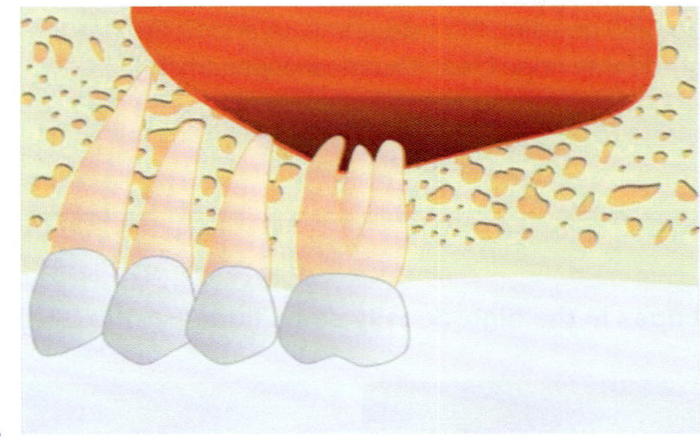
A

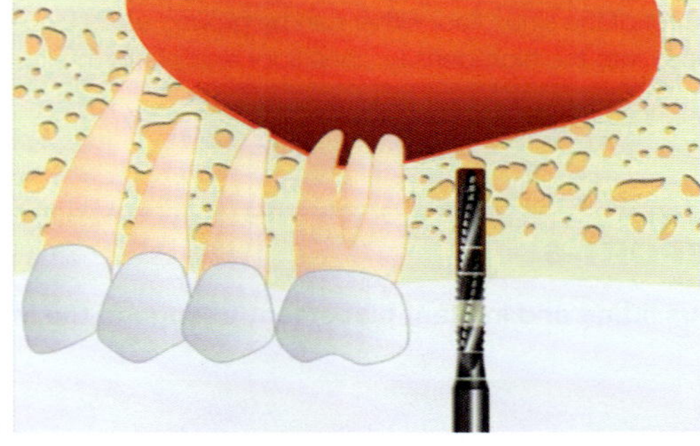
B

Fig 18.70 (A) Residual subantral bone height, which is insufficient for ideal length implant placement. (B) A pilot drill/Lindemann drill is used to prepare the implant osteotomy 1–2 mm short of sinus floor.

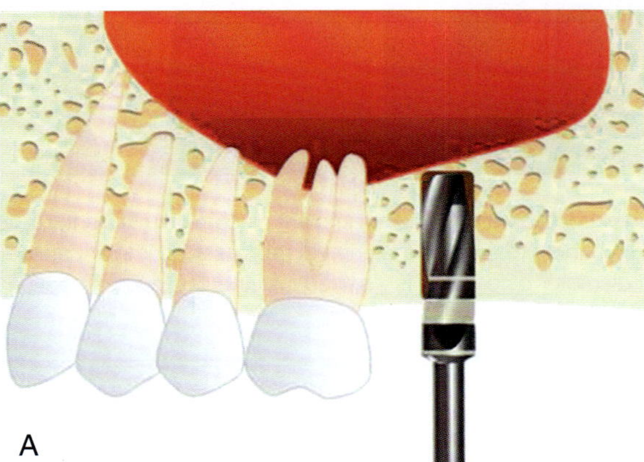
A

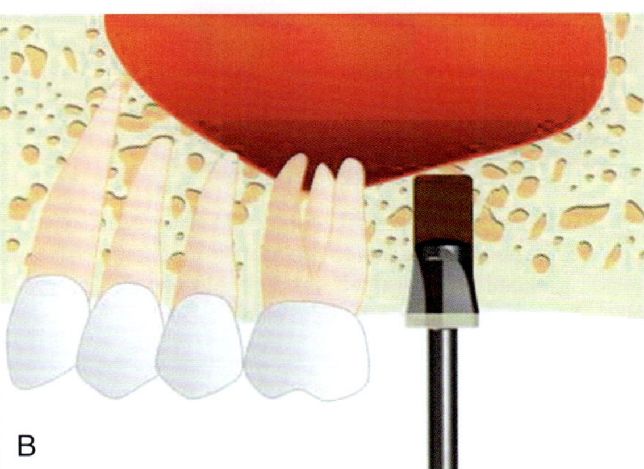
B

Fig 18.71 (A) All the osteotomy widening drills are used to the same depth. (B) A countersinking drill can be used to submerge the implant 1 mm apical to the ridge crest.

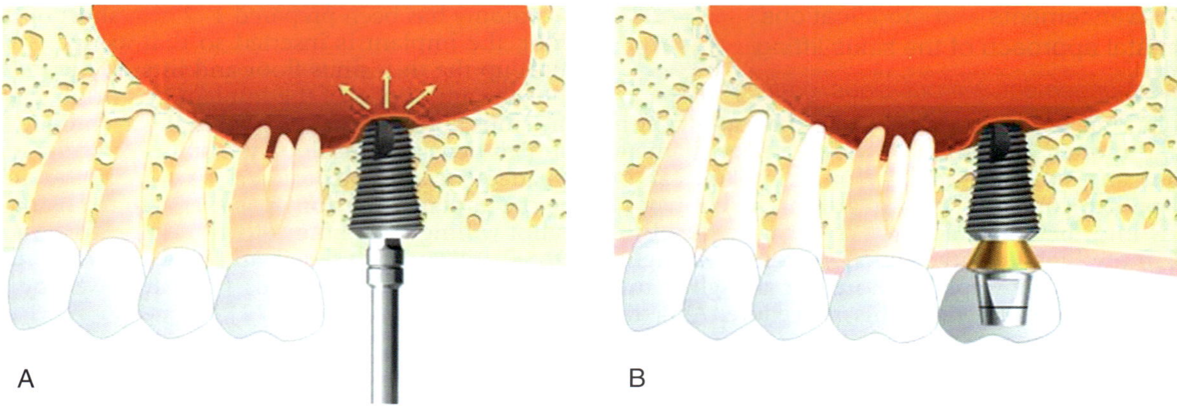

Fig 18.72 The rest of the sinus floor either can be ground using DASK or fractured up using the osteotome. (A and B) Further, the implant is inserted to engage its apex into the high-density sinus floor and platform into the high-density ridge crest (bicortical engagement).

CASE REPORT-6

Internal sinus lifting and implant placement to engage the implant apex in the high-density sinus floor (Fig 18.73A–J).

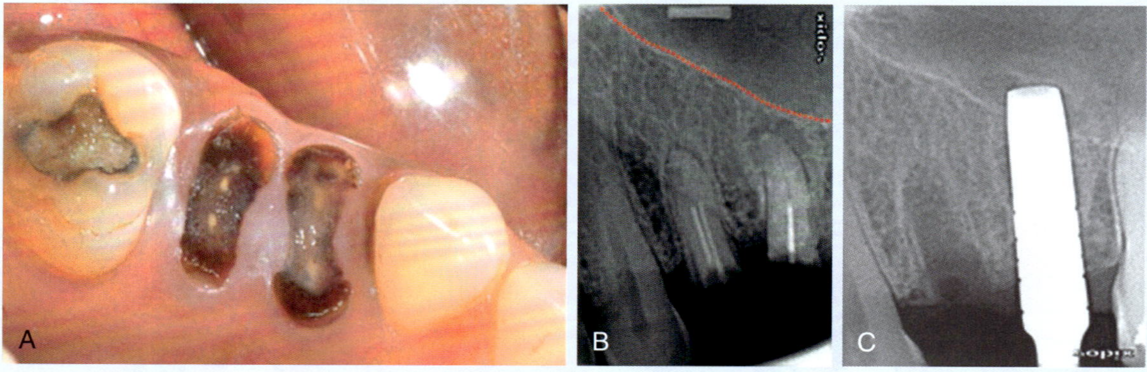

Fig 18.73 (A) Clinical view of the root stumps of left bicuspids which are to be extracted with immediate implant placement. (B) Dental radiograph showing limited bone height apical to the root stumps (especially in second bicuspid), to engage the immediately inserted implant apex. (C) The root stumps atraumatically extracted using periotomes and a large 4.2 mm diameter osteotome is inserted into the posterior extraction socket and gently tapped to fracture up the hard sinus floor.

CASE REPORT-6—cont'd

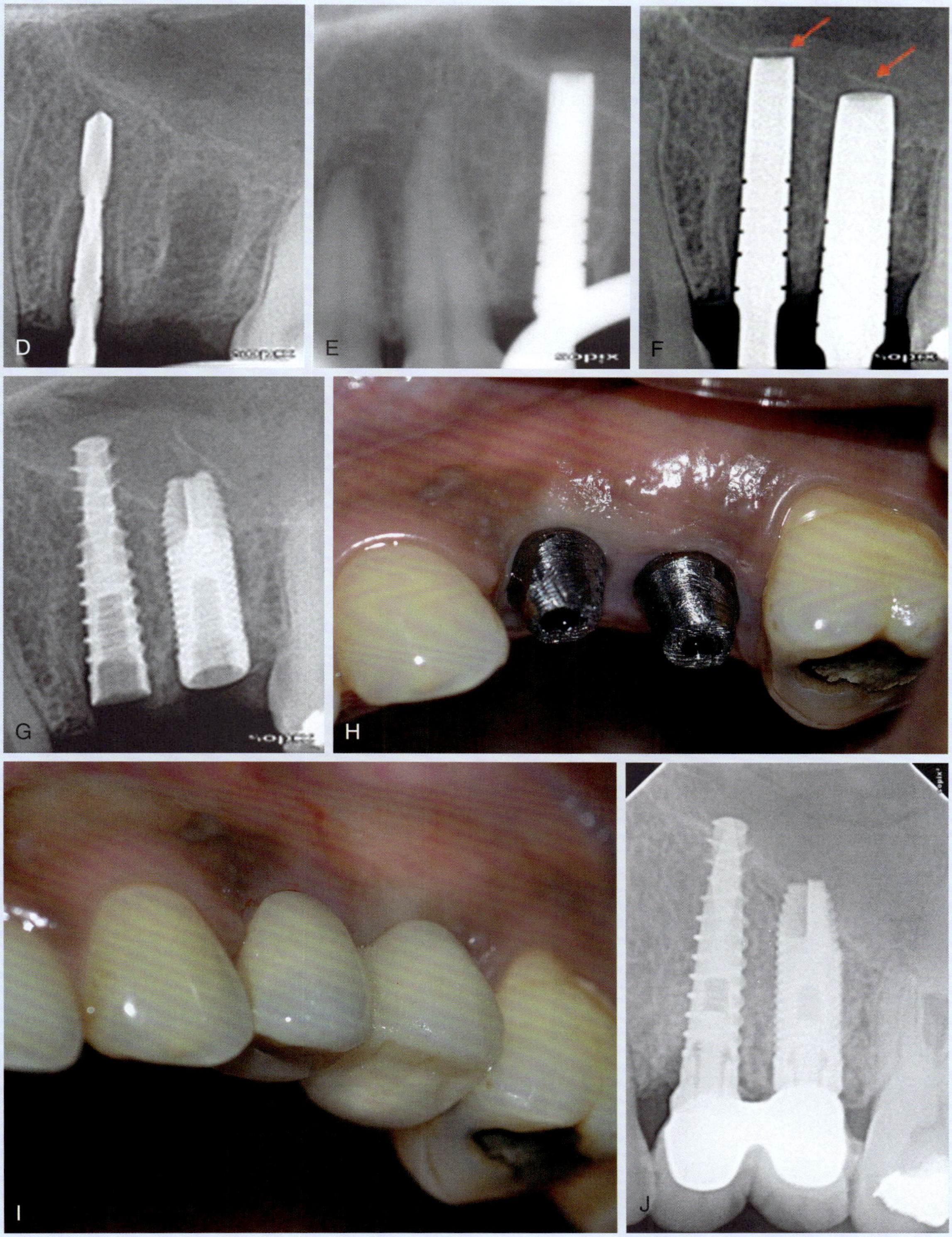

D E F G H I J

Fig 18.73, cont'd (D) The implant osteotomy is prepared through the anterior socket just 2 mm short of sinus floor. (E) Further a final drill diameter osteotome used in a similar fashion to fracture up the sinus floor. (F) Both the osteotomes can be seen in the radiograph reaching beyond the sinus floor with fractured sinus floor bony pieces *(red arrows)* tenting up the elevated sinus membrane. (G) Both the implants are inserted to engage their apex into the high density sinus floor and their platform into the ridge crest (bicortical engagement), to achieve high initial implant stability (30–35 Ncm) which is quite necessary for optimal implant success in the low-density posterior maxilla. (H and I) Implants are uncovered and restored after 4 months. (J) Postloading radiograph 6 months after the implant insertion shows new bone regeneration in the elevated sinus. Even though no bone graft material was used to fill the elevated sinus floor, the reason for the new bone formation is that the implant apex kept tenting the elevated membrane and provided the space for new bone growth.

Sinus lifting with crestal approach using DASK (grinding up technique)

Sinus lifting and grafting with the crest approach can be effectively and safely done using the Dentium Advanced Sinus Kit (DASK), which contains the special diamond-coated burs for grinding up the sinus floor to reach the membrane without damaging or perforating the same. Then a special set of sinus-lifting instruments is used to easily and safely lift up the Schneiderian membrane.

Step by step diagrammatic presentation of the grinding up technique using DASK is shown in Figs 18.74–18.78.

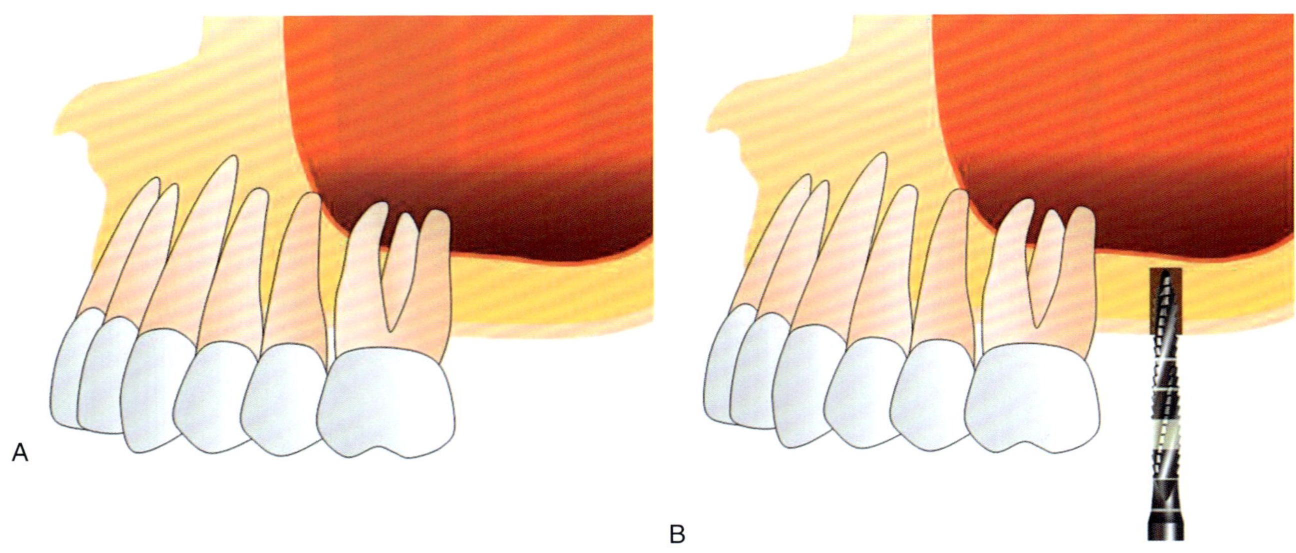

Fig 18.74 (A) Subantral bone which is inadequate (4–6 mm) in height for adequately long implant placement. (B) Pilot drilling is done 2 mm short of the sinus floor.

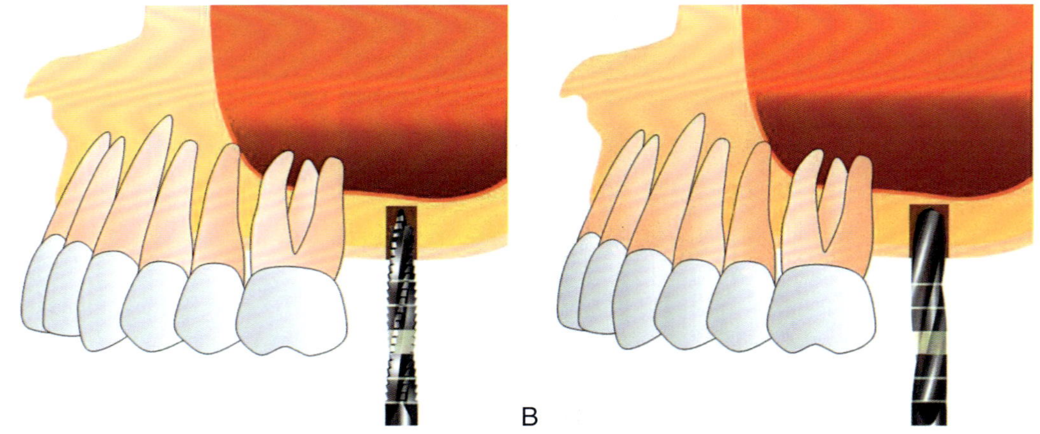

Fig 18.75 (A and B) All osteotomy widening drills are used to the same depth (2 mm short of sinus floor).

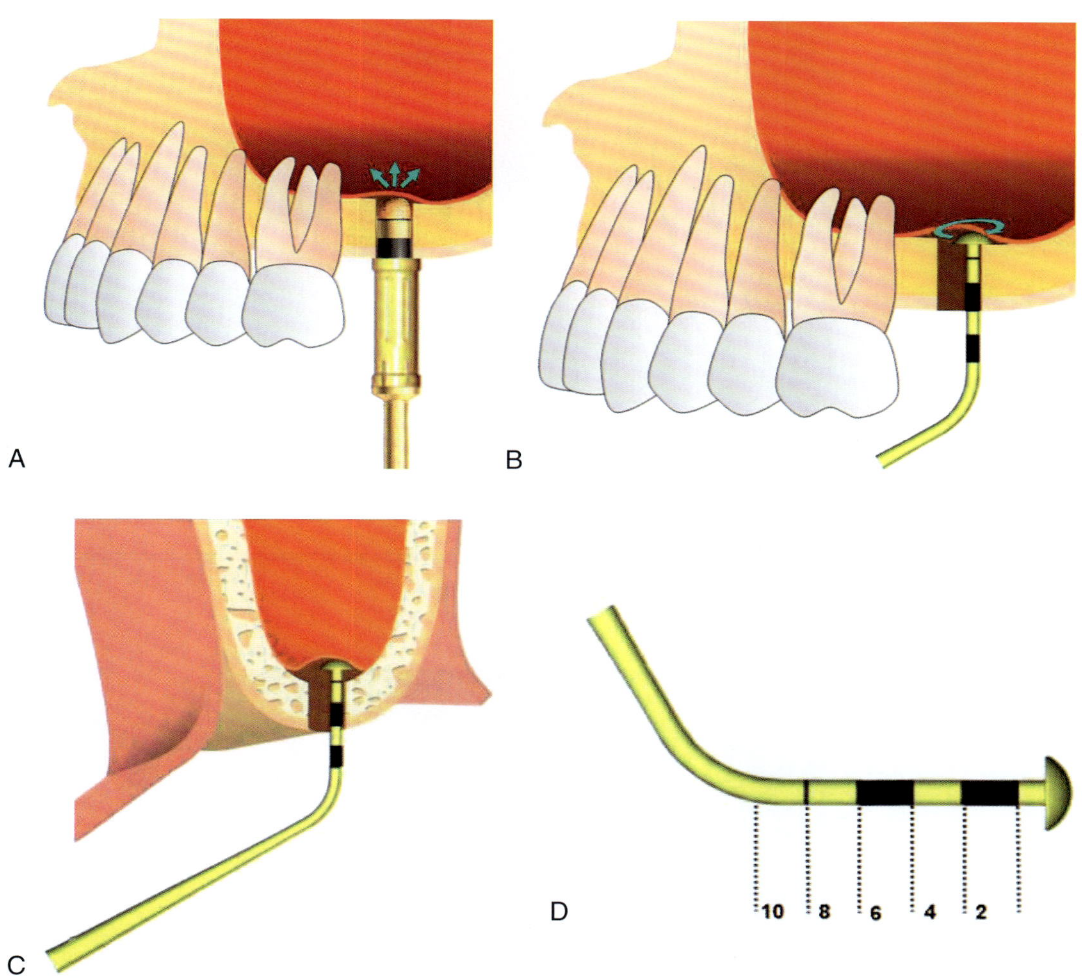

Fig 18.76 (A) After completing the osteotomy preparation for the implant 2 mm short of sinus floor, a diamond-coated bur from DASK is used to grind the rest of the subantral bone, to reach the Schneiderian membrane. (B–D) A sinus elevation probe with its umbrella-shaped tip is used for lifting the sinus membrane to the desired height.

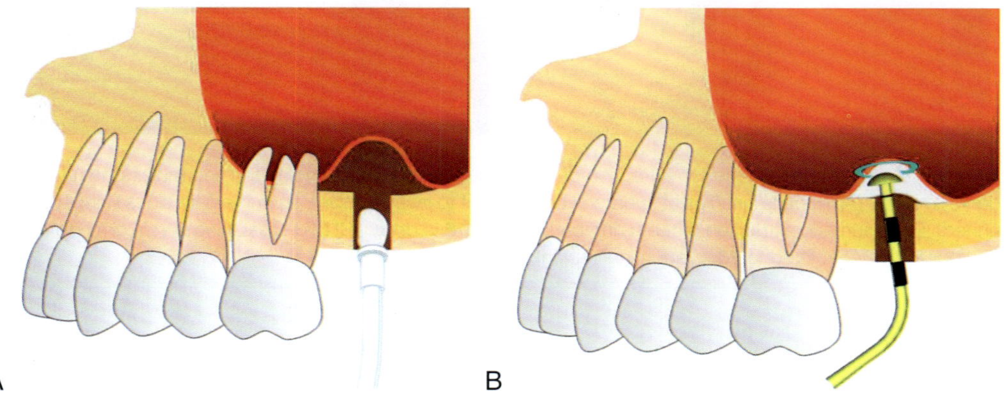

Fig 18.77 (A and B) Elevated sinus space is grafted using HA Scaffold (70%) + β-TCP (30%) – Osteon graft which also helps in further lifting the membrane.

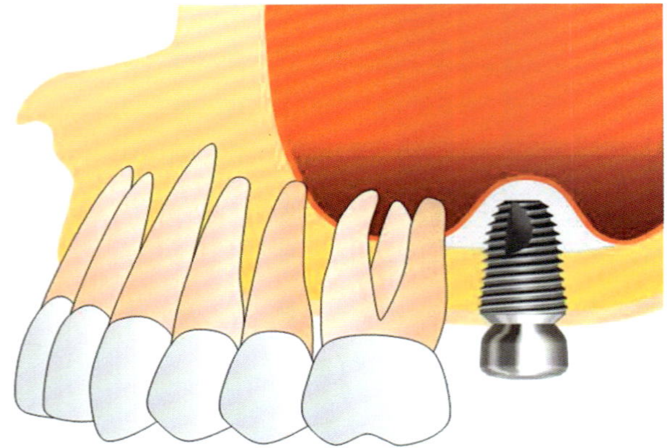

Fig 18.78 After the elevated sinus floor has successfully been grafted, the implant is inserted.

CASE REPORT-7

Sinus lifting with subcrestal approach using DASK (Figs 18.79–18.82).

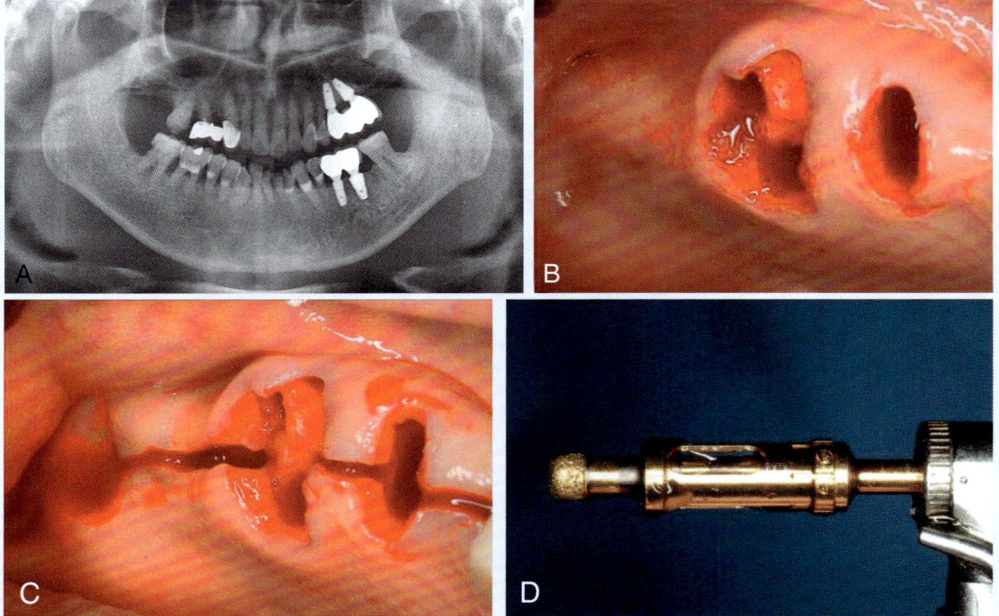

Fig 18.79 Preoperative radiograph shows need for extraction of right maxillary second premolar and first molar, and replacement of teeth numbers 14–17 with dental implant. (A) There is insufficient subantral bone height to insert implant, so immediate sinus lifting with the crestal approach using DASK is planned. (B) Atraumatic extraction of teeth numbers 15 and 16 is done. (C) Mid-crestal incision is given to expose the ridge crest. (D) Diamond-coated bur from DASK fitted to 20:1 reduction implant handpiece.

CASE REPORT-7—cont'd

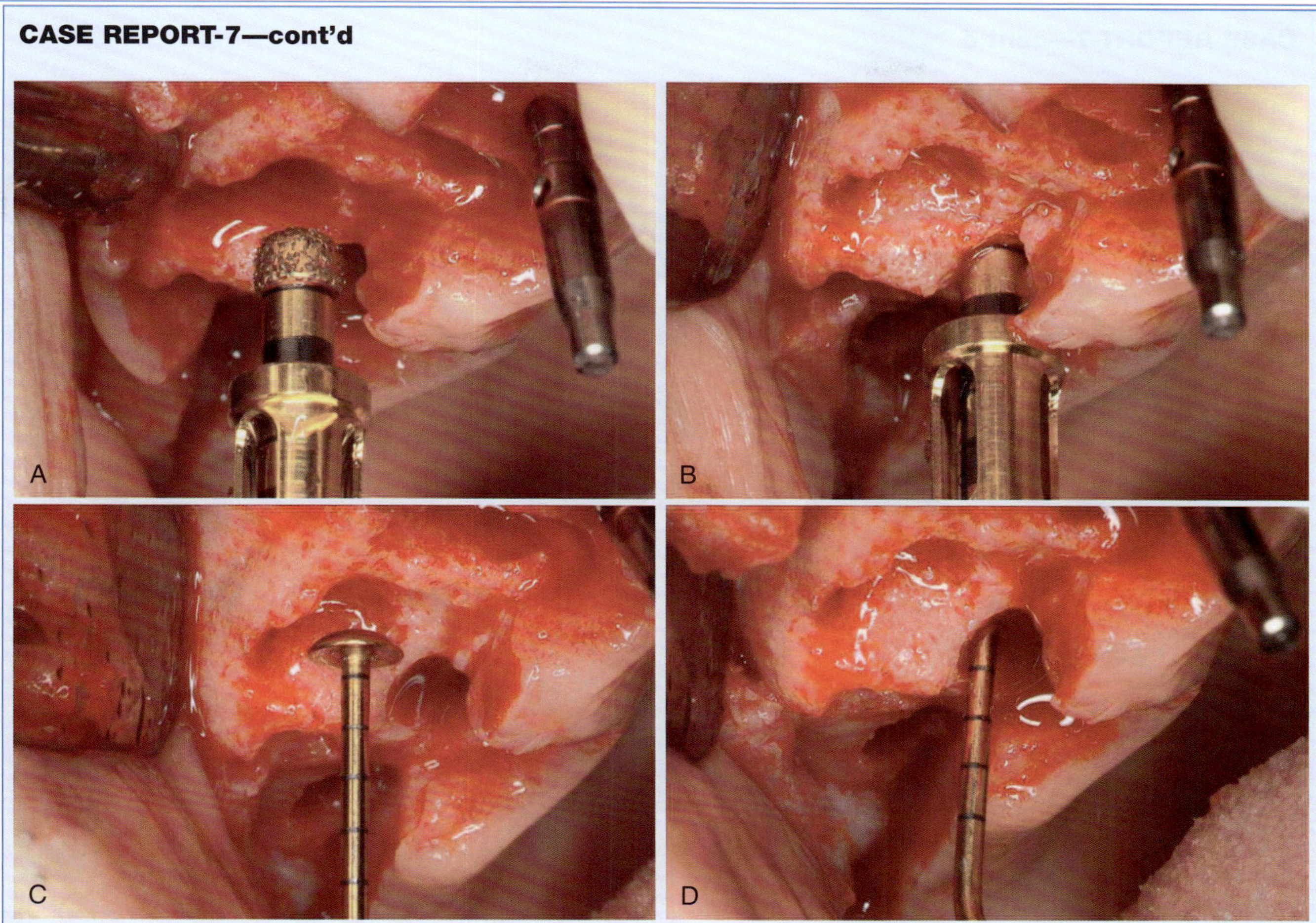

Fig 18.80 (A and B) Diamond bur from the DASK kit is used to grind the sinus floor. (C and D) Then the sinus elevator is used to elevate the sinus membrane.

Continued

CASE REPORT-7—cont'd

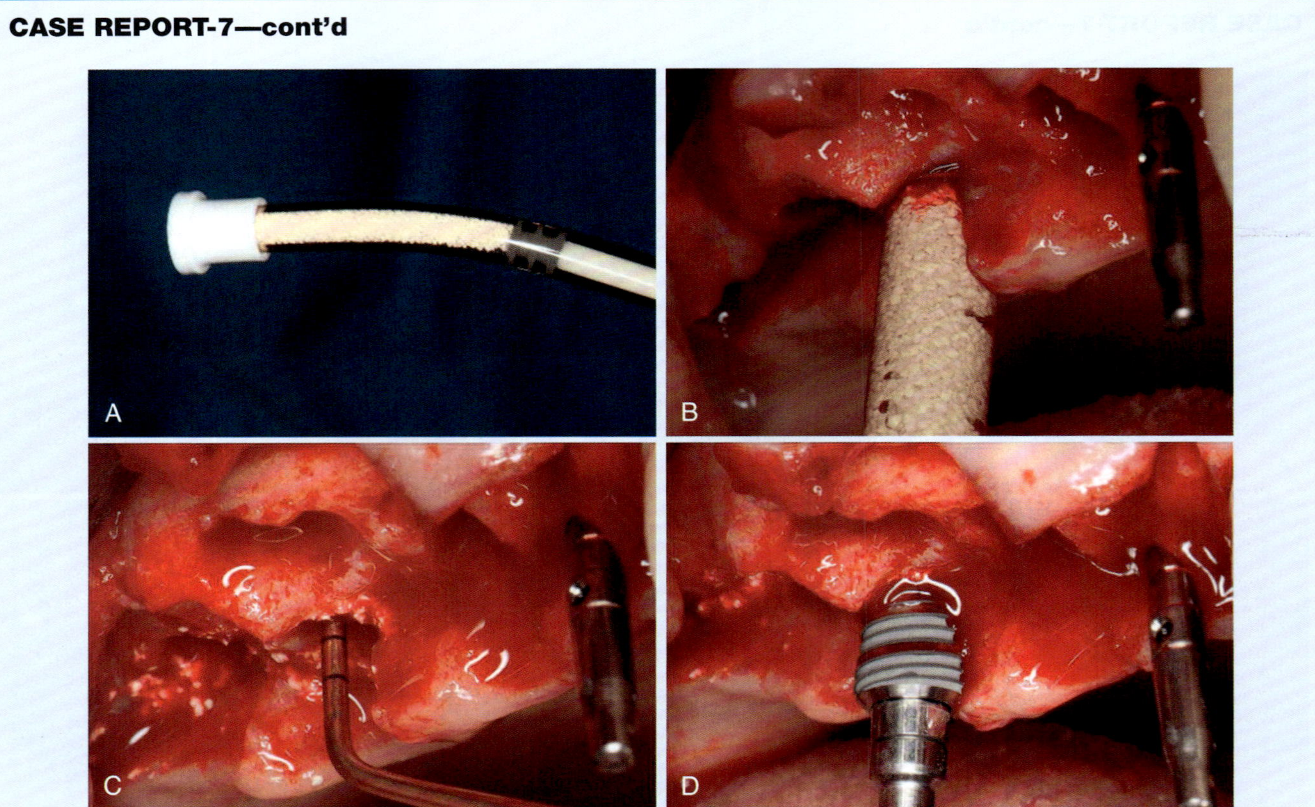

Fig 18.81 (A and B) Osteon graft is filled into the lifted sinus cavity. (C) Osteon graft can be packed into the elevated sinus floor space using the sinus elevator. (D) SuperLine Dentium implant is inserted.

CASE REPORT-7—cont'd

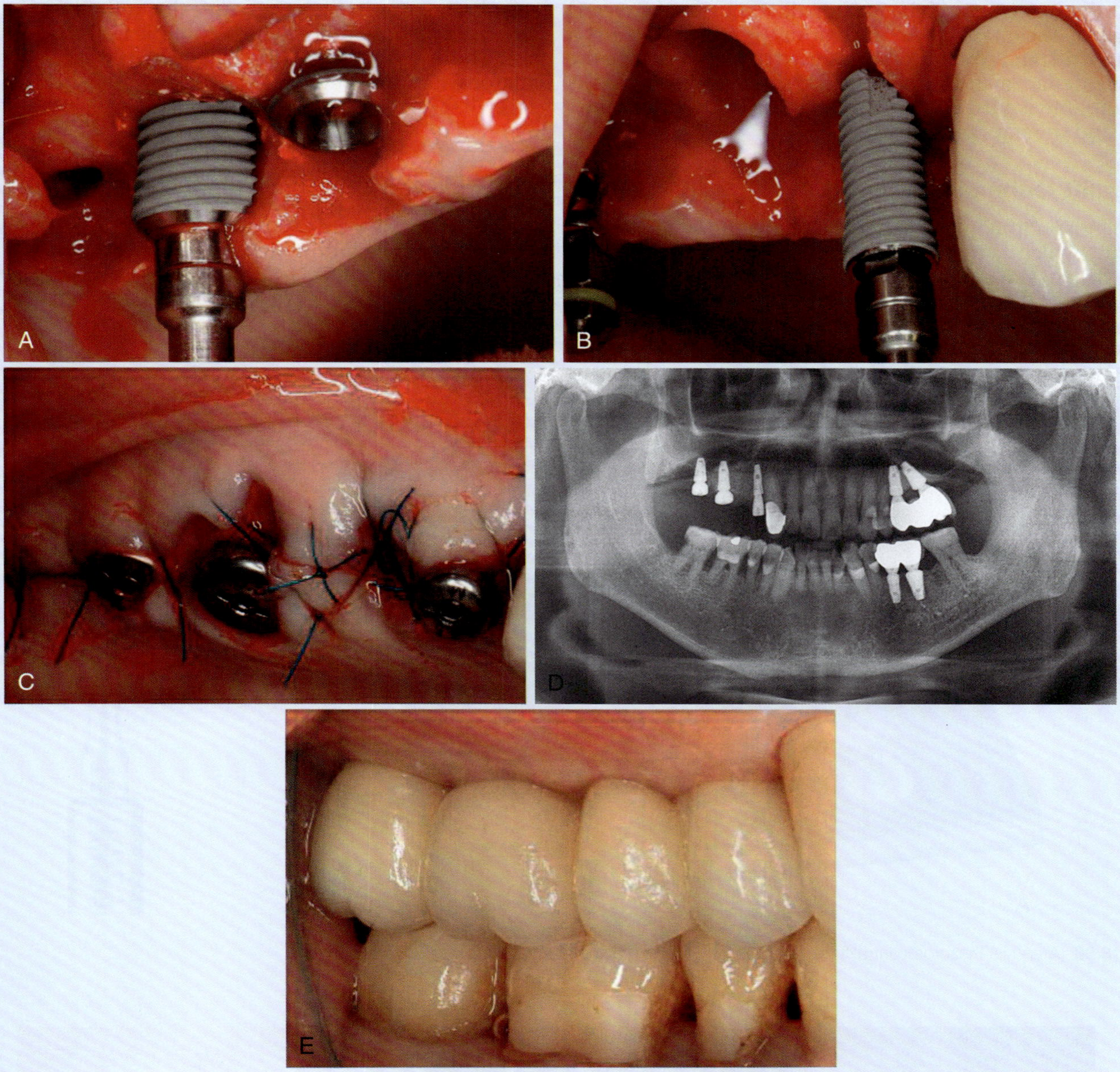

Fig 18.82 (A and B) Two more implants are inserted for teeth numbers 15 and 17. (C) The inserted implants achieved adequate initial stability so healing abutments were inserted and the flap sutured for nonsubmerged implant healing. (D) Post-sinus-lifting and implant insertion radiograph. (E) Implants are restored after 4 months.

Hydraulic sinus-lift technique

This technique was invented by Chen in 2005. The sinus membrane is lifted by controlled water pressure in this technique. A crestal incision is made, exposing the crestal ridge of the maxilla. An osteotomy is initiated with a sinus drill, and water pressure is used to gently elevate the schneiderian membrane from the sinus floor. The sinus membrane is further elevated by filling in the graft material and the implant is inserted.

Intralift technique

The most popular hydraulic sinus lift is the intralift technique, which is performed using the piezotome intralift kit (Setlec, France). This kit contains various bone grinding diamond tips which are sequentially used to grind up the subantral bone to reach the sinus membrane without tearing it. The kit also contains a special tip, which is then used to deliver a controlled jet of saline to lift up the sinus membrane (Fig 18.83A and B). It is specially designed for minimally invasive and safe sinus lifting by the crestal approach. Several diamond-coated tips of increasing diameters (from 1.35 to 2.80 mm) are designed to drill and gradually widen the access canal to the schneiderian membrane. The sterile spray cools down the tips to avoid any rise in temperature, which could lead to tissue damage. The membrane elevation is achieved by means of microcavitation using the TKW5 tip.

Advantages of the intralift technique

1. Minimally invasive technique
2. Safe and fast technique
3. Selective cut – cuts only bone without any injury to soft tissues including sinus membrane
4. Haemostatic effect – minimum bleeding during the surgery
5. Fast healing
6. Minimal failure risk.

Diagrammatic presentation of intralift operatory protocol is shown in Figs 18.84–18.87.

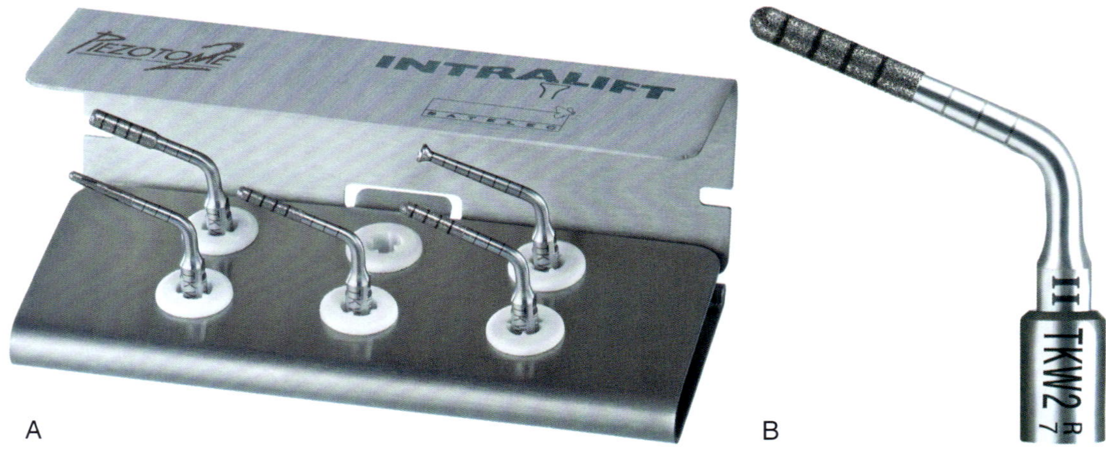

Fig 18.83 (A and B) Piezotome intralift kit from Setlec containing different intralift tips.

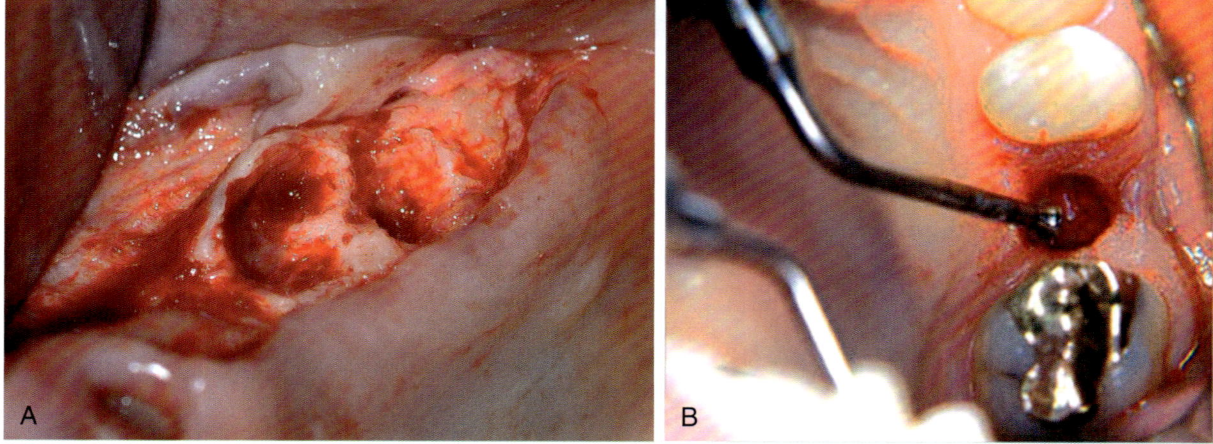

Fig 18.84 (A) Ridge crest can be approached with flap technique or (B) with soft tissue punch technique.

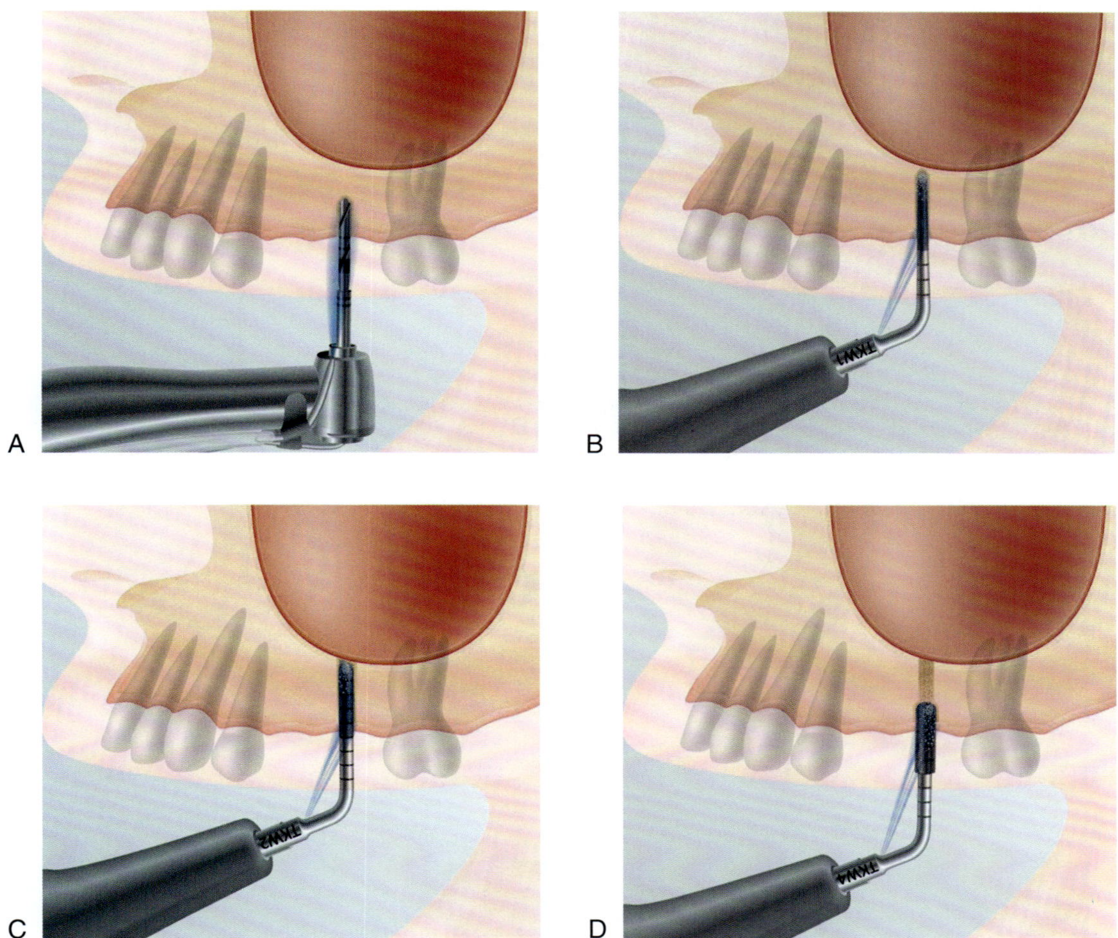

Fig 18.85 (A); If the subantral bone height is more than 3 mm and high in density, drilling should be started with a 2 mm pilot drill of any implant system to reach 2 mm short of sinus floor if subantral bone is less than 3 mm or low in density, drilling should be done with (B) TKW1 (1.35 mm) tip to reach 2 mm short of the sinus floor. (C) TKW2 (2.1 mm) tip is used to further widen the osteotomy and grind the sinus floor to reach the membrane. These tips do not cut or damage the soft tissue including the sinus membrane, unless if they are forcefully pushed up to tear the membrane. (D) A TKW4 (2.8 mm) tip is then used to widen the crestal half of the osteotomy.

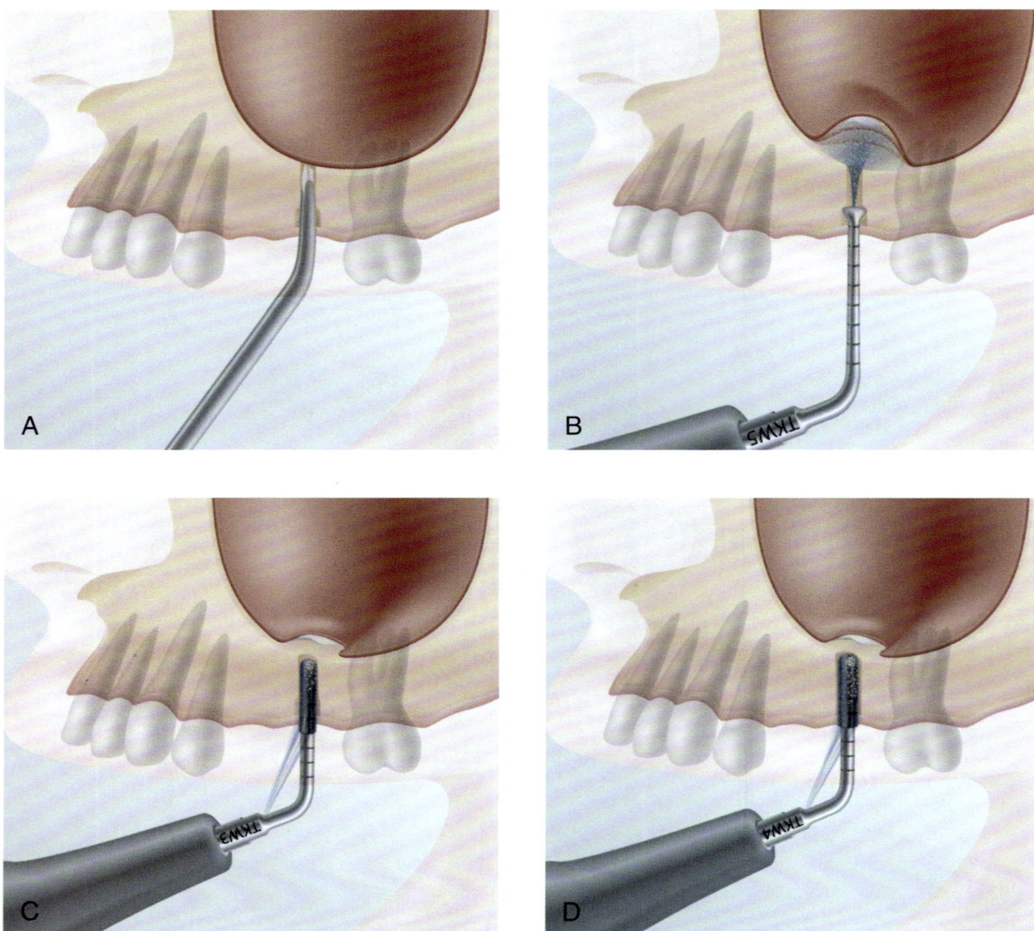

Fig 18.86 (A) A resorbable collagen membrane or plug (Collaplug, Zimmer Dental) is inserted through the osteotomy to prevent sinus membrane rupture during its hydraulic lift. (B) A TKW5 (2.8 mm) tip is inserted into the prepared osteotomy limited to the crestal half, which then delivers a jet of sterile saline to elevate the sinus membrane. A TKW5 (2.8 mm) tip is a noncutting tip that delivers sterile irrigation spray right up to the end, used for Schneiderian membrane elevation by means of microcavitation. The membrane elevation is achieved gradually, by using a series of successively increasing rates of irrigation flow. (C and D) Once the sinus membrane has been detached and elevated from the sinus floor, the osteotomy is further widened using TKW3 (2.35 mm) and TKW4 (2.8 mm) tips. This osteotomy is wide enough to insert a regular diameter (3.5–4 mm) implant but if the insertion of a wider diameter implant is planned, the osteotomy can be further widened at this stage, using the widening drills of the particular implant system.

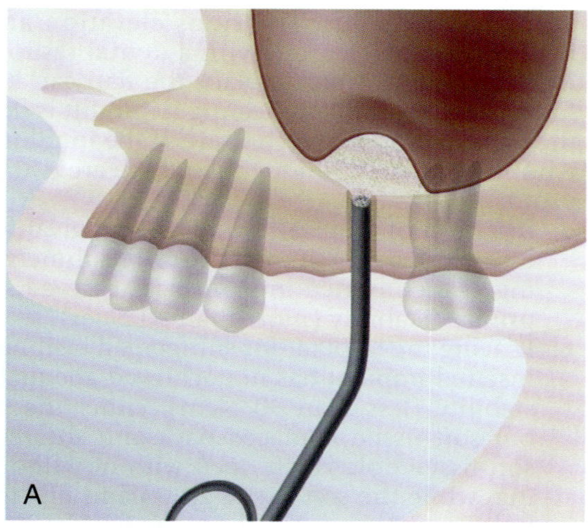

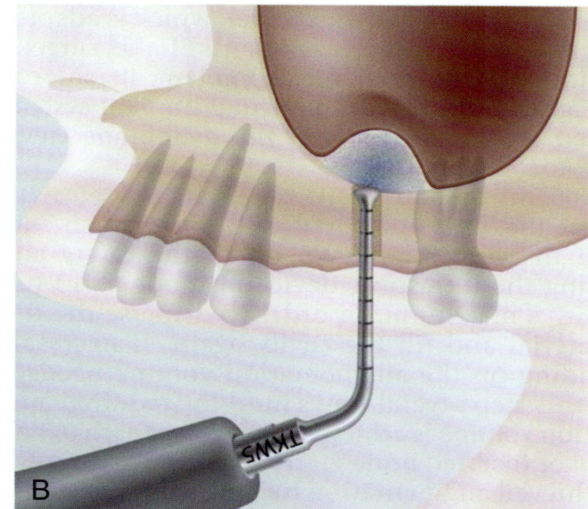

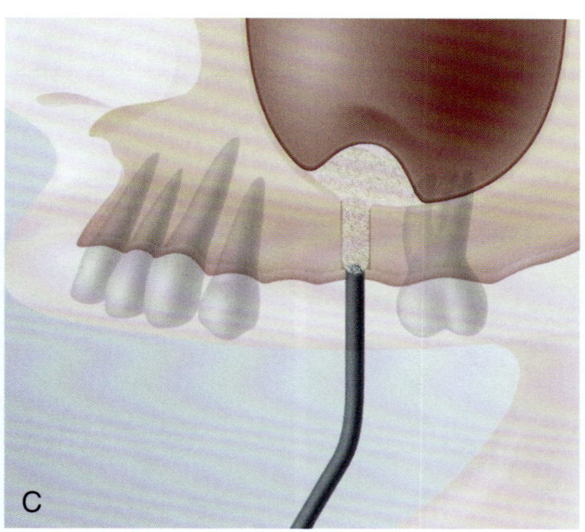

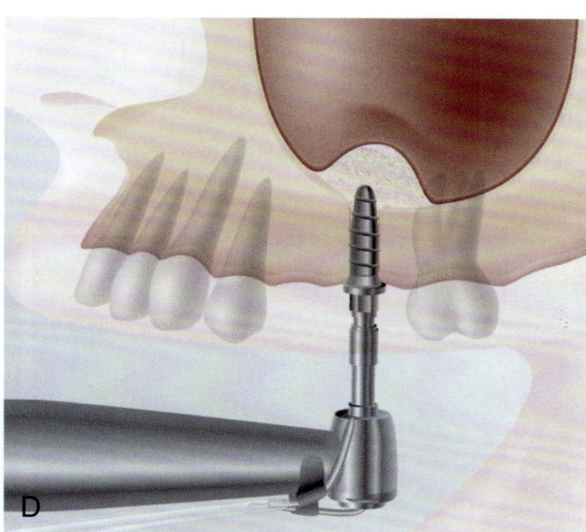

Fig 18.87 (A) The particulated graft is introduced through the osteotomy using graft carrier and (B) a TKW5 tip is used to disperse the graft into the elevated sinus floor. (C) Then the graft can be further added and (D) implant is inserted.

Key points

1. Each intralift tip is used at a particular recommended mode and saline irrigation rate of the piezosurgery machine (Table 18.1).
2. The TKW5 should be used at mode 2 or 3. Start the elevation procedure with a 40 ml/min saline flow rate and increase the flow slowly to 50–60 ml/min. Stay for maximum of 5 s at each stage.
3. When elevating the membrane with saline irrigation using the TKW5 tip, a blunt periodontal probe can be used to evaluate the height of membrane elevation after each flow step. The dentist can also verify its resiliency (elasticity) by gently tambourine the membrane with the blunt probe.
4. A collagen sponge shaped by hand, can be inserted in the cavity as a safeguard and a precautionary measure against rupture of the sinus membrane. The collagen sponge is used as a buffer before osseous filling of the elevated sinus floor. In contact with blood, the collagen sponge swells and immediately adapts to the membrane.

Table 18.1 The running mode and irrigation rate of saline at the time of using various intralift tips

INSERT TIPS	MODE	IRRIGATION RATE (ml/min)
TKW1	1	80
TKW2	1	80
TKW3	1	80
TKW4	1	80
TKW5	2 or 3	40 for 5 s 50 for 5 s 60 for 5 s
TKW5 for compacting filling material in elevated sinus	4	40 max. for 3–7 s

5. The cavity diameter drilled is 3 mm, which is adapted to a 3.5–4 mm diameter implant. If the surgeon needs to use a bigger diameter implant, he/she can use a bigger rotary drill of particular implant system, to widen the osteotomy after the membrane elevation protocol.
6. Place 0.5 ml of bone graft material in the cavity. Then use the 'plug and spray' technique which consists of inserting the TKW5 tip in the cavity and activating the ultrasonic device in mode 4, 10 ml/min, 3–7 s maximum, in order to disperse the filling material and fill the cavity again. If necessary (depending on the augmentation volume needed) repeat this step several times until the required augmentation volume is achieved. On average each 0.5 ml portion of inserted bone graft results in minimum 2 mm achieved augmentation height. The dentist may then measure with a probe to evaluate that how far the augmentation material has been inserted into the maxillary sinus. The sinus elevation and grafting can also be checked with a dental radiograph.
7. After insertion of the implant the flap can be closed for submerged implant healing if intralift is done with the incision and flap technique. If the intralift is done with the punch technique then there are two possible protocols:
   a. Insertion of gingival former – a gingival former is inserted over the implant for nonsubmerged healing, if the inserted implant has achieved adequate primary stability (more than 30 Ncm).
   b. Leaving the implant for submerged healing – if the inserted implant has not achieved adequate initial stability (less than 30 Ncm), either the punched out soft tissue is placed back and sutured or the soft tissue hole is left open with or without suturing, while the soft tissue grows and fills the small hole in 2–3 days. Till then, the patient is asked to keep it clean using a very soft brush.

CASE REPORT-8

Sinus elevation using intralift and implant placement (Figs 18.88–18.95).

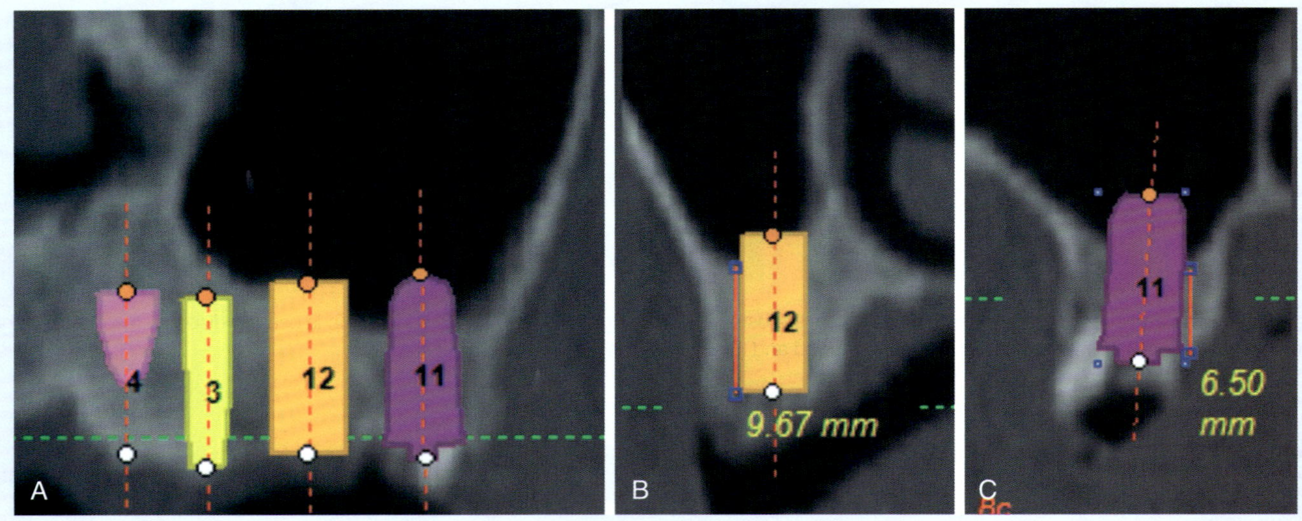

Fig 18.88 The intralift procedure was planned for 2 posterior implants (anterior implant 5 × 12 mm, posterior implant 6 × 12 mm). The dental CT image shows 9.67 mm subantral bone height at the first implant site and 6.5 mm at the second implant site. (A–C) Posterior implant site also shows the presence of root stumps, which need to be extracted at the time of sinus lift and implant placement.

CASE REPORT-8—cont'd

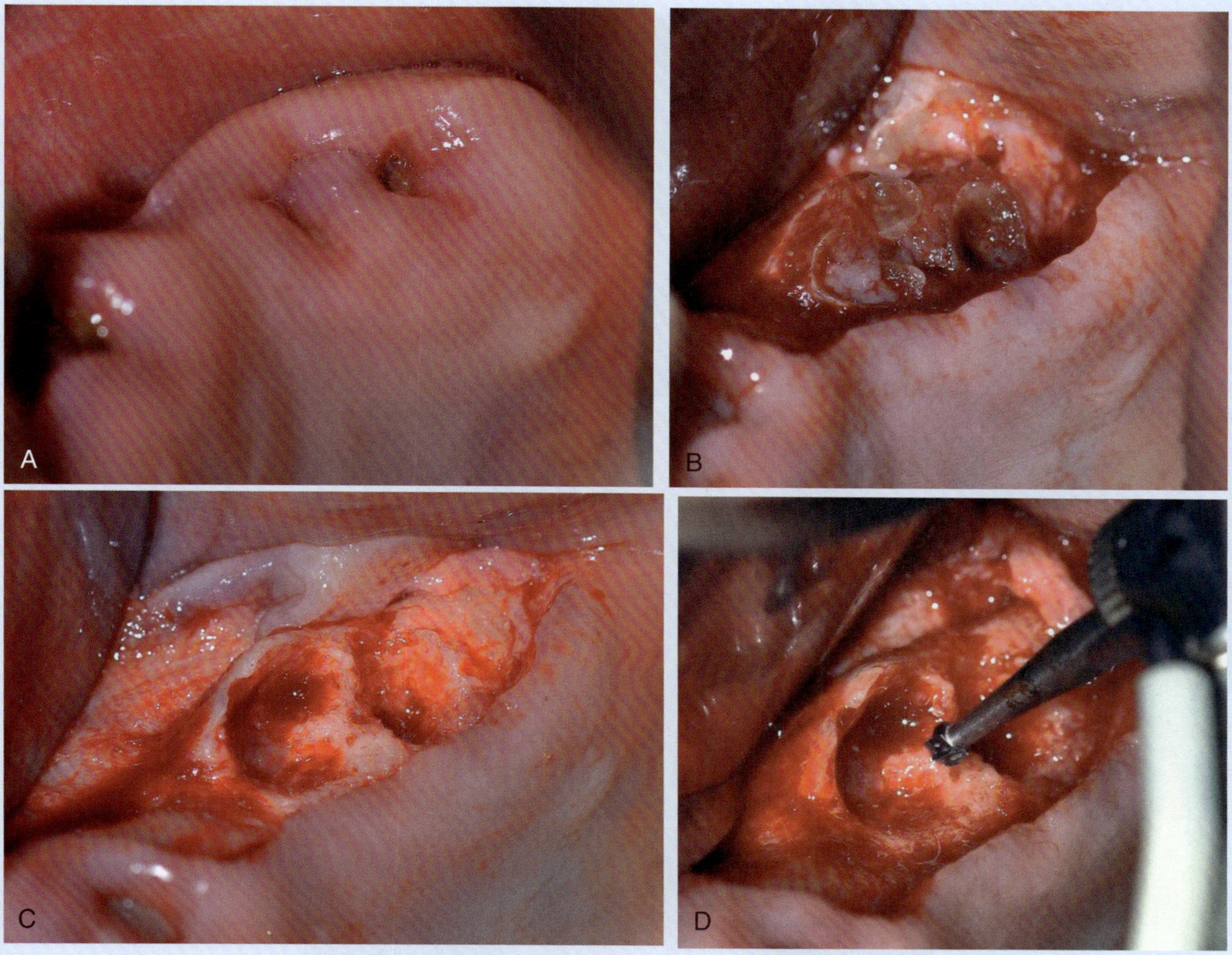

Fig 18.89 (A) Clinical view of the ridge before surgery. (B) Flap is elevated to expose the ridge crest and root stumps. (C) The root stumps are extracted, all the granulation tissue is curetted out and the socket is irrigated with parenteral form of clindamycin to kill residual pathogens before the start of drilling in the bone. (D) A small round carbide bur is used to mark the implant osteotomy sites just by punching through cortex.

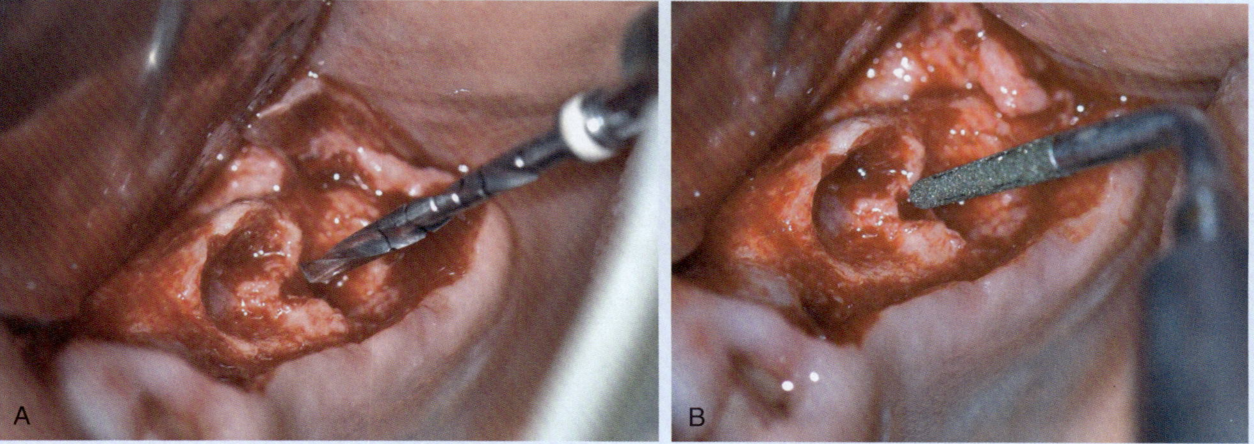

Fig 18.90 (A) The pilot drill is used to prepare the osteotomy sites 3–4 mm short of sinus floor. (B) The TKW1 tip is then used to prepare the osteotomy site to reach 2 mm short of the sinus membrane.

Continued

CASE REPORT-8—cont'd

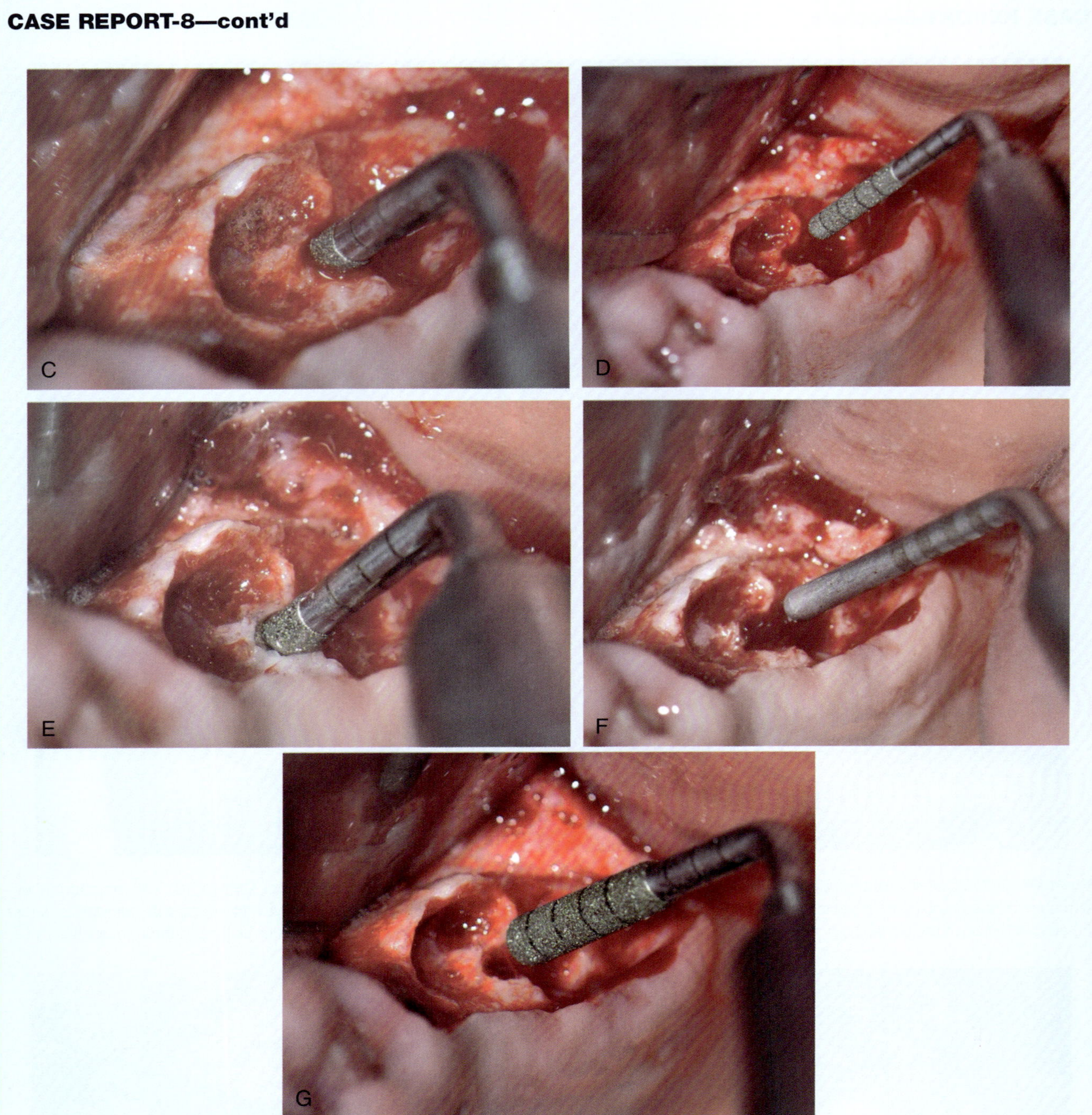

Fig 18.90, cont'd (C) The TKW1 tip can be seen going deep to reach close to the sinus membrane. (D and E) The TKW2 tip is used to widen the osteotomy sites and to grind the sinus floor to reach the schneiderian membrane. (F) Once the TKW2 tip reaches the membrane, the soft consistency of the membrane and its timbering effect can be carefully felt, either with the same tip or using a blunt probe. This can also be further checked with the dental radiograph. (G) The TKW4 tip is used then to widen the osteotomy to a depth of only 3–4 mm.

CASE REPORT-8—cont'd

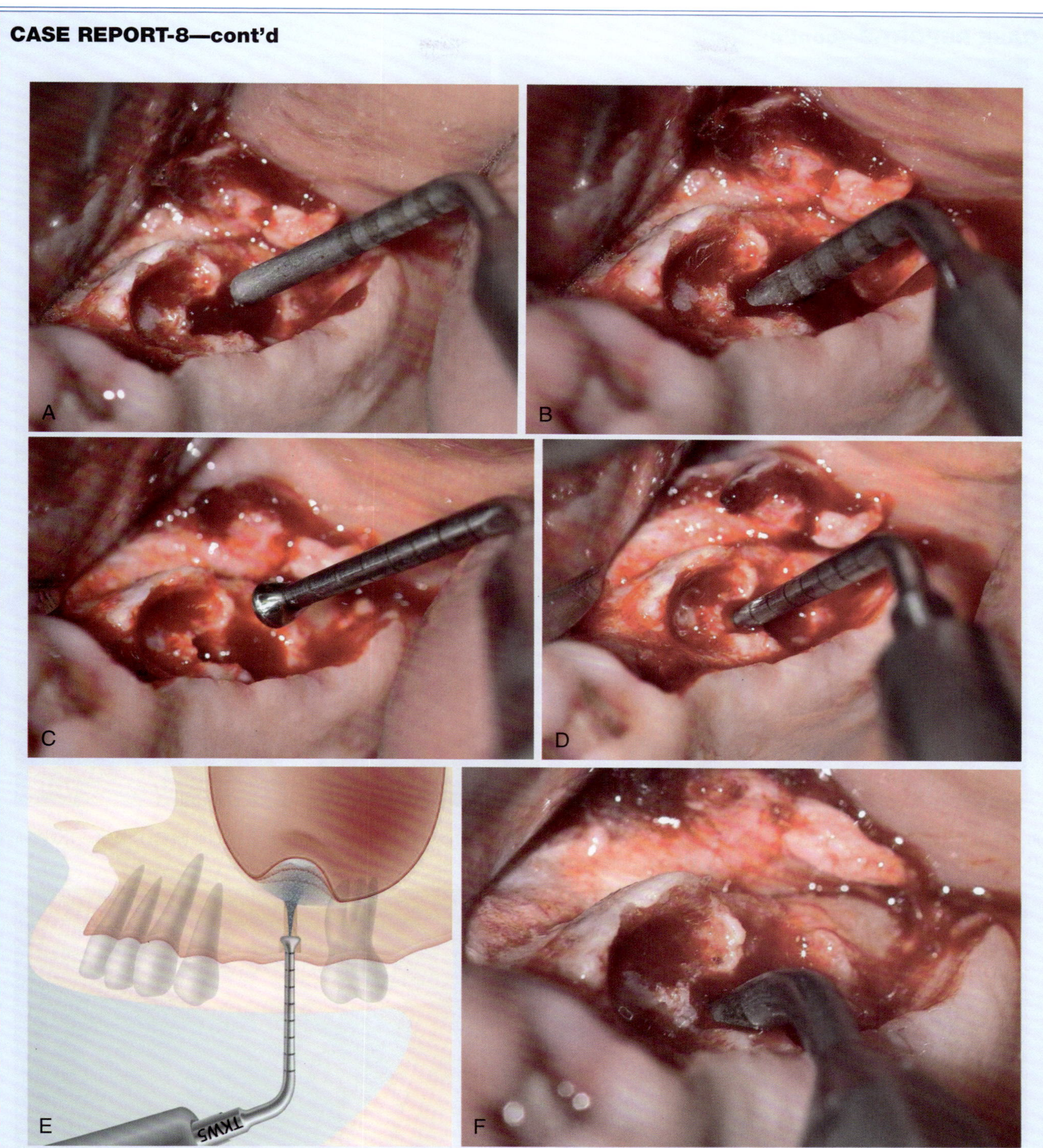

Fig 18.91 (A and B) Insertion of blunt probe before membrane elevation shows only 7 mm of bone depth. The TKW 5 tip that delivers sterile irrigation spray right up to the end, is inserted in the osteotomy, limited to the depth prepared with the TKW4 tip, and used for Schneiderian membrane elevation by means of microcavitation. (C–E) The membrane elevation is achieved gradually by a successive increase of irrigation flow rate (mode 2 or 3 with saline flow 40 ml/min for 5 s, 50 ml/min for the next 5 s and if required 60 ml/min for next 5 s). The blunt depth probe is again inserted to check the height of membrane elevation, which can be seen now as 16 mm (F). This indicates that 9 mm of membrane elevation has been achieved.

Continued

CASE REPORT-8—cont'd

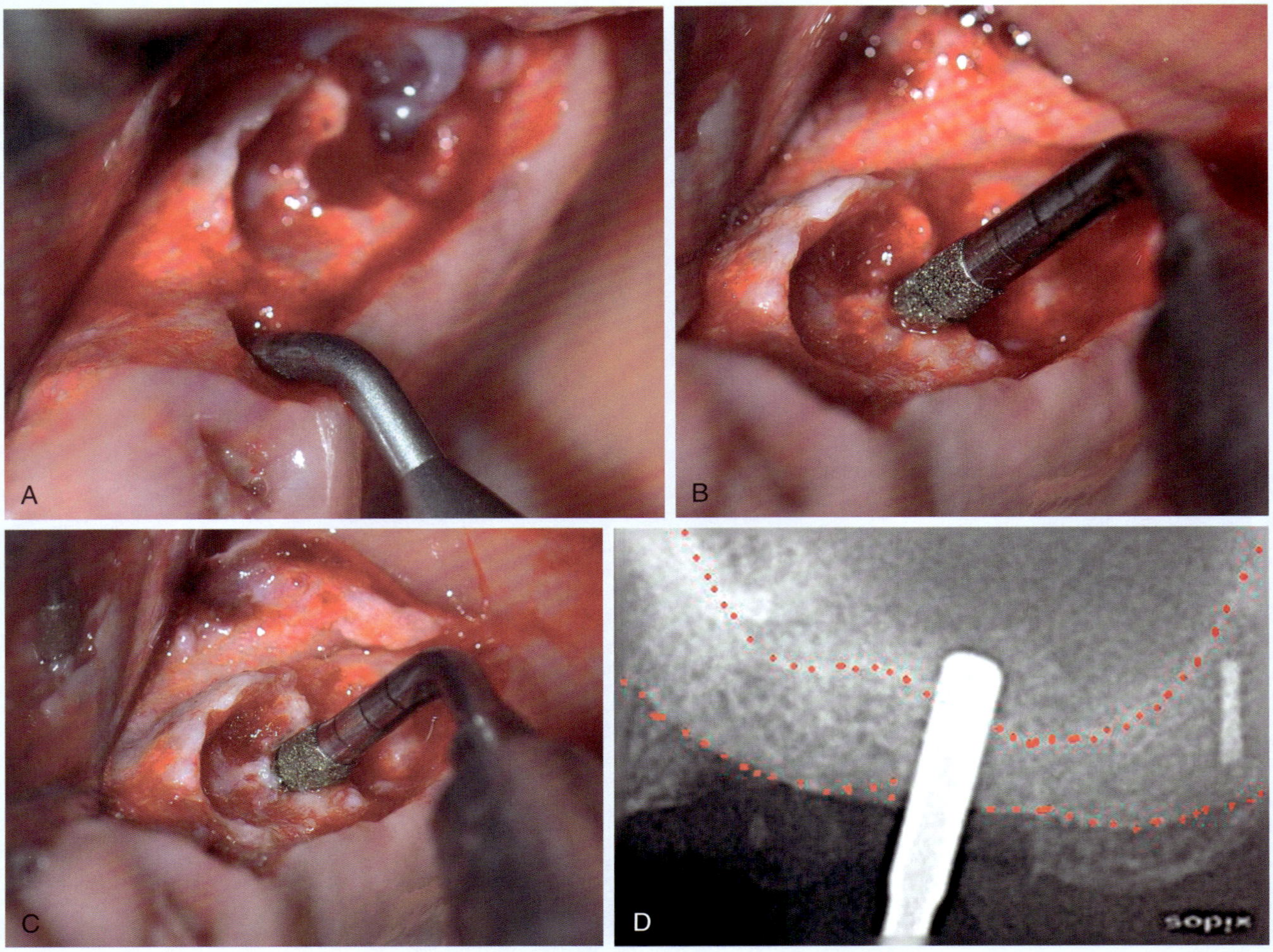

Fig 18.92 (A) A similar procedure is performed for the anterior site, which also shows achievement of 16 mm height. (B–D) Now the TKW3 and TKW4 tips are used to widen the osteotomy to the complete depth.

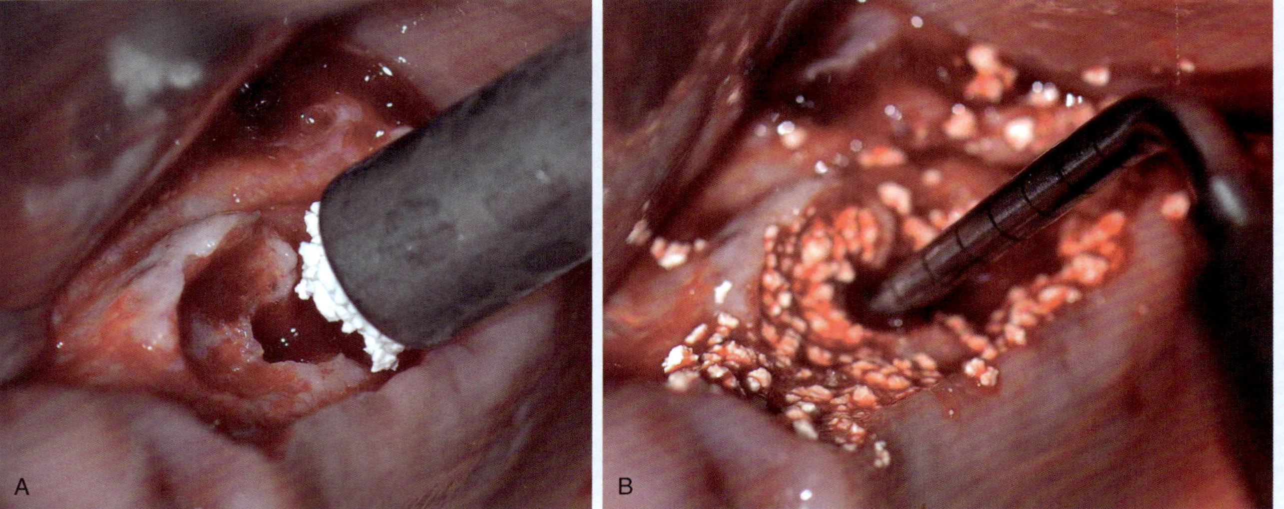

Fig 18.93 (A and B) The small particle-sized (0.4–0.9 mm) synthetic hydroxyapatite graft material mixed with clindamycin antibiotic is introduced through the osteotomy, using graft carrier and the TKW5 tip to disperse the graft into the elevated sinus floor and it is compacted as the top layer underneath the elevated sinus membrane.

CASE REPORT-8—cont'd

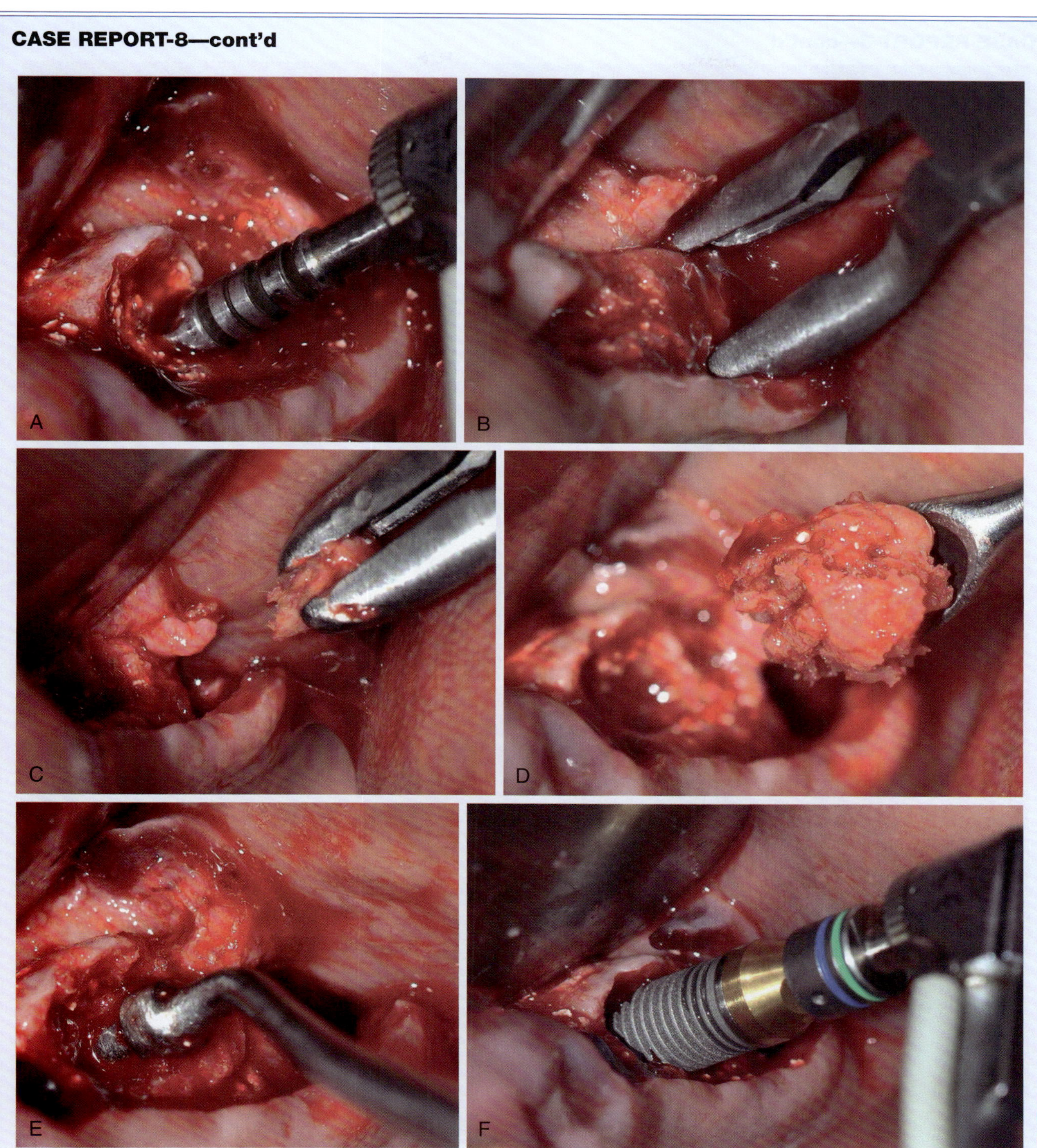

Fig 18.94 (A) The osteotomy sites are further widened using the rest of the osteotomy widening drills of the BioHorizons implant system without or with minimum saline flow. (B and C) The autogenous bone is harvested from the maxillary tuberosity using the bone rongeur and (D and E) it is used to fill rest of the elevated sinus floor space. (F) The 5 × 12 mm and 6 × 12 mm Maestro implants are inserted into their respective osteotomies.

Continued

CASE REPORT-8—cont'd

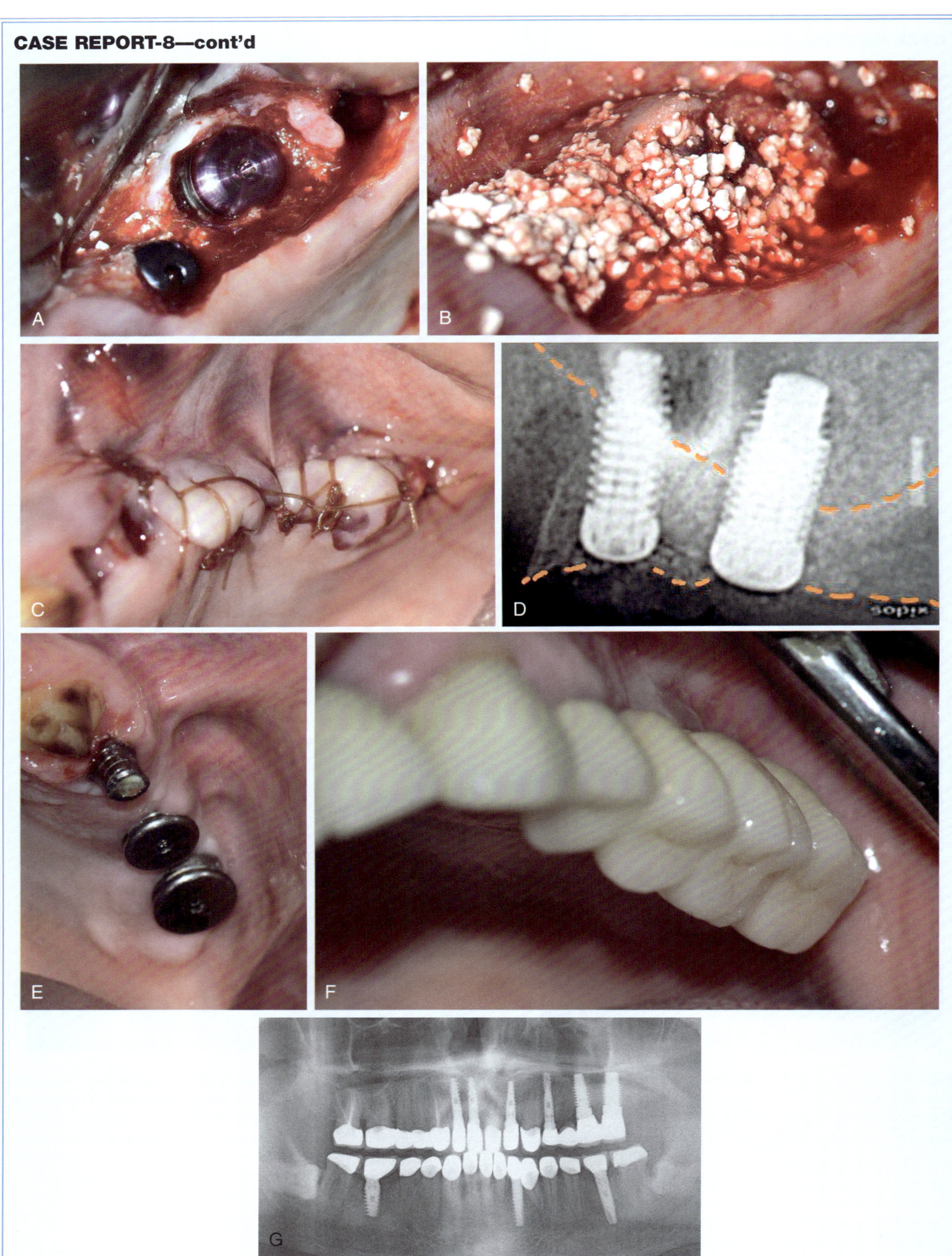

CASE REPORT-8—cont'd

Fig 18.95 The primary stability of more than 35 Ncm is achieved for both the implants. (A and B) As the posterior implant was placed in a fresh extraction socket, the synthetic HA graft was used to fill the small peri-implant spaces. (C) The periosteum is released and the flap sutured back with primary closure. (D) Postimplantation radiograph shows a noticeable amount of sinus elevation and grafting. (E and F) Implants are uncovered and restored after 4 months. Other implants were also inserted. (G) The panoramic radiograph 1 year after implant restoration shows consolidated grafted bone in the sinus and stable bone around the implants.

CASE REPORT-9

Sinus elevation grafting using intralift kit and delayed implant insertion (Fig 18.96A–D).

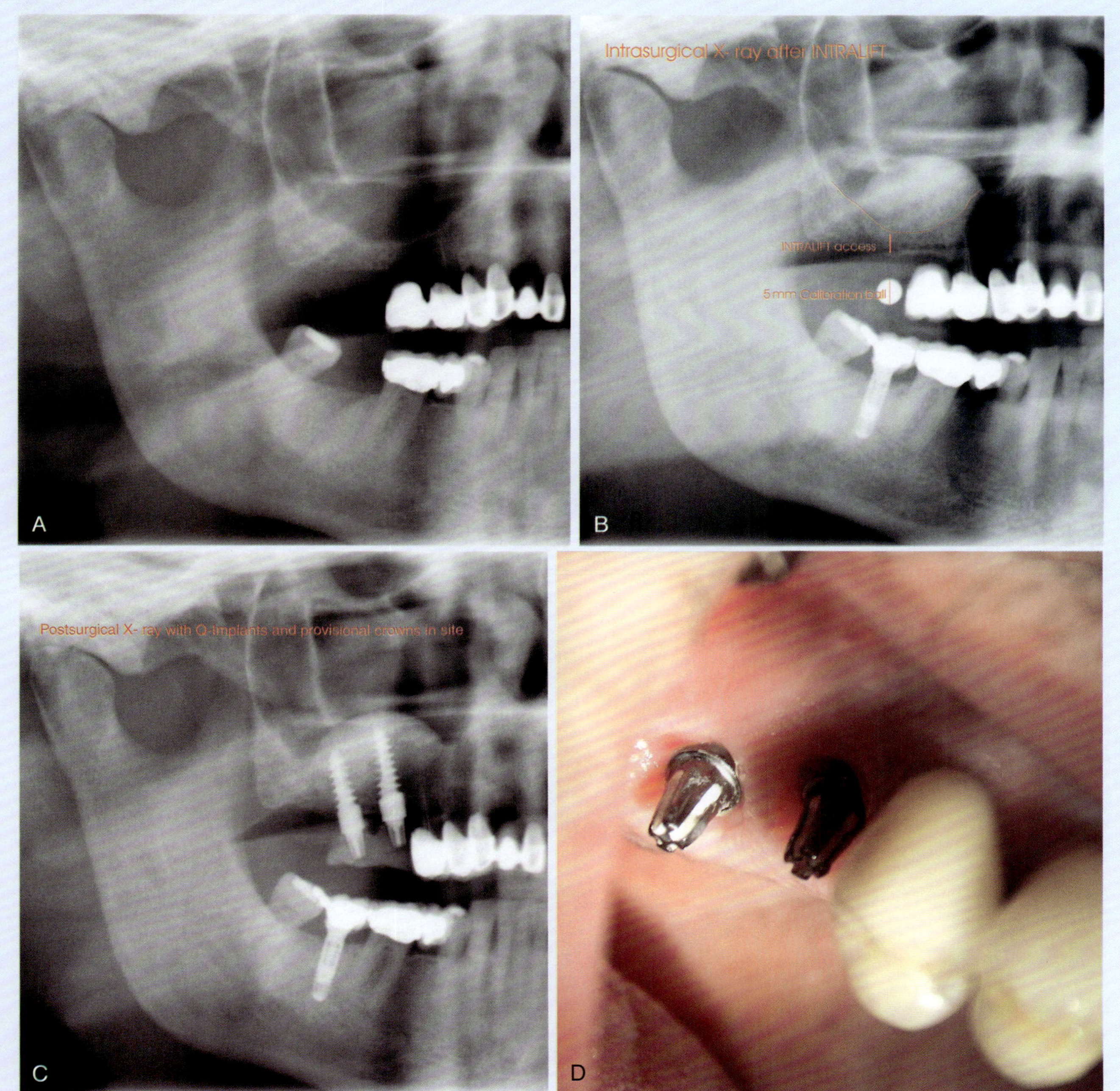

Fig 18.96 (A) Preoperative radiograph shows only 3 mm subantral bone height. (B) Postintralift radiograph shows a large degree of sinus lifting and grafting (approx. 16 mm). (C and D) Implants are inserted after the graft maturation period of 6 months.

CASE REPORT-10

Bilateral sinus elevation and grafting using intralift kit and delayed implant placement to support a full-arch fixed prosthesis (Figs 18.97–18.101).

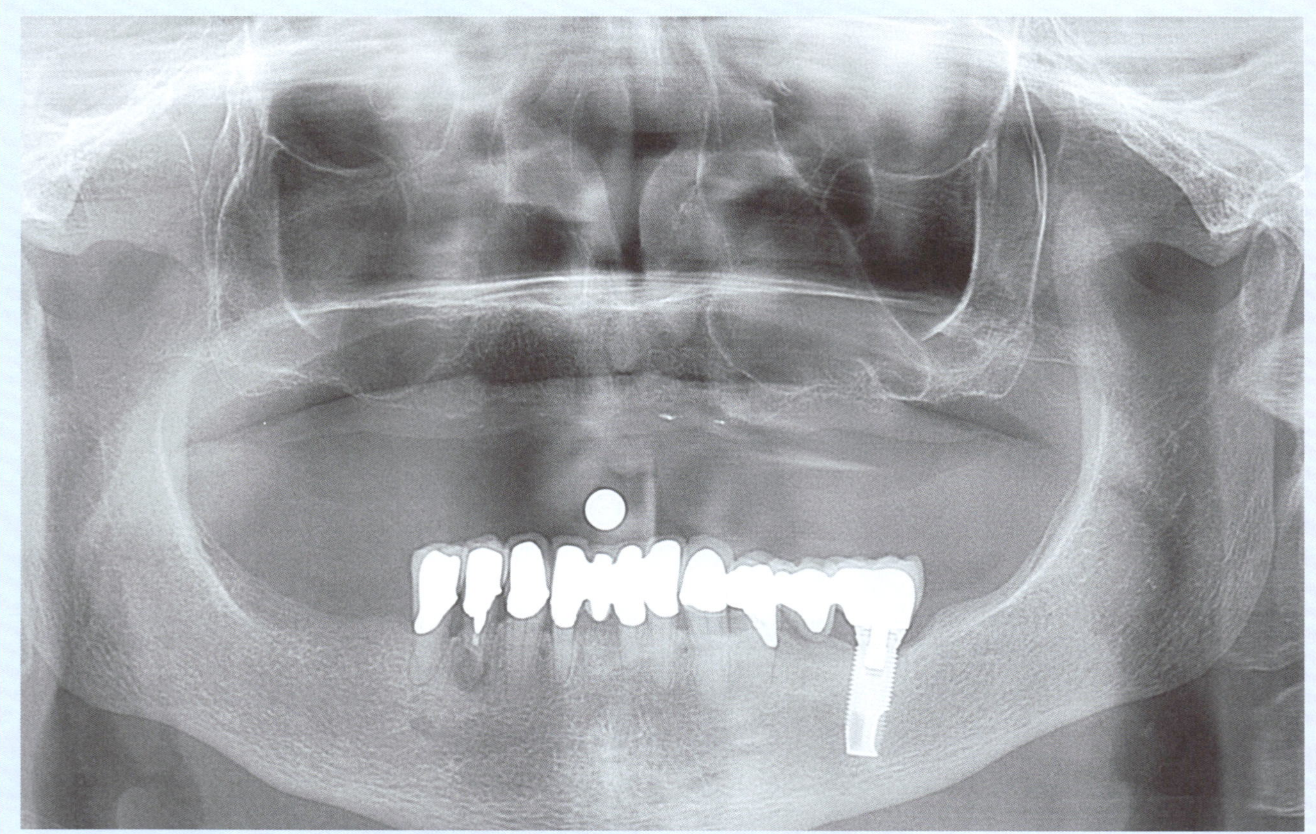

Fig 18.97 Preoperative radiograph shows the bilateral presence of very little subantral bone.

CASE REPORT-10—cont'd

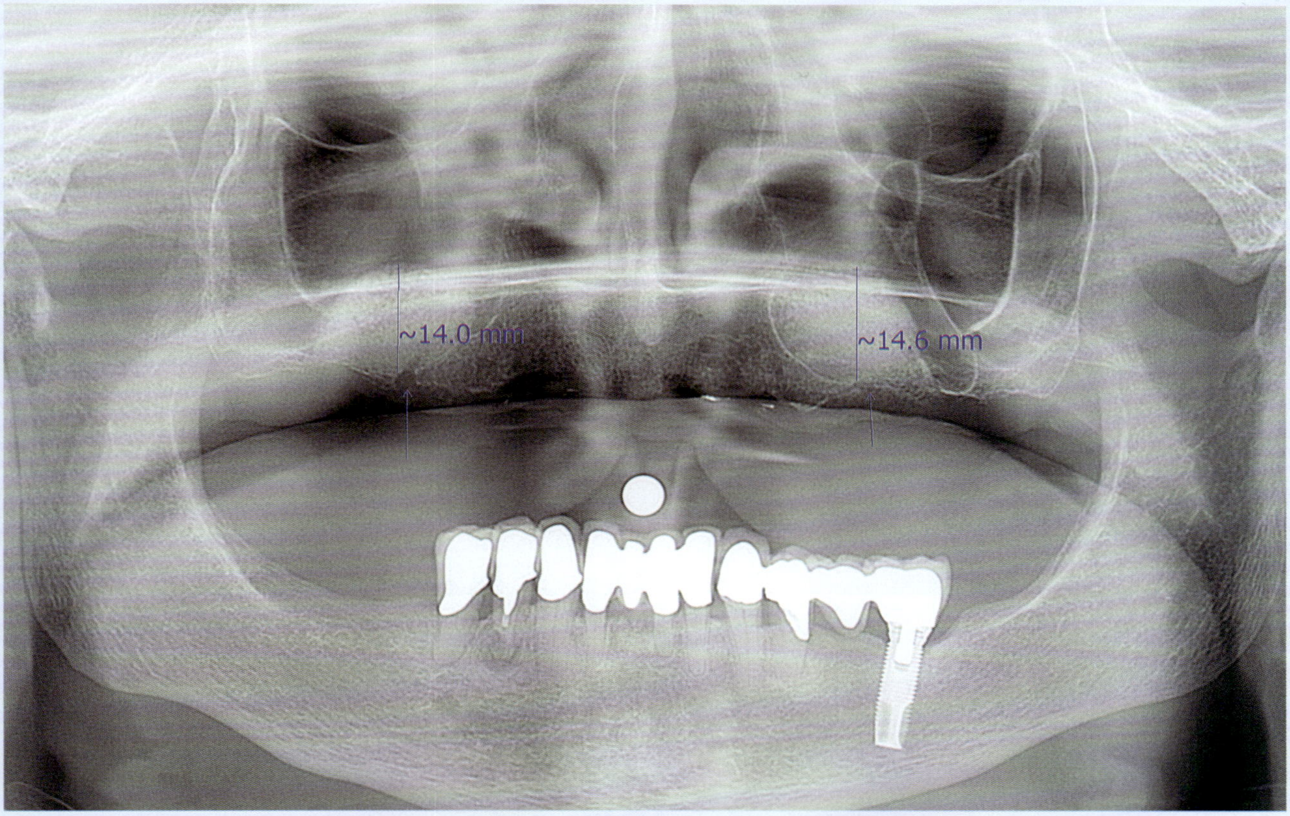

Fig 18.98 Postintralift radiograph shows that a large degree of bilateral sinus elevation and grafting has been achieved.

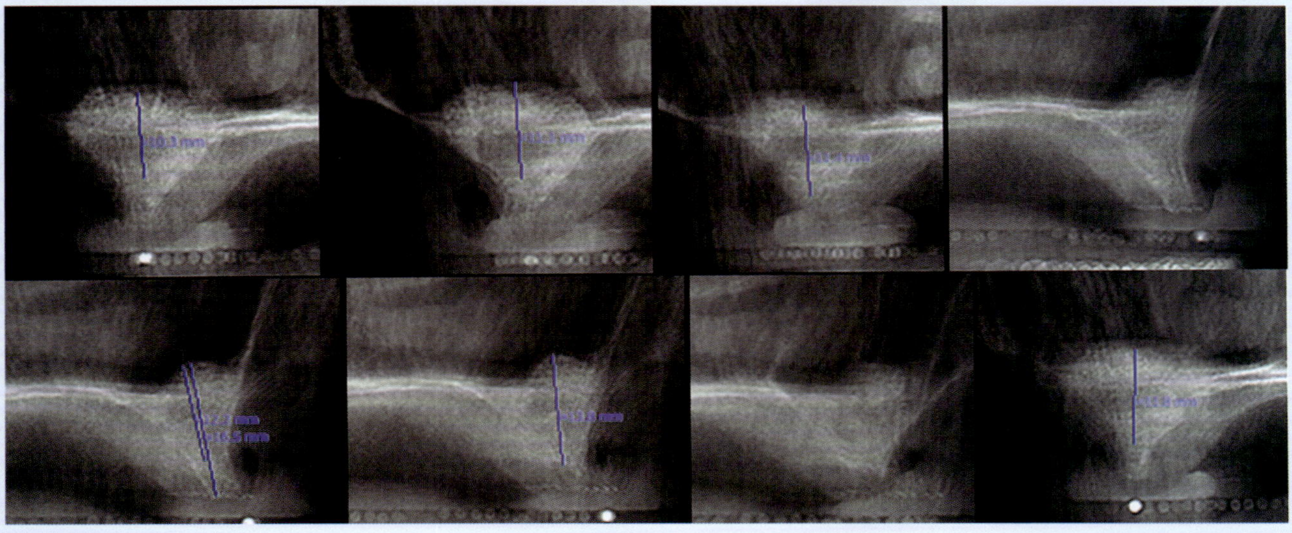

Fig 18.99 Postintralift dental CT cross-sectional scans show three-dimensional sinus membrane elevation and grafted sinus floor.

Continued

CASE REPORT-10—cont'd

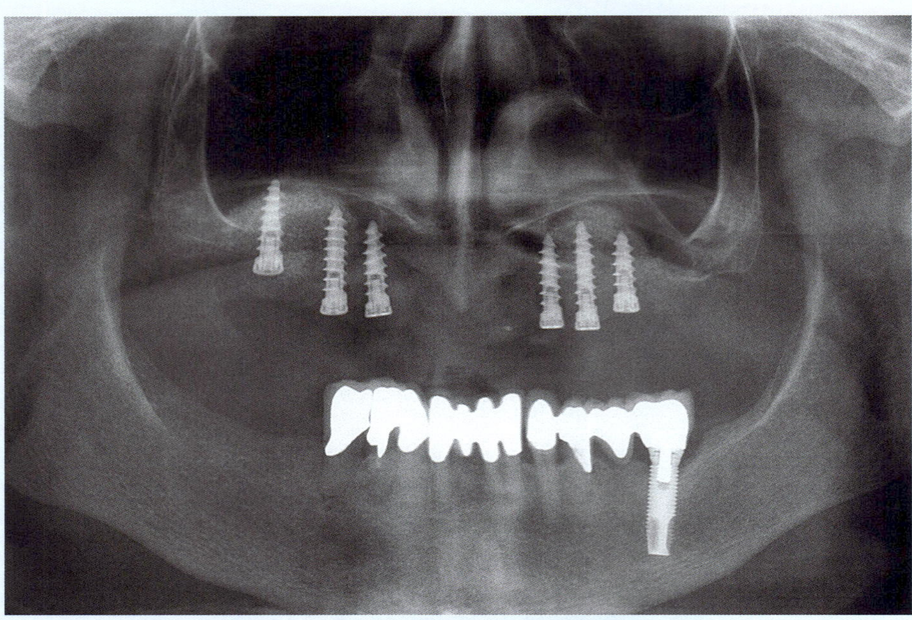

Fig 18.100 Implants are inserted after graft maturation period of 6 months.

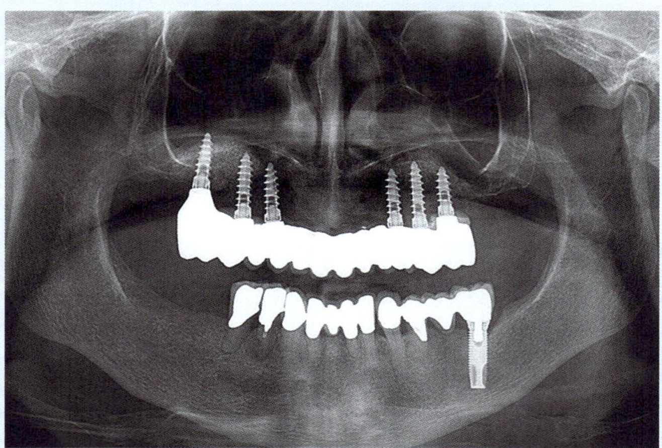

Fig 18.101 Implants are restored after healing period of 4 months to support a full-arch fixed prosthesis.

Frequently asked questions about the intralift technique

Why is the intralift technique the safest technique?

The sinus membrane tolerates high pressure loadings when pressure is evenly distributed on the entire membrane but the membrane is very sensitive to tearing forces. Conventional open or internal sinus-lift procedures always exert high tearing forces on the membrane, resulting in punctures or rips. Since the intralift is a non contact procedure exerting only pressure forces on the sinus membrane by ultrasonic activated fluid so that the danger of ripping the membrane is minimized.

Although a blind technique, is intralift sufficiently predictable?

The augmentation process takes place through the initial trepanation creating an almost perfect 'dome' in the axis of the trepanation. Each 0.5 ml portion of inserted bone graft results in a minimum of 2 mm achieved augmentation height, the bone graft perfectly surrounding the implant.

How can I know that the elevation is correctly performed?

Use a periodontal probe to measure how far the bone material has been inserted into the maxillary sinus and compare with a preoperative radiograph.

Are there any risks of membrane rupture? If so, how should the procedure be continued?

In case the membrane is punctured initially with the pilot drill or TKW1 (check with 'nose blow' test), a small piece of collagenous sponge should be placed into the trepanation before proceeding with the hydrodynamic ultrasonic detachment of the membrane (using the 'TKW5' tip). Since no tearing forces are exerted on the membrane, the puncture will not widen or rip. Insertion of the bone graft has then to be performed very gently, and a control radiograph is mandatory prior to insertion of the implant. Heavy rips of the membrane can only occur when using TKW5 tip in mode 1 (maximum power) and fluid flow superior to 40 ml/min.

How long does the irrigation (saline solution) stay in the sinus floor after the membrane is lifted using TKW5? How does the membrane behave once the irrigation solution is evacuated?

Most of the water will automatically come out of the preparation socket and the rest will be 'pressed out' while filling in the osteotomy with augmentation material. The saline has no (negative) effect, so the question and doubts over small saline volumes that may be residual in the sinus is superfluous. Once the water has been evacuated, the membrane comes back naturally to its original position. Once the membrane is detached, it will adapt to the quantity of inserted bone graft.

What would you do to protect the membrane from perforation if a bigger implant body (e.g. 4.5 mm) is used along with drills of a particular implant system after the use of TKW4 tip (2.8 mm)?

Before placing an implant the **intralift** should be successfully done. After augmentation the preparation of the implant site is possible. Drilling can be performed without any irrigation and at only 200 rpm. If the membrane is elevated successfully and enough material is placed prior to the insertion of the implant, a collagenous sponge can again be placed into the socket for a buffer effect. If an implant with a round shape is used, it will (after successful membrane elevation is completed) hold the membrane like a tent. In the author's experience, it is almost impossible to perforate the membrane after the sinus mucosa has been elevated successfully (even though no augmentation material is placed). To achieve a higher primary stability when the bone height is reduced, it is recommended that the implant preparation is under dimensional (stopped one bur before the last preparation bur).

What should be done if there is a large bone augmentation to perform?

Large augmentations can be performed through the 3 mm trepanation with the 'plug and spray' technique. The bone graft will get evenly dispersed under the membrane. Alternatively, additional trepanations can be drilled after primary augmentation with a minimum 1.5 ml graft, and additional grafts can be placed through these additional trepanations.

What are the risks for the patient?

Beside the general risks of augmentative surgery/external and internal sinus lift, there are no specific risks in the intralift technique.

Is it true that a quicker bone reformation is observed?

Since the intralift (when applied by the gingival punch) is a minimally invasive procedure, it is not traumatic for the human body. Leaving the periosteum fully intact, it was observed that the healing process started when surgery was finished and took about 1 month.

Is it true that it is a very slow technique?

The detachment of the membrane takes a maximum of 12 × 5 s. The most time-consuming part in the entire procedure is the filling with bone graft through the 3 mm trepanation. Depending on the bone graft type used, the filling time varies. Application of jelly-like or spongeous bone grafts may help to speed up the process. After few cases, the practitioner will be able to gain a lot of time (about 30–40%). A quick learning curve does exist for the usage of ultrasonics in bone surgery applications. According to Dr Wainwright, an internal sinus lift with intralift will take about 20 min for the whole procedure.

In the case of an implant superior to 4 mm, should the trepanation be enlarged before or after the bone filling procedure?

The preparation of the implant site should be performed after bone filling/intralift augmentation, because after 'bone height' is increased and the space is filled with augmentation material, a violation of the membrane is not possible. After preparation with the drills (with no irrigation and slowly) the material that might be excavated again during drilling procedure is collected and re-plugged again.

How should the enlargement of the trepanation hole be performed without disorganizing sinus bone filling?

In the superior maxilla, one possible technique is not to use irrigation in combination with the drilling protocol. The preparation for desired implant diameter should be done at low speed – 175 rpm. One effect is that very vital bone is collected in the drills; the other benefit is that you have a perfect view of the operative-field and the question of the augmentation material dissipating with irrigation is answered. There are numerous articles on low speed drill protocol, i.e. Eduardo Anitua in Spain, 80–100 rpm.

Postoperative instructions to the patient after the sinus-lift procedure

Activities

1. Do not blow your nose for the next 4 weeks.
2. Be sure to sneeze with your mouth is open.
3. Do not spit or drink with straws.
4. You should avoid flying in a pressurized aircraft or scuba diving because it may increase sinus pressure.
5. You can take a decongestant to help reduce the pressure in your sinuses.
6. You should not play musical instruments that require you to blow or blow up balloons; avoid any other activity that increases oral or nasal pressure.

Antibiotics

All prescribed antibiotics are to be taken as directed in order to prevent infection.

Oral hygiene

During the first 24-h period, do not spit or rinse. This can disturb a blood clot or open the wound, which can prolong bleeding and hinder healing. After the first 24-h period, you can rinse with 1/2 teaspoon of salt in a cup of warm water at least four to five times a day, especially before bed and after meals. Do not brush your teeth near the surgical site for 48 h. Be sure to be very gentle when brushing. Also, be gentle when coughing up phlegm.

Smoking

Smoking significantly increases the possibility of implant failure.

Prosthesis or night guards

Until your postoperative appointment, you should not use flippers, partial dentures, or full dentures.

Postoperative complications

Please visit the implant surgeon, if you experience any of the following:

- If you experience an unusual flow of liquids or air between your nose and mouth.
- If small graft particles begin discharging from your nose.
- If there is an increase of nasal or sinus congestion near the surgical site.
- If you notice an increase in swelling (after 3 days) on your cheek, mouth, or below the eyes.

Complications after sinus graft surgery and their management

Membrane perforation/tearing

This is the most common complication of sinus grafting and occurs in 10–35% of cases. Membrane perforation occurs more commonly in smokers and in the sinuses with anatomical variants such as the presence of septa. Careful access to the sinus membrane and thereafter its careful elevation from the all the bony walls of the sinus using the appropriate armamentarium may reduce the chances of its tearing. Sinus membrane perforation usually does not affect the sinus if the procedure is aborted and flap is sutured back, as it results in regeneration of the membrane in few weeks time and thereafter it can be re-accessed for the sinus grafting procedure. The membrane tearing may result in the loss of graft into the sinus which in turn may take infection.

Management

If the tear or perforation of the membrane occurs during its elevation, the continuation of the sinus elevation procedure is modified. The sinus membrane should be elevated off the bony walls of the antrum all around the perforation and then a dry piece of collagen barrier membrane should be placed to cover the perforation; the sinus is then continued to be grafted as planned and the implant is inserted (Figs 18.102 and 18.103).

Large polyp

If a large polyp is seen in the sinus it should be curetted out before performing the sinus grafting procedure.

Mucous retention cyst

If any mucous retention cyst is seen in the sinus, it should be punctured and drained. Usually, implant placement should be delayed in these cases. If an immediate implant is planned, the region should be flushed with parenteral form of clindamycin after puncturing the mucous retention cyst. Then the sinus grafting and implant placement in the usual fashion can be carried out (Fig 18.104A–I).

Bleeding

Profuse bleeding can occur from the buccal flap tissue if the posterior superior artery gets severed by the vertical incision or by the rotary bur used to prepare the lateral sinus

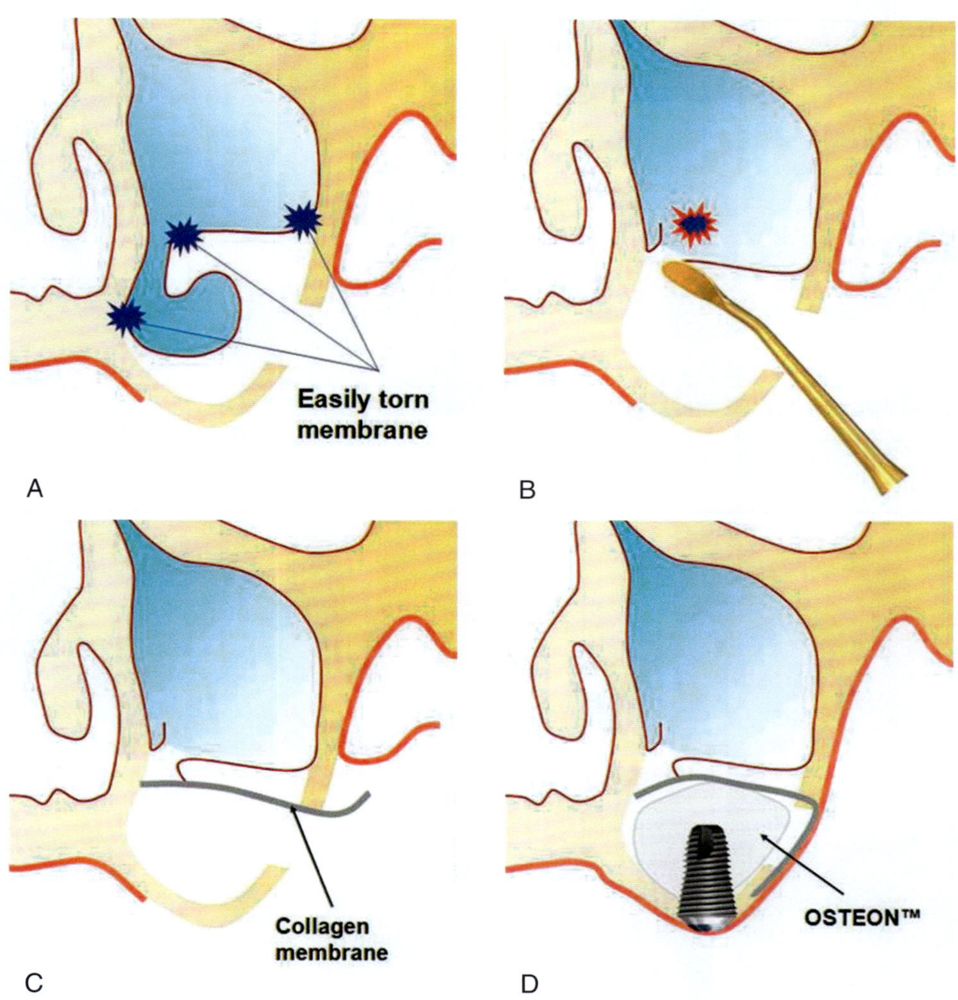

Fig 18.102 If the tear or perforation of the membrane occurs during its elevation, the continuation of the sinus elevation procedure is modified. (A–D) The sinus membrane should be elevated off the bony walls of the antrum all around the perforation and then a dry piece of collagen barrier membrane should be placed to cover the perforation; the sinus is continued to be grafted as planned and the implant is inserted.

window. Extraosseous anastomoses are formed by the infraorbital and posterior superior artery which is located 23 mm from the dentate ridge crest but can be located 10 mm from the resorbed ridge. Care should be taken not to sever these anastomoses as they bleed profusely. The haemostat can be used to stop bleeding from the severed artery.

Bleeding can also be seen when the sinus membrane is elevated from the medial wall of the sinus, which can be stopped by packing the elevated sinus cavity with a gouge piece soaked with the local anaesthetic containing adrenalin. Once the bleeding has stopped, the sinus can be grafted.

Antral septa

Antral septa are the most common osseous anatomical variant seen in the maxillary sinus. CT scans are the most accurate method to diagnose and evaluate the antral septa.

Antral septa mostly found in the middle of the sinus cavity (between second premolar and first molar region) (Fig 18.105A and B). Two separate lateral windows should be prepared to individually access both the sinus compartments and their grafting.

Incision line opening

Causes of incision line opening can be:

1. Lateral ridge augmentation performed simultaneously with sinus grafting, which increases the hard tissue volume under the flap and tension in sutures. Periosteum should be released to achieve a tension-free closure.
2. Soft tissue supported prosthesis is given before suture removal, which compresses the surgical area during function. The soft tissue supported prosthesis should be avoided during the primary healing of the soft tissue.
3. Postoperative swelling causes tension in the sutures and results in the incision line opening. Steroids can be prescribed to prevent any inflammatory

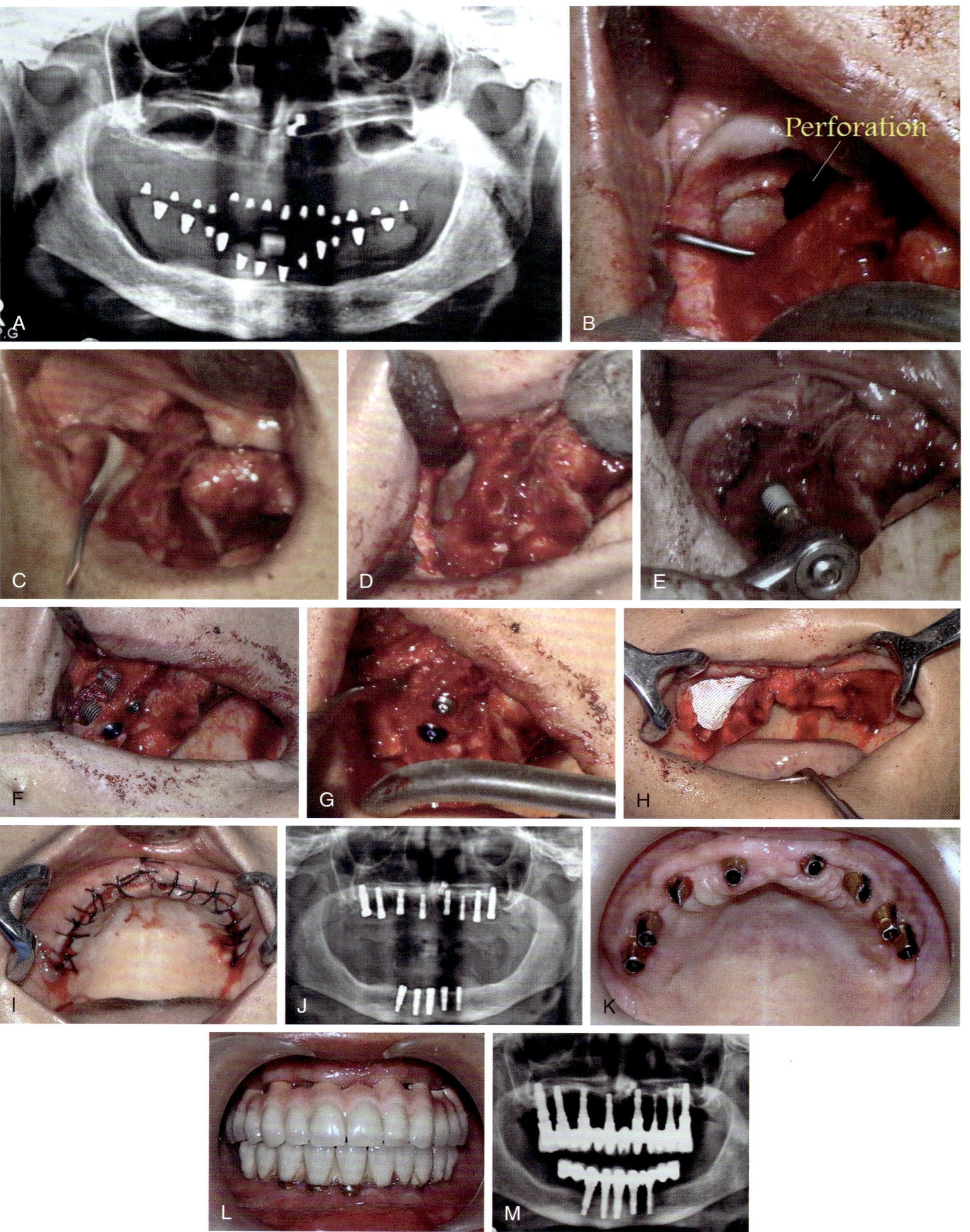

Fig 18.103 (A) Preoperative radiograph showing limited bilateral subantral bone height. (B) A large perforation has occurred in the sinus membrane during its elevation. (C and D) A resorbable collagen membrane is used to repair the perforation. (E) First the bone graft is introduced to fill the medial part of the sinus and (F) then implants are inserted. (G) Then more graft is introduced to loosely fill the sinus cavity. (H) Another collagen membrane was used to cover the window as well as the implants to avoid loss of any graft. (I) Flap sutured back with watertight sutures. (J) Postoperative radiograph shows bilateral sinus grafting and implant placement. (K and L) Implants are uncovered and restored after 10 months. (M) Radiograph 2 years after postloading follow-up.

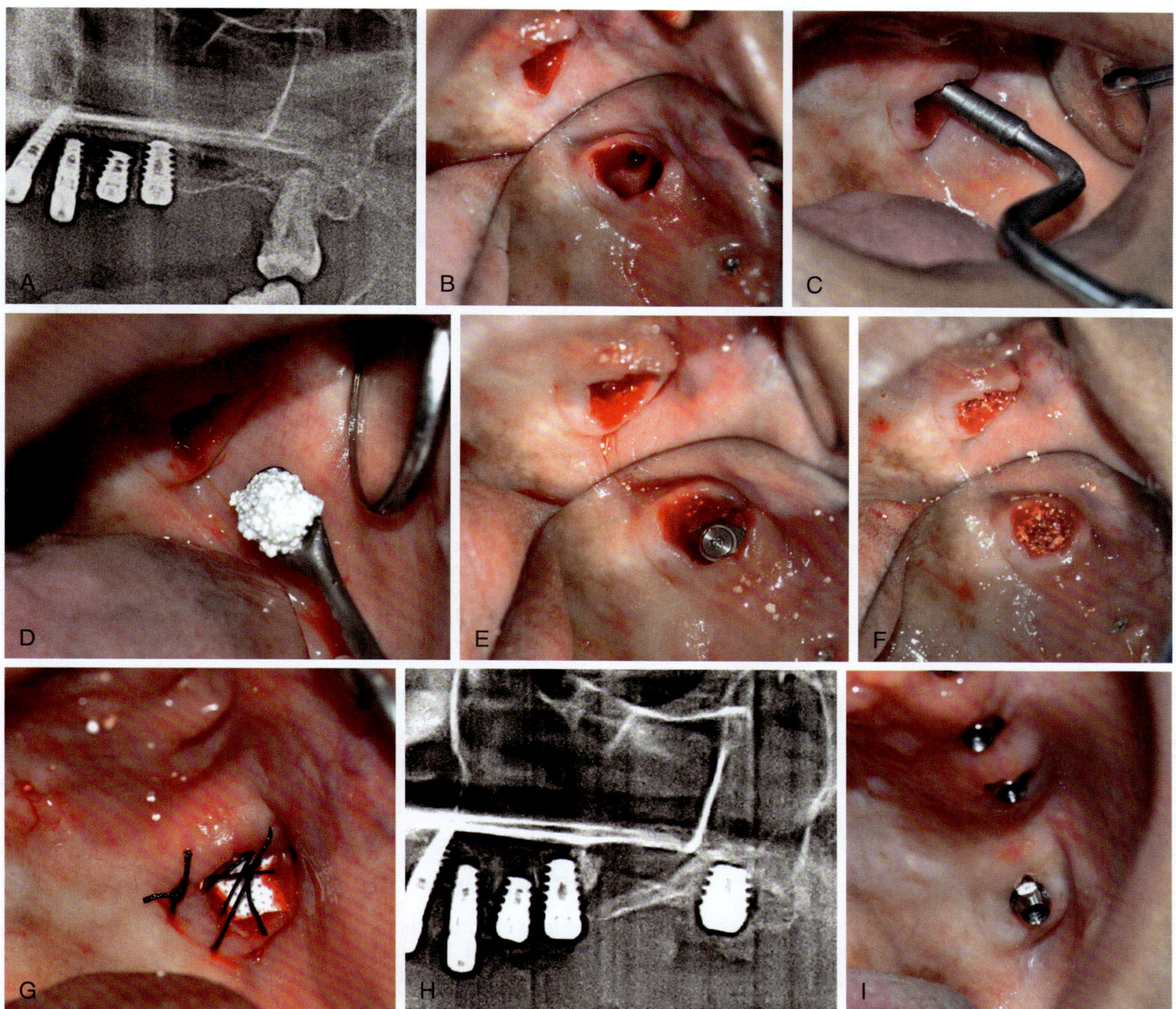

Fig 18.104 (A) Radiograph shows large mucous retention cyst in the sinus at the molar site. (B) The tooth is extracted and (C) an osteotome is used to fracture the sinus floor. The mucous retention cyst is carefully punctured and drained, using a sharp probe. The site is irrigated using the parenteral form of clindamycin. (D) Further, bone substitute is deposited into the cavity and (E) the membrane is further lifted using the same osteotome and the implant is inserted. (F) The peri-implant socket spaces are grafted and (G) site is covered with a polytetrafluoroethylene (PTFE) cytoplast membrane, which is stabilized with sutures. (H) Postimplantation radiograph shows elevated and grafted sinus and placed implant, without any visibility of the mucous retention cyst. (I) The successfully osseointegrated implant is uncovered after 4 months for restoration.

postoperative swelling. Cold dressing for 48 h post-surgery to reduce the inflammatory response, and hot fomentation after 48 h to diffuse the inflammatory fluid from the surgical site, should be done to manage the postsurgical swelling and suture breakdown.

Incision line opening does not usually affect sinus grafting; the patient should be instructed to keep the region clean by using oral rinses and soft brushes until the soft tissue heals with secondary intension. If an incision is made on the buccal aspect of the ridge for the lateral approach, suture line opening can lead to loss of sinus graft.

Neural injury

If the infraorbital nerve gets severed during surgery, the patient can feel paraesthesia in the infraorbital region, in the lateral part of the nose and over the lip on the same side. This is a very uncommon complication and even if it occurs, the sensations revert in a few weeks.

Acute maxillary sinusitis

Acute postoperative sinusitis occurs in 5–20% of sinus grafting cases. The infection starts 3–7 days after the sinus graft surgery with symptoms like headache, pain, and tenderness in the area of the maxillary sinus and rhinorrhoea.

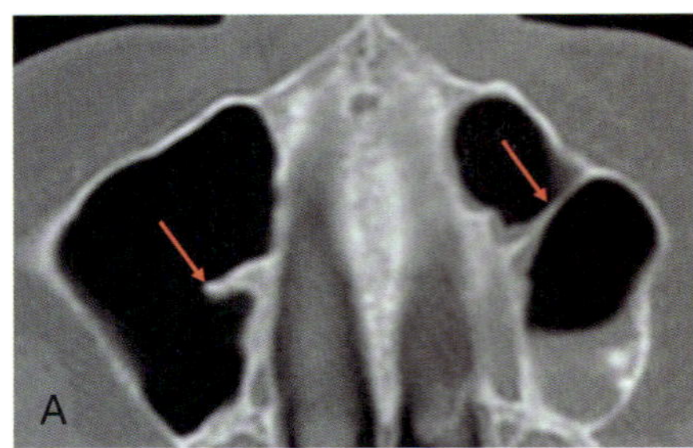

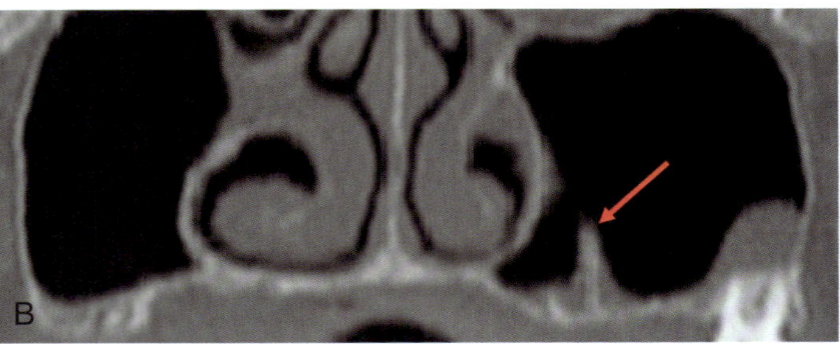

Fig 18.105 (A) Axial view dental CT scan shows a sharp osseous septa emerging from the medial wall of the right sinus cavity. A long septa completely divides the left sinus cavity into two separate compartments. (B) Panoramic view of dental CT scan showing a sharp osseous septa emerging from the floor of the left sinus cavity.

Mild postoperative infection

Symptoms:

1. Nasal discharge or nasal blockage
2. Pain and pressure in infraorbital area
3. Intraoral as well as extraoral swelling
4. Cough.

Management:

1. Amoxicillin–clavulanic acid combination (tab. Augmentin, 1000 mg one tab b.i.d. for 2 weeks)
2. Decongestant (Oxymetazoline, 0.05% for 3 days)
3. Nasal saline rinses.

Moderate to severe postoperative infection

Symptoms:

1. Severe headache
2. High-grade fever
3. Swelling in periorbital region with ocular symptoms like diplopia, proptosis
4. Altered mental status
5. Infraorbital hyperaesthesia.

Management

1. Moxifloxacin, 400 mg one tablet b.i.d. for two weeks
2. Medrol dosepak, 4 mg, as directed
3. Nasal saline rinses.

The patient should be referred to ENT surgeon if the condition does not improve with antibiotics within 4–5 days.

Penetration of the implant apex into the sinus

If the implant has perforated the sinus membrane and its apex penetrates into the sinus; it can be a source of periodic sinusitis. But many of the newer studies have shown that if the implant apex penetrates into the sinus 2 mm or less, the membrane gets regenerated and covers it within few weeks; and if it has penetrated more than 2 mm, then being sterile material it does not usually cause any problem, but further clinical trials need to be done to evaluate the long term effect of the implant apex exposed in the sinus cavity.

Oroantral fistula

It may develop postoperatively, especially if the patient has a history of infection. If it is small, it will close spontaneously with systemic antibiotics and oral hygiene care (chlorhexidine mouth rinses). If the fistula is larger than 5 mm, it requires surgical closure.

Overfilling of the sinus

Care should be taken not to overfill the sinus, as it can block the ostium. Because the ostium is situated at a very high position, most cases of sinus overfilling do not cause any complications.

Summary

Sinus elevation is a procedure that is very commonly being performed. The techniques and approaches described in this chapter should be performed only after the proper hands-on training, to avoid postoperative complications. Meticulous diagnosis and treatment planning should be done for the sinus grafting cases, to evaluate the presence of any septa, sinus thickening, chronic sinus infections, mucous cysts, appropriate approach for sinus membrane lifting and the nature and volume of the bone graft required to graft the sinus floor. Usually, the internal sinus elevation procedure should be preferred for cases where a small height of sinus elevation is required. The lateral approach should be preferred for the cases where a large area and height of the sinus membrane needs to be elevated. For the lateral approach, if performed using rotary bur, the large-diameter diamond bur should be preferred over the carbide bur, to avoid the tearing of the membrane. The oval window should be prepared for the lateral approach, because the membrane can tear during elevation at the corners of the rectangular osseous window. Before start elevating the membrane, the osseous window should be tapped using the back of the mouth mirror handle, to fracture the small and thin bridges between the osseous window and the surrounding bone. The use of piezotome or DASK kit obviously offers several advantages to perform safe and efficient sinus lifting.

Summer's technique can be effectively used to stabilize the implant apex in the high-density sinus floor and also to elevate and graft the sinus with the subcrestal approach. In several cases where the sinus floor is irregular in height, it becomes difficult to perform the osteotome technique, as at one part the osteotome reaches close to of sinus floor, but on other margin can be well short of floor which resulted in difficulty in fracturing up the sinus floor and same time gives lot of mental trauma to the patient. In such cases the DASK kit or intralift obviously offer several advantages for easy and safe lifting of the sinus membrane. A careful evaluation of the lifted sinus membrane is mandatory before starting the graft of the sinus floor, as any tear in the membrane that has already occurred, may result in the loss of the graft in the sinus cavity and postoperative sinus infection.

Further Reading

Woo I, Le BT. Maxillary sinus floor elevation: review of anatomy and two techniques. Implant Dent 2004;13(1):28–32.

Chackartchi T, Iezzi G, Goldstein M, et al. Prospective, intra-individual controlled clinical, micro-computerized tomography and histomorphometric study. Clin Oral Implants Res 2011;22(5):473–80.

Valentini P, Abensur DJ. Maxillary sinus grafting with an organic bovine bone: a clinical report of long-term results. Int J Oral Maxillofac Implants 2003;18(4):556–60.

Tadjoedin ES, de Lange GL, Bronckers ALJJ, et al. Deproteinized cancellous bovine bone (Bio-Oss) as bone substitute for sinus floor elevation. J Clin Periodontol 2003;30:261–70.

De Souza Nunes LS, De Oliveira RV, Holgado LA, et al. Immunoexpression of Cbfa-1/Runx2 and VEGF in sinus lift procedures using bone substitutes in rabbits. Clin Oral Implants Res 2010;21(6):584–90; Epub 2010 Jan 23.

Mordenfeld A, Hallmann M, Johansson CB et al. Histological and histomorphometrical analyses of biopsies harvested 11 years after maxillary sinus floor augmentation with deproteinized bovine and autogenous bone. Clin Oral Implants Res 2010; 21(9):961–70.

Galindo-Moreno P, Padial-Molina M, Fernandez-Barbero JE, et al. Optimal microvessel density from composite graft of autogenous maxillary cortical bone and anorganic bovine bone in sinus augmentation: influences of clinical variables. Clin Oral Implants Res 2010;21(2):221–7.

Pacifici L, Casella F, Ripari M. Lifting of the maxillary sinus: complementary use of platelet rich plasma, autologous bone deproteinized bovine bone. Case report. Minerva Stomatol 2003;52:471–8.

Pietursson BE, Tan WC, Zwahlen M, et al. A systematic review of the success of sinus floor elevation and survival of implants inserted in combination with sinus floor elevation. J Clin Periodontol 2008;35:216–40.

Marchetti C, Pieri F, et al. Impact of implant surface and grafting protocol on clinical outcomes of endosseous implants. Int J Oral Maxillofac Implants 2007;22(3):399–407.

Galindo-Moreno P, Moreno-Riestra I, Avila G, et al. Effect of anorganic bovine bone to autogenous cortical bone ratio upon bone remodeling patterns following maxillary sinus augmentation. Clin Oral Implants Res 2011;22(8):857–64.

Araújo MG, Lindhe J. Ridge preservation with the use of Bio-Oss® Collagen: a 6-month study in the dog. Clin Oral Implants Res 2009;20:433–40.

Hallmann M, Sennerby L, Lundgren S. A clinical and histologic evaluation of implant integration in the posterior maxilla after sinus floor augmentation with autogenous bone, bovine hydroxyapatite, or a 20:80 mixture. Int J Oral Maxillofac Implants 2002;17:635–43.

Hallmann M, Hedin M, Sennerby L, et al. A prospective 1-year clinical and radiographic study of implants placed after maxillary sinus floor augmentation with bovine hydroxyapatite and autogenous bone. J Oral Maxillofac Surg 2002;60:277–84.

Tawil G, Mawla M. Sinus floor elevation using a bovine bone mineral (Bio-Oss) with or without the concomitant use of a bi-layered collagen barrier (Bio-Gide): a clinical report of immediate and delayed implant placement. Int J Oral Maxillofac Impl 2001;16:13–21.

Cordioli G, Mazzocco C, et al. Maxillary sinus floor augmentation using bioactive glass granules and autogenous bone with simultaneous implant placement. Clinical and histological findings. Clin Oral Implants Res 2001;12:270–8.

Strietzel FP, Nowak M, et al. Peri-implant alveolar bone loss with respect to bone quality after use of the osteotome technique: results of a retrospective study. Clin Oral Implants Res 2002;13:508–13.

Jakse N, Seibert FJ, et al. A modified technique of harvesting tibial cancellous bone and its use for sinus grafting. Clin Oral Implants Res 2001;12:488–94.

Maiorana C, Redemagni M, Rabagliati M, et al. Treatment of maxillary ridge resorption by sinus augmentation with iliac cancellous bone, anorganic bovine bone, and endosseous implants: a clinical and histologic report. Int J Oral Maxillofac Implants 2000;15:873–8.

Urban IA, Lozada JL. A prospective study of implants placed in augmented sinuses with minimal and moderate residual crestal bone: results after 1 to 5 years. Int J Oral Maxillofac Implants 2010;25(6):1203–12.

Smiler DG, Holmes RE. Sinus lift procedure using porous hydroxyapatite: a preliminary clinical report. J Oral Implantol 1987;13:239–53.

Zitzmann NU, Scharer P. Sinus elevation procedures in the resorbed posterior maxilla: comparison of the crestal and lateral approaches. Oral Surg Oral Med Oral Pathol Oral Radiol Endod 1998;85:8–17.

Summers RB. Sinus floor elevation with osteotomes. J Esthet Dent 1998;10:164–71.

Misch CE. Maxillary sinus anatomy, pathology, and graft surgery. Contemporary implant dentistry. 3rd ed. Indian Reprint; ISBN: 978-81-312-1510-4.

Valentini P, Abensur D, Wenz B, et al. Sinus grafting with porous bone mineral (Bio-Oss®) for implant placement: a study on 15 patients. Int J Periodontics Restorative Dent 2000;20:245–53.

Sartori S, Silvestri M, Forni F, et al. Ten-year follow-up in a maxillary sinus augmentation using anorganic bovine bone (Bio-Oss). A case report with histomorphometric evaluation. Clin Oral Implants Res 2003;14(3):369–72.

McAllister B, Margolin M, Cogan A, et al. Eighteen-month radiographic and histologic evaluation of sinus grafting with anorganic bovine bone in the chimpanzee. Int J Oral Maxillofac Implants 1999;14.

Haas R, Mailath G, Dörtbudak O, et al. Bovine hydroxyapatite for maxillary sinus augmentation: analysis of interfacial bond strength of dental implants using pull-out tests. Clin Oral Implants Res 1998;9:117–22.

McAllister B, Margolin M, Cogan A, et al. Residual lateral wall defects following sinus grafting with recombinant human osteogenic protein-1 or Bio-Oss® in the chimpanzee. Int J Periodontics Restorative Dent 1998;18(3).

Hürzeler MB, Quiñones CR, Kirsch A, et al. Maxillary sinus augmentation using different grafting materials and dental implants in monkeys – part I. Evaluation of anorganic bovine-derived bone matrix. Clin Oral Implants Res 1997;8:476–86.

Valentini P, Abensur D. Maxillary sinus floor elevation for implant placement with demineralized freeze-dried bone and bovine bone (Bio-Oss®): a clinical study of 20 patients. Int J Periodontics Restorative Dent 1997:17.

Wetzel AC, Stich H, Caffesse RG. Bone apposition onto oral implants in the sinus area filled with different grafting materials. Clin Oral Implants Res 1995;6:155–63.

Tatum OH. Maxillary and sinus implant reconstruction. Dent Clin North Am 1986; 30:207–29.

Boyne P, James RA. Grafting of the maxillary sinus floor with autogenous marrow and bone. J Oral Maxillofac Surg 1980; 17:113–6.

Ruoff H, Terheyden H. Retrospective radiographic investigation of the long-term stability of xenografts (Geistlich Bio-Oss) in the sinus. Z Zahnärztl Impl 2009;25(2):160–9.

Becker ST, Terheyden H, et al. Prospective observation of 41 perforations of the Schneiderian membrane during sinus floor elevation. Clin Oral Implants Res 2008; 19(12):1285–9.

Degidi M, Daprile G, Piattelli A. RFA values of implants placed in sinus grafted and nongrafted sites after 6 and 12 months. Clin Implant Dent Relat Res 2009; 11(3):178–182.

Raghoebar GM, Timmenga NM, et al. Maxillary bone grafting for insertion of endosseous implants: results after 12–24 months. Clin Oral Implants Res 2001;12: 279–86.

Testori T, Wallace SS, et al. Repair of large sinus membrane perforations using stabilized collagen barrier membranes: surgical techniques with histologic and radiographic evidence of success. Int J Periodontics Restorative Dent 2008;28(1):9–17.

Maiorana C, Sigurta D, Miranda A, et al. Sinus elevation with alloplasts or xenogenic materials and implants: an up-to-4-year clinical and radiologic follow-up. Int J Oral Maxillofac Implants 2006;21(3):426–32.

Wallace SS, Froum SJ, Cho SC, et al. Sinus augmentation utilizing anorganic bovine bone (Bio-Oss) with absorbable and nonabsorbable membranes placed over the lateral window: histomorphometric and clinical analyses. Int J Periodotics Restorative Dent 2005;25:551–9.

Kahnberg KE, Ekestubbe A, et al. Sinus lifting procedure. I. One-stage surgery with bone transplant and implants. Clin Oral Implants Res 2001;12:479–87.

Block MS, Kent JN. Sinus augmentation for dental implants: the use of autogenous bone. J Oral Maxillofac Surg 1997;55:1281–6.

Del Fabbro M, Testori T, Francetti L, et al. Systematic review of survival rates for implants placed in the grafted maxillary sinus. Int J Periodontics Restorative Dent 2004;24:565–77.

John HD, Wenz B. Histomorphometric analysis of natural bone mineral for maxillary sinus augmentation. Int J Oral Maxillofac Implants 2004;19:199–207.

Wallace SS, Froum SJ. Effect of maxillary sinus augmentation on the survival of endosseous dental implants. A systematic review. Ann Periodontol 2003;8:328–43.

Chackartchi T, Iezzi G, Goldstein M, et al: Sinus floor augmentation using large (1-2 mm) or small (0.25-1 mm) bovine bone mineral particles: a prospective, intra-individual controlled clinical, micro-computerized tomography and histomorphometric study. Clin Oral Implants Res. 2011 May;22(5):473–80.

Tadjoedin ES, de Lange GL, et al. High concentrations of bioactive glass material (BioGran) vs. autogenous bone for sinus floor elevation. Clin Oral Implants Res 2002;13:428–36.

Van den Bergh JPA, ten Bruggenkate CM, et al. Anatomical aspects of sinus floor elevations. Clin Oral Implants Res 2000; 11:256–65.

Chanavaz M. Maxillary sinus: anatomy, physiology, surgery and bone grafting related to implantology. Eleven years of surgical experience (1979–1990). J Oral Implantol 1990;16:199–209.

Solar P, Geyerhofer U, et al. Blood supply to the maxillary sinus relevant to sinus floor elevation procedures. Clin Oral Implants Res 1999;10:34–44.

Summers RB. A new concept in maxillary implant surgery: the osteotome technique. Compend Contin Educ Dent 1994; 15:152–62.

Marx RE, Garg AK. A novel aid to elevation of the sinus membrane for the sinus lift procedure. Implant Dent 2002;11:268–71.

Nasal floor elevation and grafting 19

Ajay Vikram Singh

CHAPTER CONTENTS HD

Introduction

Implant therapy in the anterior maxilla is considered to be most challenging because of the high aesthetic demands of the patient and facial cantilevers. In recent years, similar to the sinus elevation procedure, nasal floor elevation and grafting has become an effective treatment modality to achieve the bone height required to place long implants and simultaneously engage the implant in the high density nasal floor to achieve adequate primary stability. Nasal floor elevation and grafting can be done to insert longer implants at the maxillary central and lateral incisors in both the dentate and the long-time edentulous severely resorbed premaxilla. This procedure can also be performed to insert implants at the canine positions, only in cases of severely resorbed premaxilla. The reason is that the nasal cavity is usually present above, medial and palatal to the canine position in the dentate position. However, a nasal recess is present behind the lateral piriform rim and comes above the apical region of the canine position once the premaxilla has resorbed palatally. Nasal floor elevation with or without grafting offers several advantages including insertion of a longer implant than planned specially in the severely resorbed premaxilla, high initial stability in the inserted implant so that it can be immediately restored to return aesthetics to the patient, etc. Further, the anterior region of the nasal floor does not contain any vital structure; so its careful elevation does not usually cause any postoperative or long-term complication.

Anatomy

The piriform aperture which ranges from 20 to 28 mm in adults is bounded below and laterally by the maxilla. The anatomical areas of concern for nasal floor elevation and grafting procedure are:

1. **Anterior nasal spine**. This is the anterior-most component and considered one of the reference points during blunt dissection and labial flap elevation to uncover the nasal floor.
2. **Inferior piriform rim**. This is another reference point and should be uncovered to access the nasal floor for elevation and grafting.
3. **Nasal floor**. Present posterior and inferior to the inferior piriform rim. It is accessed through elevating the nasal mucosa superior and posterior from inferior and lateral piriform rim.
4. **Lateral piriform rim**. The inferior piriform rim extends lateral and superior from the lateral piriform rim. The nasal mucosa should be elevated from this rim to achieve adequate height in nasal floor elevation and grafting.
5. **Nasal recess**. It is present behind the lateral piriform rim and makes a concavity in the lateral wall of the piriform aperture above the canine region of the palatally resorbed premaxilla. The nasal mucosa should be elevated at this region, especially if the nasal floor grafting is to be done for implant

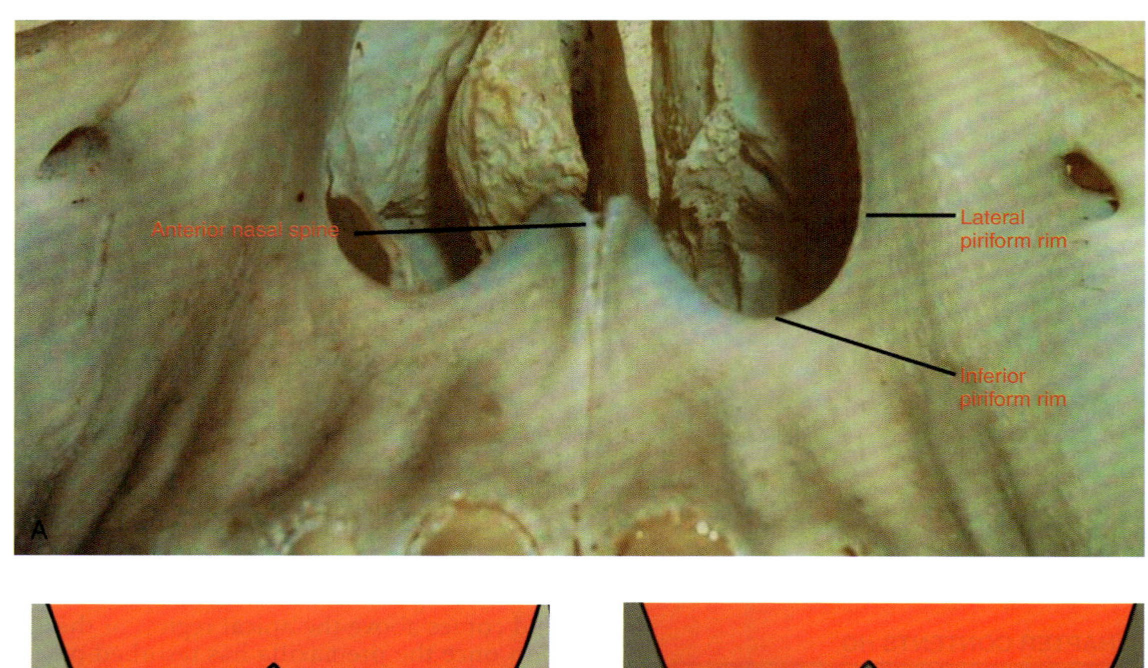

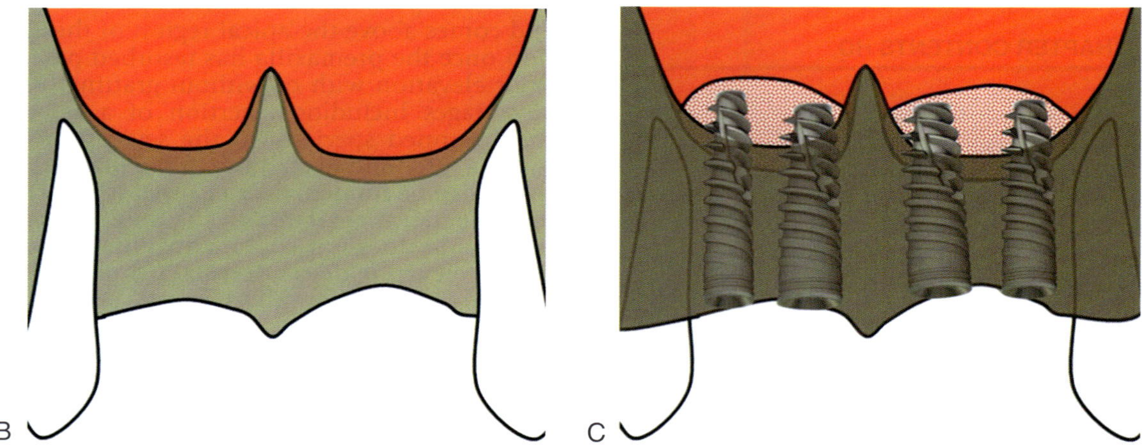

Fig 19.1 The anterior nasal spine is the anterior-most component and is considered to be the highest limit for flap elevation to uncover the inferior and lateral piriform rims and to access the nasal floor, which is usually present posterior and inferior to the inferior piriform rim. The canine root remains situated distal to the lateral piriform rim of the nose. (A–C) However, the nasal recess extends distal and behind the piriform rim to reach over the canine site of the resorbed premaxilla.

insertion at the canine position of the resorbed premaxilla (Fig 19.1A–C).

Indications

1. In the severely resorbed anterior maxilla, the nasal floor elevation and grafting can be performed to insert long implants at the central, lateral incisors as well as canine positions.
2. Anterior maxilla with poor density bone.
3. Demanding situation of placing long implant with desired stability in the anterior maxilla, e.g. all-on-4 technique, knife-edge thin premaxilla.
4. Adjuvant with sinus grafting in cases of severely resorbed maxilla to insert multiple implants for full-arch restoration.
5. Long implant placement to stabilize its apex in high-density nasal floor in cases of large osseous defect in the anterior maxilla, which is grafted simultaneously with implant placement.
6. Adjuvant with ridge splitting procedure to achieve adequate stability of the implant in the high-density nasal floor.
7. High primary stability of the implant is required with bicortical engagement to immediately restore the implant in resorbed anterior maxilla or in immediate implantation in extraction socket.

Contraindications

1. Nasal pathology.
2. Deviated nasal septum.
3. Shallow nasal floor, which may cause the patient to feel the implant apex in the nasal cavity.

Advantages

1. 3–5 mm long implant can be inserted in comparison to the usual implant placement.
2. Bicortical implant engagement – implant head is engaged in the high-density crestal bone and its apex is engaged in the high-density nasal floor.
3. The procedure excludes the need of onlay bone grafting for the severely resorbed anterior maxilla.
4. Implant can be established in hard nasal floor to achieve adequate primary stability in case of low-density bone, ridge splitting procedure, immediately grafted large osseous defect, immediate implant in extraction socket in the premaxillary region.
5. Implant can be restored immediately.
6. Less invasive procedure and can be performed under local anaesthesia.
7. Safe procedure as there are minimum chances of any serious complication related to the procedure.

Procedure

There are two techniques for performing the nasal floor grafting procedure:

1. Open technique
2. Closed technique (subcrestal approach).

Open technique

In this technique, the facial flap is elevated to expose the nasal cavity. Further, the nasal floor epithelium is carefully detached from the inferior and lateral piriform rims followed by epithelial elevation 3–5 mm distally and superiorly, using various types of sinus curettes to create a subepithelial pouch at the nasal floor. After achieving the desired height of nasal floor epithelium elevation, the implant osteotomy is prepared with the drills perforating through the nasal floor in the region where the nasal epithelium has been elevated. The nasal floor is grafted using autogenous bone and/or any bone substitutes and the implant is inserted with its apex emerging through the hard nasal bony floor. The nasal mucosa is elevated and grafted approximately 3–5 mm distally and superiorly with this technique.

CASE REPORT-1

Immediate implant with nasal floor grafting. A 50-year-old male patient referred to the author's centre for immediate replacement of his mobile maxillary central incisor. On examination, the tooth was found extremely mobile with the other adjacent teeth in good periodontal health. The marginal soft tissue on the facial aspect had receded approximately 10 mm from its position but the papillae were at the original level. The teeth were badly stained because of fluorosis and tobacco chewing. On radiographic and dental CT evaluation, a large three-walled osseous defect which nearly reached the nasal floor was visible. The tooth root was seen completely encapsulated into the fibrous tissue. The patient expressed the desire for immediate implant placement and restoration of of aesthetics on the same day. The case was found challenging in a few aspects.

Challenges in this case

1. Achieving adequate primary stability for the immediately inserted implant, as there were large 3-walled osseous defect nearly reaching the nasal floor
2. Augmentation of the large osseous defect simultaneous with the implant insertion
3. Space maintenance for the bone graft
4. Immediate restoration of the lost marginal soft tissue
5. Achieving primary closure for submerged implant healing and graft maturation
6. Immediate and long-term aesthetic restoration which should match with the fluoride-affected as well as badly tobacco-stained adjacent natural teeth.

After meticulous planning using the radiograph, dental CT imaging, and clinical pictures of the case, the following treatment plan was finally decided upon to treat the patient with implant prosthesis.

Treatment planning

Step 1: Extraction of tooth.

Step 2: Careful incision and flap elevation to expose the osseous defect and its debridement.

Step 3: Elevation of the nasal floor epithelium and nasal floor grafting.

Step 4: A long and narrow platform implant (3.75 × 18 mm) insertion within the osseous envelope and at the correct prosthetic position, stabilizing its apex in the high-density nasal floor.

Step 5: Grafting of the osseous defect using autogenous bone (harvested from the maxillary tuberosity) mixed with bone substitutes (HA + β-TCP) and plasma rich in growth factors (PRGF) extracted from the venous blood of the patient just before the implant surgery. The use of a tent screw was planned to provide adequate space for the bone graft.

Step 6: Use of nonresorbable polytetrafluoroethylene (PTFE) membrane to cover the whole grafted site, releasing the periosteum to achieve the primary closure. The grafting of the soft tissue defect with an epithelialized connective tissue graft harvested from the tuberosity region, before harvesting the autogenous bone.

Step 7: The sectioning of the root of the extracted tooth and bonding with adjacent teeth to restore the aesthetics of the patient immediately after implant insertion.

Step by step clinical presentation of the case is depicted in Figs 19.2–19.13.

Continued

CASE REPORT-1—cont'd

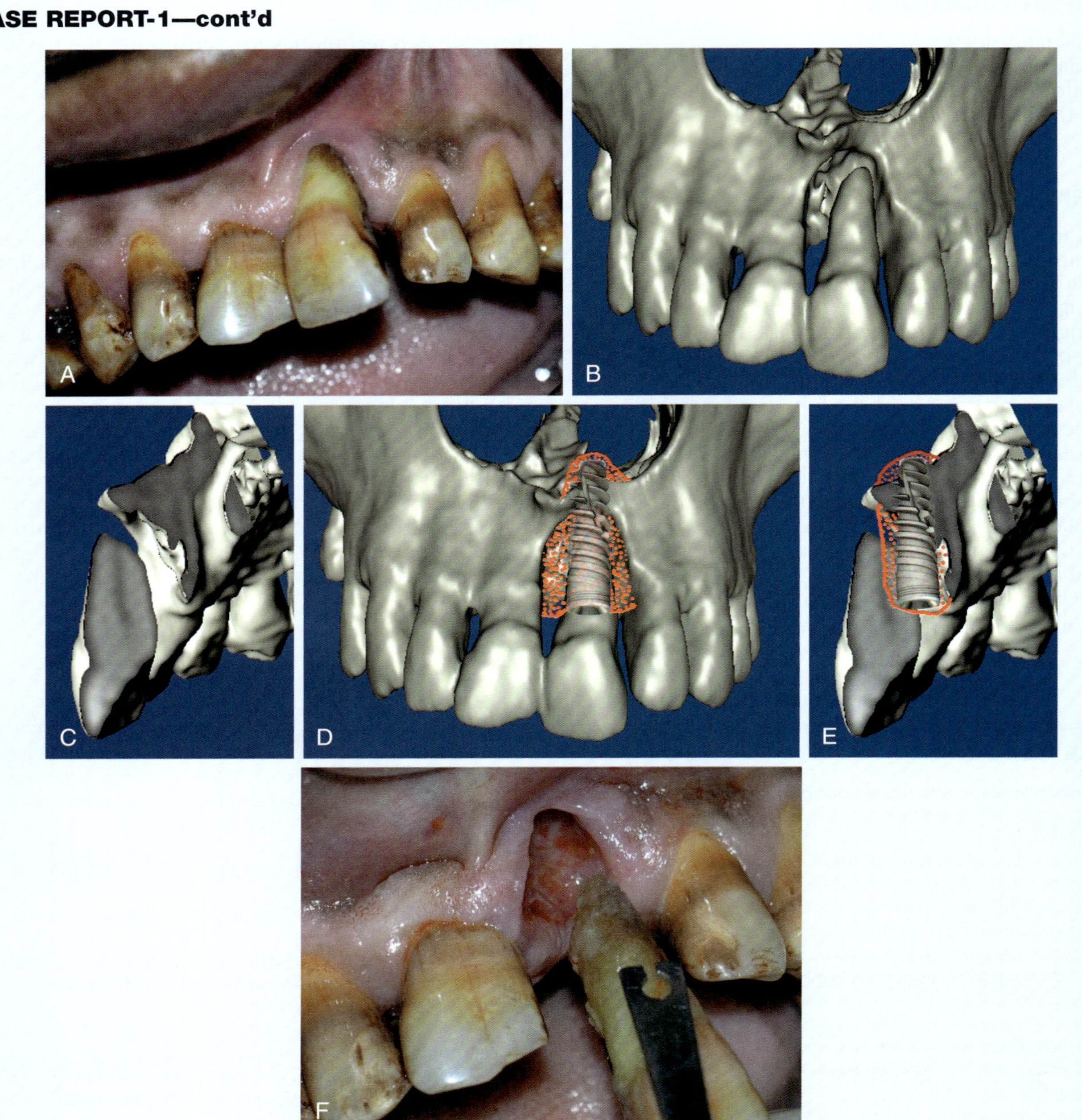

Fig 19.2 (A) Tooth number 21 with severe mobility and soft tissue recession. (B and C) Dental CT has revealed the three-dimensional loss of periodontal bone with complete soft tissue encapsulation of the root. Immediate implantation with simultaneous bone grafting is planned. (D and E) The implant apex needs to be stabilized in the high-density nasal floor to achieve adequate initial stability, thus nasal floor elevation and grafting is planned. (F) The tooth is extracted, showing the soft tissue encapsulation of the root apex.

CASE REPORT-1—cont'd

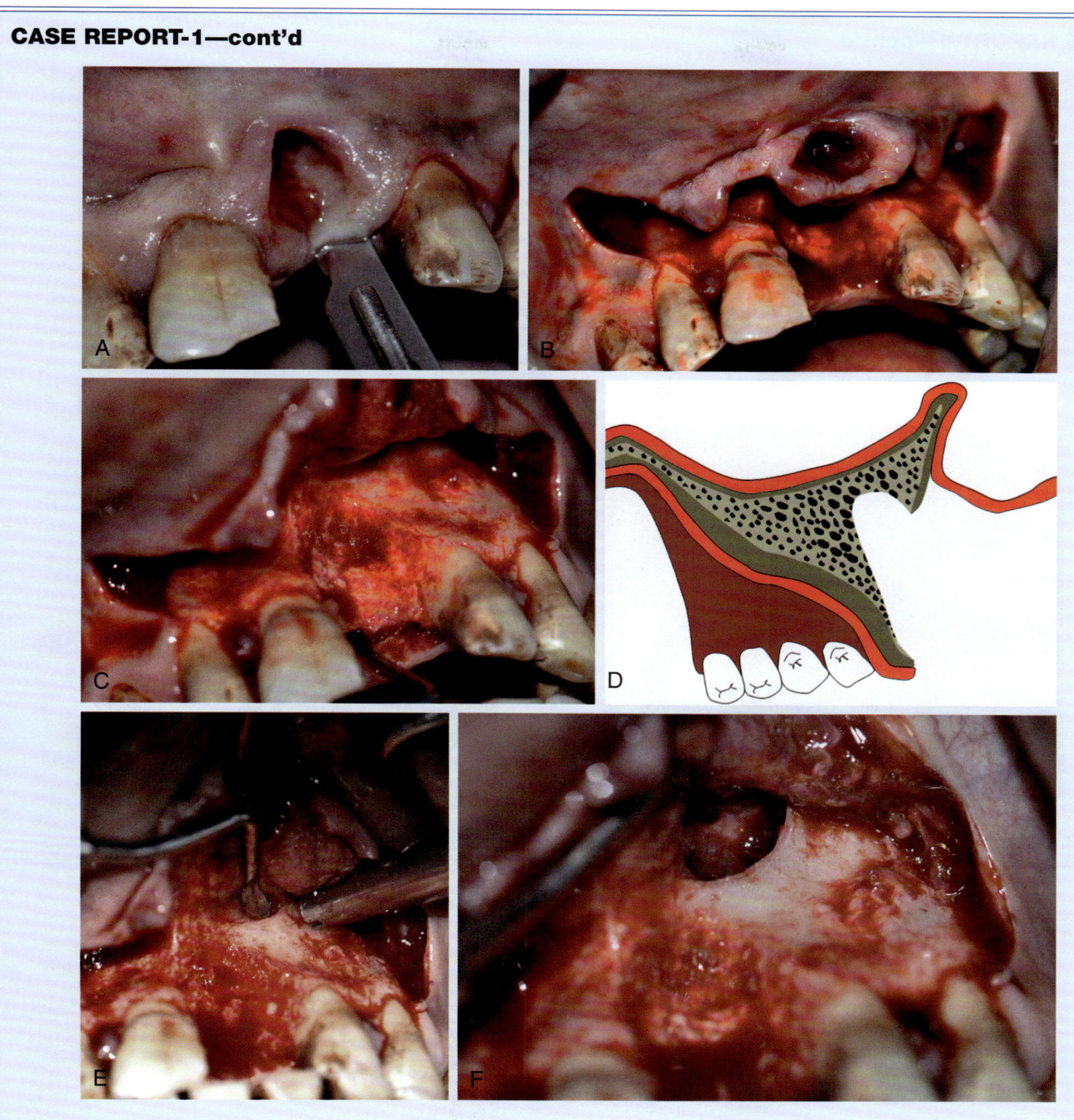

Fig 19.3 (A and B) A mid-crestal incision is given and the facial mucoperiosteal flap is elevated to include the fibrous encapsulation included in the elevated flap. (C and D) A large osseous defect can be seen at the site which looks unfavourable for immediate implant with simultaneous bone grafting because of inadequate bone volume to achieve the primary stability of the implant. (E–G) The flap is further elevated to expose the inferior piriform rim of left nasal cavity and the nasal floor epithelium is elevated using a set of sinus curettes.

Continued

CASE REPORT-1—cont'd

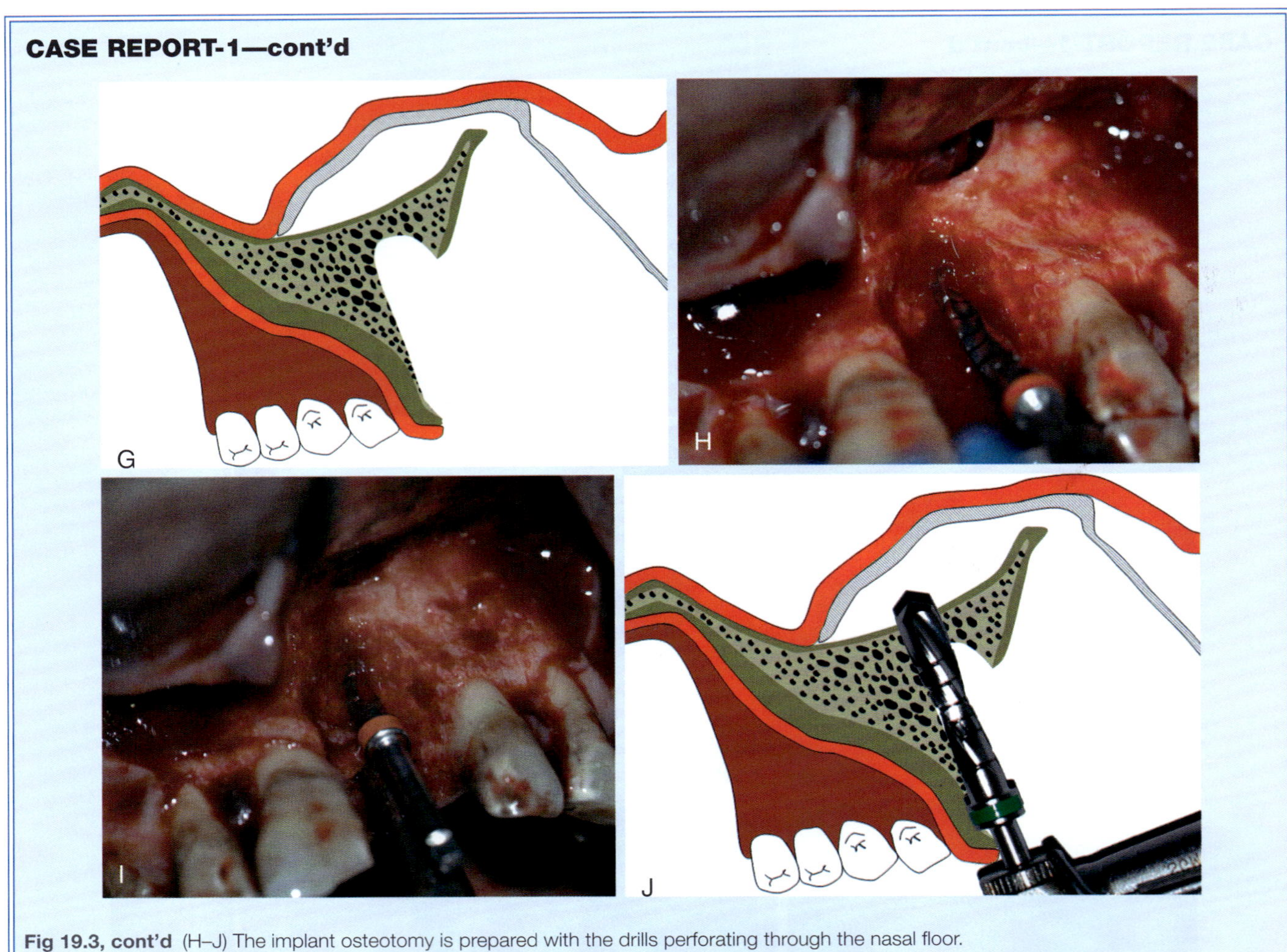

Fig 19.3, cont'd (H–J) The implant osteotomy is prepared with the drills perforating through the nasal floor.

CASE REPORT-1—cont'd

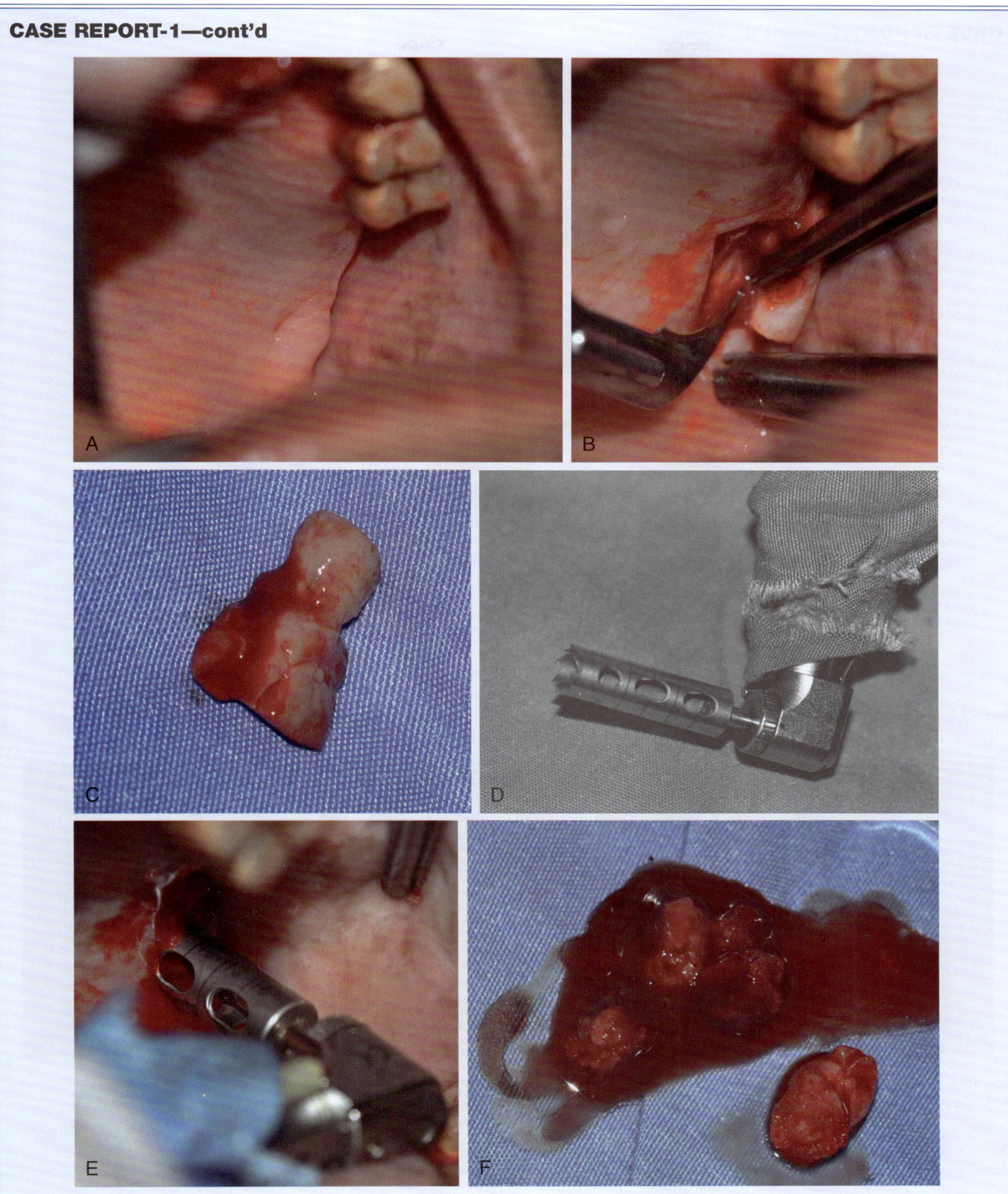

Fig 19.4 (A–C) A thick epithelialized connective tissue graft is harvested from the edentulous posterior maxillary ridge. (D–F) Further, a trephine drill is used to harvest the autogenous bone from the maxillary tuberosity.

Continued

CASE REPORT-1—cont'd

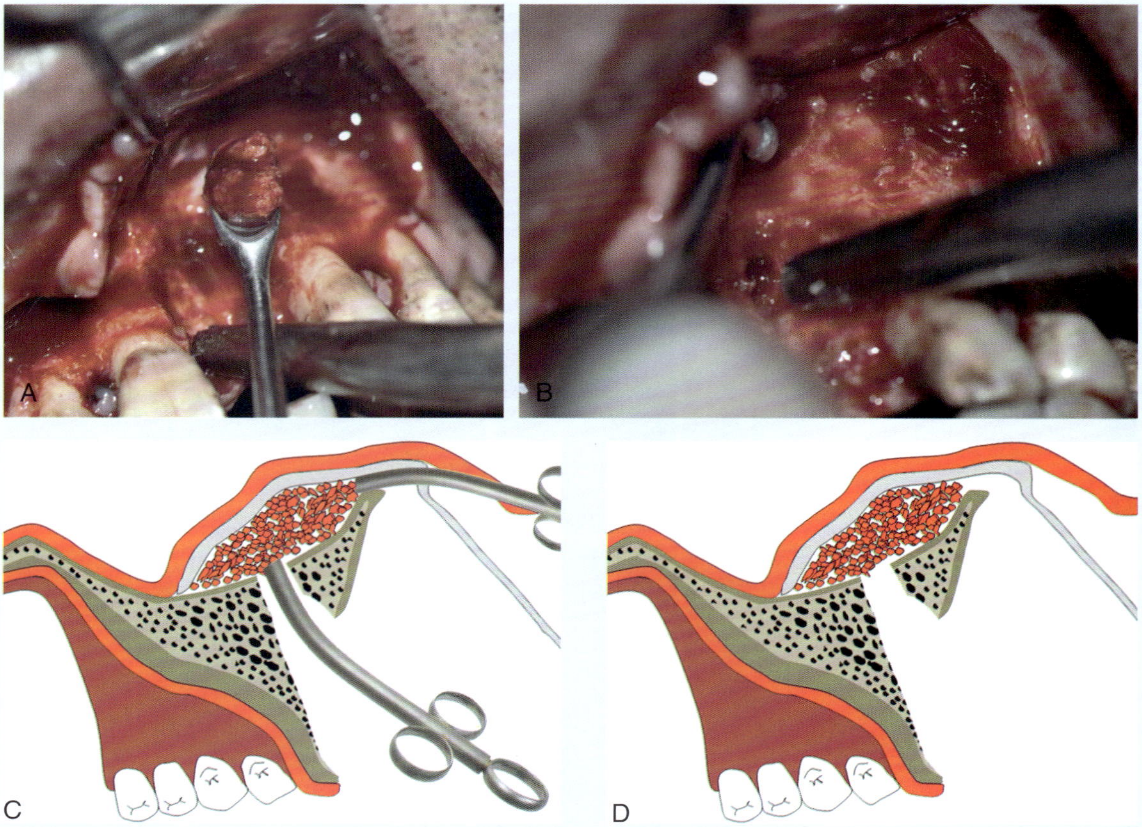

Fig 19.5 (A–D) The elevated nasal floor is grafted using the autogenous bone as the first layer through the both accesses.

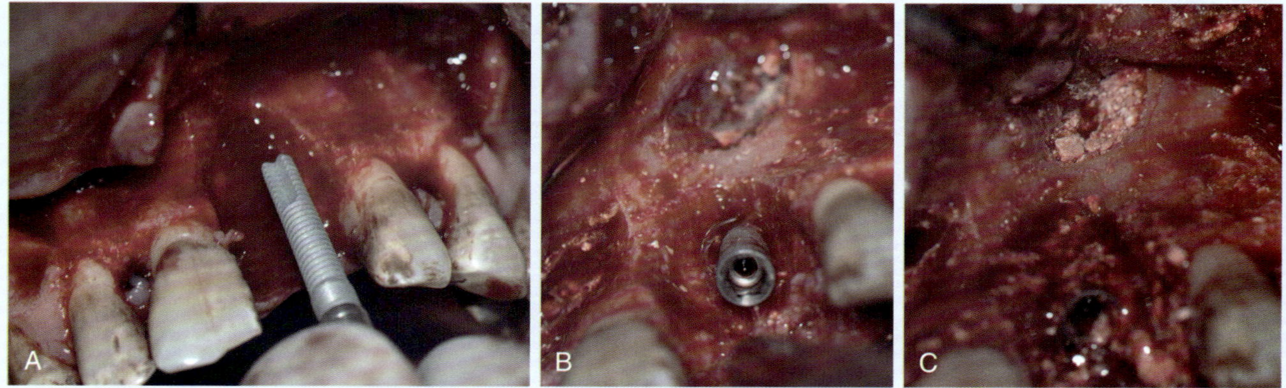

Fig 19.6 A long implant (3.75 × 18 mm) is inserted within the osseous envelope and with the implant apex emerging 5 mm through the nasal floor. High primary stability of the implant is achieved. (A–E) Following implant placement, the rest of the nasal floor is grafted using bone substitute. (F–K) A long tent screw is inserted for space maintenance underneath the barrier membrane and the osseous defect is first grafted with autogenous bone followed by bone substitute (HA + β-TCP) mixed with PRGF.

CASE REPORT-1—cont'd

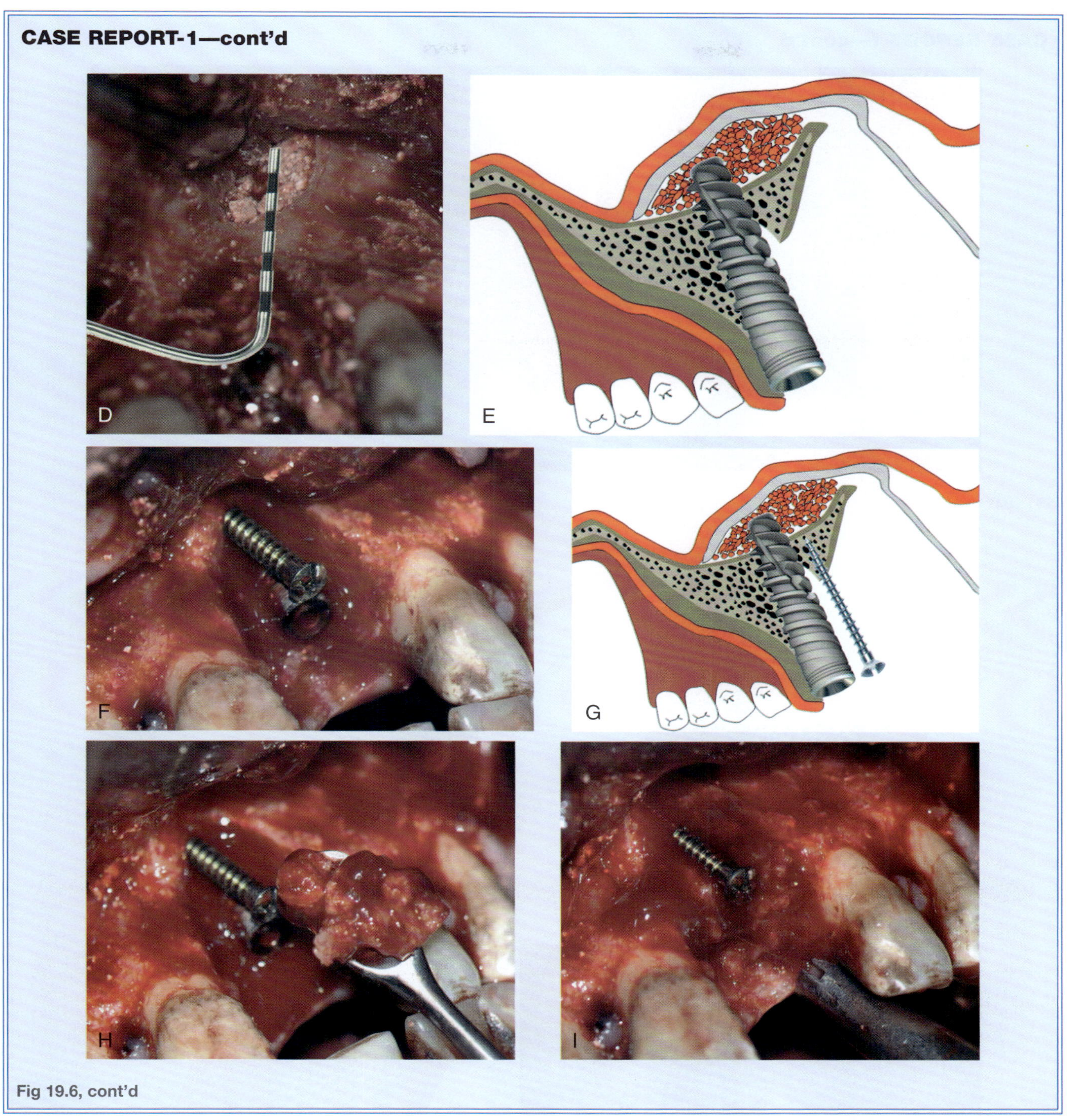

Fig 19.6, cont'd

Continued

CASE REPORT-1—cont'd

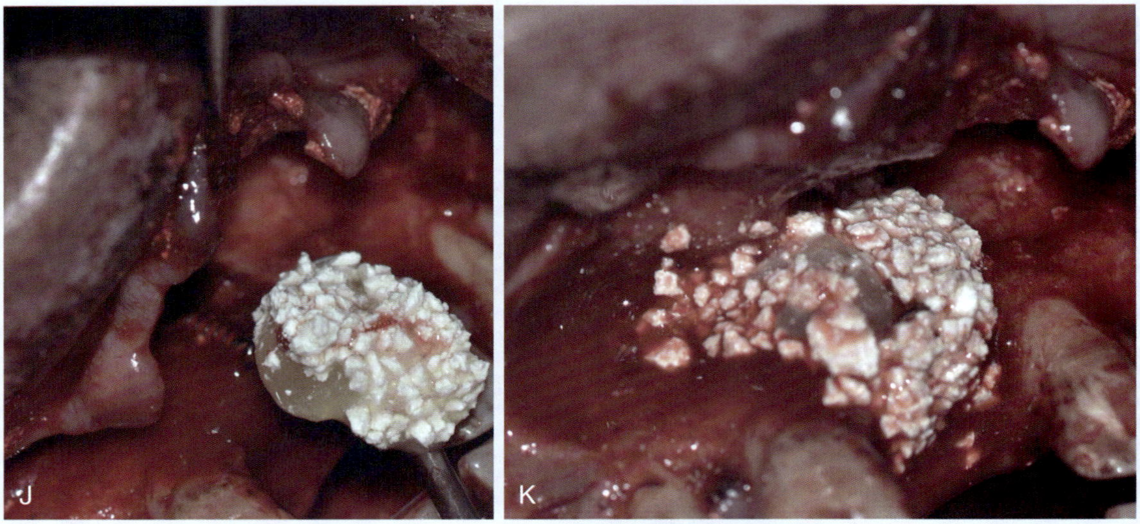

J

K

Fig 19.6, cont'd

A

B

C

D

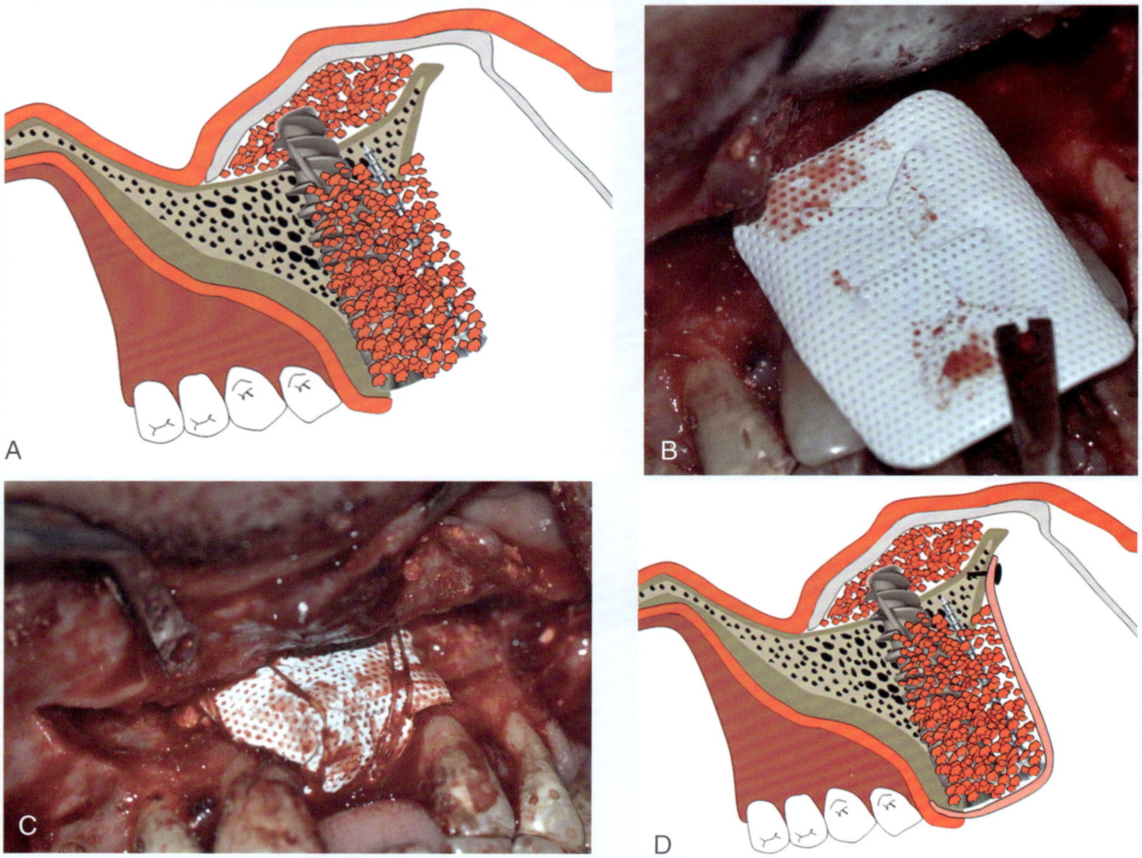

Fig 19.7 (A) Once the osseous defect has been grafted, (B and C) a titanium reinforced PTFE cytoplast barrier membrane is placed to cover the graft and stabilized with sutures. (D) The barrier membrane can also be stabilized using bone tacks.

CASE REPORT-1—cont'd

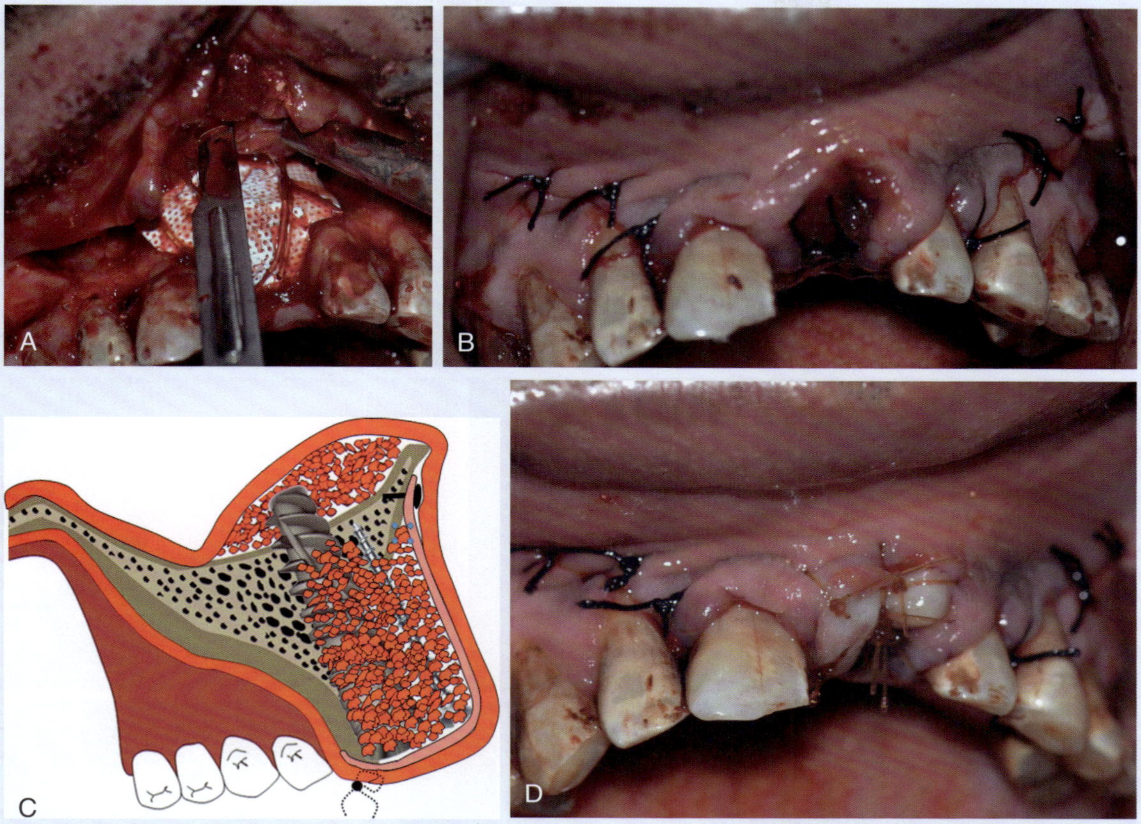

Fig 19.8 (A) A horizontal releasing incision is given through the periosteum from underneath the flap parallel to the crestal incision to release the periosteum. (B and C) The flap is coronally advanced and sutured with primary closer. (D) The soft tissue graft is sutured over the extraction site to regenerate a thick and keratinized marginal soft tissue around the final implant prosthesis.

Continued

CASE REPORT-1—cont'd

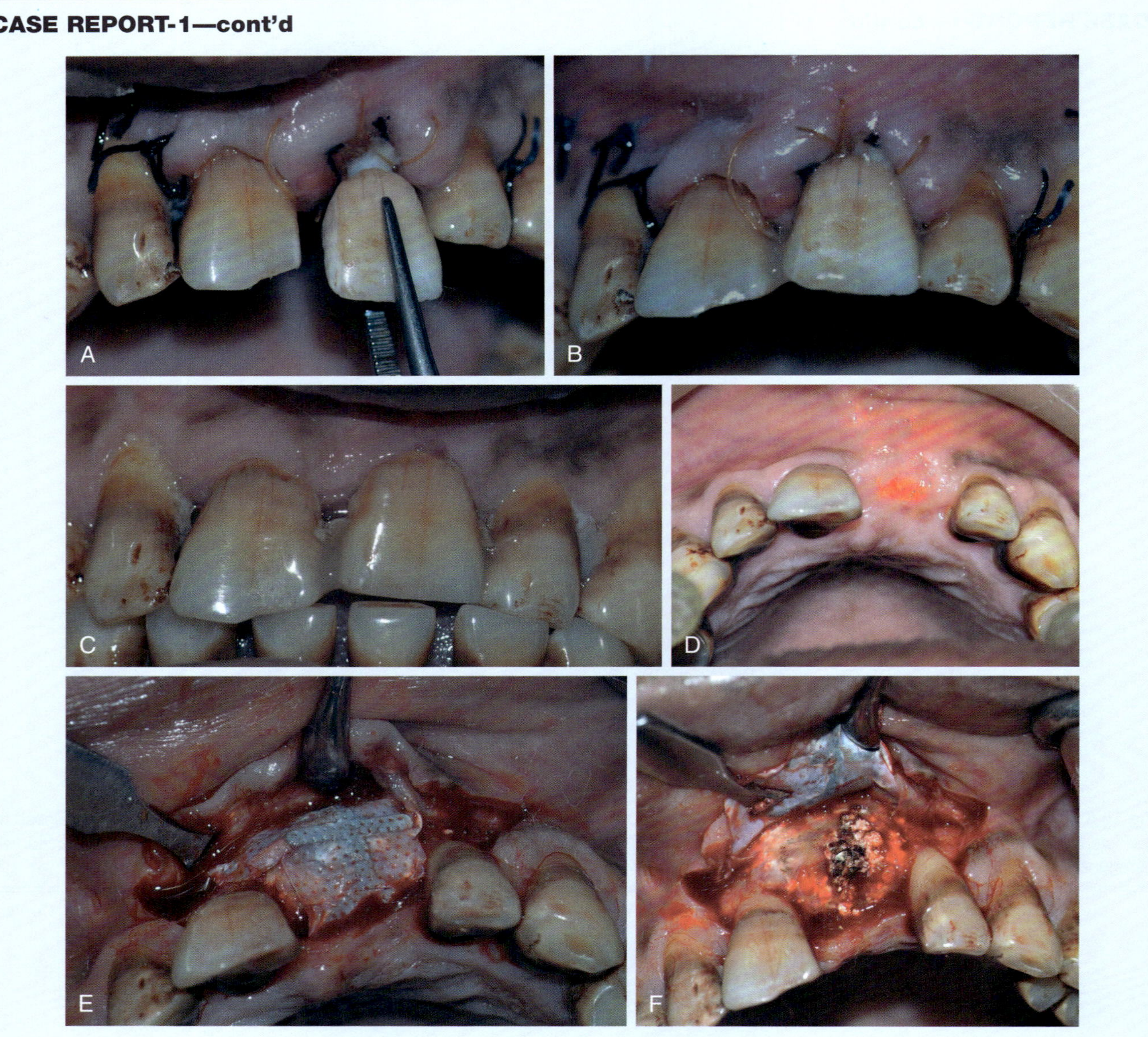

Fig 19.9 (A and B) The extracted tooth is shaped and bonded with the adjacent teeth. (C and D) The bonded tooth removed after 4 months shows healed site with acceptable ridge morphology. (E and F) The site uncovered after 4 months shows the new bone regeneration under TXT membrane.

CASE REPORT-1—cont'd

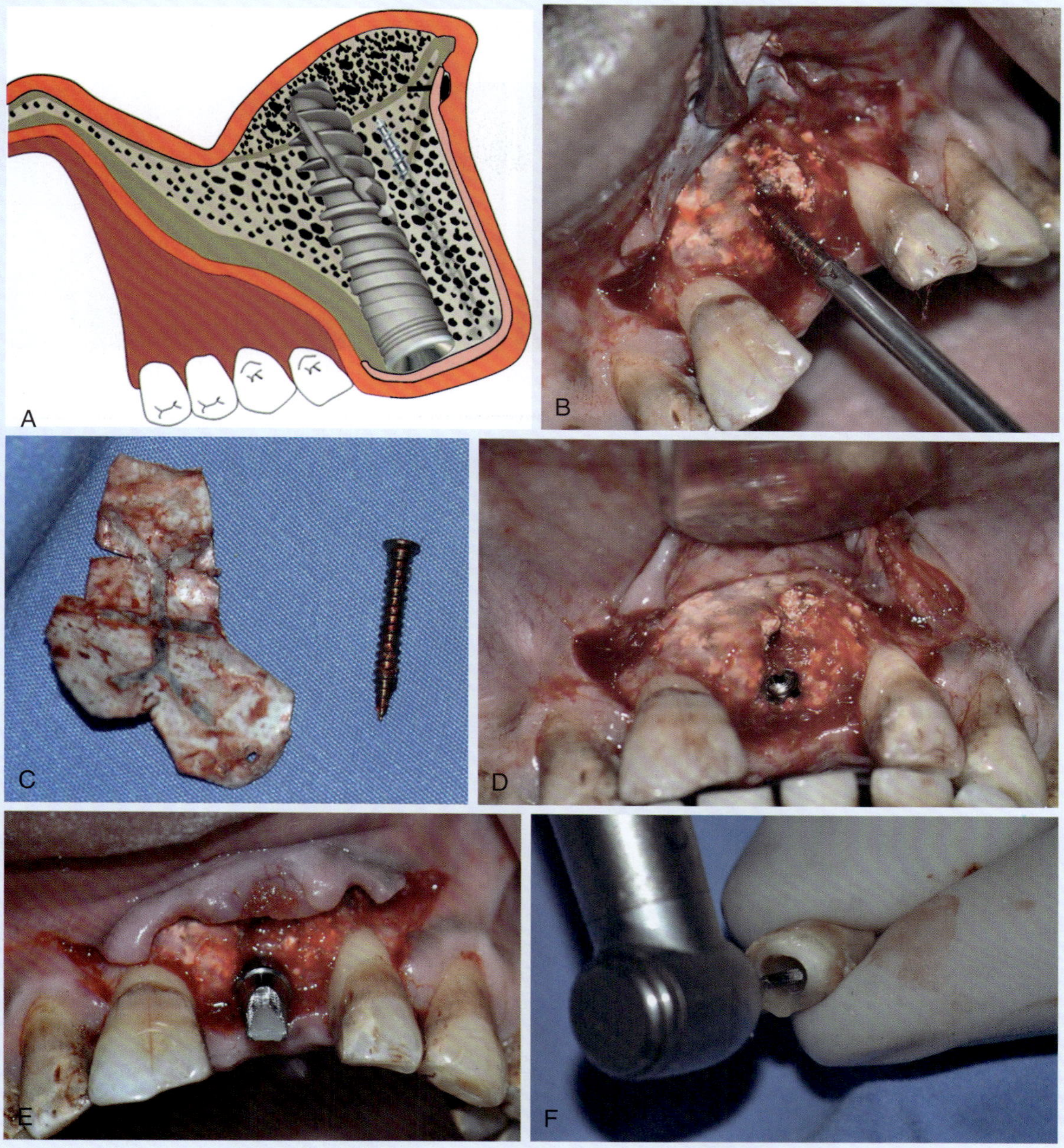

Fig 19.10 (A–E) The fixation screw and TXT membrane are removed and a straight abutment is inserted on top of the implant. (F) The patient's tooth is hollowed out to create the space for the abutment.

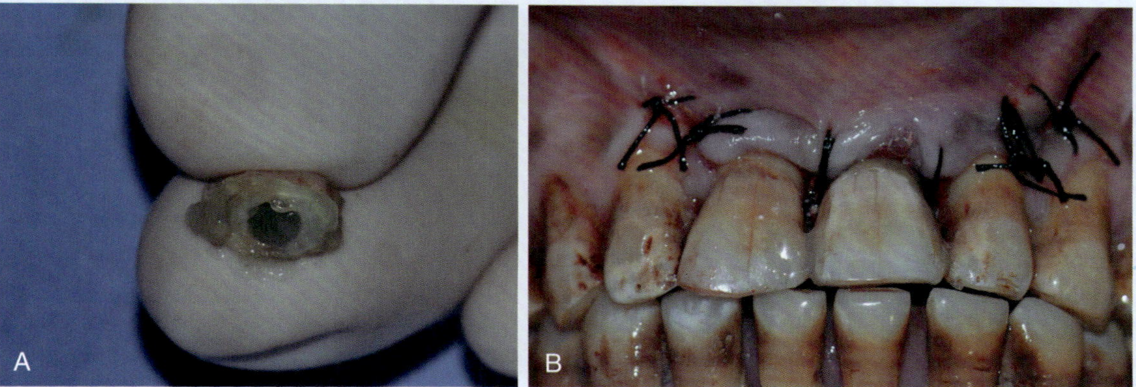

Fig 19.11 (A and B) The tooth is etched from inside and bonded over the abutment using dual cure resin cement.

Continued

CASE REPORT-1—cont'd

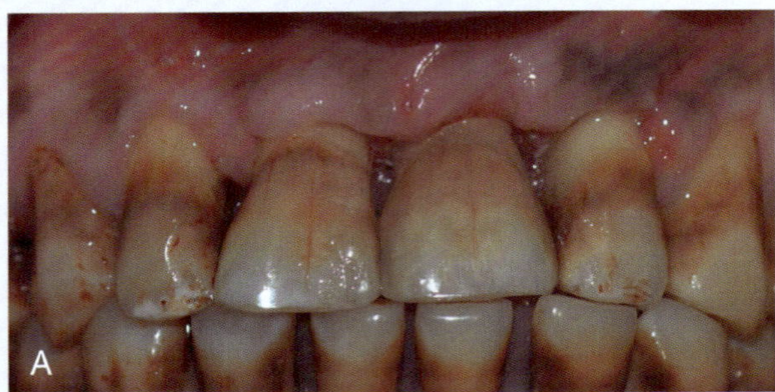

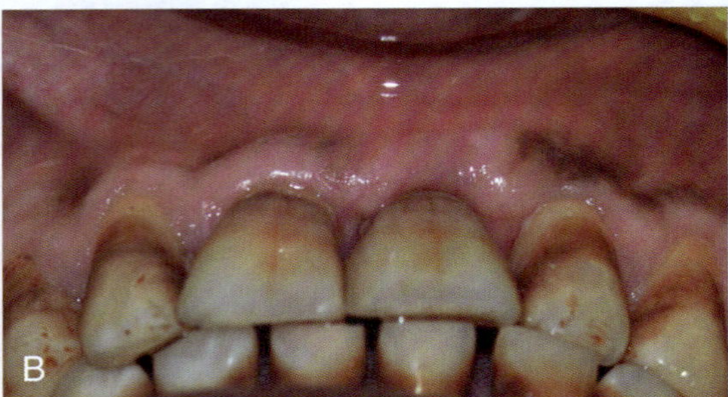

Fig 19.12 (A) Follow-up clinical views after 1 week and (B) after 1 year.

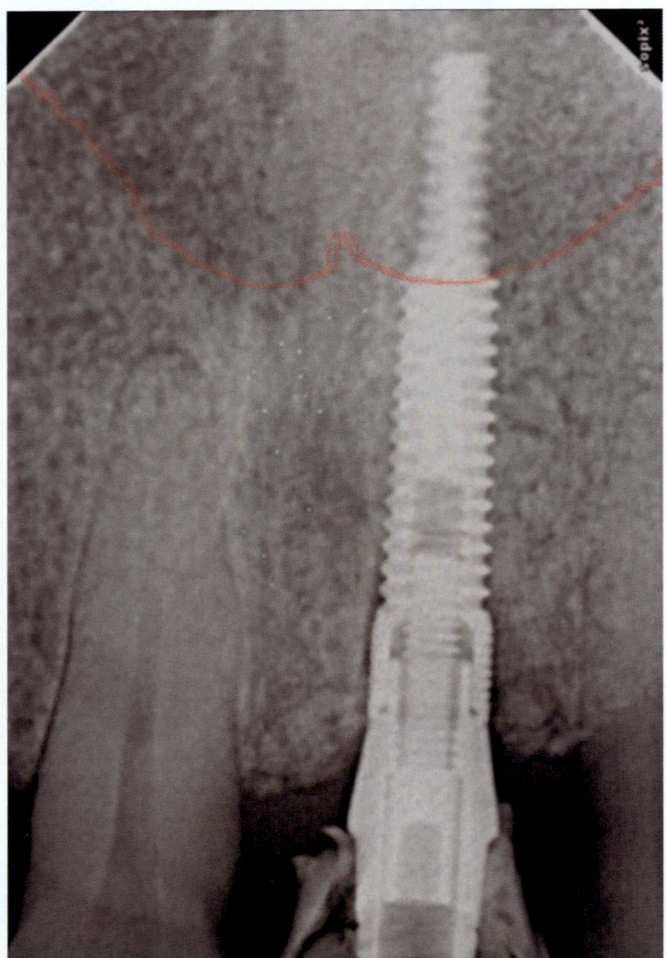

Fig 19.13 Follow-up radiograph 1 year after restoration shows homogenous bone consolidation around the implant.

CASE REPORT-2

Immediate implant with nasal floor grafting and immediate restoration (Figs 19.14–19.20).

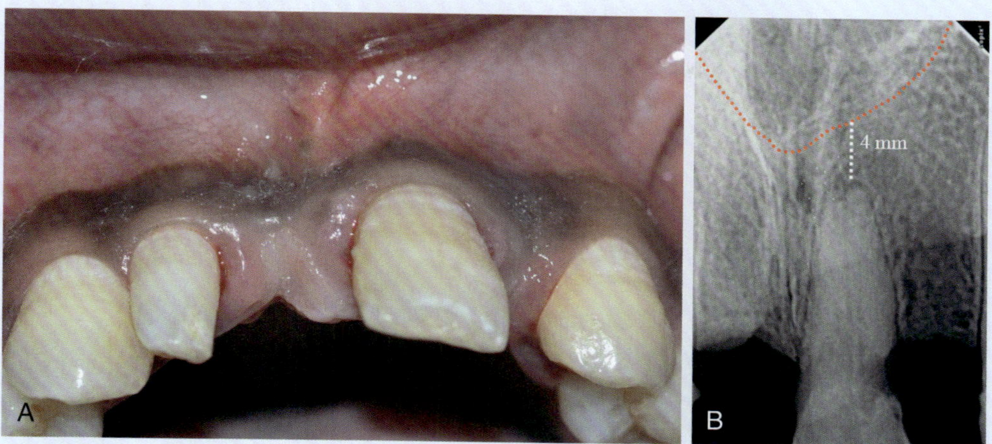

Fig 19.14 (A) Missing teeth numbers 11 and 22 and mobile tooth number 21. Extraction of tooth number and immediate implant placement is planned at tooth numbers 11 and 21 for a three-unit bridge. (B) Preoperative radiograph shows only 4 mm bone between root apex and nasal floor. For immediate restoration of the implants, insertion of the longest possible implant with its apex stabilized in the high-density nasal floor by nasal floor elevation and grafting, is planned.

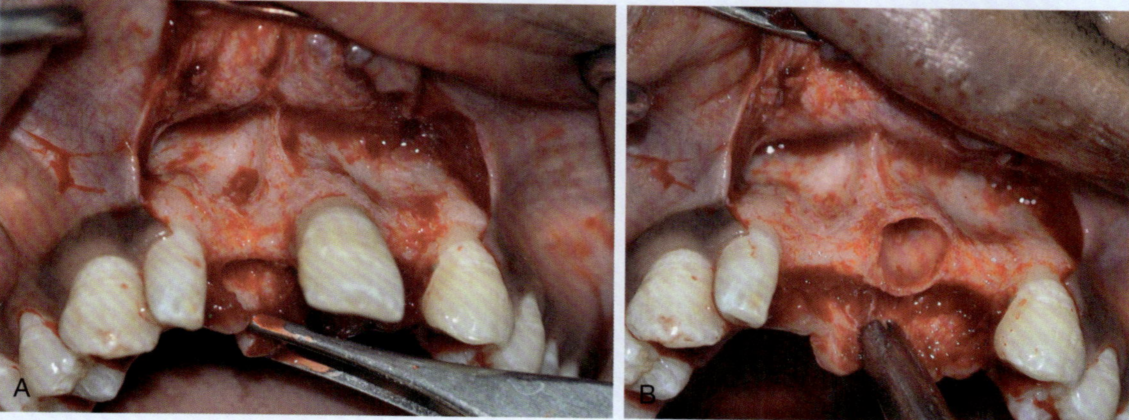

Fig 19.15 (A) Flap is elevated and (B) tooth is atraumatically extracted.

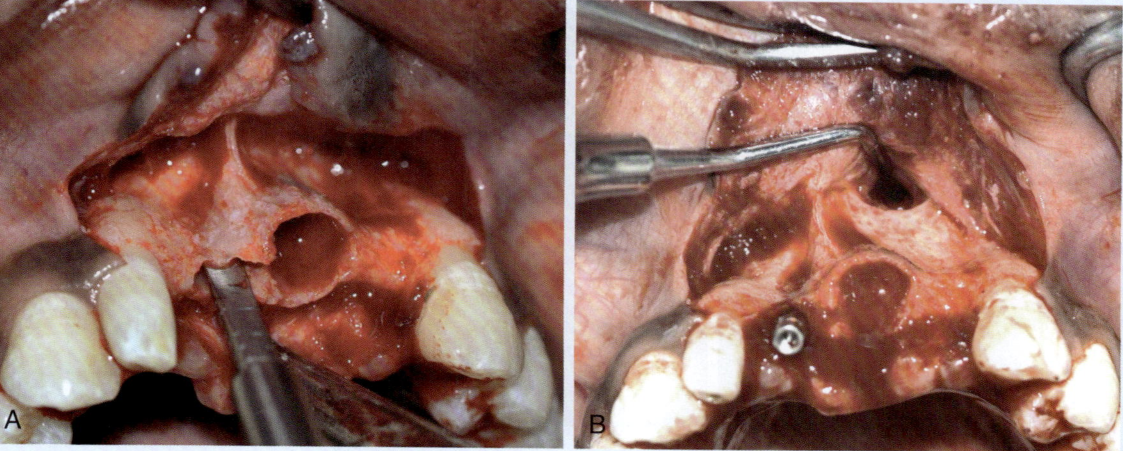

Fig 19.16 Implant (3.3 × 15 mm) is inserted at tooth number 11 after performing ridge split and expansion procedure. Inserted implant achieved high initial stability (more than 35 Ncm.). (A and B) Further, the nasal epithelium is elevated on the left side using appropriate sinus curette.

Continued

CASE REPORT-2—cont'd

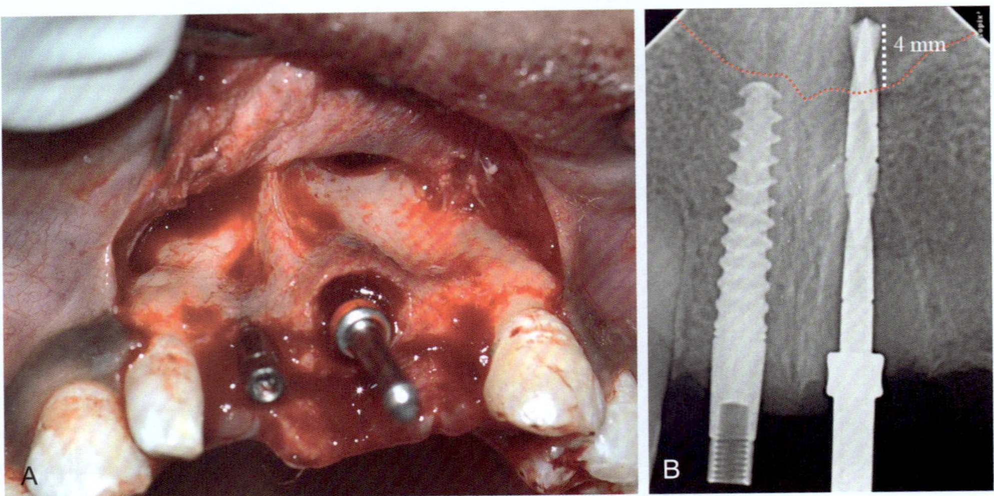

Fig 19.17 (A) After the nasal epithelium is elevated to the planned height and depth, the implant osteotomy is prepared through the socket to perforate through the high density nasal floor. (B) Radiograph shows the pilot drill 4 mm beyond the nasal floor.

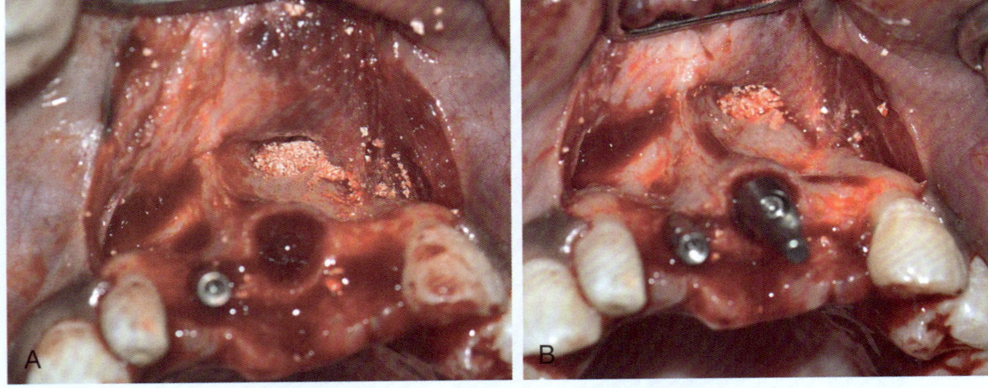

Fig 19.18 (A) Once the implant osteotomy is completed, the elevated nasal floor is grafted using bone substitute (HA + β-TCP) and (B) implant is inserted. Implant has achieved high primary stability (more than 35 Ncm.)

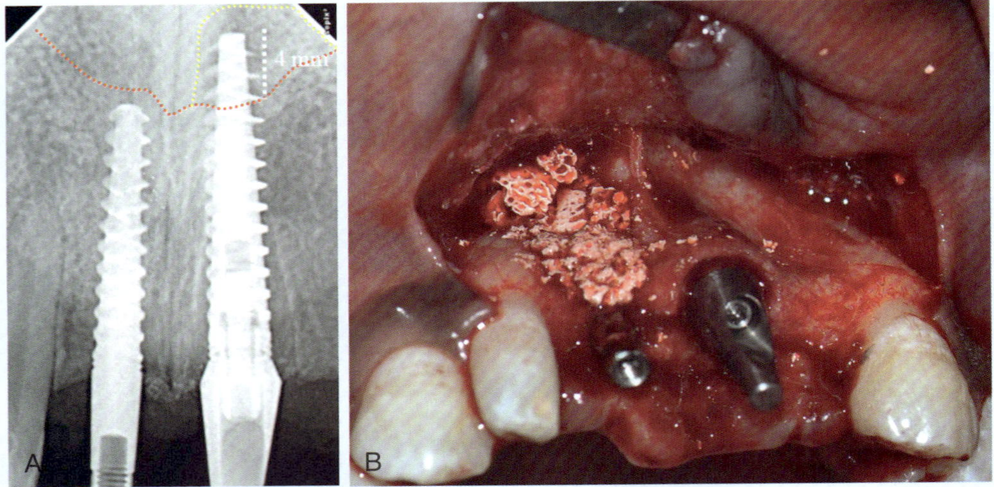

Fig 19.19 (A) Post implantation radiograph shows implant apex emerging 4 mm beyond the nasal floor and grafted nasal cavity. (B) Some amount of graft is deposited in the facial concavity to reinforce the thin facial plate and to improve the ridge morphology.

CASE REPORT-2—cont'd

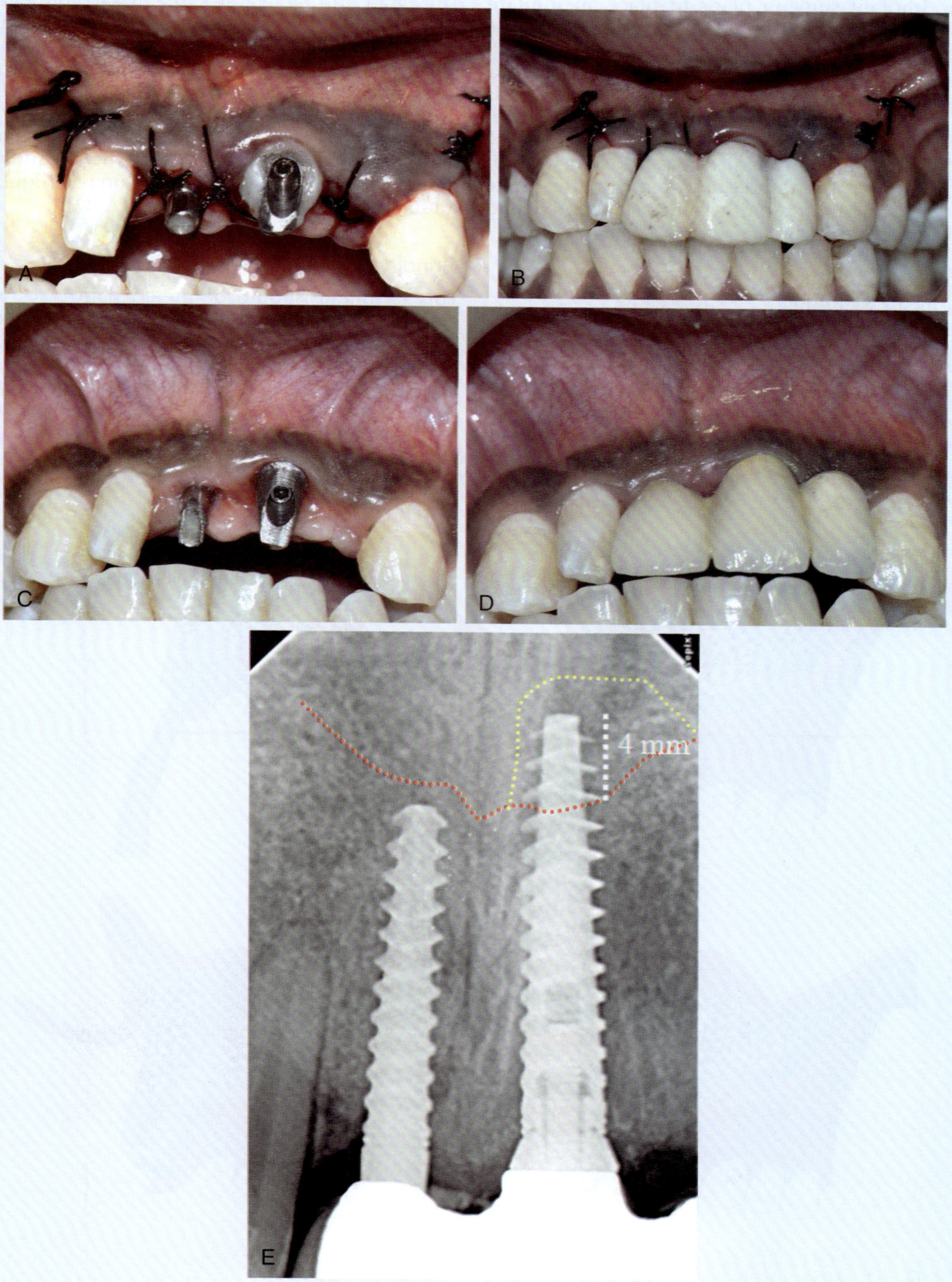

Fig 19.20 (A) Flap is sutured and (B) implants are immediately restored in function to restore the aesthetic as well as the functional demands of the patient. (C) Healing after 3 weeks. (D) Implants are restored with a definitive prosthesis after 6 weeks. (E) The radiograph 1 year after loading shows stable crestal bone level and consolidated bone graft at the nasal floor.

Continued

Closed technique (subcrestal approach)

Often the implant surgeon plans to place an implant with the flapless or by minimal flap elevation technique to minimize the soft tissue injury and post implantation complications like suture line opening, infection, etc. In such cases, a large amount of facial flap elevation is required only to access and graft the nasal floor. Therefore in such cases, the subcrestal approach can be the more appropriate and minimally invasive technique for the nasal floor elevation and grafting procedure. There are further two techniques for the subcrestal approach to the nasal epithelium:

a. Osteotome technique
b. Grinding up technique.

Osteotome technique

To perform this technique, the implant osteotomy is finished 1–2 mm short of nasal floor followed by use of an appropriate size osteotome to carefully fracture up the nasal floor. The bone substitute is introduced into the osteotomy and pushed up into the elevated nasal floor. This graft further elevates the nasal epithelium. After achieving desired nasal floor elevation and grafting, the implant is inserted with its apex emerging 3–5 mm above the nasal floor. This technique is indicated only in the cases where the nasal floor is thin and density of the nasal floor is poor to medium, so that it can be easily fractured using the osteotome. If the surgeon fails to fracture the nasal floor with controlled tapping, he/she should immediately switch over to the grinding up technique, to avoid trauma to the nasal floor (Fig 19.21A–D).

Grinding up technique

This technique should be preferred in cases with thick and high-density nasal floor and also in the cases where the mental trauma of tapping is to be avoided. To perform this technique, the osteotomy for the planned implant is finished 1–2 mm short of the nasal floor. Then, the rest of the subnasal bone is ground up using a coarse round rotary diamond bur, DASK drill, or piezo diamond tip,

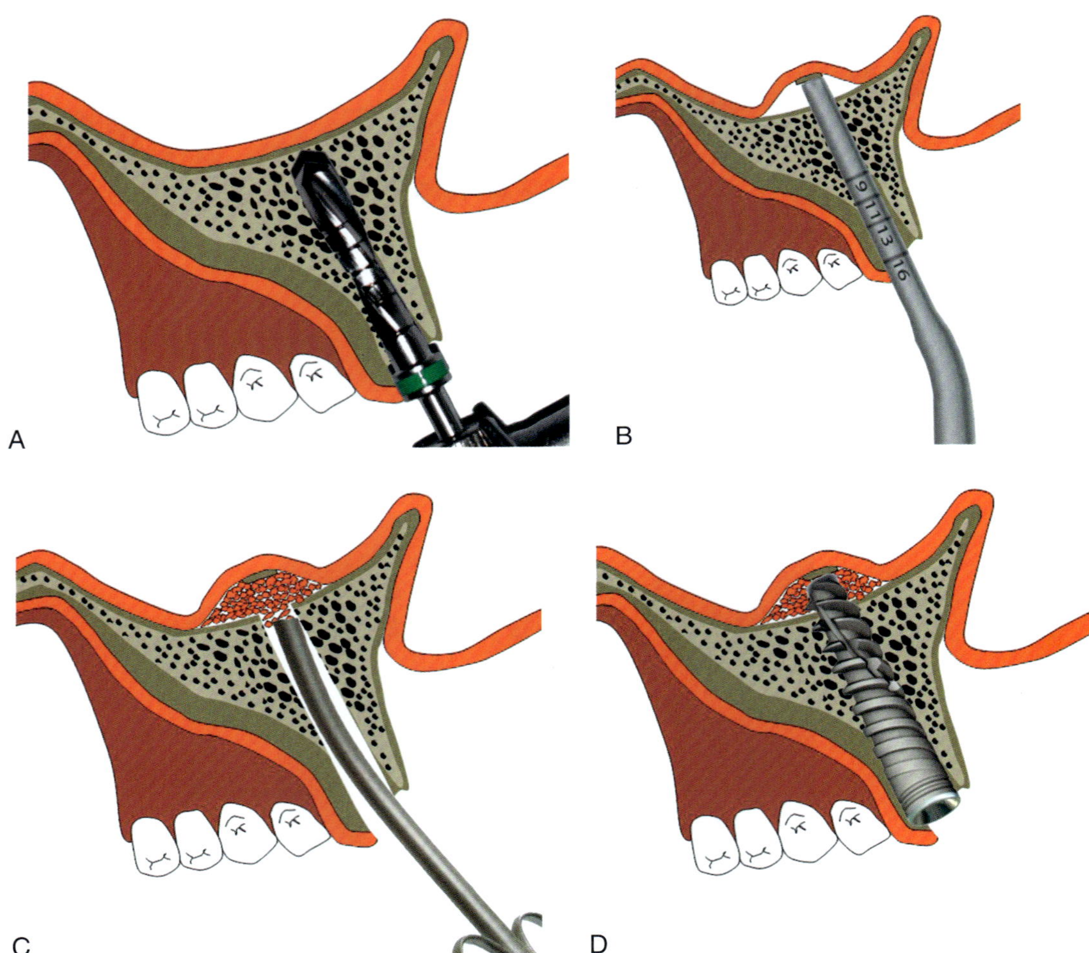

Fig 19.21 Step by step diagrammatic presentation of osteotome technique. (A) After completing the implant osteotomy preparation 1–2 mm short of nasal floor, (B) an appropriate size Summer's osteotome is used to fracture up the nasal floor. (C) Further, nasal floor elevation and grafting is achieved by filling the particulated graft through the prepared osteotomy and condensing it, using the same osteotome. (D) Once the nasal floor has been elevated and grafted, the implant is inserted in the usual manner.

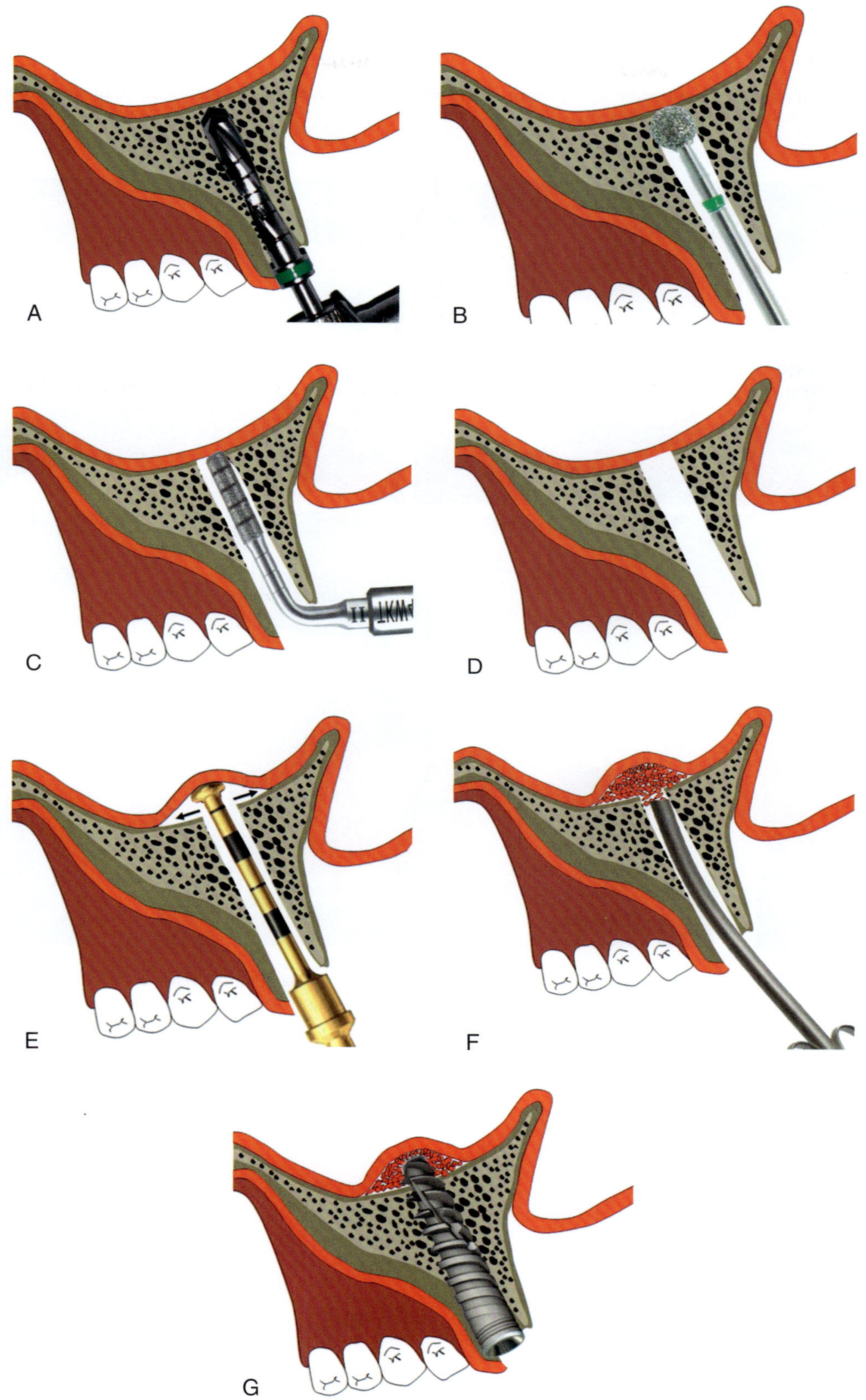

Fig 19.22 Step by step diagrammatic presentation of grinding up technique. (A) The osteotomy for the planned implant is finished 1–2 mm short of nasal floor. (B) Then, the rest of the subnasal bone is ground up using a coarse round rotary diamond bur, DASK drill, or (C) piezo diamond tips to reach the (D) nasal epithelium. (E) Further, the nasal epithelium is carefully elevated through the prepared osteotomy, using an umbrella-shaped elevator or depth probe. (F) The bone graft is introduced and pushed up to the nasal floor which further elevates the nasal mucosa. (G) Then, the implant is inserted in the usual fashion with its apex emerging into the nasal cavity which also keeps tenting the nasal epithelium and so maintains the space for new bone formation at the grafted nasal floor.

CASE REPORT-3

Immediate implant with nasal floor elevation and grafting with subcrestal grinding technique followed by immediate restoration of implants in function (Figs 19.23 and 19.24).

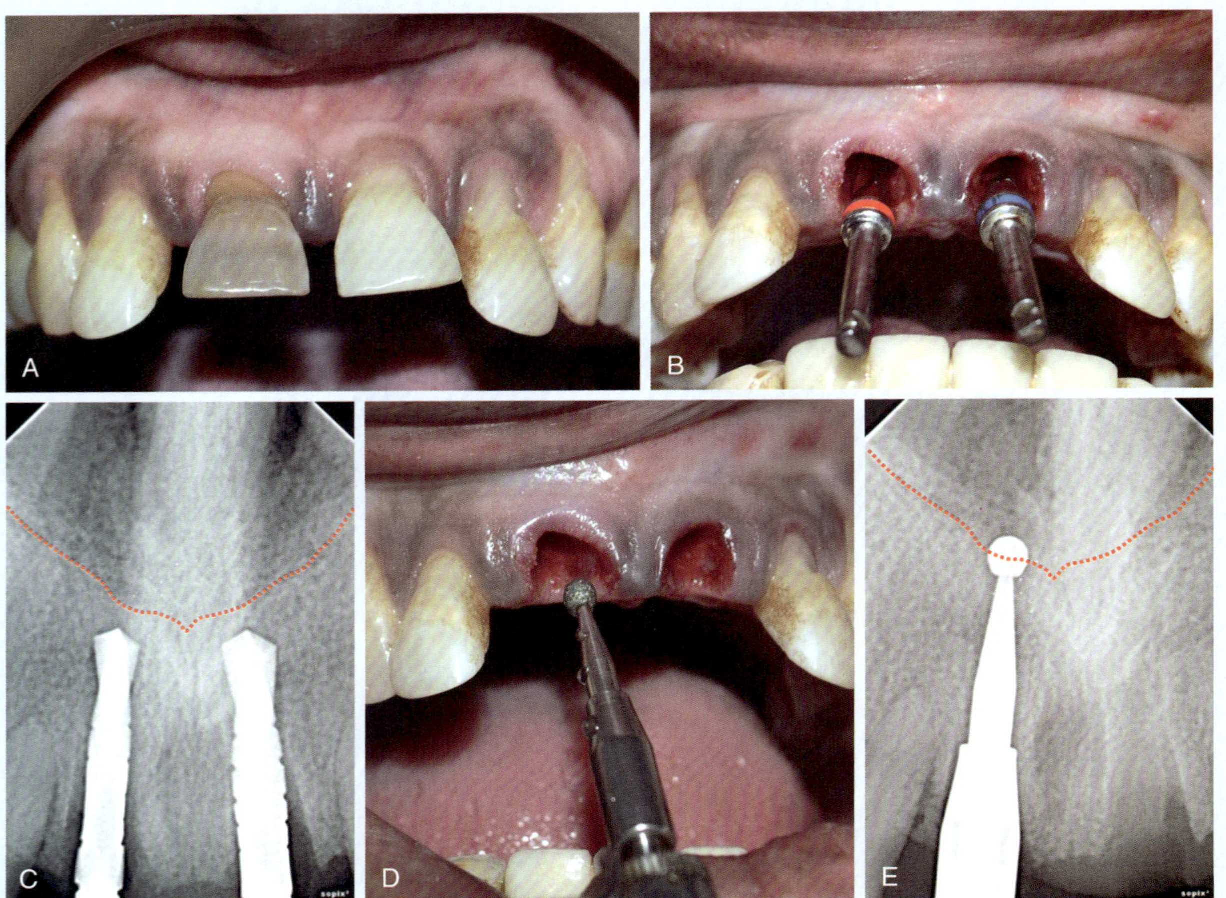

Fig. 19.23 (A) Maxillary central incisors with grade 2 mobility because of lost periodontal support. (B and C) The teeth are extracted with minimum trauma, and implant osteotomies are prepared 2 mm short of nasal floor. (D and E) A round diamond bur is then used to carefully grind up rest of the nasal floor to reach the nasal epithelium.

CASE REPORT-3—cont'd

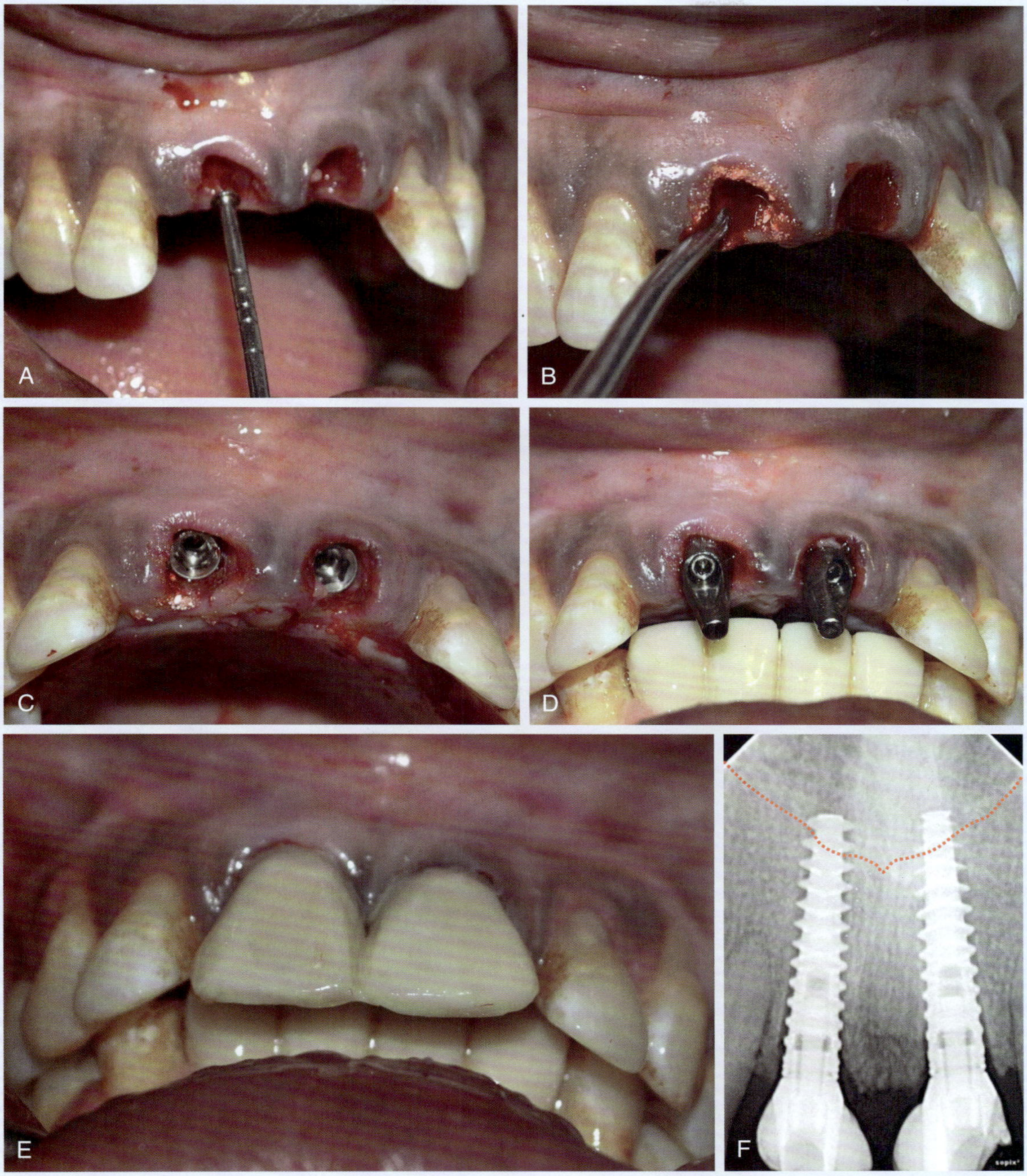

Fig 19.24 (A) After grinding up the nasal floor to reach the nasal epithelium, the depth probe with umbrella-shaped tip at its end is used to carefully elevate the nasal epithelium. (B) Further, the elevated nasal floor is grafted through the prepared osteotomy and (C) implants are inserted. (D) The abutments are placed on the top of the implants and (E) implants are restored immediately in function. (F) The post surgery radiograph shows that the apex of both implants have been well stabilized into the nasal floor.

Continued

CASE REPORT-4

Immediate implant with nasal floor elevation and grafting with subcrestal osteotome technique followed by immediate restoration of implant in function.

A 30-year-old female patient presented with soft tissue granulation on the facial aspect of the tooth number 21. The dental radiograph revealed root caries, which had grossly decayed the cervical portion of the root. Root canal therapy and the post and core approach were tried first but the canal in the apical half was found calcified, compromising the long-term survival of the tooth. So, the decision was taken to remove the tooth and follow through with immediate implant placement in the socket. The patient also requested that she would like allowed to go out after the implant surgery, with the provisional crown on the implant. So there were a few challenges in this case to achieve a predictable outcome. They are:

1. Only 3 mm of bone was present, as seen in the radiograph, between the root apex and the nasal floor. If the implant is placed with the conventional protocol, the implant should be placed 2 mm short of nasal floor. In that case, initial stability to the implant could have been inadequate to immediately restore the implant. Thus to achieve adequate implant stability, besides using adequate size implant to engage its threads along the socket walls, it was decided to perform the nasal floor elevation procedure, so that the implant apex could be stabilized in the high-density nasal floor.
2. Another challenge was the soft tissue level of the free gingiva on the facial aspect, which had shifted about 4 mm apical to the ideal position. Usually epithelialized connective tissue grafting is performed in such cases but as three-dimensional blood supply was available at the site the author decided to go with minimally invasive flapless implant surgery, supporting the soft tissue in original form and shape so that the lost tissue could be regenerated in a few weeks.

Step by step clinical case presentation is shown in Figs 19.25–19.32.

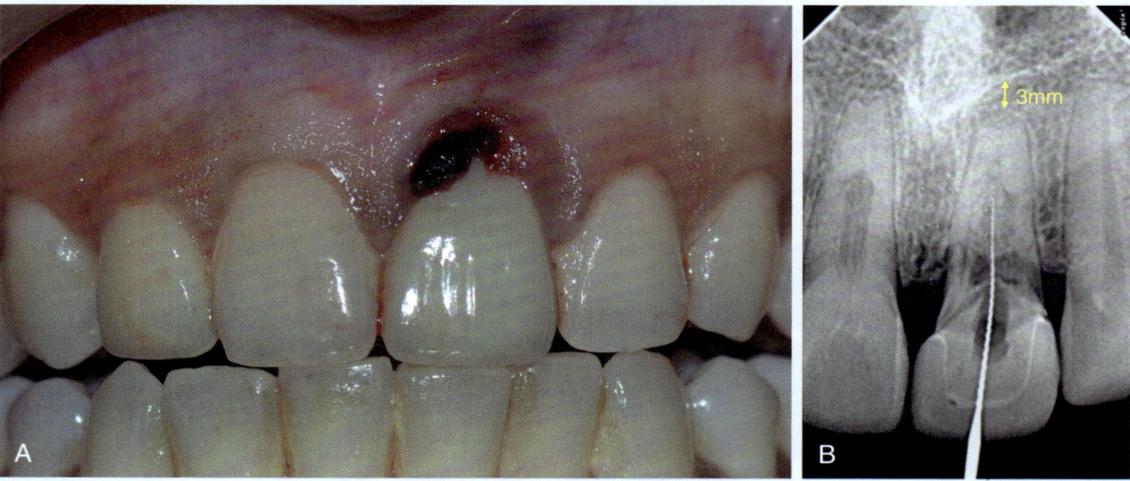

Fig 19.25 (A) Tooth number 21 with the visible soft tissue granulation at the facial aspect. (B) Radiograph revealed large root caries, calcified canal at the apical half and only 3 mm bone apical to the root.

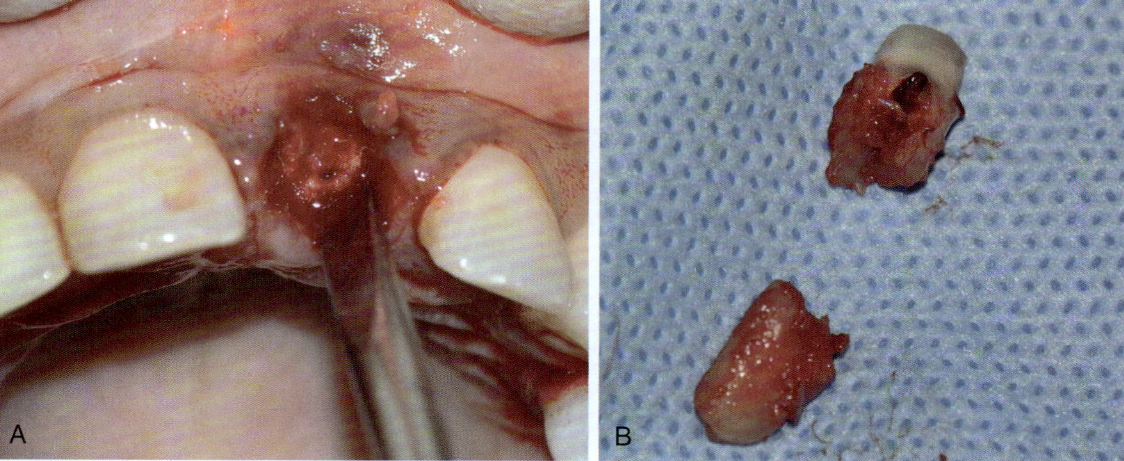

Fig 19.26 (A and B) Tooth is carefully extracted using periotomes and luxators with minimum trauma to the osseous structure and soft tissues.

CASE REPORT-4—cont'd

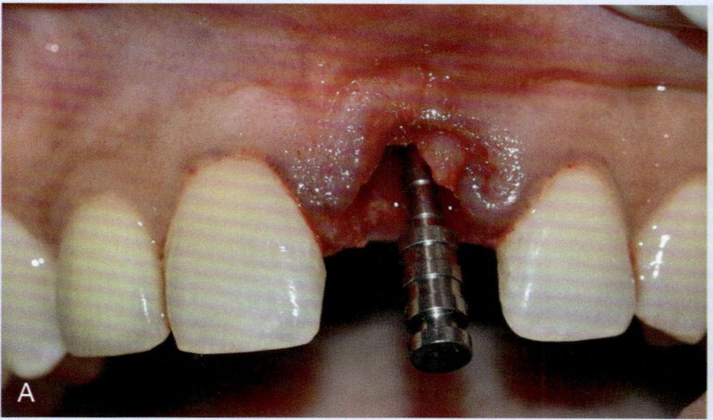
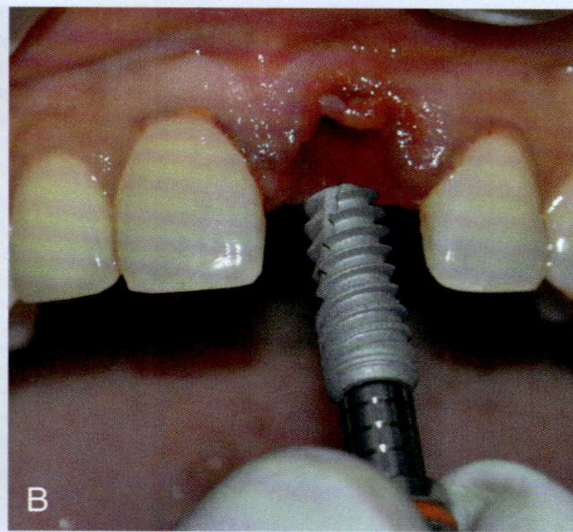

Fig 19.27 Implant osteotomy is prepared with the correct axis; nasal floor is elevated with the subcrestal socket lift technique using osteotomes (subcrestal closed osteotome technique) and a tapered 5 × 11.5 mm implant is inserted. (A and B) Implant achieved initial stability of more than 35 Ncm.

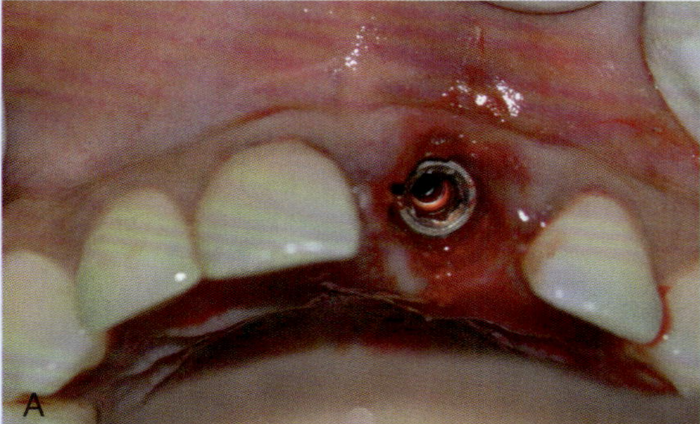
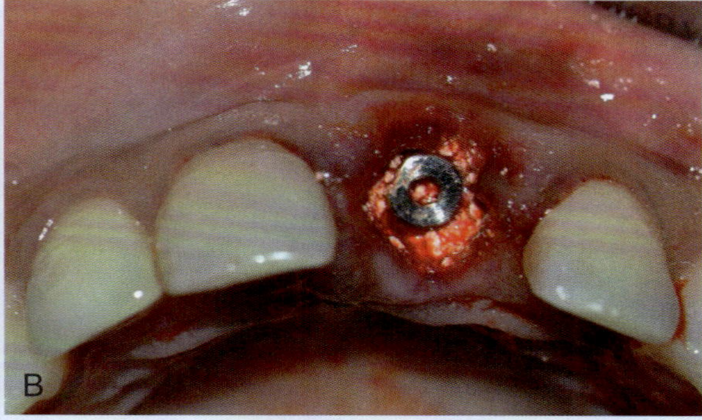

Fig 19.28 (A) Implant at the final position. (B) The peri-implant socket spaces are loosely filled using HA + β-TCP bone graft.

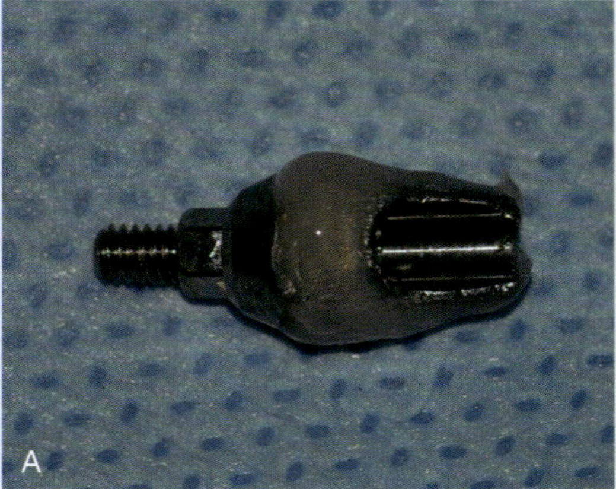
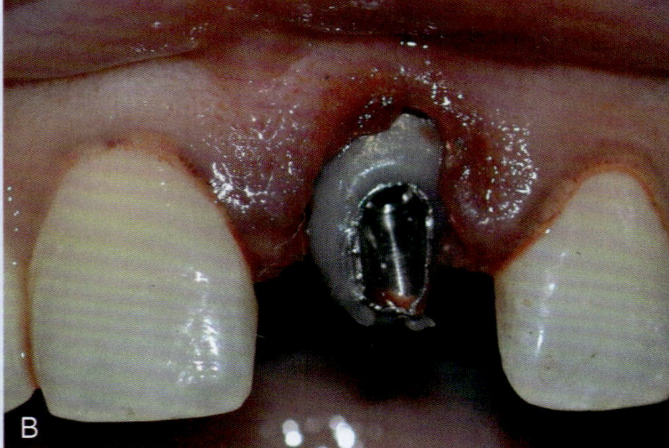

Fig 19.29 (A and B) A modified custom abutment is screwed over the implant.

Continued

CASE REPORT-4—cont'd

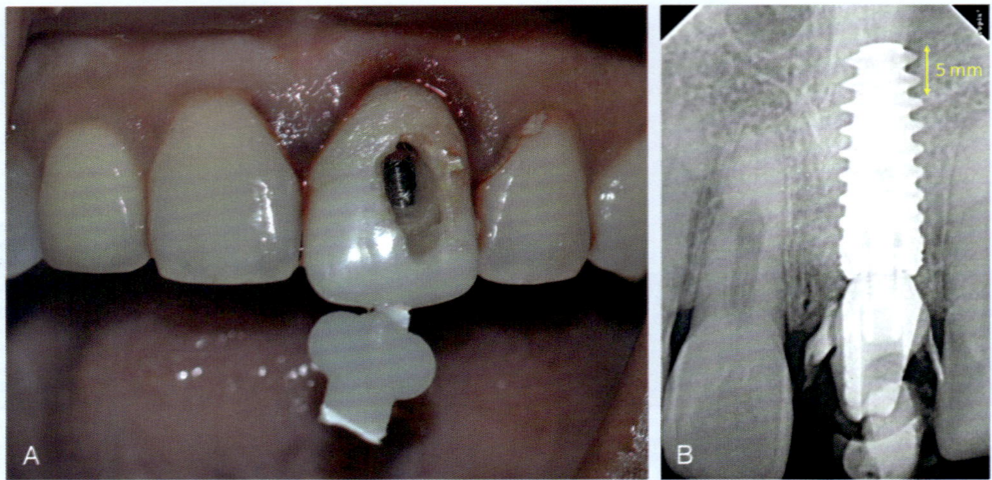

Fig 19.30 (A) A provisional crown is fixed over the abutment immediately after implant insertion and the screw hole is closed using composite. (B) Post implant surgery radiograph shows elevated nasal floor and implant apex stabilized in the nasal floor.

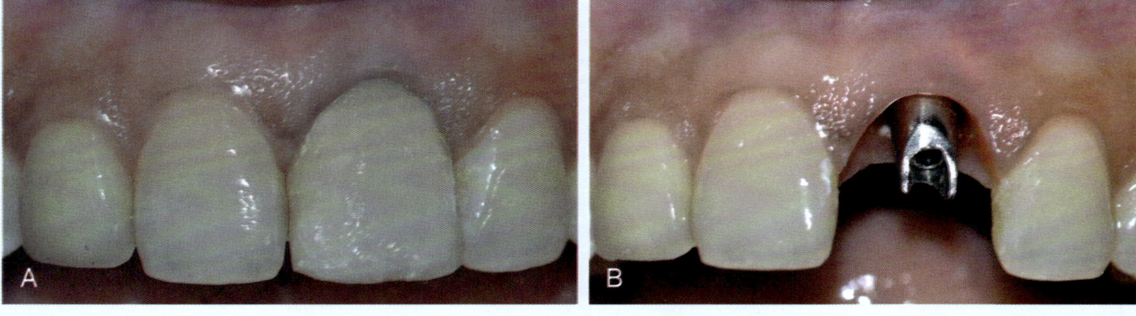

Fig 19.31 (A and B) Immediate and continued anatomical support and maintenance of the blood supply to the marginal soft tissue has regenerated it to the desired level in 6 weeks.

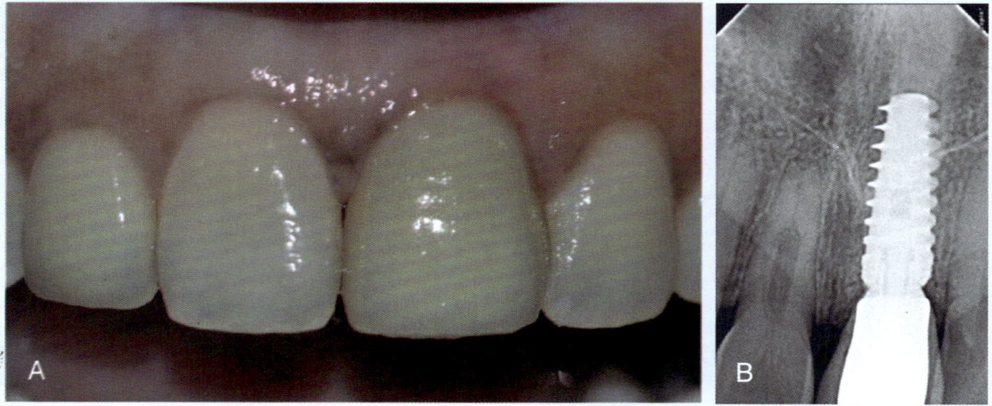

Fig 19.32 (A) The implant is restored early using a cement-retained zirconium crown. (B) The radiograph 1 year after the restoration shows stable crestal bone level and consolidated nasal floor graft.

to reach the nasal epithelium. Further, the nasal epithelium is carefully elevated through the prepared osteotomy using an umbrella-shaped elevator or depth probe. The bone graft is introduced and pushed up to the nasal floor which further elevates the nasal mucosa. Then, the implant is inserted in the usual fashion with its apex emerging into the nasal cavity, which also keeps tenting the nasal epithelium and so maintains the space for new bone formation at the grafted nasal floor (Fig 19.22A–G).

Complications

Bleeding

A strip about 1.5 mm wide covering a region of wide and long capillary loops, known as Kiesselbach's plexus, is found at the junction between the squamous epithelium of the nasal vestibule and the respiratory epithelium of the nasal cavity. This plexus extends to the lower and central part of the cartilaginous septum and is a common region for nose bleeding. Any injury to this plexus by implant drill or any instrument can lead to profuse bleeding. Nasal floor elevation and grafting is usually limited anterior to this plexus. However, if bleeding occurs, which is very rare in nasal floor grafting, it can be controlled by packing the nasal cavity for 20–30 min, with a cotton roll lightly coated with petroleum jelly. The bleeding can also be controlled using absorbable gelatin sponge (Ab Gel), electrocautery, etc.

Tearing of nasal mucosa/implant exposed in the nose

The nasal mucosa is generally thicker and more resistant to tearing, compared with the maxillary sinus mucosa. The chance of its tearing is negligible during its elevation, however it can be perforated or torn by any sharp instrument, implant drill, implant with sharp apex, etc. Nasal mucosal tearing can result in bacterial infiltration from the nasal cavity to the implant site. The torn mucosa should be sutured with watertight closure. Occasionally, the implant apex can perforate the nasal mucosa during the surgery or years later due to continuous pressure from underneath the nasal mucosa, especially in cases where the implant apex protrudes through the nasal floor without nasal floor grafting. The threaded implant apex protruding out of the nasal mucosa may capture mucosal scabs and cause foul odour or rhinosinusitis. A bone grafting of the nasal floor before implant insertion decreases this risk. However, when this occurs to a rigid implant, an implant apicoectomy can be performed to remove the protruding apex of the implant.

Implant mobility

The inserted implant can be mobile if it is not secured well with adequate initial stability. The implant may also show mobility because of retrograde pressure, if the patient places a finger in the nose. The loose implant should be removed and if not infected, another bigger diameter implant can be inserted immediately with adequate primary stability.

Maxillary sinus perforation

During the nasal floor elevation and implant insertion for maxillary canine position, the implant drill or the implant apex may inadvertently penetrate through the anterior wall of the maxillary sinus. If this occurs, either the implant insertion can be delayed or the sinus membrane can be elevated at the perforation area through the lateral approach and grafted with simultaneous implant insertion.

Summary

Nasal floor elevation and grafting can be a valuable procedure to stabilize the implant apex in the high-density nasal floor for the purposes of stabilizing the implant in immediate implant cases or in cases with large osseous defects, which are unfavourable to achieve adequate implant stability. A 3–5 mm, longer-than-usual implant can be inserted by the nasal floor elevation procedure. In several maxillary anterior implant cases, high primary stability can be achieved if the implant is stabilized in the high-density nasal floor so that the aesthetics of the patient can be immediately restored with implant-supported provisional prosthesis. Stabilizing implants in the nasal floor in full-arch cases may provide adequate stability to immediately restore the implants with a full-arch splinted prosthesis. The open technique should be preferred in the cases where the flap needs to be raised for implant insertion and also in the cases where multiple implants need to be stabilized in the nasal floor with a large volume of nasal floor grafting to place adequately long implants in the severely resorbed maxilla. The grinding up technique should be preferred in the closed subcrestal approach as it avoids inadvertent trauma to the nasal cavity and the mental trauma caused to the patient by tapping. The subcrestal approach should be preferred in the cases where flapless implant insertion has been planned. Irrespective of the approach, osteotomy preparation and nasal floor elevation should be performed carefully and should be checked with radiographs for the position of the drill or osteotome in respect to the nasal floor.

Further Reading

Mazor Ziv, Lorean Adi, Mijiritsky Eitan, et al. Nasal floor elevation combined with implant placement. Clin Implant Dent Relat Res, Volume, November, 2010.

Rubo de Rezende ML, de Melo LG, Hamata MM, et al. Particulate inlay nasal graft with immediate dental implant placement in a patient with repaired alveolar cleft: case report. Implant Dent 2008;17:332–8.

Higuchi K. Bone grafting into the nasal floor. In: Worthington P, Branemark PI, editors. Advanced osseointegration surgery, application in the maxillofacial region. Chicago: Quintessence; 1992.

Misch CM, Misch CE, Resnik RR, et al. Reconstruction of maxillary alveolar defects with mandibular symphysis grafts for dental implants: a preliminary procedural report. Int J Oral Maxillofac Implants 1992;7:360–6.

Kahnberg KE, Nystrom E, Bartholdsson L. Combined use of bone grafts and Branemark fixtures in the treatment of severely resorbed maxillae. Int J Oral Maxillofac Implants 1989;4:297.

Nkenke E, Kloss F, Whitfag J, et al. Histomorphometric and fluorescence microscopy analysis of bone remodeling after installation of implants using an osteotome technique. Clin Oral Implants Res 2002;13:595–602.

Jensen J, Krantz-Simonsen E, Sindet-Pedersen S. Reconstruction of the severely resorbed maxillary with bone grafting and osseointegrated implants – a preliminary report. J Oral Maxillofac Surg 1990;48:27–32.

Branemark PL, Adell R, Albrektsson T, et al. An experimental and clinical study of osseointegrated implants penetrating the nasal cavity and maxillary sinus. J Oral Maxillofac Surg 1984;42:497–505.

Keller EE, Tolman CE, Eckert SE. Maxillary antral-nasal inlay autogenous bone graft reconstruction of compromised maxilla: a 12-year retrospective study. Int J Oral Maxillofac Implant 1999;14:707–21.

Keller EE, Eckert SE, Tolman DE. Maxillary antral and nasal one-stage inlay composite bone graft: preliminary report on 30 recipient sites. J Oral Maxillofac Surg 1994;52:438–47.

Ivanoff CH, Grondahl K, Bergstrom C, et al. Influence of bicortical or monocortical anchorage on maxillary implant stability: a 15-year retrospective study of Branemark system implants. Int J Oral Maxillofac Implants 2000;15:103–10.

Chanavaz M. Maxillary sinus: anatomy, physiology, surgery, and bone grafting related to implantology – eleven years of surgical experience (1979–1990). J Oral Implantol 1990;16:199–209.

Jensen J, Sindet-Pederson S, Oliver AJ. Varying treatment strategies for reconstruction of maxillary atrophy with implants: results in 98 patients. J Oral Maxillofac Surg 1994;52:210.

Tatum OH. Maxillary and sinus implant reconstruction. Dent Clin North Am 1986; 30:209–29.

Lang J. Clinical anatomy of the nose, nasal cavity and paranasal sinuses. New York: Thieme; 1989.

Dahlin C, Lekholm U, Becker W, et al. Treatment of fenestration and dehiscence bone defects around oral implants using the guided tissue regeneration technique: a prospective multicenter study. Int J Oral Maxollofac Implants 1995;10:312–8.

Misch CE, Dietsh F. Endosteal implants and iliac crest grafts to restore severely resorbed, totally edentulous maxillae – a retrospective study. J Oral Implantol 1994;20:100–10.

Lundgren S, Nystrom E, Milson H, et al. Bone grafting to the maxillary sinuses, nasal floor and anterior maxilla in the atrophic edentulous maxilla: a two-stage technique. Int J Oral Maxillofac Surg 1997;26:128–434.

Immediate loading using basal implants

20

Stefan KA Ihde Antonina Ihde

CHAPTER CONTENTS HD

Introduction

The traditional procedure in dental implantology is based on the placement of large bullet-shaped implant bodies into the jawbone. The position of these implants coincides typically with the position of the former teeth in order to create an 'emerging profile'. As many patients do not provide the necessary amounts of bone in the designated position, often bone augmentations are performed. In the clinical reality however, a great many patients remain untreated or get only a partial treatment if the treatment provider offers only this traditional approach. There are several reasons for this:

1. A number of patients refuse a treatment protocol with several surgical steps and waiting times.
2. A large number of patients (e.g. smokers, medically impaired patients, patients with profound periodontal involvement) are being excluded from dental implant therapy because they do not qualify for bone augmentation procedures.
3. An increasing number of patients refuse bone augmentations, because the (true) rumour has spread, that inclusion into this treatment protocol makes the outcome unpredictable.

Hence, when using traditional dental implants, a considerable group of patients are either refused full treatment or they refuse the treatment offered. To be specific, patients with pronounced atrophy, i.e. those who would require dental implant treatment most, are left untreated. This is a unique situation in dentistry.

Today 'basal implantology' is able to address and solve all these issues and provide help for the most-compromised patient group.

Devices and insertion technique of lateral and screwable basal implants

Basal implants belong to the group of osseointegrated implants. Their common features are:

1. Cortical positioning of load transmitting implant areas

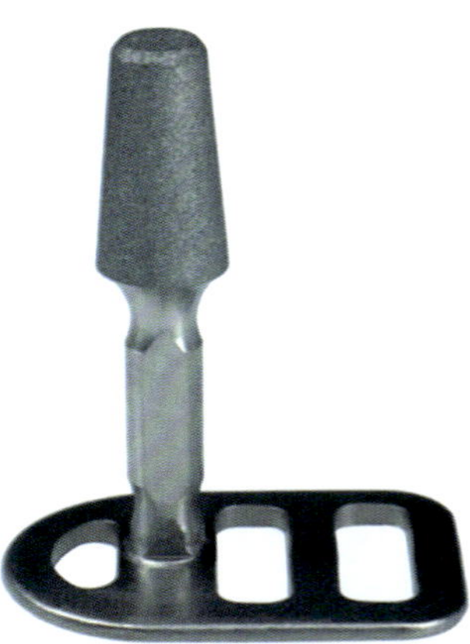

Fig 20.1 A one-piece lateral basal implant (BOI) for insertion into the basal jawbone. This implant features two bending zones along the vertical shaft. The fracture-proof design of the base plate was introduced in 2002. In this design the prosthetic construction is cemented.

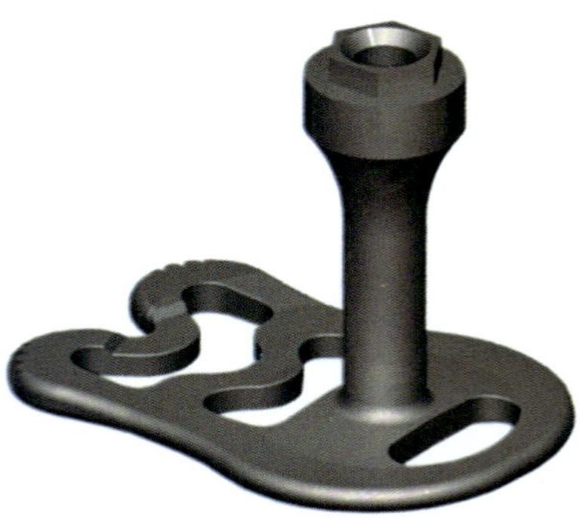

Fig 20.3 A lateral basal implant for screw-connection (TOI® IE). This type is compatible to the standard external hex 2.7 mmd. The implant provides a platform of 3.7 mm.

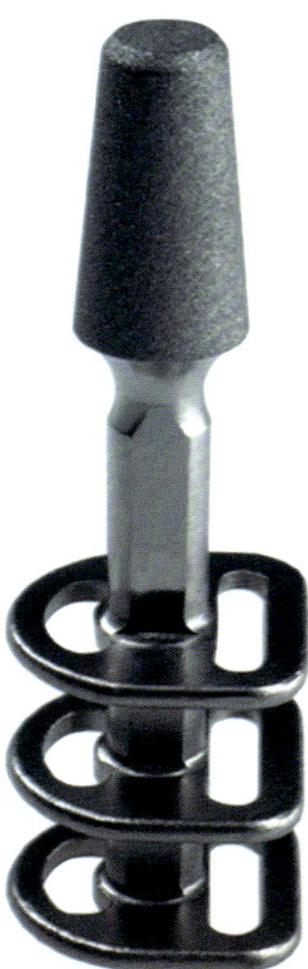

Fig 20.2 Triple BOI implant (BBB 7 H6) for multicortical anchorage. This design is frequently used in the area of the canines in both jaws. For triple base plate implants the term 'basal implant' is misleading, as of course only one or at maximum two base plates can be actually positioned in the basal bone. The surgeon should position the implant in such a way, that as many as possible base plates get engaged into the cortical bone.

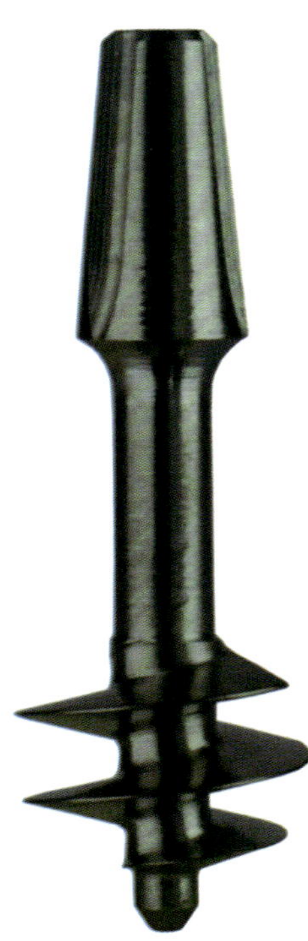

Fig 20.4 A one-piece basal screw implant (BCS®). The cortical load transmission is done through the large basal threads. These threads should be anchored in the cortical opposite to the crest. Some BCS implants provide lengthy grooves or holes in the threads for the in-growth of vessels or bone. Screwable basal implants are available in diameters 3.5–12 mm and in lengths of 10–38 mm. Load transmission along the polished vertical shaft is not required for the functioning of this type of implant. This implant features some structural elasticity, and masticatory loads are transmitted into the basal bone and into resorption-free bone areas.

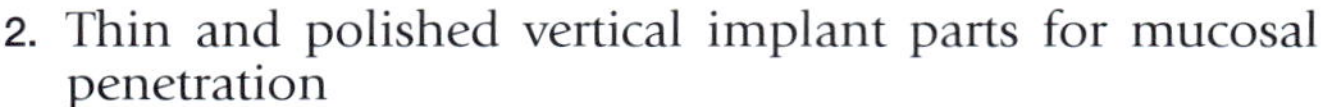

2. Thin and polished vertical implant parts for mucosal penetration
3. The usage of resorption-stable bone areas foranchorage
4. The possibility of immediate loading
5. Macro-mechanical anchorage
6. Immediate cortical osseointegration in the case of screwable basal implants (e.g. BCS®)
7. Gradual biological osseointegration (under immediate load conditions) in the case of lateral basal implants (e.g. BOI®) (Figs 20.1–20.8).

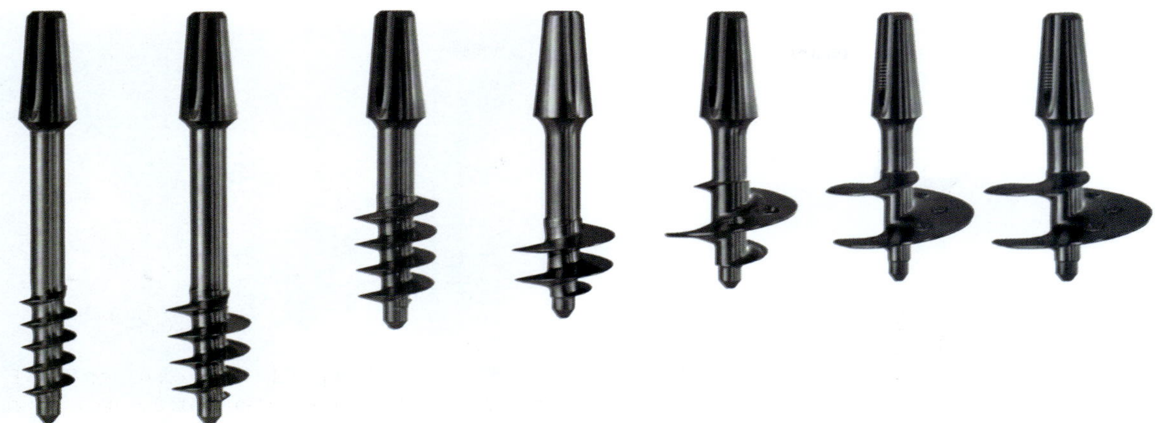

Fig 20.5 A large variety of BCS implants allow placement in all bone situations. Thereby either the width of the bone is utilized (through threads of 3.5–12 mm in width) or the height of the bone (through implants with 10–38 mm length), or both. Since only small bone cavities of 2–2.5 mm are drilled out, the threads have to compress the bone considerably. Therefore not all types of BCS implants can be inserted into the lower jaw with high mineralization (high density bone).

Insertion of screwable basal implants (tubero-pterygoid screw implants/GBC)

In the upper jaw, the opposing (second) cortical must be reached by the screw thread. The preparation is best done with a handgrip and the pathfinder drill, followed by a 2 mmd twist drill. This is the best way to find out the correct direction for the implant. To penetrate the second cortical, a tapping instrument is used (i.e. a Bein elevator). The quality of the bone can be evaluated through the sound of the taps.

In the lower jaw long tubero-pterygoid screw implants (i.e. BCS—diameter 3.5–4.6 mm; length 23–29 mm) are often used in the anterior region, while shorter but wider designs (i.e. 5.5 × 10–14 mm) are suitable in the posterior region. In many cases, the bone lateral and below the mylohyoid ridge forms an almost horizontal plate. This plate is suited perfectly as a second cortical.

Placement of lateral basal implants (BOI/TOI)

For lateral basal implants, the preparation of a full thickness flap is mandatory. Good vision on the bone surface must be given and all soft tissues including muscle attachments must be removed.

Treatment rationale in basal implantology

General comments

Conventional dental implantology has developed independently from the field of orthopaedic surgery and traumatology. In retrospective this was unfortunate, because both orthopaedic surgery and traumatology had discovered the secret of safe, immediate loading a long time ago, whereas dental implantology was still working with 'healing times', considering the importance of implant-surface alterations and bone augmentations.

The two main principles used in fracture treatment with plates and screws are bicortical or multicortical anchorage and immediate splinting of implants (Fig 20.8).

The principles of fracture treatment have been explained in textbooks. In surgical fracture treatment, immediate splinting (and thereby loading) is a pure necessity, because a second or third surgical approach through the skin and around often massive packages of muscle clearly must be avoided. In addition, every intervention is followed by massive swelling and the burdens of rehabilitation. Other than in the dental field, local resistance against infection in the long bones is poor and the occurrence of osteomyelitis is a realistic threat. Massive and long-lasting swellings occur and require intense postoperative care. In addition, such intervention requires surgery under total anaesthesia, which increases risks and costs. Hence, surgery on fractured long bones from early times aimed at one surgical intervention and immediate loading.

Another reason why 'immediate loading' was always the preferred method in traumatology and joint replacement is found in the nature of bone – immobilization quickly reduces the degree of mineralization, because the bone responds with strong remodelling both to increased and to decreased loads. Osteoporosis due to inactivity may reduce the overall mineralization of a patient's bone by 15% after 6 weeks. This is a dramatic figure and it shows how quickly bone responds. The response is invisible to our eyes.

In dental implantology, these problems are not of much concern, because resistance against infection in the jawbone and access to bone in the oral field are good. In living patients, jawbones never become inactive because even edentulous patients eat and carry out oral functions one way or another. Probably for this reason, dental patients were treated for decades, without concern of

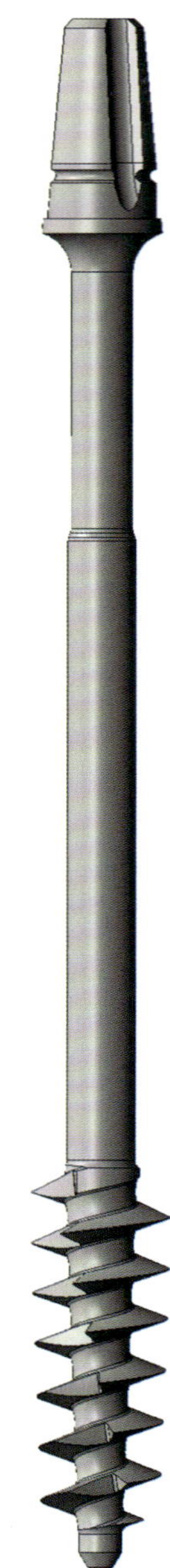

Fig 20.6 For use as zygoma implants, ZSI implants have been developed. They feature an aggressive thread for zygomatic anchorage and a bending zone near the abutment. The bending zone allows insertion from the palatal aspect of the maxillary alveolar crest and subsequent bending of the implant. This way the head reaches the crest and fits under the prosthetic construction. ZSI implants are available in lengths 35–50 mm and are used after preparing the bone with a twist drill 2.2 mm/50 mm. Both intrasinusal and extrasinusal placements are possible.

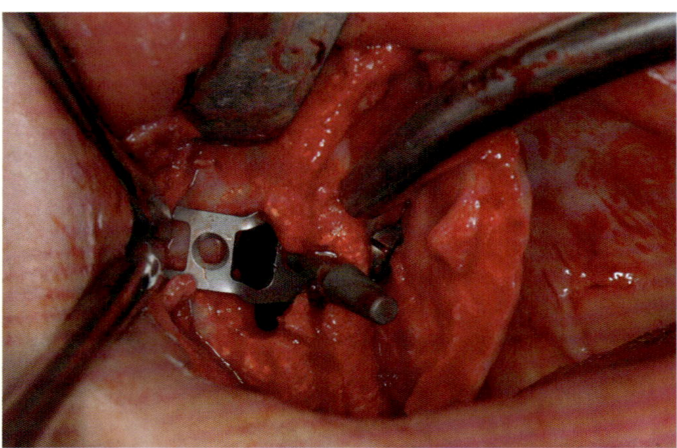

Fig 20.7 Transsinusal placement of a BOI-BAC implant, with vertical screw anchorage on the palatal bone, and before lateral screw anchorage on the lateral cortical of the maxillary sinus.

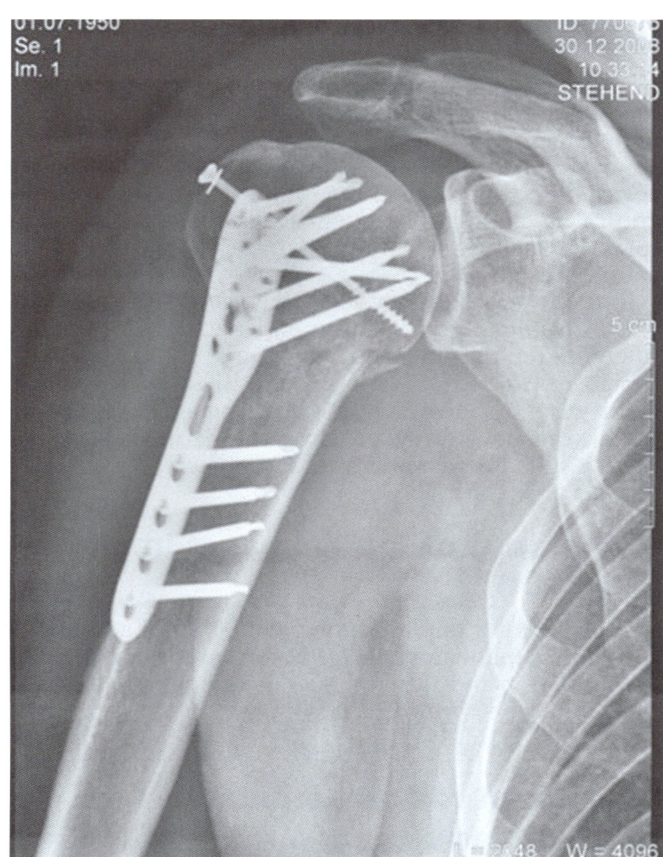

Fig 20.8 Treatment of the fracture of an upper arm in an immediate loading protocol. The positioning of the implant is strictly cortical (although some implants, due to the projection of the radiograph, seem to be without cortical anchorage). The implants are not placed parallel. The fracture plate allows immediate splinting of all implants.

infection, in two-stage protocols. It was actually increasing competition between dentists who made ‘immediate loading’ an issue. In addition, avoiding bone augmentations (including their cost and suffering) became a competitive advantage.

The ‘All-on-4’ concept and the inclusion of zygoma screw implants changed the situation a bit; however this treatment is accessible only through specialized treatment providers and involves extremely high overall costs for implants, central treatment support, and templates.

These issues have been solved by basal implantology.

The bone sets the clock

The 'healing' of bone starts 3 days after any bone surgery or fracture through a process of remodelling. Hence, within the first 3 days of surgery or fracture, a very stable type of bone becomes available. For this reason, the authors recommend insertion of the implant within this short period with prosthetic reconstruction, and recommend that it is left in place for a minimum of 6–9 months. This ensures that the remodelling ('healing') of the bone does not reduce its stability in the very critical phase before implants are splinted. During a metal try-in, the peri-implant bone around each single implant can be much more traumatized than during regular mastication while the implant is splinted.

Different ways to "osseointegration"

A few words must be spent on what is called 'osseointegration'. The term has been defined as 'direct contact between implant and bone'. The authors add that this contact must also be durable, whereas the degree of mineralization of the bony interface is not a criterion for successful osseointegration.

In the authors' view, at least three roads can lead to this desired result. Two of these roads take separate routes.

1. Traditionally, the active growth of bone towards the implant surface was considered to be the (only) way to achieve osseointegration. The process requires at least a minimal amount of space around the endosseous implant surface and it requires blood access to support the production of the **woven bone** matrix and its subsequent mineralization. Workers in the scientific field discussed the significance of specific implant surfaces and assumed that the 'healing time' could be brought down by altering or 'improving' the surfaces. All evidence presented for this theory was proved wrong. What is called the 'biologic osseointegration' definitely works, but it must be accepted that this pathway is not the only possible road. This process of gradual integration was never used in the field of orthopaedic surgery and its usage in dental implantology is unique. No rationale whatsoever supports the placement of dental implants in the worst bone available – the native spongious bone.

When observing implants after their osseointegration, it is found that mainly secondary osteons are in direct contact with the implant. These osteons have remodelled the primary woven bone or previous osteonal bone. Depending on whether direct matrix deposition as a function of woven bone takes place, or if there is direct integration through osteons, a small layer of what was called 'soft tissue' and is in fact the most peripheral collagen layer of the circumferential lamella of the osteon, is visible under the microscope. Workers in the scientific field have for decades been fighting about the question of direct bone-to-implant contact without understanding that different types of bone (woven bone, osteonal bone) yield different results when performing 'osseointegration'.

2. Orthopaedic surgeons always create direct contact between the implant and the cortical bone. Their treatment rationale coincides with the fact that defects in the cortical bone are always repaired, and consequently, implant bodies which are placed in the sphere of the corticals will be integrated almost regardless of the biocompatibility of the implant material and its surface.
3. Whenever spongious bone is compressed, its structure gets damaged and the degree of mineralization of this compressed bone is increased notably. Compression screws (e.g. single piece KOS®, or two-stage Hexacone®) utilize the stability which results out of this compression and they take advantage of the fact that the osteonal remodelling cannot have its origin in the compressed bone areas. Hence, compression screw implants like KOS and Hexacone provide grounds for a treatment protocol in immediate loading.

Treatment planning for basal implants

Diagnostics

Basal implants may be used as single tooth replacement by experienced treatment providers, but this application is not their central function. Excellent results are achieved if three or more implants are splinted in a segment or a full bridge. In selected situations two splinted implants can also be successful in an immediate loading protocol, and in a number of situations the trained implantologist can work even with single implants in this way. Although BOI implants are three-dimensional, the two dimensions shown on a panoramic radiograph are sufficient to plan a case. Three-dimensional planning is helpful to identify irregularities in the bones (i.e. leftover roots) and the true periodontal state of teeth. Often a three-dimensional exploration gives indications for additional extraction, thus making the case safer to treat and improving the overall prognosis.

Choice of implant sites

The resorption-stable areas in the jawbone are located as follows:

1. The nasal spine
2. The pterygoid plate of the sphenoid bone
3. The zygomatic bone
4. Bone caudal to the oblique line in the mandible
5. The bone of the floor of the nose
6. The laminae cribrosae of extraction sites

Depending on the pathway of past atrophy and changes in morphology, bone configurations which are not present in all patients, can be considered to be resorption-stable: the bone caudally to the attachment of the mylohyoid muscle on the lingual side of the mandible. This bone is easy to access, especially if this bone is provided (almost) horizontal. For providing additional stability in

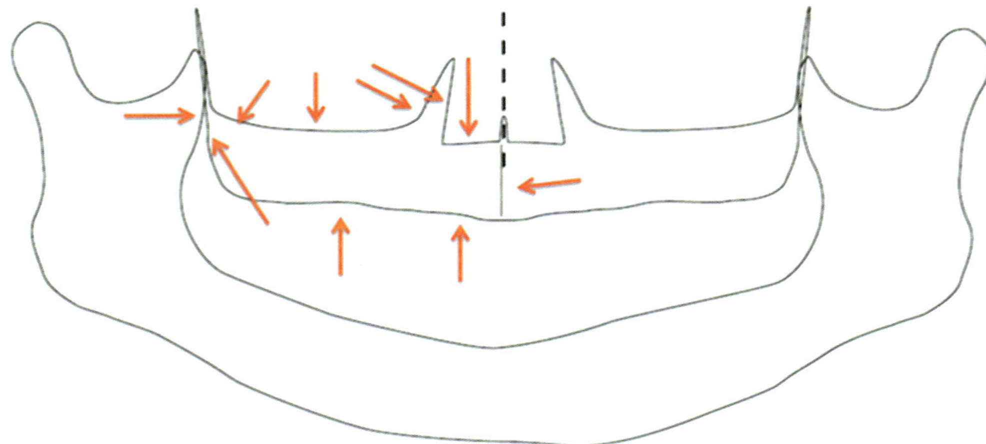

Fig 20.9 Visualization of accessible corticals in the right maxilla – besides the first (crestal) cortical all other corticals shown here can serve as second corticals. The bone in the area of the nasal spine (arrow from the right) is often through and through cortical – for this reason it is often unnecessary to reach the floor of the nose as second cortical. Note that in addition to the corticals shown here, the pterygoid plate of the sphenoid bone offers two more corticals for posterior support.

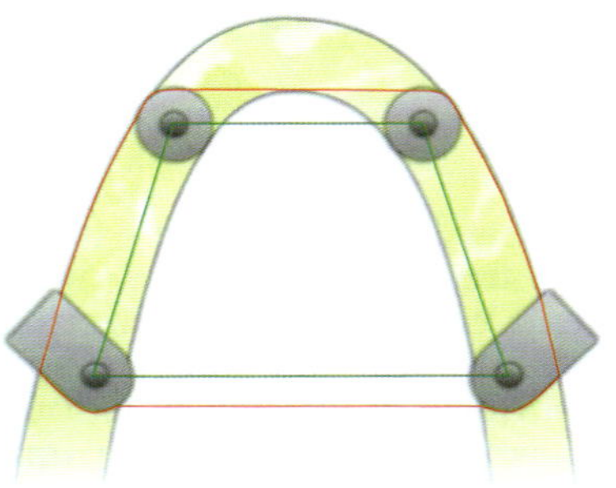

Fig 20.10 The supporting polygon around the disc plates of lateral basal implants (red circle) is much larger than the polygon marked by crestal (screw) implants (green circle). In this diagram, the implants are placed in the strategic positions of the canines and the second molars. Considering that most of the masticatory forces are exerted in the distal region, more implants in the anterior jaw will not help to cope with those forces nor will they increase the polygon significantly.

immediate loading cases, resorbable bone areas may also be used, although these areas are prone to remodelling and loss of their cortical properties (Fig 20.9).

Overall load distribution

In full bridges and in bridges following the tooth arch at least a little bit, the supporting polygon (Fig 20.10) must be considered. Lateral basal implants provide a larger supporting polygon than screwable implants. While the distal mandible usually provides enough cortical bone of high quality, the bone in the distal maxilla is poor. Hence, additional cortical support is required in the maxilla. BCS implants and (in cases of extreme atrophy) zygoma implants provide the required amount of reliable and stable cortical retention.

BCS/GBC and zygoma (ZSI) implants

Implants which are anchored both in the maxillary bone and in the sphenoid bone can anchor up to four corticals – they penetrate the crestal cortical of the maxilla, the distal cortical of the maxilla, and up to two corticals marking the pterygoid plate. The technique of placing these screws is a bit tricky to learn, because the surgeon's brain has to imagine bone regions, which are not visibly available on conventional radiographs or in the reality of the surgical intervention. In most cases, the experienced surgeon will be able to place these screws without preparing a flap, simply by palpating the medial hamulus of the pterygoid plate and by observing the anatomy of the distal maxilla. If a flapless approach fails, a small flap will reveal details of the anatomy and allow placement of this implant without problems. In some cases, the approach towards the sphenoid bone requires trespassing the maxillary sinus and even the Schneiderian membrane with the thin and polished implant. The procedure is feasible to the surgically trained dentist as well as to the oral or maxillofacial surgeon.

The usage of zygoma implants (ZSI) or BCS implants in the area of the zygomatic bone requires a profound knowledge of anatomy. Today both the trans sinusal approach and the subperiosteal approach are recognized. In any case, the implant must be anchored rigidly in the zygomatic bone and immediately splinted. In circular bridges, zygoma implants are connected to two to four anterior implants. In the lateral segment bridges, ZSI implants may be considered in combination with BCS implants and implants placed oblique, anterior to the maxillary sinus (e.g. BCS). This way stability against lateral forces stemming from all directions is obtained.

The advantage of using ZSI implants in the zygoma region compared to traditional bullet-shaped implants is that the bendable neck of the ZSI implant can be aligned with the tooth arch, even though the implant projects out of the palatal side of the crest. Although the

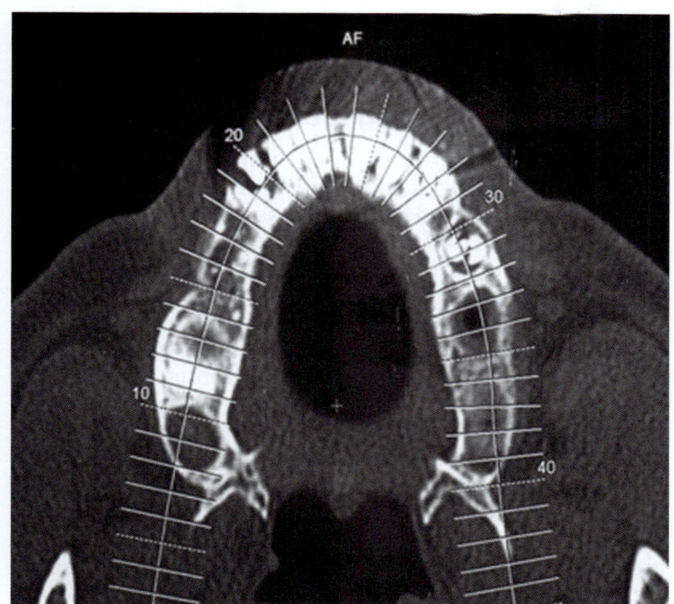

Fig 20.11 During the growth of the skull, the distance between the two pterygoid processes remains constant quite early in childhood, while the maxilla still grows. One motor of this growth are the teeth. Because the maxilla is attached to the pterygoid plate, this growth occurs in transversal direction and the maxilla becomes rounded – tubero-pterygoid screw implants are hence inserted in a medial and distal direction. After the teeth are lost, the morphology however changes. In very atrophic jawbones the direction of insertion for the tubero-pterygoid screw implant is predominantly distal, and is not or is very little directed towards the medial. Tubero-pterygoid screw implants can utilize four corticals if placed correctly – the crestal (first) and distal (second) cortical of the maxilla and the anterior (third) and posterior (fourth) cortical of the sphenoid bone. In case that the maxillary sinus is trespassed by the implant, another two corticals contribute to stability.

technique is really special and not included in general teaching in any dental speciality, it cannot be assumed, in general, that this implant technique is to be restricted to maxillofacial or oral surgeons. The technique requires profound knowledge of the anatomy of the skull. The treatment provider must be able to manage complications which may occur 'one floor higher up', and in any case full anaesthesia will often be a necessary part of the treatment plan (Fig 20.11).

Concepts for full bridges

It is recommended that implants be placed in the strategic positions of the canines and the second molars. The area of the first molars in the upper jaw is not a recommended area for implant placement, unless intrasinusal buttresses maintain bone height and provide additional triangulated cortical support. Without these buttresses, the bone in this area is prone to bidirectional resorption (maxillary expansion and alveolar atrophy) and hence should be avoided.

The placement of a BCS implant is always part of the treatment plan. Often two implants may be placed in this region. One of them will reach the distal cortical of the maxilla and often the pterygoid plate, whereas the anterior BCS utilizes the basal cortical of the maxillary sinus.

Additional implants between the canines and between the canines and tuberosity will increase overall stability and compensate in the event of error. They increase the amount of cortical anchorage and thereby improve the prognosis. Implants between the canines may be contraindicated however, when it comes to compensation of Angle class II and class III jaw relationships by means of prosthetics. In such cases, anterior implants may limit the freedom of the dentist technician, because the position of the implants is connected to the available bone between the canines, whereas the position of the teeth is better directed towards the teeth in the opposing dentition.

Concepts for unilateral bridge segments

The domain of basal implant is the distal mandible and the distal maxilla. In these areas, this technique helps patients the most. As immediately loaded constructions are typically based on at least three implants, space must be found for them.

Maxillary segments

Whenever the second and third molars are extracted, easy access for a BCS implant is given. For another posterior implant, the tuberosity is used again – either another BCS implant (e.g. 5.5 or 7 mmd) is applied or a lateral basal implant (e.g. BS 9H6 to 12H6) are placed. The area of the first molar should be left out. Anterior to the maxillary sinus, the third implant is placed. In cases where decayed and root canal treated premolars are present, these teeth should be extracted, as the prognosis of these teeth is bad and they block the access to the cortical to the nasal floor.

This concept seems rigorous. However, the authors can recommend following it without compromise. Leftover, ailing first premolars will lead to the necessity of corrective intervention sooner or later. Keep in mind that the prosthetic value of a premolar is reduced, and saving these teeth in cases where root canals are required, is often impossible. The prosthetic prognosis of canines (even if subjected to root canal treatment) is better. Therefore, we should include these teeth into an unilateral construction if needed. Another rationale for this decision is that the aesthetic outcome after singular extraction of upper canines is often unfavourable.

Mandibular segments

The treatment options in the mandible depend on the position of the nerve. In most cases, enough bone is present on top of the lower alveolar nerve. If it is not the case, the base plate of the basal implant can be placed below the nerve and can bypass the nerve with the vertical implant part. As an alternative, placement of short but wide BCS implants into the horizontal basal bone areas near the mylohyoid ridge, is an option. Distal to the mental nerve either one BAST 9/16 implant is utilized, or two implants with a smaller base plate. These are combined with at least one long BCS implant which bypasses the mental foramen and anchors in the basal mandibular bone. For this purpose, BCS implants providing a length of 20 mm and more are typically used.

Replacement of lower first molars

Decay and/or periodontal involvement is often the indication for an early first lower molar extraction. In such cases, therapy with a conventional dental implant is not immediately possible, because bone is lacking. We recommend replacing these teeth with two tilted BCS implants, one into each socket of the extracted tooth. BCS 3.5 or 3.6 mmd are the preferred ...options, the heads of the abutments are made parallel by bending the shaft. The key to success is cortical support for the basal thread of the implant. In most cases, the implant has to be inclined towards the lingual and hence the lingual cortical is used for anchorage (Fig 20.12 A–C). The width of the occlusal table should not exceed 6 mm, (i.e. the width of a premolar). This avoids off-axis loads and functional lateral excursions of the block of crowns and allows treatment in an immediate loading procedure with two implants only. If the vestibular bone is missing in one of the roots, the combination of one lateral basal implant (BOI) and one BCS implant gives a promising alternative. Note that bicortical support is necessary for the BOI implant. The rationale of using two implants to replace one tooth can be explained to the patient easily, because actually, two functional roots are replaced.

Replacement of upper second molars

When it comes to replacing the upper second molars, two implants are indicated. One implant – typically a BCS 5.5 mmd or larger – is positioned under the clinical crown of this tooth, while the second implant utilizes the bone of the tubero-pterygoid region. Both implants are splinted by the crown in an immediate loading procedure. In general, the authors do not recommend replacing a single molar by one basal implant only.

Inclusion of remaining teeth

In dental implantology the inclusion or exclusion of natural abutments into the construction has been discussed vigorously for decades. The opponents of such combinations claim that the elastic properties of teeth and implants are too different to allow such a combination, while the protagonists argue that the clinical reality is that this combination works.

The authors have found that combinations of teeth and basal implants yield good and stable results. On the other hand, they have also observed that in a considerable number of cases, decay of teeth has led to situations where bridges had to be removed and more implants were necessary. In such cases, the question of 'guarantee' is often raised by the patient. When planning the inclusion of natural teeth, the dental surgeon should ensure that the teeth are free of all decay, should not have been subject to root canal treatment, and should not have been restored with a crown. Including a second or third crown into constructions with implants is clearly not recommended, because the average lifespan of second crowns is well below 10 years, and the average lifespan of third crowns is well below 5 years. In other words, differences in elasticity (created by osseointegration of the implant and the fibrous ligament connection of the tooth) are not critical. The main concern is the expected durability of the construction.

A typical indication for successful combined construction is the replacement of chewing surfaces in the extremely atrophic distal mandible or maxilla, while all premolars are present.

The issue of these extractions and the reasons for leaving the teeth in and combining them with implants, should be discussed with the patient openly. For the treatment provider, who was taught for years to make tooth-saving efforts, it is astonishing that many patients (unexpectedly)

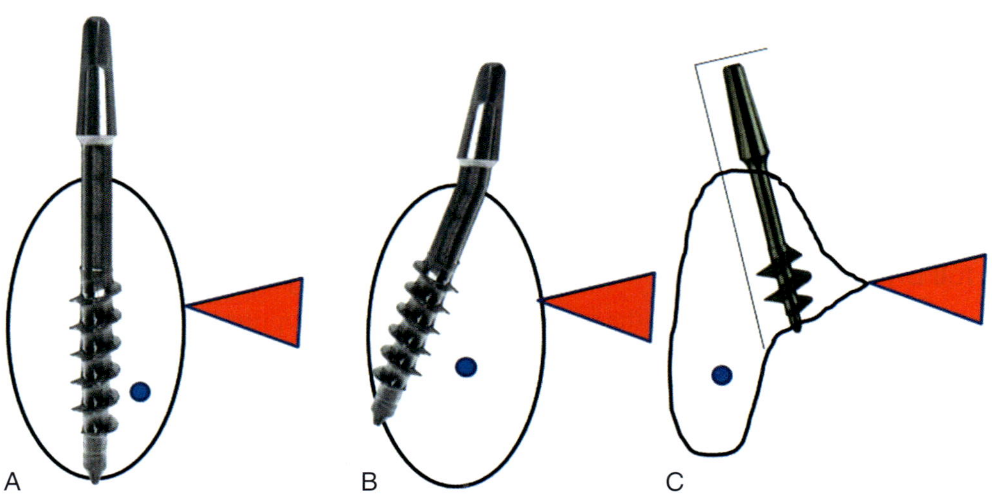

Fig 20.12 In the mandible a vast number of possibilities for the placement of BCS implants are given. (A) Usage of the crestal (first) and basal (second) cortical. (B) Usage of the highly mineralized vestibular (second) cortical with subsequent bending of the implant. (C) Quite often the bone lateral and caudal to the attachment of the mylohyoid muscle provides a suitable second cortical for the rest of a BCS implant.

want to have their teeth out, and have a clear and final switch to an implant-borne dentition.

Single tooth replacement

The use of lateral basal implants for single-tooth replacement, requires a very precise surgical approach. The reason for this is that once the horizontal osteotomy has been made, no change in height is possible; whereas a screw implant can be screwed deeper into the bone easily. This corrective step is not available for lateral implants. The only way to change the abutment height is to decide on a different implant with a longer or shorter shaft.

For replacing upper laterals and first premolars the 4T implants were developed – they feature three base plates of 5 × 7 mm and are inserted with the small side ahead. Hence, the osteotomy is prepared using a 5 mm triple cutter.

If more space is available, larger implants can be used. However, in general, triple-base plate implants are recommended. Whenever delayed or late load is planned, lateral basal implants with internal connection may be used and they heal in submerged mode.

Replacement of single teeth with single BCS implants is an option only if masticatory forces are really reduced and all loads leading to rotation are abandoned.

Contraindications

In dental literature, numerous contraindications stemming from general health problems have been discussed and should be considered. According to the authors' experience two main fields are important:

1. Patients who have undergone intravenous bisphosphonates treatment are not candidates for dental implant treatment, unless proof has been given that the function of their osteonal systems is not prevented, and remodelling can work.
2. Cases that do not allow stable mastication on both sides of the jaws and the positioning of a bilateral, equal masticatory table from 6-6 in both jaws, are not suitable for immediate loading treatment. The rationale behind this is that the chewing sides will develop quickly and the bone around implants on the chewing side will get overloaded.

The same will happen if general conditions (i.e. hemiparesis) prevents bilateral function. Therefore, such conditions are contraindications.

Disinfection and antibiotic regime

Although it has never been shown in reliable studies that antibiotic 'coverage' increases the success rates of dental implantology, administering these drugs is widely accepted. In basal implantology this is an option, especially to give moral support to the patient. Most patients are in good health and will easily cope with these drugs.

During the surgical procedure 10 g of amoxicillin (powder) may be added to the cooling liquid. This precaution is very effective because reasonable amounts of the drug really arrive and potentially work at the site of action.

In our view the use of Betadine (povidone-iodine) is extremely helpful, as it attacks bacterial fungi and viruses, across the board. It acts in less than 1 min. The authors rinse the insertion slots of lateral basal implants and the slots of crestal implants with this agent. The implants are bathed in this solution before placement, so that infections are prevented and good soft-tissue healing is achieved. The authors consider the application of Betadine to be by far more important than oral or intravenous antibiotic coverage.

Prosthetic procedures and considerations

Typically impressions are taken immediately after implant placement. The impression copings are either screwed on (for TOI IE-implants) or tapped on (for all single-piece implants with cementing abutment like BOI or BCS) prior to the normal laboratory procedures. It is recommended to try-in either the metal frame or the milling template for zirconium fabrication.

In the authors' experience the only way to keep forces on the bridge low, is to follow some quite old but valuable rules of prosthetics:

1. The plane of bite should be aligned to the Camper plane.
2. The occlusion in the distal jaws should include an occlusal equivalent of the curve of Spee.
3. During lateral movements the vertical deviation of the mandible must be symmetrical, i.e. the AFMP (angle fonctionnelle de mastication de Planas), must be symmetrical. Only this allows an equal, symmetrical, bilateral mastication.
4. The length and width of the masticatory table must be identical on both sides.
5. Wisdom teeth should be taken out.
6. The front teeth must not be in contact during occlusion or lateral grinding movements – this avoids anterior patterns of chewing and thereby extruding forces on distal implants.

The above-mentioned requirements are in fact 'nothing new'. During the authors' work on teeth and long-time integrated implants, they have learnt to overlook these demands and make compromises. Such compromises however, must not be made in immediate-loading treatment protocols on basal implants. In any case, the functional outcome will be more favourable if prosthetic workpieces are created within the framework of these rules.

The dentist's technician needs the following information for creating two full bridges on implants:

1. The vertical dimension
2. The position of the upper central incisor
3. The orientation of one of the models with respect to the skeleton
4. A bite taken in the correct vertical dimension.

With this information he/she can prepare this bridge following standard procedures for full dentures.

Although strong composites are available today, the authors still prefer to create a cast metal frame for the bridge. Metal-to-ceramic bridges are typically requested by the patients, but they are prone to ceramic chip-offs over time. Metal-to-plastic bridges with ready-made artificial teeth (either from acrylic composites or even from ceramics) are preferred by the authors, because they are easy and cheap to make and allow easier repair compared to ceramic bridges. Recently bridges from zirconium have become an alternative. If they are made from full zirconium (e.g. Prettau®) with considerable thickness, the chances of fractures are extremely low. The aesthetics of 'full zirconium' is today more than acceptable and with the appearance of CAD-production technology, the work proceeds fast and aesthetics can be planned well.

Prosthetic concepts are based on the concept that was developed for full dentures, except that teeth in the frontal zone should come in contact neither during mouth closing nor during lateral movements.

Connecting implants and prosthetics

If implants with screw connection are chosen (e.g. TOI IE), the connection between prosthetics and implants is provided by screws. The advantage of this procedure is that prosthetics may be taken off at any time and this can be useful when it comes to creating a close fit between the gums and the bridge over the years. On the other hand, it is obvious that all screw connections can fail; screws can get loose and this may result in overload on the bone around those implants, which are still rigidly connected to the bridge.

The same can happen, if temporary cements are used and the connection fails. In cases where very little bone is available, the usage of temporary cement is not recommended. Furthermore, this cement should not be used, if large sagittal discrepancies are present (Angle class II and class III), because in these cases often considerable segments of the bridge (i.e. the masticatory surfaces) are not supported by implants. The treatment provider is often tempted to use temporary cements and the following reasons are obvious:

1. Easy correction of prosthetics
2. Easy possibility to evaluate the integration of single implants under bridge (this is considered necessary by implantologists working with traditional two-stage implant systems).

The big danger associated with temporary cements is that patients may not notice if the bridge is partly loose. Patients who have had removable dentures before, will be fully satisfied with a mobile bridge which is connected only to one (mobile) implant – this situation is from their point of view, still much better compared to the previous denture. The longer the distance between their place of dwelling and the office of the treatment provider, the smaller are the chances that patients will turn up in the office to report a small problem. From this the authors have learnt that temporary cements are not suitable for patients who live far away from the dental office.

The authors have used several brands of permanent cement and conventional glass ionomer cements give good results for a number of years. However, they are technique-sensitive and they are especially sensitive to water, liquids, and blood during the process of cementation. The authors have achieved best results with Fuji Plus cement. The auto mix (capsule) variant requires extremely fast handling. If full bridges on more than six implants are cemented, two application pliers are needed and typically two nurses. The hand mix variant (powder–liquid) is slower and even large bridges can be handled with one nurse only.

Maintenance and functional grinding

In the authors' experience, very little grinding of the incorporated masticatory surfaces has been necessary, both initially and over the years – typically the situation is stable. The same cannot be expected on immediately loaded implants. Here are the main reasons:

1. Around teeth and long-time-integrated implants, the remodelling is finished and the bone morphology is stable.
2. Around freshly placed implants, especially if extractions were done simultaneously, strong remodelling takes place. This alters the shape of the bone, changes the plane of bite, and reduces total bone mass (thereby altering the vertical dimension).
3. Any remodelling which was initiated by the surgical implant placement will at the same time be influenced by the new functional situation. This additionally leads to changes in the morphology of the bone.
4. Keep in mind, that osseo integrated implants are rigidly anchored in the bone; they can neither elongate nor intrude. They have no way to compensate for changes in the way that teeth can. They have to follow all morphological changes. The masticatory surfaces mounted onto them follow the same way.

Hence on freshly placed and immediately loaded implants, frequent and larger adjustments will be necessary than on teeth or on long-time-integrated implants. The treatment provider should consider this necessity and inform the patient in time, and the initial vertical dimension chosen, should be large enough to allow such adjustments.

It is the purpose of the authors' maintenance procedure to ensure that the conditions defined earlier in this chapter will prevail throughout the period of usage of the bridge. One major problem is that although mastication can be adjusted by grinding, this consumes the vertical dimension. Hence, after years, the vertical dimension will have to be raised again. If this is neglected, the front teeth will get into an unwanted amount of contact and the pattern of chewing tends to change. This leads to three changes:

1. The functional situation changes and so does the distribution of pressure and tension areas within the jawbones.
2. The canine implant tends to become a fulcrum.
3. The distal implants are loaded on extrusion.

It is still open to discussion as to which of the three conditions is the major contributor to subsequent problems and should be discussed academically. In the clinical reality, these developments lead to fractures of implants or prosthetics and to mobilities of implants induced either by overloading or by underloading (in areas of tension). During checkups the treatment provider should ensure that all connections between implants and the bridges are tight, and in the lower distal mandible he/she should make sure that enough space between the bridge and the crest is left to allow vertical functional growth of the mandible.

Examples of such cases are shown in (Figs 20.13–20.19).

EXAMPLE CASES-

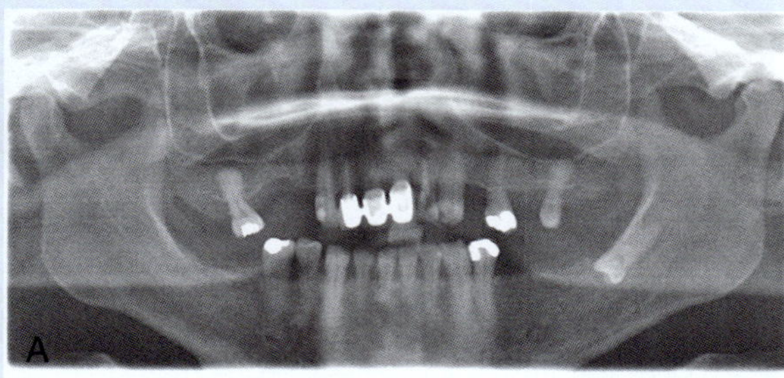

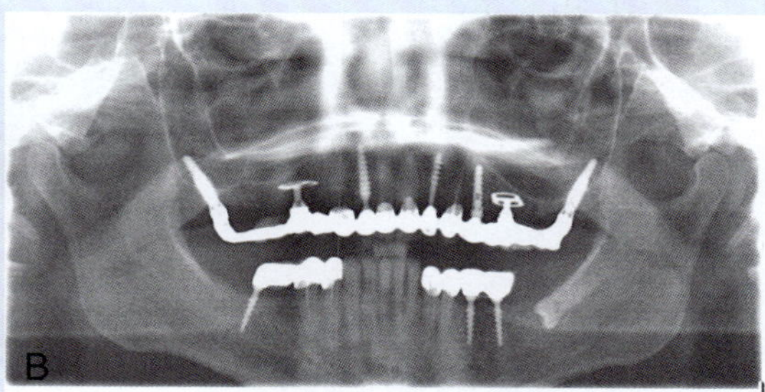

Fig 20.13 Full upper bridge on BOI (15, 25), KOS (teeth numbers 12, 22, 46, 35, and 35) and TPG (teeth numbers 18, 28) implants, placed immediately after the extraction of seven teeth in the maxilla. The upper canines were left in because the patient requested this. The bridge is connected with screws on the four distal implants and cemented in the front. (A and B) In the lower jaw, a suitable masticatory table and support was created with the help of teeth and three implants (*Courtesy:* Dr Henri Diederich, Luxembourg).

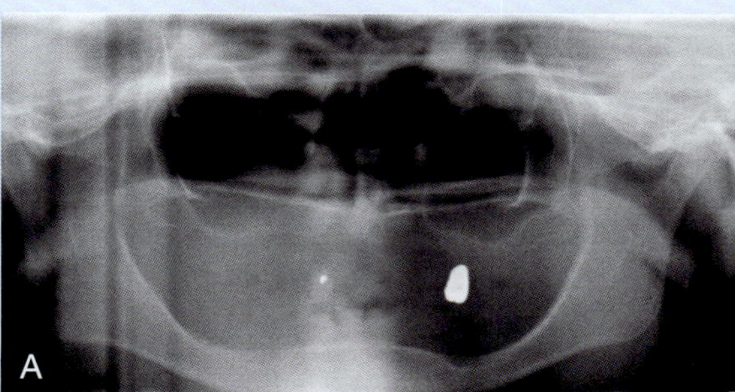

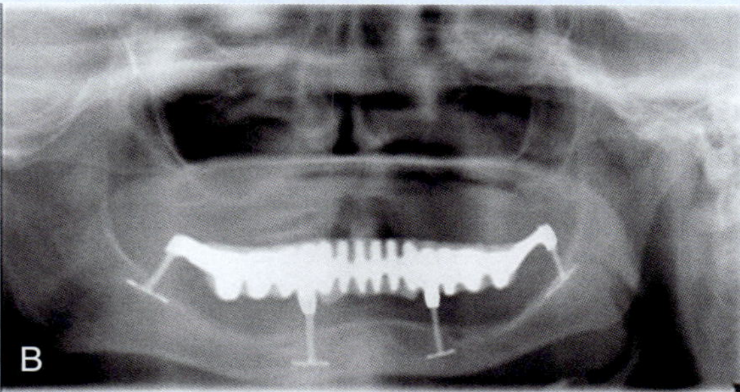

Fig 20.14 A full-arch fixed prosthesis supported by only four lateral basal implants in a severely atrophied mandibular ridge. The vertical dimension is fully reconstructed. (A) Preoperative view. (B) Postoperative view. No crater-like bone loss, no peri-implantitis. Loading of the implants within 5 days. (*Courtesy:* Ihde S, Rusak A. Case report: treatment of a severely resorbed mandible with endosseous implants in an immediate loading protocol. CMF Impl Dir 2009;1:150–153).

Continued

CASE REPORT—cont'd

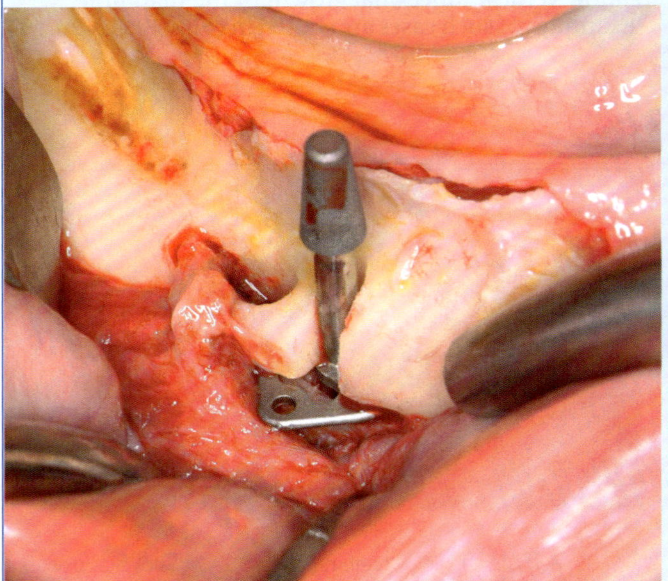

Fig 20.15 Lateral basal implant during insertion in the atrophied mandible. The base plate is positioned below the mental nerve. The nerve had been transpositioned a few millimetres towards the distal to avoid any damage.

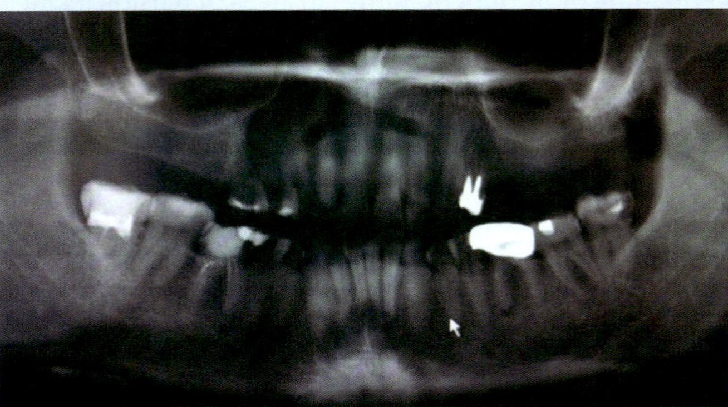

Fig 20.16 Before the upper segments can be installed, teeth numbers 38 and 48 must be extracted and 47 should be reduced in height. The tooth number 24 should be extracted right before the implants are placed. All surgical steps need to be done in one appointment. Note that a lot of adjustments are necessary in the lower jaw to allow immediate loading in the upper jaw.

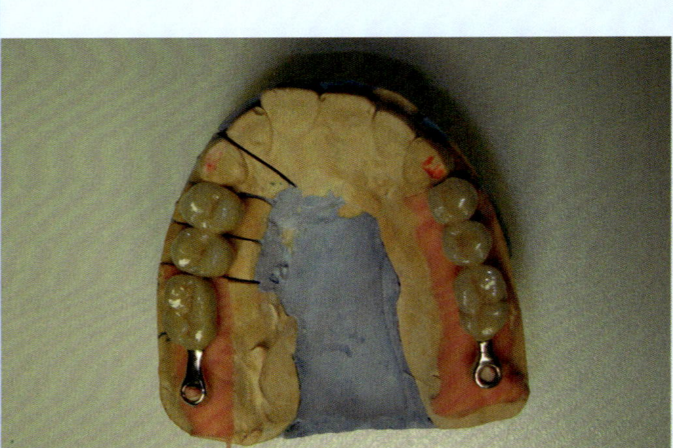

Fig 20.17 To reach an adequate vertical situation, the two premolars on the left side have to be crowned. These crowns are kept separate from the implants. To replace tooth number 16 in an immediate load protocol, three implants are necessary. For replacing two premolars and one molar on the left side, only four implants are needed. Small technical abutments are connecting the posterior implants to the constructions.

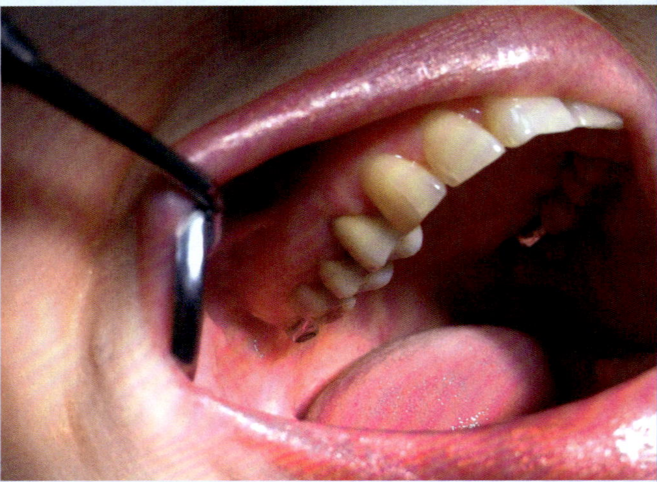

Fig 20.18 Intraoral view after fixing the prosthesis in the mouth.

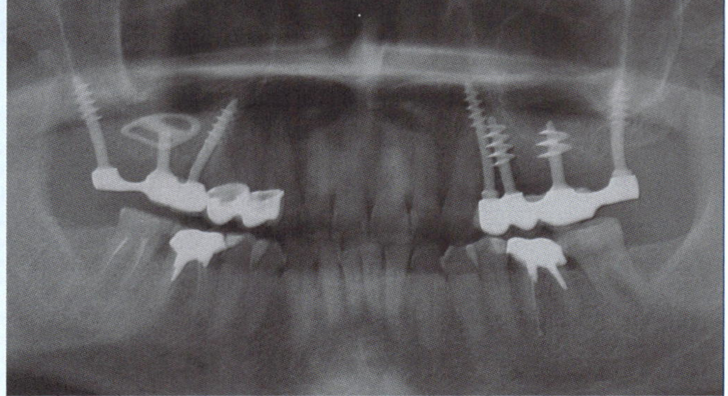

Fig 20.19 Nine months postoperative panoramic radiograph shows the uneventful integration of the implants and no bone loss at all. The extraction socket of tooth number 25 has filled with bone.

Summary

If lateral (BOI) or screwable (BCS) basal implants are utilized, the burdens of bone augmentations and waiting ('healing') time are in almost all cases excluded from dental implantology. In the concept of basal implantology, bicortical or multicortical anchorage is achieved during surgery and the prosthetic construction serves as an immediate and often permanent splint. The patients are able to return to normal masticatory function immediately. Immediate loading is not an option – for this concept, it is a necessity.

The concept of basal implantology requires profound knowledge on maxillofacial anatomy in both the resorbed and the nonresorbed states. The surgical and the prosthetic protocols have to be carried out rigorously, without compromise. Good care has to be taken not to overload the bone around single implants, even when they are splinted inside a larger prosthetic construction. All forces should be positioned inside the supporting polygon.

Basal implantology permits treating almost 100% of the patients with fixed teeth throughout their lives. The procedure is predictable and affordable; however it requires intense training of the treatment provider. Most of the traditional 'rules' of dental implantology cannot be applied – rules of orthopaedic surgery or traumatology are much more applicable to basal implantology than the rules of conventional dental implantology. They should be combined with adequate prosthetics.

Further Reading

Rüedi TP, Buckley RE, Moran CG. AO principles of fracture treatment. Stuttgart: Thieme; 2000, ISBN-10:3131174412.

Ihde S, Ihde A. Immediate loading. 2nd ed. Munich/Germany: The International Implant Foundation Publishing; 2012, ISBN 978-3-9851468-3-5.

Ihde S, Konstantinovic VS. Immediate loading of dental implants. Where is the dip? CMF Impl Dir 2007;4:137–45.

Planas P. La réhabilitation neuro-occlusale. Paris: Masson; 1982.

Ihde S, Rusak A. Case report: treatment of a severely resorbed mandible with endosseous implants in an immediate loading protocol. CMF Impl Dir 2009;1:150–3.

Full-arch fixed prosthesis: conventional approach

21

Ajay Vikram Singh   Amir Gazmawe

CHAPTER CONTENTS HD

Introduction

Patients who have lost or are losing all their teeth often show a fancy for the full-arch fixed prosthesis, which is nonremovable and can be brushed in the mouth like natural teeth. Despite being preferred by many patients, implant-retained fixed prostheses have many limitations and disadvantages. They need more surgical intervention to place more number of implants, which often need expensive and more invasive grafting procedures. First, information must be obtained to plan the case for function and aesthetics. Study models must be prepared and articulated to record and analyse the present occlusal relationship. Diagnostic wax-ups should be done and tried in the mouth to evaluate aesthetics and phonetics. Radiographs including periapicals, panoramics, and dental CT scans must be taken to evaluate the osseous support for dental implants, any present osseous defect, the sinus lining, and the mandibular canal. Interactive CT scans with radiographic guides offer detailed information on implant placement related to tooth position and aesthetics. The implant numbers and positions are decided by keeping various factors in mind, such as arch form, bone availability, bone density, number of units of the prosthesis, force factors, positions, paths of vital structures, etc. Consideration must be given to establish a comfortable, cleansable prosthesis with a stable, harmonious occlusion that also meets aesthetic and phonetic requirements. Prosthodontic procedures such as reconstruction of the vertical dimension of occlusion, aesthetic evaluation of intraoral and extraoral states, and establishing anterior guidance, must all be seriously and carefully considered in planning for an implant prosthesis.

The specific positioning of the implant in the maxilla for a maxillary implant-supported full-arch restoration is an important issue for both aesthetic and biomechanical reasons. From an aesthetic viewpoint, implants ideally should not be placed in the anterior region to avoid aesthetic compromise of the definitive prosthesis. For biomechanical reasons, implant positioning should be distributed among the posterior as well as anterior regions to decrease the potential for cantilever effects. However, occlusal forces can also be distributed away from anterior implants by balanced posterior contact during excursive movements, which decrease the loading of anterior implants. In cases with severe ridge loss in the premaxillary region, a pink porcelain design for anterior pontics can be planned to mask severe tissue loss. Cement-retained definitive prostheses rather than screw-retained alternatives can be selected, to facilitate aesthetic and occlusal considerations. It becomes often a difficult task to close the screw hole visible in the aesthetic region using a composite of an exactly blending shade. Moreover, the screw opening in the anterior for such a restoration would occupy between 30% and 50% of the occlusal surface, compromising the aesthetic result, interfering with the development of optimal occlusion and jeopardizing the axial loading principle of implants. Further, a passive fit cement-retained restoration is easy to fabricate when compared to the screw-retained full-arch metal framework. A passive-fitting framework is always preferred for an implant-supported prosthesis because the misfit of screw-retained prostheses may result in a greater level of masticatory forces being imparted to the screw-retained implant fixtures, which can cause crestal bone resorption and failure of the implants. Conversely, machine-made abutments used for the cement-retained prosthetic design result in a more passive fit. The lack of screw holes in cemented prostheses improves aesthetics and enhances the physical strength of porcelain or acrylic resin, resulting in fewer fractures. Additionally, the occlusion can be better developed to facilitate axial loading. Cement-retained implant prostheses result in reduced chair time and provide easier access where vertical space is limited. Reduced costs and complexity of components along with simpler laboratory procedures are important

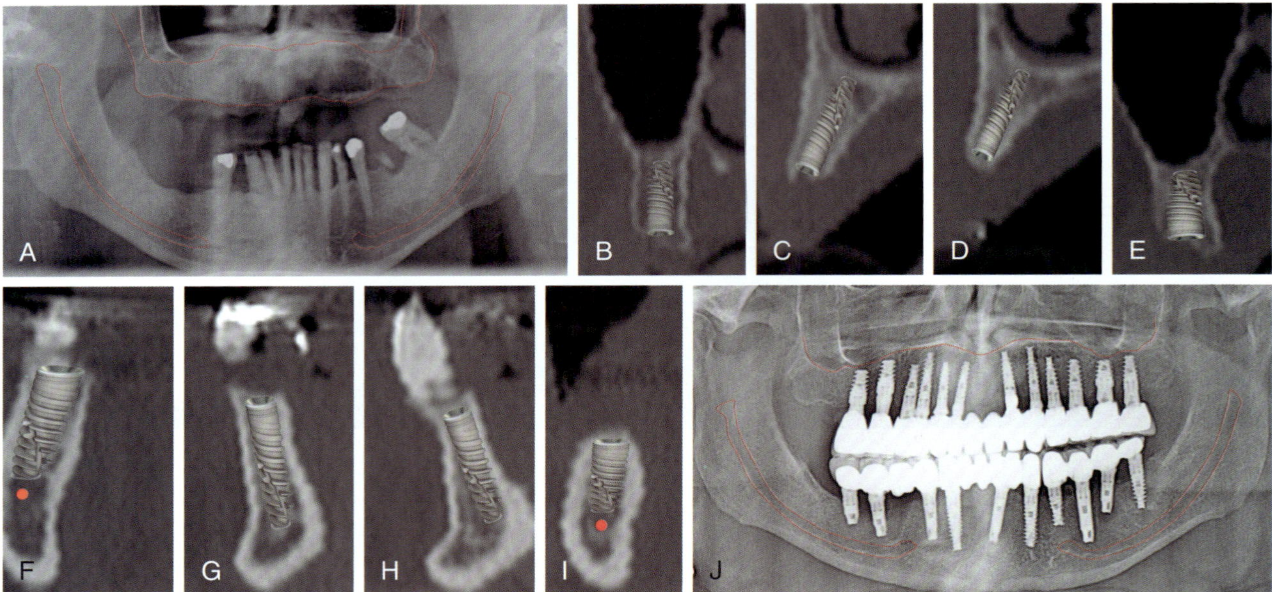

Fig 21.1 Patients often present with an adequate bone volume in the anterior as well as posterior regions of the maxilla and mandible to insert adequate number of implants with adequate size without performing any grafting procedure to provide full mouth fixed prosthesis. (A–J) Panoramic and CT scan cross-sections show adequate bone dimensions to insert adequate number of implants with ideal dimensions to support a full mouth fixed ceramic prosthesis.

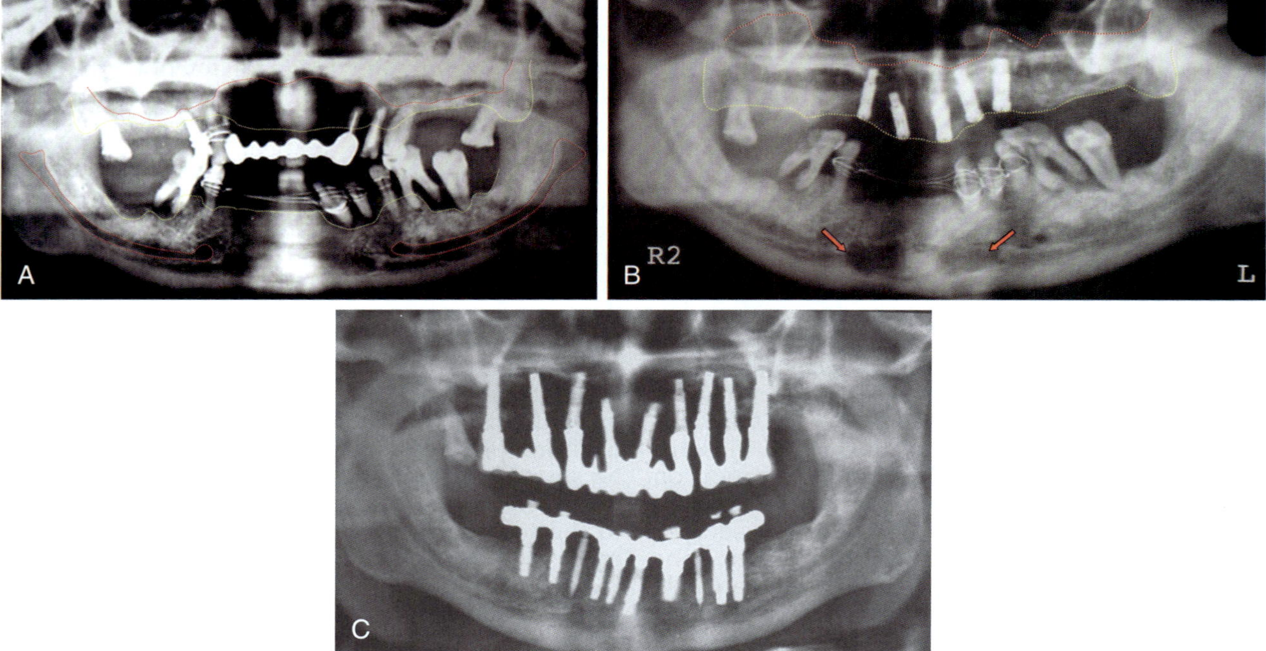

Fig 21.2 Many patients present with inadequate bone dimensions to insert adequate number of implants with adequate dimensions and thus need minor to major bone augmentation procedures to rehabilitate the patient with full mouth, implant-supported fixed prosthesis. (A) Panoramic radiograph shows inadequate bone height under the maxillary sinuses to insert implants. (B) The bilateral sinus grafting is performed using autogenous bone harvested from the mandibular symphysis (red arrows) mixed with bone substitutes to regenerate new bone dimensions in the sinuses. (C) The implants are inserted 10 months after the sinus grafting and restored after further healing period of 4 months. Thus, the case is completed in 14 months.

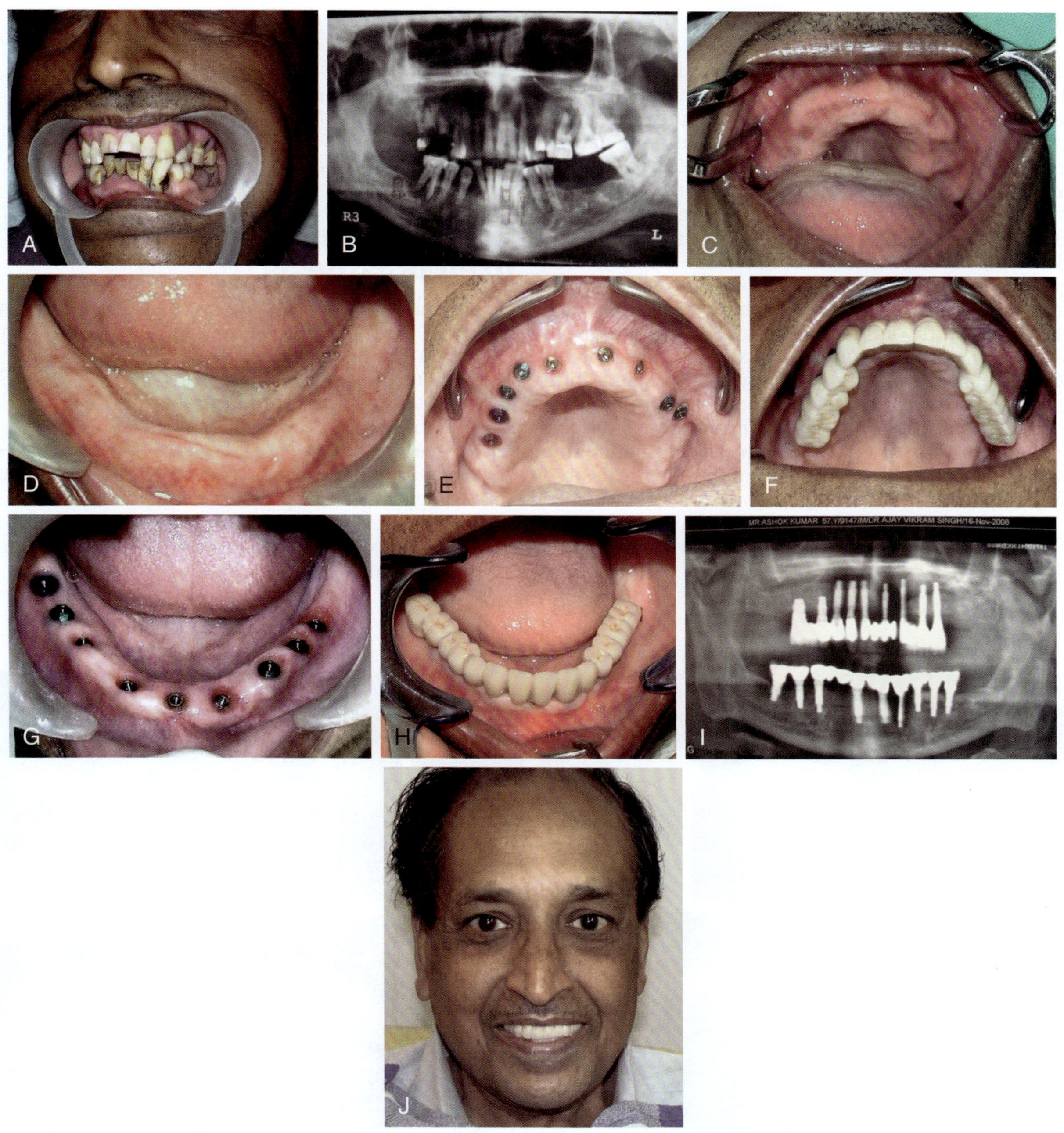

Fig 21.3 Traditional full mouth rehabilitation using implant-supported fixed ceramic prosthesis also requires placement of several implants with or without augmentation procedures. (A and B) Patient with all periodontally compromised teeth, which need extraction, and implant-supported prosthesis. (C and D) All teeth are extracted and soft relined dentures are given to the patient for 6 weeks, till all the soft tissue is healed. (E–J) Multiple implants are inserted in the upper and lower jaws to support fixed implant-supported cement-retained ceramic prosthesis.

advantages attributed to the cement-retained design. The ability of the bone-implant interface to survive under loading is a result of many factors. Though the cement-retained prosthesis offers various advantages, the screw-retained prosthesis offers retrievability and ensures that there is no cement in the peri-implant tissue. These advantages of the screw-retained prosthesis need to be considered for full-arch cases. The intraoral repairing of the fractured full-arch cemented prosthesis is very difficult and its removal may need to cut all the prostheses in the mouth and may involve the fabrication of a new prosthesis. The screw-retained hybrid prosthesis is highly preferred for full-arch cases because it is retrievable, easy to repair, light weight, offers high aesthetics because readymade acrylic teeth are used, and is cost effective.

Once all the implant numbers, dimensions, and positions have been determined to provide a fixed prosthesis, it then must be decided how the case will be provisionalized during the treatment period. Usually, a removable provisional prosthesis is preferred to avoid undue forces on the implants during the healing period, but most patients prefer a fixed provisional prosthesis over a removable one because it offers stability, aesthetics, and less interference of speech patterns. The fixed provisional prosthesis either can be fixed on the same implants if the implants have been well stabilized in the bone, or a few additional narrow diameter provisional implants can be inserted to support the provisional prosthesis. A laboratory-processed fixed provisional prosthesis offers several advantages over a chair side-produced provisional prosthesis. These advantages include improved aesthetics, smoother surface, increased strength, and reduced chair time. Conventionally, efforts are made to insert all implants maximally parallel to each other for easy seating of the prosthesis; but with the invention of newer prosthetic components, angulation problems can be easily taken care of by using various angled abutments during prosthetic reconstruction of the implants.

Full-arch implant cases present variable hard and soft tissue situations with few cases presenting with adequate amount of bone volume to insert implants with desired dimensions and at the desired positions. Many cases need bone augmentation procedures such as sinus grafting, block grafting, etc. during or before implant placements (Figs 21.1–21.4).

Advantages of full-arch fixed prosthesis

1. Psychological satisfaction of having fixed teeth.
2. More chewing efficiency.
3. Long lasting.
4. Preserves alveolar bone loss.

Disadvantages of full-arch fixed prosthesis

1. Expensive, because of the need for more implants.
2. Often needs expensive and more invasive bone augmentation procedures.
3. More technique-sensitive.
4. More specific implant placement needed.
5. Difficult to maintain.
6. Difficult to repair.
7. More and continuous forces on the implants cannot be avoided in patients with parafunctional forces (bruxism).
8. Less support to the perioral muscles when compared to overdentures.

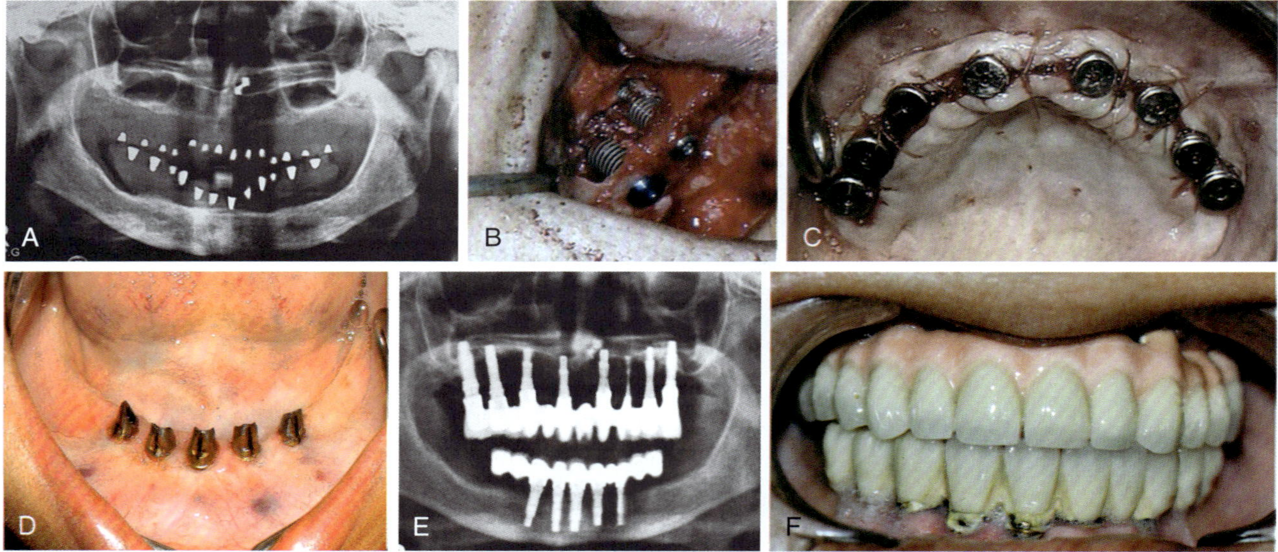

Fig 21.4 (A) Edentulous patient who has been wearing soft tissue supported dentures for more than 10 years, has lost vertical bone height in the upper and lower posterior regions. (B and C) Sinus grafting procedure is performed in posterior maxilla to insert implants in the upper full-arch. (D and E) Five implants are inserted between two mental foramina and fixed cement-retained prosthesis with distal cantilevers is fixed on lower implants. It took a complete year to give a fixed ceramic prosthesis to the patient. (F) Poor maintenance of the prosthesis by the patient lead to large amount of calculus which can be seen around the lower implants, causing various problems like frequent bleeding, soft tissue recession, and crestal bone resorption.

CASE REPORT-1

Step by step procedure for mandibular implant-supported fixed prosthesis (Figs 21.5–21.10).

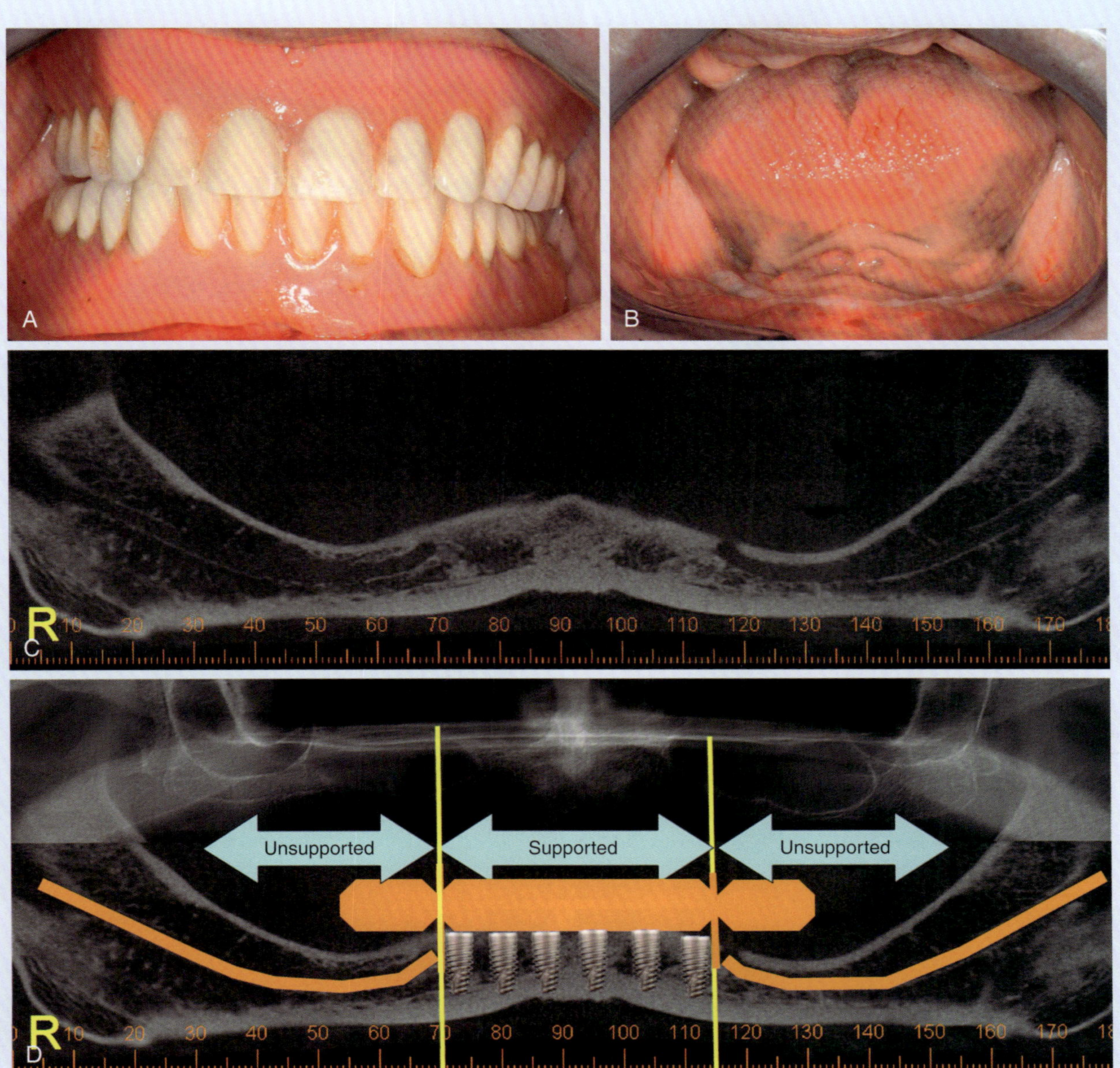

Fig 21.5 (A and B) Patient wearing soft tissue-supported dentures, complained of a retention problem with the lower denture because of age-related severe ridge resorption. The patient expressed a strong desire to have lower teeth fixed over implants. (C) The panoramic view of the mandible shows inadequate bone height above the mandibular canals to insert implants in the posterior segments. (D) Vertical bone augmentation procedures were refused by the patient, hence a fixed distal cantilevered 12-unit ceramic prosthesis, supported by 6 implants to be placed between mental foramina, is planned. Patient was advised to go for upper implant-supported ceramic prosthesis, once she was satisfied with the lower one.

Continued

CASE REPORT-1—cont'd

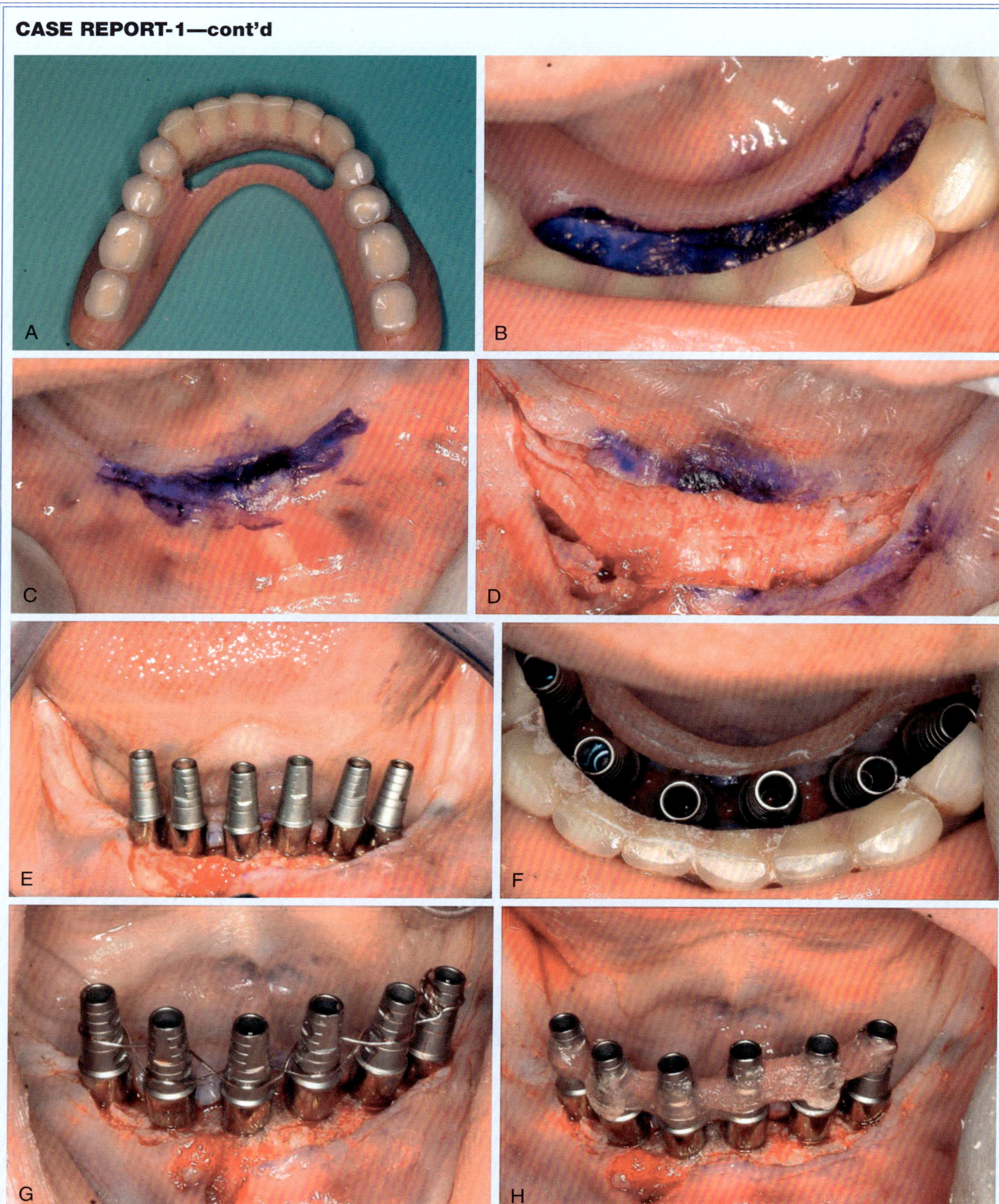

Fig 21.6 (A) Denture base is cut for prosthetically guided implant placement. (B) Denture is seated in mouth and ridge area is marked using tissue pencil. (C) Denture is removed, (D) flaps are elevated to expose the bony ridge, (E and F) and six implants are inserted between two mental foramina at the appropriate prosthetic positions. All the implants achieved adequate primary stability (more than 35 Ncm), thus an implant-supported fixed provisional prosthesis is planned to be fixed immediately on the inserted implants. (G) All the implant abutments are splinted together using a stainless steel wire, (H) which is further reinforced using the self-cure resin to firmly engage them together.

CASE REPORT-1—cont'd

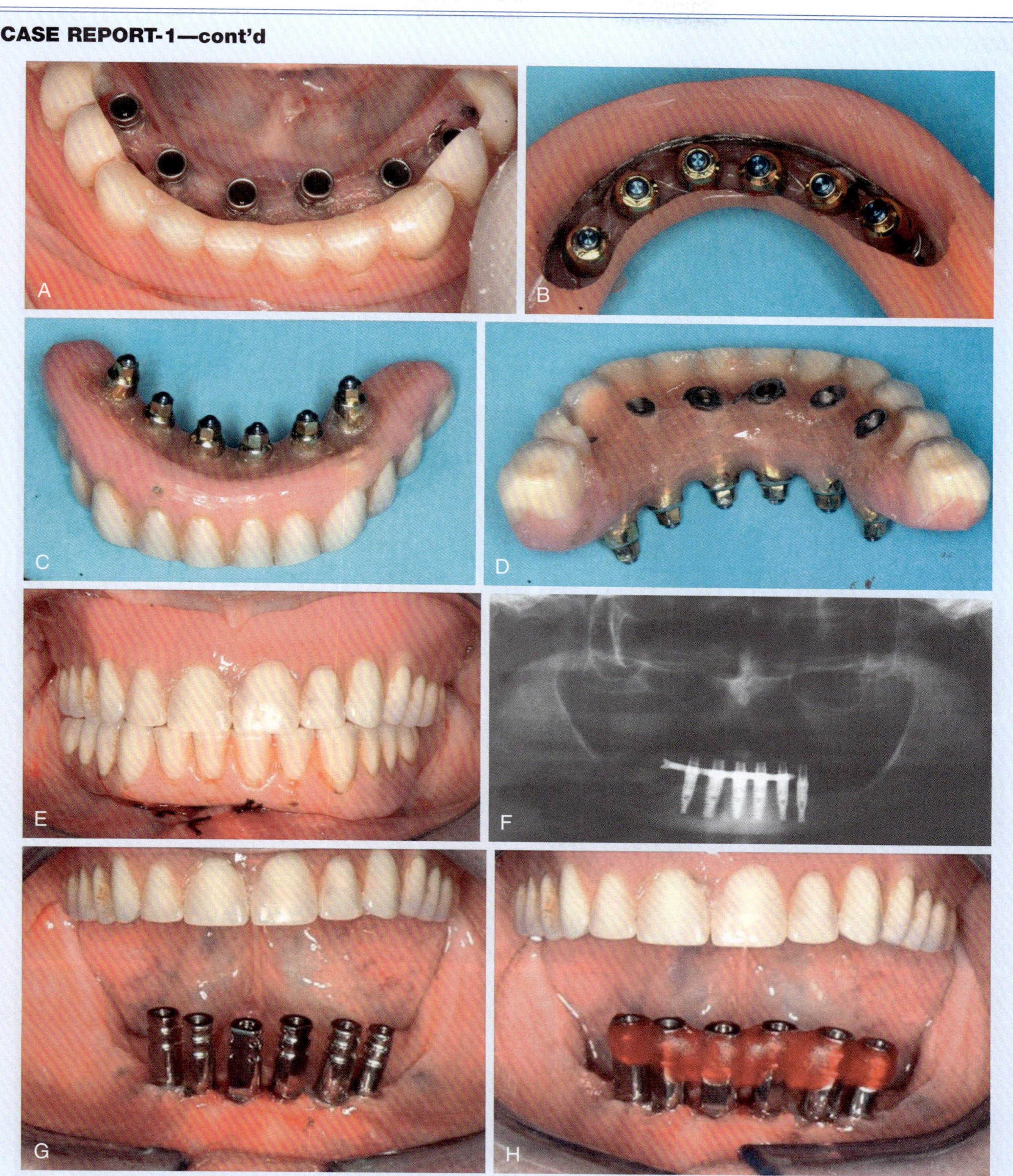

Fig 21.7 (A) Denture is passively seated in the mouth in the correct occlusion and resin is added to bond the abutments with the denture in position. (B) Once the resin gets set, the abutments along with attached denture, are unscrewed out of the mouth. (C) The resin is further added at the tissue as well as occlusal surface to fill all the peri-abutment spaces of the denture. (D) The part of the abutments occlusally emerging out of the denture has been reduced. The distal part of the denture is also reduced to limit the prosthesis up to the first molar, to minimize the cantilevering of the prosthesis. (E) Flaps are sutured and the prosthesis is screwed in the mouth. (F) Postoperative radiograph. After 3 weeks, when the soft tissue has healed, (G) prosthesis is unscrewed out from the mouth, and impression posts are inserted on top of the implants, and (H) splinted together using pattern resin.

Continued

CASE REPORT-1—cont'd

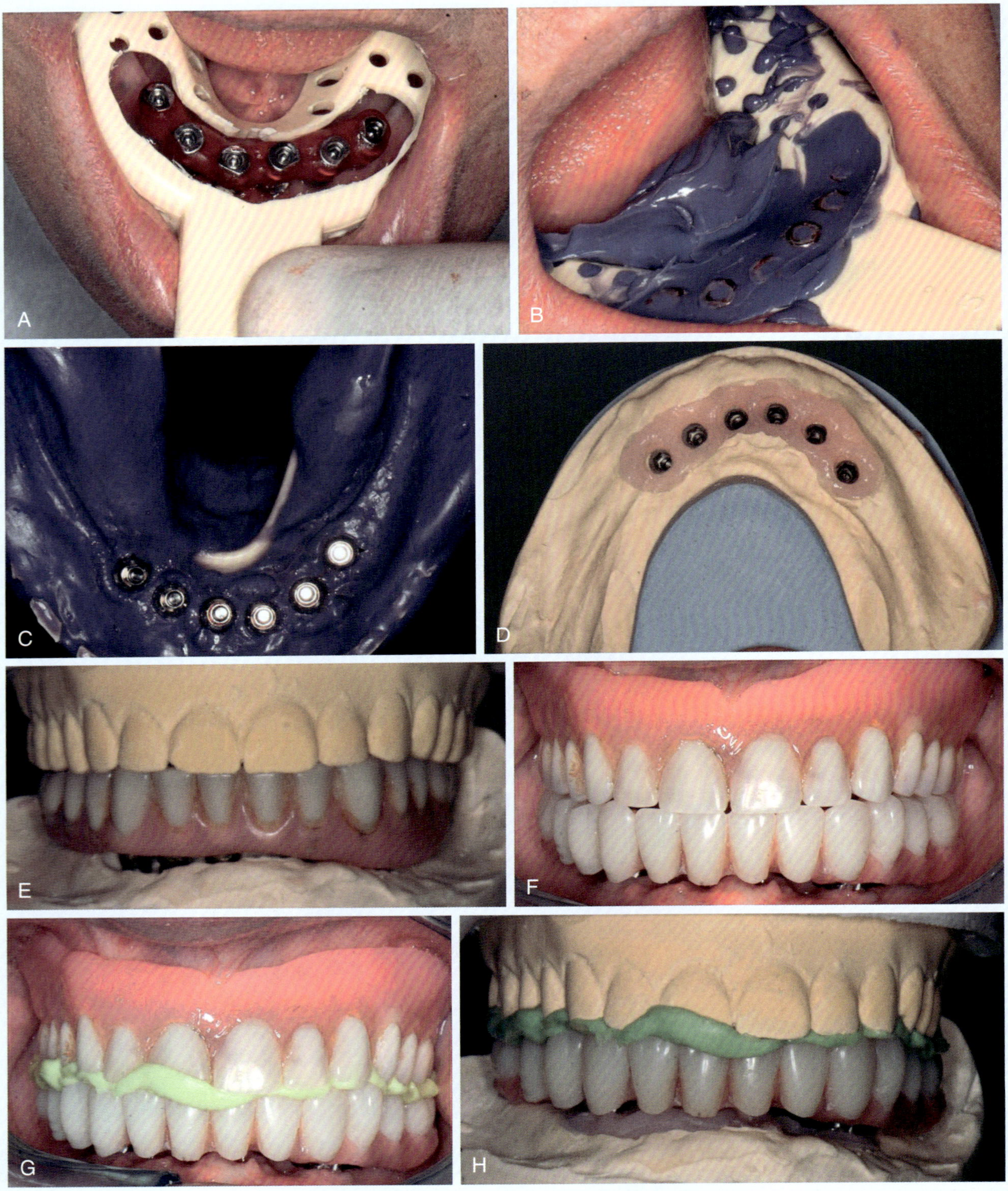

A B C D E F G H

Fig 21.8 (A–C) The custom impression tray has been modified for the open tray technique and impression is made with open tray technique using polyether impression material. (D) The working cast is fabricated, and (E) denture is fixed over the cast. (F and G) A duplicate prosthesis is fabricated for the bite registration and lab purposes, and is fixed in the mouth for bite registration. (H) The working cast is rearticulated at the correct centric position.

CASE REPORT-1—cont'd

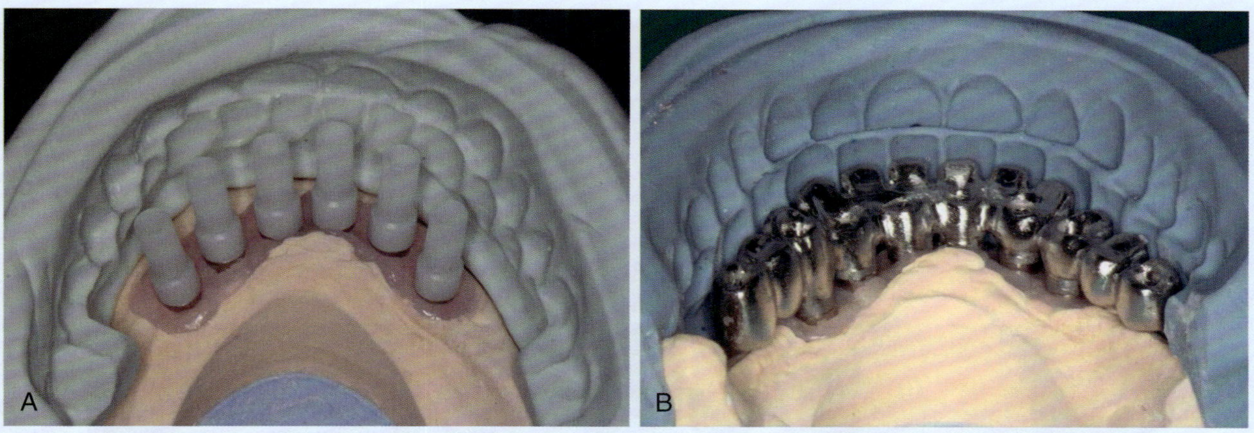

Fig 21.9 The indexing for the teeth positions and available spaces for the prosthesis is done using putty impression material. (A) The plastic abutments are fixed on top of the analogues to fabricate the screw-retained prosthesis. (B) Further, a wax pattern is prepared and a metal framework is fabricated in the laboratory leaving adequate spaces for ceramic buildup.

Continued

CASE REPORT-1—cont'd

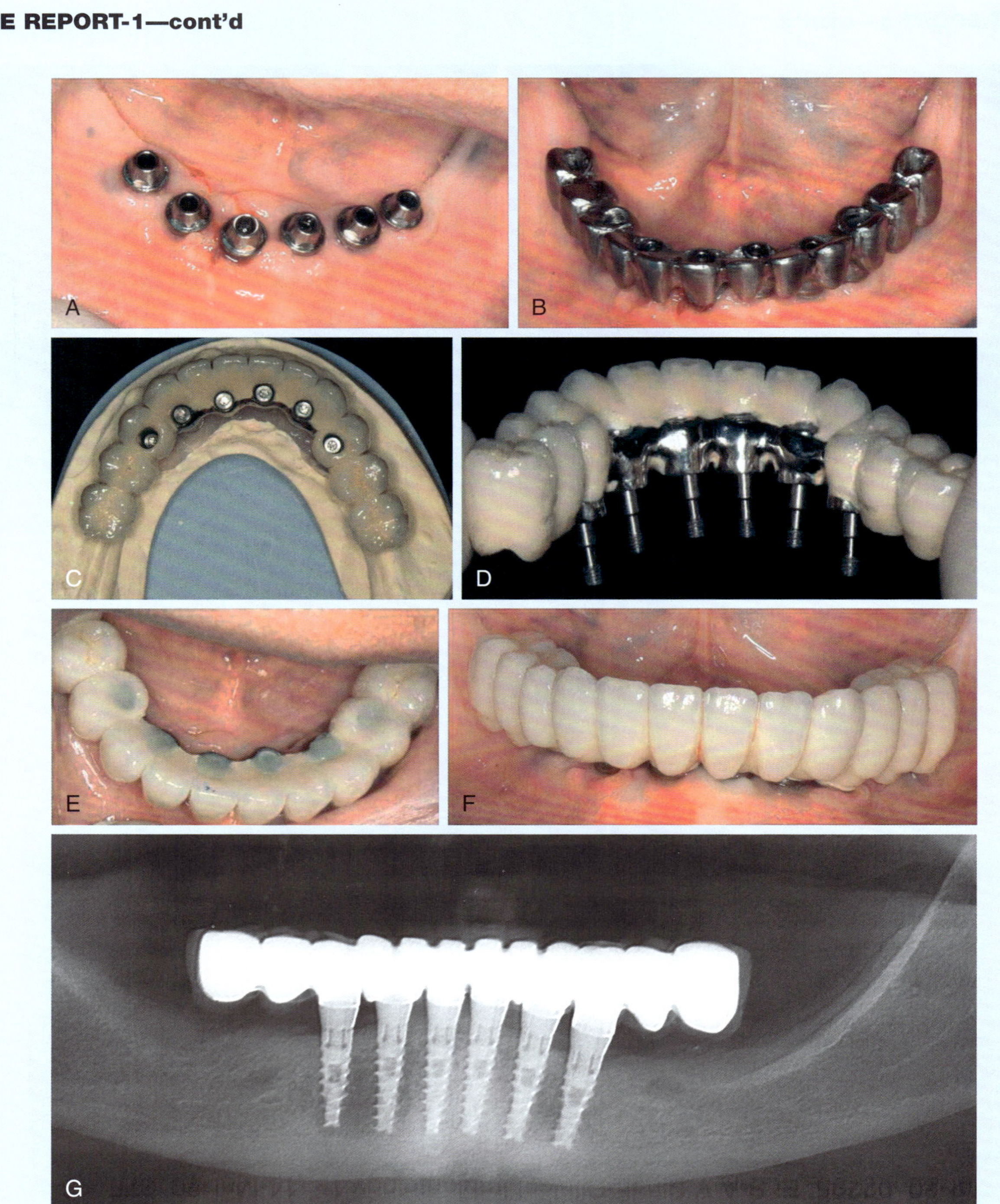

Fig 21.10 (A and B) The abutments for screw (TCT abutments) are screwed on top of the implants in the mouth and the metal framework is screwed to check its complete and passive seating over the implants. (C and D) The finally fabricated screw-retained ceramic prosthesis is screwed over the implants, the connection screws are finally tightened at the moment force of 30 Ncm using a torque ratchet, and (E and F) screw holes are sealed using flow gutta-percha and composite. (G) Post loading radiograph.

CASE REPORT-2

A 40-year-old patient presented with a partially edentulous maxilla with few mobile teeth in upper and lower arches. An implant-supported, 4-unit prosthesis was present in the mandibular right posterior region. Patient expressed the desire for the fixed full-arch prosthesis. When the panoramic radiograph and dental CT scan were evaluated, inadequate bone was present in the subantral region to insert implants without performing any sinus grafting procedure. The insertion of multiple implants only in the anterior region to support a distal cantilevered 12-unit prosthesis was planned. On right side, the sinus was extended to the canine position, so implant placement with internal sinus elevation was planned in this region. (Figs 21.11–21.17).

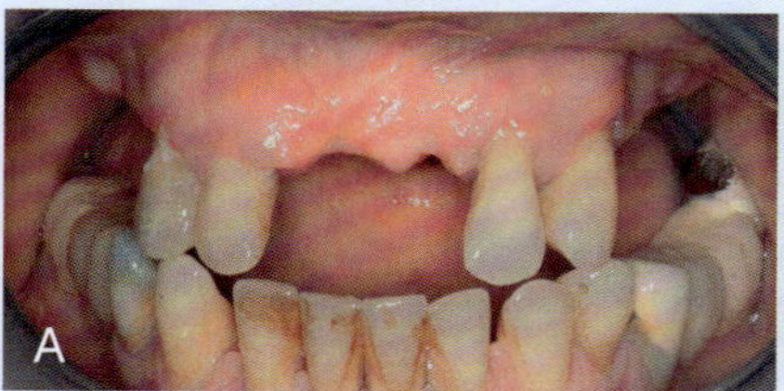

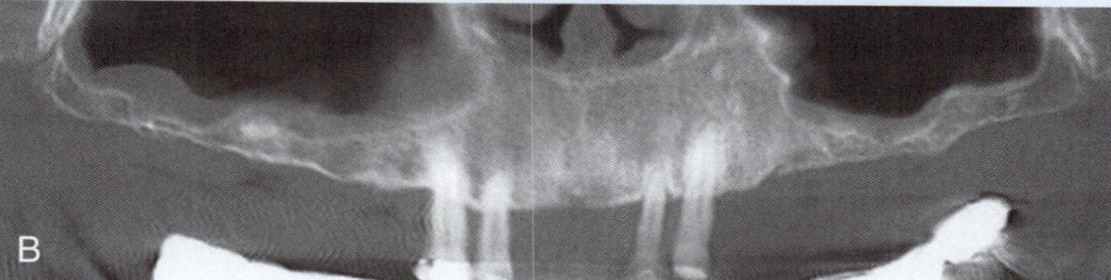

Fig 21.11 (A) Preoperative clinical view of partially edentulous maxilla. (B) The panoramic view of dental CT scan shows inadequate bone in the subantral region but adequate bone is present in the anterior maxilla to insert adequate number of implants to support a 12-unit fixed prosthesis. Distal tilting of left posterior implant is planned to reduce the length of distal cantilever, and the right posterior implants are planned to be stabilized in the high-density sinus floor by internal sinus elevation without grafting.

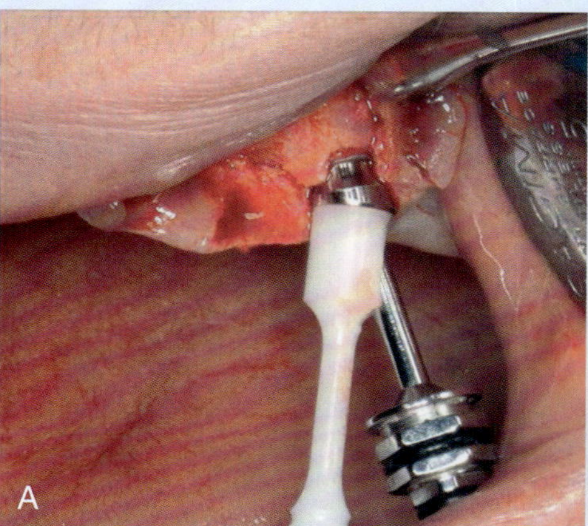

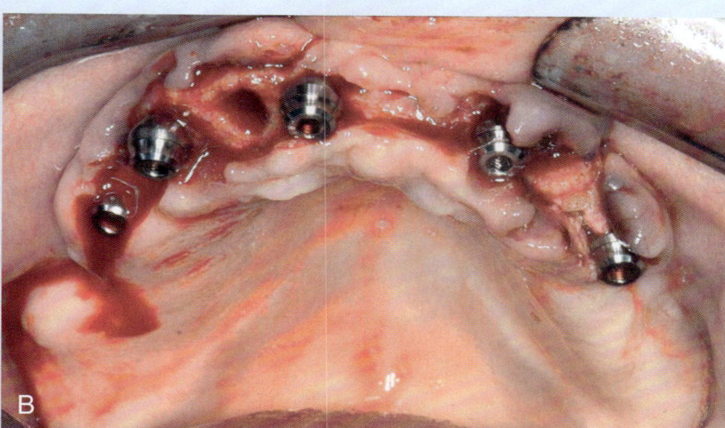

Fig 21.12 (A) Left posterior implant is distally tilted and a 30° multiunit abutment is inserted. (B) Other implants are in place with straight or 17° multiunit abutments.

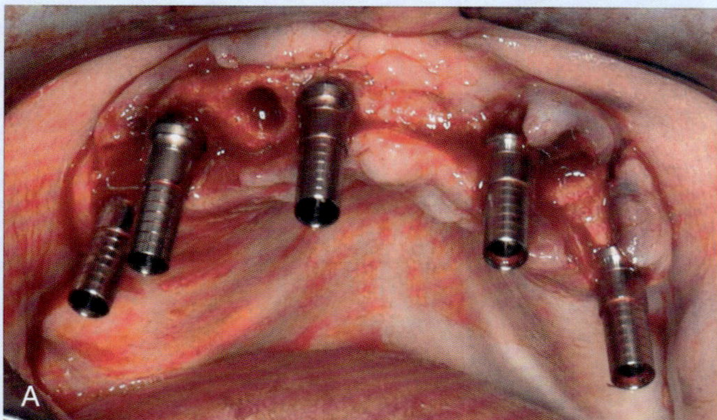

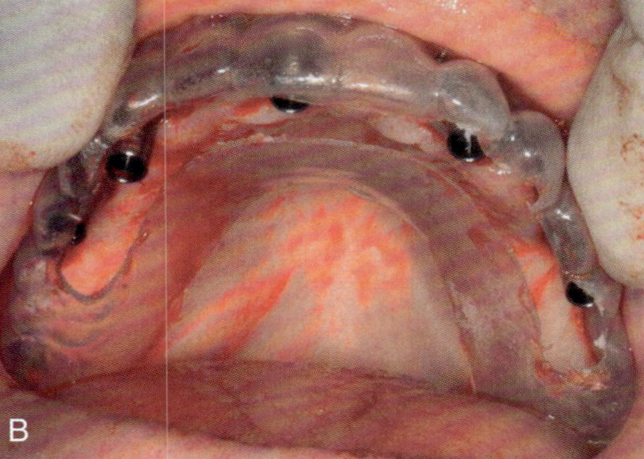

Fig 21.13 (A) Temporary titanium cylinders are placed over the multiunit abutments. (B) The prefabricated guide is tried in the mouth for its passive seating.

Continued

CASE REPORT-2—cont'd

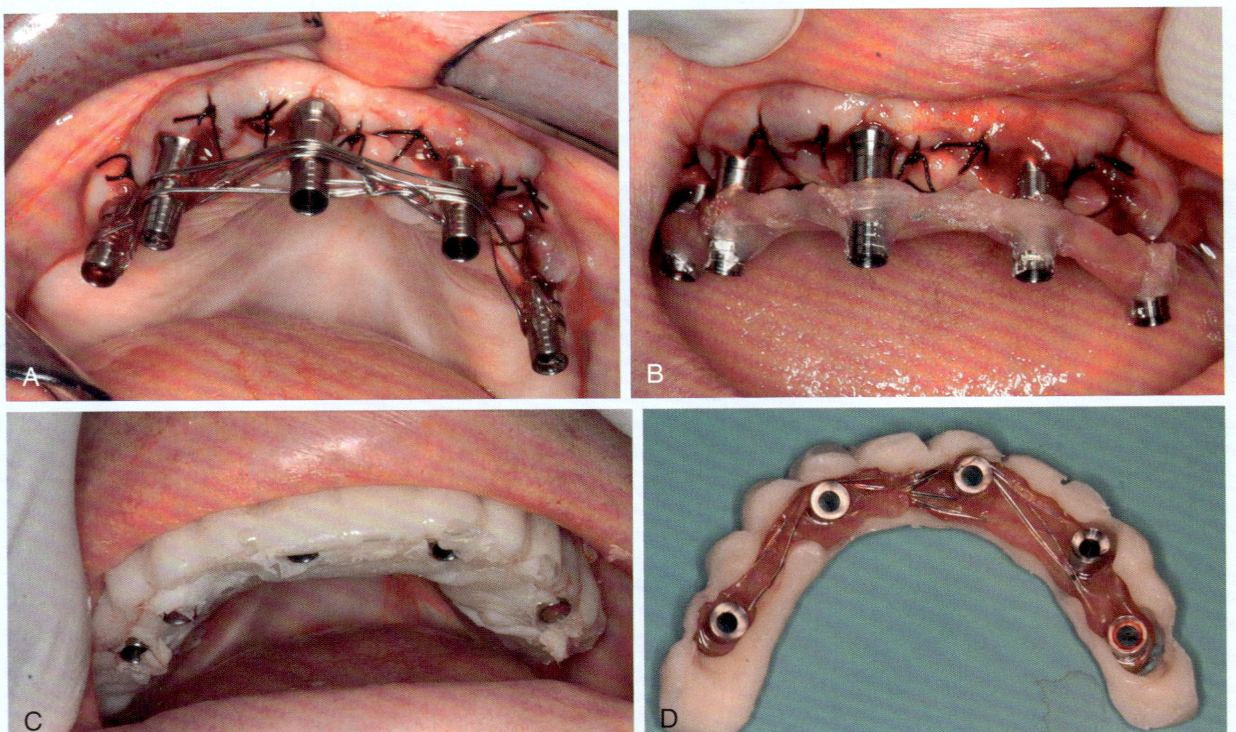

Fig 21.14 (A and B) Implants are splinted together using stainless steel wire and pattern resin and (C) the guide filled with self-cure acrylic is seated in the mouth in the correct occlusion. (D) After the acrylic gets set the prosthesis is unscrewed from the implants.

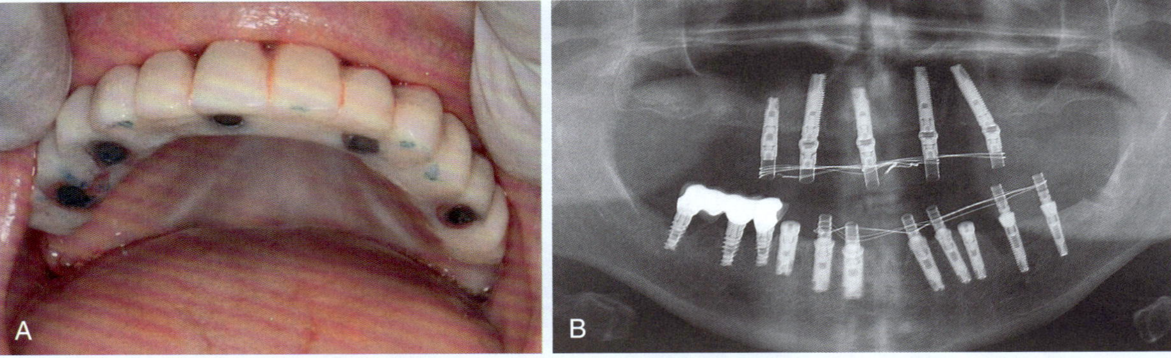

Fig 21.15 (A) The prosthesis is finished, polished, and fixed over the implants. Postimplantation radiograph shows left posterior tilted implant. The right posterior implants have been stabilized into the sinus floor. (B) All the teeth in the mandibular arch which were mobile have been extracted and multiple implants have been immediately inserted into the lower arch.

CASE REPORT-2—cont'd

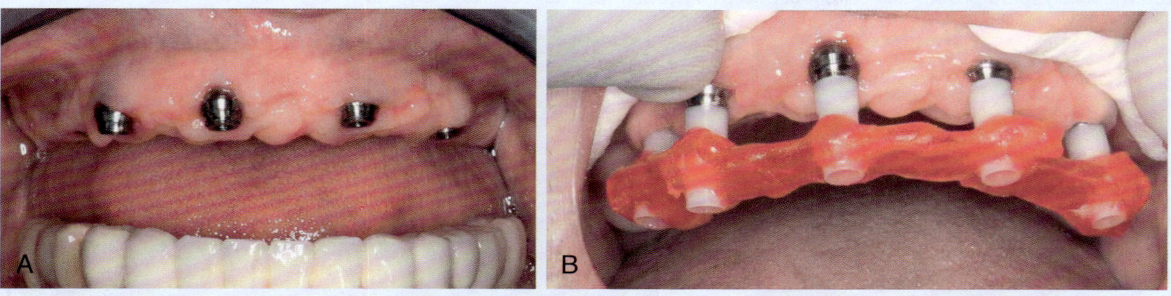

Fig 21.16 Healing at 6 weeks after implant placement. (A) The lower implants have been restored using ceramic prosthesis. (B) Castable plastic abutments splinted together using pattern resin are tried in the mouth for the complete and passive fit over the implants.

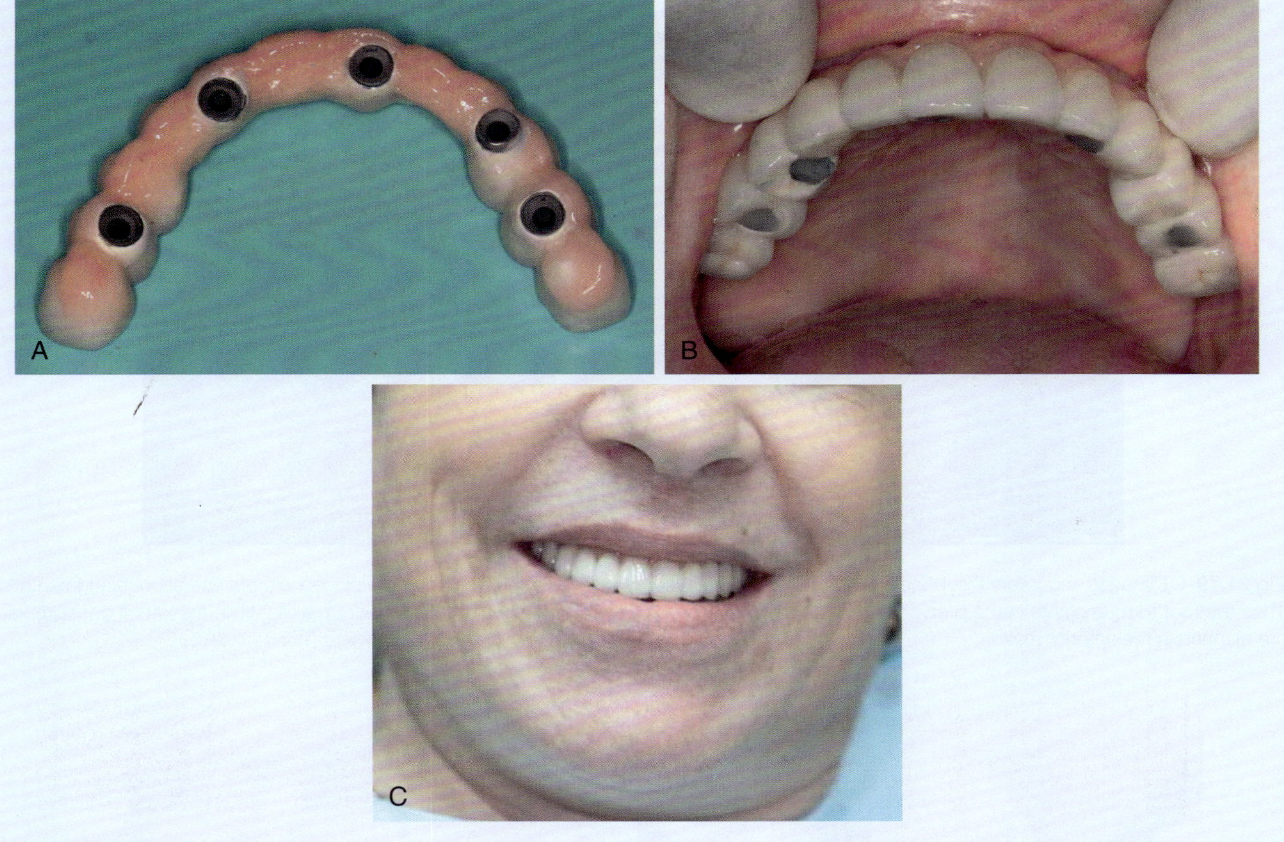

Fig 21.17 (A–C) A screw-retained ceramic prosthesis is fabricated and has been fixed in the mouth.

CASE REPORT-3

Full-arch maxillary fixed prosthesis on basal and pterygoid implants *(Courtesy: Shlomo Birshan, Israel)* (Figs 21.18–21.27).

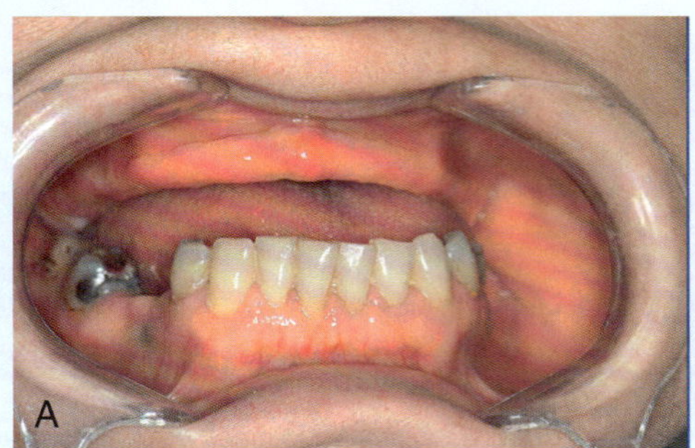

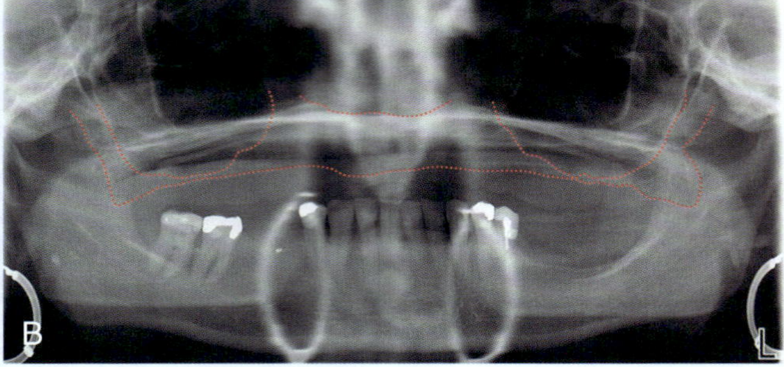

Fig 21.18 (A) Edentulous maxilla. (B) Panoramic radiograph shows inadequate subantral bone to insert implants.

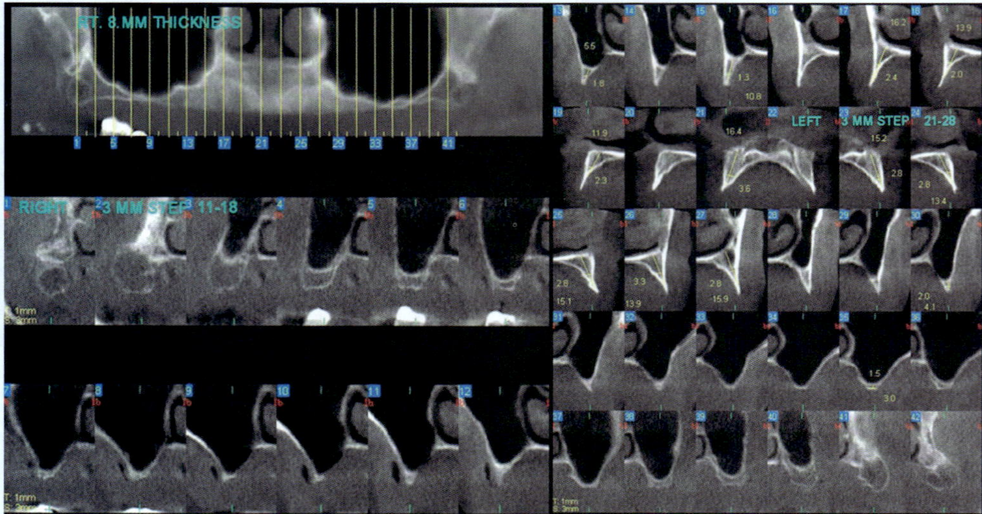

Fig 21.19 CT images show very thin bone in the anterior maxilla, where root form implants cannot be placed without lateral bone augmentation. Thus the root form implants in the pterygoid plates and maxillary tuberosity are planned in the posterior maxilla while the lateral basal implants are planned in the anterior maxilla.

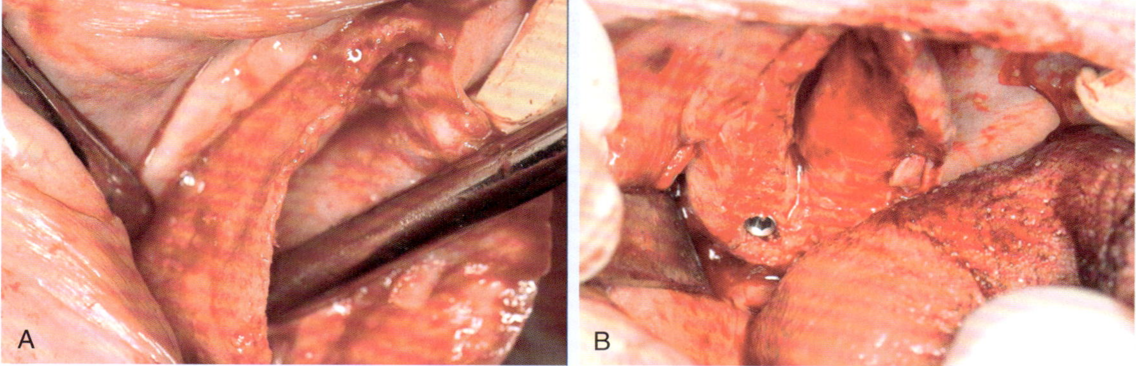

Fig 21.20 (A) Thin bony ridge can be seen after mucoperiosteum flap elevation. (B) Root form implant inserted into medial pterygoid bone can be seen.

CASE REPORT-3—cont'd

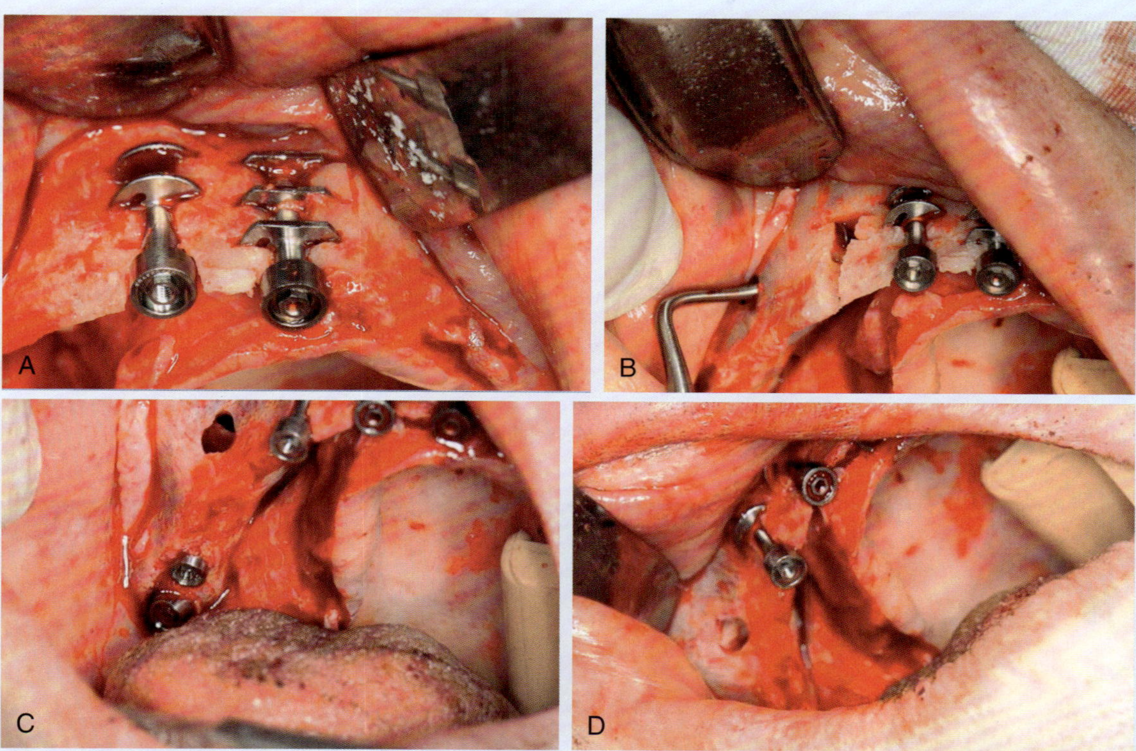

Fig 21.21 (A) After lateral osteotomy preparation using combi disc cutters, the basal implants are inserted in the anterior maxilla with high stability. (B) A small window is prepared at the lateral wall of the sinus and the anterior wall of the sinus is explored using a probe. (C and D) Small tearing in the sinus membrane is closed using PRF membrane.

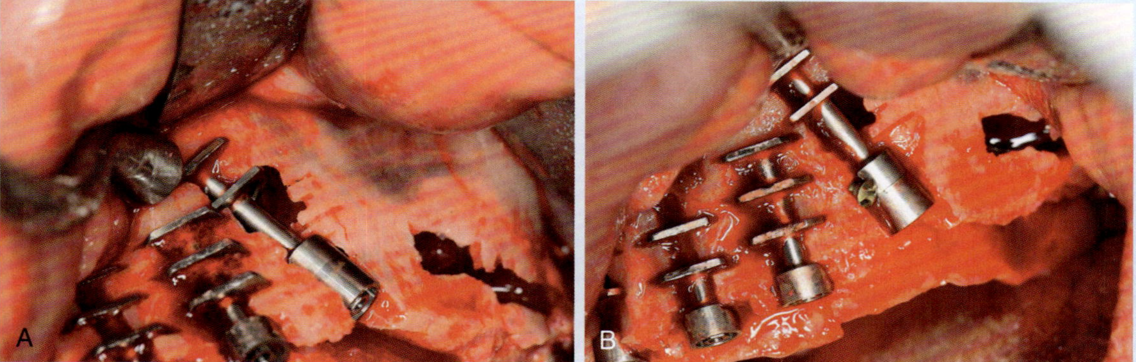

Fig 21.22 (A) The left sinus membrane is elevated with lateral window preparation and implants are inserted; but the posterior-most basal implant lost stability and could have displaced laterally before it osseointegrated. (B) Thus a long fixation screw was used to secure the implant in position and to prevent its lateral displacement.

Continued

CASE REPORT-3—cont'd

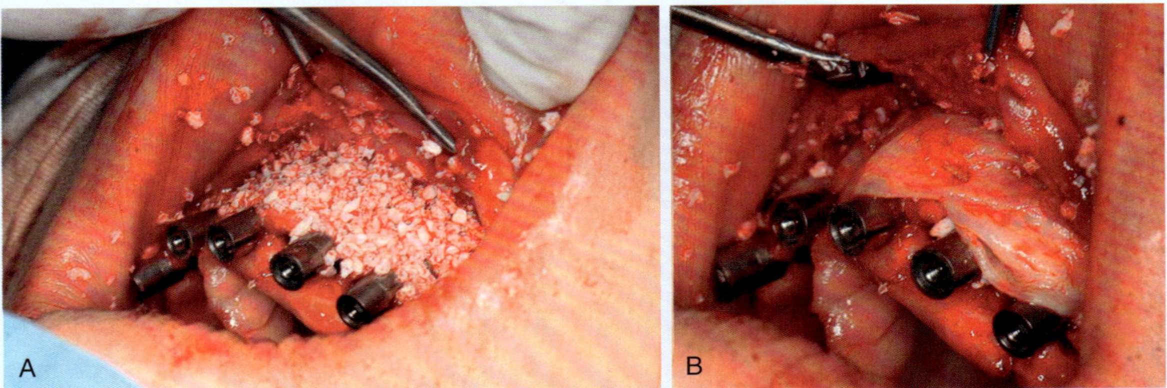

Fig 21.23 (A) The bone substitute is deposited over the implants (B) which is further covered using PRF membrane.

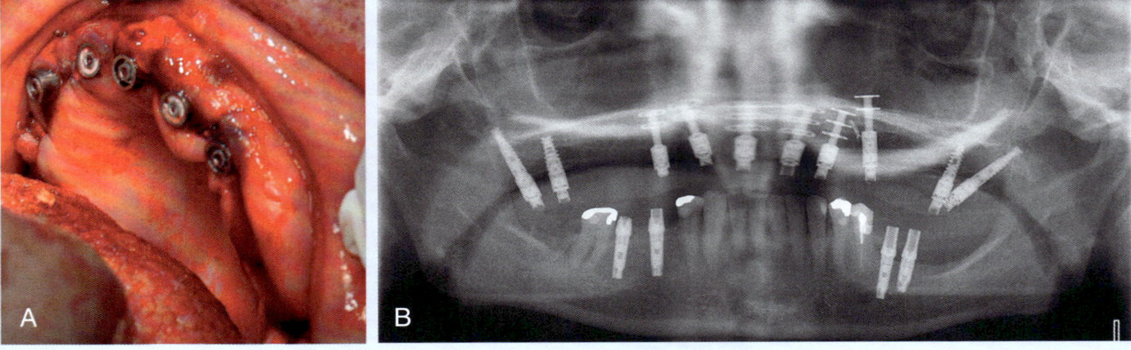

Fig 21.24 (A) The flap is sutured back. (B) Postimplantation radiograph.

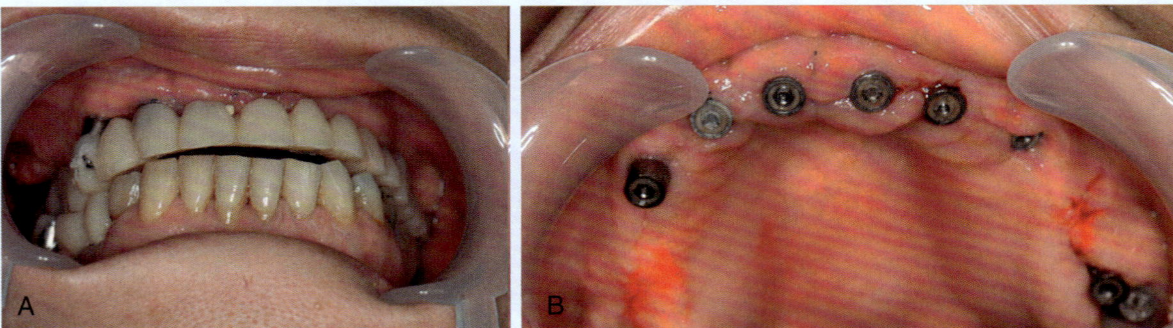

Fig 21.25 (A) A provisional acrylic prosthesis is fixed over the implants the day after implant insertion surgery. (B) Healing 3 weeks after implant placement.

CASE REPORT-3—cont'd

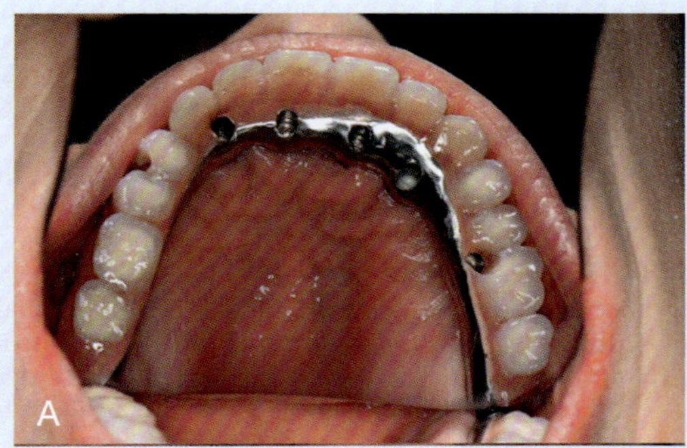

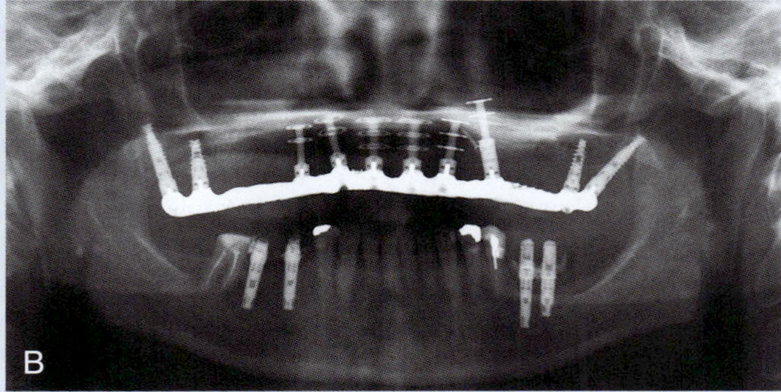

Fig 21.26 (A) A definitive prosthesis is screwed over the implants after 6 weeks. (B) Post loading radiograph.

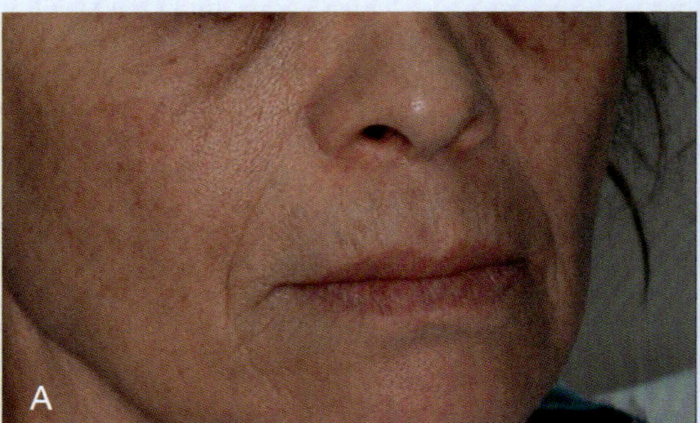

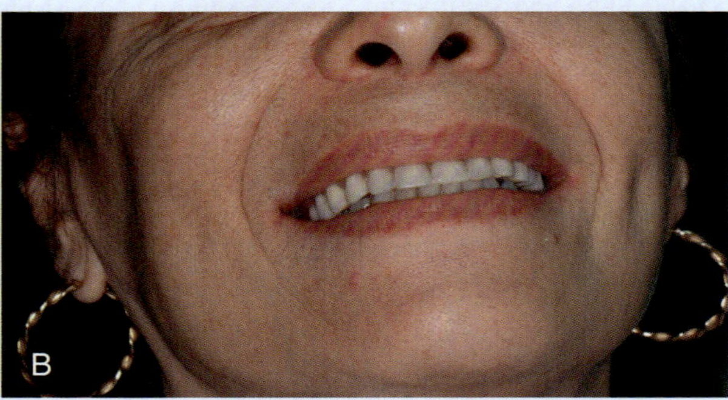

Fig 21.27 (A) The maxillofacial profile of the patient, when she was wearing a removable maxillary prosthesis and (B) after the implant prosthesis was in place.

Summary

Full-arch cases that are planned to be restored with an implant-supported fixed prosthesis need meticulous treatment planning for appropriate implant positioning and adequate number of implant insertion and provisionalization during the treatment phase. The conventional approach for full mouth rehabilitation may require the placement of a large number of implants with simultaneous bone grafting procedures. Meticulous treatment planning is required to satisfactorily treat full mouth cases because various factors, such as bone density and volume, use of adequate number of implants in correct position, arch form, the vertical dimension of occlusion, position, form, and the material of the future prosthesis, provisionalization of the case during the treatment phase, etc. contribute substantially to the success of the treatment. The long-term proven success of osseointegrated implants is known to depend on bone type and volume, implant positioning in respect of the future prosthesis, force factors, and the design of the superstructures for distributing masticatory and functional loads to the implants. The failure of implant superstructures is typically attributed to fracture of abutments or connection screws, porcelain fracture, and fracture of the cantilevered area of the prosthesis. Optimal three-dimensional positioning of the implants considering various factors such as arch form, force factors, and type of final prosthesis, allows for a long-term aesthetic and functional outcome of the implant-supported prosthesis. Conventionally, implants have been placed maximally parallel to each other but the invention of newer prosthetic tools such as angled abutments and multiunit abutments has simplified prosthetic reconstruction of implants which are not parallel to each other. A screw-retained prosthesis offers the advantages of retrievability and no cement in the peri-implant soft tissue but fabrication of passive screw-retained prosthesis requires accurate implant impression transfer and adequate laboratory support, where the technician has expertise in fabricating the passively seated, screw-retained implant superstructure using plastic abutments. The cement-retained prosthesis is easy to fabricate and passively seat over implants. It also avoids the problem of screw holes displaying into the aesthetic region.

Note: Various step by step surgical and prosthetic procedures for full mouth rehabilitation with fixed implant-supported prosthesis are described in Chapter 22, Full-arch fixed prosthesis: 'All-on-4'/'All-on-6' approach.'

Further Reading

Misch CE. Screw-retained versus cement-retained implant-supported prostheses. Pract Periodont Aes Dent 1995;7:15–8.

Carlson B, Carlsson GE. Prosthodontic complications in osseointegrated dental implant treatment. Int J Oral Maxillofac Implants 1994;9:90–4.

Weinberg LA. The biomechanics of force distribution in implant-supported prostheses. Int J Oral Maxillofac Implants 1993;8:19–31.

Misch CE, Bidez MW. Implant-protected occlusion: a biomechanical rationale. Compend Contin Dent Educ 1994;15:1330–43.

Heydecke G, Boudrias P, Awad MA, et al. Within-subject comparisons of maxillary fixed and removable implant prostheses: patient satisfaction and choice of prosthesis. Clin Oral Impl Res 2003;14:125–30.

Lundgren D, Falk H, Laurell L. The influence of number and distribution of occlusal cantilever contacts on closing and chewing forces in dentitions with implant-supported fixed prostheses occluding with complete dentures. Int J Oral Maxillofac Implants 1989;4:277–83; 21.

Rungcharassaeng K, Kan JY. Fabricating a stable record base for completely edentulous patients treated with osseointegrated implants using healing abutments. J Prosthet Dent 1999;81:224–7.

Celletti R, Pameijer C, Bracchetti G, et al. Histologic evaluation of osseointegrated implants restored in nonaxial functional occlusion with pre-angled abutments. Int J Perio Rest Dent 1995;15:563–73.

Arvidson K, Bystedt H, Frykholm A, et al. 3-year clinical study of Astra dental implants in the treatment of edentulous mandibles. Int J Oral Maxollofac Implants 1992;7:321–9.

Hebel KS, Gajar RC. Cement-retained versus screw-retained implant restorations: achieving optimal occlusion and esthetics in implant dentistry. J Prosthet Dent 1997;77:28–35.

O'Roark WL. Improving implant survival rates by using a new method of risk analysis. Int J Oral Maxillofac Implants 1991;8:31–57.

Branemark PI. Osseointegrated implants in the treatment of the edentulous jaw experience from a 10-year period. Stockholm: Amquist and Wesell Internate; 1997.

Adell RE, Lekholm UJ, Rockler BI. A 15-year study of osseointegrated implants in the treatment of the edentulous jaw. Int J Oral Surg 1981;10:387–416.

Misch CE. Contemporary implant dentistry. St Louis: Mosby-Year Book Inc; 1993, pp. 651–685.

Jemt T, Linden B, Lekholm U. Failures and complications in 127 consecutively placed fixed partial prostheses supported by Branemark implants: from prosthesis treatment to first annual check up. Int J Oral Maxillofac Implants 1992;7:40–4.

Jemt T, Lekholm U. Oral implant treatment in posterior partially edentulous jaws: a 5-year follow-up report. Int J Oral Maxillofac Implants 1993;8:635–40.

Ogiso M, Tabata T, Kuo PT, et al. A histologic comparison of the functional loading capacity of an occluded dense apatite implant and the natural dentition. J Prosthet Dent 1994;71:581–8.

Kallus T, Bessing C. Loose gold screws frequently occur in full-arch fixed prostheses supported by osseointegrated implants after 5 years. Int J Oral Maxillofac Implants 1994;9:169–78.

Tischler M. Full-arch fixed prosthetics supported by dental implants and natural teeth: planning, provisionalization, treatment sequences: two case examples: dentistrytoday.com September 2004.

Nalbandian S, Lawrence B. Full-arch implant-supported 12-unit zirconia bridge. Australian Dental Practice 180–186, May/June 2007.

Full-arch fixed prosthesis: 'All-on-4™'/'All-on-6' approach

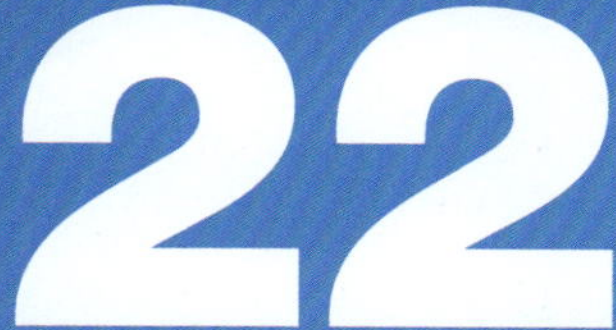

Ajay Vikram Singh   Sunita Singh

CHAPTER CONTENTS HD

Introduction

The conventional full-arch fixed implant-supported prosthesis often needs placement of several implants (8–12) to support a 12- to 14-unit fixed prosthesis. Moreover, the patients who come to the implant dentist for the full-arch implant-supported prosthesis usually present the loss of ridge volume especially in the maxillary and mandibular posterior regions, which limits the insertion of the implant with adequate dimensions without prior bone augmentation. The long-term edentulism of the posterior maxilla or replacement of lost maxillary molars and premolars other than the implant prosthesis, may result in lowering of the sinus floor because of the pneumatization of the sinus. In several cases, it results in the presence of inadequate subantral bone height to insert the implant. Thus, in several cases that need the full-arch implant prosthesis, the sinus augmentation procedure needs to be performed to regenerate the desired bone dimensions. However, this procedure may take 6–8 months before implants can be inserted. Moreover, the density of the bone in this region is usually poor and may require subgingival healing of the inserted implants for a further 6–8 months before they are loaded to support fixed prostheses.

So restoring the maxilla with fixed full-arch implant-supported prosthesis offers several disadvantages such as the need for sinus grafting procedures in some cases, delayed implant placement, a long time span (6 months to 1 year) to restore the case, multiple surgical interventions, more complications, a long period of wearing a provisional prosthesis (usually removable), high cost of the procedure, etc.

Similarly, the full-arch implant-supported mandibular prosthesis needs the insertion of 6–10 implants. The presence of mental foramina limits long implant placement only in the anterior mandibular region and often the bone available above the mandibular canals in the posterior mandible is found inadequate for the insertion of an adequately long implant. This results in the possibility of the placement of only 5–6 implants in the mandibular anterior region and a fixed prosthesis with long distal cantilevered extensions, which can be placed to a limited extent to avoid future complications. The onlay grafting to generate bone volume in the posterior mandible needs a lot of surgical interventions, a long time span to complete treatment, more complications, increased cost, etc.

To overcome these problems and to restore the full-arch cases immediately after graftless implant insertion, Dr Paulo Malo at the Malo Clinic, Lisbon, Portugal invented the 'All-on-4™' implant procedure. In 1993, he performed the pilot study to establish the All-on-4™ standard protocol. Since 1998, when the NobelSpeedy implant (Nobel Biocare, India) was developed, he published many retrospective studies about All-on-4™ for maxillary and mandibular rehabilitation.

All-on-4™ is a graftless implant placement procedure for restoring the edentulous jaw by tilting posterior implants for utilizing maximum amount of bone and stabilizing them in highest possible bone density. The tilting of posterior implants reduces the length of posterior cantilevering of the prosthesis. Moreover, it allows long implant placement and the insertion of the implant apex in the high-density anterior maxilla or anterior mandible, to achieve adequate primary stability for immediate loading on the implants, using a provisional splinted acrylic prosthesis. Hence, this facilitates optimal support for an acrylic prosthesis that can be immediately fixed over

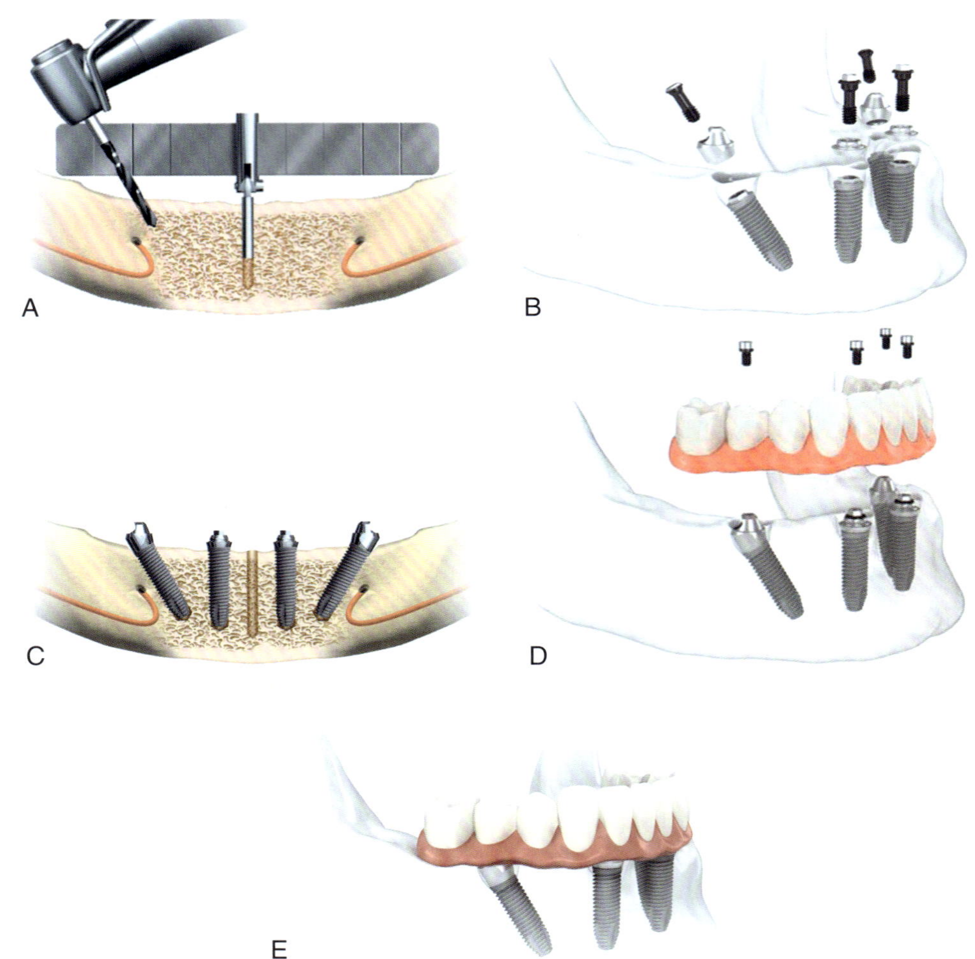

Fig 22.1 Flaps are elevated to expose the bony ridge, and the mental foramina are located. An osteotomy of approximately 10 mm depth in the midline is prepared using a φ 2 mm twist drill and the All-on-4 guide is correctly placed in this midline osteotomy. The posterior osteotomies are prepared to the appropriate depth and tilted distally to the maximum angle of 45°. (A) The posterior osteotomies are prepared in such a manner that the posteriorily tilted implants are placed minimum 2 mm anterior to the inferior alveolar nerve. The osteotomies for the anterior implants are prepared in the usual manner. (B and C) After placing all the four implants, the straight or 17° multiunit abutments are placed on top of the anterior implants whereas the 30° multiunit abutments are inserted over the posterior tilted implants. Multiunit abutments of appropriate collar height should be selected for each implant and should be tightened to 15 Ncm using torque ratchet. (D and E) Immediate provisional and later on definitive hybrid prosthesis are fixed over these implants using fixation screws. *(Courtesy: Nobel Biocare, India).*

the inserted implants to restore aesthetics and function within a few hours of implant insertion surgery. All-on-4™ is based on Nobel Biocare's pioneering 'Immediate Function' capability.

To perform this technique, a total of four implants are inserted with the back implants tilted up to 45°, often in close approximation to the inferior and anterior wall of maxillary sinus in the upper jaw and superior and anterior to the inferior alveolar nerve and mental foramina in the mandible, to take maximum advantage of existing bone by inserting long implants and firmly stabilizing their apex in high-density anterior bone. A fixed standardized surgical guide is used to correct implant placement. Both flap and flapless (guided) approaches are compatible with the technique. Special components are developed to correct the prosthetic angulation of the tilted implants as well as to immediately restore the implants in function. If necessary, a cantilever can also be added to the final prosthesis. The skilled approach of tilting the posterior implants avoids expensive, time-consuming, and more invasive grafting procedures like sinus grafting, block grafting, etc.

Step by step diagrammatic presentation of All-on-4™ in the mandible is shown in Fig 22.1A–E.

Step by step diagrammatic presentation of All-on-4™ in the maxilla is shown in Fig 22.2A–D

All-on-6 technique

Because of graftless implant placement and immediate loading, the All-on-4™ technique is very successfully being performed by many dentists and has gained high popularity among implant dentists as well as patients. The only limitation with this technique is that prosthesis with only limited number of teeth (10–12 units) can be

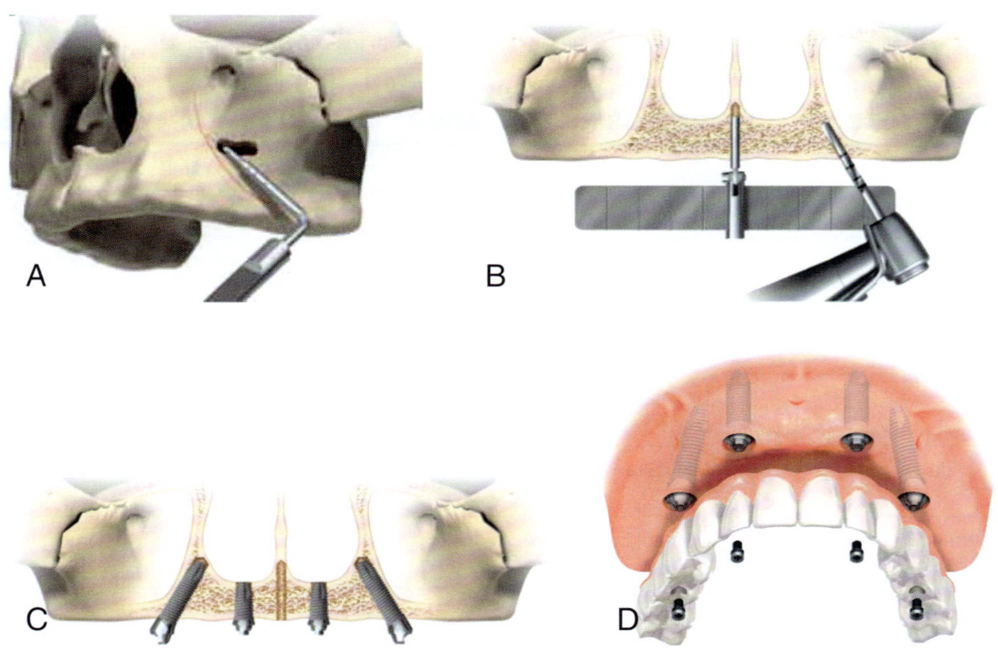

Fig 22.2 Flap is elevated to expose the bony ridge as well as lateral wall of the maxillary sinus. A small opening on the lateral wall of the sinus is prepared where the anterior wall of the sinus is expected. Further, the anterior wall of the maxillary sinus is explored by using a probe through this opening. (A) The lateral window is extended if necessary and position of the anterior wall is marked using a sterile pencil. An osteotomy approximately 10 mm depth is prepared in the midline using a φ 2 mm twist drill and the All-on-4™ guide is correctly placed in the midline osteotomy. (B) The osteotomies for the posterior implants should be started as posterior as possible to minimize the cantilever and allowing approximately 4 mm distance from the sinus. The posterior osteotomies are prepared to the appropriate depth and tilted to the maximum angle to the 45°, so that the posteriorly tilted implants are placed a minimum 2 mm anterior to the anterior wall of the sinus. Two implants at the most-anterior position are placed in the usual manner. (C) The 17° or straight multiunit abutments are placed on the anterior implants whereas the 30° multiunit abutments are placed on the posterior implants. (D) Immediate provisional and later on definitive hybrid prosthesis are fixed over the implants using fixation screws *(Courtesy: Nobel Biocare, India).*

fixed over these four implants. Further, the loss of any one implant reverts the entire procedure to the initial stage.

To avoid such problems and also for the patients who express the desire for a 14-unit prosthesis, two more implants can be inserted posterior to the posterior wall of the sinus in the maxillary tuberosity and tilted anteriorly at 45° to minimize the length of the unsupported bridge framework between two distal implants. The severely resorbed posterior maxilla with a large volume of posterior expansion of the sinus often does not leave enough bone volume in the tuberosity region to place an implant of an adequate size. In such cases, the implant is inserted in the tuberosity with the apex of the implant at the junction of the pyramidal process of the palatine bone and the pterygoid process of the sphenoid bone. The implant placed would then engage all three bone segments that constitute this region. The implant placement in the tuberosity with its apex engaging the medial pterygoid process of sphenoid bone is the most preferred option because it allows the multicortical engagement of the implant to achieve adequate initial stability for the implant.

To perform the All-on-6 procedure in the mandible, the two straight implants should be inserted usually at the first or second molar site but if inadequate ridge height above the mandibular canal does not allow placement of implants in the molar region, then the short and wide implant can be inserted at the angle of the mandible (into the buccal shelf area) tilted anteriorly at 30–45°.

With the few advantages, there are also several disadvantages with All-on-6 procedures such as increased cost, need of a highly skilled approach to correctly place implants in pterygoid process, difficult approach for the insertion and restoration of posterior implants, need of a skilled technician to fabricate the prosthesis, and problems in oral hygiene maintenance in the back region.

Comparative features of the traditional versus All-on-4™/All-on-6 approach

Advantages of the All-on-4™/All-on-6 technique

1. Vast numbers of the edentulous patients can be treated with the technique.
2. Being a graftless and immediate loading technique, it is more acceptable to patients.
3. Fewer implants are inserted.
4. Fixed teeth can be given on four implants to patients for whom sinus grafting/nerve transpositioning procedures are contraindicated.

Table 22.1 Comparison of the graftless All-on-4™/All-on-6 approaches with the conventional full-arch implant procedure

COMPARATIVE FEATURE	TRADITIONAL APPROACH FOR RESTORING FULL-ARCH	ALL-ON-4™/ALL-ON-6 APPROACH
Sinus grafting	May be required	Not required
Only grafting	May be required	Not required
No. of implants	More no. of implants are inserted	Less no. of implants are needed
Immediate fixed restoration in function	May not be possible	Possible
Surgery	More invasive	Less invasive
Surgical steps	May require multiple surgical steps like grafting procedures, implants insertion, uncovery, etc.	Only one surgical step, i.e. implant insertion
Time span needed to deliver the final prosthesis	May take 6 months to 1 year	Can be completed in a few weeks
Sinus pathology contraindicating the grafting and implant placement	May not be possible	Possible
Patient's acceptance	Less	More
CT guided implant placement	Possible in selective cases	Possible in most cases

5. Lower cost of the treatment compared to the traditional implant-supported full-arch fixed prosthesis which often needs bone grafting, more implants, multiple surgical steps, etc.
6. Long tilted distal implant can be maximally stabilized by utilizing high-density bone of the anterior region. Placement of longer implants, enhancement of the area of interaction between bone and implant, and also primary anchorage.
7. A greater distance between implants, allowing the elimination of cantilevers in the prosthesis, which results in better load distribution.
8. By reducing the number of implants to four, each implant can be placed without interfering with the adjacent implants.
9. The placement of implants in residual bone, avoiding more complex techniques of bone graft and/or sinus lift.
10. Immediate loading is done in most of the cases so that the patient gets at least provisional fixed teeth on the day of implant placement for aesthetics and function.
11. It can be performed by implant surgeons who are not very expert at performing procedures like sinus grafting, block grafting, nerve transpositioning, etc.
12. Only one surgical step is required (no implant uncovery).
13. The high success rate of the procedure (as shown in the various studies).
14. Treatment completed in very short period of time (in a few weeks) whereas the traditional technique may however take years to complete treatment.

Disadvantages of the All-on-4™/All-on-6 technique

1. It cannot be performed in patients presenting with large osseous defects in the anterior region, which needs grafting procedures to regenerate new bone before All-on-4™ implant placement.
2. Extraction of firm, healthy teeth is mandatory, if any are present in the anterior jaw.
3. Reduction of bone crest causes increased soft tissue height which in turn leads to increased pocket depth around the abutment, more chances of bacterial growth, and peri-implantitis.
4. With the All-on-4™, only the 10- to 12-unit prosthesis is delivered over the four implants, and often patients request the addition of more posterior teeth to maximize chewing efficiency and improve the overall maxillofacial prosthesis.
5. Oral hygiene: Maintenance of the hybrid prosthesis is often difficult for some patients and they need regular visits to the dentist for its cleaning.

Indications

1. Edentulous patients who need fixed implant-supported prosthesis – maxillary, mandibular or both.
2. Patients with partial maxillary/mandibular edentulism with only few intact natural teeth in the anterior region.
3. Patients with worn out dentition which needs extraction and replacement of all teeth.
4. Patients with periodontally compromised mobile teeth which need extraction and replacement.
5. Edentulous or partially edentulous patients with very limited subantral bone height in the posterior maxilla.
6. Edentulous or partially edentulous patients with very limited bone height above the mandibular canals in the posterior mandible.
7. Edentulous patients with maxillary sinus pathologies contraindicating the sinus grafting procedure.
8. Patients with adequate volume of healthy bone in the maxillary and mandibular anterior region to place implants.

9. Implant overdenture cases with severe ridge resorption – tilting posterior implants give more support to the denture and prevent soft tissue abrasion and further bone loss in the posterior region.

Contraindications

1. Patients with inadequate bone volume in the maxillary and mandibular anterior region to place implants.
2. Anterior wall of the sinus is located far anterior to the usual position, contraindicating tilting of the posterior implants to reach the second premolar or first molar position (Fig 22.3).

Key points for successful All-on-4™/All-on-6 implant therapy

1. Meticulous treatment planning to see the position and path of anterior, inferior, and posterior wall of maxillary sinus.

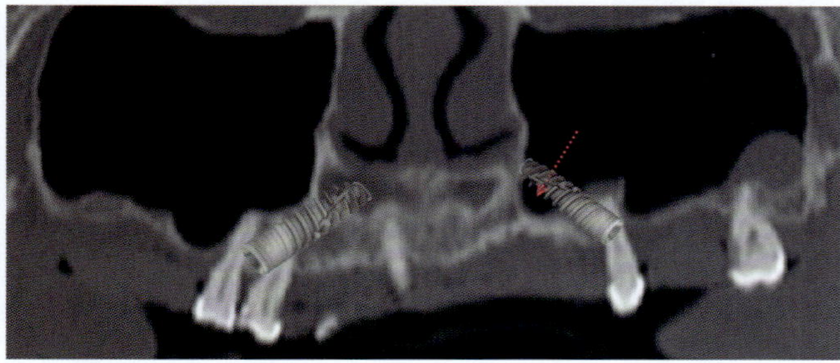

Fig 22.3 The left maxillary sinus has been overexpanded anteriorly (red arrow), contraindicating the placement of the tilted implant at the far posterior position.

2. Dental CT planning if possible, to see the possible placement of the implants with desired dimensions and their three-dimensional positioning for the best possible prosthesis.
3. Placement of longest possible implants and stabilization in the cortical bone such as nasal floor, basal bone of the anterior mandible, pterygoid process, etc. to achieve high primary stability.
4. Tilting of the posterior implants using the All-on-4™ guide to avoid extreme tilting which may result in parallelism problems during restoration.
5. Selection of multiunit abutments with proper collar height and angulation.
6. Sequential radiographs with the drill into the osteotomy during initial osteotomy preparation for posterior implants, to evaluate the direction of the drilling in respect to vital structures such as the sinus wall and the mandibular canal.
7. Placement of the implants with minimum diameter of 3.3mm at the anterior positions and 3.75–4.2mm for the posterior positions to avoid problems such as connection screw loosening and implant body fracture.
8. Adequate vertical ridge reduction before implant placement to avoid the display of the unaesthetic transition line of prosthesis and ridge tissue when the patient smiles (Fig 22.4A–D).

Management of complications

1. **Over or inadequate tilting of the posterior implants.** It can be avoided with accurate treatment planning and use of the All-on-4™ guide available from Nobel Biocare.
2. **Perforation through the inferior or anterior wall of the sinus.** It can be avoided by proper exploration of the anterior wall of the sinus. Pilot drilling should

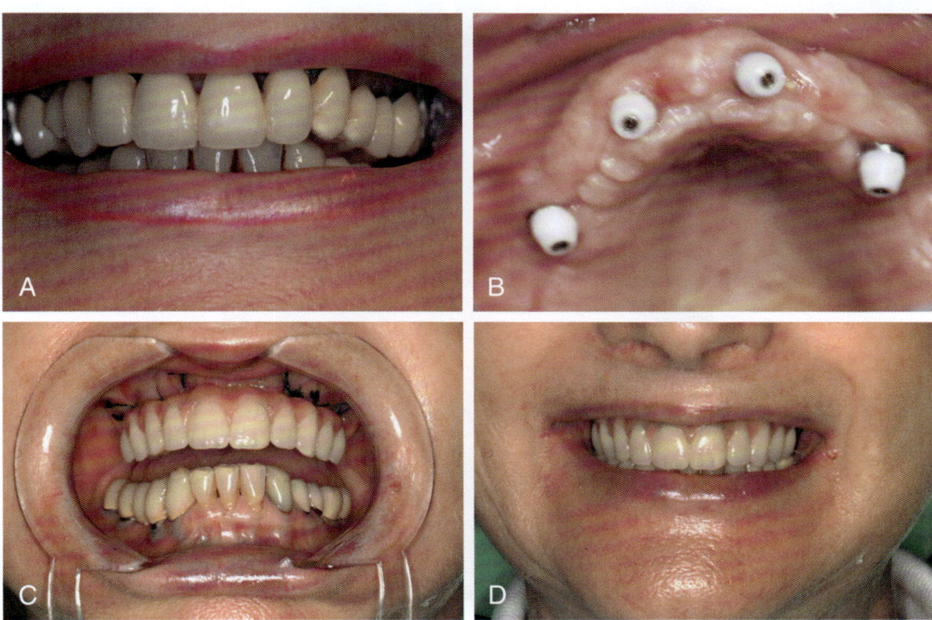

Fig 22.4 (A) Unaesthetic gingival line with the old prosthesis is visible during the smile. A planned vertical ridge reduction before the implant placement results in nonvisibility of the transition line of the final All-on-4™ implant prosthesis, when the patient smiles. (B–D) This gives a natural appearance to the All-on-4™ prosthesis. *(Courtesy: Saad Zemmouri, Morocco)*.

CASE REPORT-1

Step by step procedure for All-on-6 in the maxilla (Figs 22.5–22.19).

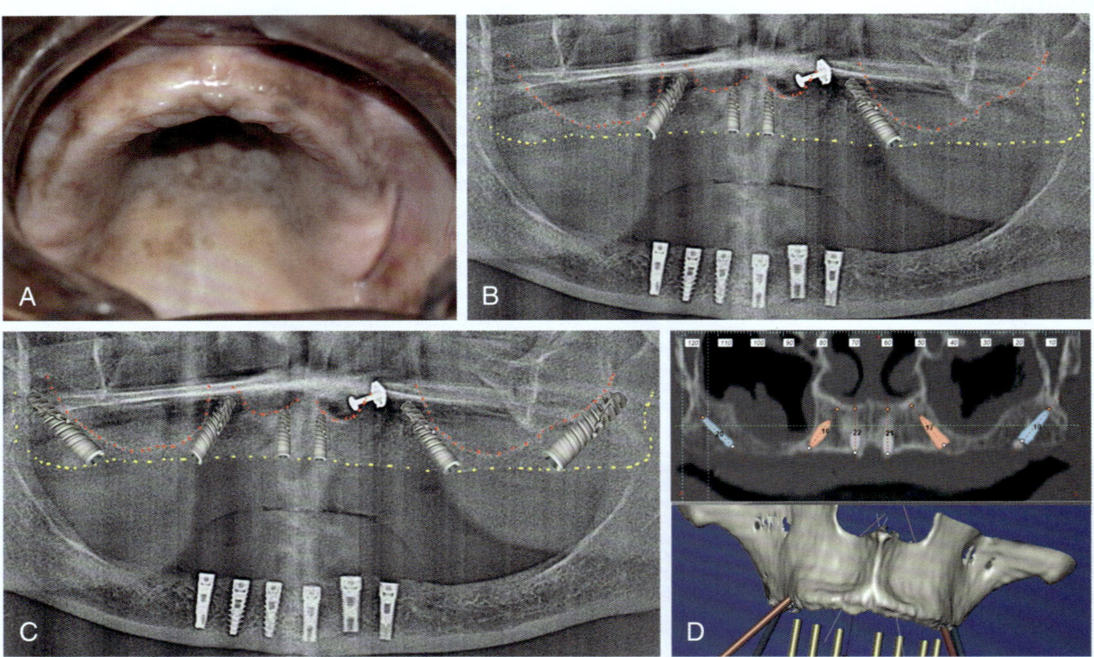

Fig 22.5 (A) Edentulous maxilla. (B) The panoramic radiograph shows adequate bone for All-on-4™ (C) as well as All-on-6 procedure. (D) The dental CT scan shows sinus membrane thickening, contraindicating sinus grafting procedure. Adequate amount of bone is luckily present bilaterally posterior to the sinus to insert adequate size implants, but needs to be laterally condensed to achieve adequate stability for the inserted implants.

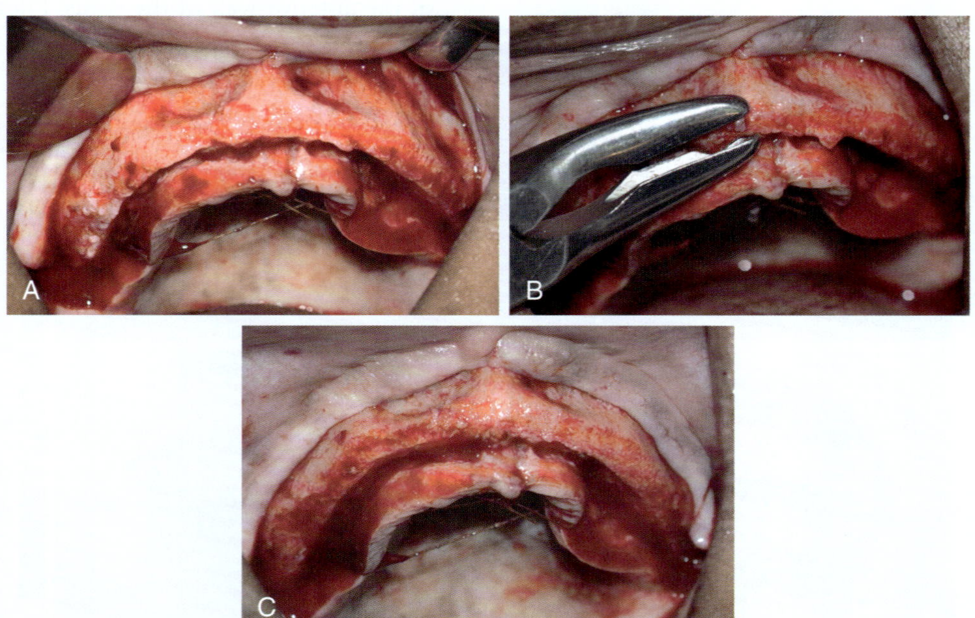

Fig 22.6 (A) Mucoperiosteal flaps are elevated to expose the bone ridge as well as the facial wall of the ridge and (B and C) planned amount of vertical ridge reduction is done using a bone rongeur to achieve the wide ridge crest to place implants with adequate diameters as well as to shift the transition line of the future prosthesis and ridge tissue apical to the high smile line of the patient.

CASE REPORT-1—cont'd

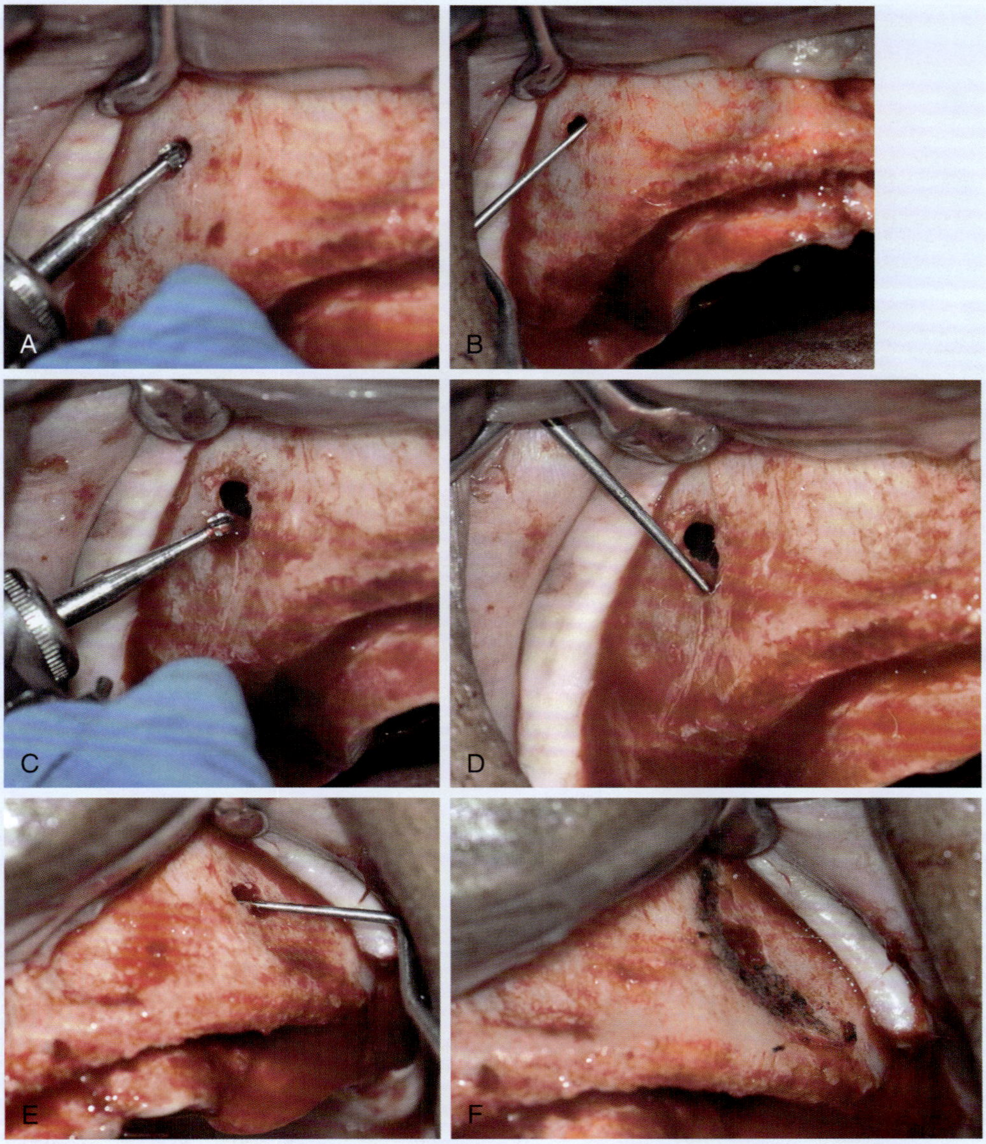

A B C D E F

Fig 22.7 (A) A small opening at the lateral wall of the right sinus is prepared using a round carbide bur. (B) The anterior wall of the sinus is explored using a probe. (C) The opening is extended to appropriately explore (D) the complete path of the anterior wall of the sinus. (E) The anterior wall of the left sinus is also explored in the same way and (F) it is marked using a sterile HB pencil.

Continued

CASE REPORT-1—cont'd

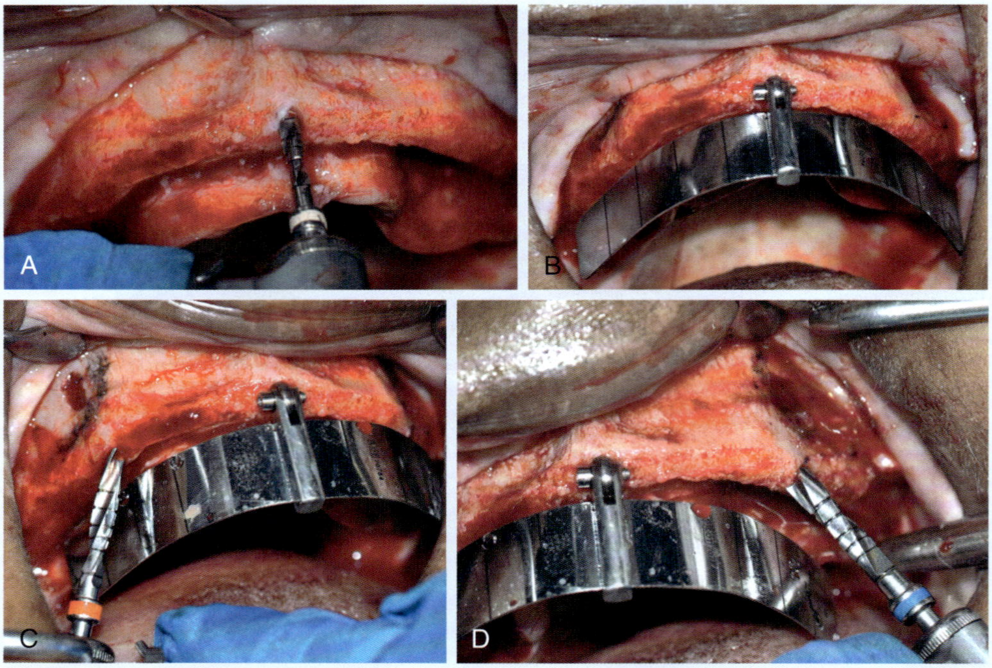

Fig 22.8 (A) An osteotomy is prepared using 2.0 mm pilot drill in the midline and (B) the All-on-4™ guide (Nobel Biocare, India) is placed. (C and D) The osteotomies are prepared for the posterior implants angled at the 45° and just anterior to the anterior wall of the sinus.

CASE REPORT-1—cont'd

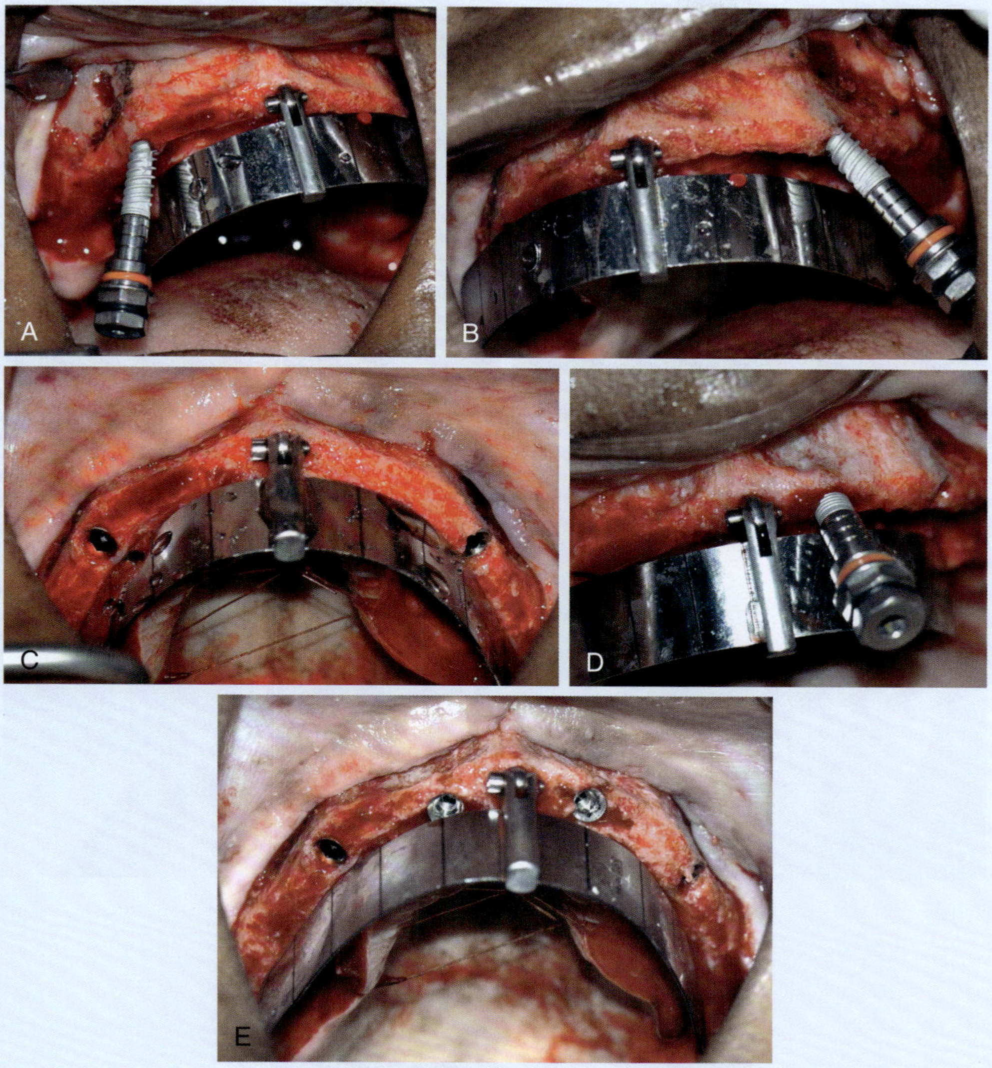

A B C D E

Fig 22.9 (A–C) The posterior implants are installed at the 45° and just anterior to the anterior wall of the sinus. (D and E) Two implants are placed at the anterior positions.

Continued

CASE REPORT-1—cont'd

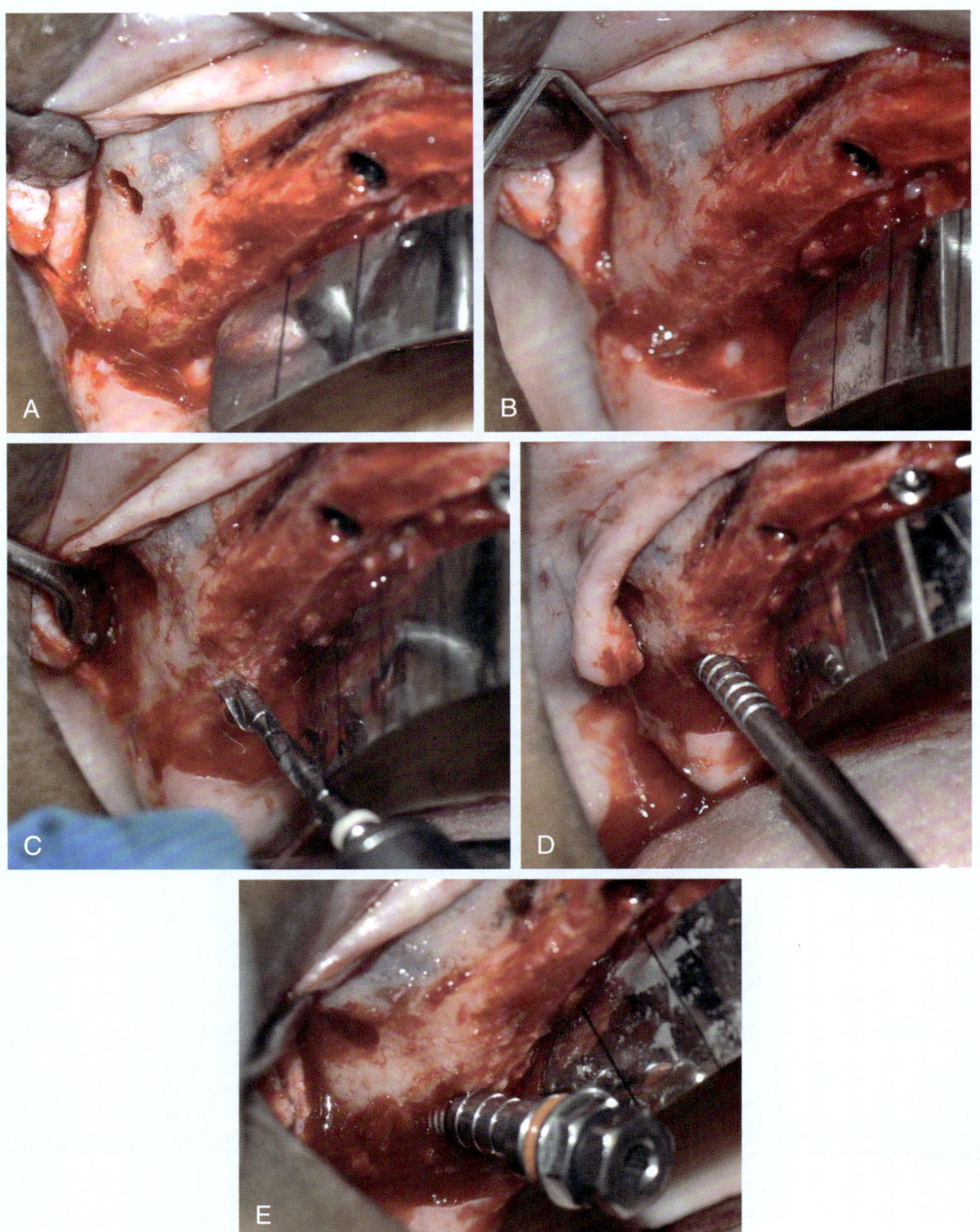

Fig 22.10 (A and B) Posterior wall of the right sinus is explored by preparing another small opening through the lateral wall and (C) the osteotomy is prepared using pilot drill at 45°, just posterior to the posterior wall of the sinus. (D) The osteotomes are then sequentially used for lateral bone condensation to improve the bone density around the implant. (E) The implant which is tilted at 45° is installed.

CASE REPORT-1—cont'd

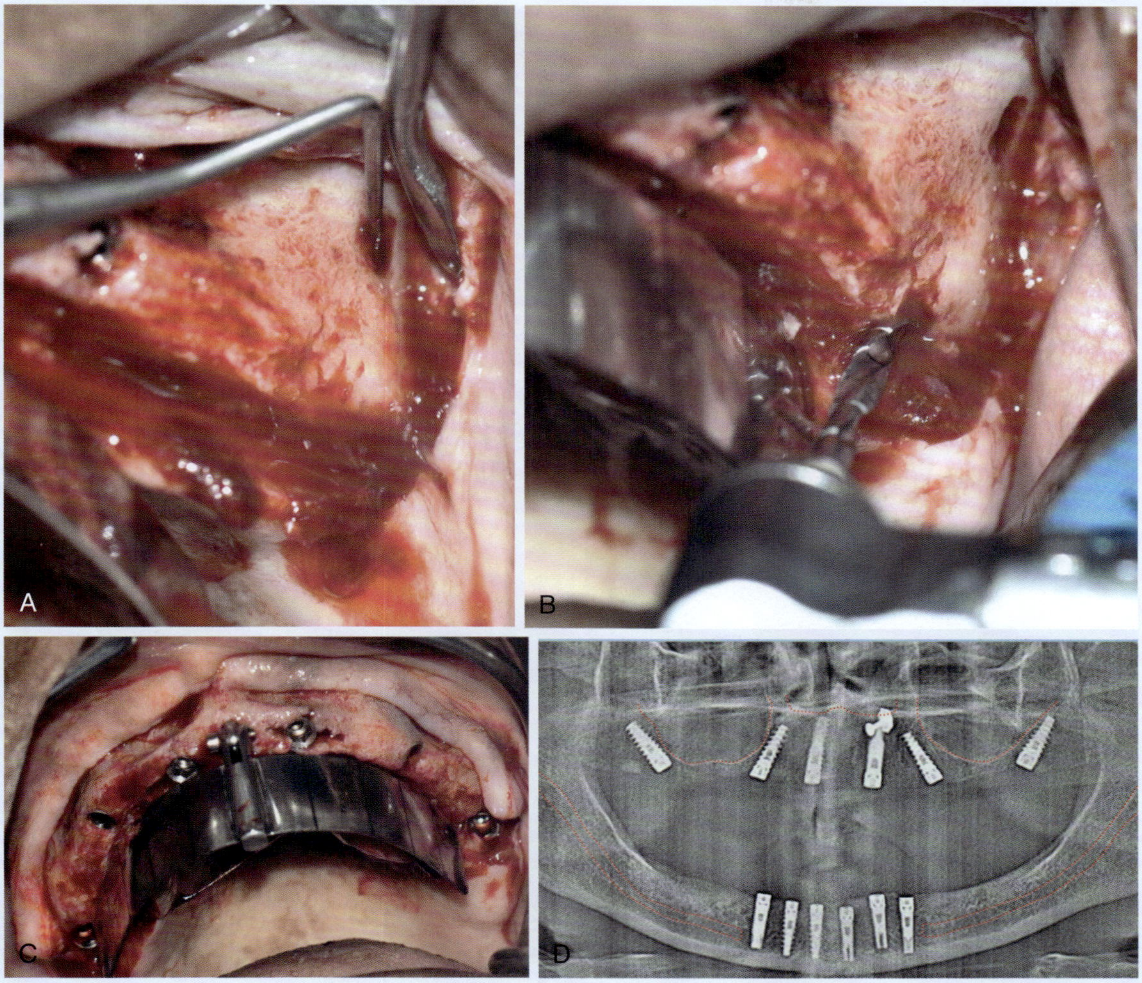

Fig 22.11 (A–C) Posterior wall of the left sinus is also explored in the same fashion and implant is inserted. (D) Postimplantation radiograph shows accurate placement of all six implants.

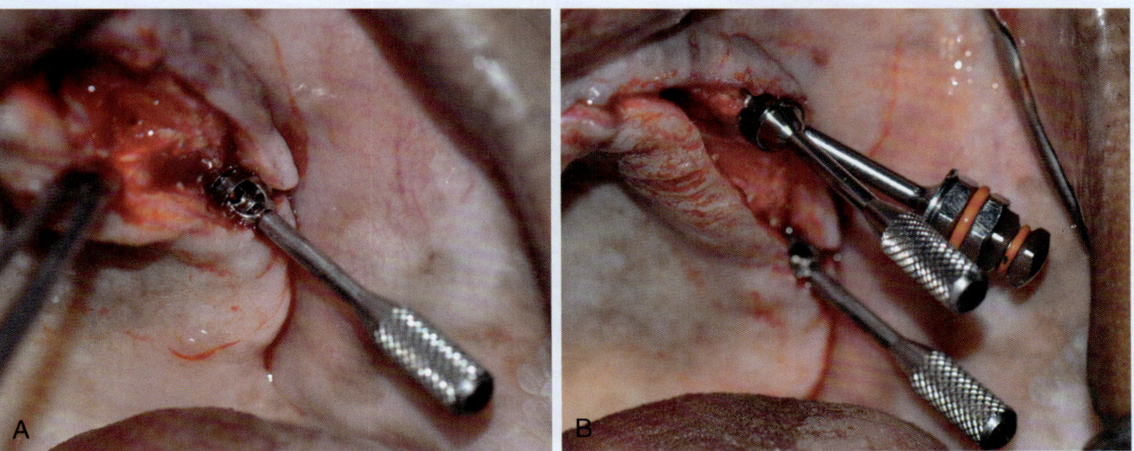

Fig 22.12 (A–C) The 30° multiunit abutments are placed on top of the all four posterior implants whereas the 17° multiunit abutments are placed on top of the both anterior implants.

Continued

CASE REPORT-1—cont'd

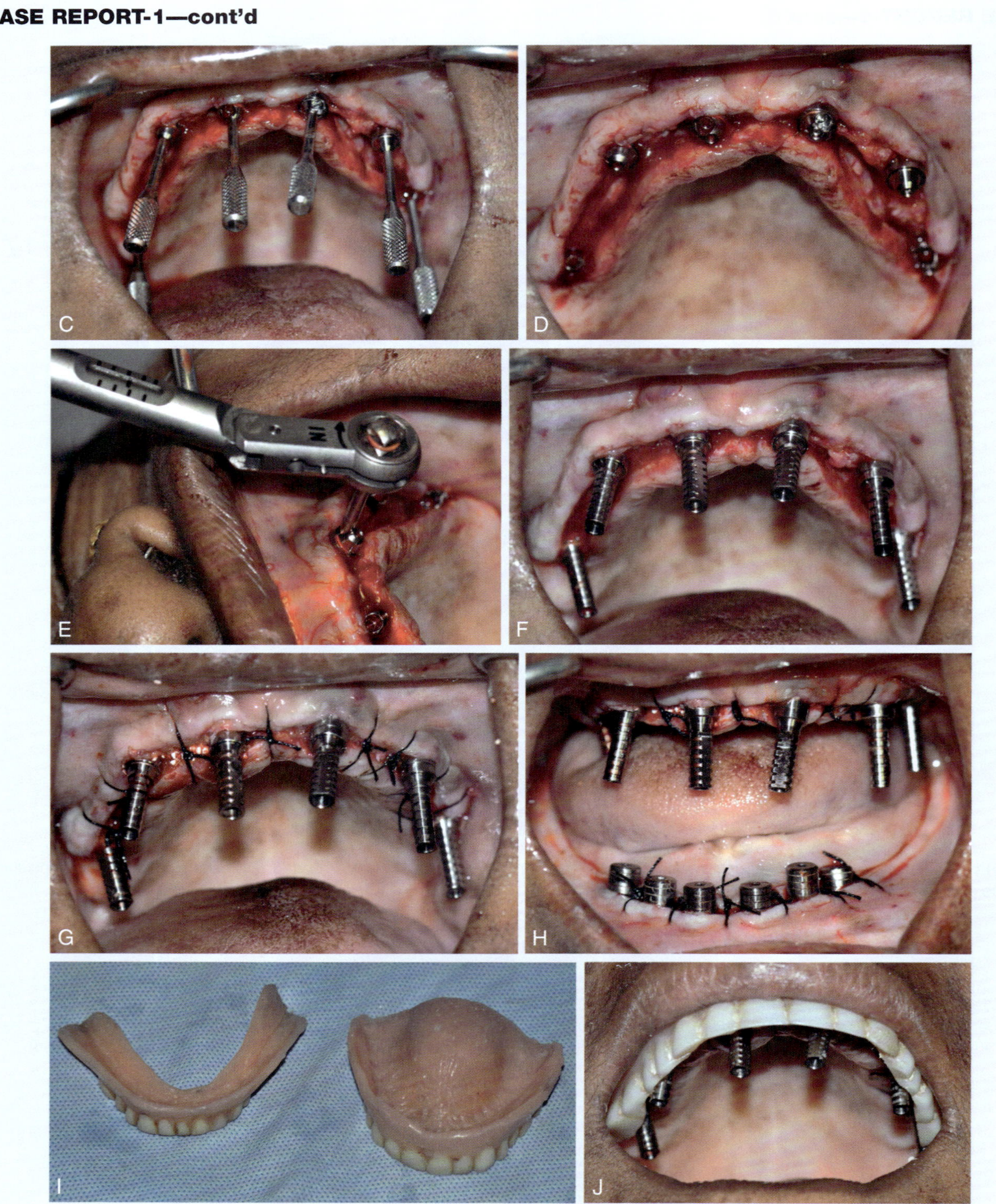

Fig 22.12, cont'd (D) Abutment mounts are removed and (E) the abutment screws are tightened at 15 Ncm using a torque ratchet. (F) The temporary titanium cylinders are screwed on top of the multiunit abutments using the connection screw and (G) flap is sutured. (H) Lower implants are also uncovered and healing abutments are inserted. (I) The patient's old dentures. (J) Upper denture is prepared and tried in the mouth for its passive seating through the abutments.

CASE REPORT-1—cont'd

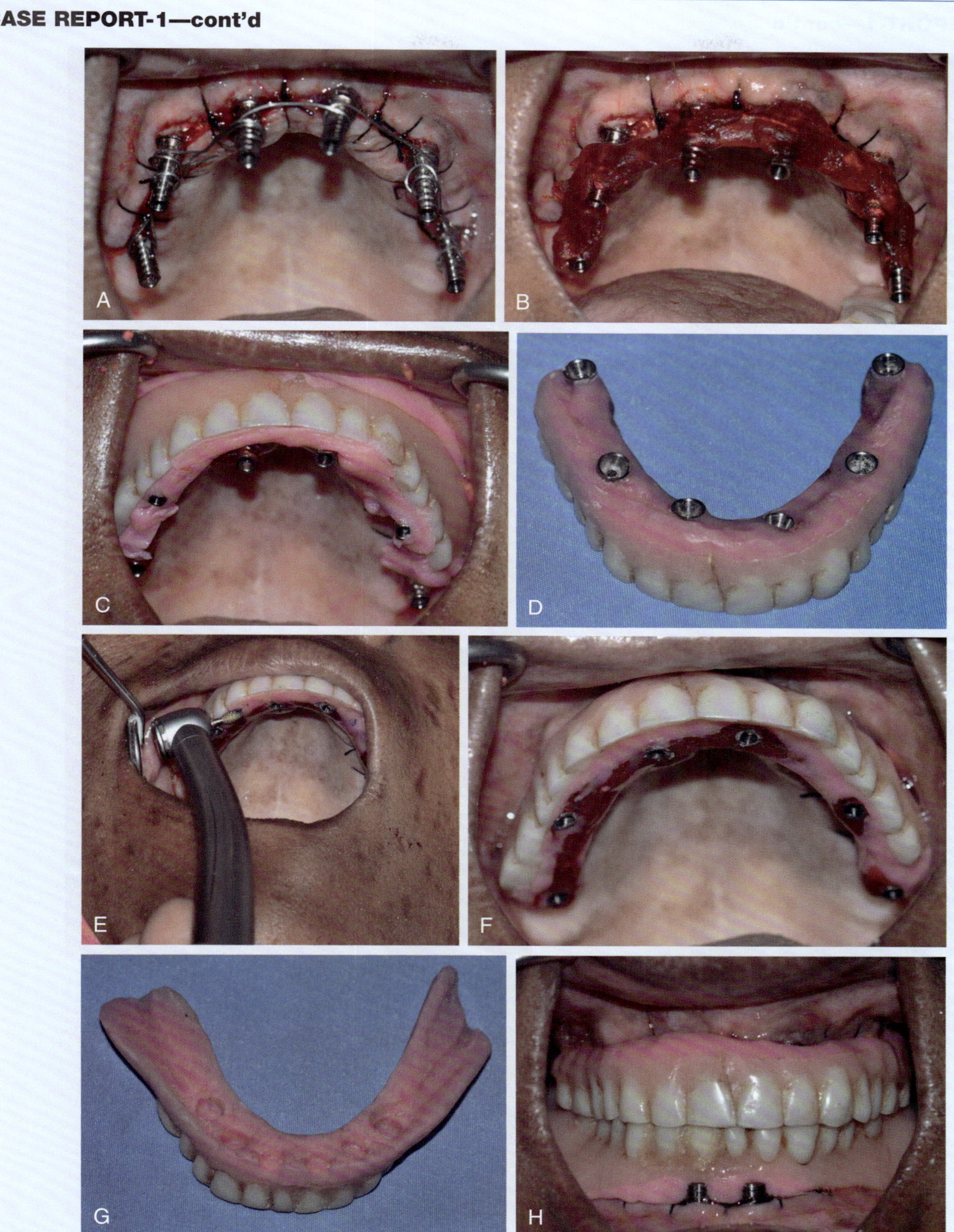

Fig 22.13 (A and B) All the abutments are splinted using a stainless steel wire, which is further reinforced using pattern resin. (C) The self-cure acrylic is mixed, filled into the denture which is accurately seated in the mouth at the correct position. (D) After the acrylic has set, the connection screws of the abutments are unscrewed and the denture along with the abutments is removed from the mouth. The prosthesis is finished, polished, and fixed over the multiunit abutments. (E and F) All the necessary occlusal adjustments are made in the mouth. (G) Relined lower denture. (H) Upper fixed and lower removable provisional prosthesis delivered on the same day as All-on-6 surgery.

Continued

CASE REPORT-1—cont'd

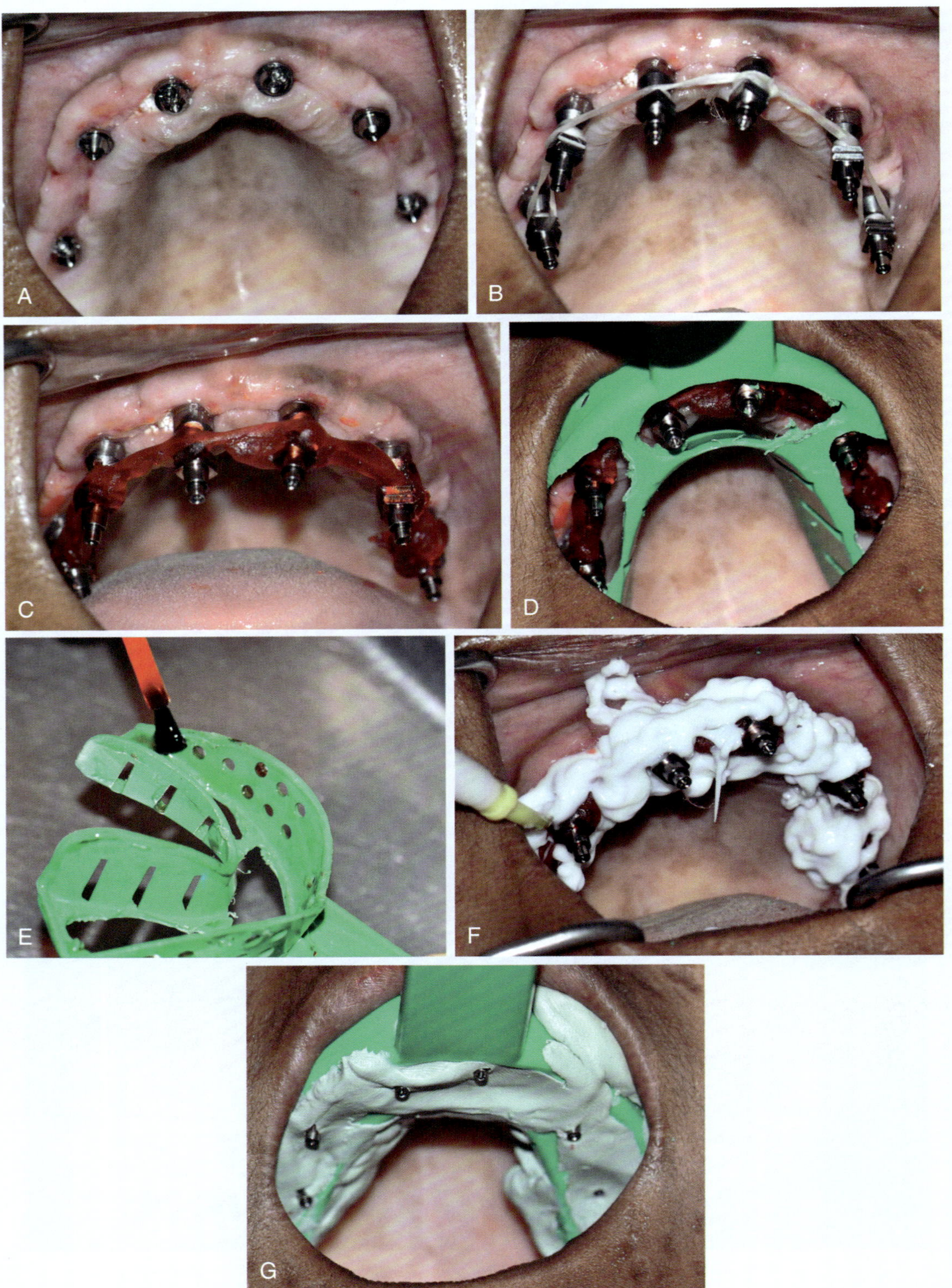

Fig 22.14 (A) Healing after 6 weeks, when the provisional prosthesis is removed for the impression procedure. (B) The open tray impression abutments are placed over the multiunit abutments and splinted using dental floss and (C) further reinforced using the pattern resin to avoid any movement of the abutments in respect to each other during the impression transfer. (D) A custom tray is prepared and tried in the mouth for its passive seating. (E) Tray is painted with tray adhesive. (F) The light body impression material is appropriately flowed under and all around the impression abutments and (G) the tray filled with putty is accurately seated in the mouth.

CASE REPORT-1—cont'd

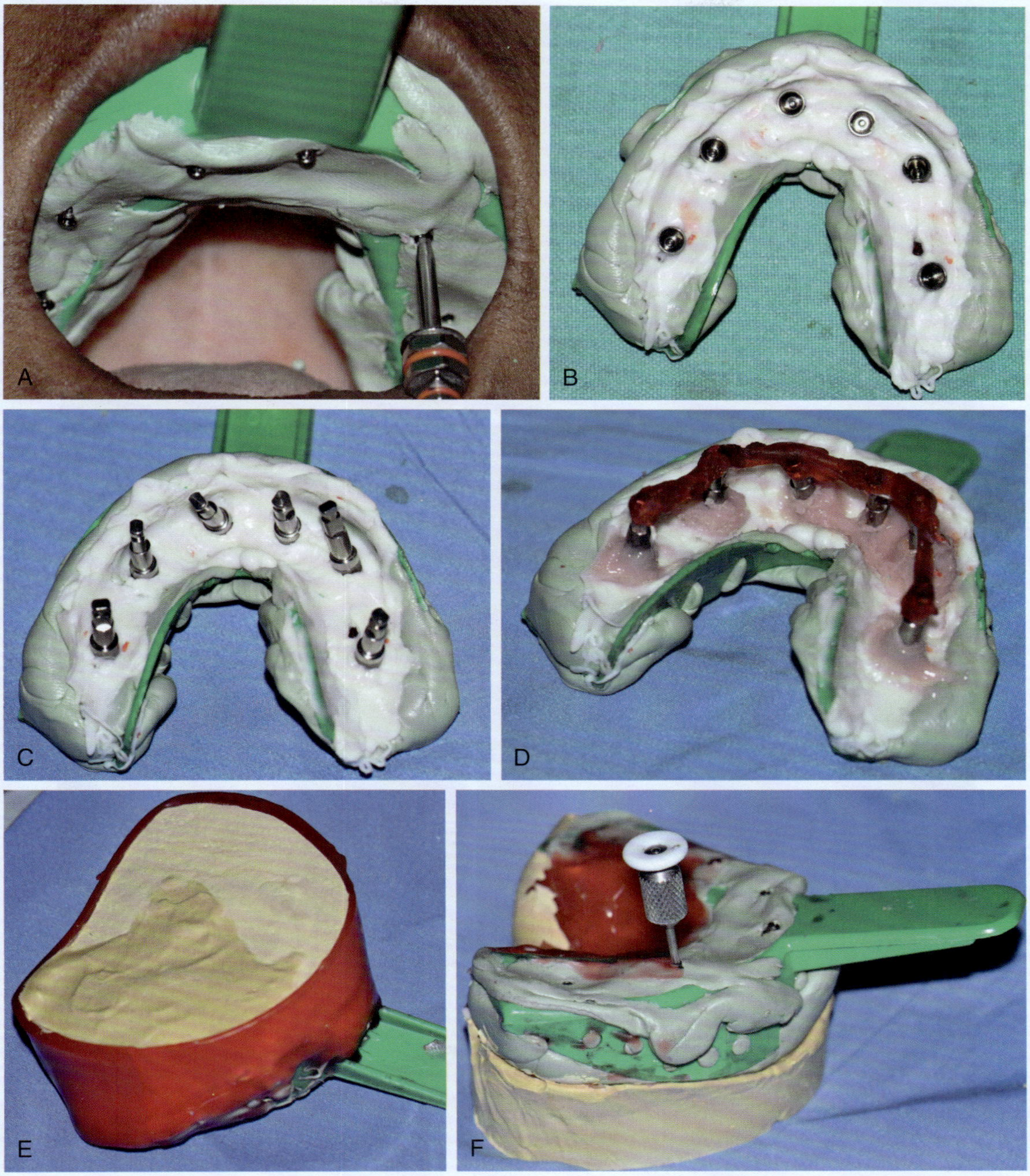

A B C D E F

Fig 22.15 (A) The long fixation screws, emerging out of the impression, are unscrewed (B) before removing the impression from the mouth. (C) The abutment analogues are assembled with the impression abutments. The abutment analogues are splinted together using pattern resin to avoid their micromovements in the stone plaster during the prosthetic steps in the laboratory. (D) The soft tissue replicating material is poured around the abutment analogue connections. (E) The impression is further poured using hard stone plaster. (F) The fixation screws are again unscrewed before removing the impression from the working cast.

Continued

CASE REPORT-1—cont'd

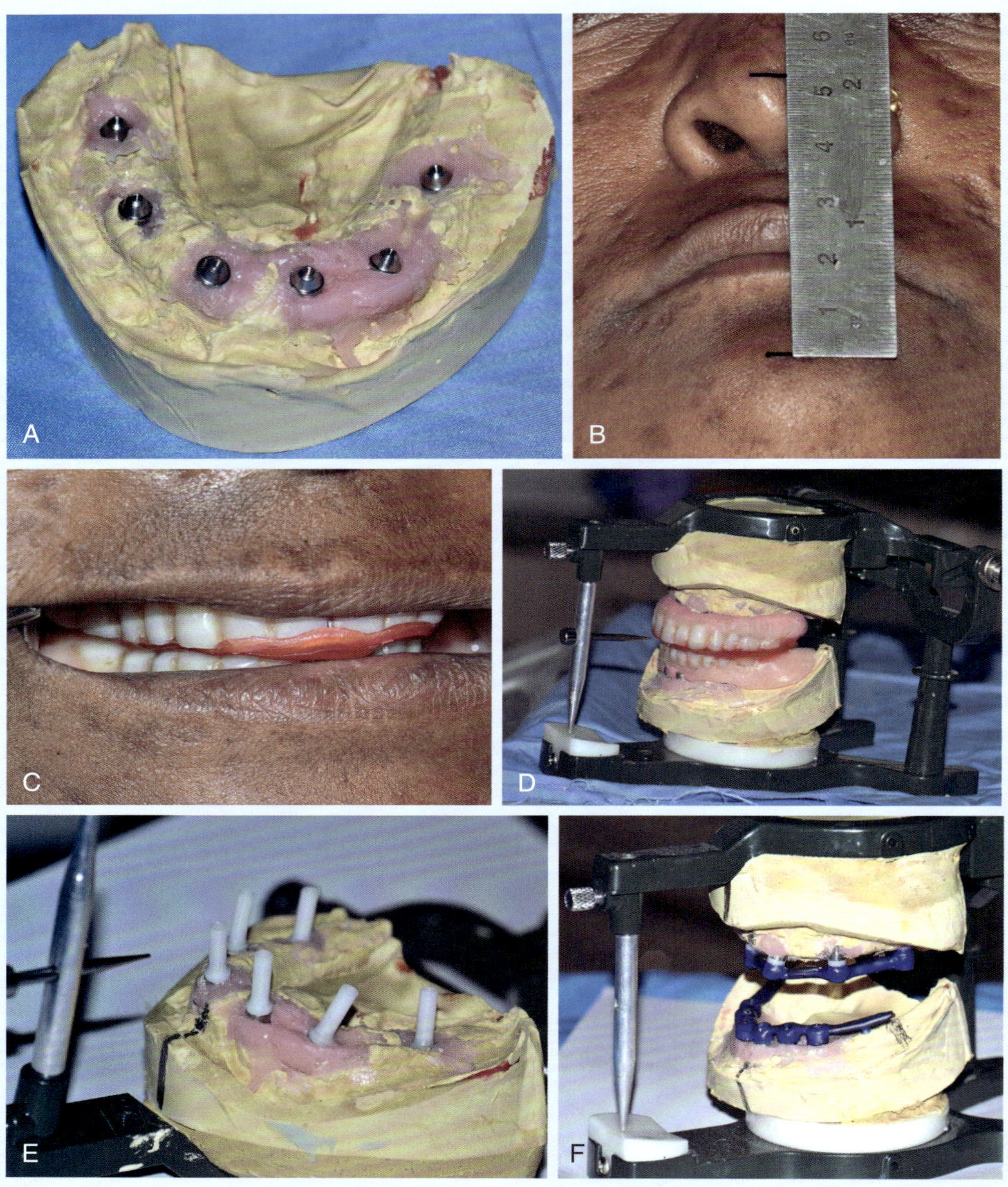

Fig 22.16 (A) The abutment analogues in the working cast. (B) The vertical height of occlusion is recorded at the centric position and (C) bite registration is done using the old prosthesis. (D) The final working casts are mounted on the articulator at the similar maxillo-mandibular relation. (E) The castable plastic abutments are screwed over the abutment analogues using fixation screws. (F) The wax pattern is prepared to fabricate a cast bar framework for upper and lower prosthesis.

CASE REPORT-1—cont'd

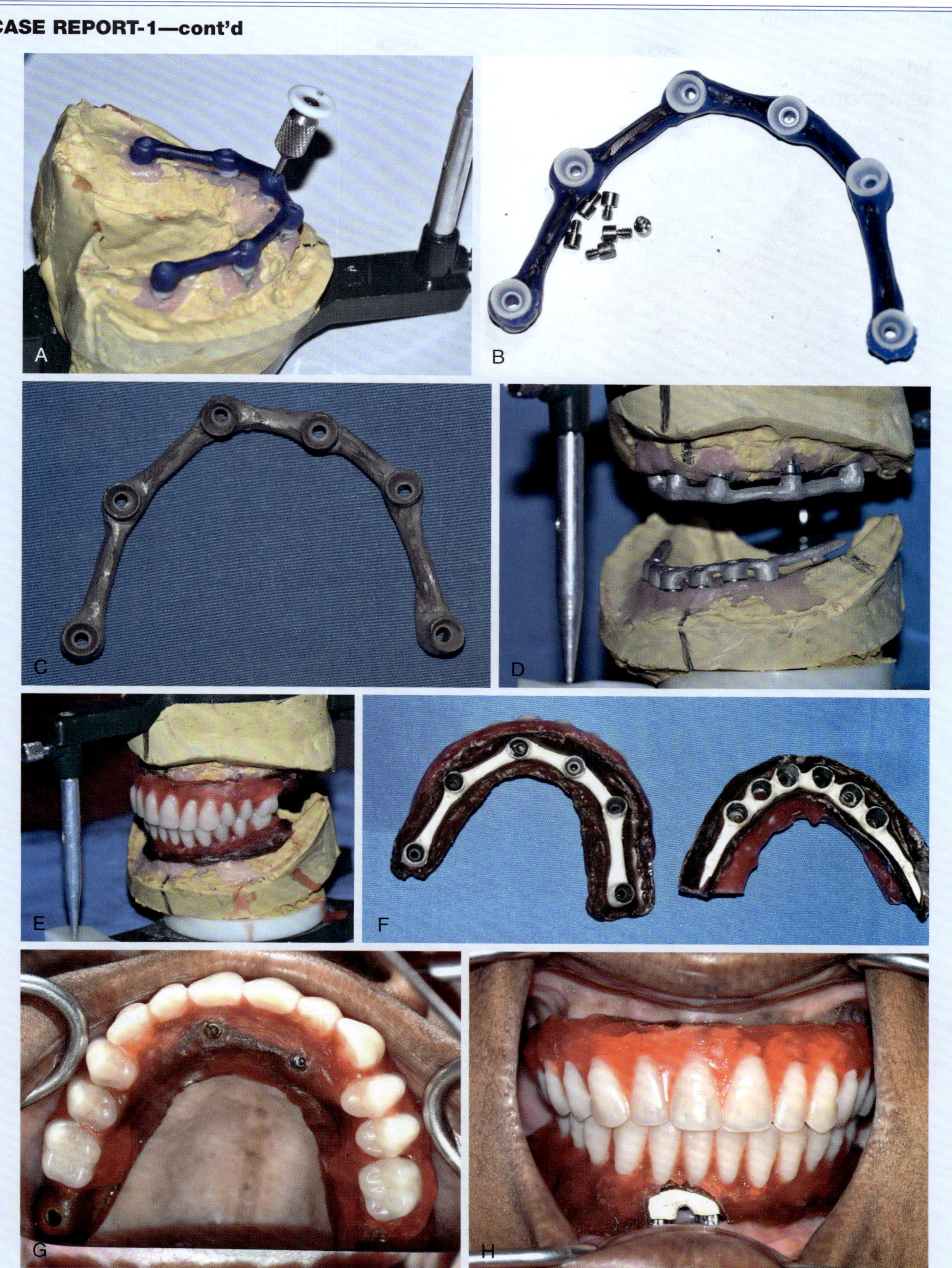

Fig 22.17 (A and B) The fixation screws are unscrewed and the wax pattern along with castable abutments are removed from the cast. (C) The fixation screws are separated and the whole wax pattern along with castable abutments is cast to fabricate a bar of the Ni–Cr or titanium metal, (D) which is screwed over the working casts. The ceramic wash opaque can be used over the bar to avoid metal display through the thin acrylic. (E) The base plate is adapted over the bar and the teeth setting is done in the usual fashion. (F–H) The upper and lower bar framework along with teeth setting are tried in the mouth to check the passive seating of the bar as well as the occlusion.

Continued

CASE REPORT-1—cont'd

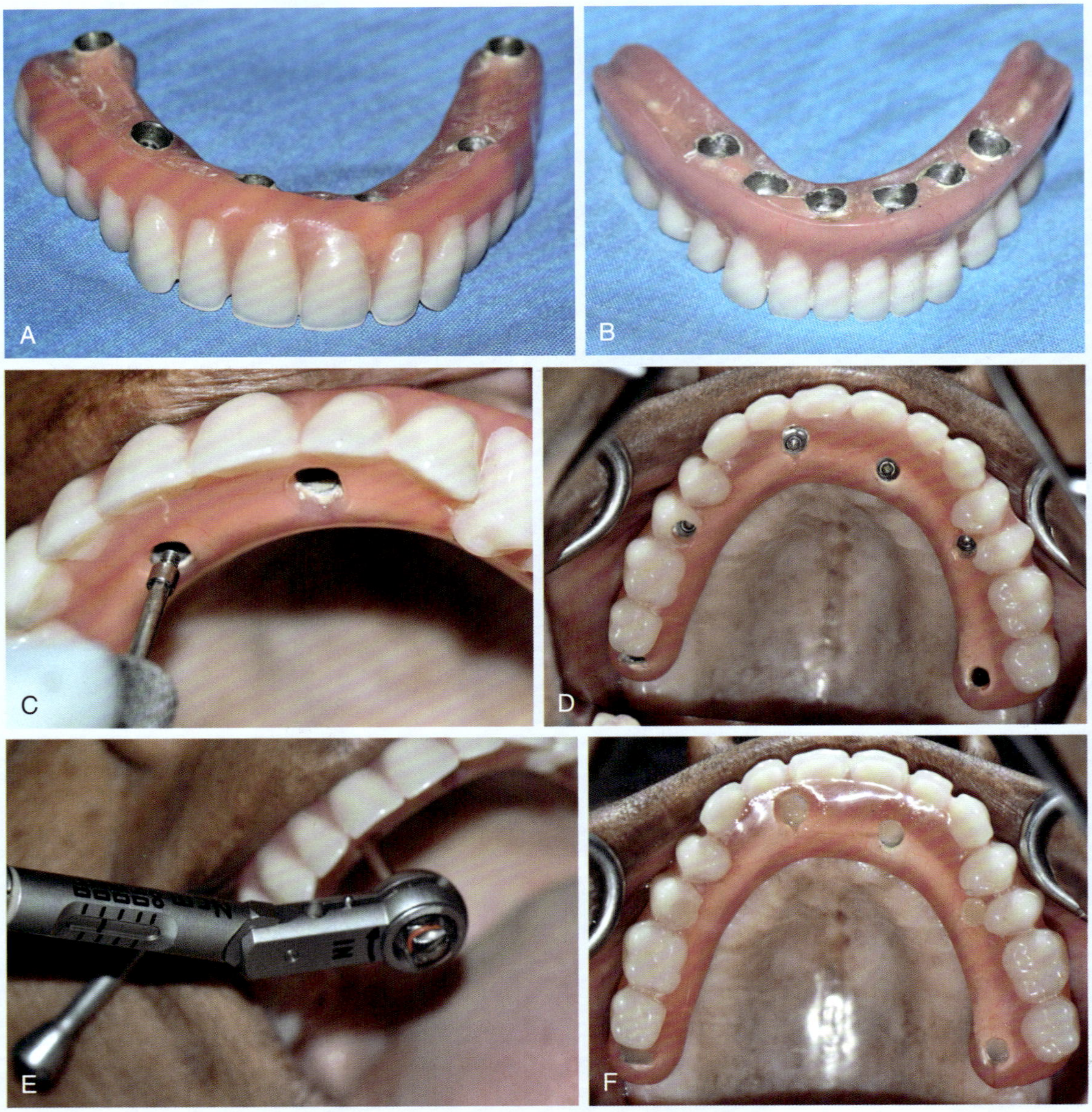

Fig 22.18 The finally acrylized upper and lower hybrid prosthesis. (A and B) A cement-retained hybrid prosthesis is fabricated for the lower arch. (C and D) The upper prosthesis is seated over the multiunit abutments and screwed using the fixation screws. (E) The torque ratchet is used to finally tighten the fixation screws at the moment of 15 Ncm. (F) The screw holes are filled with gutta-percha and covered over with flowable composite. The final 14-unit All-on-6 prosthesis is fixed in the mouth.

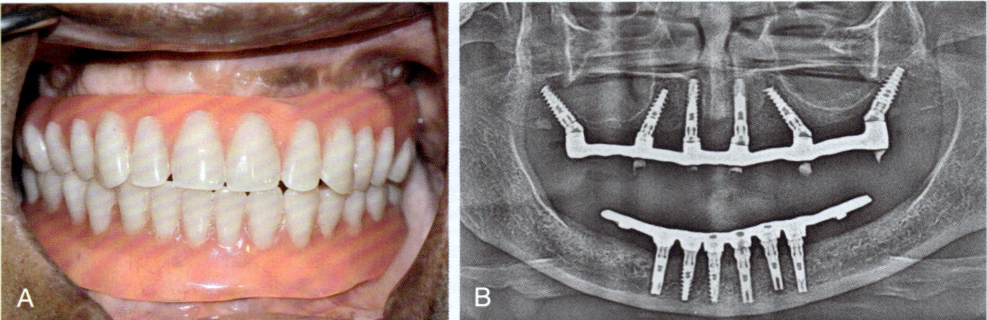

Fig 22.19 (A) Final upper and lower hybrid prosthesis in the mouth and (B) post loading radiograph. All implants showed stable crestal bone level when radiographically evaluated one year after loading.

CASE REPORT-2

All-on-6 implant procedure for both arches with pterygoid implants in the posterior maxilla (Figs 22.20–22.35).

A 50-year-old male was referred to the author for full mouth rehabilitation with bilateral sinus grafting. On examination, the patient was fit for implant as well as sinus grafting surgeries. On discussion, the patient expressed the desire for immediate restoration of his aesthetics with a fixed prosthesis as he was a speaker at business meetings and conferences and could not manage with the removable prosthesis. He also desired to complete the treatment in the shortest possible time span without much grafting and long waiting periods. Conventional implantation obviously required the sinus grafting procedure with delayed implant placement after the graft maturation period of a minimum of 6 months. It further required, 6 months of subgingival healing for the implants could also be necessary. So all in all, the case could have been completed only in more than 1 year and with multiple surgical steps. To minimize surgical steps, avoid the sinus grafting procedure, for immediate restoration, and to finish the treatment in a short span of time, the All-on-6 technique was planned for this case.

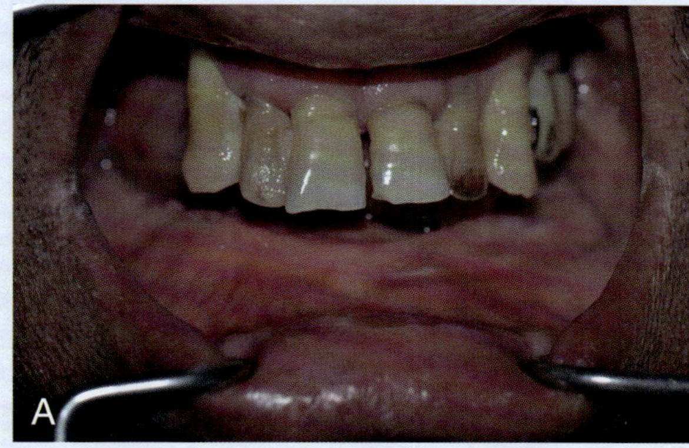

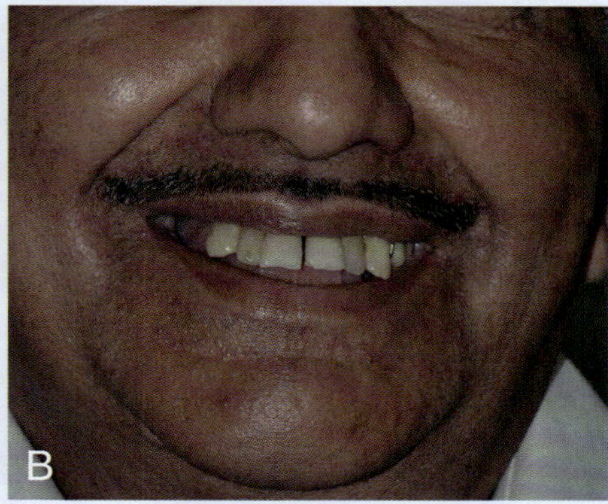

Fig 22.20 (A) A-50-year old male presented with severely resorbed mandibular ridge (he wore a removable ridge-supported denture); and a few teeth in the upper jaw were present, most of them were mobile and needed extraction. (B) On smiling, the patient did not show the marginal gingiva and so did not need any ridge reduction for the maxillary bone during the implant placement surgery.

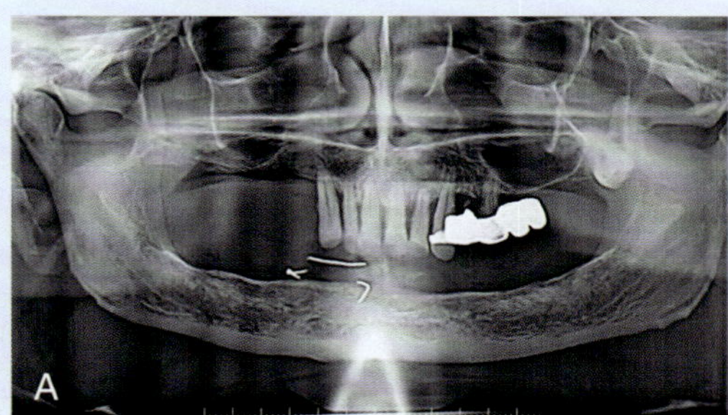

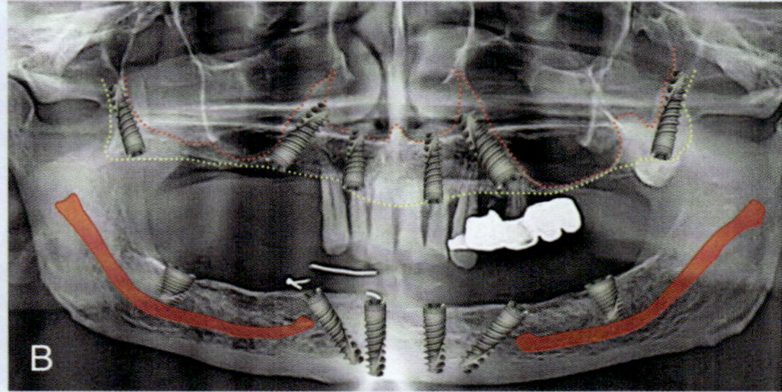

Fig 22.21 Panoramic radiograph shows that hardly any bone is available bilaterally under the maxillary sinuses. A minimum amount of bone is available bilaterally posterior to the sinuses to insert the posterior-most implants. Moreover, an impacted maxillary third molar was also seen on left side, which could hinder placement of implant in the tuberosity. The ridge in the anterior region of the maxilla as well as mandible looked adequate for the insertion of four implants with distal tilting of the posterior implants. The placement of only four implants (All-on-4™) would have resulted in the possibility of a 10- to 12-unit prosthesis but the patient expressed the desire for a 14-unit prosthesis for both arches and that needed the addition of two more implants in the posterior region. Thus for the maxilla, the placement of two additional implants in the maxillary tuberosity with their engagement in the medial pterygoid process was planned. For the mandible, the addition of two more implants with large diameter and short length (5 × 8 mm) in the posterior mandible (in the buccal shelf region) were planned. (A) Immediate extraction of impacted maxillary molar was planned before the placement of implant in the pterygoid process. (B) The panoramic radiograph with the simulated implants shows the planned positions and angulations of all the implants.

Continued

CASE REPORT-2—cont'd

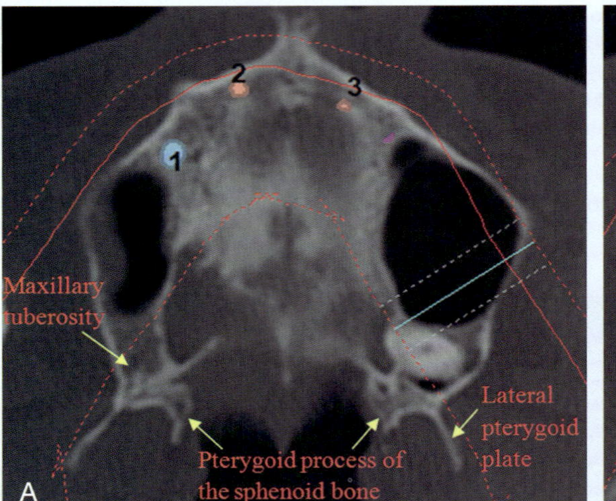

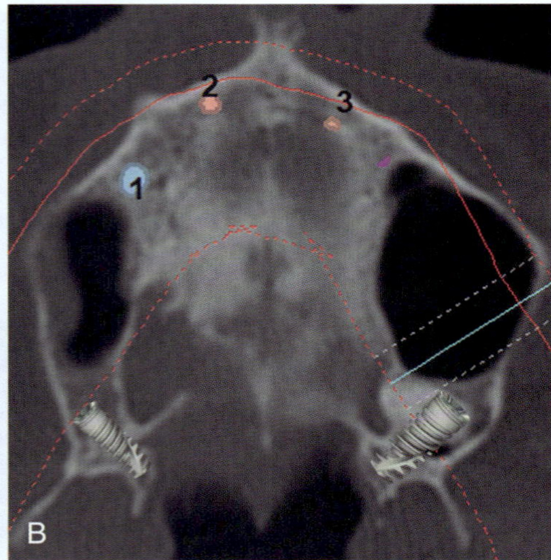

Fig 22.22 (A) The axial view of the dental CT scan shows the location and direction of the pterygoid process of the sphenoid bone in respect of the maxillary tuberosity and (B) the planned axial position and direction of the posterior implants.

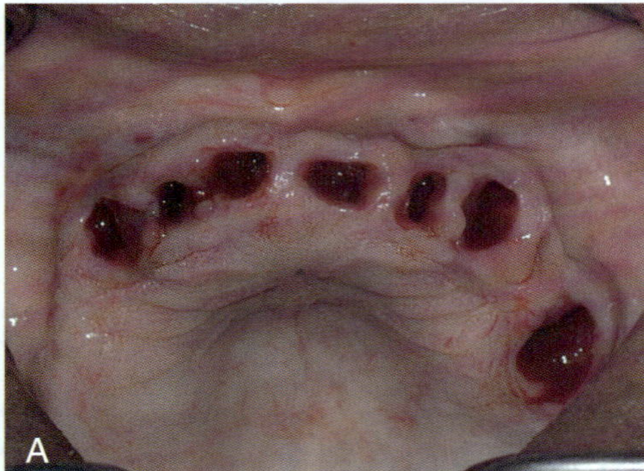

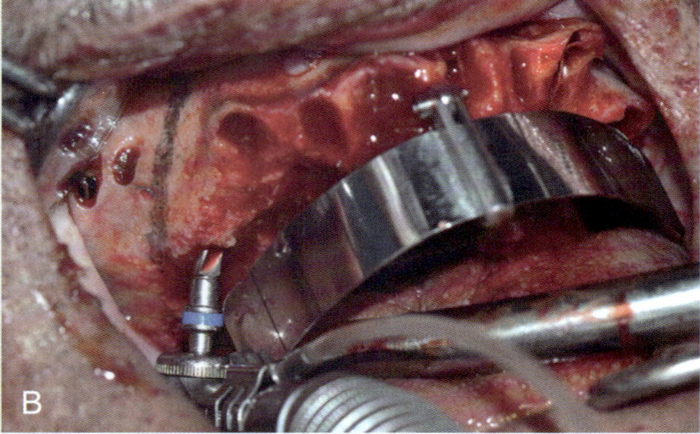

Fig 22.23 (A) All the front maxillary teeth were pulled out and mucoperiosteal flaps were elevated to expose the maxillary ridge as well as the lateral wall of the sinus. The anterior wall of the sinus was bilaterally explored and marked by preparing a small opening through the lateral wall of the sinus. (B) The All-on-4™ guide was seated in the mouth and implant osteotomies were prepared with distal tilting of the posterior implants at 45°.

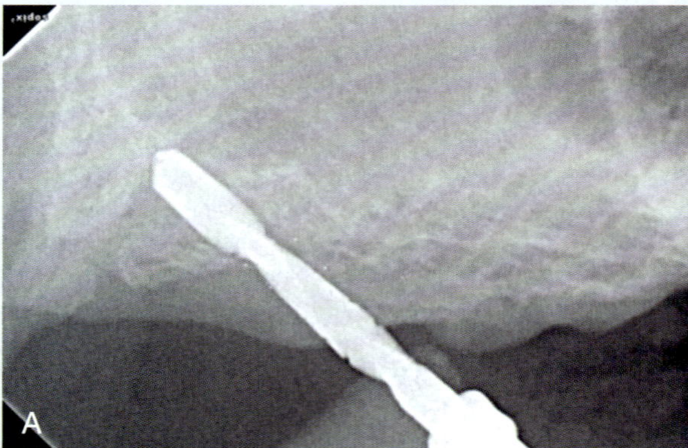

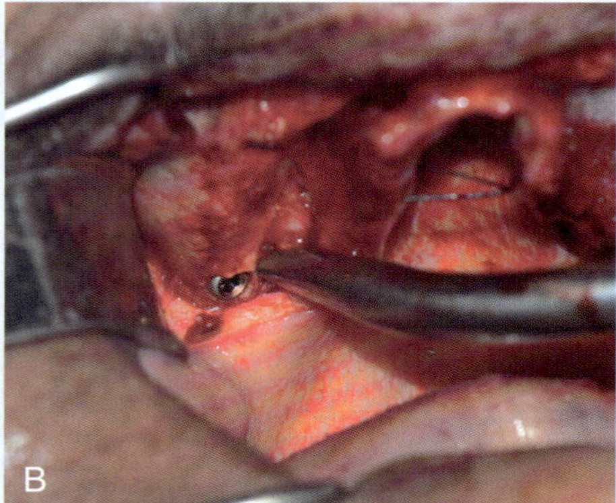

Fig 22.24 The osteotomy for the right posterior-most implant was prepared through the maxillary tuberosity and right up to the medial pterygoid process of the sphenoid bone. (A) The direction of the drill in respect of the posterior wall of the sinus was assessed by taking step by step radiographs during osteotomy preparation. (B) The pterygoid implant in place. The inserted implant achieved primary stability of more than 35 Ncm.

CASE REPORT-2—cont'd

Fig 22.25 (A and B) The impacted third molar on the left side was extracted and implant osteotomy was prepared through the extraction socket and (C) the implant was inserted in the medial pterygoid process. As the implant apex had been inserted into the high-density medial pterygoid process, the inserted implant achieved primary stability of more than 35 Ncm. (D) But the finally inserted implant showed a large peri-implant extraction socket space at its cervical third which needed to be grafted.

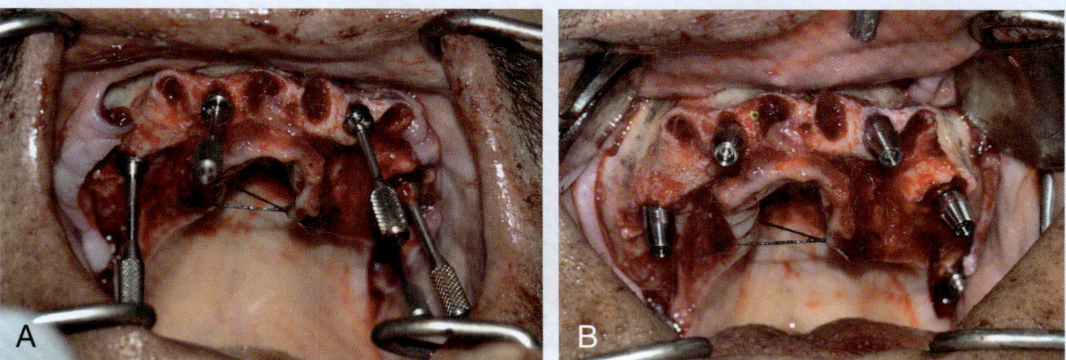

Fig 22.26 All implants were inserted at their planned positions with high primary stability. The apexes of all four anterior implants were stabilized into the high-density nasal floor to achieve high primary stability. (A) The appropriate multiunit abutments were inserted on all six implants. (B) Further, the abutment mounts were removed and healing abutments were inserted on top of all the multiunit abutments.

Continued

CASE REPORT-2—cont'd

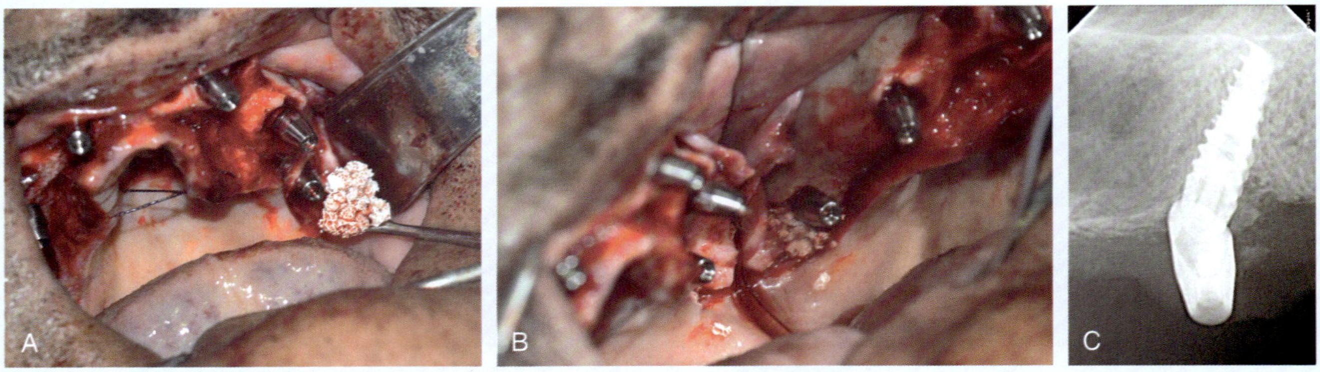

Fig 22.27 (A and B) The peri-implant socket spaces around the left pterygoid implant were grafted using bone substitute. (C) The post implant radiograph shows accurate implant insertion and grafting.

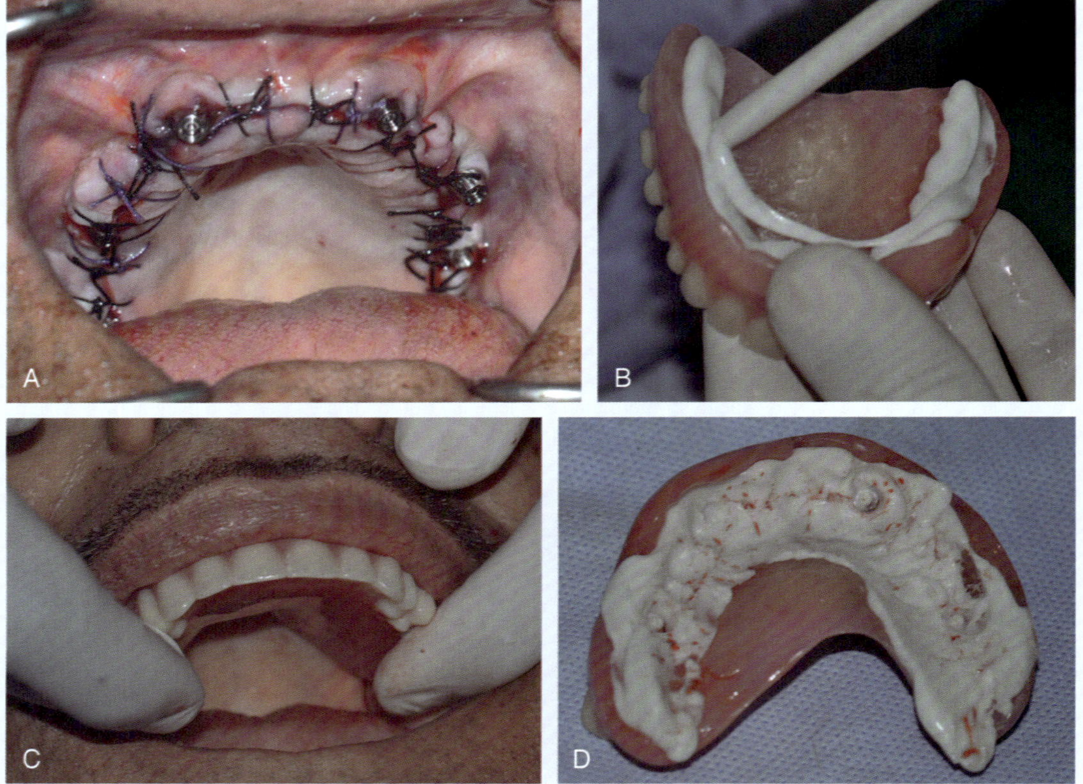

Fig 22.28 (A) The flap was sutured with the healing abutments emerging out of the tissues. (B–D) The indexes of the implant positions were transferred to the prefabricated denture using the light body silicon impression material.

CASE REPORT-2—cont'd

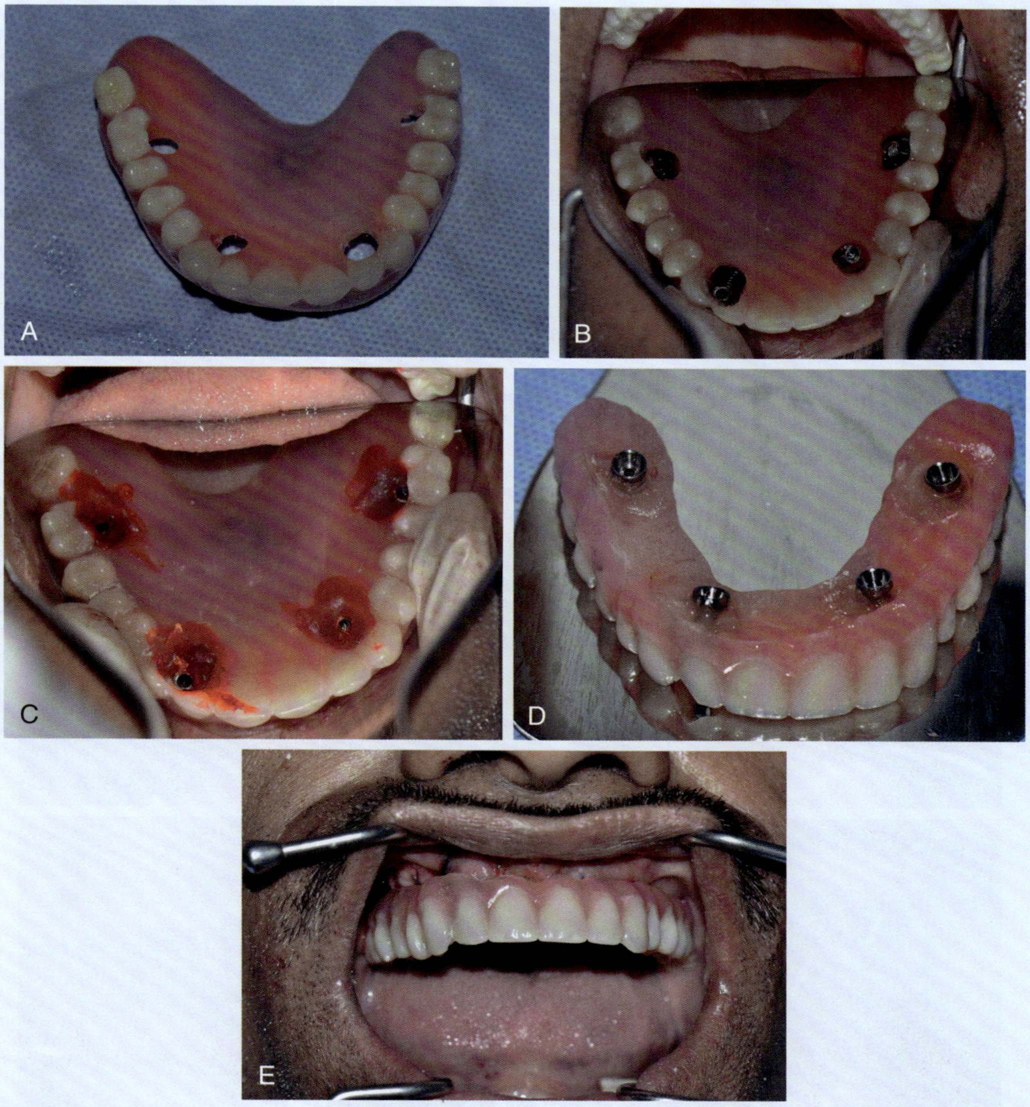

A B C D E

Fig 22.29 (A) The holes were prepared through the denture at the indexed positions. The healing abutments of four anterior implants were removed and replaced with the titanium cylinders. (B) The denture was seated at the correct position with the titanium cylinders emerging out of the holes. (C) The pattern resin was carefully filled around the titanium cylinders and once it had set in the mouth, the titanium cylinders were unscrewed to remove the denture from the mouth. Self-cure acrylic was filled into the deficiencies around the cylinders. (D and E) The palatal extension of the denture was removed and the denture was finished, polished and screwed in the mouth over the four anterior implants. The patient was recalled on the next day for the insertion of the lower implants.

Continued

CASE REPORT-2—cont'd

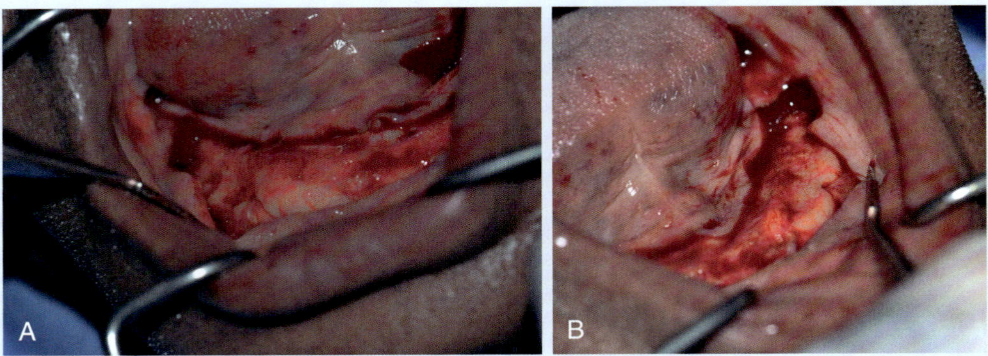

Fig 22.30 (A and B) For the lower arch, the mucoperiosteal flap was elevated to expose the ridge and the mental foramina were bilaterally explored.

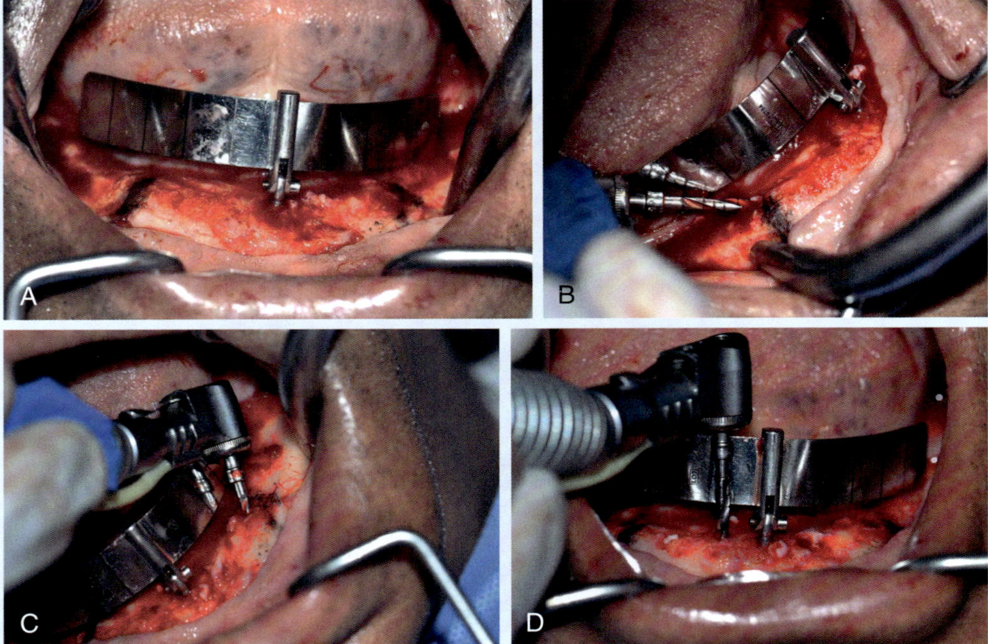

Fig 22.31 (A) The position of the mental foramina was marked on the ridge using a sterile HB pencil and the All-on-4™ guide was seated in mouth. (B and C) The osteotomies for the two posterior implants were prepared with distal tilting and keeping final drill position 2 mm anterior to the mental foramina. (D) The straight osteotomies for two anterior implants were prepared.

CASE REPORT-2—cont'd

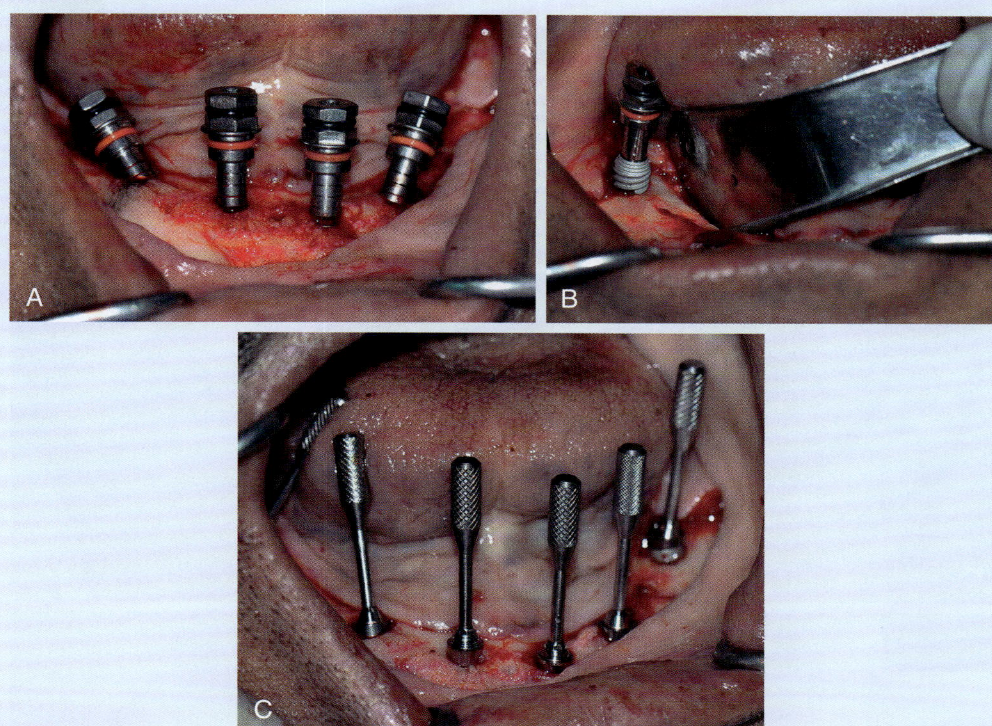

Fig 22.32 (A) Four anterior implants at their final positions with distal tilting of the two posterior implants at 45° to the long axis. (B) Two implants were placed at the most-posterior positions (into the buccal shelf region). (C) The appropriate multiunit abutments were inserted on the top of all the implants.

Continued

CASE REPORT-2—cont'd

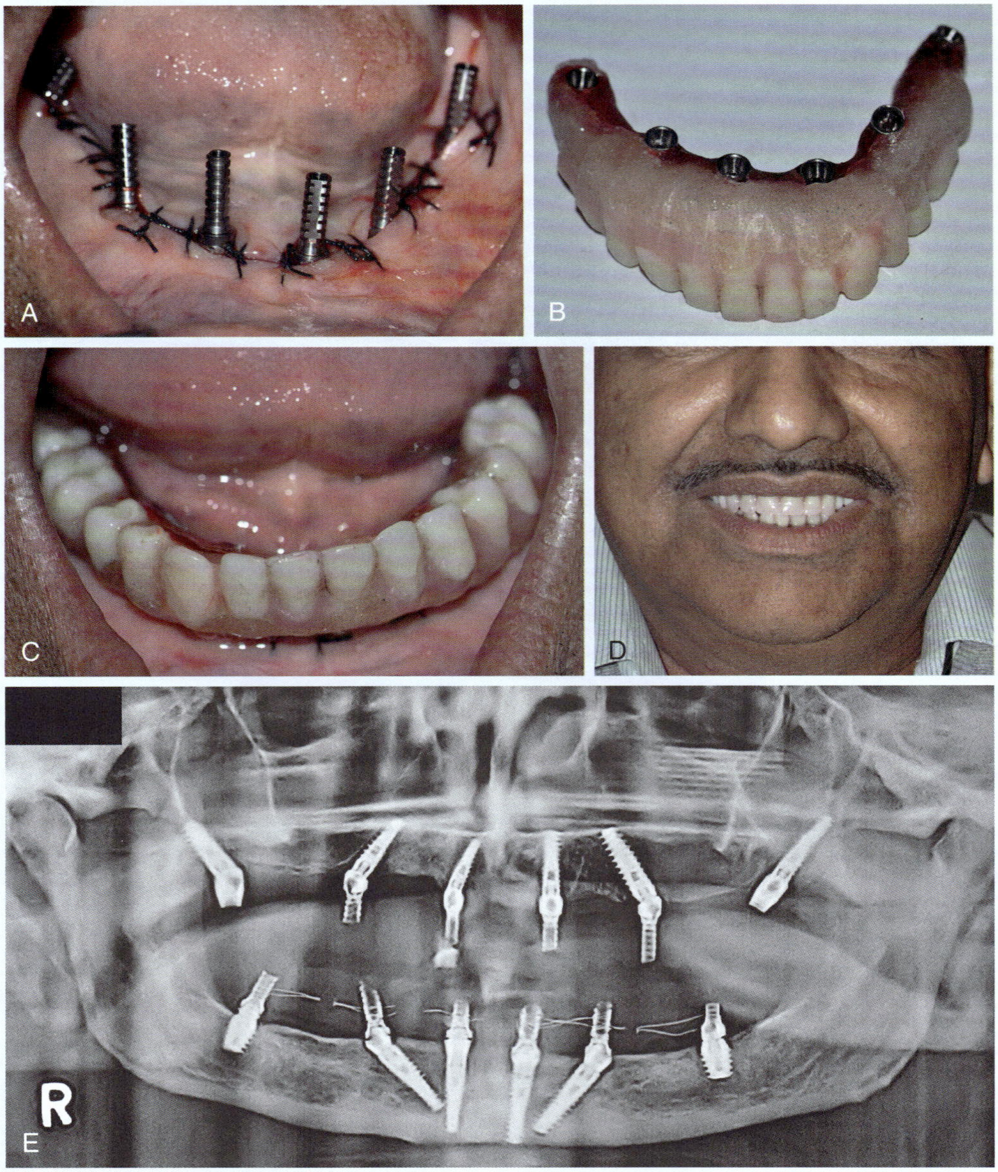

Fig 22.33 (A) Temporary titanium cylinders were placed on top of the multiunit abutments. The prefabricated lower denture was prepared and seated in the mouth with the cylinders emerging out of the holes prepared in the denture. Further, the cylinders were connected to the denture using pattern resin and removed from the mouth along with the cylinders. (B) The denture was finished, polished, and (C) screwed over lower six implants. (D) Maxillofacial view of the patient after the upper and lower provisional prosthesis were fixed in the mouth. Patient was rehabilitated with fixed prosthesis in 2 days. (E) Postimplantation radiograph shows that all the implants have been inserted at the desired positions.

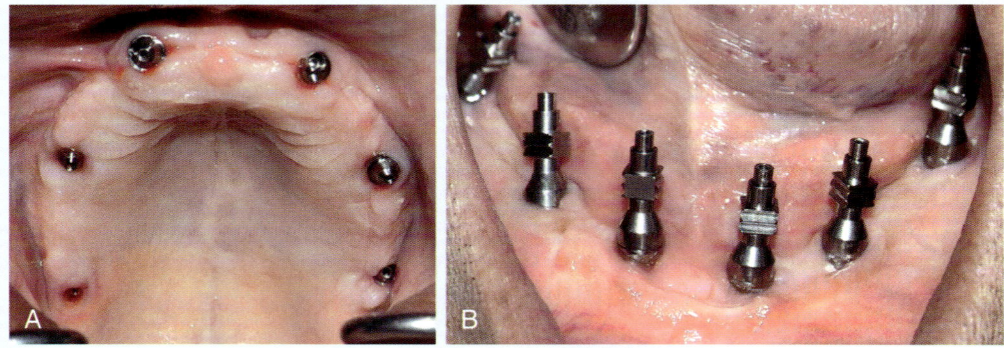

Fig 22.34 (A and B) The healing of the tissue as seen on removing the provisional prosthesis after 4 months for prosthetic procedures. The impression procedures, bite registration, and try-in for the definitive prosthesis were done in the same way as described in the Case Report-1.

CASE REPORT-2—cont'd

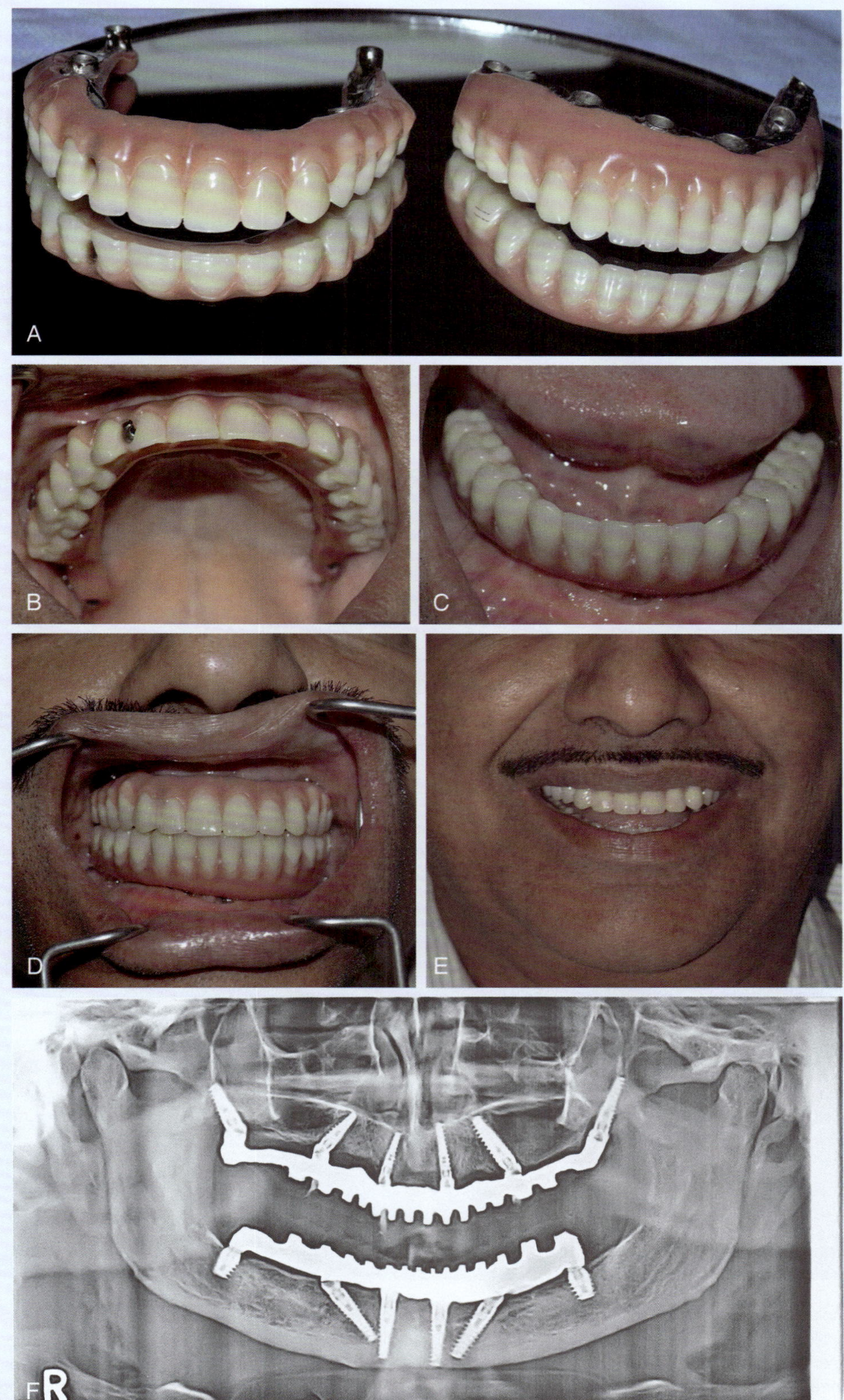

Fig 22.35 (A) Upper and lower screw-retained final prosthesis. (B) Upper prosthesis after fixing over the implants. (C) Lower prosthesis after fixing over the implants. (D) Finally fixed upper and lower prosthesis in occlusion. (E) Maxillofacial view of the patient after rehabilitation. (F) Post loading radiograph showing accurately performed All-on-6 procedure with pterygoid implants in the posterior maxilla.

Continued

CASE REPORT-3

CT guided flapless placement of four implants with distal tilting of posterior implants (Figs 22.36–22.40).

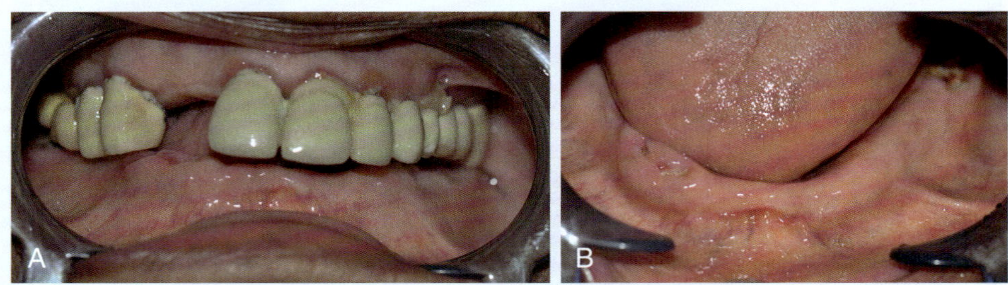

Fig 22.36 (A and B) A 78-year-old female patient presented with upper intact dentition and a missing lower one and desired to have fixed teeth for the lower arch.

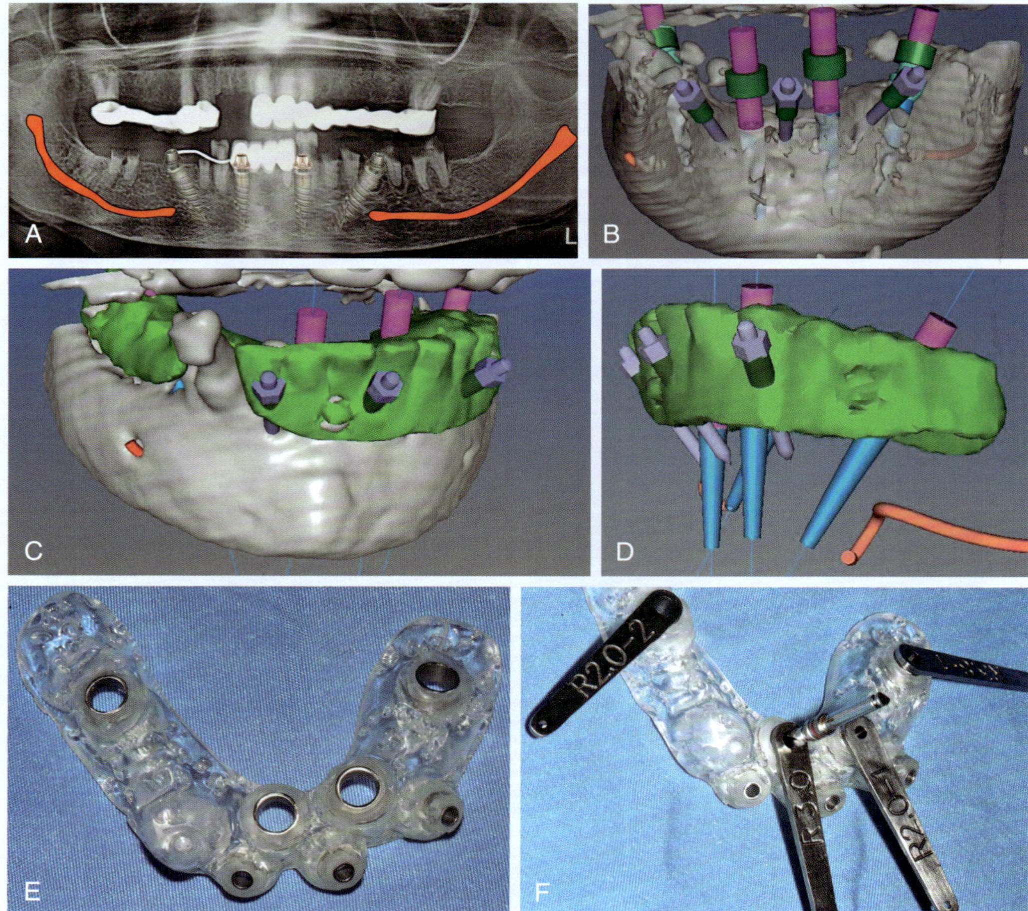

Fig 22.37 (A) Four implants to support a 12-unit fixed hybrid prosthesis is planned; the posterior implants needed to be tilted up to 45° to minimize the length of distal cantilevers. Keeping the patient's age in mind, the minimal invasive CT guided flapless implant placement procedure is planned. (B–D) The implant dimensions, their positions and angulations are planned using the dental CT planning software and the files are exported to the CAD/CAM milling centre (Pink city cera dental Lab, Jaipur). (E) Using the exported files, the CAD/CAM centre fabricated an accurate soft tissue-supported implant insertion guide. (F) The special sleeves are used to accurately drill for a particular implant.

CASE REPORT-3—cont'd

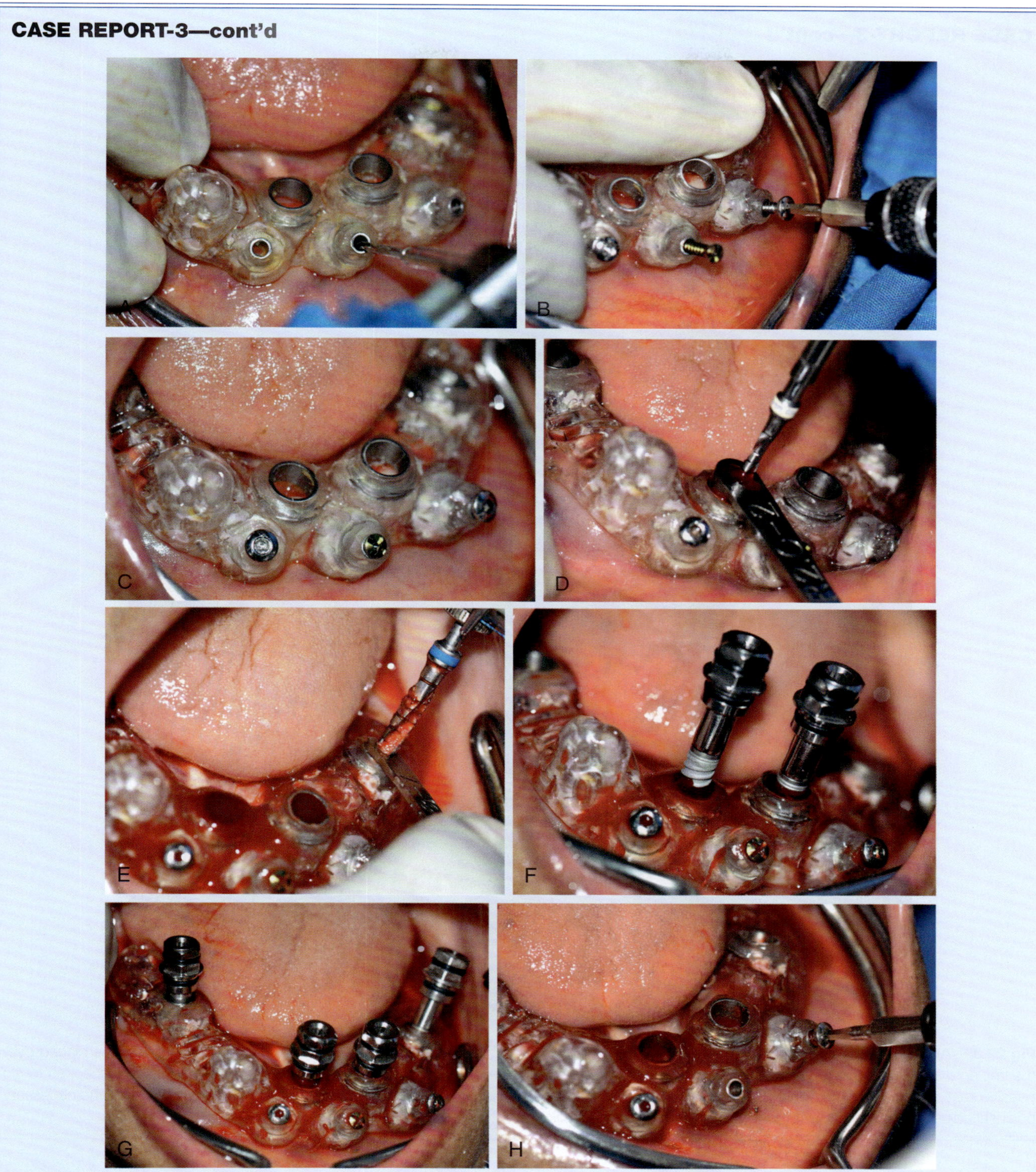

Fig 22.38 (A–C) The guide is accurately seated over the soft tissue ridge and immobilized using long fixation screws. (D and E) The implant osteotomies are prepared through the guide using special sleeves and (F and G) implants are inserted. (H) The guide is removed after all the implants have been installed.

Continued

CASE REPORT-3—cont'd

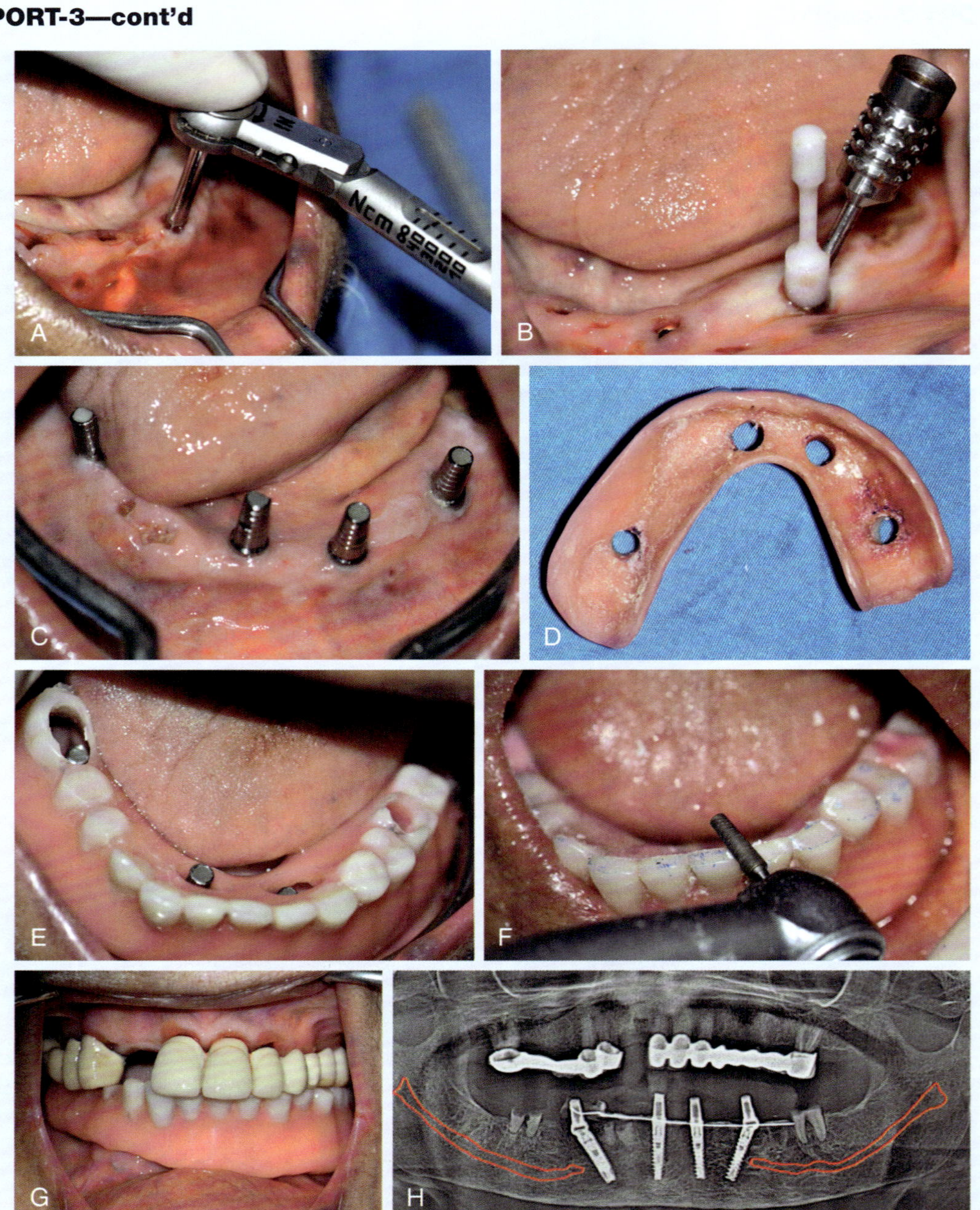

Fig 22.39 (A) All the implants attained primary stability more than 35 Ncm. (B) The appropriately selected multiunit abutments are placed over the implants and (C) straight abutments are fixed on top of multiunit abutments. (D) The patient's old denture is prepared and (E) checked for its passive seating in the mouth. (F and G) The provisional prosthesis is fixed over the implants on the same day of implant placement and necessary occlusal adjustments are made in mouth. (H) Post implantation radiograph.

CASE REPORT-3—cont'd

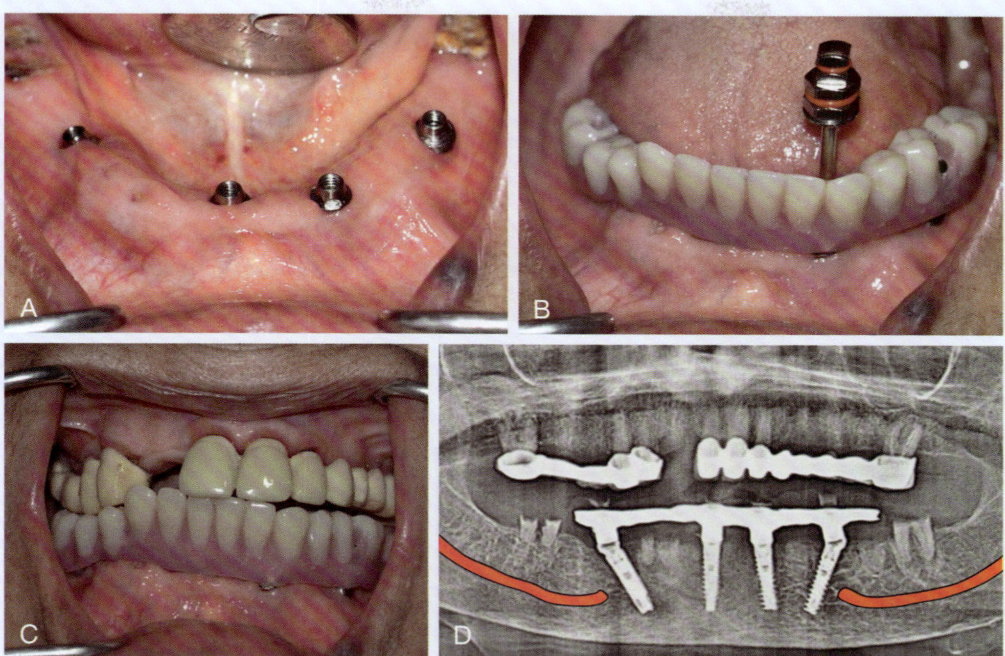

Fig 22.40 (A) Healing after 6 weeks, when provisional prosthesis is removed for the final prosthetic procedures. (B and C) Twelve-unit hybrid prosthesis, which is fixed on four implants. (D) Post loading radiograph.

CASE REPORT-4

Full mouth rehabilitation using tilted implant concept *(Courtesy: Amir Gazmawe, Israel).* (Figs 22.41–22.50).

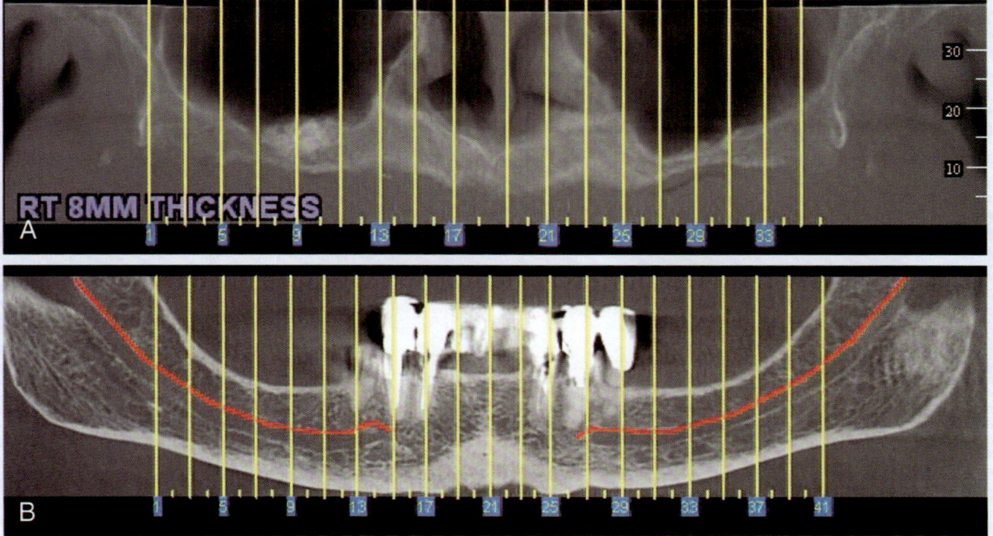

Fig 22.41 (A and B) Panoramic CT images of the maxilla and mandible showing inadequate bone height in the subantral region and over the mandibular canal to insert adequately long implants without performing any bone augmentation procedure. Four implants in the anterior region of each arch are planned with distal tilting of posterior implants to minimize the distal cantilevers.

Continued

CASE REPORT-4—cont'd

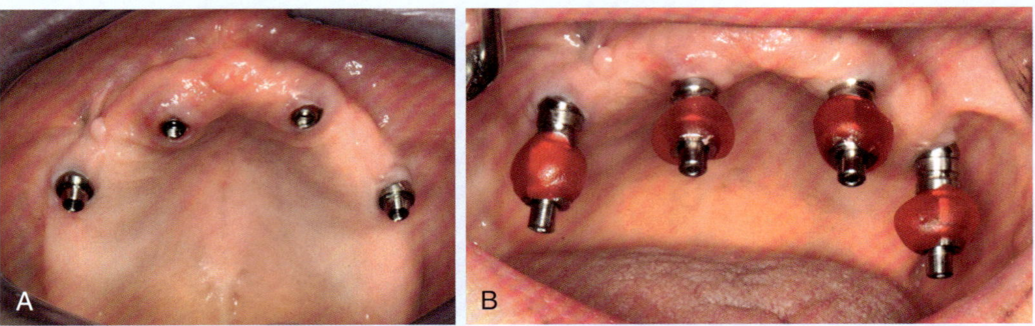

Fig 22.42 (A) Four implants in place with multiunit abutments. (B) Open tray impression abutments placed on top of the multiunit abutments.

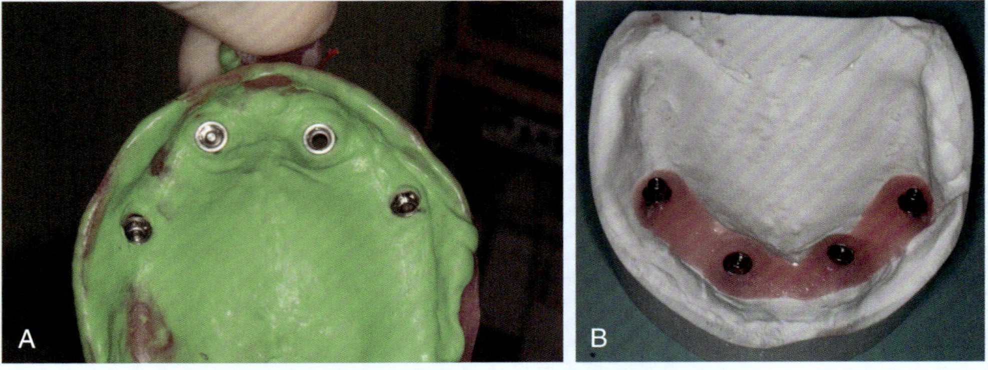

Fig 22.43 (A) Abutment level implant impression and (B) final working cast with abutment analogues.

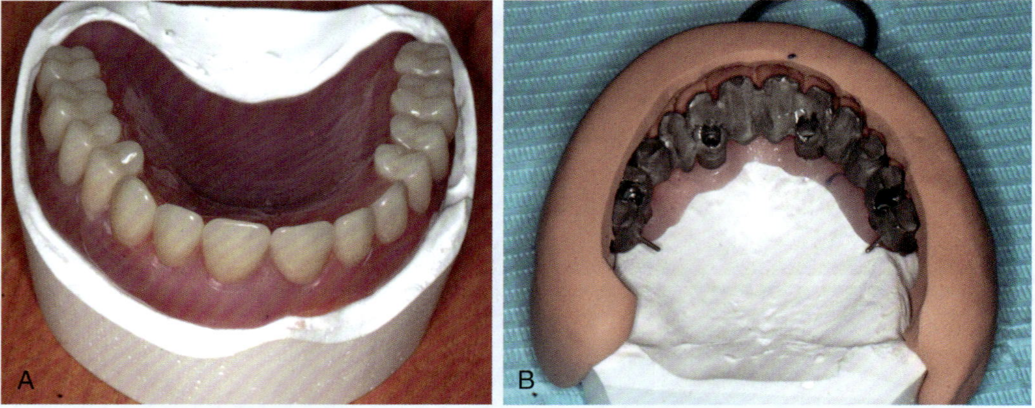

Fig 22.44 (A and B) Patient's old denture is seated over the cast and a teeth index is made using silicon putty, which is used to cast the metal framework at the ideal position.

CASE REPORT-4—cont'd

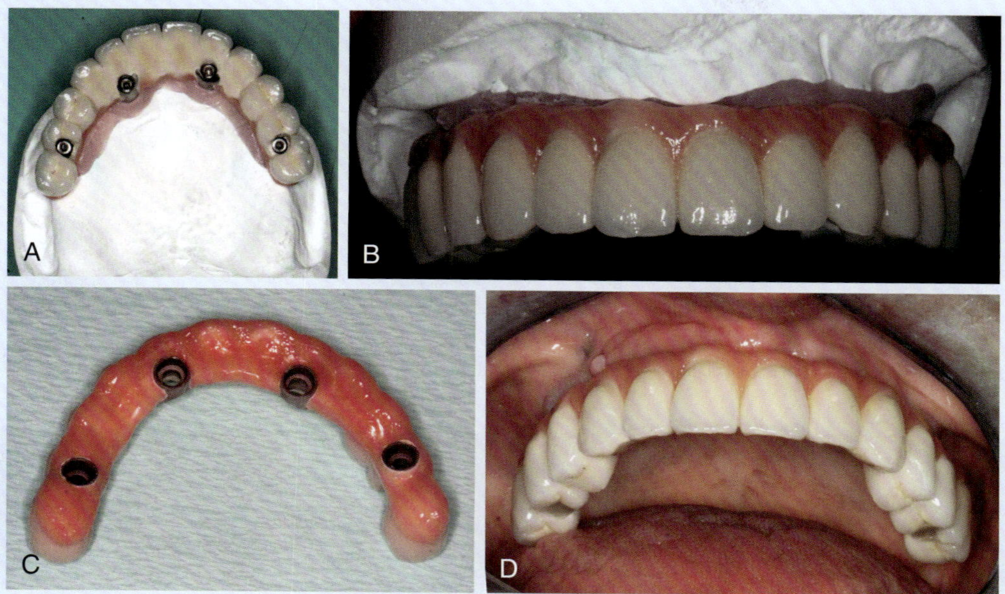

Fig 22.45 (A–D) The final screw-retained ceramic prosthesis, which is screwed over the upper implants.

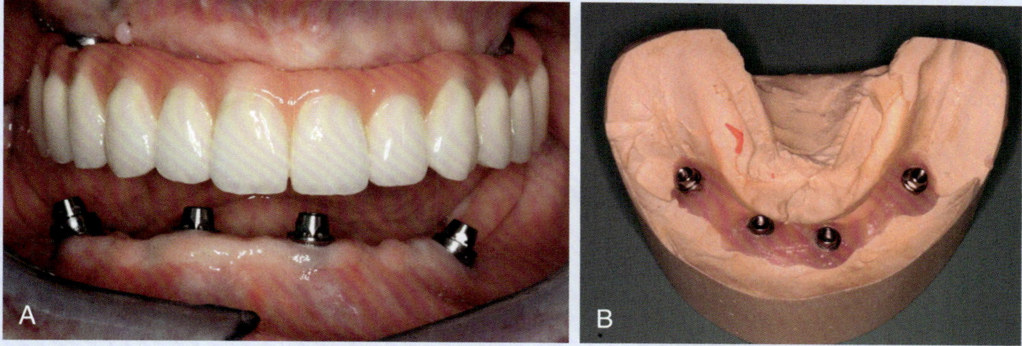

Fig 22.46 (A) Four implants are placed in the lower arch with distal tilting of posterior implants. (B) The impression is made and working cast is prepared in the same way as mentioned before.

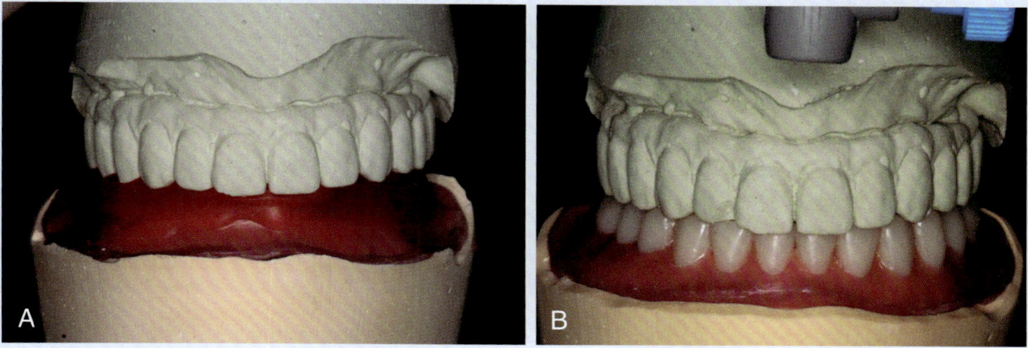

Fig 22.47 (A) Jaw relation is recorded and casts are mounted on the articulator at the centric position. (B) The tooth setting is done in ideal occlusion.

Continued

CASE REPORT-4—cont'd

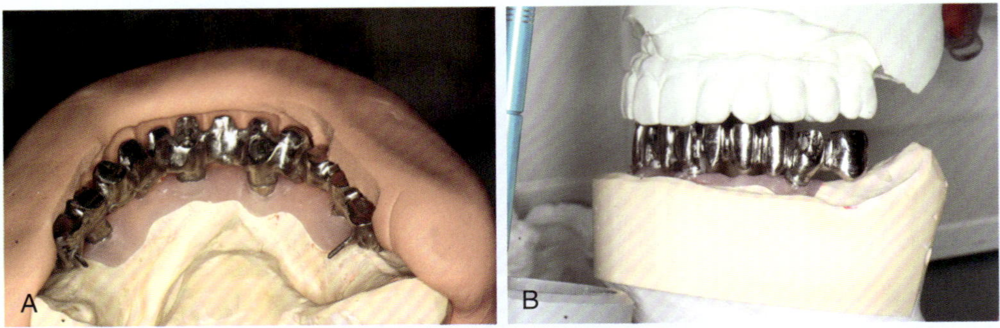

Fig 22.48 (A and B) Teeth indexing is done using silicon putty and the metal framework of an ideal shape and position on the cast.

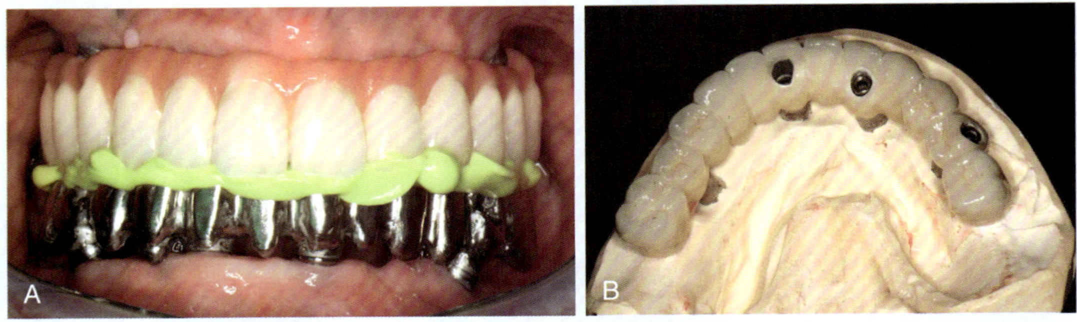

Fig 22.49 (A) The metal formwork is screwed over the implants and bite registration is done. (B) The final screw-retained ceramic prosthesis on the cast.

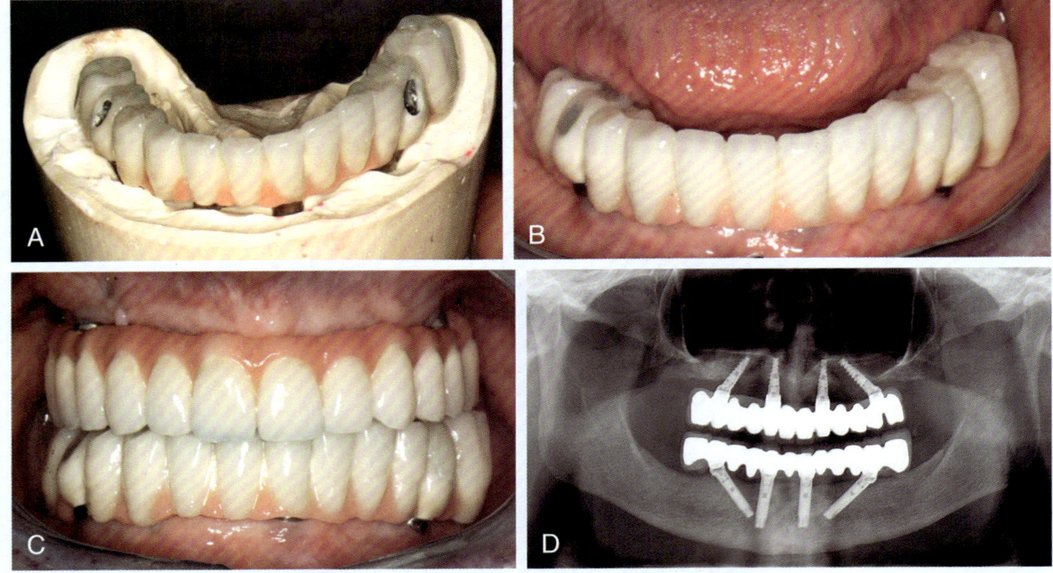

Fig 22.50 (A and B) Final prosthesis is screwed in the mouth. (C) Upper and lower final prosthesis in the mouth. (D) Post loading radiograph.

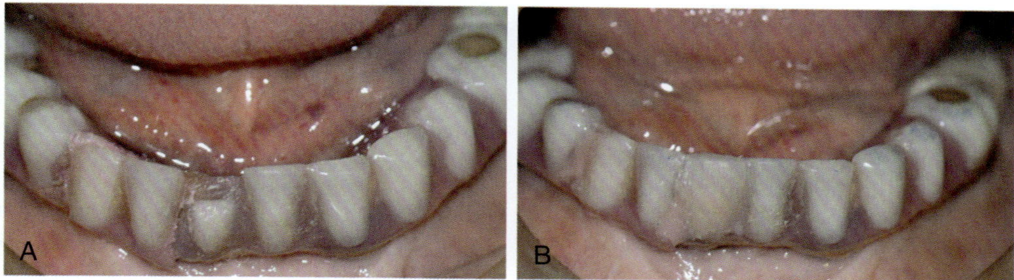

Fig 22.51 (A) Traumatic fracture of a tooth from the All-on-4™ hybrid prosthesis, (B) repaired in the mouth using acrylic.

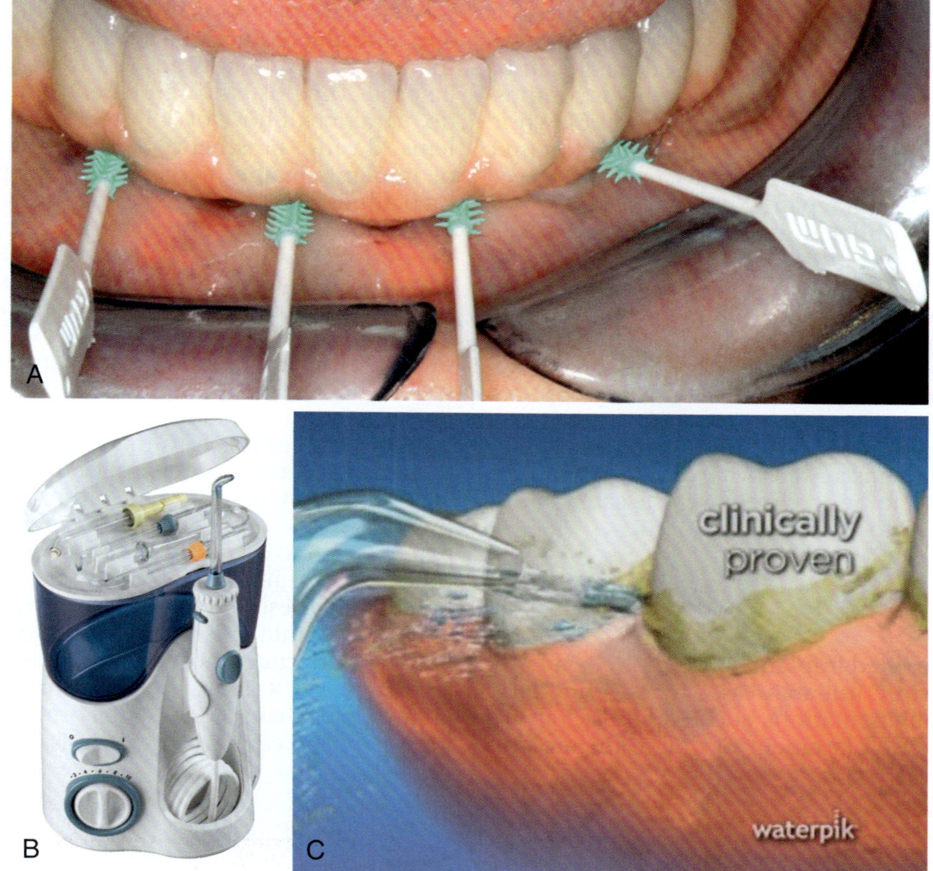

Fig 22.52 (A) Interdental brushes should be used to clean the tissue surface of the All-on-4/All-on-6 prosthesis. (B and C) The waterpik is a new invention and very useful to clean full-arch implant prosthesis as it offers multiple water jets, as well as flossing and brushing tips to reach the difficult areas under and over the prosthesis.

begin a minimum of 4 mm anterior to the sinus, evaluated with a radiograph. If the pilot drill has perforated the sinus cavity, it should be evaluated with a radiograph and the osteotomy preparation should be redirected to the planned direction, avoiding the enlargement of the perforation. The path of the anterior wall of the sinus should be marked on the facial wall using a sterile pencil, so that it can be visualized when drilling for implants.

3. **Nerve injury during posterior implant placement in the mandible.** It can be avoided by properly exploring the mental foramina and starting drilling a minimum of 4 mm anterior to it. The presence of the anterior loop should be clearly evaluated in the radiographs, dental CT scan and/or inserting a blunt explorer in the mental foramina. If the anterior loop is present, the implant should be positioned a minimum of 2 mm anterior to the anterior loop. For instant radiographic evaluation after flap elevation, a pilot drill is placed over the facial plate anterior to the mental foramina and a radiograph is taken to evaluate the appropriate direction anterior to the loop. If nerve injury has already been occurred, osteotomy preparation is redirected to the correct direction and the implant is placed. If patient

complains of any paraesthesia on the chin and lip of the side involved, proper measures should be taken to manage the paraesthesia (for more information about 'management of nerve injury' refer to in the Chapter 24 'Complications and management').

4. **Fracture of distal cantilevers of the provisional all acrylic bridge.** This is the most common complication in the All-on-4™ technique and it can be avoided by avoiding distal cantilevers in the acrylic prosthesis or by using high-strength pattern resin as the base of the acrylic bridge. This complication is very uncommon in All-on-6 procedures as it does not usually require the distal cantilevers.
5. **Fracture of teeth from the definitive prosthesis.** Usually a screw-retained hybrid or ceramic prosthesis is used as the final prosthesis in All-on-4™ or All-on-6 techniques, hence if it is a hybrid prosthesis it can be easily repaired in the mouth using acrylic or composite (Fig 22.51A and B). In case of big fractures of hybrid prostheses or if the ceramic chips off from the ceramic prosthesis, the prosthesis can be unscrewed/retrieved from the implants and repaired in the laboratory.
6. **Food impaction under the prosthesis.** Besides normal teeth brushing, interdental brushes should be regularly used by the patient to clean the tissue surface of the denture. The waterpik is a new invention and very useful in the cleaning of such prostheses. The prosthesis can be unscrewed from the mouth and polished in the laboratory as and when required (Fig 22.52A–C).
7. **Wearing out of the teeth of hybrid prostheses.** The prosthesis can be unscrewed from the implant and a new set of teeth can be acrylized over the same framework in the laboratory.

Summary

In several cases, the tilted implant concept can be an ultimate option to restore full-arch cases by avoiding large volume of bone augmentations such as sinus grafting, block grafting etc. The placement of only four implants with distal tilting of the posterior implants usually allows the fixing of a restoration with a 12-unit prosthesis, which offers several advantages such as immediate loading in most cases using an all acrylic bridge, minimized distal cantilevering, placement of posterior implants longer than usual with higher stability, and less invasive procedure because only one surgery is done to insert implants. For a few patients who desire complete arch prosthesis, two additional implants can be added in the posterior region such as in the tuberosity and/or medial pterygoid process in the maxilla and in the buccal shelf region in the mandible to support a 14-unit prosthesis. The accurate exploration of the anterior wall of the sinus in the maxilla and mental foramina in the mandible is mandatory to place posterior implants at the desired positions and with the required distal tilting. To appropriately tilt the posterior implants an All-on-4™ Malo guide should be used. The posterior implants should be tilted distally up to a maximum of 45° to avoid parallelism problems during prosthetic construction. The placement of implants in the medial pterygoid process may need meticulous treatment planning using dental CT scan and skilled surgical approach to install the implant at the desired position and angulation. Often the implants placed in the pterygoid process show extreme angulation in respect to the other implants; to restore such cases, flat connection abutments can be used for the pterygoid implants in place of multiunit abutments. In the All-on-6 technique, the teeth set should end well anterior to the posterior-most implants to avoid cheek bite problems and for easy approach to the posterior-most connection screw. An accurate impression transfer with the open tray technique is mandatory to avoid prosthetic passive seating errors. The posts should be splinted together using pattern resin to avoid their movement in respect to each other during impression transfer. The screw-retained hybrid prosthesis should be preferred over the cement-retained ceramic prosthesis because of many advantages. It is cost effective, more aesthetic, light weight, easy to repair, and retrievable. Long-term maintenance and regular follow-up visits to the dental office are required for the long-term success of the prosthesis as well as implants.

Further Reading

Malo P, Nobre M, Lope A. The use of computer-guided flapless implant surgery and four implants placed in immediate function to support a fixed denture: preliminary results after a mean follow-up period of thirteen months. J Prosthet Dent 2007; 97(6 Suppl):86–95.

Maló P, Rangert B, Dvärsäter L. Immediate function of Brånemark implants in the aesthetic zone: a retrospective clinical study with 6 months to 4 years follow-up. Clin Implant Dent Relat Res 2000;2:138–46.

Krekmanov L, Kahn M, Rangert B, et al. Tilting of posterior mandibular and maxillary implants of improved prosthesis support. Int J Oral Maxillofac Implants 2000;15:405–14.

Adell R, Eriksson B, Lekholm U, et al. A long-term follow-up study of osseointegrated implants in the treatment of totally edentulous jaws. Int J Oral Maxillofac Implants 1990;5:347–59.

Balshi TJ, Wolfinger GJ. Immediate loading of Brånemark implants in edentulous mandibles. A preliminary report. Implant Dent 1997;6:83–8.

Schnitman DA, Wohrle PS, Rubenstein JE, et al. Branemark implants immediately loaded with fixed prosthesis at implant placement: ten year results. Int J Oral Maxillofac Implants 1997;12:495–503.

Duyck J, Van Oosterwyck H, Vander Sloten J, et al. Magnitude and distribution of occlusal forces on oral implants supporting fixed prostheses: an in vivo study. Clin Oral Implants Res 2000;11:465–75.

Van Steenberghe D, Glauser R, Blomback U, et al. A computed tomographic scan-derived customized surgical template and fixed prosthesis for flapless surgery and immediate loading of implants in fully edentulous maxillae: a prospective multicenter study. Clin Implant Dent Relat Res 2005;7(Suppl. 1):S111–20.

Ericsson I, Randow K, Nilner K, et al. Early functional loading of Brånemark dental implants: 5-year clinical follow-up study. Clin Implant Dent Relat Res 2000;2:70–7.

Branemark PI, Svensson B, van Steenberghe D. Ten year survival rates of fixed prostheses on four to six implants Ad Modum Branemark in full edentulism. Clin Oral Implants Res 1995;6:227–31.

Fortin Y, Sullivan RM, Rangert B. The Marius implant bridge: surgical and prosthetic-rehabilitation for the completely edentulous upper jaw with moderate to severe resorption: a 5-year retrospective clinical study. Clin Implant Dent Relat Res 2002;4:69–77.

Aparicio C, Perales P, Rangert B. Tilted implants as an alternative to maxillary sinus grafting: a clinical, radiographic and periotest study. Clin Implant Dent Relat Res 2001;3:39–49.

Maló P, Rangert B, Nobre M. "All-on-Four" immediate function concept with Brånemark System implants for completely edentulous mandibles: a retrospective clinical study. Clin Implant Dent Relat Res 2003;5:S2–9.

Chow J, Hui E, Liu J, et al. The Hong Kong Bridge protocol. Immediate loading of mandibular Brånemark fixtures using a fixed provisional prosthesis: preliminary results. Clin Implant Dent Relat Res 2001;3:166–74.

Maló P, Rangert B, Nobre M. "All-on-4" immediate-function concept with Brånemark System implants for completely edentulous maxilla: a 1-year retrospective clinical study. Clin Implant Dent Relat Res 2005;7:S88–94.

Rosen A, Gynther G. Implant treatment without bone grafting in edentulous severely resorbed maxillas: a long-term follow-up study. Oral Maxillofac Surg 2007;65:W10–1016.

Mal P, Rangert B, Nombre M. 'All on Four' immediate function concept with Branemark System implants for completely edentulous maxilla: a 1-year retrospective clinical study. Clin Implant Dent Relat Res 2003;7(Suppl. 1):588–94.

Davo Rodriguez, Malevez C, Rojas J. Immediate Function in atrophic upper jaw using Zygoma implants. J Prosthet Dent 2007; (Submitted).

Tulasne JF. Osseointegrated fixtures in the pterygoid region. In: Worthington P, Branemark PI, editors. Advanced osseointegration surgery. Applications in the maxillofacial region. Chicago, USA: Quintessence Publ. Co, Inc; 1992. p. 182–8.

Graves SL. The pterygoid plate implant: a solution for restoring the posterior maxilla. Int J Periodontics Restorative Dent 1994;4:512–23.

Parel S, Branemark PI, Ohrnell LO, Svensson B. Remote implant anchorage for the rehabilitation of maxillary defects. J Prosthet Dent 2001;86:377–81.

Vrielinck L, Politis C, Schepers S, Pauwels M, Naert I. Image-based planning and clinical validation of zygoma and pterygoid implant placement in patients with severe bone atrophy using customized drill guides. ; Preliminary results from a prospective clinical follow-up study. Int J Oral Maxillofac Surg 2003;32:7–14.

Hirsch J-M, Henry P, Andreasson L, et al. A clinical Evaluation of the Zygoma Fixture. One-year follow-up at 16 clinics. J Oral Maxillofac Surg 2004;9(Suppl):22–9.

Aparicio C, Arevalo X, Ouzzani W, Granados C. A retrospective clinical and radiographic evaluation of tilted implants used in the treatment of severely resorbed edentulous maxilla. Appl Osseointegrat Res 2003;1:17–21.

Randow K, Ericsson I, Nilner K, Peterson A, Glantz PO. Immediate functional loading of Brånemark dental implants. An 18-month clinical follow-up study. Clin Oral Implants Res 1999;10:8–15.

Brånemark PI, Engstrand P, Öhrnell LO, et al. A new treatment concept for rehabilitation of the edentulous mandible. Preliminary results from a prospective clinical follow-up study. Clin Implant Dent Relat Res 1999;1:2–16.

Örtorp A, Jemt T. Clinical experience of CNC-milled titanium frameworks supported by implants in the edentulous jaw: a 3-year interim report. Clin Implant Dent Relat Res 2002;4:104–9.

Peto R, Pike MC, Armitage P, et al. Design and analysis of randomized clinical trials requiring prolonged observation of each patient: II. Analysis and examples. Br J Cancer 1977;35:1–39.

Petersson A, Rangert B, Randow K, Ericsson I. Marginal bone resorption at different treatment concepts using Brånemark dental implants in anterior mandibles. Clin Implant Dent Relat Res 2001;3:142–7.

Chaushu G, Chaushu S, Tzohar A, Dayan D. Immediate loading of single tooth implants: immediate versus nonimmediate implantation. A clinical report. Int J Oral Maxillofac Implants 2001;16:267–72.

Hui E, Chow J, Li D, Liu J, Wat P, Law H. Immediate provisional for single-tooth implant replacement with Brånemark System: preliminary report. Clin Implant Dent Relat Res 2001;3:79–86.

Esposito M, Hirsch JM, Lekholm U, Thomsen P. Failure patterns of four osseointegrated oral implant systems. J Materials Science Materials in Medicine 1997(Suppl 8):843–7.

Soft tissue grafting in implantology

23

Ajay Vikram Singh

CHAPTER CONTENTS HD

Introduction

The soft tissue around the restored implant prosthesis plays a big role in the long-term maintenance and longevity of restored implants. Many research papers have been published to describe the role of soft tissue for long-term maintenance of the implant. Based on research and the clinical experience of experienced periodontists and implantologists, the presence of an adequate zone of thick, nonmobile and keratinized soft tissue around the implant prosthesis is paramount to resist marginal tissue recession and peri-implant inflammation. An absolute minimum 3-mm thick zone of nonmobile and keratinized marginal soft tissue should be present to make a peri-implant soft tissue seal, resistant to recession and peri-implant infections. If it is not present, the surgeon should perform the soft tissue grafting procedure to generate a thick, stable, and keratinized marginal soft tissue zone around the implant (Fig 23.1A and B).

Disadvantages of the thin, mobile, and nonkeratinized marginal soft tissue

1. Unable to protect the peri-implant tissues from injury
2. Unable to resist the pull of muscles

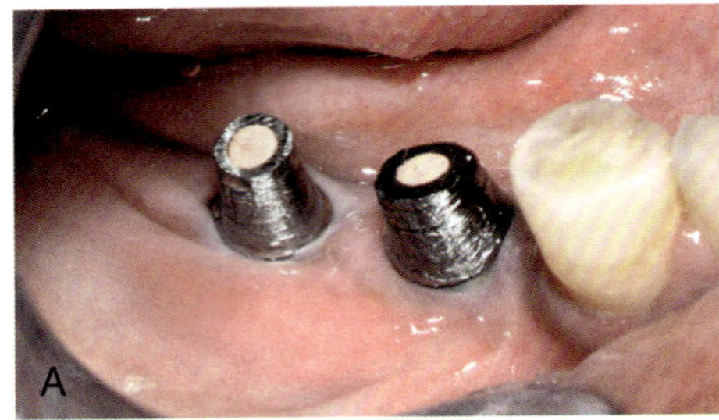

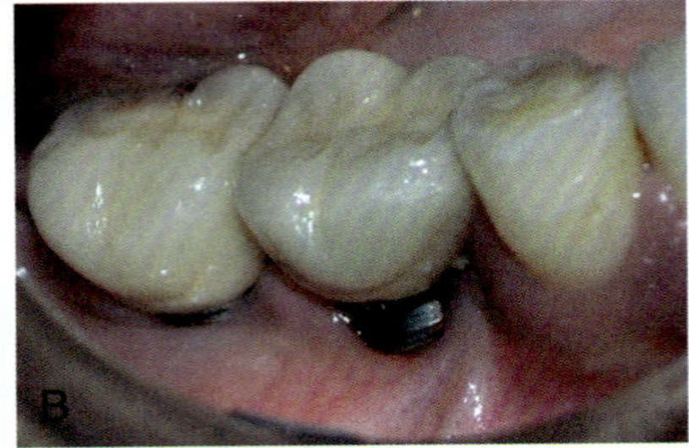

Fig 23.1 (A and B) A thin, mobile, and nonkeratinized marginal soft tissue is less resistant to the muscle pull and recession, which may result in recurrent peri-implantitis and subsequent peri-implant bone loss.

3. Leads to more recession and attachment loss from inflammation
4. Mobile margin resulting in more plaque
5. Poor soft tissue aesthetics with the implant prosthesis in the aesthetic region.

Advantages of the thick, nonmobile, and keratinized marginal soft tissue

1. Protects the peri-implant tissues from injury and infection
2. Resists the pull of muscles
3. Resistant to marginal soft tissue recession
4. Better plaque control
5. Adequate soft tissue aesthetics.

Soft tissue grafting in implant therapy creates a stable peri-implant soft tissue environment by providing an adequate zone of thick, keratinized, and nonmobile soft tissue with intimate adaptation to the emerging implant superstructures. This results in the maintenance of a biological soft tissue seal, and hence, reduction in the incidence of peri-implantitis. Additionally, it provides adequate soft tissue to craft and achieve natural soft tissue architecture for natural aesthetics, and emerging harmonious implant restoration.

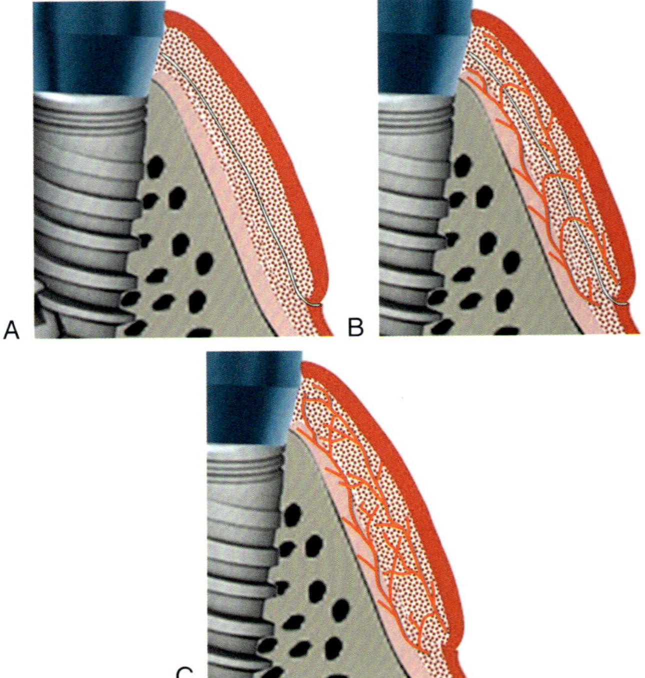

Fig 23.2 (A) Three phases of free soft tissue graft healing – initial phase, (B) revascularization phase and, (C) tissue maturation phase.

Surgical principles of soft tissue grafting

Graft size

The donor site should provide an adequate sized graft to regenerate the required soft tissue dimensions at the recipient site. The adequate size graft not only facilitates immobilization at the recipient site but also receives adequate peripheral circulation from the surrounding recipient site in cases of exposed implant abutment coverage.

Graft uniformity

Graft with a uniform surface facilitates intimate adaptation to the recipient site.

Graft thickness

Grafts with thickness of more than 1.25 mm are preferred when used to cover an avascular surface like the exposed implant abutment at its centre portion. The graft first gets necrosed over this avascular surface and is gradually taken over by the granulation tissue from the periphery to form a scar. The thicker graft is better able to maintain physical integrity during this process, which may take 4–6 weeks. Thus, a full thickness or a thick split thickness graft should be preferred for soft tissue grafting around the dental implant.

Graft vascularization

The free graft (epithelialized connective tissue graft) initially survives with plasmatic circulation and subsequently receives vascularity from the recipient site when capillaries from the recipient site grow and invade the soft tissue graft. Hence, the recipient site should provide adequate vascularity to the graft. When the recipient site has a partially avascular surface like the exposed implant abutment, a thick and large sized graft should be preferred to receive vascularity from the surrounding vascular surface of the recipient site.

Graft adaptation

The graft should intimately be adapted to the underlying recipient surface at the time of operation, which results in a thin layer of exudates between the graft and the recipient bed and achieves a 'plasmatic circulation' for the initial survival of the graft. Inadequate adaptation of the graft causes a thick exudative layer or blood clot at the interface, which may hamper plasmatic circulation and may lead to graft rejection. To achieve adequate graft adaptation over the recipient bed, the graft should have a uniform surface and should be compressed for a few minutes before and after suturing, using moist cotton to eject the blood and extra exudates from the interface to achieve intimate contact of the two surfaces. The recipient site should be uniformly prepared to enhance the intimate adaptation of the graft. The periosteum is considered an excellent recipient surface for the free graft as it provides close adaptation and rich blood supply to the overlying free graft.

Adequate haemostasis

Adequate haemostasis must be obtained at the recipient site because active haemorrhage may prevent intimate adaptation of the graft to the recipient bed. It also facilitates the formation and maintenance of a thin fibrin layer at the graft–recipient surface interface, providing the physical attachment of the graft to the recipient bed and also helping in the establishment of plasmatic circulation between two surfaces, which nourishes the graft before its vascularization.

Graft immobilization

The closely adapted graft should be firmly immobilized onto the recipient bed using multiple interrupted sutures. Mobility of the graft during initial healing, can hamper its nourishment through plasmatic circulation or can disrupt newly forming blood vessels that supply the graft. This may result in excessive shrinkage or sloughing of the graft. The free graft should not be sutured to the surrounding mobile muscular tissue, which can pull the graft during muscle movement. It should be sutured to the underlying periosteum of the recipient bed and the surrounding nonmobile attached tissue.

Healing of free grafts

A free graft, which has been secured onto a connective tissue recipient bed shows three phases of healing (Fig 23.2A–C).

Initial phase (0–3 days)

An intimate adaptation of the graft to the recipient site at the time of surgery leads to:

1. The formation of a thin layer of exudates between graft and recipient bed.
2. Establishment of 'plasmatic circulation' from the recipient site to the graft to provide initial nourishment to the graft.

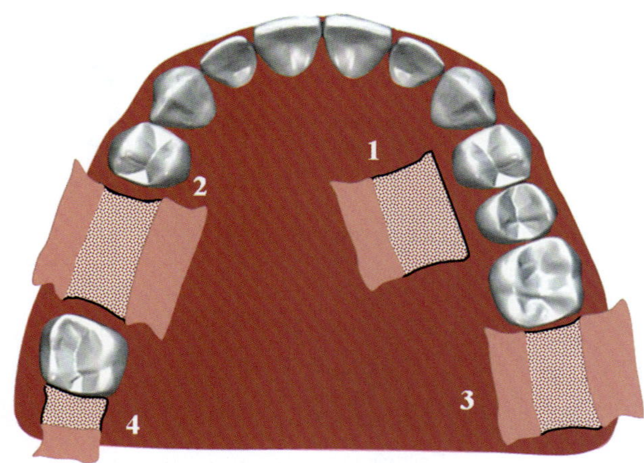

Fig 23.3 Possible donor sites for soft tissue graft – palate mesial to the first molar (1) posterior ridge areas (2), and maxillary tuberosity (3 and 4).

Revascularization phase (2–11 days)

1. Anastomoses occurs between blood vessels of the graft and recipient bed (after 4 to 5 days).
2. Circulation gets re-established in the pre-existing graft vessels.
3. Capillary proliferation within the graft results in the regeneration of dense blood vessels into the graft.
4. Fibrous union between graft and recipient tissue occurs.
5. Re-epithelialization over the graft gets established mainly by proliferation from the adjacent tissues.
6. If a free graft is placed on a root or implant surface, apical migration of epithelium on this surface takes place at this time.

Tissue maturation phase (11–42 days)

1. Gradual reduction of the number of blood vessels occurs in the graft.
2. After 14 days, the vascular system appears normal.
3. Epithelium forms a keratin layer.

Time for soft tissue grafting-usually the soft tissue grafting is preferred at the stage of implant uncovery, but soft tissue grafting can be performed at any stage such as-

1. Prior to implant placement
2. At the same time as implant placement
3. At the time of implant uncovery – most preferred stage
4. After prosthetic insertion.

Keys to success

1. Adequate preparation of the recipient site
2. Selection of an adequate donor site
3. Meticulous preparation of the graft
4. Precision in placement of the graft

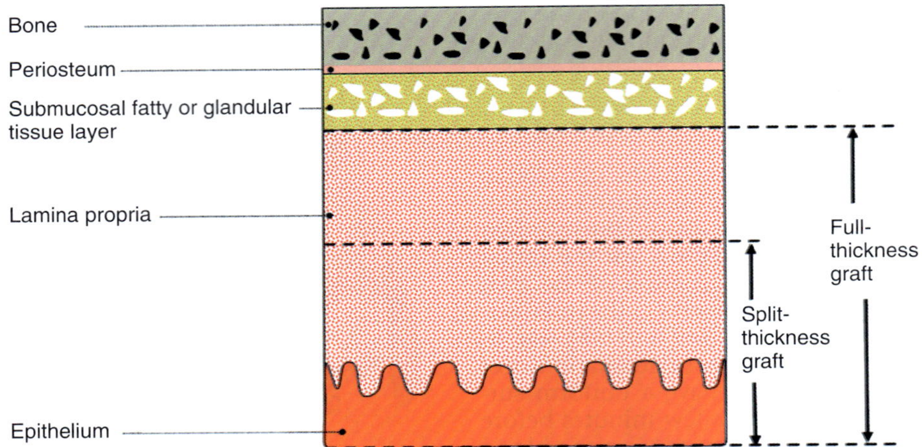

Fig 23.4 A cross-section of the hard palate in the region of maxillary first molar region shows different layers of soft tissue over the palatal bone. Sullivan et al classified the gingival grafts as split-thickness grafts or full-thickness grafts. A full-thickness graft includes all the lamina propria with the epithelium but a split-thickness graft includes only a partial thickness of the connective tissue with the epithelium. A split thickness graft can be further classified as thin, intermediate, and thick depending on the thickness of the connective tissue (1/4, 1/2, or 2/3) harvested with the overlying epithelium. The fatty or glandular tissue is not harvested with the mucosal graft.

5. Obtaining adequate haemostasis
6. Intimate adaptation of the graft
7. Adequate immobilization of the graft with suturing
8. Postoperative care of the graft for 3–4 weeks.

Possible donor sites for graft harvesting

The richest autogenous source of connective tissue or epithelialized, connective-tissue intraoral graft is the palate, but in selective cases the epithelialized connective-tissue graft can also be harvested from the edentulous ridge area of the maxilla or mandible and also from the maxillary tuberosity (Fig 23.3). Sullivan et al classified gingival grafts as split thickness gingival grafts or full thickness gingival grafts. A full thickness graft includes all the lamina propria with the epithelium, but a split thickness graft, includes only the partial thickness of the connective tissue with the epithelium. A split thickness graft can be further classified as thin, intermediate, and thick depending on the thickness of the connective tissue (1/4rth, 1/2, or 2/3rd of total thickness) harvested with the overlying epithelium. The fatty or glandular tissue is not harvested with the mucosal graft (Fig 23.4).

Armamentaria and materials required

1. Micro Adson forceps
2. Artery forceps
3. Micro scissor
4. Straight and angled surgical blade handles
5. Micro needle holder
6. Micro elevators
7. Soft tissue punch
8. Retractors
9. Surgical blade numbers 11, 12, and 15
10. Suture material (4-0 with reverse cutting edge needle)
11. Collagen sponge (Fig 23.5A–D).

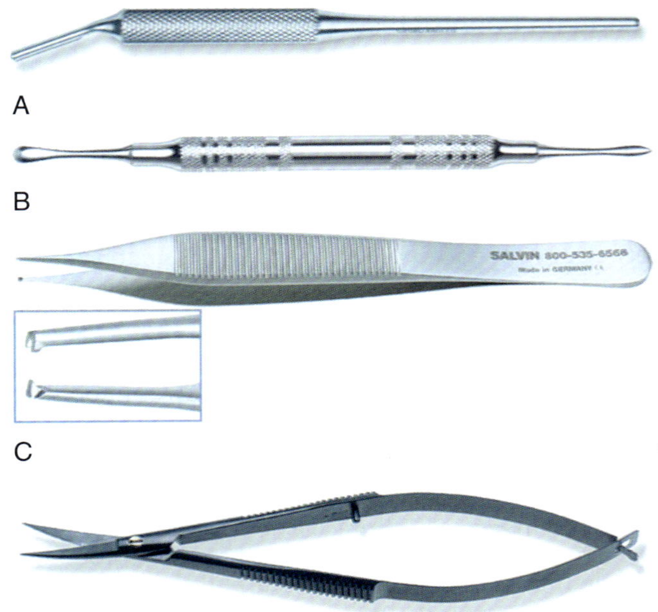

Fig 23.5 (A) Angled surgical blade handle, (B) micro elevator, (C) Micro Adson forceps, (D) micro scissors (*Courtesy: Salvin Dental Specialities, USA*).

Technique-1 – Epithelialized connective tissue graft or free gingival graft technique

A partial thickness or full thickness epithelialized connective tissue graft can be harvested from the palate.

Indications

1. For increasing the zone of keratinized tissue around the implant for ease of maintenance.

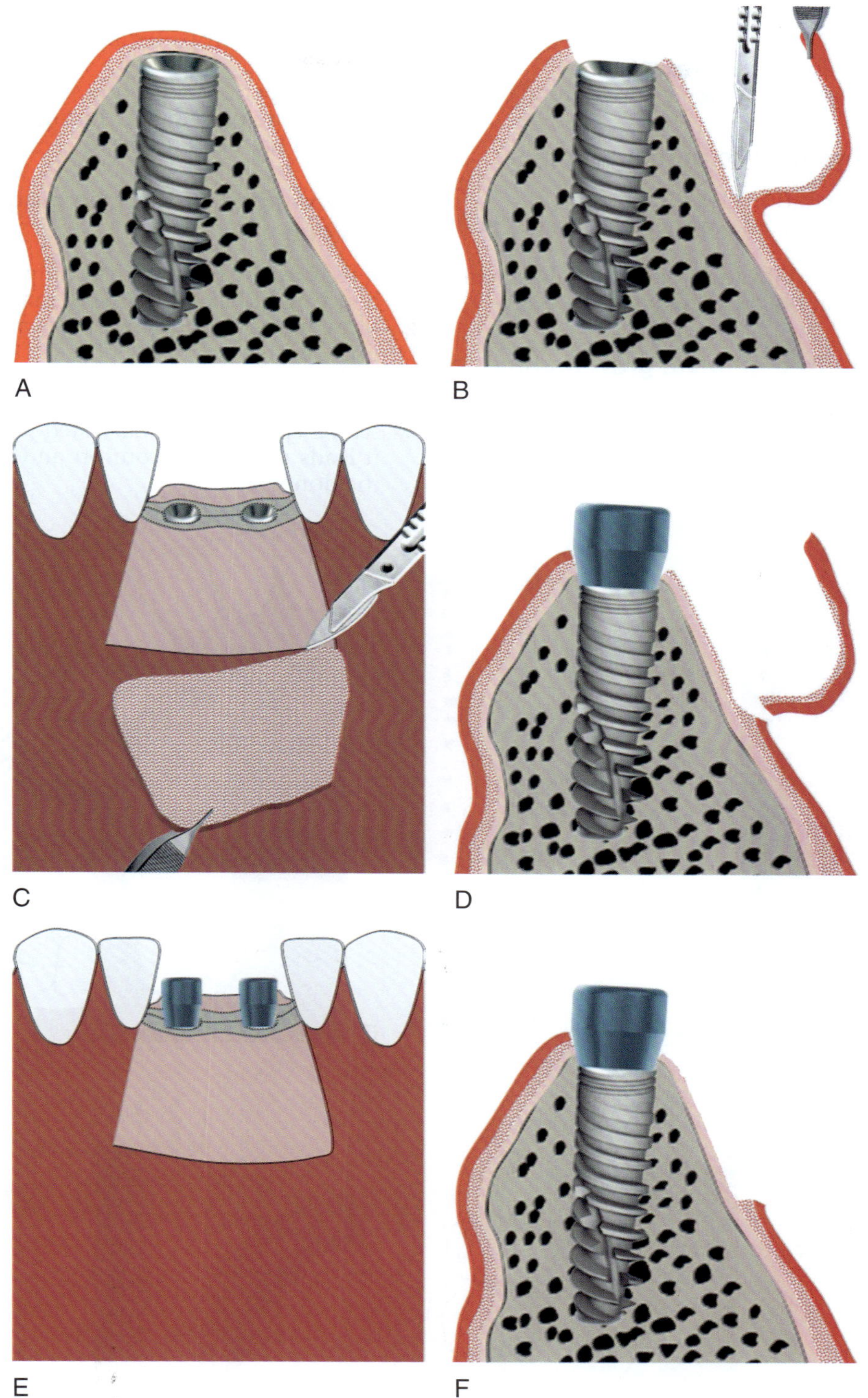

Fig 23.6 A horizontal incision is made, using surgical blade number 15, just coronal to the desired soft tissue augmentation. Vertical incisions are then extended apically from the lateral aspects of the horizontal incision. All three incisions are made perpendicular to the existing soft tissue surface to create butt joint with the free gingival graft. All the incisions are limited to the mucosa and should not cut the underlying periosteum. (A and B) The sharp dissections are made apically to elevate all the mucosal tissue, leaving the periosteum intact to the bone. (C and D) The resultant flap is usually excised. (E and F) All the residual remnants of the connective tissue or muscle attachments are removed using a soft tissue nipper or sharp soft tissue scissors to create a rigid periosteal recipient bed. If performed at the time of implant uncovery, the implant is exposed and a gingival former is inserted. Haemostasis is obtained by compressing the site with a moist cotton pack for few minutes.

2. For increasing the soft tissue thickness around the implant.
3. To obtain implant abutment coverage.
4. To obtain the exposed root coverage of a natural tooth.

Step by step diagrammatic presentation

1. **Recipient site preparation** (Fig 23.6A–F)
2. **Harvesting epithelialized connective tissue graft** (Fig 23.7A–E)
3. **Adaptation and immobilization of epithelialized connective tissue graft at the recipient site** (Fig 23.8A–D).

Advantages of the free gingival graft technique

1. Relatively easy to perform when compared to other soft tissue grafting procedures.
2. A large area can be grafted.
3. Thickens tissue and regenerates a keratinized epithelium.
4. It can be performed using acellular dermal matrix (AlloDerm®) in patients who resist harvesting autogenous graft.
5. It can be performed at any stage, before or at the time of implant placement, during uncovery or after the implant has been restored.

Disadvantages of the free gingival graft technique

1. It receives the nourishment only from the periosteum, hence, it takes a long time to maturate.
2. More prone to suture breakdown and graft mobilization during the healing phase.
3. Colour mismatch of maturated grafted site and the surrounding soft tissue.
4. As the epithelium is harvested with connective tissue, it leads to more discomfort and long healing time at the donor site.

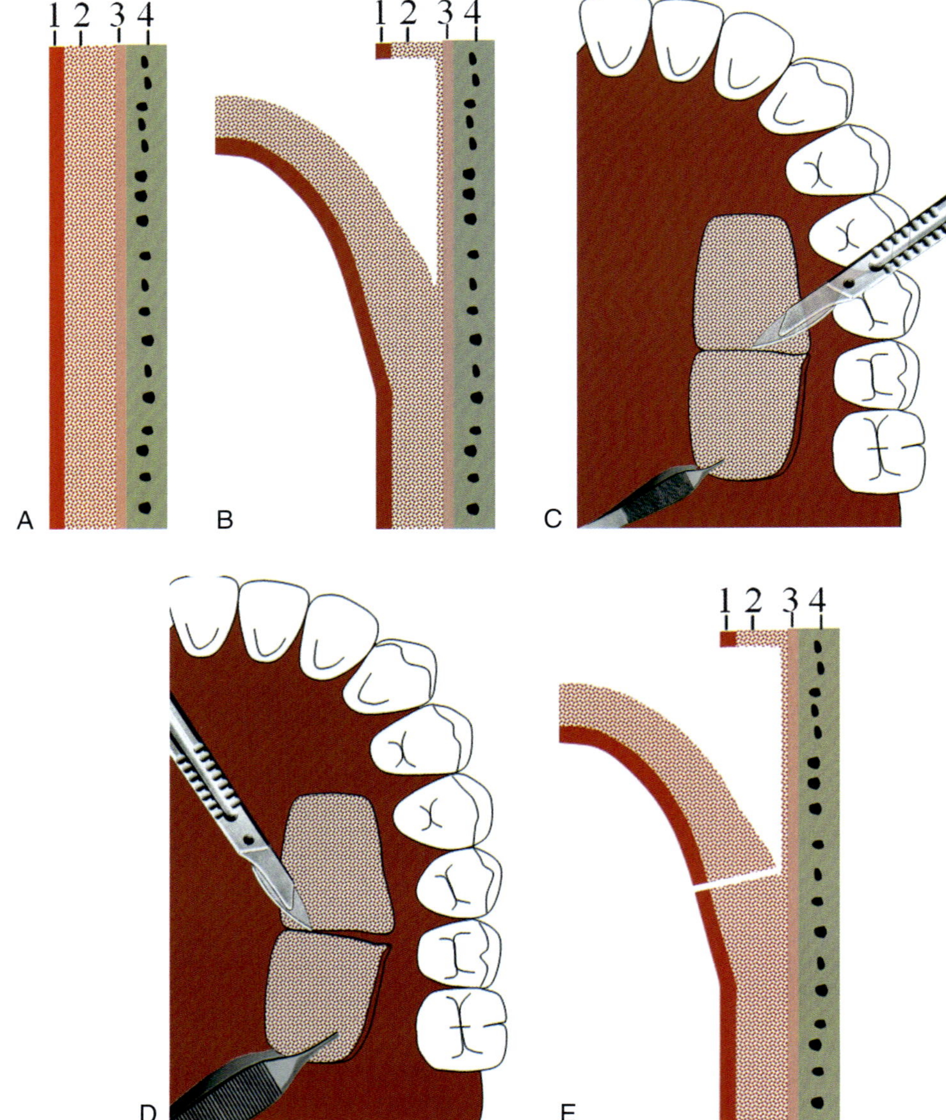

Fig 23.7 Rectangular-shaped horizontal incisions, limited to the connective tissue, are made using a number 15 blade at the hard palate in the premolar region leaving 2–3 mm marginal gingiva. (A–C) The sharp dissections are made to elevate a full thickness or partial thickness free gingival graft, leaving the glandular tissue behind, attached to the periosteum. (D and E) The resultant flap is removed and immediately transferred to the prepared recipient site.

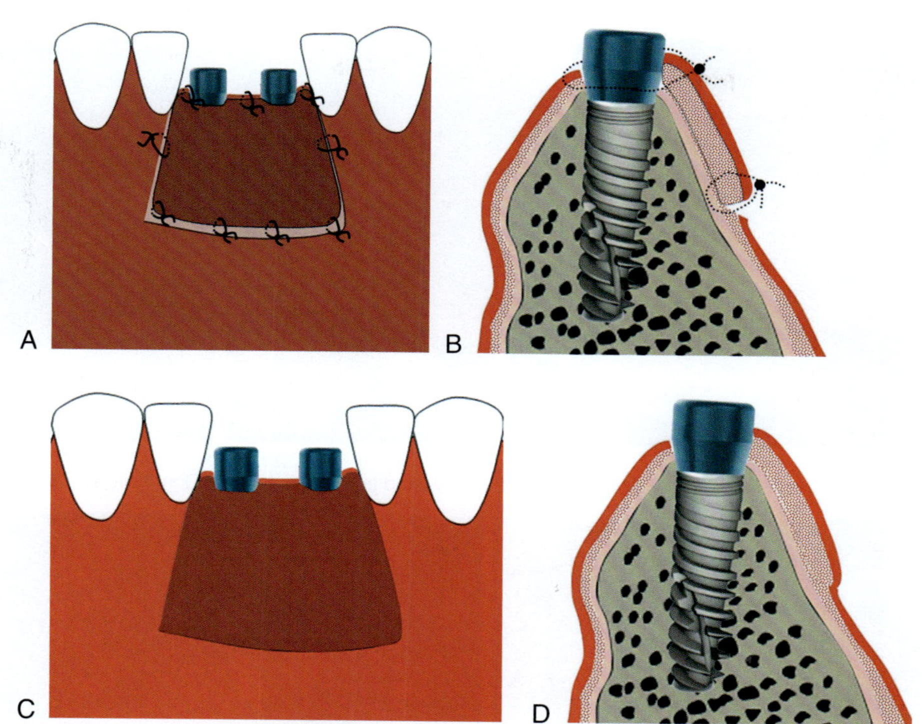

Fig 23.8 Free gingival graft is shaped to accurately fit at the prepared recipient site. (A and B) Once the haemostasis is obtained at the recipient periosteum bed, the graft is adapted and sutured with the periosteum and surrounding nonmobile tissue using 4-0 chromic gut sutures. Once immobilized with sutures, the graft should be compressed using a moistened saline sponge for 10–12 min, to squeeze out extra blood from the interface and to achieve intimate contact between the two surfaces, to form a thin fibrin clot at the interface. The patient is instructed not to brush the site for 3 weeks. Sutures are removed after 10–13 days. (C and D) The graft through the different stages of its regeneration, slowly maturates into a thick keratinized soft tissue at the site and this procedure may however take 8–10 weeks.

CASE REPORT-1

Use of epithelialized connective tissue palatal graft (free gingival graft) to regenerate thick, nonmobile, and keratinized marginal soft tissue zone around the implants (Figs 23.9–23.12).

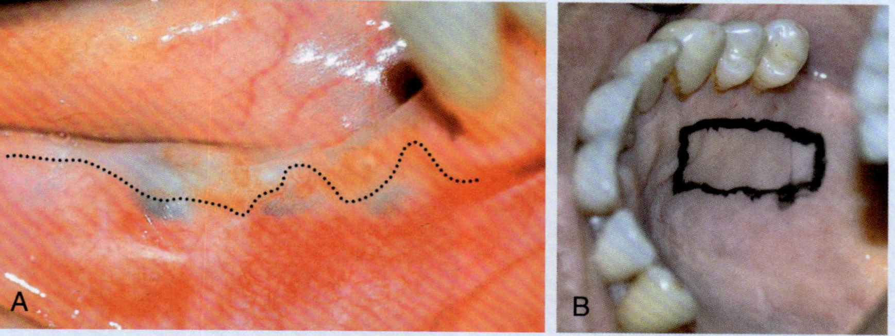

Fig 23.9 (A) Thin, mobile, and nonkeratinized soft tissue over the implants can be seen at the uncovery phase. (B) A full thickness epithelialized connective tissue palatal graft (free gingival graft) is planned to regenerate a zone of thick, nonmobile, and keratinized marginal soft tissue around the implants.

Continued

CASE REPORT-1—cont'd

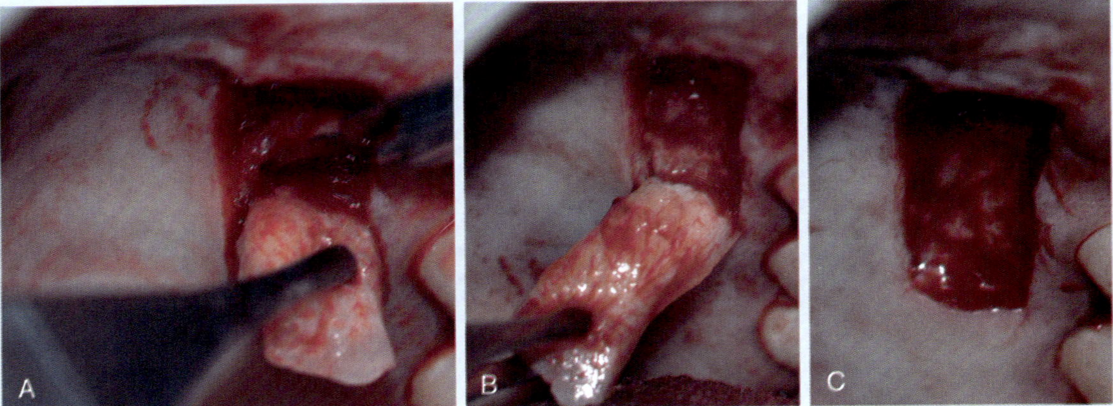

Fig 23.10 (A and B) An adequate size full thickness free gingival graft is harvested from the palate. (C) Donor site after graft has been harvested.

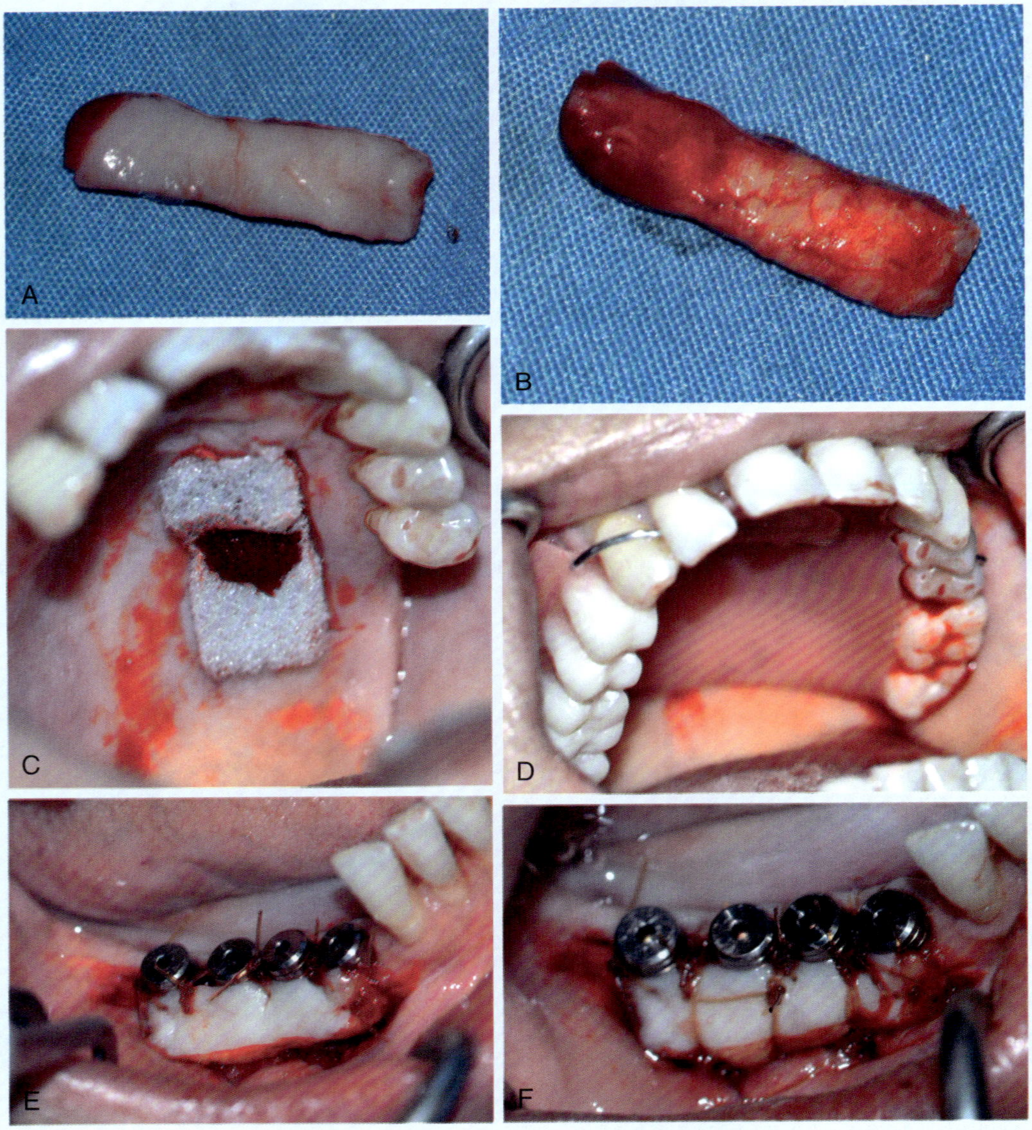

Fig 23.11 (A) Epithelial surface of the graft. (B) Connective tissue surface of the graft. (C) Haemostasis is achieved at the donor site by compression with moistened cotton for few minutes and an absorbable gelatin sponge is placed at the site. (D) A prefabricated acrylic template is seated over the site to control bleeding and minimize discomfort. (E) The graft is immediately transferred to the prepared recipient periosteal bed and immobilized by suturing first with the attached gingiva and (F) then with the underlying periosteum.

CASE REPORT-1—cont'd

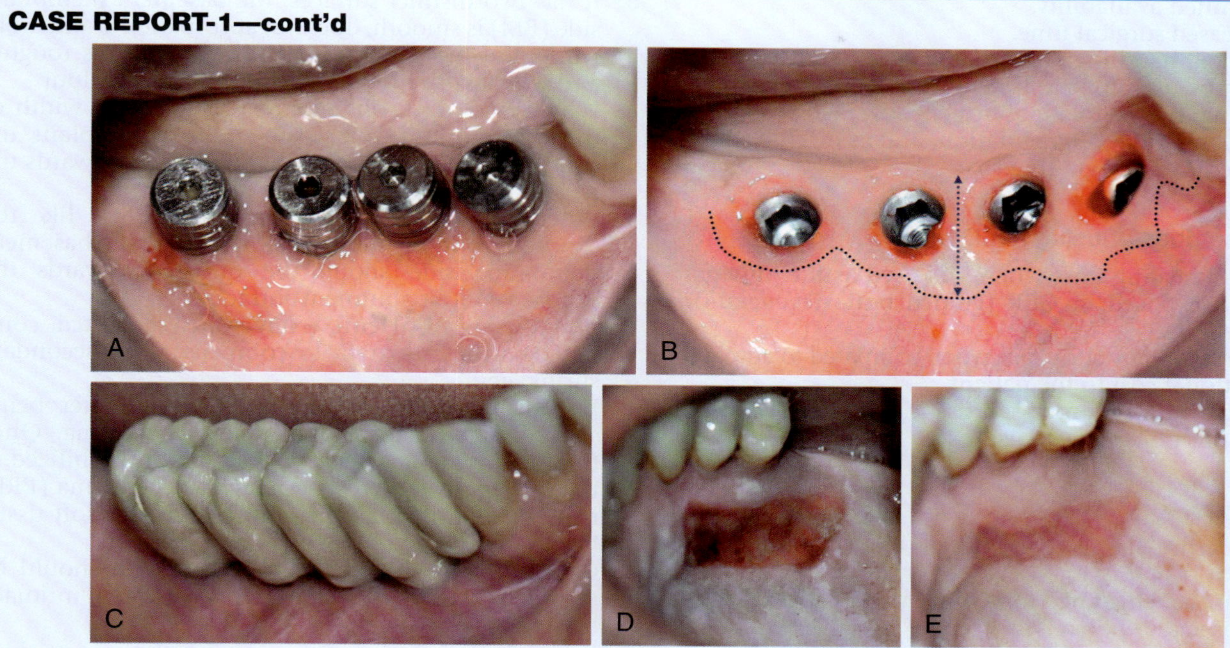

Fig 23.12 (A) The site after 2 weeks shows capillary proliferation and re-epithelialization. (B) The site after 8 weeks shows regeneration of a thick, nonmobile, and keratinized zone of marginal soft tissue around the implants which is more resistant to the recession, muscle pull, and peri-implantitis. (C) Implants are restored. (D) The healing of the donor site after 2 weeks and (E) 4 weeks.

Grafting using acellular dermal matrix (AlloDerm® membrane)

AlloDerm® (LifeCell Corporation, Branchburg, NJ, USA), is a donated human soft tissue that is processed to remove the dermal cells, leaving behind a regenerative collagen matrix. It has successfully been used as an alternative to the autogenous epithelialized palatal graft.

AlloDerm® allows clinicians to perform soft tissue regeneration procedures without the discomfort and second-site morbidity often associated with palatal tissue harvesting. Because it is available in unlimited quantities, treatment of all necessary areas can be accomplished with fewer procedures than would be possible with palatal harvesting.

AlloDerm® is ideal for patients who either lack adequate harvestable tissue or prefer not to undergo a palatal harvest. Widely used in root coverage procedures, AlloDerm® has demonstrated clinical and aesthetic results equivalent to palatal tissue. It may also be used for free gingival grafting, soft tissue ridge augmentation, and as a cell-occlusive barrier for bone grafting. It is available in two thickness ranges: 0.9–1.6 mm (AlloDerm) and 0.5–0.9 mm (AlloDerm GBR) to suit specific applications.

Processing of AlloDerm®

AlloDerm® is composed of freeze-dried skin allograft, which is processed to remove all the immunogenic cellular components like epidermis and dermal cells, leaving only a useful acellular dermal matrix that is used for soft tissue grafting purposes.

During the proprietary processing, a buffered salt solution gently separates the epidermis from the basement membrane. Many cell types within the dermis are then solubilized and washed away using a patented series of nondenaturing detergent washes.

The tissue matrix is then preserved using a patented freeze-drying process that prevents damaging crystal formations, thereby retaining the critical biochemical and structural components needed to maintain the tissue's natural regenerative properties. The graft is then ready for rehydration and implantation to help the human body begin its tissue regeneration process.

How AlloDerm® works

AlloDerm® provides a matrix consisting of collagens, elastin, blood vessel channels, and proteins that support revascularization, cell repopulation and tissue remodelling. When the graft is left exposed, as in guided bone regeneration or a free gingival graft, the AlloDerm matrix will support epithelial migration through creeping substitution across the basement membrane.

After placement, the patient's blood infiltrates the AlloDerm graft through retained vascular channels, bringing host stem cells that bind themselves to the proteins in the matrix. Significant revascularization can begin as early as 1 week after implantation.

The host cells respond to the local environment and the matrix is remodelled into the patient's own tissue, in a fashion similar to the body's natural cell attrition and replacement process.

Advantages of using AlloDerm®

1. Elimination of donor site.
2. Only one surgical site, hence more comfortable for the patient.

3. Unlimited availability.
4. Decreased surgical time.
5. Excellent handling properties.
6. It can be used for multiple purposes like free gingival grafting, root/implant abutment coverage procedures, soft tissue ridge augmentation, and as a cell-occlusive barrier for bone grafting.

Disadvantages of using AlloDerm®

1. Longer healing time when it is used as the only graft or left exposed in GBR (guided bone regeneration) procedures.
2. More secondary shrinkage when compared to autograft.
3. Additional cost to the patient.
4. Being a human processed tissue, some patients have religious objections to using it.

Key points

1. AlloDerm® has a 2-year shelf life when stored in 1–10°C (34–50°F).
2. It must be rehydrated for a minimum of 10 min before it is used.
3. It has two distinct surfaces: the basement membrane side (BM) is smooth, does not absorb blood, and looks white; but the connective tissue side (CT) is rougher and will absorb blood and changes to red colour.
4. When used as an only graft to increase the width of thick, keratinized, soft tissue around an implant, the connective tissue side should be oriented towards the recipient site.
5. When used to cover an avascular surface like the exposed root or implant abutment, the basement membrane side should be oriented towards the exposed root or abutment surface.
6. When using AlloDerm, a larger area is grafted, compared to the autograft, to compensate for secondary shrinkage.
7. If possible, AlloDerm should be used after being soaked in nonactivated, platelet-rich plasma. Once the membrane has been sutured and immobilized at the recipient site, activated platelet-rich plasma (PRP) is used topically over the graft to enhance soft tissue healing.
8. Once immobilized at the site, AlloDerm should be pressed with a moist saline sponge to obtain intimacy between the two surfaces.

CASE REPORT-2

Regeneration of thick, nonmobile, and keratinized marginal soft tissue using the dermal matrix (Alloderm®) (Figs 23.13 and 23.14).

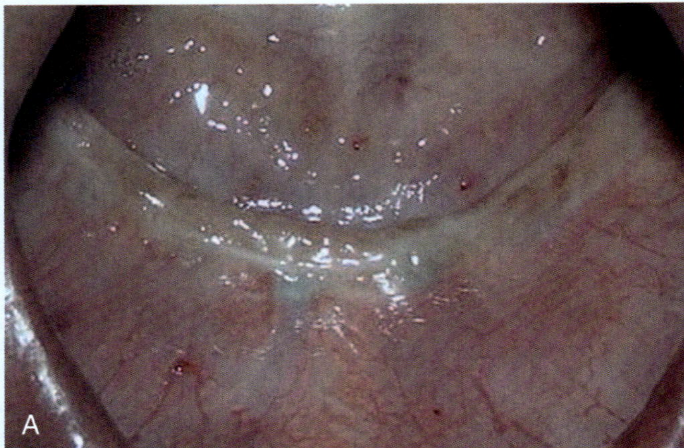

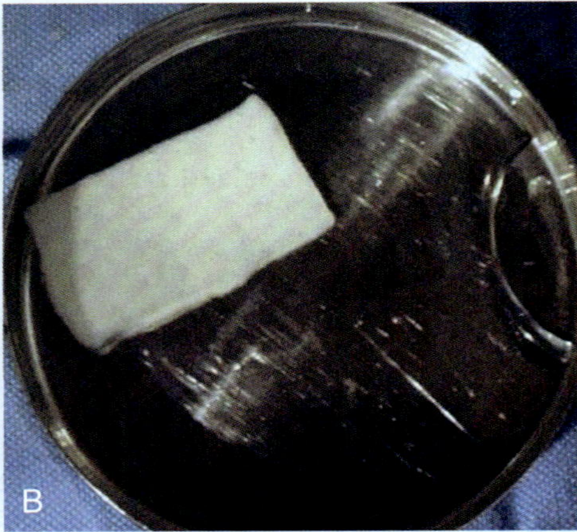

Fig 23.13 (A) Presence of an inadequate band of keratinized marginal soft tissue over the ridge can be seen at the time of implant uncovery. (B) AlloDerm® membrane.

CASE REPORT-2—cont'd

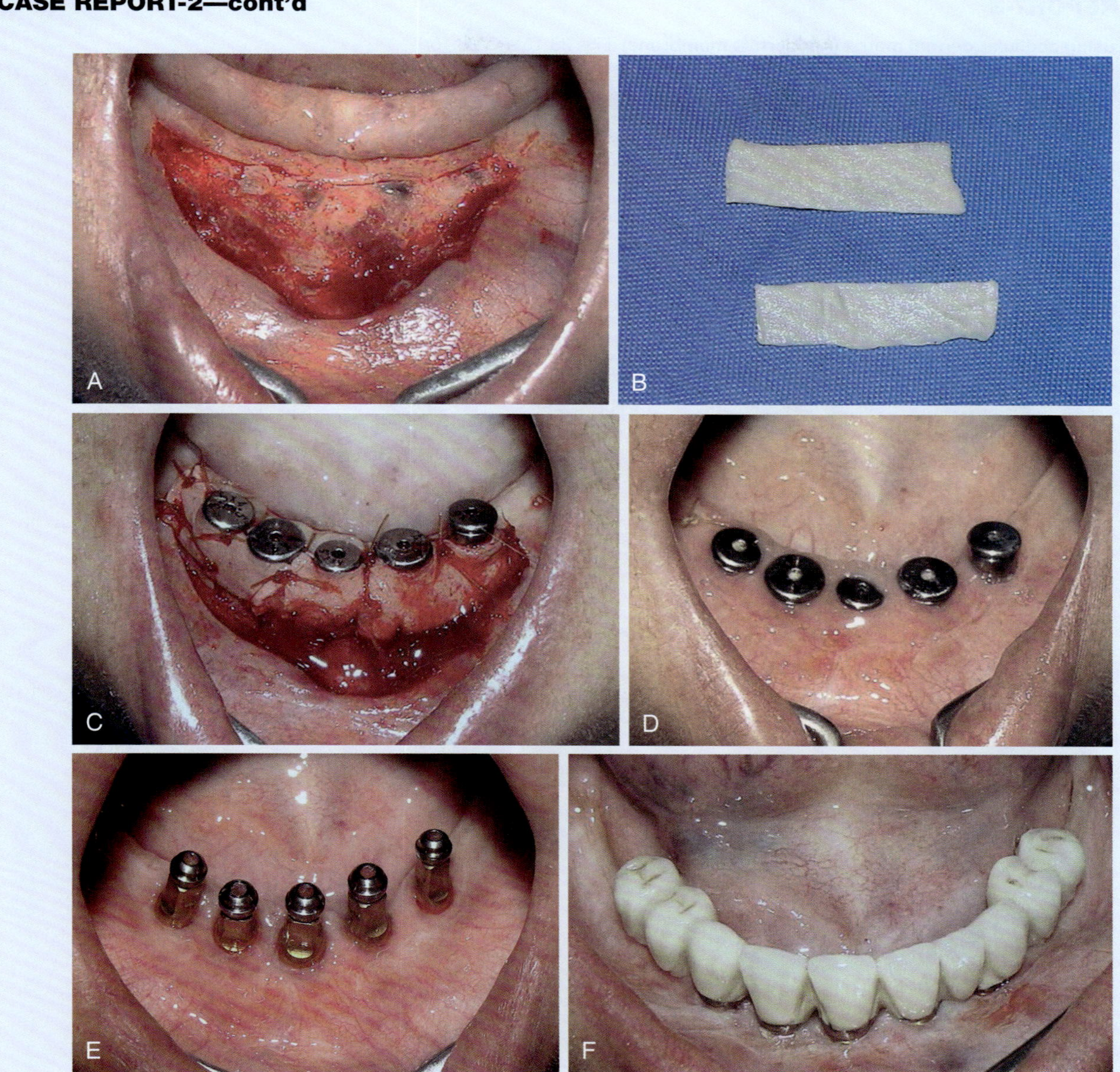

Fig 23.14 (A) A horizontal incision is made at the junction of mobile and stable tissue, the keratinized soft tissue band present at the ridge crest is shifted to the lingual and blunt dissections are given to prepare a rigid periosteal bed at facial aspect. (B) The membrane is cut into two pieces and (C) sutured to immobilize at the recipient site after gingival formers have been inserted on top of the implants. (D) Site after 2 weeks is showing newly generated thick, nonmobile, and keratinized soft tissue collar around the implants. (E and F) Implants are restored 6 weeks after the soft tissue grafting.

CASE REPORT-3

Grafting using acellular dermal matrix (Alloderm® membrane) (Figs 23.15 and 23.16).

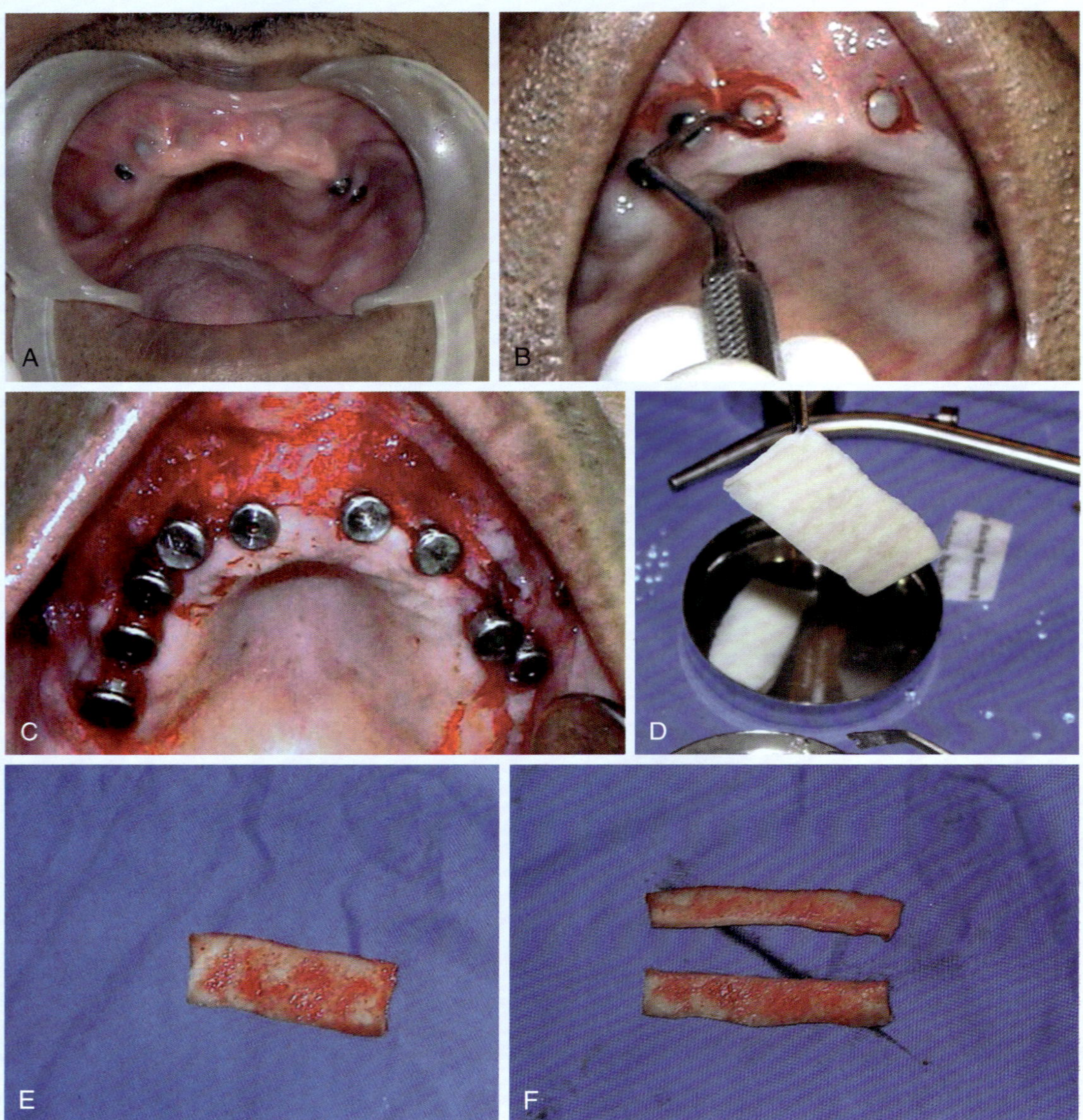

Fig 23.15 (A) Thin, nonkeratinized and mobile marginal soft tissue can be seen at the implant site during implant uncovery stage. (B) Implants are uncovered using soft tissue punch and the gingival formers are inserted. (C) Blunt dissections have been made to remove all the nonkeratinized mobile tissue and muscle fibres, leaving behind a firm, attached periosteum. (D and E) AlloDerm® membrane is washed in saline, soaked in the patient's blood to identify its connective tissue surface as it soaks blood and becomes red. (F) The membrane is cut into two surfaces to graft a large surface area.

CASE REPORT-3—cont'd

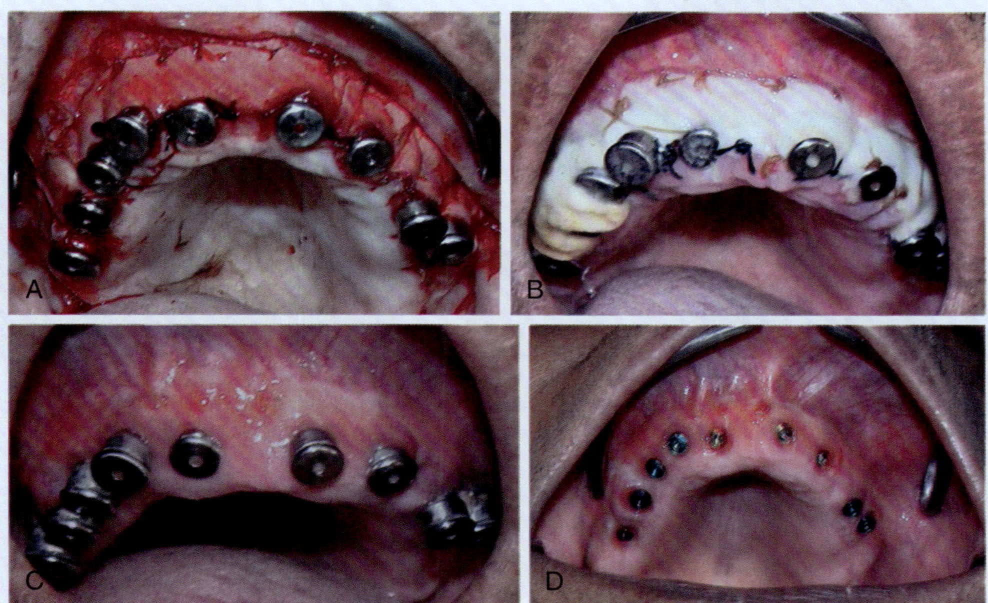

Fig 23.16 (A) The membrane is immobilized over the recipient periosteal bed using 4-0 chromic gut sutures. (B) The membrane gets slowly resorbed and (C and D) regenerates a new keratinized, thick and stable marginal soft tissue band around the implants.

Technique-2 – Subepithelial connective tissue graft technique

In 1982, Langer and Calagna introduced this technique for the enhancement of anterior soft tissue aesthetics. A subepithelial connective tissue graft is harvested from the palate and used for localized ridge augmentation, exposed root coverage, or exposed implant abutment. A subepithelial connective tissue pouch is created at the recipient site and the connective tissue graft is positioned between the periosteum and a partial thickness cover flap. This technique offers several advantages over the free gingival graft.

Advantages

1. Less invasive procedure.
2. Excellent colour matching with the adjacent tissue.
3. Less technique-sensitive.
4. Graft receives dual blood supply both from the underlying periosteum as well as from the overlying host tissue.
5. The graft achieves better stability at the host site.
6. Less postoperative care is required compared to the free gingival graft.
7. More predictable results.

Step by step diagrammatic presentation

1. **Host site preparation** (Figs 23.17 and 23.18).
2. **Harvesting the connective tissue graft from the palate.** There are two techniques to harvest the connective tissue from the palate:
   a. **Open approach** (Fig 23.19A–D)
   b. **Closed approach** (Figs 23.20 and 23.21).
3. **Suturing connective tissue graft over the host site** (Fig 23.22A–F).

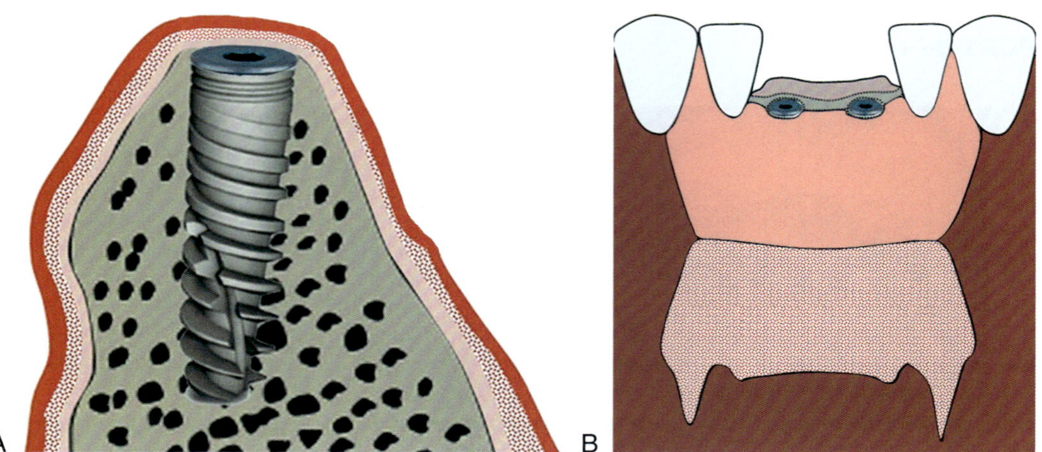

Fig 23.17 (A) A thin connective tissue layer is seen between the epithelium and periosteum at the crestal and the facial aspect of the implant. (B) A partial thickness flap, leaving the periosteum intact, is elevated to uncover the implants as well as the facial aspect of the ridge.

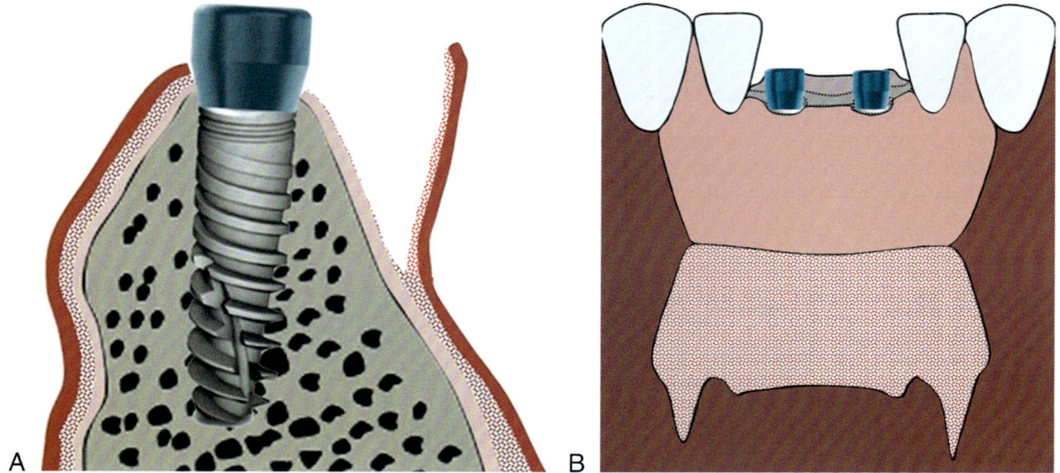

Fig 23.18 (A and B) The cover screw is replaced with healing abutments.

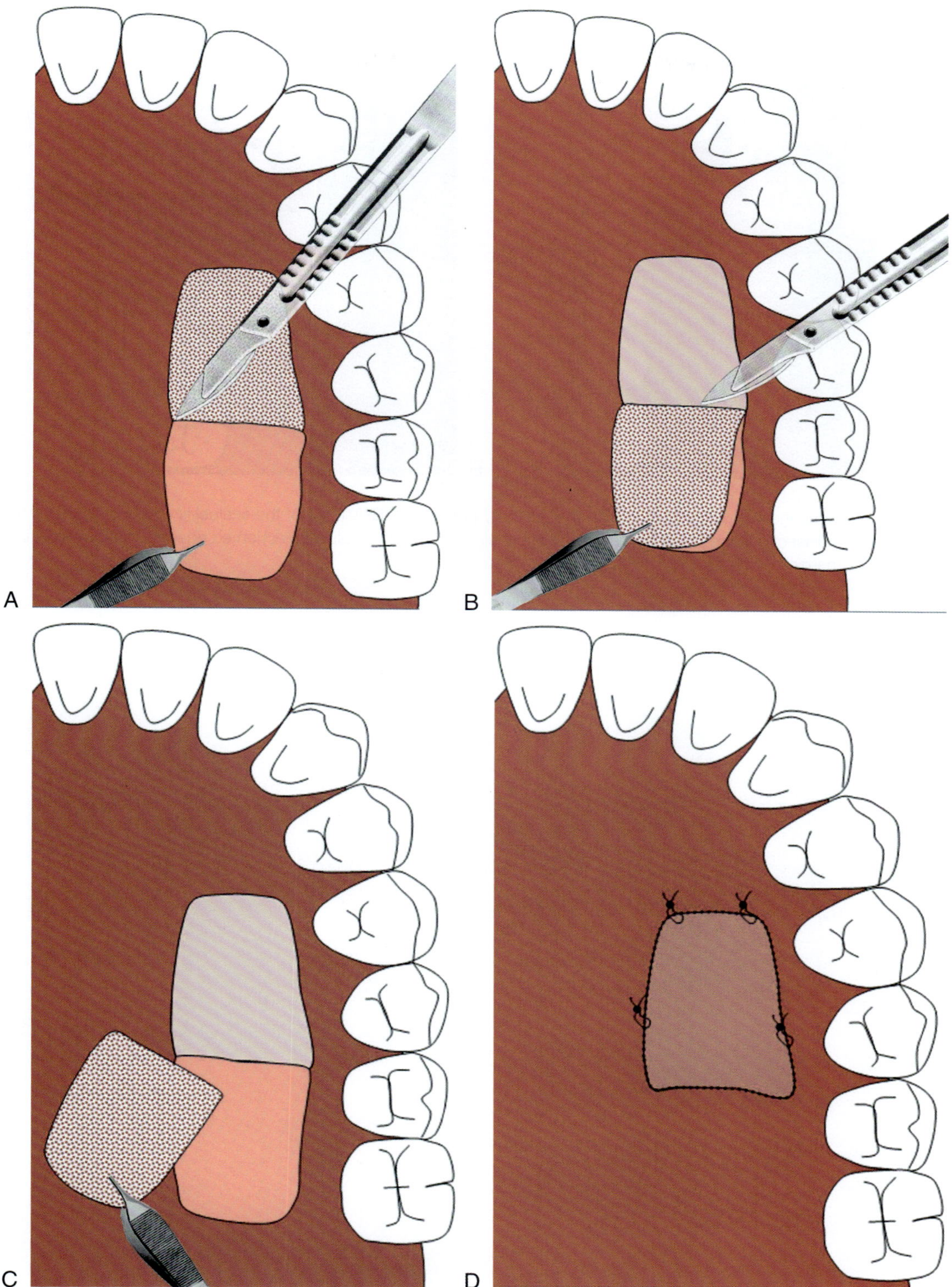

Fig 23.19 (A) An incision is given through the palate epithelium and a sharp dissection is made to elevate the epithelium. (B and C) Once the underlying connective tissue is exposed, sharp dissections are made to harvest the thick connective tissue layer, leaving the fatty tissue (glandular) layer attached to the periosteum. (D) Haemostasis is achieved and the epthelium is sutured back.

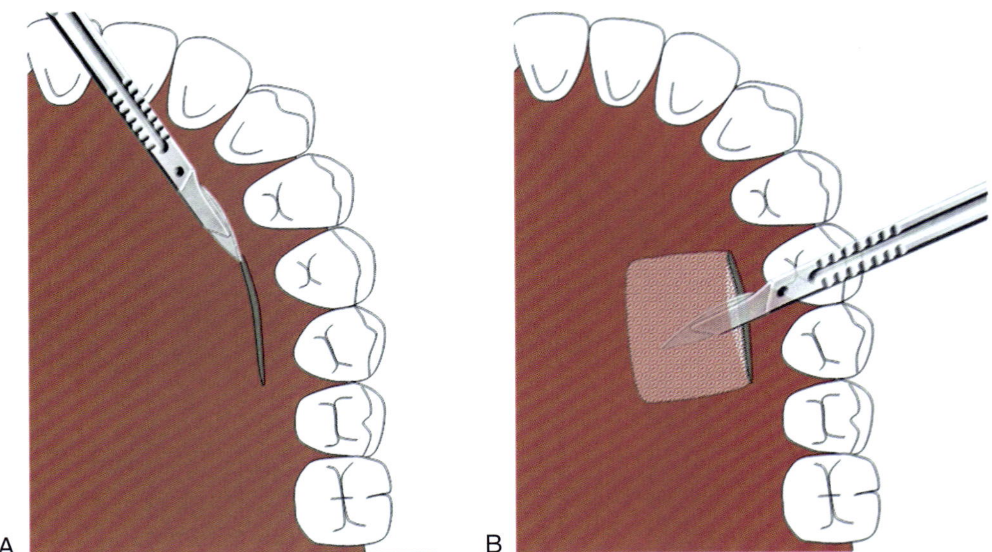

Fig 23.20 (A) A sharp and deep incision is made medial to the maxillary premolars. (B) The tip of the scalpel is reoriented parallel to the surface of the palatal tissue, and sharp dissections are made to create a subepithelial pouch. The scalpel is reoriented again to make vertical incisions through the connective tissue at all margins of the pouch.

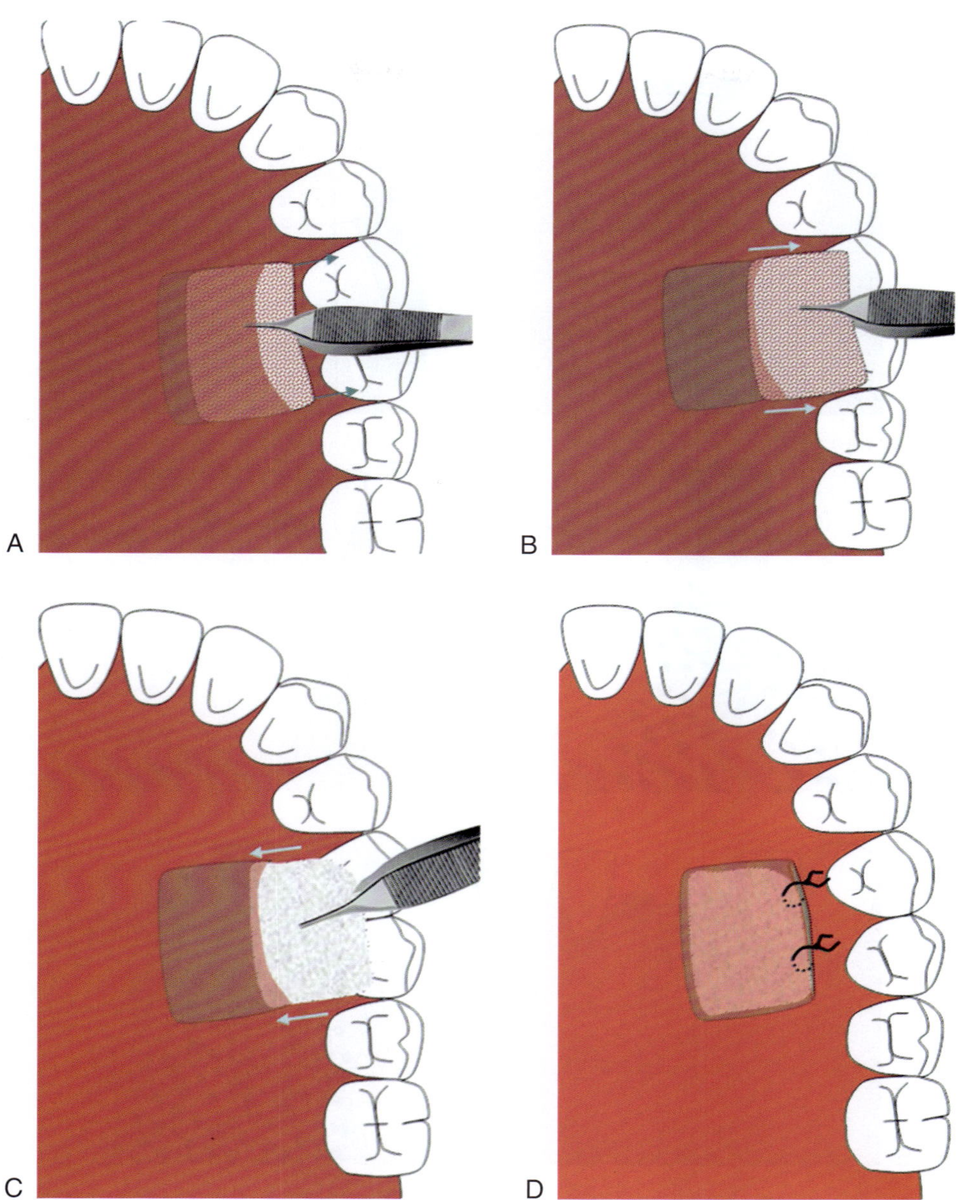

Fig 23.21 (A and B) The subperiosteal dissection is then performed using a small periosteal elevator and the connective tissue is removed from the pouch using Adson tissue forceps. (C) A piece of absorbable collagen (Collaplug) is then inserted into the pouch to obtain haemostasis and fill the dead space. (D) The incision line is sutured using 4-0 chromic suture.

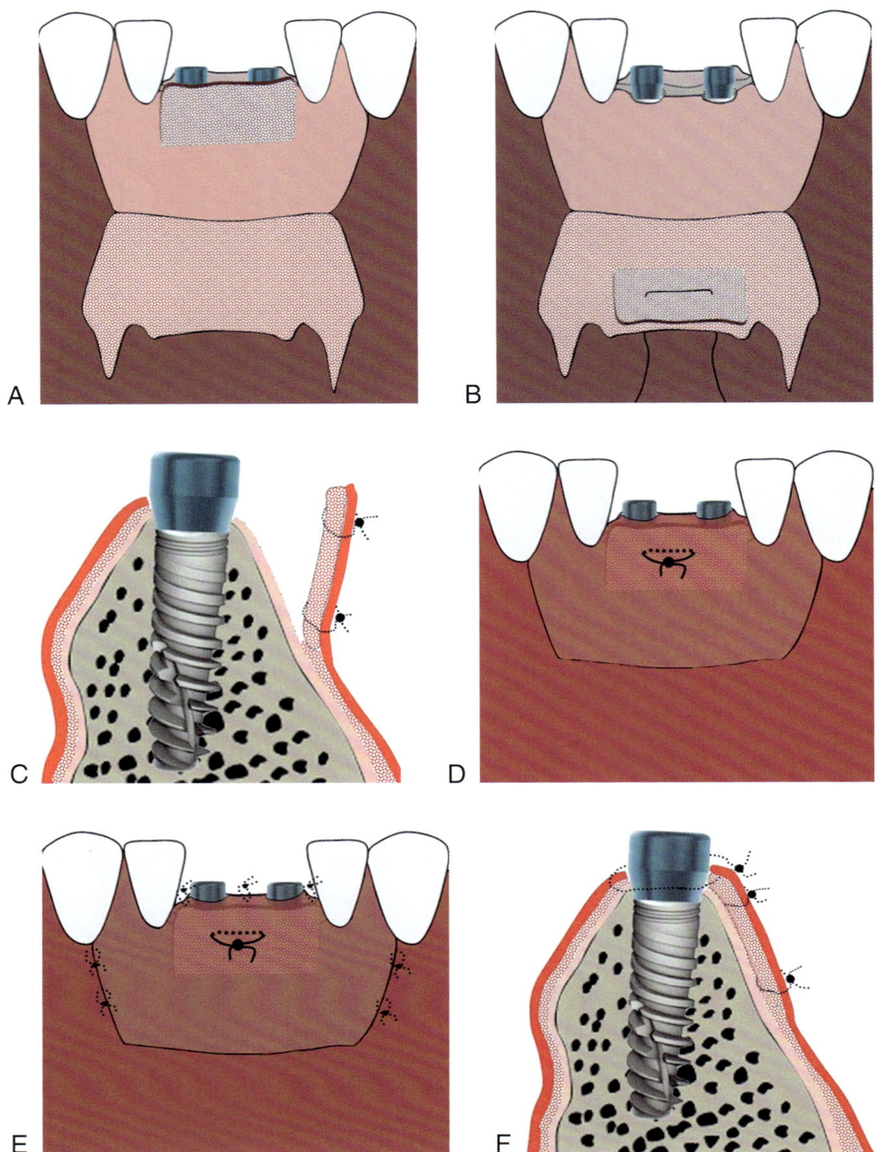

Fig 23.22 (A–C) The connective tissue graft is shaped, adapted at the host site and sutured with the flap. (D–F) The flap is repositioned and sutured back.

CASE REPORT-4

Connective tissue grafting to enhance soft tissue emergence around implant restoration (Figs 23.23–23.27).

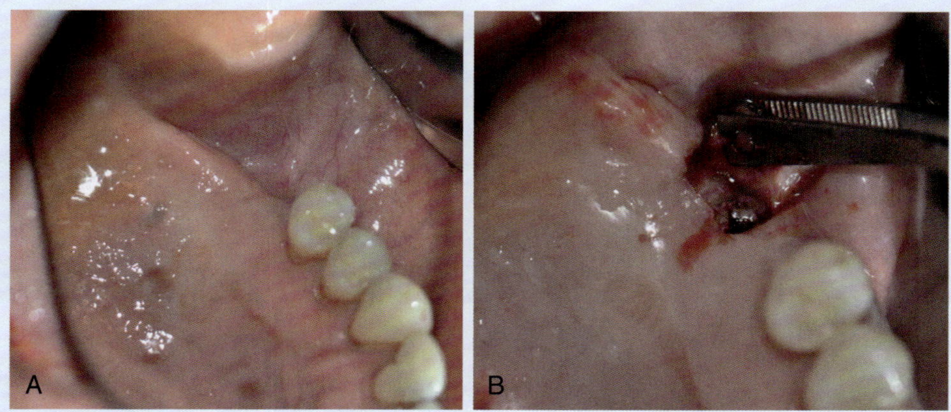

Fig 23.23 (A) Inadequate amount of facial soft tissue before the uncovery of an implant at the first molar site. (B) A partial thickness flap is elevated to expose the implant.

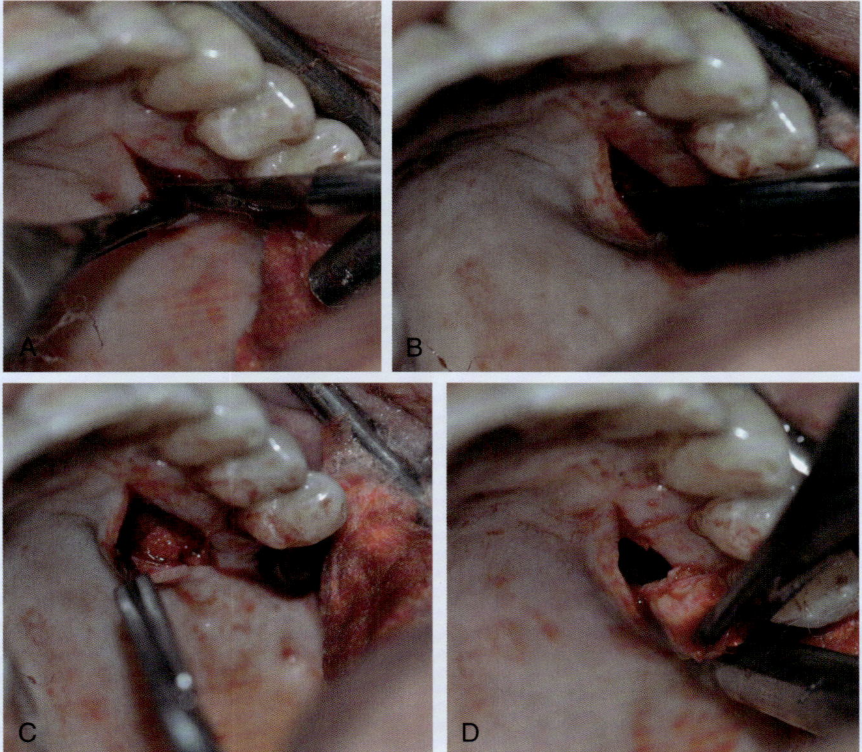

Fig 23.24 (A–C) A vertical incision is given at the palate, medial to the premolars, and a subepithelial pouch is created by giving sharp dissections through the subepithelial layer. (D) The underlying connective tissue is harvested from the pouch.

Continued

CASE REPORT-4—cont'd

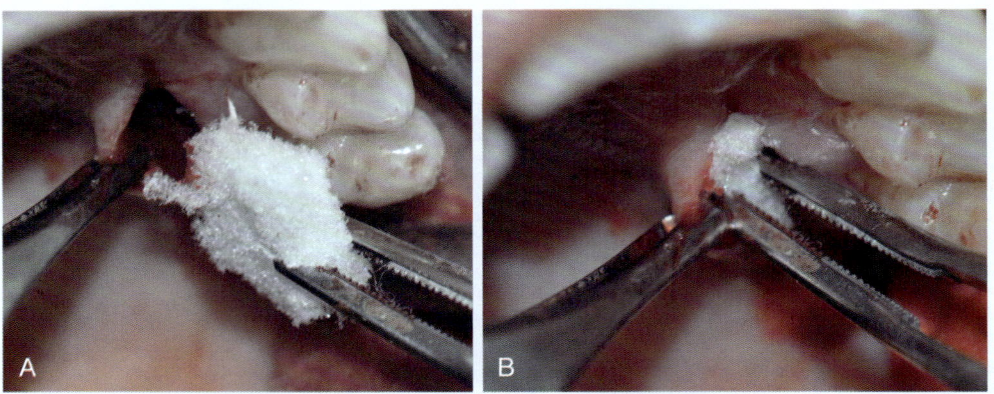

Fig 23.25 (A and B) A small piece of collagen sponge is inserted to achieve haemostasis and to fill the dead space.

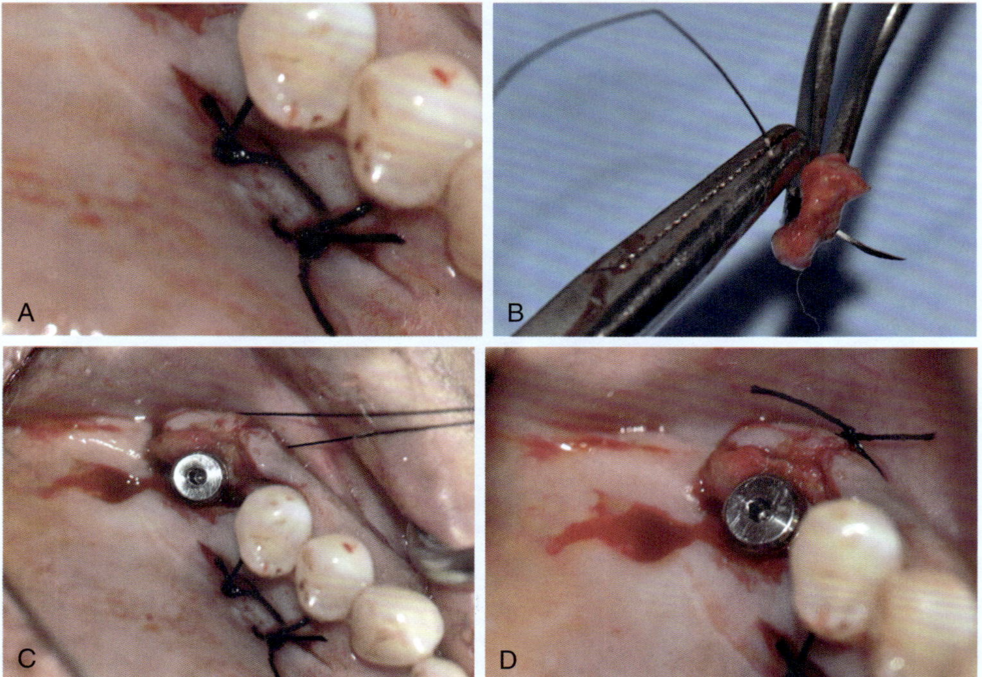

Fig 23.26 (A) The incision line is sutured with primary closure. (B-D) The connective tissue is adapted at the recipient site and sutured underneath the facial flap.

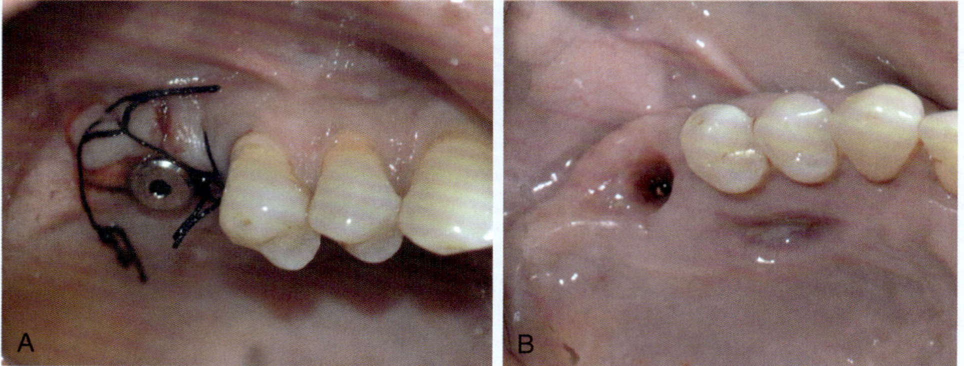

Fig 23.27 (A) The flap is sutured to achieve close approximation. (B) The healing after 4 weeks shows regeneration of a thick soft tissue layer on the facial aspect of the implant.

Technique 3 — Subepithelial pouch technique

The pouch technique is performed to achieve horizontal as well as vertical soft tissue augmentation, to cover the exposed implant and/or abutment and to achieve an aesthetic soft tissue emergence profile around the implant restoration.

Step by step diagrammatic presentation is shown in (Figs 23.28–23.30).

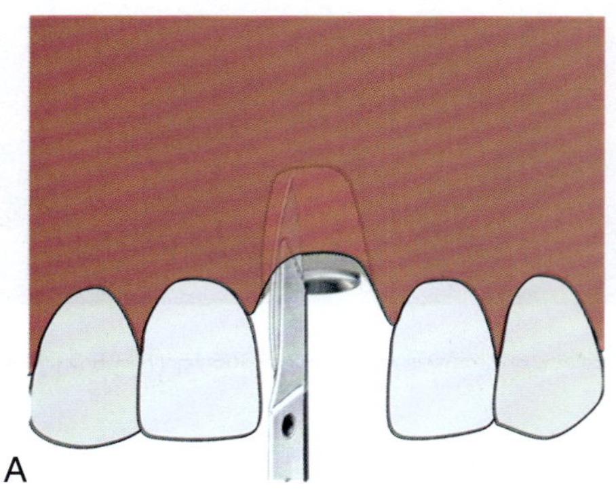

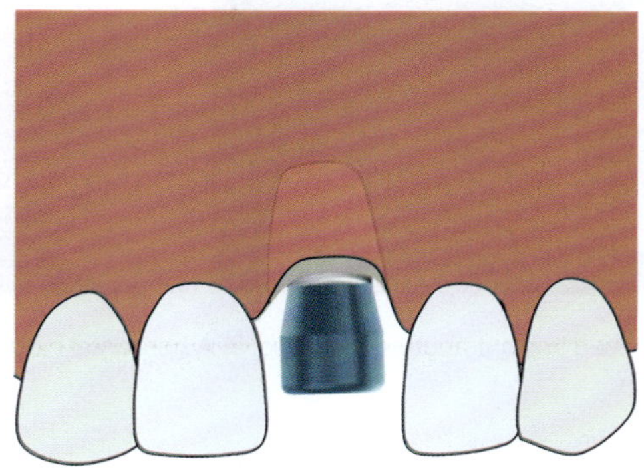

Fig 23.28 (A and B) A partial thickness subepithelial pouch is created to the desired apical extension.

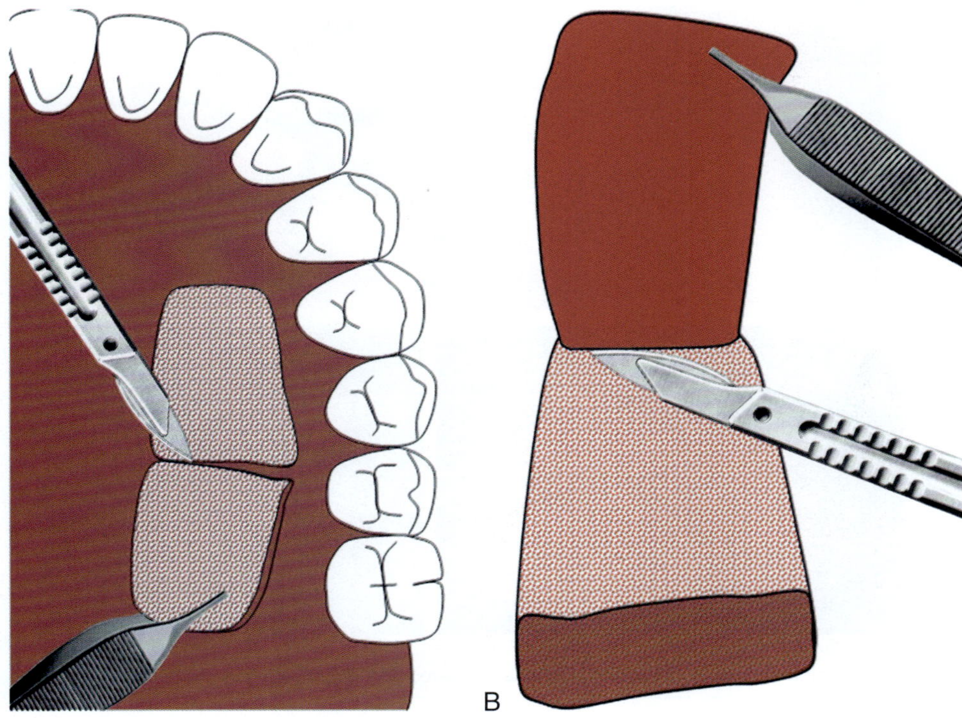

Fig 23.29 (A) An epithelialized connective tissue graft is harvested from the palate. (B) The epithelial layer is scraped out from the area of the graft, which is planned to be placed underneath the subepithelial layer into the pouch.

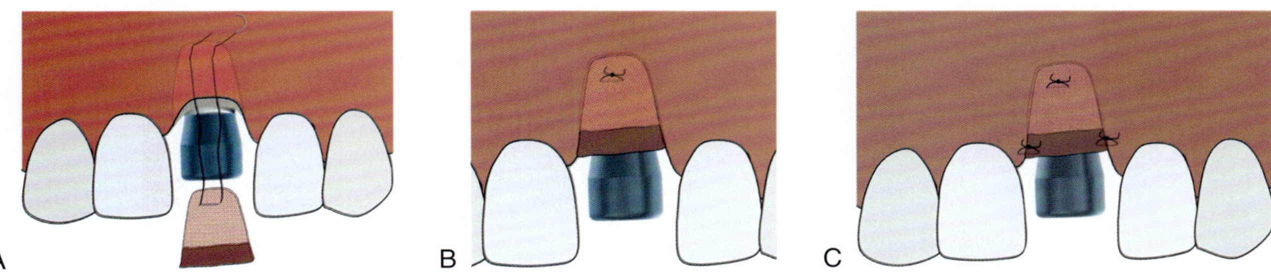

Fig 23.30 (A–C) The graft is transported to the pouch and sutured to immobilize it into the pouch.

CASE REPORT-5

Subepithelial connective tissue graft to cover the exposed abutment (Figs 23.31–23.34).

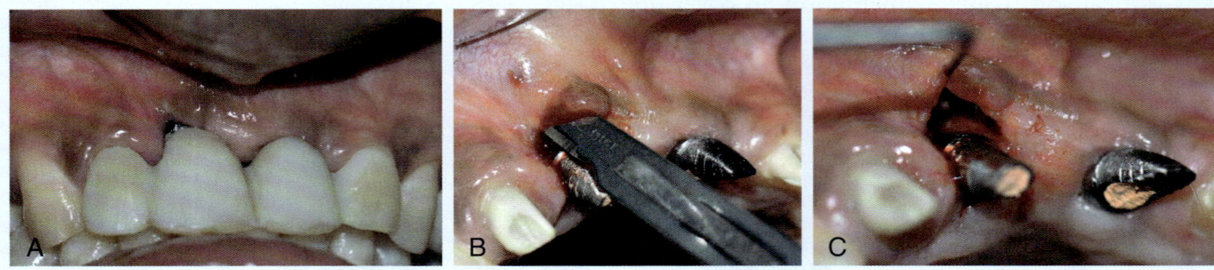

Fig 23.31 (A) Exposed implant abutment. (B and C) A horizontal incision is made parallel to the facial surface to create a partial thickness, subepithelial pouch.

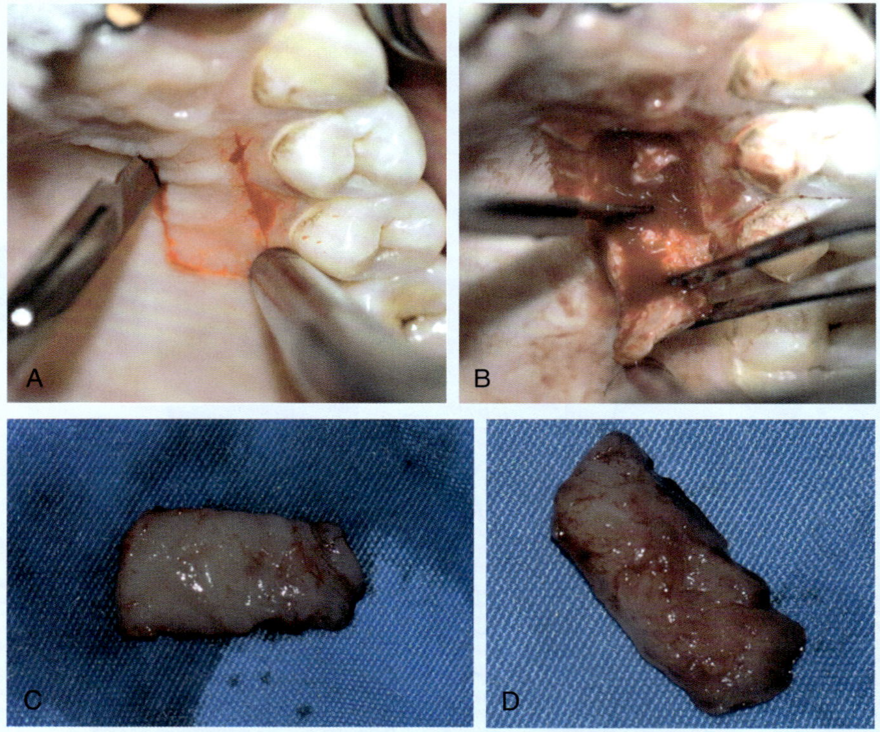

Fig 23.32 (A–D) A full thickness epithelialized connect tissue graft is harvested from the palate.

CASE REPORT-5—cont'd

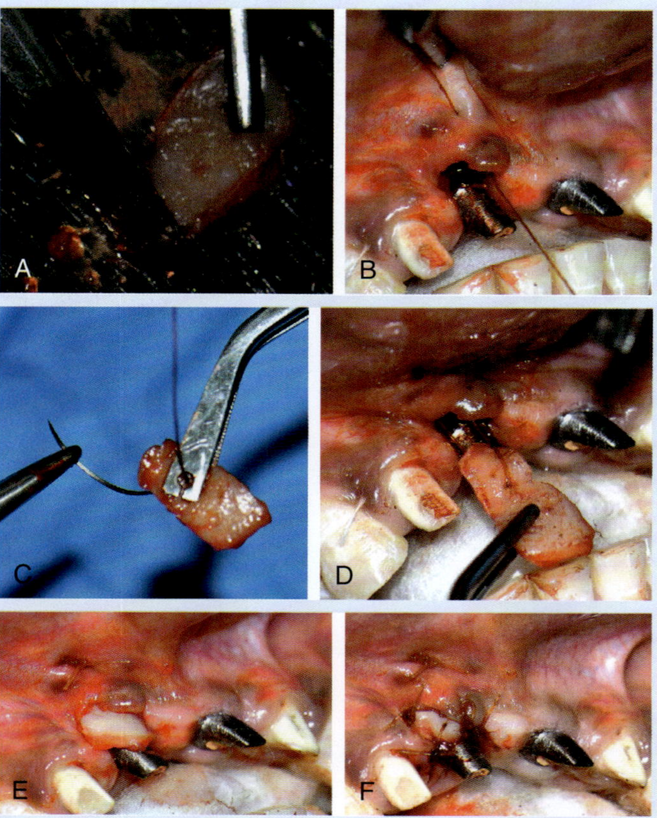

Fig 23.33 (A) The epithelium is scraped out from the three quarters of the graft using a number 15 surgical blade. (B–E) The connective tissue portion of the graft is transported into the pouch and secured with a suture. (F) The crestal part of the graft is further stabilized using 4-0 chromic sutures.

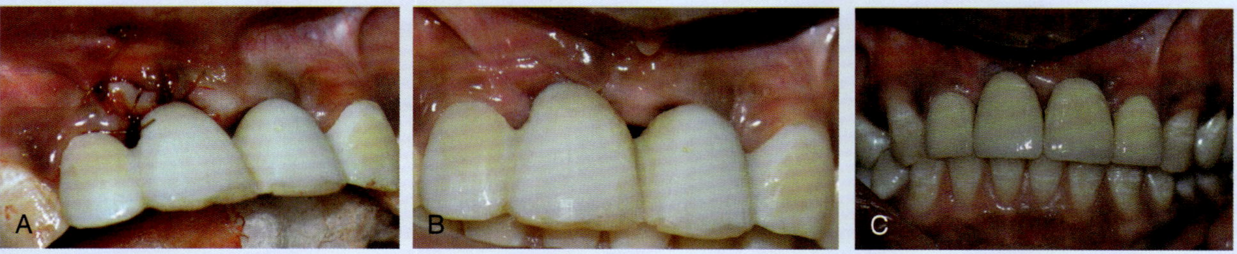

Fig 23.34 (A and B) A thick soft tissue regeneration can be seen over the exposed abutment after 4 weeks. (C) Implants are restored using zirconia crowns.

Technique-4 – Modified palatal roll technique for dental implants

This technique was first described by Abrams in 1980 to be used in periodontology and later modified by Scharf and Tarnow in 1992. Reikie described the application of this technique in implantology, in 1995. A partial thickness flap is elevated at the palatal aspect of the implant site, and the underlying connective tissue is reflected and rolled back to position under the thin facial tissue. This provides adequate soft tissue to achieve a healthy and aesthetic emergence profile for the implant prosthesis. This technique was first used in the maxillary anterior region but lack of thick palatal soft tissue and the presence of neurovascular tissue have limited the use of this technique in the maxillary anterior region, although it can be used to correct small soft tissue defects. This technique can be successfully used for implants in the maxillary region posterior to the canine, to correct small to moderate soft tissue defects (Figs 23.35–23.38).

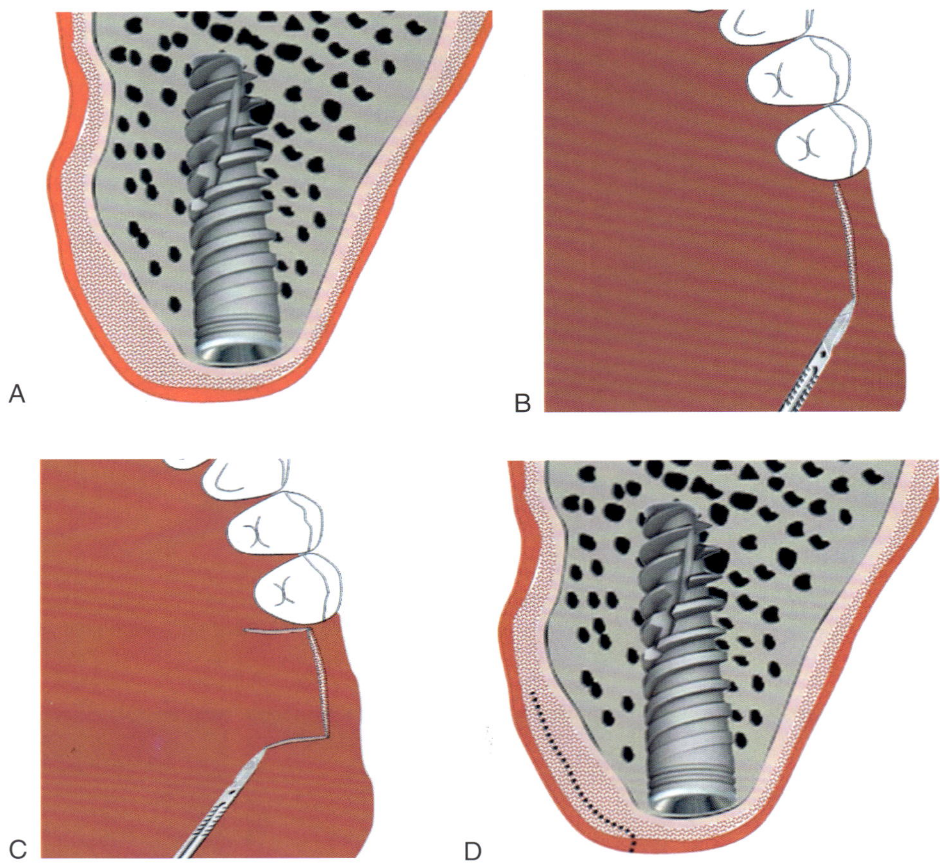

Fig 23.35 (A) Inadequate soft tissue thickness on the facial aspect, which needs to be grafted to regenerate a thick soft tissue to achieve an aesthetic emergence profile on the facial aspect of the implant prosthesis. (B) A shallow mid-crestal incision is made through the epithelium. (C and D) Two shallow vertical incisions are given on the palatal aspect.

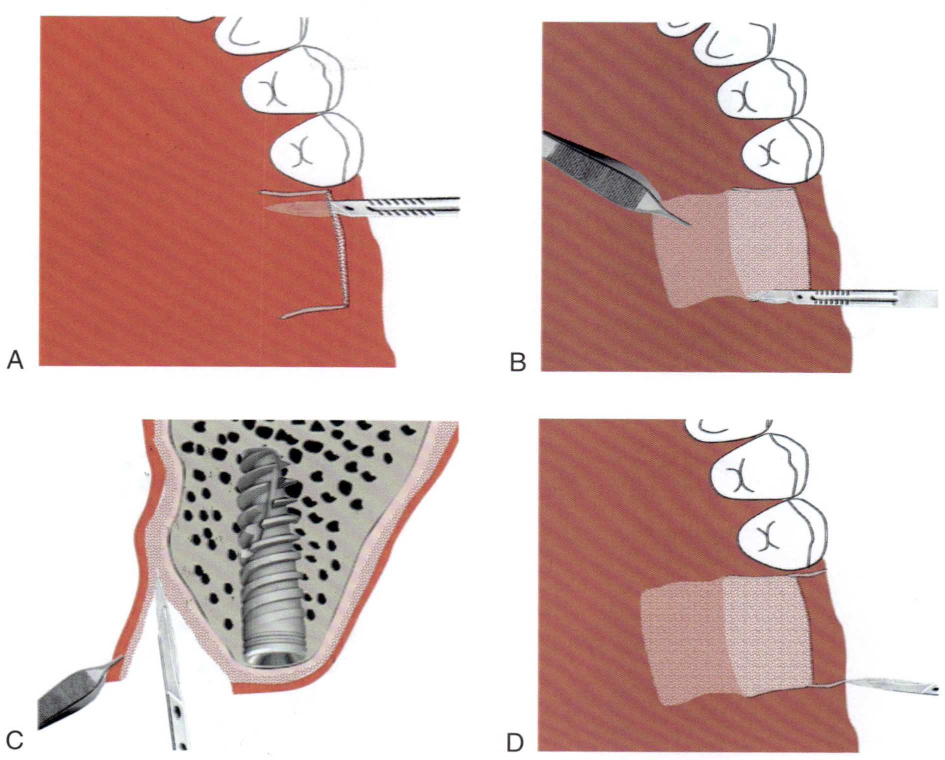

Fig 23.36 (A –C) Blunt dissections are used to elevate a split thickness palatal flap. (D) Further, two deep vertical incisions are made on the facial aspect.

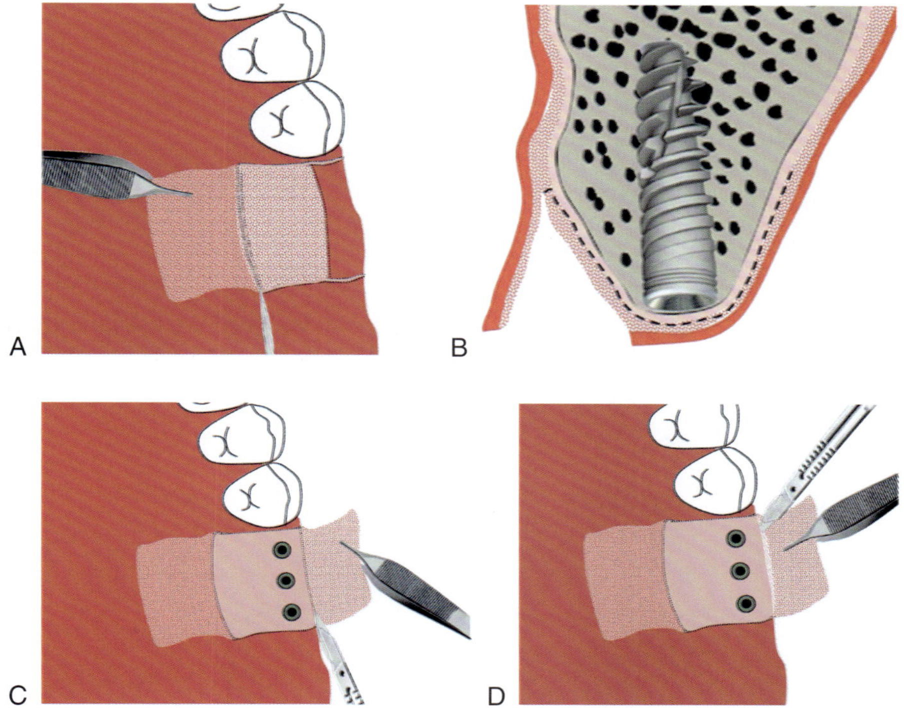

Fig 23.37 (A) The facial vertical incisions are extended to the palatal aspect to the same depth, followed by one horizontal incision at the most distant part of the palatal extension. (B and C) The blunt dissections are again used to elevate the supraperiosteal connective tissue layer. (D) The flap is further elevated from the facial aspect to the planned apical extension.

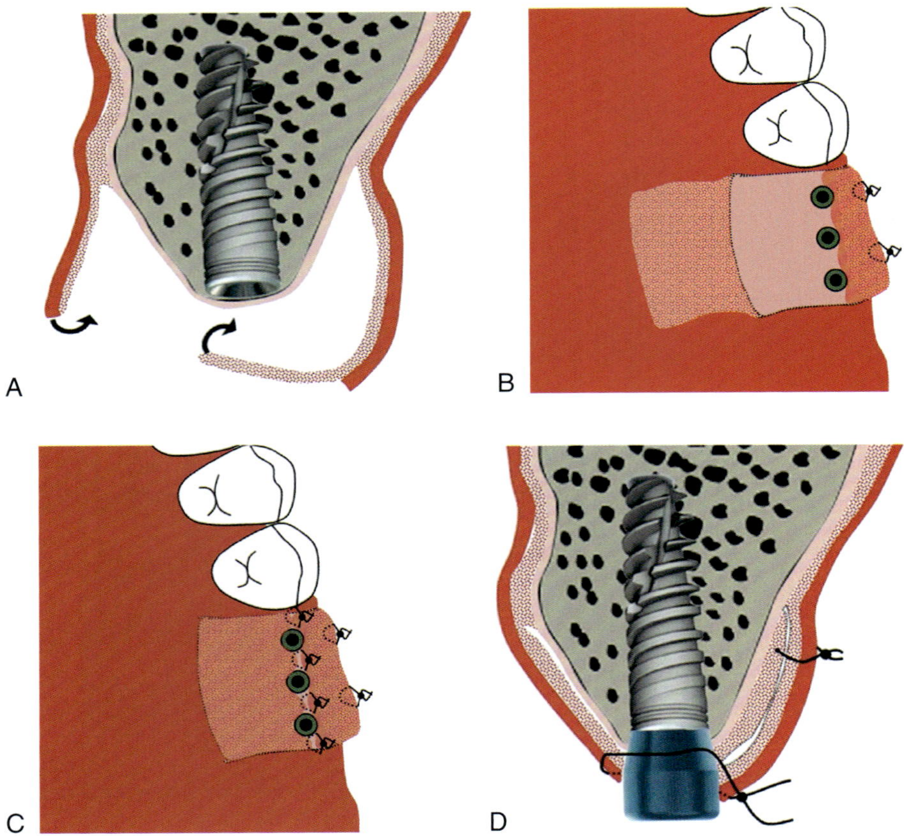

Fig 23.38 The elevated connective tissue layer is rolled back and placed under the facial flap. (A and B) Further, it is immoblized with sutures. (C and D) The healing abutments are inserted to the uncovered implants and flaps are sutured back.

CASE REPORT-6

Enhancement of the soft tissue emergence around implants using a modified roll back technique (Figs 23.39 and 23.40).

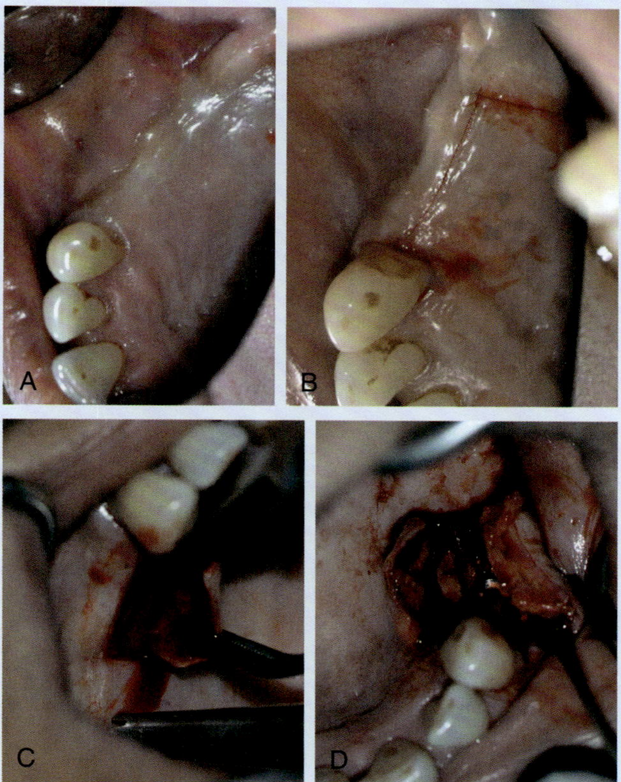

Fig 23.39 (A) Inadequate amount of soft tissue thickness can be seen on the facial aspect of the ridge showing a large facial concavity in ridge morphology. (B) A shallow mid-crestal horizontal and two vertical incisions are made on the palatal aspect. (C) Blunt dissections are given to elevate the partial thickness palatal flap, leaving behind the thick connective tissue layer attached to the periosteum. (D) Vertical incisions are made on the facial aspect and blunt dissection is again used to elevate a supraperiosteal connective tissue layer.

CASE REPORT-6—cont'd

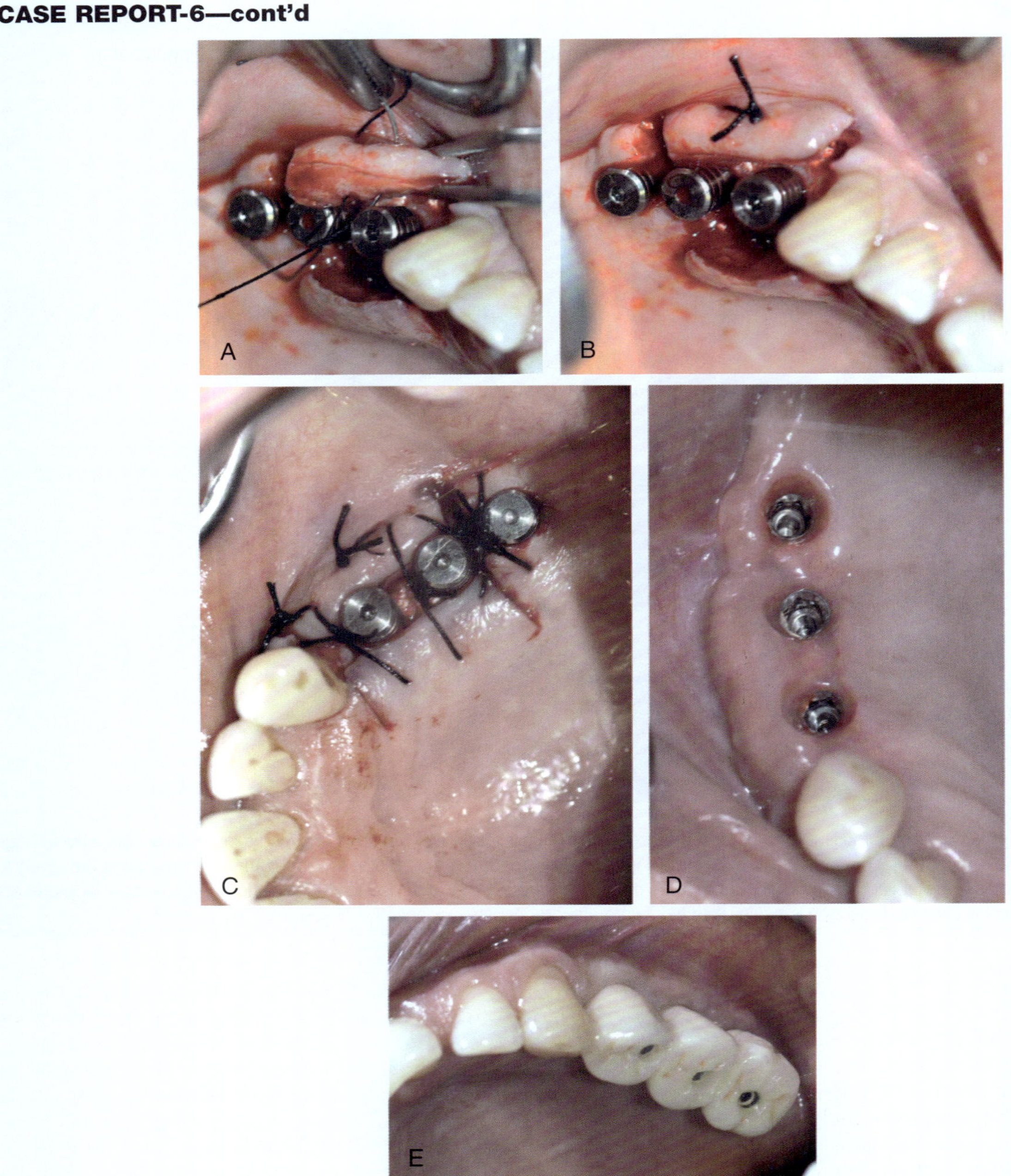

Fig 23.40 The healing abutments are inserted on top of the implants. (A and B) The connective tissue layer is rolled back, placed under the facial flap and immoblized with suture. (C) The flaps are further sutured using multiple inturpted sutures. (D) The healing after 3 weeks shows a thick amount of soft tissue regeneration on the facial aspect of the implants. (E) This not only provides adequate soft tissue for an aesthetic emergence profile but also avoids the dark buccal corridor.

Post-surgical instructions

Brushing/flossing

Both grafted and donor sites should not be brushed/flossed for an initial 3 weeks after soft tissue grafting surgery. The patient should use an antibacterial oral rinse (chlorhexidine gluconate 0.12%) 2–3 times a day for 3–4 weeks. It is important to rinse very gently as vigorous rinsing may disturb the grafted site visually.

Lip pulling

The patient should be instructed not to pull out his/her lip or cheek to look at the graft. The inner portion of the lip may be attached to the graft to enhance the blood supply, thus pulling of lip or cheek may destabilize the graft, and graft rejection may occur. Excessive movement of the lips or pressure on the cheeks or lips should also be avoided.

Discomfort

An anti-inflammatory analgesic medication, such as ibuprofen or diclofenac, should be prescribed along with antibiotics and multivitamins for 3–5 days after surgery.

Smoking

Tobacco smoking decreases polymorphonuclear leukocyte activity, resulting in a lower rate of chemotactic migration and reduced phagocytic activity, which contribute to decreased resistance to inflammation, infection, and impaired soft tissue healing potential. Hence, the patient should be instructed not to smoke for 3–4 weeks after surgery, because it can prevent the union of the graft to the host site, which may result in failure.

Exercise

The patient should refrain from any physical activity for 2–3 days after surgery.

Sutures

The patient should be instructed to keep the tongue away from playing with the stitches, which hold the graft in place.

Never remove or disturb any tissue at the grafted area. The graft generates new maturated tissue after passing through a few resorption and regeneration stages. Hence, it is expected that the graft may not look very pretty during the first 2 weeks after surgery.

Diet

The patient should not bite foods like sandwiches, burgers, etc. for the first 2–3 weeks after surgery. Soft cold foods are best on the day of the surgery. A soft diet during the first week after the surgery is recommended. Crunchy foods, carbonated drinks and alcohol should not be consumed during the first week.

Emergency

The patient should be instructed to visit the dentist for any emergency.

Summary

Soft tissue plays an important role in the long-term survival of the implant. A thick, stable and keratinized marginal tissue is more resistant to muscle pull, recession and peri-implantitis. The techniques of soft tissue augmentation described in this chapter have specific indications and should be performed as necessary in the particular case. The epithelialized connective tissue graft harvested from the palate is the most common autogenous soft tissue graft used to augment medium to large soft tissue defects. When harvesting this graft from the palate, a careful approach is required to successfully harvest the graft with adequate size and thickness. The partial thickness or full thickness graft can be harvested leaving the fatty tissue layer attached to the periosteum. A prefabricated stent can be used to harvest a graft of the desired dimensions. When harvesting the autogenous graft from the palate, the most posterior incision should not be extended beyond the first molar, to avoid injury to the anterior palatine vessels, which may result in profuse bleeding during the procedure. The bleeding which usually occurs during the graft-harvesting procedure can be prevented by applying pressure on the site for 3–5 min using moist cotton. After the soft tissue has been harvested, haemostasis can be achieved by using the collagen sponge placed into the donor site and a prefabricated acrylic plate is seated in mouth covering the donor site. The patient have to wear this plate for 2–3 weeks to avoid any injury (which can result in profuse bleeding), to the donor site during the healing period. This plate also avoids painful and burning sensations at the donor site. The harvested graft should be immediately transferred to the host site, which has been prepared before harvesting the graft. This maintains the cell vitality of the transplanted graft.

The acellular AlloDerm can be a good option for patients who resist providing their own tissue and also for dentists who are not highly skilled to harvest an autogenous soft tissue graft. The connective tissue graft can be used for implant cases with aesthetic soft tissue defects to improve soft tissue emergence for implant restorations. The connective tissue graft can be harvested from the palate with the open or the closed technique and can be grafted either at the time of implant insertion surgery or during uncovery. Careful preparation of the recipient bed and adaptation of the graft is paramount for the success of the procedure.

Further reading

Palacci P. Optimal implant positioning and soft-tissue considerations. Oral Maxillofac Surg Clin North Am 1996;8:445–452.

Grunder U. Stability of the mucosal topography around single-tooth implants and adjacent teeth: 1-year results. Int J Periodontics Restorative Dent 2000;20:11–7.

Mehlbauer Michael J, Greenwell Henry. Complete root coverage at multiple sites using an acellular dermal matrix allograft. Compendium 2005;21:727–33.

Hirsch, et al. A 2-year follow-up of root coverage using subpedicle acellular dermal matrix allografts and subepithelial connective tissue autografts. J Periodontol 2005;76:1323–8.

Gapski, Parks, Wang. Acellular dermal matrix for mucogingival surgery: a meta-analysis. J Periodontol 2005;76:178–86.

Jemt T. Restoring the gingival contour by means of provisional resin crowns after single implant treatment. Int J Periodontics Restorative Dent 1999;19:20.

Scar A. Soft tissue and Esthetic considerations in implant dentistry. Quintessence Publishing Co. 2003, ISBN 0-86715-345-7.

Griffin TJ, Cheung WS, Zavras AI, et al. Postoperative complications following gingival augmentation procedures. J Periodontol 2006;77:2070–9.

Hertel RC, Blijdorp PA, Baker DL. A preventive mucosal flap technique for use in implantology. Int J Oral Maxillofac Implants 1993;8:452–8.

Bengazi F, Wennstro¨m JL, Lekholm U. Recession of the soft tissue margin at oral implants. A 2-year longitudinal prospective study. Clin Oral Implants Res 1996;7:303–10.

Jemt T. Regeneration of gingival papillae after single implant treatment. Int J Periodontics Restorative Dent 1997;17:326–33.

Palacci P, Nowzari H. Soft tissue enhancement around dental implants. Periodontology 2000, 2008;47:113–32.

Kamalakidis S, Paniz G, Kang KH, et al. Nonsurgical management of soft tissue deficiencies for anterior single implant-supported restorations: a clinical report. J Prosthet Dent 2007;97:1–5.

Kan JY, Rungcharassaeng K, Umezu K, et al. Dimensions of peri-implant mucosa: an evaluation of maxillary anterior single implants in humans. J Periodontol 2003;74:557–62.

Israelson H, Plemons JM. Dental implants, regenerative techniques, and periodontal plastic surgery to restore maxillary anterior aesthetics. Int J Oral Maxillofac Implants 1993;8:555–61.

Woodyard, et al. The clinical effect of acellular dermal matrix on gingival thickness and root coverage compared to coronally positioned flap alone. J Periodontol 2004;75:44–56.

Aichelmann-Reidy, Yukna, Evans, et al. Clinical evaluation of acellular allograft dermis for the treatment of human gingival recession. J Periodontol 2001;72:998–1005.

Luczyszyn, Papalexiou, Novaes Jr , et al. Acellular dermal matrix and hydroxyapatite in prevention of ridge deformities after tooth extraction. Implant Dent 2005;14(2):176–84.

Cummings, Kaldahl, Allen. Histologic evaluation of autogenous connective tissue and acellular dermal matrix grafts in humans. J Periodontol 2005;76:178–86.

Froum, Cho, Elian, et al. Extraction sockets and implantation of hydroxyapatites with membrane barriers, a histologic study. Implant Dent 2004;13(2):153–64.

Novaes Jr , Souza. Acellular dermal matrix graft as a membrane for guided bone regeneration: a case report. Implant Dent 2001;10(3):192–5.

Berglundh T, Lindhe J. Dimension of the peri-implant mucosa. Biological width revisited. J Clin Periodontol 1996;23:971–3.

Fowler, Breault, Rebitski. Ridge preservation utilizing an acellular dermal allograft and demineralized freeze-dried bone allograft: part I. A report of two cases. J Periodontol 2000;71:1353–9.

Palacci P. Optimal implant positioning and soft tissue considerations. Oral Maxillofac Surg Clin North Am 1996;8:445–52.

Henderson R, et al. Predictable multiple site root coverage using an acellular dermal matrix allograft. J Periodontol 2001;72:571–82.

Santos, Goumenos, Pascual. Management of gingival recession by the use of a acellular dermal graft material: a 12-case series. J Periodontal 2005;76:1982–90.

Paolantonio, Dolci, Esposito, et al. Subpedicle acellular dermal matrix graft and autogenous connective tissue graft in the treatment of gingival recessions: a comparative 1-year clinical study. J Periodontol 2002;73:1299–307.

Palacci P, Ericsson I, Engstrand P, et al. Optimal implant positioning and soft tissue management for the Branemark system. Chicago: Quintessence Books; 1995.

Strub JP, Garberthuel TW, Grunder U. The role of attached gingiva in the health of peri-implant tissues in dogs. 1. Clinical findings. Int J Periodontics Restorative Dent 1991;11:317–33.

Henderson, Greenwell, Drisko, et al. Predictable multiple site root coverage using an acellular dermal matrix allograft. J Periodontol 2001;72:571–82.

Sullivan RM. Perspectives on aesthetics in implant dentistry. Compend Contin Educ Dent 2001;22:685–92.

Complications and management

24

Ajay Vikram Singh Sunita Singh

CHAPTER CONTENTS HD

Introduction

Scientific literature has evidenced that implant therapy obtains a success rate greater than 90%. With the increasing acceptance of dental implantation as a viable tooth replacement therapy, complications and failure rates have also increased proportionately. Complications and failures in implant dentistry can range from minor to major, reversible to irreversible, and problematic to detrimental. As a result, these clinical problems cause frustrations and disappointments for patients and dental professionals and cast doubts on the success of dental implant therapy. These problems can have many different levels of undesirable consequences that may lead to compromised or less than optimal clinical results for the patients, nonproductive wasted clinical chair time, extra financial burden to the patient and dentist, create antagonistic tension in

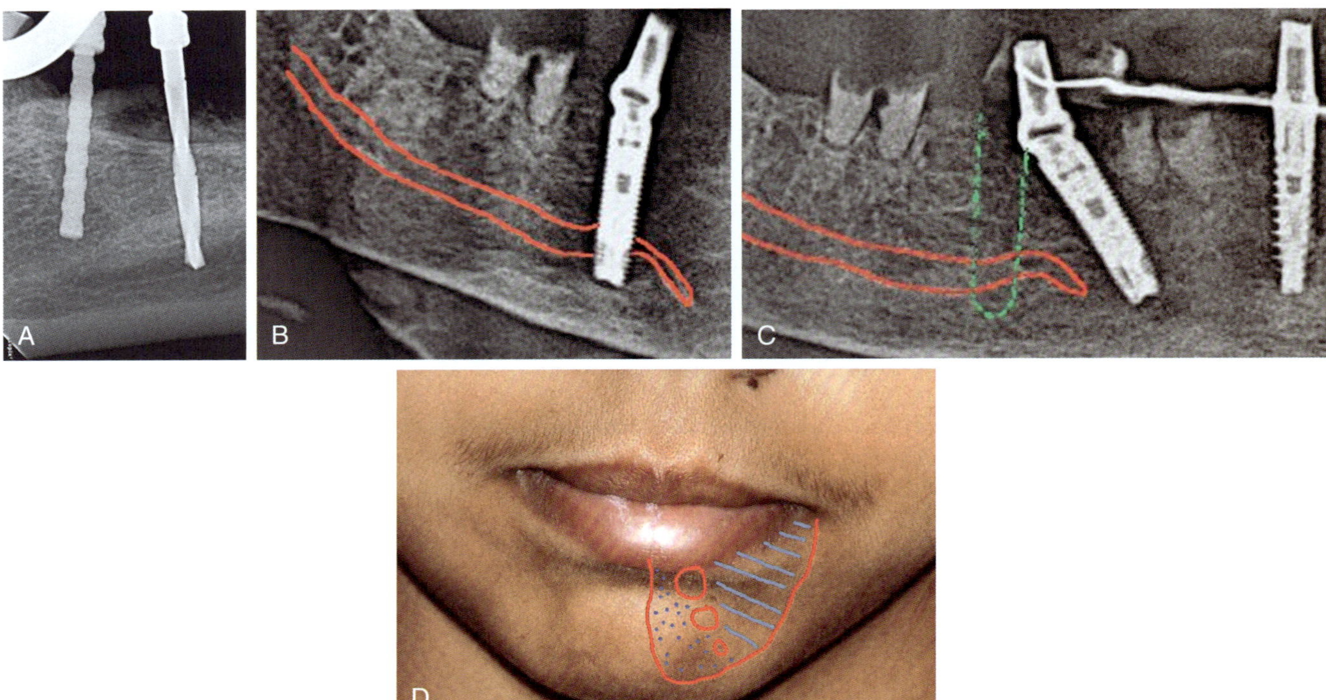

Fig 24.1 (A) Radiograph showing the pilot drill encroaching at the nerve. Further drilling reaching the same depth must be avoided and an implant with shorter length should be inserted. (B and C) If the post implantation radiograph shows that the implant has been placed through the mandibular canal, the implant should immediately be removed and another short length implant inserted or the same implant inserted with different angulation if possible, to avoid nerve injury. (D) If the patient complains of neurosensory dysfunction on the second day of surgery, the areas of anaesthesia, paraesthesia, and dysaesthesia should be marked differently on the patient's lower jaw and photographed for future comparisons of recovery.

patients, and ultimately affect the reputation of the dentist and the profession. Complaints to regulatory colleges and litigations involving implant dentistry have also increased over the past decade. Understanding the various complications and failures in implant dentistry can lead to prevention, early detection, and better management of implant cases. A range of possible surgical and prosthetic problems, their prevention, and management are described below.

Complications

Nerve injury

Many implant surgeons decide the final implant length only by referring to the dental or panoramic radiograph. These radiographs usually show some degree of magnification, which may result in nerve injury during implant placement if the longest implant is placed with reference to the radiograph without considering the magnification factor. Moreover, the radiographs often do not show the clear path of the mandibular canal, which can also be a cause of misdiagnosis and nerve injury. The mandibular canal is the most important vital structure that should be taken care of during implant insertion in the mandibular posterior region. The path of the canal should be clearly evaluated to assess the bone height available to insert the implant. The presence of the anterior loop should also be evaluated when inserting the implant in the mandibular premolars and canine region. For cases with limited bone height above the mandibular canal, dental CT scan should be used to plan for the implant with appropriate dimensions. However, the implant should be placed minimum 2–3 mm short of the mandibular canal (Fig 24.1A–D).

Prevention and management

1. Detailed radiographic and CT planning to evaluate the exact path of the mandibular canal.
2. Length of the planned implant should be 2-3 mm less than the height of the bone present above mandibular canal (3.0 mm safety distance) (Fig 24.2).
3. If the case has been planned using only the panoramic radiograph, the 25% magnification of the radiograph should be reduced from the bone height measured above the canal in the radiograph. For example, if the panoramic radiograph shows 15 mm bone height above the canal, the actual bone height can be only 12 mm and after deducting another 3 mm as the safety distance, only a 9 mm long implant should be chosen for placement. However, if the dental CT scan, which shows the actual bone dimensions, shows 15 mm bone height above the mandibular canal, the surgeon can place a 12 mm long implant.
4. In the case of limited bone height above the mandibular canal, a radiograph should be taken after pilot drilling short of 3 mm from the planned implant depth, to reconfirm the canal position in respect to the implant length (Fig 24.3).

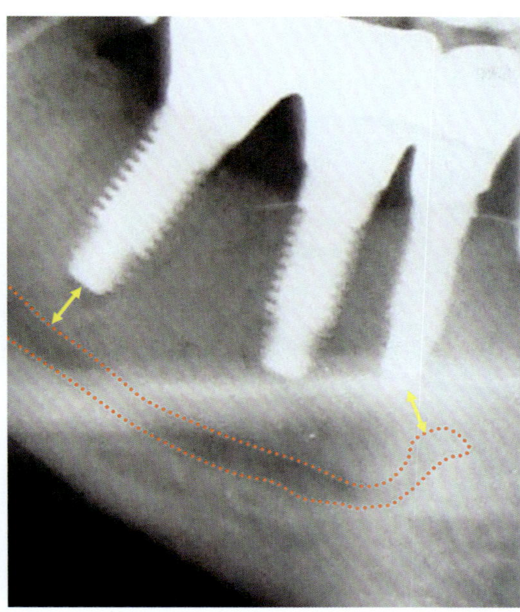

Fig 24.2 Implants should be inserted a minimum 2–3 mm short of the mandibular canal.

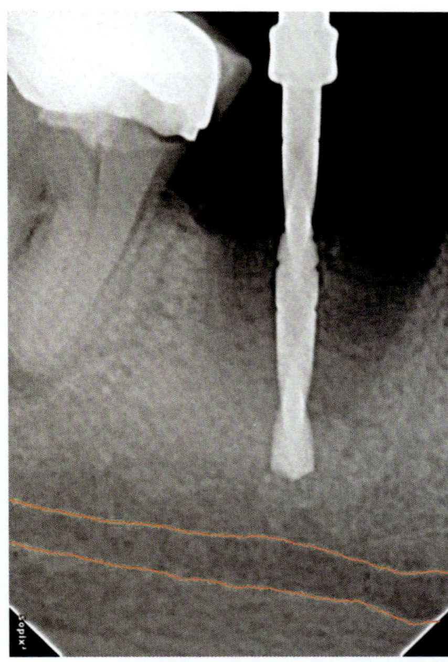

Fig 24.3 The dental radiograph with pilot drill into the osteotomy is taken to assess the distance from mandibular canal.

5. If the osteotomy has been prepared and the implant has been placed with its apex just touching the canal, the patient should be recalled two days after surgery and enquired if there is any altered sensation over the chin and lower lip of the same side. If the answer is "Yes", then either the implant should be unscrewed 1.0 mm to release the pressure from the nerve or it can be removed and replaced with a shorter length implant. The patient may, however, take 2–4 months to recover from the paraesthesia.

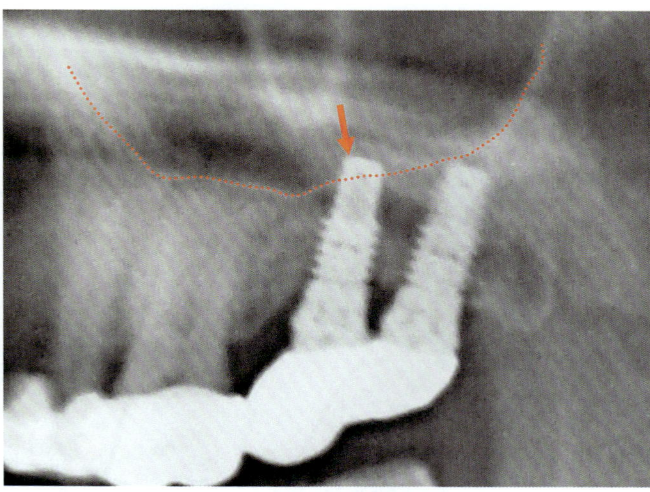

Fig 24.4 The radiograph shows the implant apex penetrating into the sinus. The implant has been in normal function for 5 years and the patient has not presented any clinical or radiographic signs and symptoms of sinus pathology.

If the implant surgeon has severely injured or crushed the nerve, it may require microsurgical repair of the nerve, if the paraesthesia is not recovered by therapeutic measures. The nerve injury may produce short-term or even protracted paraesthesia (abnormal sensation without being unpleasant or painful) or dysaesthesia (unpleasant or painful sensation) to the patient over the lip and chin of the side.

Treatment to recover the altered nerve functions

1. **Drug therapy.** The following drugs should be prescribed to the patient:
   - Vitamin B_1 – facilitates nerve injury metabolism.
   - Vitamin B_6 – regulates neural activities.
   - Vitamin B_{12} – enhances protein synthesis of neural cells, neural fibres and myelin formation.
   - Vitamin E – improves local circulation.
   - ATP tablets – 20 mg – 2 tab. (enteric) t.i.d – facilitates nerve injury metabolism.
   - Steroids (dexamethasone) – relieves oedematous compression and inflammation around the nerve).
2. **Physical therapy.** Warm compressions and massage of the paralysed area facilitate nerve restoration and relieves neural pain.
3. **Microsurgical repair.** If the altered nerve sensations have not even started recovering in 2–3 months, the patient should be referred to a surgeon who has expertise in performing microsurgical repair of the neural tissues. To microsurgically repair the crushed nerve, the mesial and distal ends of the nerve bundles are located, the crushed part of the nerve is resected, two to three nonresorbable sutures are placed to approximate the ends, and a collagen membrane is wrapped around the repaired nerve for predictable nerve tissue regeneration.

Dr WL Gore and Dr Flagstaff used a polytetrafluoroethylene (PTFE) tube to repair the inferior alveolar and

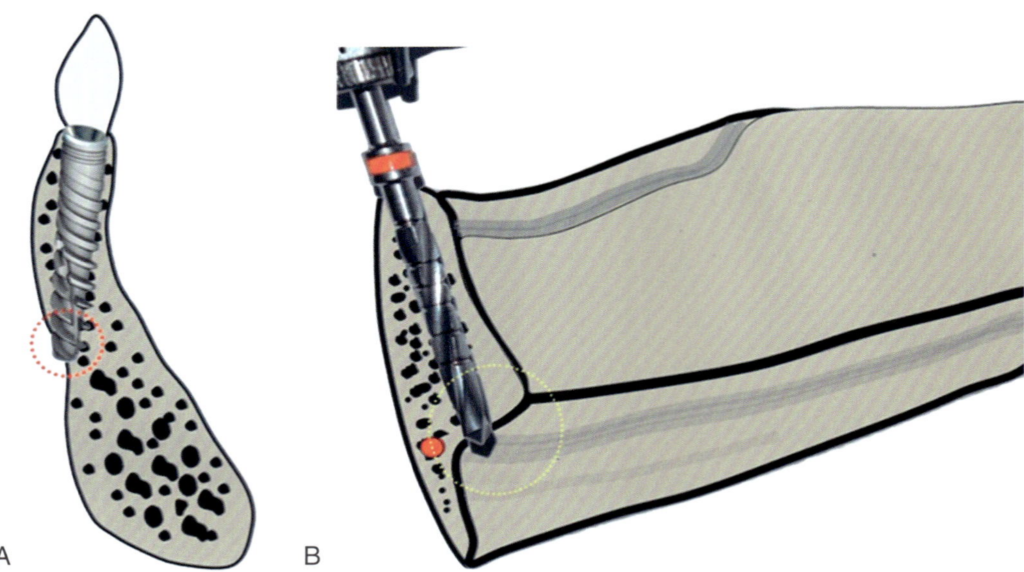

Fig 24.5 The anterior mandible is the area where the bony ridge maximally changes its axial direction through the different stages of bone resorption. (A) One should carefully evaluate the bony ridge topography to avoid any dehiscence through the lingual cortical plate during osteotomy preparation. (B) Care must also be taken to avoid the penetration through the submandibular fossa which is located below the mylohyoid line and also into the sublingual space in the anterior mandible where the sublingual artery is located. Inadvertent penetration of these lingual plates can be avoided by appropriately directing the pilot drill towards the buccal and monitoring the area with digital contact on lingual aspect while drilling.

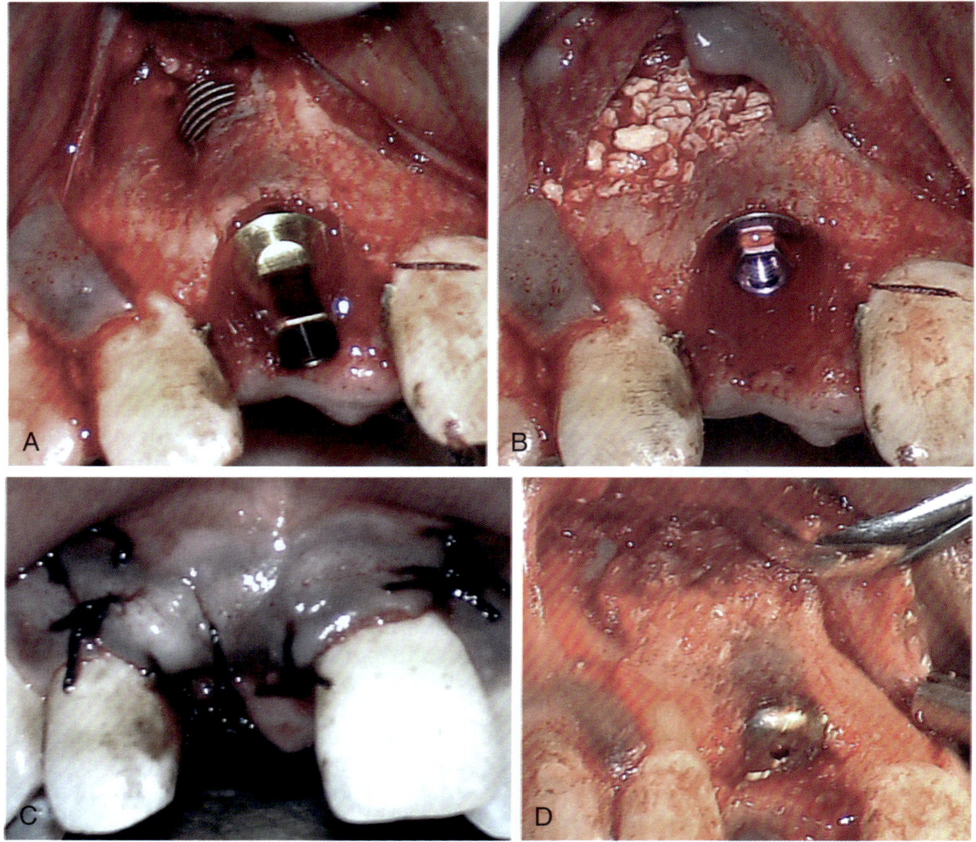

Fig 24.6 (A) A fenestration through the labial cortical plate can be seen with the implant thread exposure. (B and C) The site is grafted using Bio-Oss (xenograft) graft material and the flap is sutured back without using any barrier membrane. (D) The implant is uncovered after 4 months showing new bone formation at the grafted site.

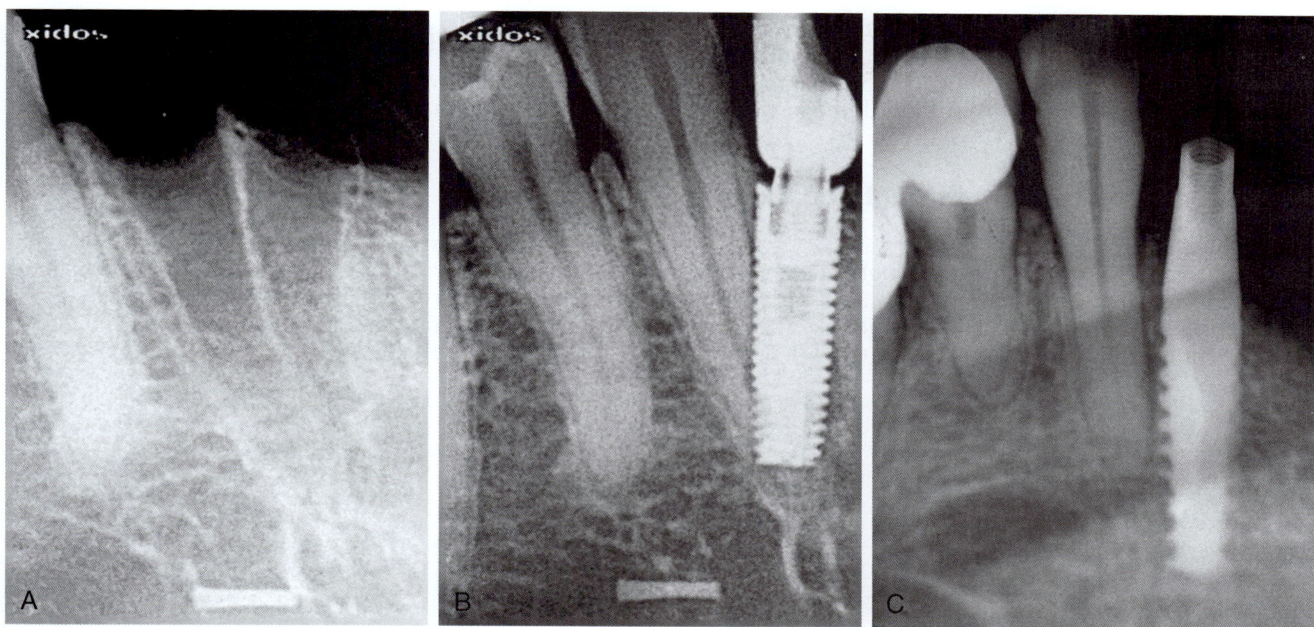

Fig 24.7 (A and B) Implant placed at the site of the madibular lateral incisor has penetrated through the canine root. (C) Implant encroaching the periodontal ligaments of the adjacent tooth.

lingual nerve. Proximal and distal ends were placed in the PTFE tube and secured using 8-0 nylon sutures. The procedure was performed in a total of seven patients and only two patients recovered from the paraesthesia.

Maxillary sinus perforation

The implant surgeon may inadvertently perforate the sinus floor during implant placement in the maxillary posterior region. If there is only a small perforation with the pilot drill, osteotomy preparation can be continued 2 mm short of the sinus floor and the implant can be placed. Small perforations spontaneously heal and do not cause any problem to implant healing. If a large perforation has been made into the sinus membrane, the surgeon can abort the implant placement and close the flap, and re-enter after it is healed in 3–4 months. Alternatively, the sinus membrane can be elevated with the lateral approach, the perforation can be repaired using resorbable collagen membrane and the implant can be placed in the same sitting. According to the traditional concept, if the implant perforates the sinus membrane and penetrates the sinus, it can be a source of periodic sinusitis. Recent studies have shown that if the implant apex has penetrated into the sinus 2 mm or less, the membrane regenerates and covers it within few weeks; and even if it has penetrated more than 2 mm, being a sterile material it does not usually cause any problem. However, further clinical trials and scientific evidence are required to prove that implant apex penetration in the sinus is safe and does not cause any long-term complication to the sinus cavity or impede implant survival (Fig 24.4).

Dehiscence/perforation through the lingual cortical plate

Perforation through the palatal cortical plate in the maxilla is very rare because of its high density and favourable topography. When the perforation occurs through the lingual cortical plate of the mandible, it is often difficult to elevate the lingual flap to such an extent as to expose the perforation (especially if it has occurred deep apically), and to graft the perforation. The appropriate way is to abort the implant placement and leave the site to heal, with or without grafting the already prepared osteotomy. Implant placement can be attempted again once the site has healed. Though very rare, a life-threatening haemorrhage may happen with the perforation of the lingual cortical plate when drilling for mandibular implants. The drill may traumatize two major arteries: (i) the lingual artery (which supplies the tongue) and its terminal branches called sublingual arteries supplying the lingual and gingival aspects of the anterior cortical plate of the mandible and (ii) the facial artery, which runs under the base of the mandible in the second molar region. Significant internal bleeding from these arteries in the floor of mouth may result in a life-threatening haemorrhage, which causes swelling of the floor of mouth and tongue, and respiratory obstruction. When such a haemorrhage is noticed, the tongue should be pulled out and pressure placed along the inner and inferior aspects of the body of the mandible. One should also compress the site with one finger intraorally over the site and another finger placed extraorally, compressing the two fingers together. A haemostatic agent should be placed into the osteotomy and the patient should immediately be transported to the hospital where a team of surgeons can ligate the injured vessels, give an endotracheal intubation, or perform an emergency tracheotomy (Fig 24.5A and B).

The risk of lingual plate perforation or fenestration, due to lingual concavity, in an edentulous posterior mandible in the region of second premolar or first molar was found to be only 0.053% if a regular 3.75 mm diameter tapered implant was used. In the presence of significant lingual concavity in the posterior mandible, a smaller regular diameter implant with a stepped taper design should be considered, to avoid potential fatal damage of the vital structures.

Dehiscence/perforation through the facial cortical plate

Any dehiscence or perforation through the facial cortical plate during osteotomy preparation can be grafted using autogenous bone and/or bone substitutes, after implant placement in the same sitting (Fig 24.6A–D).

Drilling through the root of the adjacent tooth

Drilling in the wrong direction or the presence of inclined roots of the adjacent tooth may inadvertently cause this complication (Fig 24.7A–C).

Prevention

Meticulous treatment planning using radiographs and CT images and careful osteotomy preparation in three-dimensionally correct directions, which can be evaluated with the radiograph after the drilling to partial depth, can avoid this complication.

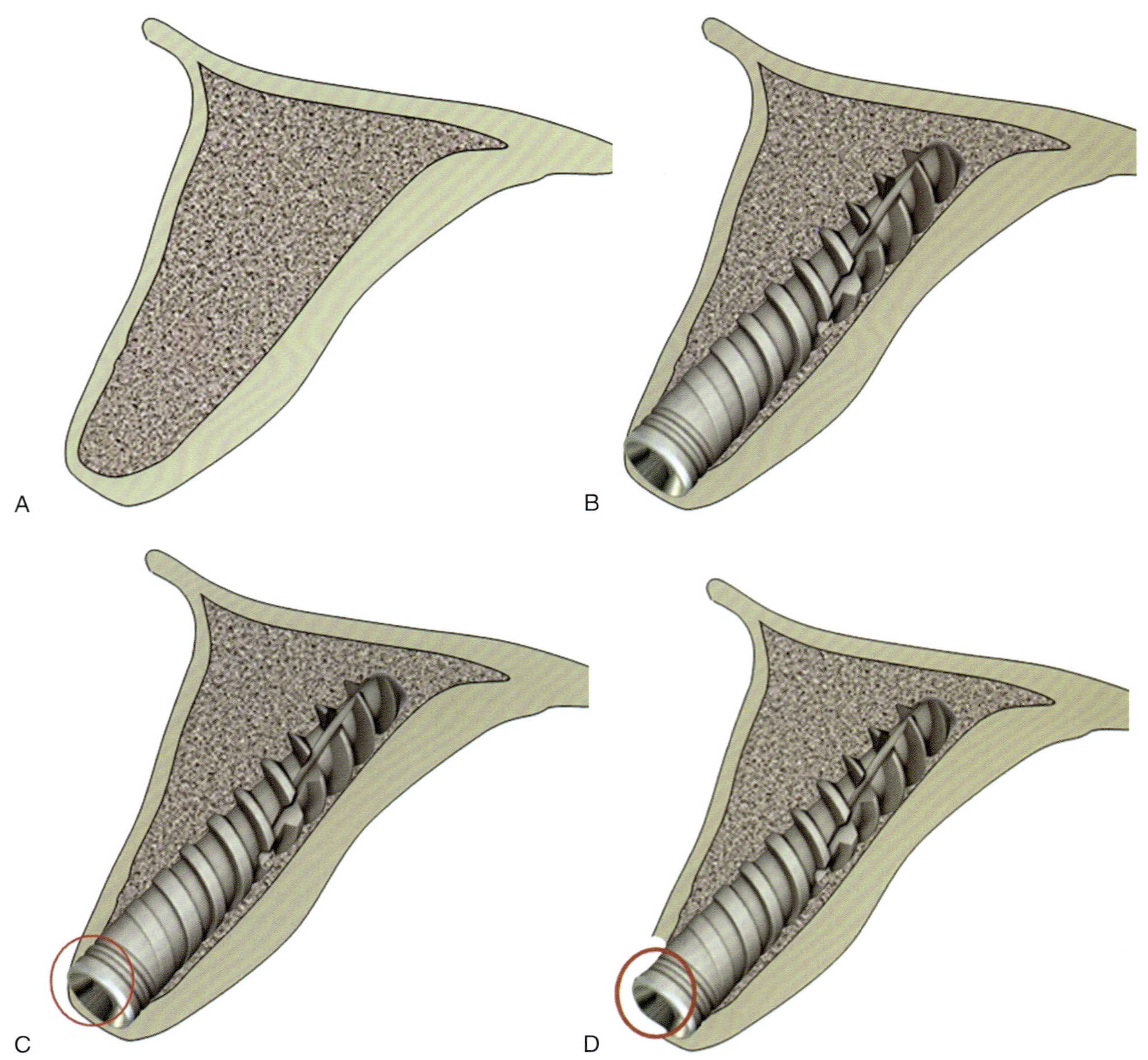

Fig 24.8 (A) The cross-section of anterior maxilla before implant insertion (B) implant placement in the incorrect direction, (C) causing thin labial cortical plate at the crestal region, (D) which fails to survive and gets resorbed.

Management

The management of this complication depends on the severity of injury to the adjacent tooth that occurs during implant placement.

1. **Encroachment only at the root apex.** If the pilot drill has only encroached at the root apex, further osteotomy should be prepared in the correct direction and the implant should be placed. If the tooth becomes symptomatic, root canal therapy should be done in a follow-up visit.

If the implant has been placed encroaching the root apex, root canal therapy should be done in the same sitting using only sterile saline for root canal irrigation. The root canals should be obturated at the same sitting.

2. **Perforation through the apical third.** Osteotomy should be prepared in the correct direction and the implant placed. Root canal therapy with simultaneous resection of the perforated root apex should be done with the lateral approach and the area should be grafted in the same surgical sitting using any bone substitute.
3. **Perforation through the middle third.** The osteotomy should be prepared in the correct direction and the implant should be inserted. The tooth should be extracted and socket grafted in the same surgical sitting, using any bone substitute.

Off-axis implant placement

Off-axis implant placement not only results in a challenging situation for prosthetic rehabilitation but also causes the resorption of thin bone at the crestal region, which leads to bone defects and soft tissue recession (Figs 24.8 and 24.9).

Management

The implant should be removed and the same or a new implant should be reinserted at the correct axis. (Figs 24.10–24.14).

Inappropriate three-dimensional implant positioning in the aesthetic region

The implant positioning should be three-dimensionally accurate in the aesthetic region to achieve optimal hard and soft tissue aesthetics. When adjacent teeth are present with the gingival collar at the correct position, the implant should be placed in such a way that its platform is finally positioned 2–3 mm apical to the imaginary line connecting the cementoenamel junction (CEJ) of two adjacent teeth, to achieve the adequate emergence profile through the soft tissue. If soft tissue recession has already occurred on the adjacent teeth, the implant platform should be positioned 2–3 mm apical to the gingival zenith. The implant platform should also be placed 1–1.5 mm palatal to the imaginary line connecting the CEJ of two adjacent teeth (Fig 24.15A–D).

Implants too close to each other

If two adjacent implants are placed very close to each other, the thin bone (less than 3 mm) present between two adjacent implants fails to survive because of lack of nutrient supply and gets resorbed (Fig 24.16A and B).

Incomplete seating of the prosthesis

Incomplete seating of the prosthesis on the abutment creates a subgingival gap, which may retain plaque and lead to chronic inflammation of the peri-implant tissues. This may also lead to instability of the marginal gingival tissues and in cases with the thin soft tissue biotype, may lead to recession or small fenestrations within the peri-implant tissues (Fig 24.17).

Causes of improper seating of the prosthesis onto an abutment

1. Resistance from peri-implant tissues or entrapment of soft tissue between the abutment–crown margins during prosthesis seating.
2. Premature interproximal contacts on the adjacent teeth.

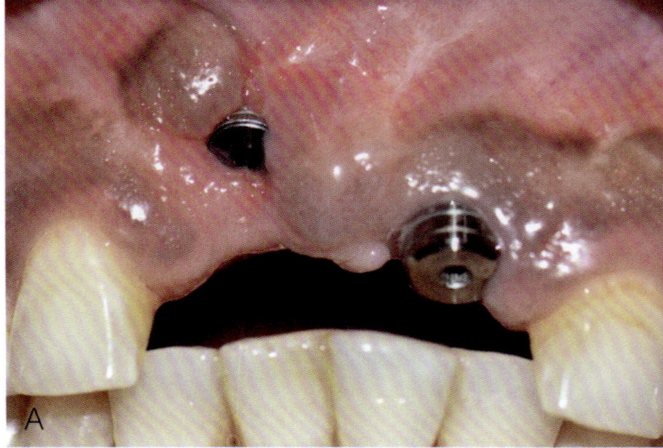

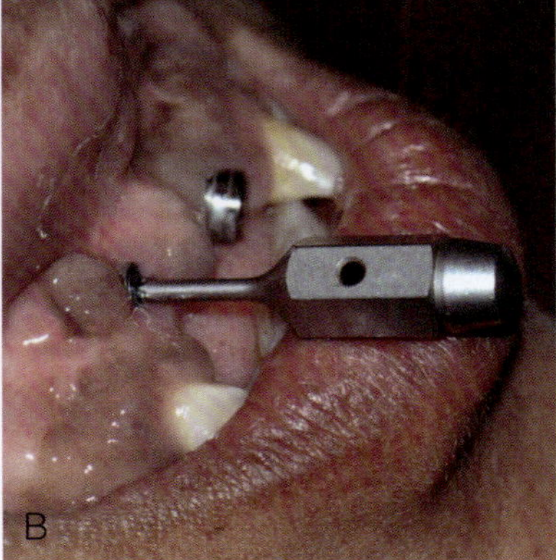

Fig 24.9 (A) The implant placed in the wrong axis resulted in loss of thin hard and soft tissue on the labial aspect if restored, (B) it will lead to a very unaesthetic prosthesis.

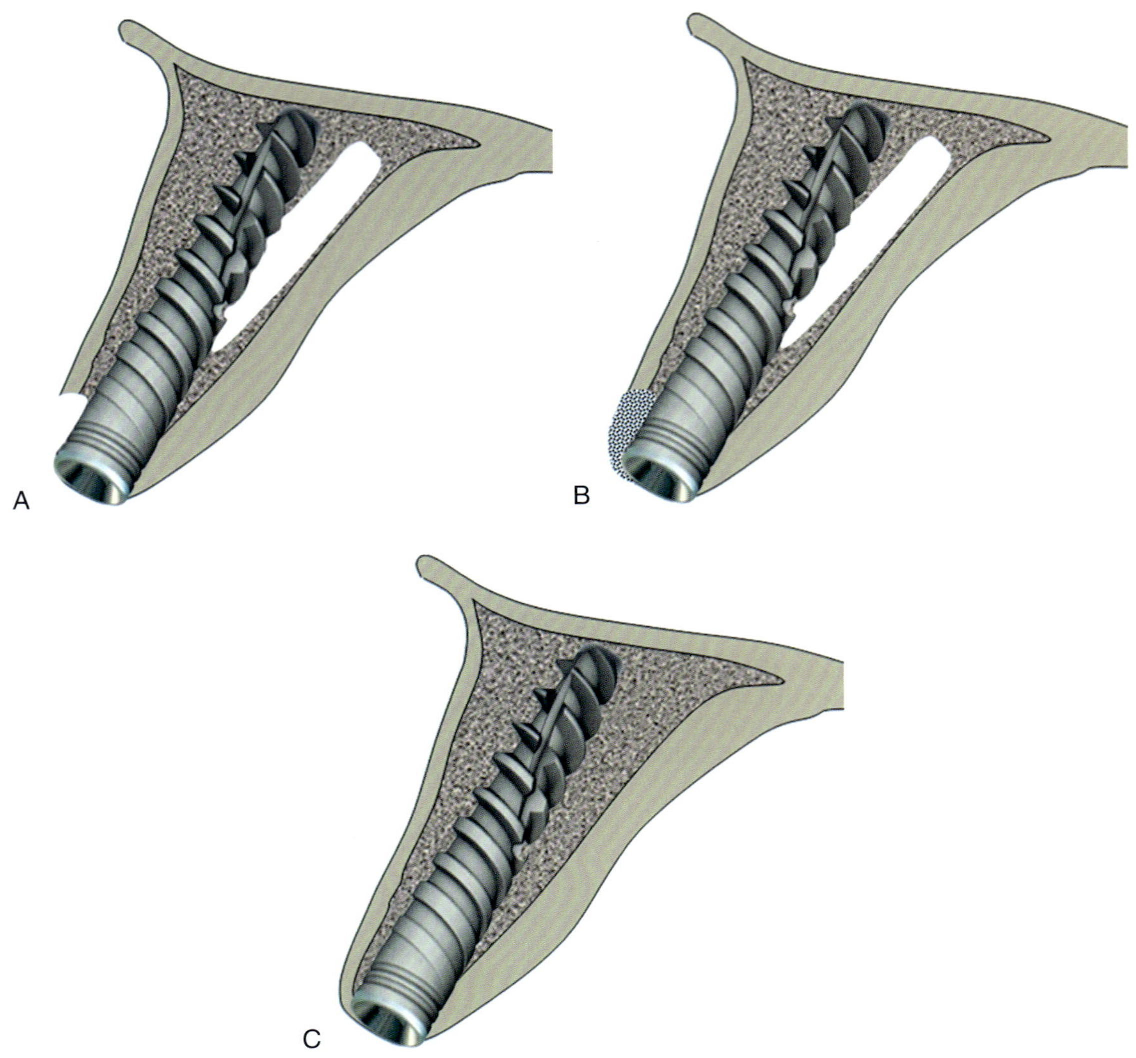

Fig 24.10 The implant can be removed and osteotomy prepared in the correct direction. (A) The same or a new implant is inserted. (B and C) The bone defect is grafted using autogenous or synthetic graft material and the flap is sutured back for submerged healing for a minimum of 4 months, which allows new bone formation at the area of the defect and implant to get osseointegrated.

3. Incorrect orientation and seating of the abutment on the implant.
4. Inaccurate impression recording, transfer, and prosthesis fabrication.

Prevention and management

1. Accurate impression recording, transfer, and prosthesis fabrication.
2. The abutment should be transferred to the implant with the same orientation as on the working cast.
3. Crown seating should be checked visually and confirmed with a radiograph, prior to final cementation.
4. When the surrounding soft tissue is preventing complete seating of an implant crown, it should be carefully trimmed to completely seat the prosthesis onto the abutment.

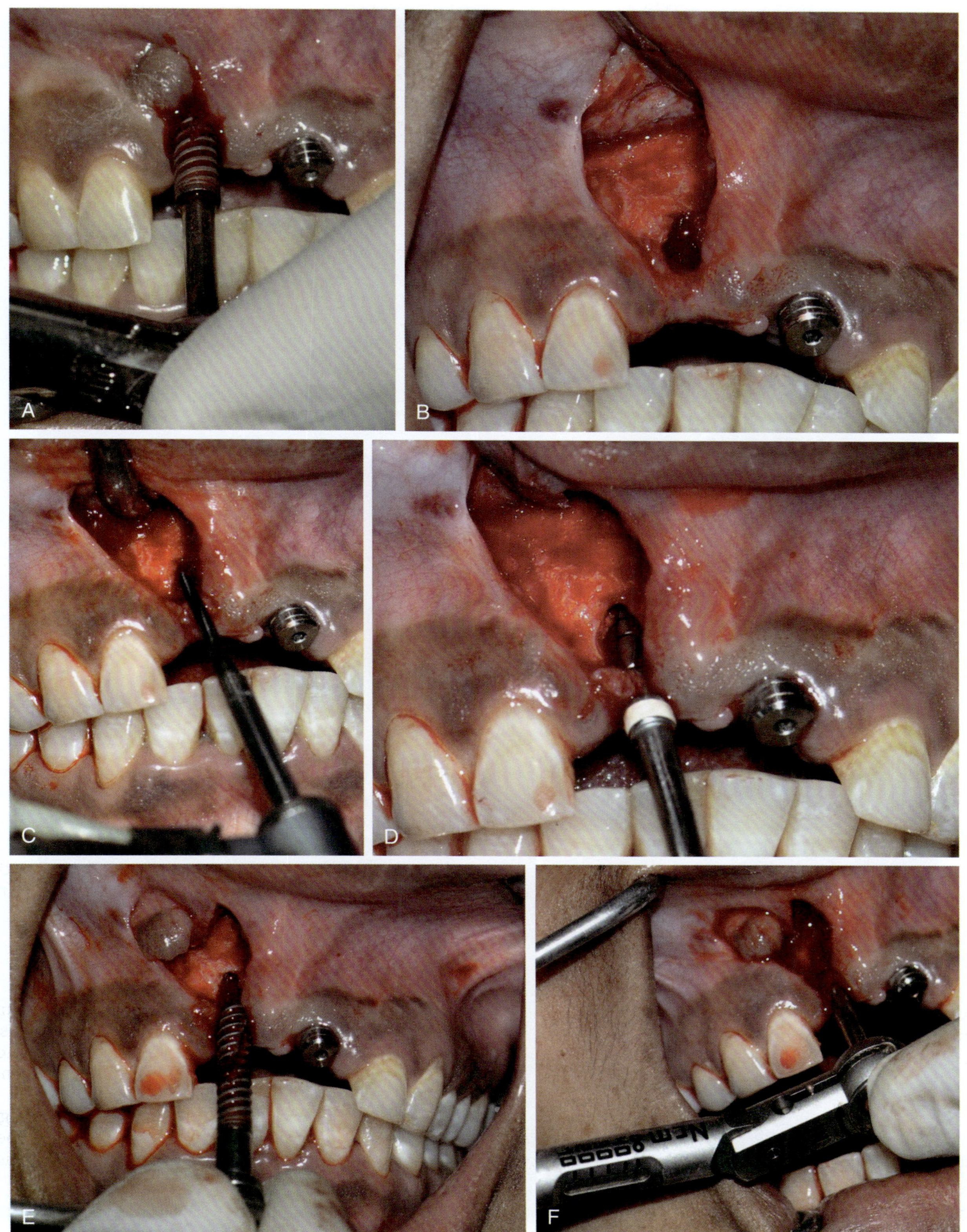

Fig 24.11 (A) The osseointegrated implant is removed using the ratchet. A papilla preservation flap is elevated to expose the implant site. (B) A bone defect is visible, which developed after the loss of thin labial cortical plate at the crestal region because of incorrect implant angulation. (C) A side-cutting Lindemann drill is used to drill the hard and thick palatal cortical plate and (D) the osteotomy is prepared in the correct direction using implant drills. (E) The same implant is reinserted with the correct angulation. (F) An adequate primary stability of the implant is achieved.

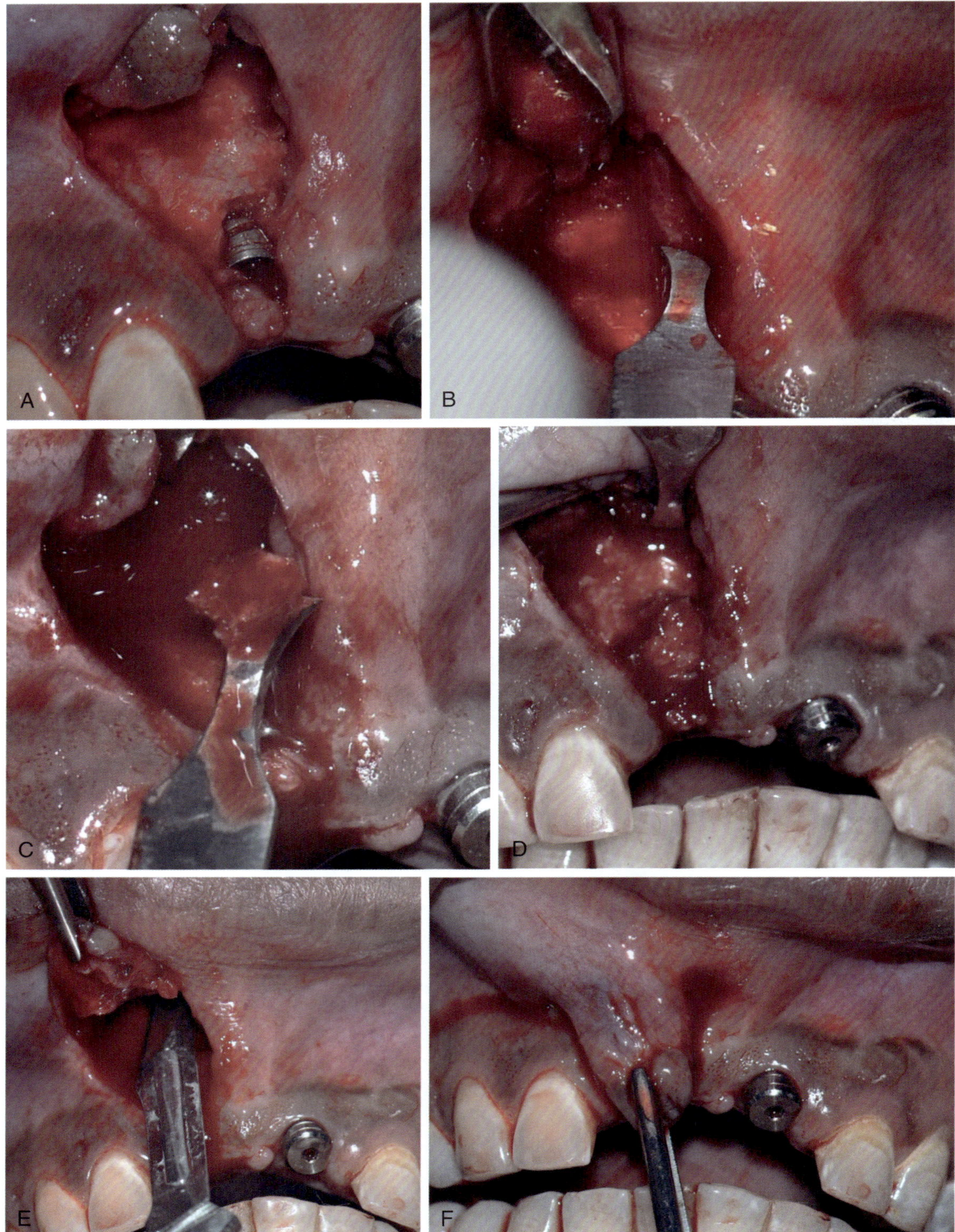

Fig 24.12 (A) The labial bone defect can be seen around the implant neck area; changing the implant direction has provided adequate room to graft the defect. (B–D) Autogenous bone is harvested from the subnasal region using a sharp chisel and used to graft the defect. (E and F) Releasing incisions are made through the periosteum of the flap to coronally advance it to achieve primary closure.

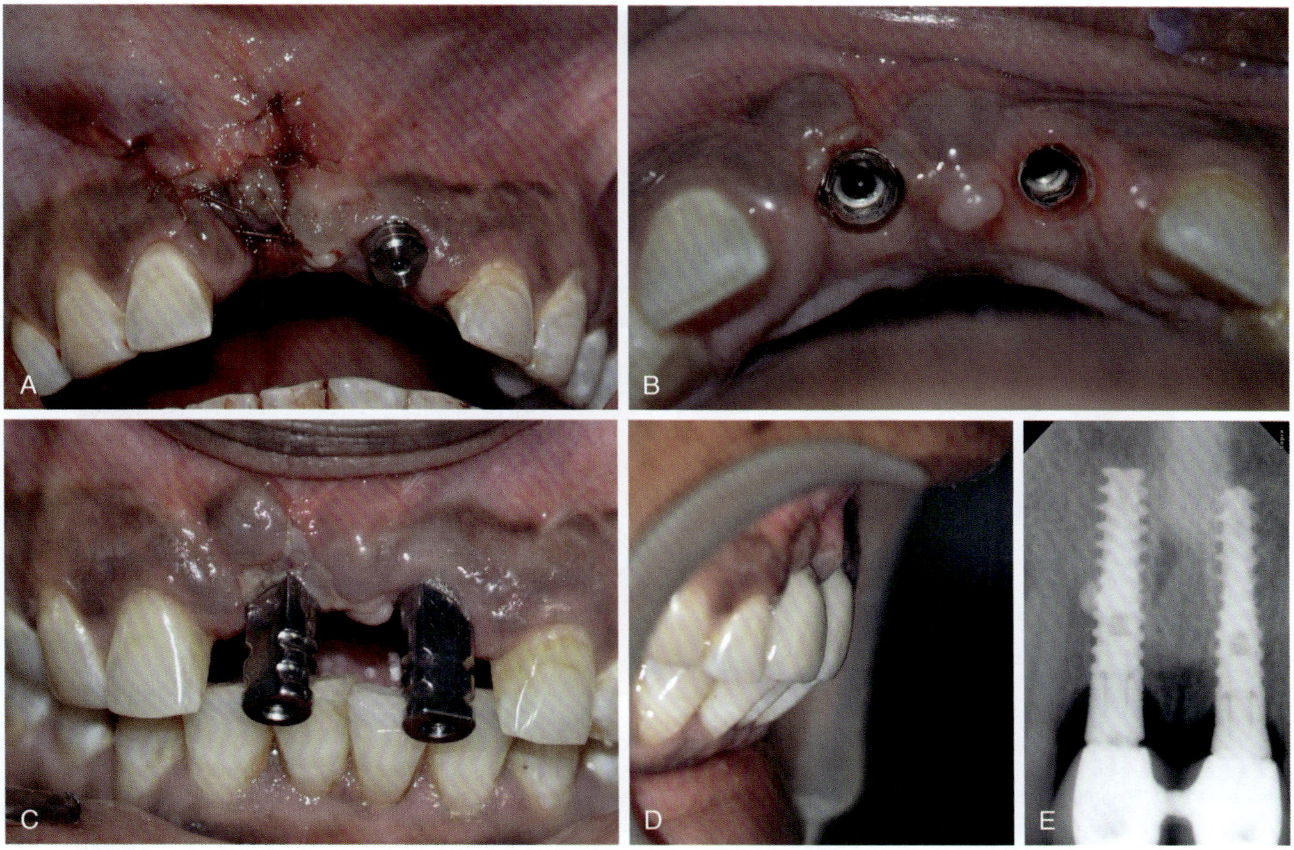

Fig 24.13 (A) The flap is sutured back with the primary closure and the site is allowed to heal for 4 months. (B and C) The implant uncovered using tissue punch shows the correct axis of the implant. (D) The implants are restored with an aesthetically acceptable prosthesis. (E) Postloading radiograph. Though, these implants are in function since 2 years with stable crestal bone level but removal and immediate reinsertion of the same implant in the same patient need further clinical trials.

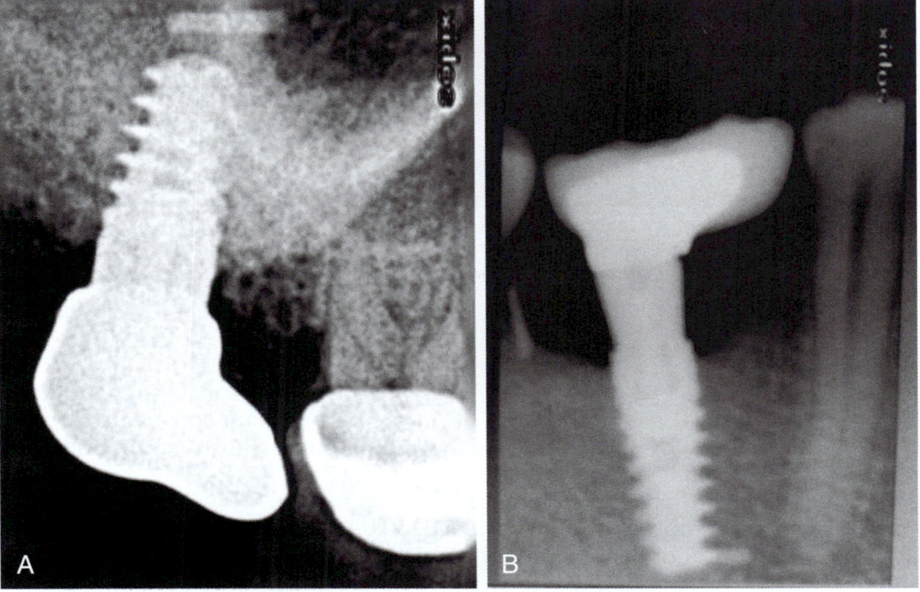

Fig 24.14 (A and B) The implants at the posterior sites if placed off-axis, may result in cantilevered prosthesis over the implant.

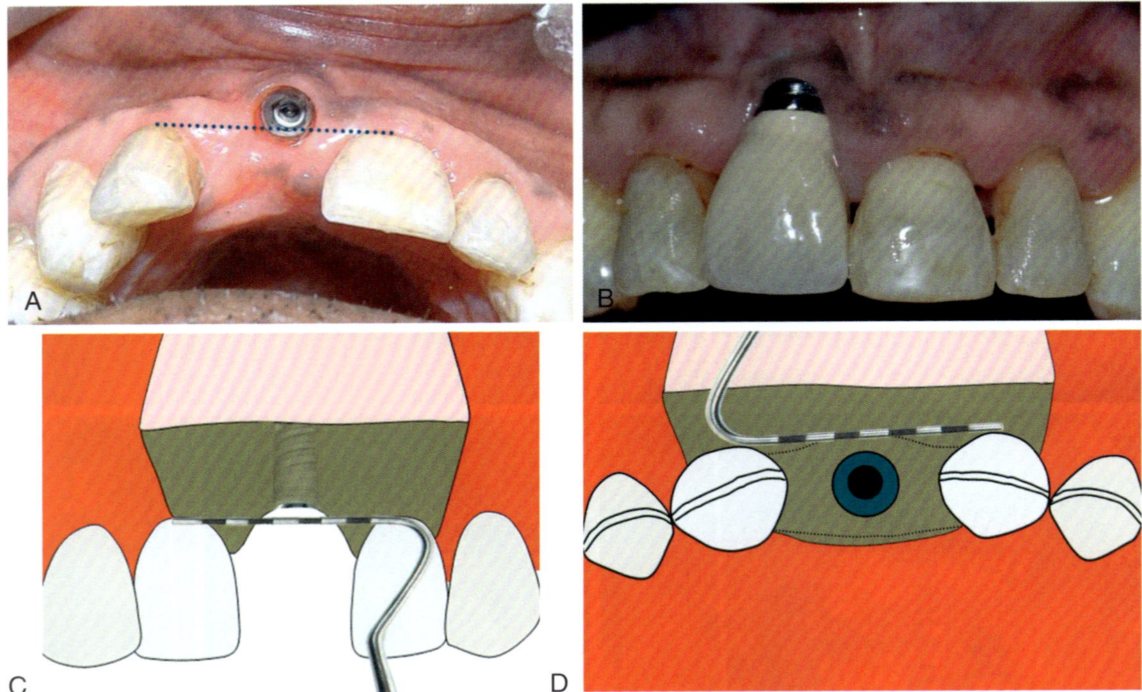

Fig 24.15 (A and B) Implant has been placed far facial and apical to the ideal position in the aesthetic region. (C) To achieve adequate aesthetic outcome, the implant should be positioned 2–3 mm apical to the imaginary line connecting the CEJ of two adjacent teeth or 2–3 mm apical to the gingival zenith. (D) The implant platform should also be placed 1–1.5 mm palatal to the imaginary line connecting the CEJ of two adjacent teeth.

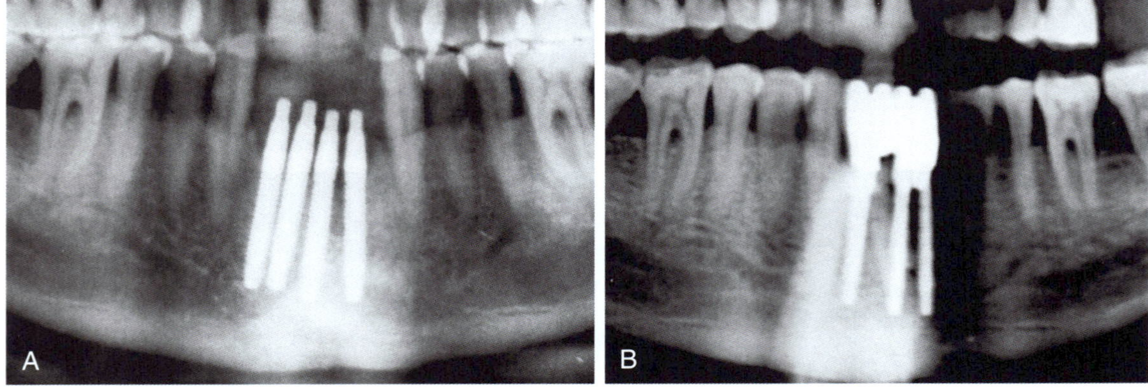

Fig 24.16 (A) Four implants placed to replace four mandibular incisors resulted in three implants very close to each other. (B) One implant is removed and the others are restored with a 3-unit bridge. These implants have been in function for 5 years without any noticeable crestal bone resorption.

Luting cement retention into the peri-implant soft tissue

Implant abutment–crown margins which are typically subgingival, pose a significant challenge when excess cement is removed following crown cementation to the implant abutment. This may be further compounded by the fact that the peri-implant tissues are tightly adapted to the newly placed implant crown, making it difficult to negotiate the subgingival area. Radiographic evaluation should always be accompanied with careful clinical evaluation of the peri-implant tissues to see if any excessive cement is present in the soft tissue. The retention of the cement in the peri-implant soft tissue may lead to recurrent pain, swelling, soft tissue inflammation, and crestal bone resorption (Fig 24.18).

Prevention

1. Avoid placing the implant abutment–crown margin interface deeper than 2–3 mm subgingivally, by selecting a final abutment with appropriate collar height; if it is any deeper, removal of excess cement becomes very difficult without surgical access.

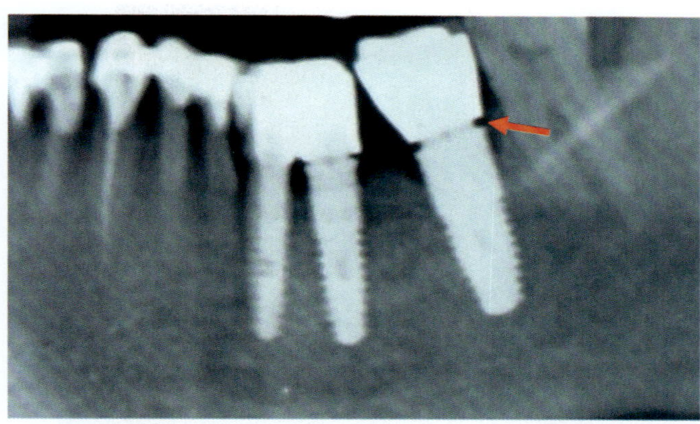

Fig 24.17 The incomplete seating of the prosthesis onto the abutment.

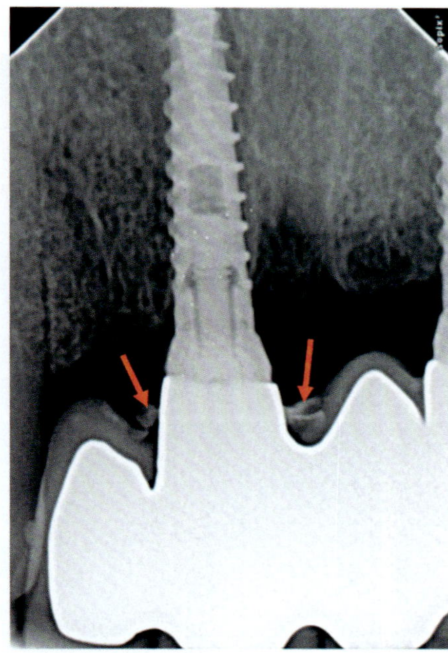

Fig 24.18 Luting cement retention in the peri-implant soft tissue can be seen in the radiograph.

2. excessive amount of cement should not be used as excess cement gets expelled comparatively deeper subgingivally, if compared to the conventional margins associated with routinely fixed crowns placed on prepared natural teeth. This is because, the implant does not have any connective tissue attachment which can prevent the cement expulsion deep into the peri-implant soft tissue.
3. Use radiopaque luting cements that can be visualized in the radiograph.
4. Using dual-cure resin cements which set quickly; the excess part can be easily removed from the deep subgingival area using a fine probe.

Management

The presence of residual cement often results in bleeding on probing, oedematous soft tissue, pain, exudate from the gingival sulcus, slight discomfort, etc. within 3–4 months of completion of the prosthesis. Occasionally the area remains asymptomatic even for years following the completion of the prosthesis. The acute inflammation associated with the presence of excess subgingival cement may also lead to crestal bone loss. Thus, the impacted cement should be identified in time and removed so as not to jeopardize the long-term health of the implant. If excess cement is removed within 3–4 months post restoration, it is possible to see reversal of crestal changes radiographically. Removal of excess subgingival cement involves anaesthetizing the peri-implant tissues with local anaesthetic and then using a periodontal curette to carefully negotiate the sulcus until the tip of the instrument makes contact with the cement. The implant surgeon should aim to get the tip of the instrument below the deposit so that a coronal sweeping action will dislodge the cement and remove it from the sulcus. In most cases, the tissues around the implant get softened and more pliable due to the associated inflammation, and while this assists with instrumentation of the subgingival areas, care needs to be taken to minimize trauma to the peri-implant tissues. This is particularly important in patients with a thin biotype and with implants in the aesthetic zone, where tissue trauma may lead to unsightly recession of the marginal peri-implant tissues. Furthermore, care should be taken to minimize scratching of the implant abutment surface during removal of the subgingival cement. When possible, plastic implant scalers should be used; however, these will often be insufficient to remove adherent excess cement. Fine-tipped periodontal curettes, such as a Mini-Five or similar curettes, used judiciously are often a better alternative.

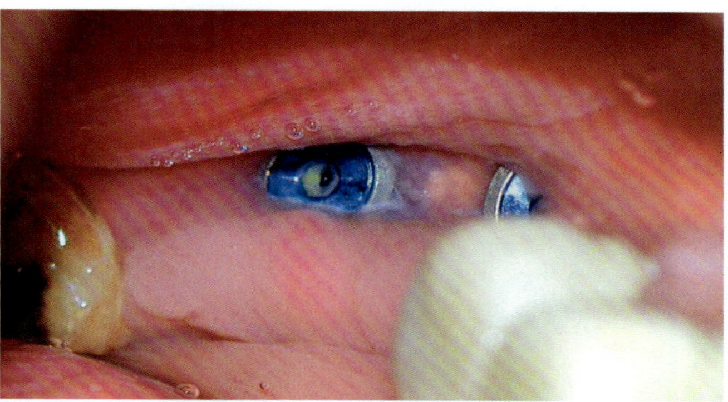

Fig 24.19 Suture line opening may result in cover screw exposure to the oral environment; the surgeon should not attempt to re-suture the flap but allow it to heal by the process of secondary intention. The patient should be instructed to keep the area very clean with the mouth rinses, soft brushes, etc. so that the tissue grows from the flap margins and covers the implant. If the implant is deep-seated, the deep soft tissue may collect food particles, which are quite difficult to clean and may cause infection to the implant. In such cases the cover screw should be replaced with a long gingival former. The implant surgeon can also irrigate the site twice a day with an antibiotic solution (e.g. injectable form of clindamycin) which raises the concentration of the antibiotic at the local site and prevents chances of infection to the implant till the soft tissue gets healed.

Suture line opening

The open suture line should not be re-sutured but the patient should be instructed to keep it clean, as it heals by secondary intention in 2–3 weeks (Fig 24.19).

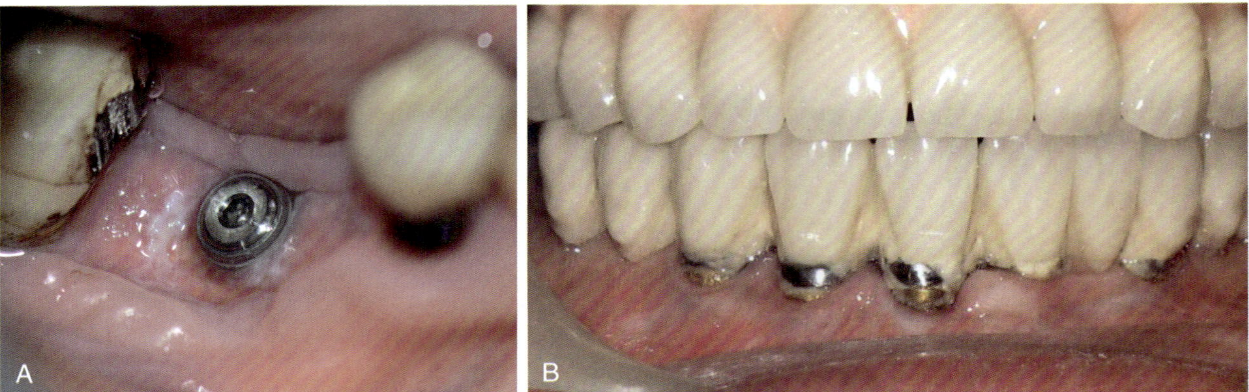

Fig 24.20 (A) Suture line opening resulted in the loss of graft and soft tissue recession, which has caused implant thread exposure to the oral environment. (B) The soft tissue with thin biotype receding with peri-implantitis and muscle pull.

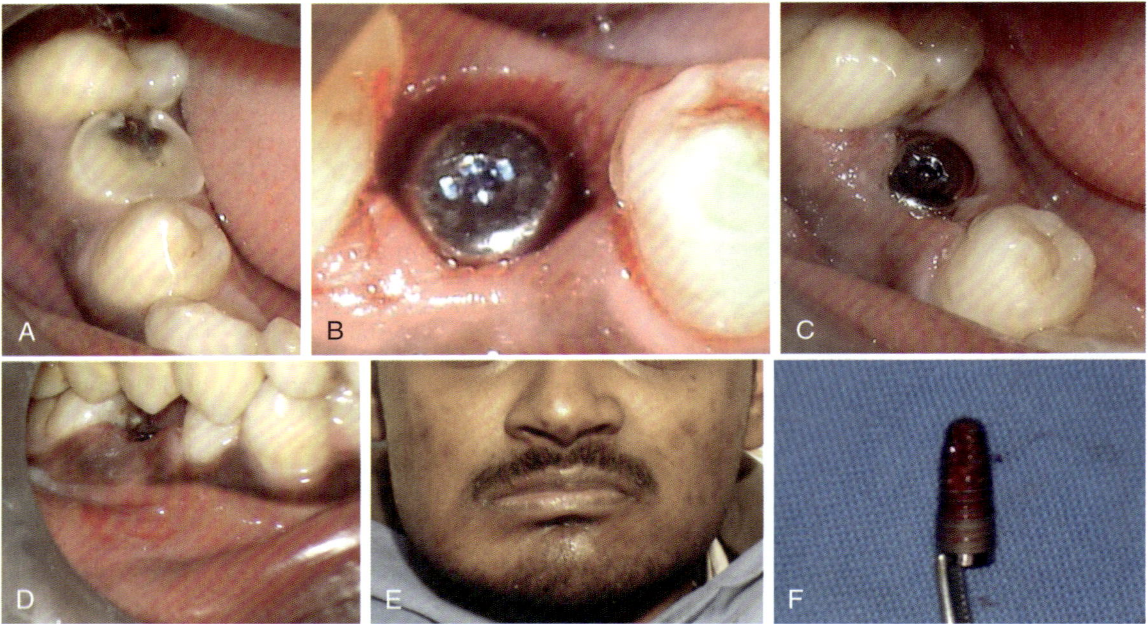

Fig 24.21 (A and B) The infected tooth is extracted and replaced by immediate implant. All measures were taken to prevent postoperative infection, such as prophylactic oral antibiotics, curetting out all the granulation tissue from the socket and irrigation of the socket with antibiotic solution before implant placement. (C) Normal soft tissue healing was seen at the second day after surgery (D) but the patient came again after 3 days with severe throbbing pain and swelling in the implant region. (E) Extraoral swelling could also be noticed. All attempts, such as injectable antibiotics and analgesics failed to reduce the pain and swelling because once the implant has received infection, it starts acting as a nonresorbable foreign body structure. (F) After the implant was removed the pain and swelling subsided within 24 h and the site healed under regular oral antibiotics.

Implant thread exposure

Exposure of implant threads in the oral environment may cause the collection of plaque over the exposed rough surface of the implant, which may further cause peri-implantitis and loss of peri-implant hard and soft tissue.

Causes of implant thread exposure

1. Suture line opening and loss of graft in cases where simultaneous bone grafting has been performed with implant placement (Fig 24.20A).
2. Soft tissue recession following crestal bone resorption.
3. More superficial implant placement.
4. Thin mobile soft tissue recedes with muscle pull (Fig 24.20B).

Management

If soft tissue healing has not covered the exposed implant threads, the threads should either be covered using soft tissue grafting with or without simultaneous bone grafting, or adequate grinding and polishing should be done

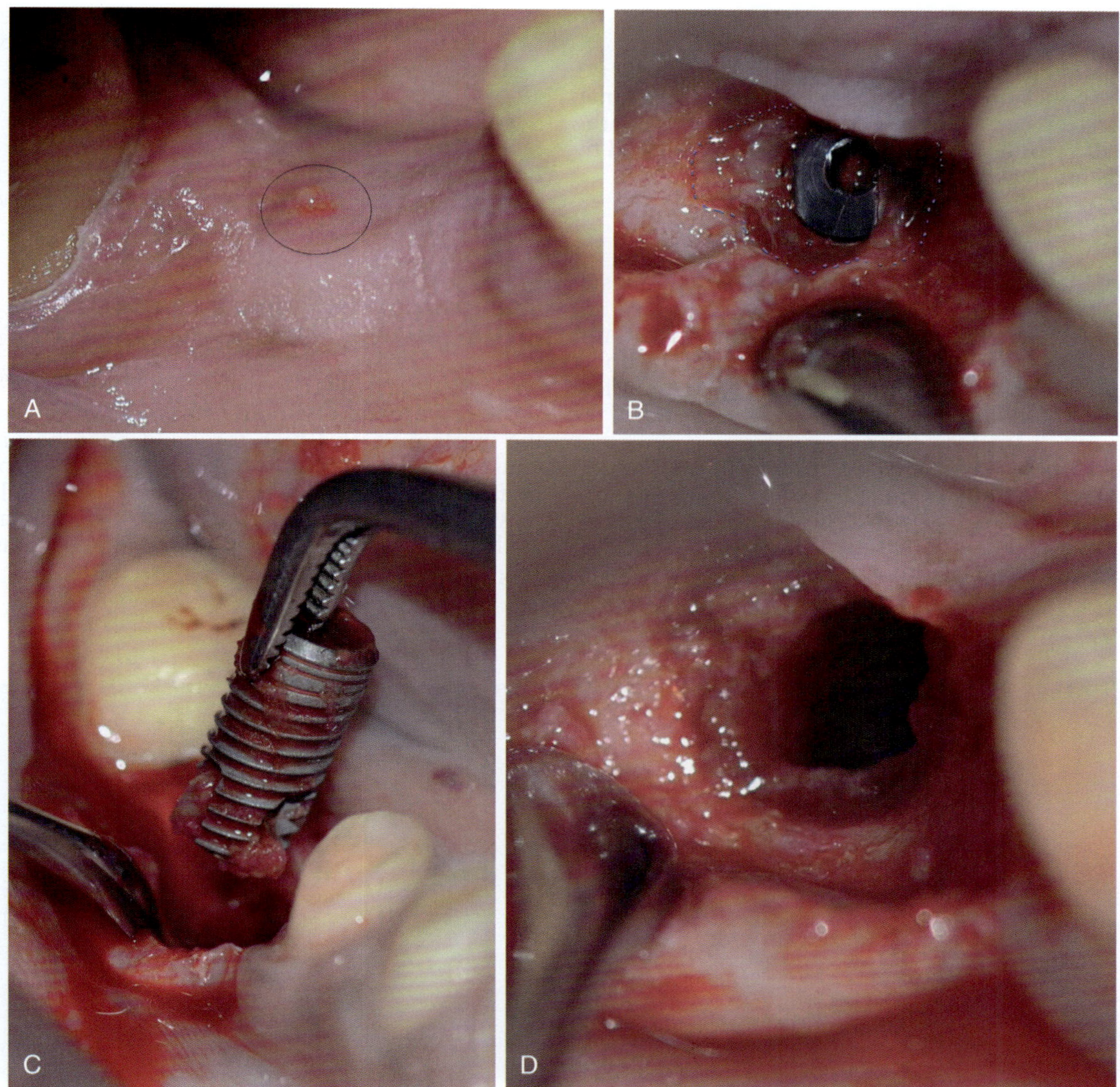

Fig 24.22 (A) A soft tissue boil at the implant site was seen during implant uncovery with a little discharge but no symptoms of pain or swelling. (B) A large amount of granulation tissue can be seen surrounding the implant indicating fibrous integration and failure of implant. (C) The implant should be removed and (D) all the granulation tissue should be curretted out. The flap is sutured back. A new implant can be inserted after the site heals in 6–8 weeks.

to make the surface very smooth, to prevent any plaque collection or peri-implantitis.

Post implantation infection

If the infection is limited to the soft tissue, a small gum boil will be noticed over the implant site. It can be punctured using a sharp probe and irrigated with chlorhexidine solution or citric acid. It heals and the pain subsides within 24 h. If there is continuous purulent discharge and severe pain which is not relieved by oral analgesics, the infection has reached to the bone–implant body interface. In such cases, the implant surgeon should immediately remove the implant and prescribe some good antibiotic like tab Augmentin 1000 mg twice a day for 5–7 days. A new implant can be inserted when the site gets healed in 6 weeks (Fig 24.21A–F).

Implant failure

1. **Post implant insertion.** If the implant fails within a few days after insertion, the causes may be infection, pressure necrosis, premature loading over inadequately stabilized implant etc.
2. **During implant uncovery.** If the implant fails to osseointegrate, a fibrous tissue grows between implant surface and surrounding bone, which often granulates and gets infected. It may sequestrate through the overlying soft tissue and often remains asymptomatic (Figs 24.22 and 24.23).
3. **After prosthetic loading.** If the implant fails after it is loaded in function, the causes may be either poor osseointegration, as in case of extremely low-density bone, or because the implant has been restored with the prosthesis with extremely offset occlusal loading.

Pressure necrosis

If the implant has been inserted into the high-density D1 or D2 type bone and screwed at a very high torque, it may lead to pressure necrosis of the surrounding bone and the patient will complain of continuous pain not relieved by analgesics, for weeks after the surgery.

Prevention

1. Use of new drills when drilling into high-density bone.
2. Drilling at higher speed and with maximum amount of chilled saline irrigation flow to cool down the bone.
3. Use of final drill with the diameter only 0.2 mm less than the implant diameter (e.g. 3.65 mm final drill for a 3.75 mm diameter implant).
4. Using the bone tap to prepare threads in the bone to accommodate implant threads.
5. Application of ice packs on the facial skin over the implant site and mouth rinsing with cold water for 48 h after implant placement.
6. Injectable/oral steroids (Dexona inj. just after surgery and tab. Decadron 4 mg once a day for the next 3 days) to reduce postoperative inflammation.

Treatment

If pain with the same intensity persists even after 1 week, the implant should be removed and another new implant inserted after 6 weeks (Fig 24.24A–C).

Osseointegrated implant removal on unscrewing cover screw/gingival former

If the cover screw or gingival former has been screwed to the implant using a high torque, it often becomes difficult to remove it at the implant uncovery or prosthetic phase. If it is removed at high torque, the implant itself may come out with the cover screw/gingival former, especially if the implant has been placed in poor-density bone (Fig 24.25).

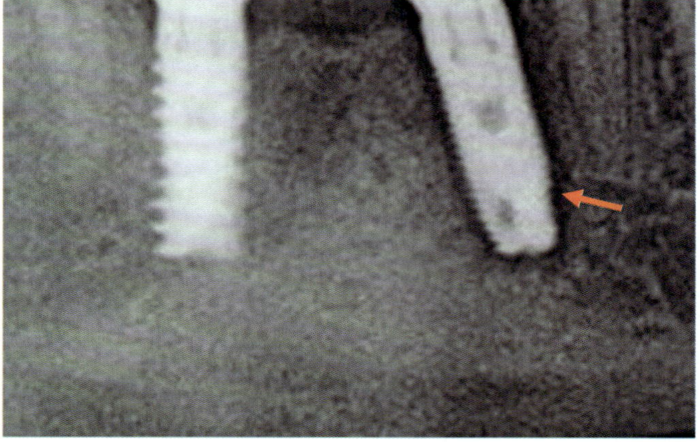

Fig 24.23 In the radiograph, A radiolucent lining can be seen around the implant which has failed to osseointegrate with the bone.

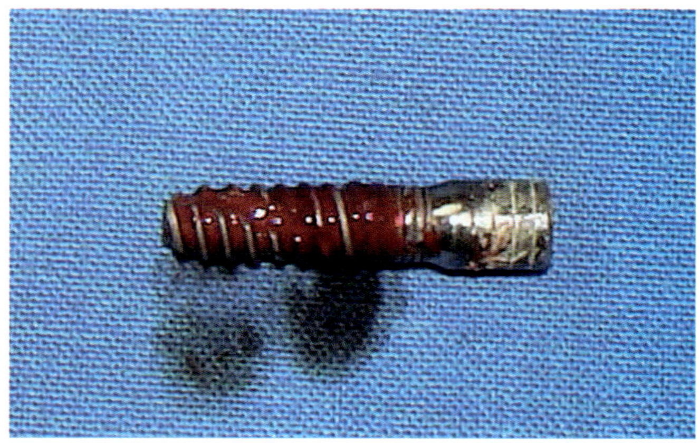

Fig 24.25 Osseointegrated implant, which has come out attached to the gingival former on its removal at high torque.

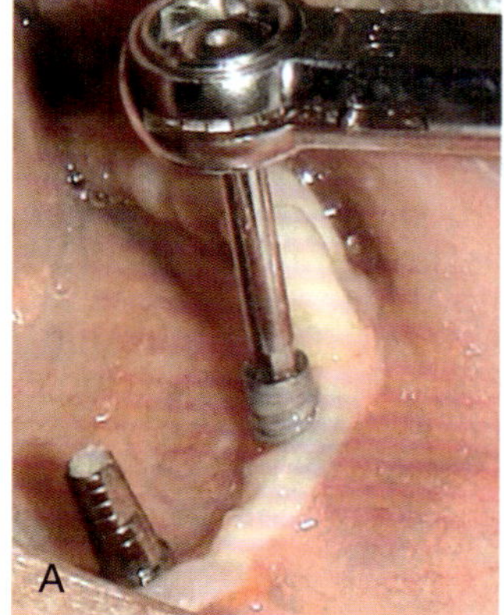

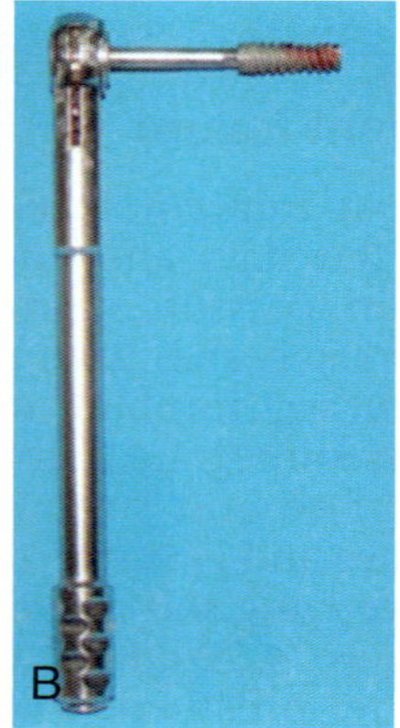

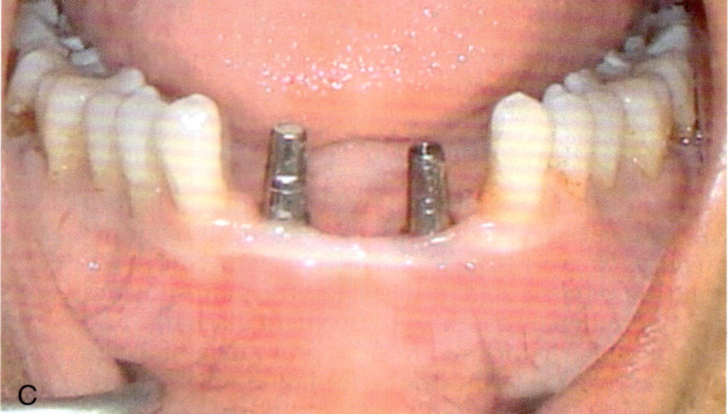

Fig 24.24 Patient complained of sharp, shooting pain in the left implant region which persisted even after 2 weeks following implant insertion. (A and B) The implant is removed using a hand ratchet and (C) another implant is inserted after 2 months. Pain subsided within 12 h of implant removal.

Crestal bone resorption

Crestal bone resorption is one of the most common problems in dental implantology.

Causes

1. Occlusal forces on the implant prosthesis are off-axis to the implant.
2. Implant with a wider platform is placed into the narrow crestal bone (Fig 24.26A).
3. Plaque collection – peri-implantitis.
4. Compromised (thin, unstable, and not keratinized) peri-implant soft tissue.

Prevention

1. Placement of two implants for the large mesiodistal space of a missing molar.
2. Implant placement along the axis of the future prosthesis (prosthetically guided implant placement).
3. Use of implant with platform switching feature (Figure 24.26B).
4. Fabrication of the implant prosthesis with narrow occlusal table (buccolingual).
5. Oral hygiene maintenance to prevent plaque collection and peri-implantitis.
6. Soft tissue grafting for compromised soft tissue around the implant prosthesis.

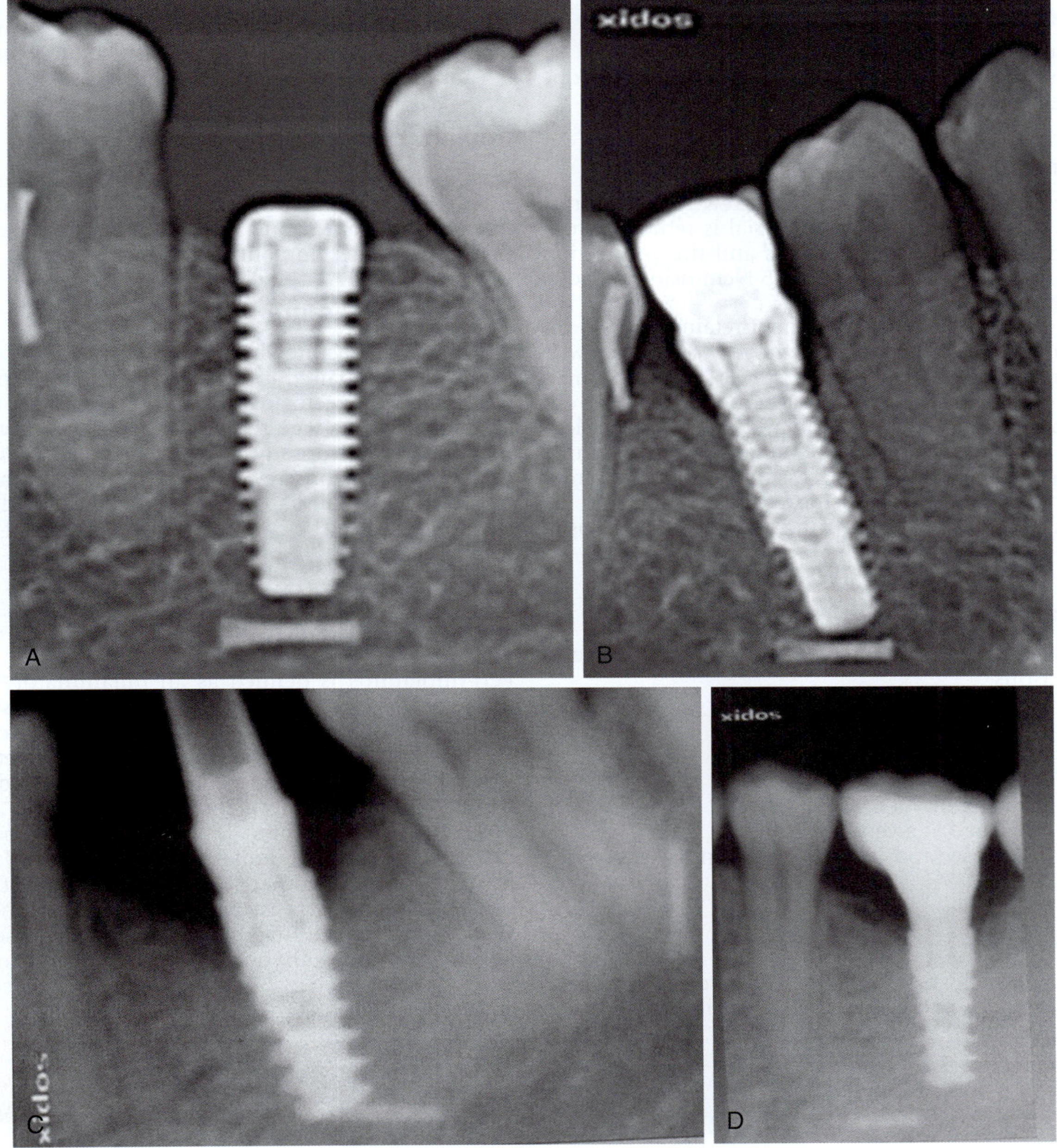

Fig 24.26 (A and B) Crestal bone resorption around the implant 1 year after implant loading. (C and D) Bone has grown around the implant platform at 1 year following implant loading, because of the platform-switching design of the implant.

Management

1. Identification and correction of the cause.
2. Bone grafting to regenerate new bone.

Connection screw loosening

Connection screw loosening is commonly encountered in implant practise.

Causes

1. Screw tightened at inadequate moment force without using torque ratchet before fixing the final prosthesis.
2. Offset/cantilevered occlusal forces.

Prevention

1. Minimize offset forces over the prosthesis.
2. Final screw tightening at 30–35 Ncm using the torque ratchet (Fig 24.27).

Management

1. If the connection screw of the screw-retained prosthesis gets loose, the filling material is removed from the screw hole in the prosthesis and the connection screw is tightened again at 30–35 Ncm using a torque ratchet.
2. If the connection screw of cement-retained prosthesis gets loose, the prosthesis is removed, or the screw is re-tightened and the same prosthesis or a new prosthesis is fixed on top of the abutment. Alternatively, the connection screw Location and direction are identified with radiographs and a small hole is prepared through the prosthesis to access the connection screw. The screw is re tightened using a torque ratchet and the access hole is closed using gutta-percha and composite (Fig 24.28).

Connection screw fracture

Though rare, it is encountered in clinical practise due to several reasons.

Causes

1. Weak screw material.
2. Manufacturing defect in the screw.
3. Screw tightened at a very high torque.
4. Screw is loose and gets broken under transverse forces.

Management

The dentist should first try to retrieve the broken screw and if this is not successful, the whole implant can be removed and immediately replaced with another implant of similar or larger dimensions. Thus in cases of connection screw breakage there are various options to solve the problem.

Option-1. The broken screw should be located using the magnification loop or surgical microscope and vibrated using a scaler tip. If the screw gets loosened, it can be removed using a long and sharp probe.

Option-2. The broken screw should be located using the magnification loop or surgical microscope and a horizontal grove should be carefully prepared into the screw, using the high speed turbine. An appropriate screwdriver is then used to unscrew and retrieve the broken screw (Fig 24.29A–J).

Option-3. If the screw cannot removed by any means, the implant can be removed and immediately replaced by another implant (Fig 24.30A–E).

Implant body fracture

It happens (rarely) if a small diameter implant is inserted for an oversized prosthesis with extreme offset forces. The fractured implant should be removed using the trephine drill and another implant inserted.

Prosthesis fracture

The cause of fracture should be corrected and the prosthesis either repaired or replaced. The hybrid prosthesis which has resin teeth are easy to repair in the mouth using composite resin (Fig 24.31A and B). The screw-retained prosthesis offers an advantage over the cement-retained one, as it can be unscrewed from the implants and easily repaired in the laboratory. The cement-retained prosthesis often needs to be cut down for easy removal from the implant.

Peri-implantitis

Peri-implantitis is defined as an inflammatory reaction with the loss of supporting bone in the tissues surrounding a functioning implant. Peri-implantitis is characterized by bleeding/suppuration on probing, together with loss of supporting bone. Cross-sectional studies have demonstrated that prevalence varies between 28% and 56%. The peri-implantitis lesion exhibits histopathological features that are similar, but not identical, to those in periodontitis. Similar to periodontitis, the treatment of peri-implantitis must be based on infection control. Under these conditions, progression of the disease may be arrested and subsequently, lost peri-implant tissues may be regenerated by bone augmentation and soft tissue grafting procedures.

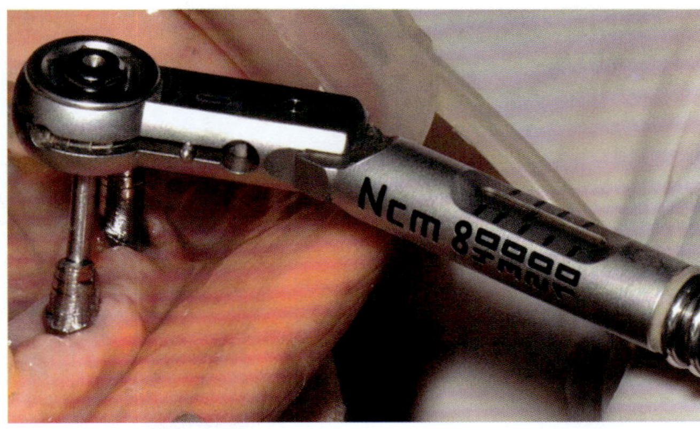

Fig 24.27 Connection screw of the implant abutment or prosthesis should be tightened at 30–35 Ncm using the torque ratchet, before fixing final prosthetic to avoid future screw loosening.

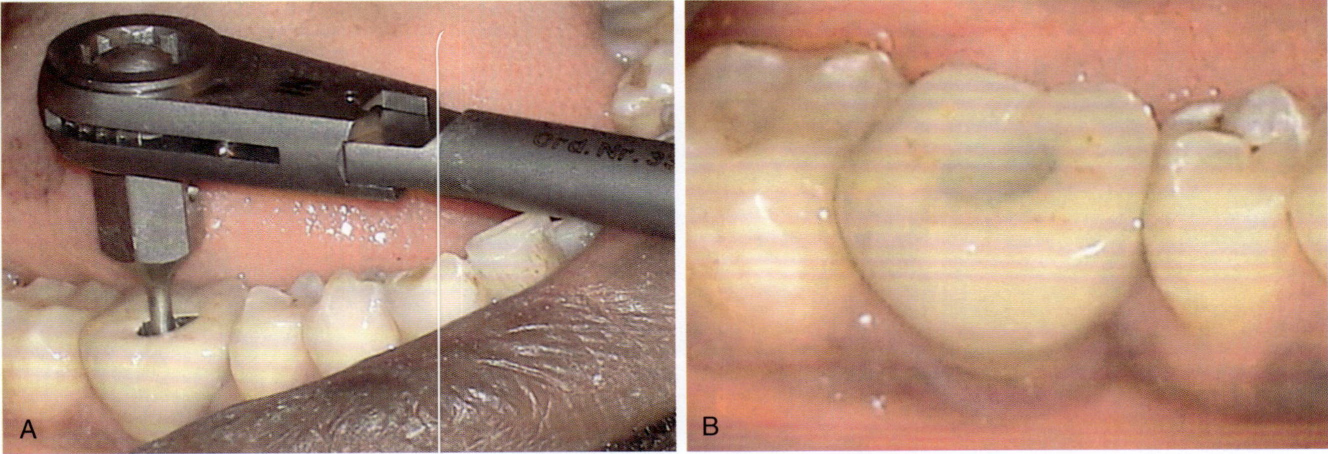

Fig 24.28 Patient reported with connection screw loosening 1 year after implant restoration. (A) An access hole is prepared through the cement-retained prosthesis to locate the connection screw and the screw is re-tightened using the torque ratchet. (B) The access hole is filled using gutta-percha and composite.

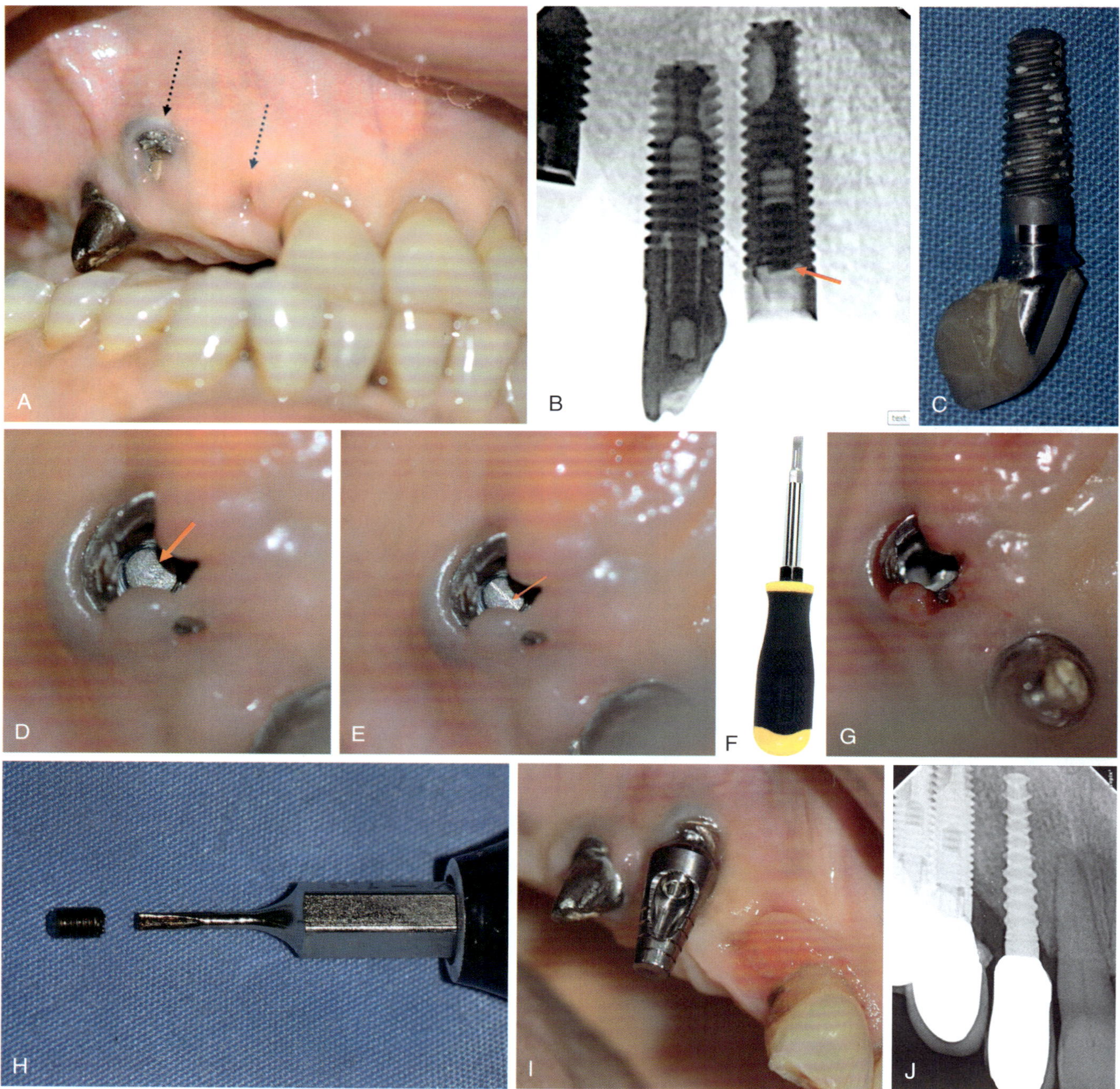

Fig 24.29 (A–C) Fractured connection screw of the implant and postloading failure of the osseointegrated implant from the anterior site because of implant loading with extreme off set occlusal forces. (D and E) The fractured part of the screw is visualized into the implant connection and a high speed turbine with a long straight fissure carbide bur is used to carefully prepare a horizontal groove into the screw under magnification (surgical microscope). (F–H) An appropriate screwdriver is then used to unscrew the broken part of the screw from the implant and (I) the abutment is fixed to the implant. (J) Another implant is inserted at the anterior site and implants are restored.

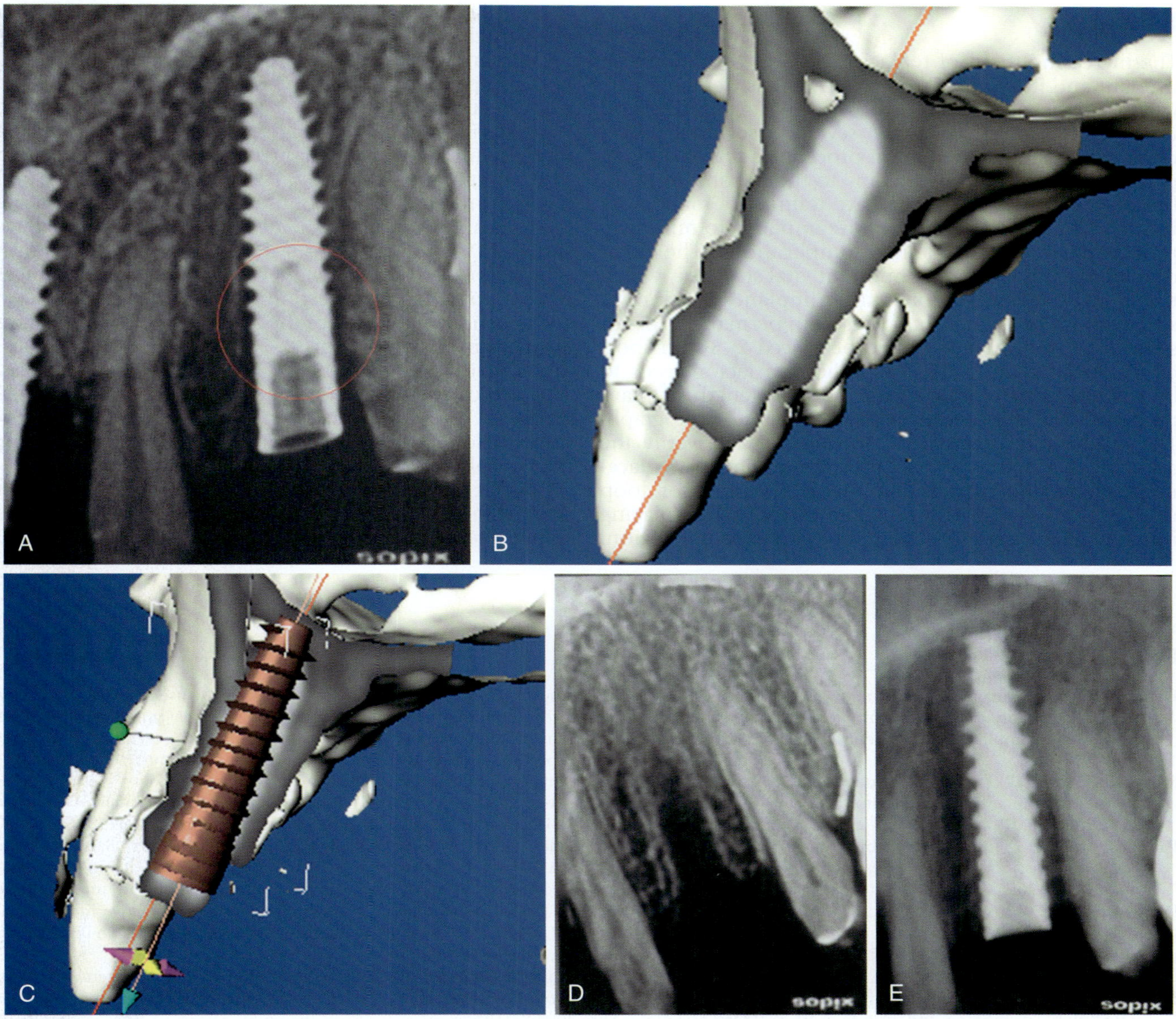

Fig 24.30 (A) Fractured screw in the implant. (B and C) When the broken screw could not be removed after making all the efforts, CT planning was done and (D) the implant was removed using the hand ratchet and (E) immediately replaced with a longer and wider implant.

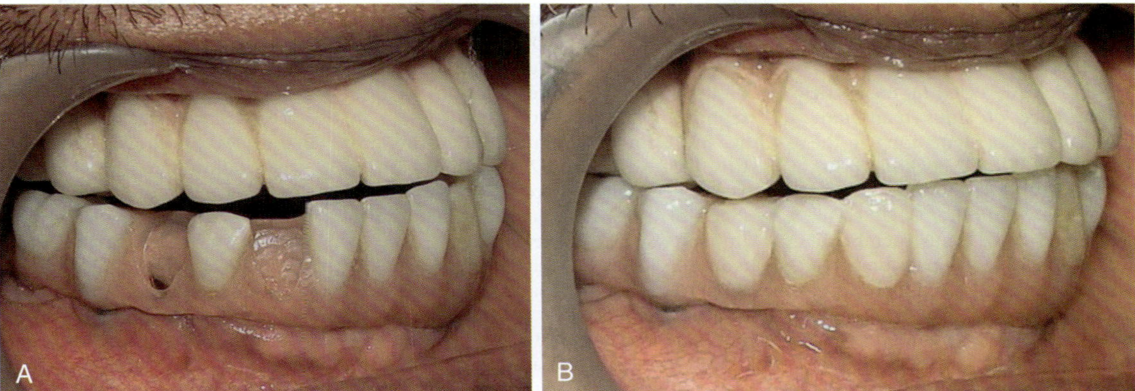

Fig 24.31 (A) The hybrid prosthesis on the lower implants has lost two resin teeth, (B) which have easily been repaired in the mouth using composite resin of a similar shade.

Summary

The increasing trend of replacing the lost tooth with an implant and its worldwide acceptance, has tremendously increased the number of dentists who are placing and restoring implants. Moreover, several associated procedures like bone augmentation procedures are also being practised to provide this therapy to the maximum number of patients. A comprehensive training is mandatory for the dentist to place and restore implants to minimize postoperative or postloading complications. The mandibular canal is the most important vital structure, which needs to be taken care off during implant insertion, as severe injury to the nerve may result in permanent loss of sensation. The implant should be placed 2–3 mm short of mandibular canal. The magnification factor needs to be calculated to plan the final implant length, if planning with the peri-apical or the panoramic radiograph. The radiograph after partial drilling can also verify the available bone for further drilling and implant placement above the mandibular canal. The anterior loop of the canal should also be taken care of when placing implants in the mandibular premolars and canine region. The implants should also be placed 2 mm short of other vital structures, such as the sinus floor, the nasal floor, etc. An implant with adequate dimensions should be inserted and also positioned at the prosthetically correct position and direction.

All sterilization and disinfection measures should be implemented during implant insertion surgery to avoid post implantation infection. If the implant after insertion has become infected, it should be removed and the site left to heal under antibiotic coverage. Several studies have shown that an oral rinse for 30 s with 0.12% chlorhexidine before the implant surgery, may reduce the chances of post implantation infection to a large extent.

The connection screw of the abutment should be tightened at a moment force of 30–35 Ncm using a mechanical driver (torque ratchet), before fixing the final prosthesis. This avoids the occurrence of screw loosening to a large extent. If the luting cement has spilt out into the peri-implant soft tissue pocket, it should be verified with the radiograph and removed to avoid peri-implantitis.

Postoperative care and follow-up visits after implant therapy are important for long-term maintenance of implant restorations.

Further Reading

Danesh-Meyer M. Diagnosis and management of commonly encountered problems with cemented implant crowns. Dent Pract 2006:142–48.

Mombelli A, Lang NP. The diagnosis and treatment of peri-implantitis. Periodontol 2000 1998;17:63–76.

Park S-H, Wang H-L. Implant reversible complications: classification and treatments. Implant Dent 2005;14:211–20.

Fugazzotto PA, Wheeler SL, Lindsay JA. Success and failure rates of cylinder implants in type IV bone. J Periodontol 1993;64:1085–7.

Shin HI, Sohn DS. A method of sealing perforated sinus membrane and histological finding of bone substitutes: a case report. Implant Dent 2005;14:328–35.

Kim S-G, Mitsugi M, Kim B-O. Simultaneous sinus lifting and alveolar distraction of the atrophic maxillary alveolus for implant placement: a preliminary report. Implant Dent 2005;14:344–8.

Ardekian L, Oved-Peleg E, Peled M, et al. The clinical significance of sinus membrane perforation during augmentation of the maxillary sinus. J Oral Maxillofac Surg 2006;64:277–82.

Proussaefs P, Lozada J, Rohrer MD, et al. Repair of the perforated sinus membrane with a resorbable collagen membrane: a human study. Int J Oral Maxillofac Impl 2004;19:413–20.

Jung JH, Choi BH, Li J, et al. The effects of exposing dental implants to the maxillary sinus cavity on sinus complications. Oral Surg Oral Med Oral Pathol Oral Radiol Endod 2006;102:602–5.

Van Steenberghe D, Lekholm U, Bolender C, et al. Applicability of osseointegrated oral implants in the rehabilitation of partial edentulism: a prospective multicenter study on 558 fixtures. Int J Oral Maxillofac Implants 1990;5:272–81.

Ayangco L, Sheridan PJ. Development and treatment of retrograde peri-implantitis involving a site with a history of failed endodontic and apicoectomy procedures: a series of reports. Int J Oral Maxillofac Implants 2001;16:412–7.

Nakamura N, Mitsuyasu T, Ohishi M. Endoscopic removal of an implant displaced in the maxillary sinus; a technical note. Int J Oral Maxillofac Surg 2004;33:195–7.

Varol A, Turker N, Basa S, et al. Endoscopic retrieval of dental implants from the maxillary sinus. Int J Oral Maxillofac Implants 2006;21:801–4.

Cheung WW. Risk management in implant dentistry. Hong Kong Dent J 2005;2:58–60.

Oh T-J, Joongkyo Y, Wang H-L. Management of the implant periapical lesions: a case report. Implant Dent 2003;12:41–6.

Klinge B, Hultin M, Berglundh T. Peri-implantitis. Dent Clin N Am 2005;49:661–76.

Garg AK, Reddi SN, Chacon GE. The importance of asepsis in dental implantology. Implant Soc 1994;5; 8e11.

Tolman DE, Keller EE. Management of mandibular fractures in patients with endosseous implants. Int J Oral Maxillofac Implants 1991;6:427–36.

Tiwana K, Morton, Tiwana PS. Aspiration and ingestion in dental practice: a 10-year institutional review. JADA 2004;135:1287–91.

Parel SM, Funk JJ. The use and fabrication of a self-retaining surgical guide for controlled implant placement; a technical note. Int J Oral Maxillofac Implants 1991;6:207–10.

Blustein R, Jackson R, Godar D, et al. Use of splint material in the placement of implants. Int J Oral Maxillofac Implants 1986;1:47–9.

Berglundh T, Persson L, Klinge B. A systematic review of the incidence of biological and technical complications in implant dentistry reported in prospective longitudinal studies of at least 5 years. J Clin Periodontol 2002;29:197–212.

Shaffer MD, Juruaz DA, Haggerty PC. The effect of periredicular endodontic pathosis on the apical region of adjacent implants. Oral Surg Oral Med Oral Pathol Oral Radiol Endod 1998;86:578–81.

el Askary AS, Meffert RM, Griffin T. Why do dental implants fail? Part I. Implant Dent 1999;8:173–85.

Worthington P. Injury to the inferior alveolar nerve during implant placement: a formula for protection of the patient and clinician. Int J Oral Maxillofac Implants 2004;19:731–4.

Sharawy M, Misch CE, Tehemar S, et al. Heat generation during implant drilling: the significance of motor speed. J Oral Maxillofac Surg 2002;60:1160–9.

Albrektsson T, Branemark PI, Hansson HA, et al. Osseointegrated titanium implants. Requirements for ensuring a long-lasting direct bone-to-implant anchorage in man. Acta Orthop Scand 1981;52; 155e170.

Heller AA, Shankland WE II. Alternative to the inferior alveolar nerve block anesthesia when placing mandibular dental implants posterior to the mental foramen. J Oral Implantol 2001;27:127–33.

Nazarian Y, Eliav E, Nahlieli O. [Hebrew] Nerve injury following implant placement: prevention, diagnosis and treatment modalities. Refuat Hapeh Vehashinayim 2003;20:44–50.

Kraut RA, Chahal O. Management of patients with trigeminal nerve injuries after mandibular implant placement. JADA 2002;133:1351–4.

Wu PB, Yung WC. Factors contributing to implant failure. Hong Kong Dent J 2005;2:12–8.

McDermott N, Chuang S, Dodson T, et al. Complications of dental implants: identification, frequency, and associated risk factors. Int J Oral Maxillofac Implants 2003;18:848–55.

Moy PK, Medina D, Aghaloo TL, et al. Dental implant failure rates and associated risk factors. Int J Oral Maxillofac Implants 2005;20:569–77.

Jabero M, Sarment DP. Advanced surgical guidance technology: a review. Implant Dent 2006;15:135–42.

Tarnow DP, Cho SC, Wallace SS. The effect of inter-implant distance on the height of inter-implant bone. J Periodontol 2000;71:546–9.

Tarnow DP, Magner AW, Fletcher P. The effect of the distance from the contact point to the crest of bone on the presence or absence of the interproximal dental papilla. J Periodontol 1992;63:995–6.

de Oliveira RR, Novaes A Jr, Taba M Jr, et al. Influence of inter-implant distance on papilla formation and bone resorption: a clinical-radiographic study in dogs. J Oral Implantol 2006;32:218–27.

Givol N, Taicher S, Chaushu G, et al. Risk management aspects of implant dentistry. Int J Oral Maxillofac Implants 2002;17:258–62.

Quirynen M, Gijbels F, Jacobs R. An infected jawbone site compromising successful osseointegration. Periodontol 2000 2003;33:129–44.

Daylene Jack-Min Leong et al. Implant Dent 2011;20(36):363.

Lioubavina-Hack N, Lang NP, Karring T. Significance of primary stability for osseointegration of dental implants. Clin Oral Impl Res 2006;17:244–50.

Sussman HI. Tooth devitalization via implant placement: a case report. Periodontal Clin Investig 1998;20:22–4.

Ercoli C, Funkenbusch PD, Lee HJ, et al. The influence of drill wear on cutting efficiency and heat production during osteotomy preparation for dental implants: a study of drill durability. Int J Oral Maxillofac Implants 2004;19:335–49.

Olson RA, Fonseca RJ, Osbon DB, et al. Fractures of the mandible: a review of 580 cases. J Oral Maxillofac Surg 1982;40:23–8.

Hegedus F, Diecidue RJ. Trigeminal nerve injuries after mandibular implant placement-practical knowledge for clinicians. Int J Oral Maxillofac Implants 2006;21:111–6.

Day RH. Microneurosurgery of the injured trigeminal nerve. Oral Maxillofac Surg Knowledge Update 1994;1:91–116.

Goodacre DJ, Rungcharassaeng K, Kan JY, et al. Clinical complications with implants and implant prostheses. J Prosthet Dent 2003;90:121–32.

Kalpidis CD, Konstantinidis AB. Critical hemorrhage in the floor of the mouth during implant placement in the first mandibular premolar position: a case report. Implant Dent 2005;14:117–24.

Balshi TJ. An analysis and management of fractured implants: a clinical report. Int J Oral Maxillofac Implants 1996;11(5):660–6.

Goodacre CJ, Kan JY, Rungcharassaeng K. Clinical complications of osseointegrated implants. J Prosthet Dent 1999;81(5):537–52.

Goodacre CJ, Bernal G, Rungcharassaeng K, et al. Clinical complications with implants and implant prostheses. J Prosthet Dent 2003;90:121–32.

Longoni, Longoni S, Sartori M, et al. Lingual vascular canals of the mandible: the risk of bleeding complications during implant procedures. Implant Dent 2007;16:131–8.

Chen S, Darby I. Dental implants: maintenance, care and treatment of peri-implant infection. Aust Dent J 2003;48(4):212–20.

Flanagan D. Important arterial supply of the mandible, control of an arterial hemorrhage, and report of a hemorrhagic incident. J Oral Implantol 2003;29:165–79.

Bartling R, Freeman K, Kraut RA. The incidence of altered sensation of the mental nerve after mandibular implant placement. J Oral Maxillofac Surg 1999;57:1408–10.

Leonhardt Å, Dahlèn G, Renvert S. Five-year clinical, microbiological, and radiological outcome following treatment of peri-implantitis in man. J Periodontol 2003;74:1415–22.

Adell R, Lekholm U, Rockler B, et al. A 15-year study of osseointegrated implants in the treatment of the edentulous jaw. Int J Oral Surg 1981;10; 387e416.

Schwarz MS. Mechanical complications of dental implants. Clin Oral Implants Res 2000;11(Suppl. 1):S156–8.

Jung RE, Pjetursson BE, Glauser R, et al. A systematic review of the 5-year survival and complication rates of implant-supported single crowns. Clin Oral Implants Res 2008;19:119–30.

Ellies L, Hawker P. The prevalence of altered sensation associated with implant surgery. Int J Oral Maxillofac Implants 1993;8:674–9.

Misch CE. Contemporary implant dentistry, 2nd ed. St. Louis: Mosby; 1999:373.

Daylene Jack-Min Leong, et al. Implant Dent. 2011;20(36):363.

Index

A

B

F

G

H

I

J

K

L

M

N

O

P

R

S

T

U

V

W

X

Z